Histology
Cell and Tissue Biology

Histology
Cell and Tissue Biology

Fifth edition

Edited by

Leon Weiss, MD

Grace Lansing Lambert Professor of Cell Biology
Department of Animal Biology
University of Pennsylvania

Elsevier Biomedical
New York • Amsterdam • Oxford

Cover Illustration is Figure 28-17 (color plate 18).

Copyright 1977, 1973, 1966 by McGraw-Hill, Inc. All rights reserved.
Copyright 1954 by McGraw-Hill, Inc. All rights reserved.

© 1983 by Elsevier Science Publishing Co., Inc. All rights reserved.
Second Printing, 1983.

Published by:
Elsevier Science Publishing Co., Inc.
52 Vanderbilt Avenue, New York, New York 10017

Sole distributors outside the USA and Canada:
Scientific and Medical Division of Macmillan Press, Ltd.
London and Basingstoke, UK

Library of Congress Cataloging in Publication Data

Main entry under title:

Histology.

 Includes bibliographies.
 1. Histology. I. Weiss, Leon.
QM551.H663 1983 611'.018 82–18218
ISBN 0–444–00716–4

Manufactured in the United States of America

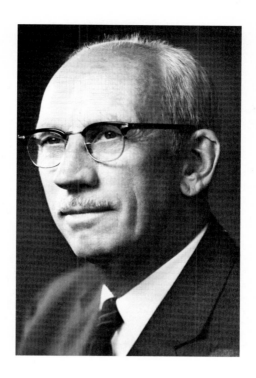

With deep affection
We dedicate this book to
ROY O. GREEP
great endocrinologist and experimental biologist,
preeminent educator, wise friend, and gentle man:
Founder and Editor of HISTOLOGY.

Contents

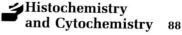

The Exocrine Pancreas and Salivary Glands 749

James D. Jamieson

Islets of Langerhans 774

G. Eric Bauer

The Respiratory System 788

Sergei P. Sorokin

The Ear   1177
Åke Flock

Introduction

If there was a time when Histology could be viewed as being out of the main stream of science and medicine, that time is past. My colleagues and I offer this comprehensive text, HISTOLOGY, and believe it has fair claim on students of Medicine and Biology.

This edition, primarily intended for courses in Histology in medical schools and graduate schools, should be useful in the study of the other basic biomedical sciences and, beyond that, in clinical medicine. Indeed, so close have the basic and clinical sciences grown that what the medical student learns from this text will be used in Physiology, Immunology, Pathology, and Pharmacology and be discussed at the patient's bedside on clinical rounds. For example, the division of lymphocytes into T and B cells and their subgroups by the labeling of distinctive cell surface molecules is intrinsic to our histological account of lymphatic tissue. This material is also an essential part of Immunology and Pathology and the student will need it in working up patients with leukemia or lymphoma.

Knowledge of the endocrine system has been enormously expanded and made more rational, as we show in this edition of HISTOLOGY, by the application of immunocytochemical methods that disclose the presence of specific hormones in specific cells. Hormones, whose presence there was unexpected, have been discovered in the islet tissue of the pancreas. Systems, such as the *enteroendocrine system*, have been newly recognized. These basic findings quickly enter the clinical domain and knowledge of them is re-quired for the rational management of diabetes, thyrotoxicosis, and other endocrinopathies. Further examples of the convergence of the basic and clinical sciences can readily be drawn from every chapter in this book.

HISTOLOGY in this, its Fifth Edition, continues to have as its plan the presentation of the microscopic and submicroscopic structure of the body at a comprehensive level but without undue detail. We depend upon bright field microscopy and transmission electron microscopy and, in addition, call upon a large number of morphological, biochemical, and physiological techniques in order to present a complete and coherent picture of our subject. These techniques include histo- and cytochemistry, autoradiography, scanning and high voltage electron microscopy, freeze-fracture-etch, tissue culture, and a variety of cell disruption and separation techniques. We cover human tissue; but, since much of the material we deal with has an experimental basis, we turn where appropriate to experimental animals.

While we have shortened the text in many places in this edition, in other places new information has caused us to expand it. The chapter on the pancreas has been divided into two chapters: Exocrine Pancreas (and Salivary Glands) and Islets of Langerhans. A new chapter on the Heart is offered. Every chapter, moreover, is introduced by a list of its sections' headings and the sections are presented in a sequence logical for each tissue. By these arrangements, and a full table of contents and index, the student may go efficiently to the page needed in the book. We provide whole chapters—as those on teeth, placenta, heart, pineal, and the special senses—that may not be used in some Histology courses. While these chapters add to the length and to the value of HISTOLOGY, they clearly do not add to the required reading load of students in those courses. We hope that our book will serve students in both long courses and short courses.

My colleagues and I write at a time, long anticipated by histologists, when it is being demonstrated in system after system that the structure of tissues is not arbitrary. Tissue structure is rather the morphologic expression of the interactions of diverse cells tightly regulated by immediate, short-range, and long-range factors—including the functions of the cells themselves. The structure and the functions of tissues are entirely interdependent and neither can be understood without the other. The study of such cellular interplay represents a significant expansion of cell biology into the biology of tissues. Because this expansion is at the heart of our exposition, we have subtitled this edition of HISTOLOGY, *Cell and Tissue Biology*.

With this edition Elsevier Science Publishing Company, Inc., assumes the publishing of HISTOLOGY. I have been heartened by the confidence of Charles Ellis, President of Elsevier, and John Lawrence, Head, Biomedical Publications, who enlisted this book and has guided its publication, and appreciate their decision to publish texts in the basic medical sciences. Barbara Conover, Director of Editing, coordinated the venture. Edmée Froment, Art Director, designed the entire book. Virginia Kudlak dummied it. Barbara Rowe, who worked out of my office, gathered and inventoried the manuscript. I have followed these dedicated book women in the intricate work needed to turn a complex heavily illustrated manuscript into a book. If this volume has the physical quality and presence to justify its claim as a definitive work, it is due to them.

I am grateful for the advice and generosity of Robert McGraw of the McGraw-Hill Book Company, who, when unable to continue publishing HISTOLOGY, materially aided me in transferring the elements of this book to its new publisher.

I thank Robert Marshak, my Dean at the School of Veterinary Medicine at the University of Pennsylvania, for his effective support of the basic sciences and his encouragement of this text. I am indebted to Michael Sorrell, Patricia McManus, Joyce Knoll, Fern Tablin, Lillian Maggio, and Karen Young—my laboratory colleagues who critically read the manuscript. Robert Walker's advice on the organization of chapters and on the clarity of exposition was invaluable.

Roy Greep created this multi-authored text and brought it to maturation. He remains a cherished friend and advisor. This book is dedicated to him.

I am proud of my colleagues, the authors of this book, who with magnanimity and profound scholarship have written chapters of exceptional quality. This book has bound us together. I hope that our solidarity and common purpose confers a unity on this work evident to the reader. I thank Alan Tartakoff, who revised the section of the Golgi Complex in Chapter 1, and I remain indebted to James Lake for his treatment of ribosomes in Chapter 1.

The National Institutes of Health, the National Science Foundation, and other granting agencies have supported the research that brought Histology to its present exciting and important state. Any success that we have in conveying this excitement and in stimulating young scholars we offer as tribute to these agencies.

Leon Weiss

Contributors

Eric G. Bauer, Ph.D.
Department of Anatomy, University of Minnesota, Minneapolis, MN 55455

Richard J. Blandau, M.D., Ph.D.
Department of Biological Structure, University of Washington, School of Medicine, Seattle, WA 98195

Ruth Ellen Bulger, Ph.D.
Department of Pathology and Laboratory Medicine, The University of Texas Health Science Center, Houston, TX 77025

W. Maxwell Cowan, M.D., Ph.D.
Salk Institute of Biological Studies, San Diego, CA 92212

Martin Dym, Ph.D.
Department of Anatomy, Georgetown University, Washington, DC 20007

Åke Flocke, Ph.D.
Department of Physiology II, Karolinska Institutet, Stockholm, Sweden

Geraldine F. Gauthier, Ph.D.
Department of Anatomy, The University of Massachusetts Medical School, Worcester, MA 01605

Burton D. Goldberg, M.D.
Department of Pathology, New York University School of Medicine, New York, NY 10016

M.R.C. Greenwood, Ph.D.
Department of Biology, Vassar College, Poughkeepsie, NY 12601

Eva Griepp, M.D.
Departments of Cell Biology and Pediatrics, New York University School of Medicine, New York, NY 10016

Nicholas S. Halmi, M.D.
Department of Anatomy, Mount Sinai Hospital School of Medicine, New York, NY 10029

James D. Jamieson, M.D., Ph.D.
Department of Cell Biology, Yale University School of Medicine, New Haven, CT 06510

Webster S.S. Jee, Ph.D.
Department of Pharmacology, Division of Radiobiology, University of Utah, College of Medicine, Salt Lake City, UT 84112

Patricia Johnson, Ph.D.
Department of Biology, Vassar College, Poughkeepsie, NY 12601

Albert L. Jones, M.D.
Cell Biology Section, Veterans' Administration Hospital, San Francisco, CA 94121

Edward G. Jones, M.D., Ph.D.
Department of Anatomy and Neurobiology, Washington University School of Medicine, St. Louis, MO 63110

Toichiro Kuwabara, M.D.
National Eye Institute, National Institutes of Health, Bethesda, MD 20014

John A. Long, Ph.D.
Department of Anatomy, University of California School of Medicine, San Francisco, CA 94112

Marion R. Neutra, Ph.D.
Department of Anatomy, Harvard Medical School,
Boston, MA 02115

Helen A. Padykula, Ph.D.
Department of Anatomy, The University of
Massachusetts Medical School, Worcester, MA 01605

Dorothy R. Pitelka, Ph.D.
Cancer Research Laboratory, University of California,
Berkeley, Berkeley, California 94720

John T. Potts, Jr., M.D.
General Medical Services, Massachusetts General
Hospital, Boston, MA 02114

Wilbur B. Quay, Ph.D.
Department of Anatomy, Division of Biochemistry,
Department of Human Biological Chemistry and
Genetics, The University of Texas Medical Branch,
Galveston, TX 77550

Michel Rabinovitch, M.D.
Department of Cell Biology, New York University
School of Medicine, New York, NY 10016

Edith Robbins, Ph.D.
Department of Cell Biology, New York University
School of Medicine, New York, NY 10016

Maya Simionescu, Ph.D.
Institute of Cellular Biology, #8 Hasdev Street,
Bucharest 70646, Rumania

Nicolae Simionescu, M.D.
Institute of Cellular Biology, #8 Hasdev Street,
Bucharest 70646, Rumania

Sergei P. Sorokin, M.D.
Department of Physiology, Harvard University School
of Public Health, Boston, MA 02115

Elinor Spring-Mills, Ph.D.
Departments of Anatomy and Urology, State
University of New York, Upstate Medical Center,
Syracuse, NY 13210

Kurt S. Stenn, M.D.
Department of Pathology, Yale University School of
Medicine, New Haven, CT 06510

Lois W. Tice, M.D.
Laboratory of Experimental Pathology, NIAMDD,
National Institutes of Health, Bethesda, MD 20014

Hershey Warshawsky, Ph.D.
Department of Anatomy, McGill University School of
Medicine, Montreal, P.Q., Canada H3C 3G1

Leon Weiss, M.D.
Laboratory of Experimental Hematology and Cell
Biology, Department of Animal Biology, University of
Pennsylvania, School of Veterinary Medicine,
Philadelphia, PA 19104

Histology

Cell and Tissue Biology

Fifth edition

Plate 1

2–12 Periodic acid Schiff (PAS) reaction, rhesus monkey uterine luminal epithelium. Polysaccharide–protein complexes have been localized in these columnar epithelial cells by the PAS reaction. The nuclei are stained with hematoxylin (basic or cationic dye). Note the PAS-positive pink cytoplasmic areas in apical cytoplasmic projections and below the nuclei. This PAS reactivity represents glycogen stores, as substantiated by characteristic ultrastructure. The proteoglycans of the extracellular matrix of the underlying connective tissue are PAS-positive.

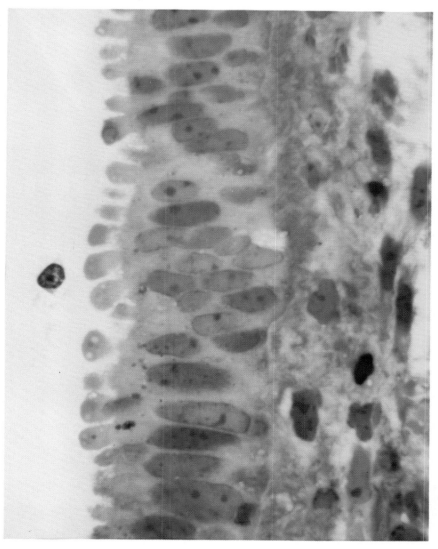

Plate 2

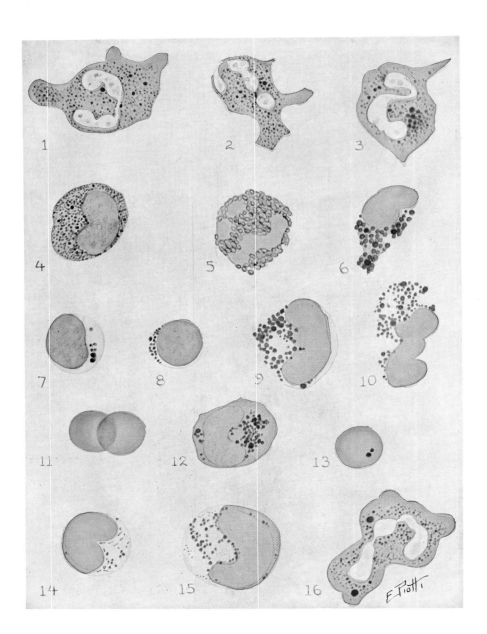

Plate 3

11–4 Human blood cells stained supravitally. All cells are from the same individual and are drawn to the same scale. Cells 1–13 are stained with neutral red only (granules and phagocytic vacuoles). Cells 14–16 are stained with neutral red and Janus green (mitochondria). (Preparation Courtesy of E. Tompkins.)

1. Polymorphonuclear neutrophil stained for 20 min at 37°C. The small dots are the specific, refractive granules, which appear brown-red or gray, depending on focus. Unlike phagocytic vacuoles, these do not change with time. The pseudopodia are usually free of the streaming granules. The larger droplets represent the phagocytic vacuoles. There are few of these in a normal neutrophil within this period of time.

2. A neutrophil from the same field after the film had been at room temperature for 1 h. Phagocytosis is slight at the lower temperature, and there is little change in the vacuoles.

3. The same cells as in 2 after the film had been at room temperature for 2 h. The number of lobes of the nucleus has changed somewhat as the result of ameboid movements. The cell has become toxically injured after long exposure and is phagocytizing abnormally.

4. Myelocyte film stained at 37°C for 1 h. There are no ameboid movements and little phagocytosis. The specific granules are more refractive and stain more on the acid side than the granules of polymorphonuclear neutrophils.

5. Polymorphonuclear eosinophil from the same film as 4. The granules are highly refractive, and the intensity of their color consequently varies with focus. They are large, rice-shaped, and fairly uniform in size. They are straw-colored when freshly stained but gradually take on an apricot tint with exposure. Eosinophils rarely contain phagocytic vacuoles.

6. Polymorphonuclear basophil. The granules are large, round, very uniform, and highly refractive; the intensity of staining therefore varies with focus. The granules stain a deeper crimson than phagocytic vacuoles or than the granules of any other cells of the blood. The nucleus rarely shows lobing, and the cells are practically never phagocytic.

7. Intermediate-sized lymphocyte from same film as 4 after the film stood at room temperature for 1 h. The cytoplasm is very clear and contains few phagocytic vacuoles. There are many fewer phagocytic vacuoles than in monocytes and they are arranged indiscriminately. Lymphocytes should rarely be confused with monocytes. Double staining with Janus green also serves to differentiate the two types (see 13 and 14).

8. Small lymphocyte from same film as 7 after the film stood at room temperature for 2 h.

9. 10. Monocytes from the same film after it stained for 5 min at 37°C, and 1 h and 2 h, respectively, at room temperature. Monocytes vary constantly in shape and degree of phagocytosis, depending on ameboid movement. They have the greatest number of phagocytic vacuoles of all blood cells and no granules. The vacuoles vary in size and change position constantly. They increase in both size and number with time of exposure.

11. Two normal erythrocytes. They do not stain. Their color is due entirely to their content of hemoglobin.

12. Monocyte from same film as 9 and 10. The cell is somewhat younger than those in 9 and 10, less ameboid, and tends to aggregate the phagocytic vacuoles into rosette formation.

13. Erythrocyte from same film as 12. The cell is younger than those in 11 and contains reticulum, which was stained with neutral red.

14. Lymphocyte stained with neutral red and Janus green (compare with 7). Janus green inhibits phagocytosis somewhat. The mitochondria stain blue-green, are definitely rod-shaped, and tend to cluster toward the nucleus. They are larger than the mitochondria of monocytes.

15. Monocyte stained with neutral red and Janus green. Phagocytosis has been inhibited somewhat. The mitochondria are smaller than those in lymphocytes and more scattered (compare with 14).

16. Polymorphonuclear neutrophil stained with neutral red and Janus green. The mitochondria are the size of those in monocytes but are less abundant. Janus green is soon toxic to cells, and this cell shows the toxic action in the form of unusual phagocytic vacuoles.

Plate 4

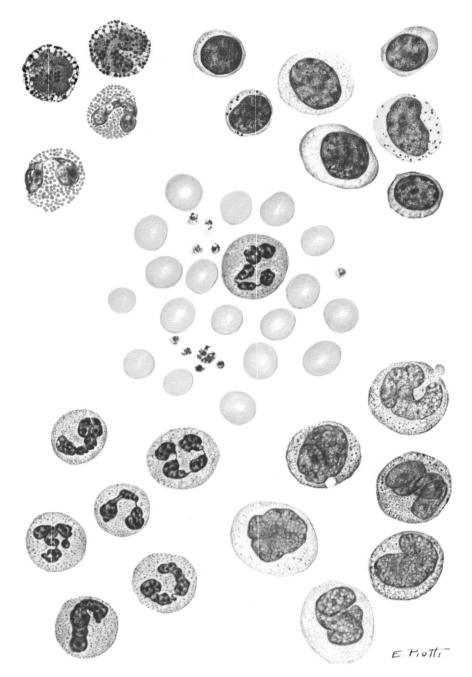

11–5 Cells from a smear preparation of normal human blood. Wright's stain. In the center, adult red corpuscles, blood platelets, and a polymorphonuclear neutrophil. At left above, two polymorphonuclear basophils and two polymorphonuclear eosinophils. At right above, three large and four small lymphocytes. At left below, polymorphonuclear neutrophils. At right below, six monocytes.

Plate 5

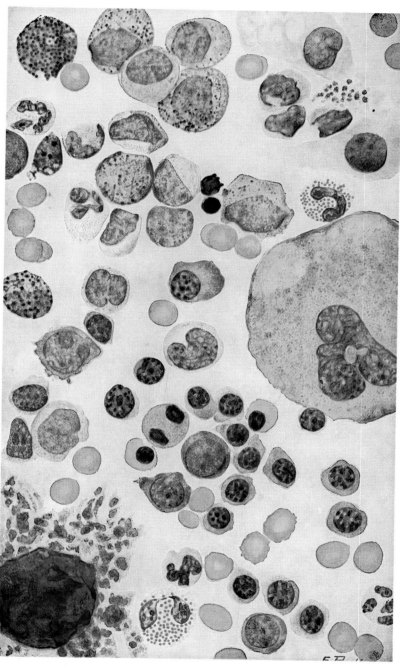

Cells from bone marrow.

Cells from spleen.

Cells found in circulating blood.

12–5 Composite plate of blood cells. **A,** eosinophilic myelocyte; **B,** myelocyte; **D,** blast form; **E,** basophilic leukocyte; **F,** small lymphocyte; **G,** medium-sized lymphocyte; **H,** large lymphocyte; **I,** blast form; **J,** basophilic erythroblast; **K,** megakaryocyte; **L,** eosinophilic leukocyte; **M,** neutrophilic leukocyte; **O,** polychromatophilic erythroblast; **P,** platelets; **Q,** reticulum cell; **R,** monocyte; **S,** plasma cell.

Plate 6

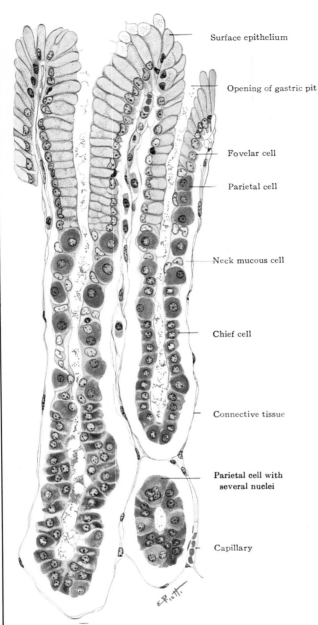

Surface epithelium

Opening of gastric pit

Fovelar cell

Parietal cell

Neck mucous cell

Chief cell

Connective tissue

Parietal cell with several nuclei

Capillary

19–11 Drawing of two gastric glands of the adult
human stomach. Four cell types are evident
in the epithelium: the surface mucous cell (extending
down into the pits), the neck mucous cell, the
acidophilic parietal (or oxyntic) cell, and the
basophilic chief (or zymogenic) cell. The epithelium
has shrunk away from the underlying basement
membrane and connective tissue. Zenker fixation;
eosin and methylene blue.

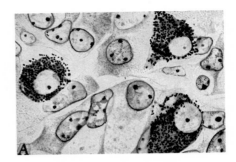

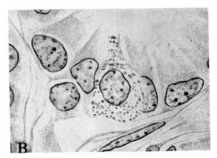

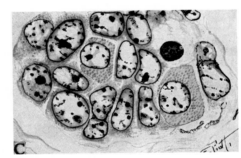

19–12 Reactions of granules in argentaffin
cells from the small intestine of a pig.
A. Fixed in alcohol-formalin-acetic acid;
stained by Bodian silver method. **B.** Fixed in
acetone; stained by Gomori method for acid
phosphatase. **C.** Fixed in Zenker-formalin;
stained with eosin and methylene blue.
× 1,200. (Courtesy of G. B. Wislocki and
E. W. Dempsey.)

Plate 7

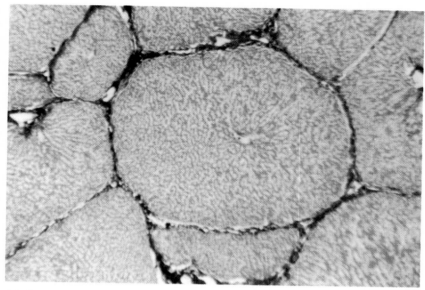

20–7 Low-power photomicrograph of a section of pig liver, showing a classic lobule. Mallory-Azan.

20–8 Low-power photomicrograph of a section of human liver, illustrating boundaries of a classic lobule. Mallory-Azan.

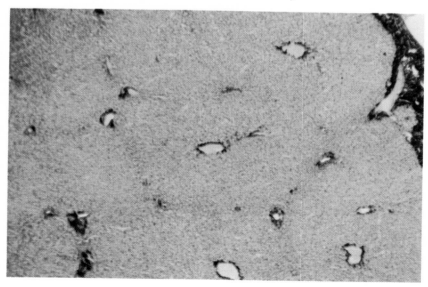

Plate 8

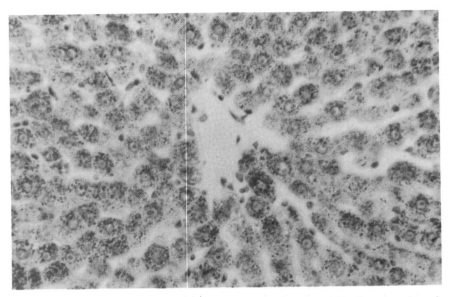

20–12 Glycogen deposits within the parenchymal cells are stained red by Best's carmine. The quantity of glycogen within the cells varies with the time interval after the last meal and the position of the cell in the lobule. Glycogen is not preserved in routine histological preparations. Rat liver. Carnoy's fixative. Hematoxylin and Best's carmine.

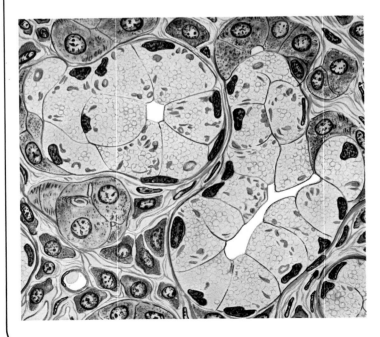

21–19 Section of the sublingual gland of a 30-year-old man. The mucus-secreting cells are stained blue; the serous cells are gray. Zenker fixation; iron-hematoxylin and Mallory's connective tissue stain.

Plate 9

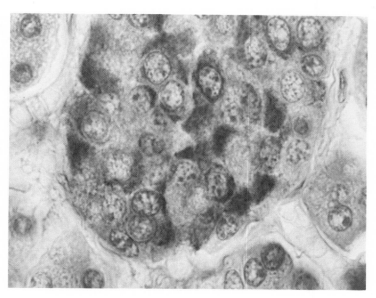

22–1 Photomicrograph of a human pancreatic islet stained with aldehyde fuchsin and Ponceau counterstain. Insulin secretory vesicles of the B cells are stained purple, whereas other islet cells and surrounding acinar cells are red-pink. A delicate reticular fiber layer borders the islet. × 1,000. (Courtesy of A.-M. Carpenter.)

23–12 Ganglion cells of the pulmonary plexus near the tracheal bifurcation of a hamster. PAS-lead hematoxylin. × 90.

23–13 Tracheal mucosa of a rat showing a brush cell **(arrowhead)** in the epithelium. PAS-lead hematoxylin. × 800.

23–16 Epithelium, fiber systems, and glands on the dorsal aspect of the trachea in a mouse. Resorcin-fuchsin, toluidine blue, and alcian green. × 175.

23–17 Tracheal smooth muscle of a mouse inserting on the elastic skeleton just deep to the thick longitudinal fibers. Resorcin-fuchsin, hematoxylin, and alcian green. × 300.

23–20 The peripheral airway (greenish) with its accompanying pulmonary artery (red) on the left, and together with the pulmonary vein (blue) on the right, as these structures appear in casts. (From Lauweryns, J. 1962. De Longvaten. Brussels: Ed. Arscia.)

23–24 Bronchial epithelium of the human lung. Alcian blue and hematoxylin. × 250.

Plate 10

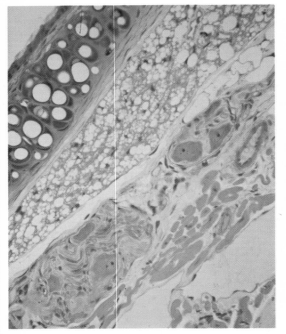

Figure 23–12

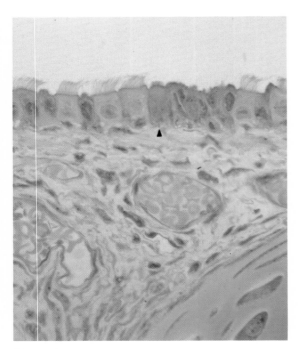

Figure 23–13

Figure 23–16

Figure 23–17

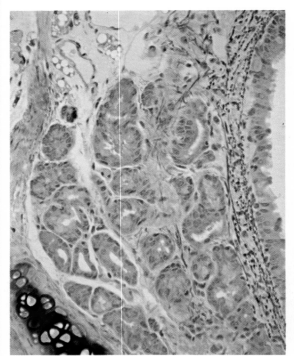

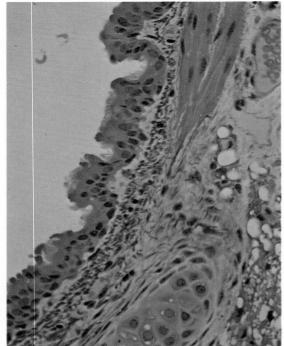

Plate 11

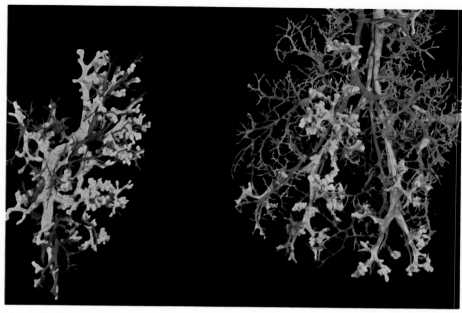

Figure 23–20

Figure 23–24

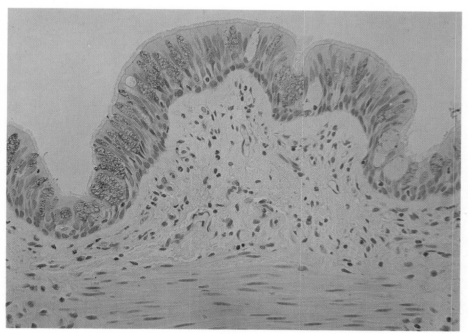

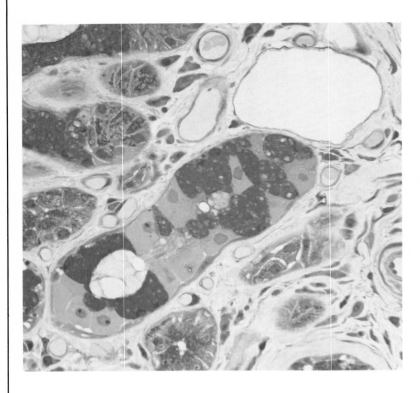

23–30 Secretory acini and intermediate duct of a human bronchial gland, showing the principal cell types present: serous (stippled purple), mucous (magenta overall), oncocytes (pale grayish), and myoepithelial (lying along basement membrane). PAS-lead hematoxylin. × 420.

23–38 Prussian blue–stained iron particles in the bronchus of a mouse, located in macrophages on the surface and in the connective tissue as well as in the epithelium in-between. Basic fuchsin. × 1,100.

23–37 Hamster bronchiole showing predominance of nonciliated bronchiolar cells, one with many secretory granules. PAS-lead hematoxylin. × 1,200.

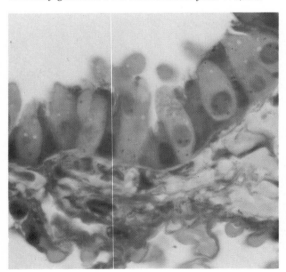

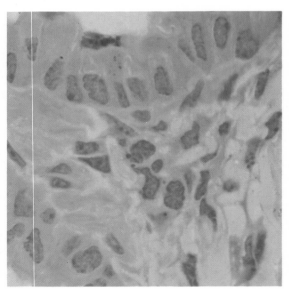

Plate 13

23–39 Human bronchial epithelium showing a small-granule cell with basally located secretory matter **(arrowhead),** as well as globule leukocytes (foamy cytoplasm) and other more usual epithelial cells. PAS-lead hematoxylin. × 2,000.

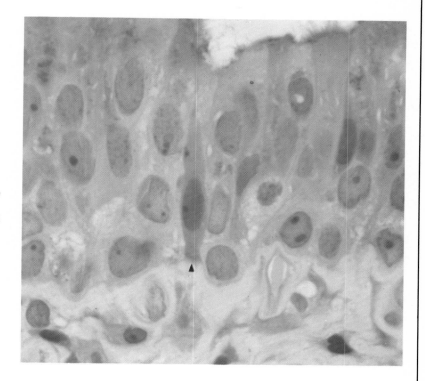

23–40 Small-granule cells (left of center) in the bronchial epithelium of a hamster; all are PAS-positive and two have lead hematoxylin–stained granules. × 900. (From Sorokin, S., and Hoyt, R. F., Jr. 1978. Anat. Rec. 192:245.)

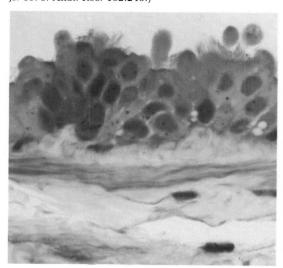

23–42 Heterophil leukocytes (pink) in migration through the epithelium at the origins of right and left bronchi in a hamster lung. PAS and hematoxylin. × 900.

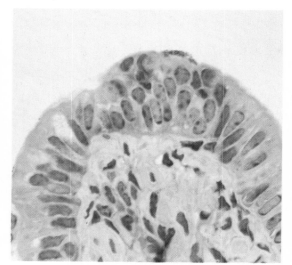

Plate 14

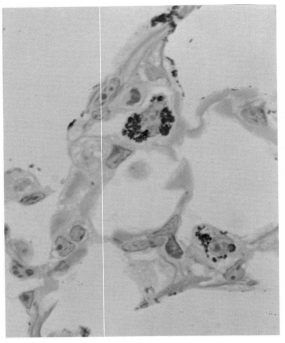

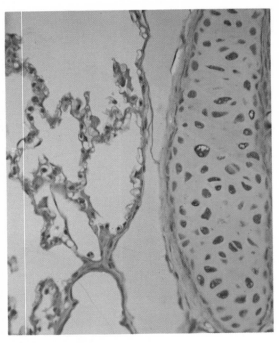

23–64 Alveolar macrophages ingesting inhaled iron oxide particles (Prussian blue) deposited in alveoli of a mouse's lung. × 1,100. (From Sorokin, S., and Brain. J. 1975. Anat. Rec. 181:581.)

23–75 Lymphatic collecting vessel with funnel-shaped valve alongside the bronchus of a cat. PAS-lead hematoxylin. × 250.

23–73 Diagram showing the interrelationships among the airways, the vascular systems, and the lymphatic networks of the lung. (After diagrams of W. S. Miller and J. Lauweryns.)

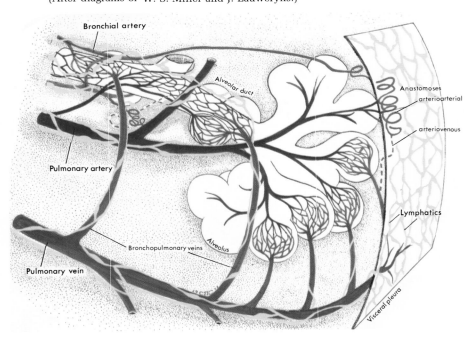

Plate 15

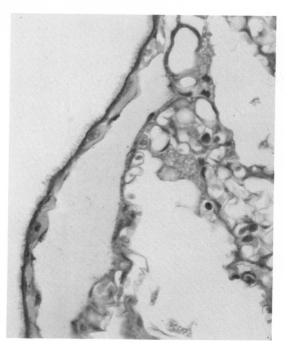

23-76 Pleural lymphatic vessel and prominent brush border of mesothelial cells in a cat's lung. PAS-lead hematoxylin. × 450.

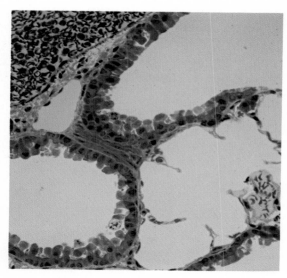

23-77 Cross section of a lymphatic vessel (upper left) near a branching point of the airway in a mouse. Prussian blue and iron hematoxylin. × 275.

23-81 Mast cell beneath pleura in a guinea pig's lung. Leukocytes within blood vessels, a great alveolar cell (foamy cytoplasm), and the squamous pleural mesothelium are nearby. Toluidine blue. × 1,500.

23-80 Subepithelial lymphoid tissue along the deep lymphatic pathway at a branching of the main bronchus in a mouse's lung. Iron-containing macrophages (Prussian blue) are within. × 120.

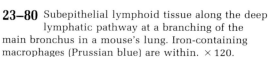

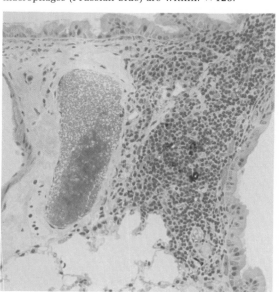

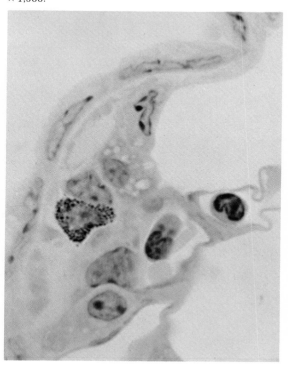

Plate 16

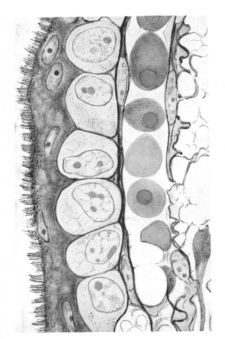

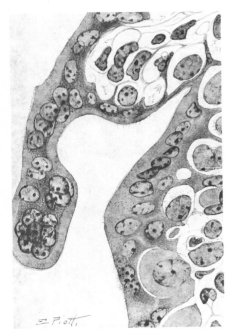

Figure 27–22

Figure 27–23

Figure 27–36

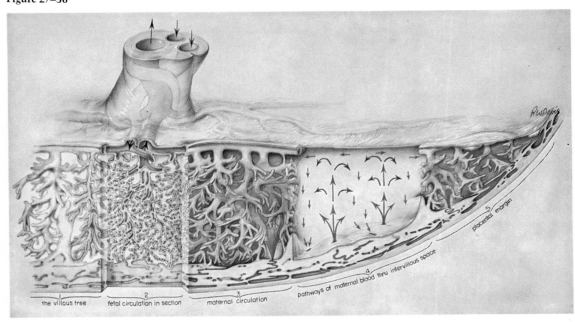

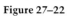

the villous tree   fetal circulation in section   maternal circulation   pathways of maternal blood thru intervillous space   placental margin

Plate 17

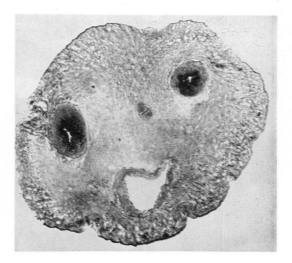

A

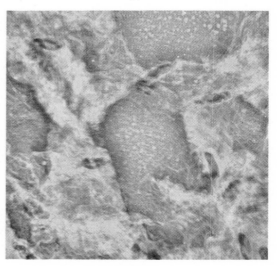

B

27–22 Drawing illustrating the structure of the human placental villus at 3 months of gestation. The trophoblast consists of an internal layer of large clear chromophobic Langhans' cells and a superficial layer of darkly stained syncytial trophoblast. The free surface of the syncytium, bordering the intervillous space, possesses a microvillous border. The Langhans' cells rest on a basement membrane. Note the difference in the size of the nuclei of the cellular and syncytial trophoblast. A capillary, containing nucleated fetal erythrocytes and lined by endothelial cells, is closely applied to the trophoblast. Mallory's connective tissue stain. × 1,520. (Courtesy of G. B. Wislocki and H. S. Bennett.)

27–23 Drawing of a section of human placental villus at 13 weeks. On the left, a tab composed exclusively of syncytium protrudes from the surface of the villus. There is marked cytoplasmic basophilia in the syncytium at the level of the nuclei, which indicates a high content of ribonucleoprotein. In the cytoplasm of the Langhans' cells there are only traces of basophilia. Methylene blue. × 1,140. (Courtesy of E. W. Dempsey and G. B. Wislocki.)

27–36 Structural organization and blood circulation in the human placenta. **Panel 1** illustrates the treelike form of a stem villus (fetus cotyledon), its origin at the chorionic plate, its branches in the intervillous space, and its anchorage to the basal plate. **Panel 2** shows the CO_2-rich blood of the umbilical arteries entering the villous tree and being returned to the fetus in oxygenated form via the umbilical vein. In **panels 3** and **4** maternal blood is shown entering the intervillous space through open-ended uteroplacental arteries. It enters in spurts and is driven toward the chorionic plate; then, as maternal pressure lessens, lateral dispersion occurs. Maternal blood drains into numerous venous openings along the basal plate. **Panel 5** illustrates the peripheral portion of the intervillous space, which consists of a series of interrupted pools or lakes. (From Harris, J. W. S., and Ramsey, E. M. 1966. Contrib. Embryol. 38:45.)

27–41 Human umbilical cord at full term stained with toluidine blue. **A.** The umbilical vein is the lower single vessel with a relatively thin wall and large lumen. The two upper vessels are the umbilical arteries with their thick walls and constricted lumina. The intense metachromasia of the ground substance of the mucous connective tissue is evident. × 6. **B.** Higher-power view of part A. Lakes of metachromatic mucous ground substance fill the interstitial spaces in the unstained collagenous framework. Only the orthochromatic nuclei of the fibroblasts are evident. × 500. Frozen dried section fixed with formalin-ether vapor. (Courtesy E. H. Leduc and G. F. Odland.)

Plate 18

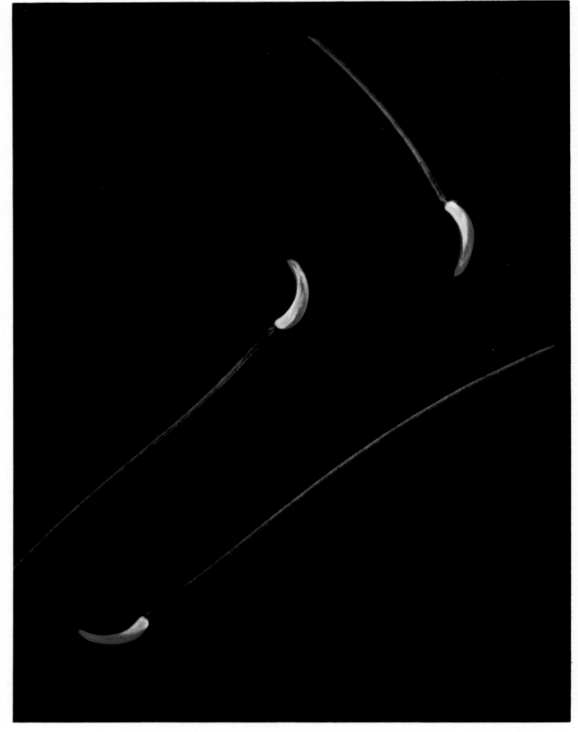

28–17 These hamster sperm have been stained with a fluorescent aminoacridine dye. The lysosomal enzymes of the acrosome stain red, the nucleus stains yellow, and the tail stains blue. (Courtesy of A. C. Allison.)

Plate 19

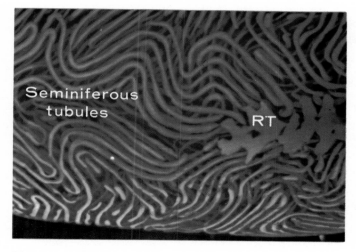

28–42 "Microfil," a compound used for microvascular injections, was introduced into the lumen of the rete testis of this rat's testis, using a 30-gauge needle. The lumina of the rete testis and the seminiferous tubules were filled with the compound. The rest of the tissue was cleared with methyl salicylate. Note the irregular outline of the superficial rete and the gentle undulating parallel pattern of the seminiferous tubules.

28–44 This preparation is similar to Fig. 28–42. The lumina of the ductuli efferentes contain the "microfil."

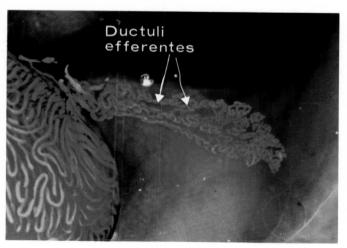

Plate 20

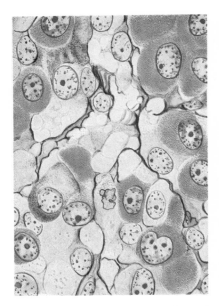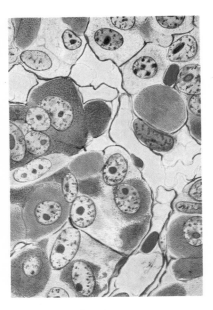

29–12 Anterior lobe of the cat hypophysis. **A.** Anestrous female.
Orange acidophils, basophils **(blue),** and chromophobes
(light blue) can be seen. **B.** Last week of pregnancy. Note presence of
numerous red carmine cells. Modified azan stain. (Drawn from
preparations of A. B. Dawson.)

The Cell

Leon Weiss

General Properties

The cell is the unit of living structure. The tissues that form the body consist entirely of cells and of extracellular material elaborated by cells. The cell, moreover, can carry out an independent existence whereas none of its constituents can do so. Indeed, an entire phylum, the Protozoa, is unicellular, and isolated metazoan cells may be maintained in tissue culture.

Most mammalian cells are microscopic, although in some instances they reach macroscopic visibility. The limits of cell size are exemplified by bacteria or bacteria-like organisms, which may be less than 1 μm in their largest dimension, and by avian egg cells, measured in centimeters (Table 1–1).

A cell is a complex, aqueous gel made of protein, carbohydrate, fat, nucleic acids, and inorganic material. Protein alone or in combination with fat, as lipoprotein, or with carbohydrate, as glycoprotein, mucoprotein, or proteoglycan, constitutes the substantive structural element both of the cell and of extracellular substances. Enzymes, large molecules that catalyze metabolic reactions, are proteins. Products and secretions of cells may be proteins. Carbohydrate is the major source of energy in mammalian cells. Among the principal carbohydrates are glucose, a monomeric utilizable form, and glycogen, a polymeric storage form. Carbohydrates built into complexes with protein may play a role in linking cells together, are major components of extracellular tissues, are significant structural elements within cells, and serve as distinctive receptors on the cell surface. Fat, too, may be a source of energy to the cell. Moreover, fatty acids, which constitute the principal storage form of fat, provide the cell with efficient depots of energy. Lipids have major structural properties. Phospholipids and sphingolipids are important in the structure of biological membranes, making them preferentially permeable to fats; they also control the orientation and mobility of proteins in the membranes.

Inorganic materials occur in cells in a variety

TABLE 1–1 Equivalent measurements

10 angstroms (Å) =	1 millimicrometer (mμm) or 1 nanometer (nm)
10,000 angstroms =	1 micrometer (μm)
1,000 microns =	1 millimeter (mm)
10 millimeters =	1 centimeter (cm)
100 centimeters =	1 meter (m)

of combinations. They may be associated with enzymes and with other proteins or fats, or they may be free of organic chemicals. They influence the adhesiveness and other physical properties of cells and extracellular materials in many different ways. Thus calcium contributes to the rigidity of bone; to the adhesiveness of the constituents of the subcellular particles, the ribosomes; to the capacity of cells to aggregate; and to the capacity of muscle to relax.

One of the achievements of microscopic anatomy is the ability to induce selective chemical reactions that reveal the location of different chemical moieties in tissue prepared for examination under the microscope. Chapter 2 is devoted to histochemistry, the term given to this division of histology, and histochemical findings are presented throughout this book.

There are two major classes of cells: prokaryotes and eukaryotes. *Prokaryotes*, exemplified by bacteria, contain nucleoprotein that may be segregated in the protoplasm as a *nuclear body* or *nucleoid* but is not enveloped in membrane. In *eukaryotes*, represented by fungi and higher forms, a true membrane-bounded nucleus is present. In fact, the eukaryotic cell is distinguished by well-developed membrane systems that not only envelope the nucleus but compartmentalize many cellular functions such as protein and steroid synthesis (the membranes of endoplasmic reticulum), respiration (the membranes of mitochondria), and secretion (the membranes of the Golgi complex).

The nucleus is typically a prominent ovoid structure lying near the center of the cell (Figs. 1–1 and 1–2). In it are chromosomes that contain *deoxyribonucleic acid (DNA)*, which encodes the genetic information. With the microscope, DNA appears as densely stained particles termed, in aggregate, *chromatin*. A nucleus may contain one or more *nucleoli*, typically spherical structures representing specialized modifications of chromosomes. There are several forms of a second type of nucleic acid, *ribonucleic acid (RNA)*. RNAs read the genetic code built into DNA and then play the central role in synthesizing the proteins encoded in the DNA. RNAs, themselves encoded in the DNA, are generated in the nucleus and are distributed in both nucleus and cytoplasm. Their complex structures and functions are discussed below.

The nucleus is surrounded by cytoplasm, the realm of protoplasm that expresses most differentiated cellular functions. The cytoplasm contains many highly organized, distinctive organ-

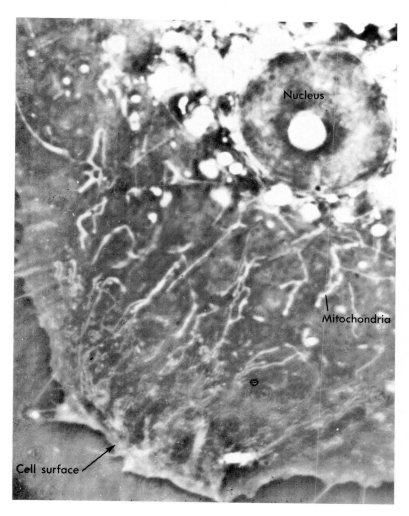

1–1 Hela cells, living in tissue culture; phase-contrast photomicrograph. Hela cells were derived by Dr. George Gey from a carcinoma of the uterine cervix explanted in tissue culture. They are maintained as a cell strain in tissue culture and used in a variety of experimental procedures. The cell border is ruffled and in places retracted, resulting in spinelike processes. The nucleus is spherical, surrounded by refractile clear bodies. Mitochondria are evident as irregular linear structures. × 1200. (From the work of Dr. G. Gey.)

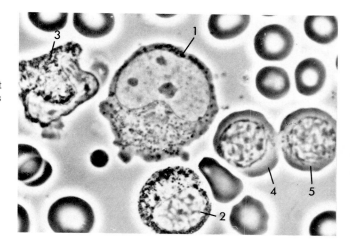

1–2 Human bone marrow cells, phase contrast microscopy. Developing white blood cells are present. They are myelocytes (*1* and *2*) and a metamyelocyte (*3*). Developing erythroblasts are also present (*4* and *5*) as are mature erythrocytes (unnumbered). See Chap. 12. × 1300. (From the work of G. A. Ackerman.)

4

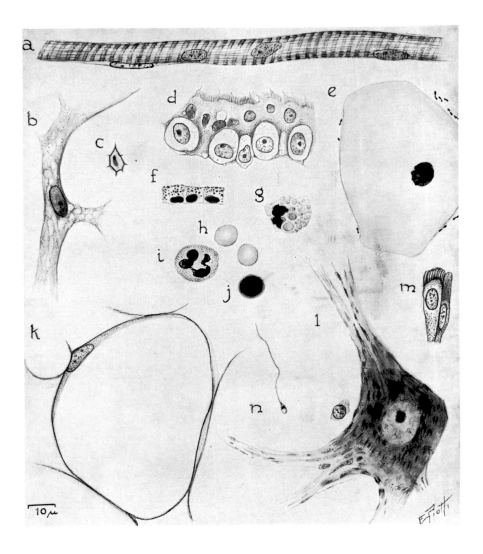

1–3 Variety of cells from the human body. **a,** portion of a striated muscle fiber. **b,** fibroblast from the umbilical cord. **c,** osteocyte within a bone lacuna. **d,** portion of the placental chorion, showing syncytial trophoblast and underlying cytotrophoblast cells. **e,** squamous epithelial cell and bacteria from a vaginal smear. **f,** three pigmented epithelial cells from the first layer of the retina. **g,** macrophage in bone marrow, which has ingested masses of blood pigments. **h,** two red blood cells. **i,** polymorphonuclear neutrophil; and **j,** small lymphocyte, all from a blood smear. **k,** fat cell from loose connective tissue. **l,** large motor neuron and adjacent small glial cell (process not revealed) from a hypoglossal nucleus in the medulla. **m,** adjacent ciliated and secretory epithelial cells from the oviduct. **n,** mature spermatozoon from semen. Cells a and d are multinucleate; g is binucleate; e has a pycnotic nucleus; c, f, j, and n have dense nuclei; the nucleus of l is extremely vesicular; i has a lobulated nucleus; the nuclei of a, g, and k are displaced by the cell contents. Some of the cells are rounded or polygonal, but a is extremely elongate, b and c have short processes, and the neuron in l has long processes (cut off here). The syncytium in d has a brush border; one cell in m has cilia; n has a flagellum. Cells a and l display cytoplasmic fibrils; f, pigment granules; g, phagocytized masses; l, specific granules; k, a space left by dissolved fat; j and the neuron in l, conspicuous amounts of cytoplasmic basophilia. [The diameter of the red blood cells (approximately 7.5 µm) provides a useful measure of the other cells.] All × 700. (Prepared by H. W. Deane and E. Piotti.)

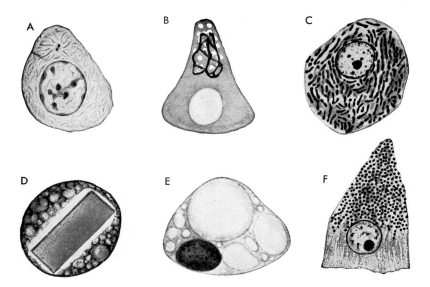

elles. These organelles include mitochondria, lysosomes, the Golgi apparatus, endoplasmic reticulum, centrioles, microtubules, microfilaments, ribosomes, secretory granules, and other structures that will be considered below. In addition, the cytoplasm contains such simple structures as glycosomes and lipid vacuoles. The cytoplasm is limited by a membrane called the *cell membrane, plasma membrane,* or *plasmalemma* (Figs. 1–2 to 1–5).

In metazoan or multicellular organisms, cells show marked specialization (Figs. 1–3 to 1–5). We speak of these cells as differentiated. In mammals cells vary in shape and size, exemplified by anucleate discoid pigmented blood cells 7 μm in diameter and branched nerve cells whose processes may reach a meter or more in length. Cell types may display pronounced internal variation. Striated muscle cells are packed with cross-banded filaments that slide on one another causing cellular contraction. Adipose cells are distended with fat, and secretory cells are filled with secretory granules. Osteoclasts may contain 25 or more nuclei, interstitial cells of the testis are packed with smooth endoplasmic reticulum, parietal cells of the stomach have rich infoldings of plasma membrane, renal tubular cells and brown fat contain extraordinarily large numbers of mitochondria, and immature erythrocytes are unusually rich in ribosomes. Keratinocytes in the skin may lose virtually all of their organelles and become scalelike structures packed with tough keratin filaments. So much has been

1–4 Various cytoplasmic organelles and cell inclusions. Because of their specific physical and chemical properties, these objects are not generally demonstrated by routine methods and are rarely revealed together. **A.** Cytocentrum in a cell of grasshopper testis, showing paired centrioles. **B.** Golgi material in a pancreatic cell of guinea pig, as demonstrated with osmic acid fixation. [Redrawn from Cowdry, E. V. (ed.) 1932. Special Cytology, 2d ed. New York: Paul B. Hoeber.] **C.** Mitochondria in a hepatocyte of a dog, stained with hematoxylin. (Weatherford.) **D.** Crystal within the nucleus of a hepatocyte of a dog. (Weatherford.) **E.** Spaces in a young fat cell left by dissolved fat. **F.** Secretory granules in a human pancreatic cell. Below and lateral to the nucleus lies ergastoplasm.

learned of the functions of the various cell constituents, in fact, that the function of a cell may be inferred from knowledge of its subcellular constituents. Indeed, such variations in cell structure and function constitute the backbone of this book.

The diversely differentiated cells that make up the complex metazoan body have clearly established a division of labor: the functions of the body are divided among them. Keratinocytes of the skin combine to form a tough protective barrier facing the outside environment. Erythrocytes of the blood, having developed chromoprotein pigment, carry the respiratory gases O_2 and CO_2. Muscle cells contract, nerve cells conduct, and bone cells provide a stable skeleton. The cells of the eye permit vision; those of the ear,

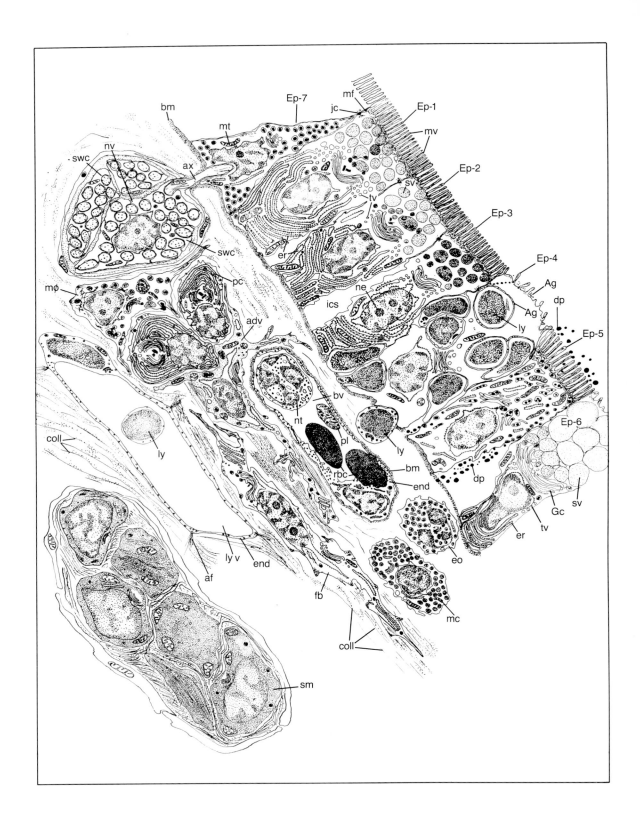

1–5 This drawing depicts a variety of cell types organized into an "imaginary" tissue that includes features of the gastrointestinal tract.

A major feature is the presence of epithelial cells lying side by side forming a surface that faces on a lumen. On their basal surface the epithelial cells rest upon a basement membrane **(bm).** (Epithelium is discussed in Chap. 3.) These epithelial cells (Ep–1 to Ep–7) are bound together by junctional membranous complexes (Chap. 3) near their luminal or apical surface, while at their lateral surfaces below the junctional complexes **(jc)** the cells diverge somewhat, creating intercellular space **(ics).** Epithelial cells Ep–1 to Ep–3 are secretory cells. They produce membrane-bounded secretory vesicles **(sv)** and release them at the luminal surface. These cells contain those cell organelles associated with secretion, viz: nucleoli **(ne)** euchromatin, endoplasmic reticulum **(er),** transport vesicles **(tv),** Golgi complex **(Gc),** and condensing, storage, and secretory vesicles. See discussions of these organelles in this chapter and discussion of secretion in Chaps. 3, 20, and 21. The apical surface of each of these cells bear microvilli **(mv).** Microfilaments **(mf)** form a terminal web beneath the microvilli and extend into them, conferring a contractile capacity upon them. Ep–5, also a secretory cell, produces mucous. Its secretory vesicles accumulate in the apical portion of the cell, but they are a good deal larger than those of Ep–1 to Ep–3 and they tend to coalesce. The Golgi complex is particularly well developed. Note that the outer nuclear membrane in the secretory cells is part of the endoplasmic reticulum and that the nuclear cisterna is dilated. The basal and lateral aspects of the cells may contain mitochondria **(m),** which are often "pocketed" by infoldings of the basal and lateral plasma membrane. Ep–1 is an absorptive cell that takes up substances in the lumen, often modifying them, transports them across the cell, and releases them to the subjacent tissues where they may be metabolized or picked up by blood or lymphatic vessels and carried to metabolic centers such as the liver. Droplets **(dp)** at the luminal surface are taken through the microvillous border and enter the cell (endocytosis) in pinocytic vesicles (p. 52). These are conveyed to the lateral margin of the cell where they are released (exocytosis). They then travel extracellularly through the basement membrane to the subjacent connective tissue. Ep–4 is a highly specialized cell, the M cell, which is part of the immune system (Chap. 19). Lymphocytes **(ly),** small immunologically competent cells that are responsible for such immunological processes as antibody formation, regularly enter and leave the M cell, lying in "pockets" of plasma membrane on its basal and lateral surfaces. The M cell takes up foreign material (antigen) from the lumen and conveys it, via pinocytotic vesicles, to the lymphocyte-containing pockets. M cells thereby present antigen to the lymphocytes initiating an immune response (Chap. 11). Ep–7 is a truncated epithelial cell resting upon the basement membrane but not reaching to the lumen. It contains granules that, on release, can influence the activity of nearby cells. A type of endocrine or paracrine cell, it may be part of the APUD system (see text). Note that it is penetrated by an axon **(ax)** that emerges from a small nerve **(nv).** The nerve consists of a large cell, Schwann cell **(swc),** whose cytoplasm carries many nerve fibers.

A stratum of connective tissue (Chap. 4) underlies the epithelium. It supports the epithelium and contains nerves, blood vessels **(bv),** lymphatic vessels **(lyv),** and free cells as macrophages **(mφ),** plasma cells **(pc),** fibroblasts **(fb),** eosinophils **(eo),** and mast cells **(mc).** Connective tissue is characterized by abundant extracellular substance. This extracellular material often includes strong, supporting collagen fibers **(coll).** The various cell types present in the connective tissues confer certain capacities on the tissue: plasma cells, antibody production; macrophages, phagocytosis; fibroblasts, collagen formation; eosinophils, phagocytosis, antiparasitic and antiinflammatory actions; mast cells, inflammation. Consult Chap. 4 (Connective Tissues) and Chap. 11 (Blood) for discussion. The blood vessel is a capillary whose wall is made of an endothelial cell **(end)** lying upon a basement membrane and an "outside" cell or adventitial cell **(adv)** (see Chap. 10). The capillary contains blood cells: a neutrophil **(nt),** red cells **(rbc),** and a platelet **(pl).** The wall of the lymphatic capillary consists of endothelium alone **(end).** The vessel contains a lymphocyte **(ly)** and its lumen is kept patent by the anchoring filaments **(af)** attached to the outside of the endothelium (Chap. 15).

Peripheral to the connective tissue layer is a fascicle of smooth muscle **(sm),** which imparts contractile functions to the tissue.

hearing; those of kidney, excretion, and so on, as this book attempts to show. Implicit in such differentiation is the formation of tissues of diverse cells to effect these functions. Nerves conduct impulses, but they form a complex tissue. Included in this tissue are fibroblasts that produce collagen to support the nerve cells, glial cells to insulate them, endothelial cells to form blood vessels to carry blood to them, and other nerves to connect with them. Thus, specialized cells exist with other specialized cells forming specialized tissues that carry out specialized functions. The dominant or distinctive cells in such tissues are recognized as *parenchyma* (e.g., the nerve cells in nervous tissue) whereas the supporting cells can be designated as *stroma*. The *vasculature*, another essential "service" part of a tissue, may be included with the stroma.

It is further implicit in the existence of the diverse tissues working together to constitute a structurally and functionally coherent body that there are integrating systems. The classic integrating systems are the nervous system (Chap. 8) and the endocrine system (Chap. 21), which coordinate such complex events as reproduction, respiration, locomotion, etc. Histology is undergoing a revolution—no other term will do—because as additional actions of the classic systems are being newly discovered, hitherto unknown integrating systems are simultaneously being recognized. For example, a fair number of substances long known as regulators in other systems are now being uncovered as neural mediators as well. Prolactin, newly discovered as a central nervous system neurotransmitter has been known for years as a hormone produced in the pituitary gland and targeting the mammary glands where it induces the production and release of milk. There are, moreover, systems of *paracrine secretion* wherein peptides released by cells lying within a tissue govern the activity of other cells in that tissue. In contrast to the *endocrine system* in which hormones released from an endocrine organ typically travel some distance via the blood stream to reach a target organ, paracrine secretion is released and diffuses locally to affect local cells. Thus, paracrine cells in the epithelium of the gut release peptides that regulate motility, absorption, and secretion of nearby cells in the gut wall (Chap. 19). Some of these paracrine cells are fired by connecting nerves. A common characteristic of a subpopulation of such secretory cells in the gastrointestinal, respiratory, and several other systems is that they form their peptides or other low-molecular weight agents by taking up amine precursors and decarboxylating them. These types of cells have therefore been collectively termed the *APUD system* (Amine Precursor Uptake and Decarboxylation), further discussed in Chaps. 19 and 29. Still another network of cells with regulatory function is that of T lymphocytes, as discussed in Chaps. 11, 12, and 14. T lymphocytes have a controlling role over lymphocytes, macrophages, and related cells in inflammation and immune reactions. They may have a rather broad role in regulating cellular differentiation in other contexts.

Despite pronounced variations in cell structure, most cells do have much in common. Before exploring the general features of cells, we shall first consider some techniques widely used by morphologists.

Microscopy

In the most common types of microscopy of biological material, light or electrons are sent through a slice of tissue. The light or electrons are modified by the tissue as they pass through it. This modification contains information inherent in the specimen, and the function of the lens systems in any microscope is to amplify and convert that information to a form, an *image*, discernible by eye.

The human eye is sensitive to the contrast of light and dark and to differences in color. A light train may be represented as electromagnetic sine waves, color being a function of wavelength and intensity a function of amplitude. To render visible the disturbance in the light train induced by a biological preparation, the light must be modified in color or intensity. Some wave frequencies must be absorbed more than others so that the preparation will be seen to contain materials of different colors, or there must be a change in the amplitude of a wave so that the preparation will be seen to consist of dark and light parts. Thus, if the rim of a nucleus is darker than the surrounding structure, the nucleus is delineated and can be recognized (Figs. 1–3 and 1–4). If such structures as mitochondria or glycosomes can be distinctively colored, they can be recognized. Perhaps the primary role of the microscope is to permit the identification of different structures within tissues. Beyond such simple identification, however, there is considerable physical, chemical, and ultrastructural information inherent in tissues that can be revealed by specialized methods of microscopic analysis. These methods depend on various types of microscope, which we shall now consider.

Bright-field Microscopy

The bright-field microscope is a complex optical instrument consisting of three lens systems, a stage on which to place the preparation, and controls to permit focus.

The light is focused on the preparation by the condenser lens system. It passes through the specimen, where it is modified, and this modified beam enters the objective lens system. An image is formed in the focal plane of the objective. In that image lies whatever resolution the instrument is capable of providing. The bright-field microscope is theoretically capable of resolving points approximately 0.2 μm apart. The ocular or eyepiece then magnifies the image formed by the objective, presenting it to the eye as a visible magnified image.

The primary purpose in staining histological preparations is to induce differential absorption of light so that various structures may be seen in distinguishing colors. Staining has expanded from this elementary function until it has become possible to stain many chemical compounds selectively and specifically (Chap. 2).

Phase-contrast Microscopy

Although unstained tissue does not absorb light, it does affect light by retarding some wave trains more than others. Thus light may enter a specimen in phase, that is, with peaks and troughs of the component sine waves in register. However, the components of the specimen, having different optical densities, retard the sine waves differentially, putting them out of phase with one another. These phase differences are not perceivable by the eye. The function of the phase microscope is to convert phase differences into amplitude differences by matching the retarded waves with out-of-phase waves so as to cancel or diminish the amplitude of the retarded waves. The phase microscope thus permits one to observe considerable detail in unstained material and hence is suited to the study of living cells (Figs. 1–1 and 1–2).

Dark-field Microscopy

The dark-field microscope is also able to provide contrast in unstained material. Its effectiveness depends on excluding the central light train that comes into the objective from the condenser in the conventional bright-field microscope. Instead, the specimen is illuminated by light coming in from the side. Should there be objects of greater optical density than their surroundings in the field, such as bacteria moving in a fluid medium, they will deflect light into the microscopic objective and appear as light objects against a dark background. Little or no internal structure of the lighted particles is revealed. This technique has largely been superseded by phase-contrast microscopy.

Interference Microscopy

The interference microscope provides not only contrast in unstained preparations but additional information on the physical properties and the submicroscopic organization of tissue. Like the phase microscope, the interference microscope relies on phase differences induced in transmitted light by differences in optical densities in the parts of the biological preparation. However, the interference microscope is a quantitative instrument in which the light trains subject to phase retardation are compared with a reference beam. Because the optical density and phase retardation are in proportion to specimen mass, the mass of different components of the cell may be calculated.

Fluorescence Microscopy

The fluorescence microscope depends on exciting the emission of visible light in a specimen irradiated with ultraviolet light. Certain biological substances, such as vitamin A, are *autofluorescent;* that is, they can absorb light of one frequency and emit light of another. In practice, light within one frequency range, usually in the ultraviolet spectrum, is focused on the specimen, care being taken to protect the observer's eyes from this damaging radiation. This light is absorbed by certain structures in the specimen, which then emit light within the visible range, the wavelength of the emitted light depending on the chemical nature of the emitting substance. Although the autofluorescence of materials like

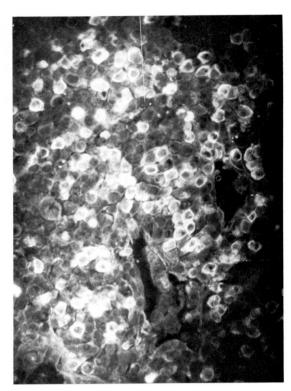

1–6 Fluorescence microscopy. A lymph node of a rabbit in the fourth day of a secondary antibody response to the antigen bovine serum albumin. The antibody, which has been tagged with a fluorescent tracer and is white in this photomicrograph, is present in the cytoplasm of plasma cells and lymphocytes. The nuclei are seldom stained and are present as negative (dark) images. See Chaps. 2 and 15. × 500. (From the work of A. H. Coons.)

vitamin A permits the use of this microscope with unstained material, the value of the technique is enormously enhanced by staining the tissue with fluorescent reagents (see Fig. 1–6 and Chaps. 2, 15, and 16).

Ultraviolet Microscopy

The ultraviolet microscope, like the fluorescence microscope, is built around the use of ultraviolet light instead of visible light. Its optical system is usually made of quartz, which efficiently transmits ultraviolet light. The image-bearing ultraviolet light coming from the ocular of the ultraviolet microscope is recorded on a photographic film, because ultraviolet light is both invisible

and damaging to the eye. The value of the ultraviolet microscope lies in the fact that certain highly significant cellular structures, notably those containing nucleic acids, absorb ultraviolet light of specific wavelengths and can therefore be demonstrated. Because the wavelength of ultraviolet is shorter than that of visible light, this microscope offers somewhat higher resolution than the bright-field microscope.

Polarizing Microscopy

The polarizing microscope permits one to determine whether biological materials have different refractive indices along different optical axes. Such materials are *birefringent* or *anisotropic*. They are able to convert a beam of linear polarized light to elliptical polarized light, one axis of which can be transmitted by an analyzer and visualized. In the polarizing microscope, light is polarized below the stage of the microscope by a Nicol quartz prism or other suitable polarizer. The polarizer is made of material capable of transmitting only polarized light in one plane or axis. By rotating the analyzer, the polarization of the light transmitted by the specimen may be determined and any change from the character of polarization of the source detected. Substances incapable of affecting polarized light are termed *isotropic*. For biological material to change linear to elliptical polarized light, submicroscopic particles that are asymmetric must be present, and these particles must be oriented in an ordered nonrandom manner. Thus, the ability of biological material to change linear to elliptical polarized light indicates that its submicroscopic structure consists of oriented asymmetric molecules.

Filaments, fibers, and linear proteins are typically birefringent. Lipoprotein complexes, such as those composing membranes, may display complex polarizing properties. Typically, the orientation of the lipid molecules, and hence their rotation of polarized light, is at right angles to that of the protein component. Polarization optics have been fruitfully applied to the study of muscle, connective tissue fibers, cell membranes, and the achromatic mitotic apparatus (Fig. 1–7).

Transmission Electron Microscopy

The transmission electron microscope (TEM), in contrast to light microscopes, uses a beam of electrons in place of a beam of light. Additional

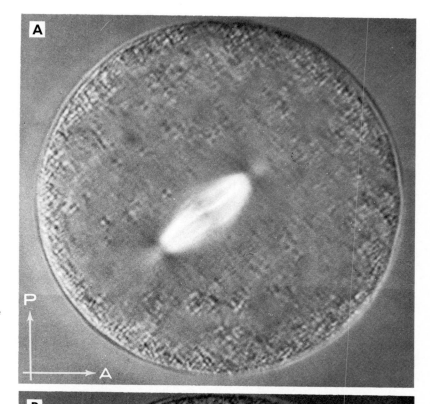

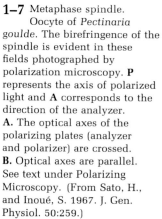

1–7 Metaphase spindle.
Oocyte of *Pectinaria goulde*. The birefringence of the spindle is evident in these fields photographed by polarization microscopy. **P** represents the axis of polarized light and **A** corresponds to the direction of the analyzer.
A. The optical axes of the polarizing plates (analyzer and polarizer) are crossed.
B. Optical axes are parallel. See text under Polarizing Microscopy. (From Sato, H., and Inoué, S. 1967. J. Gen. Physiol. 50:259.)

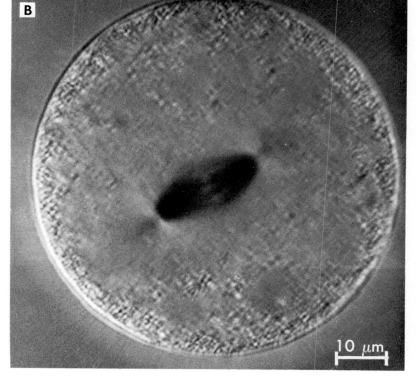

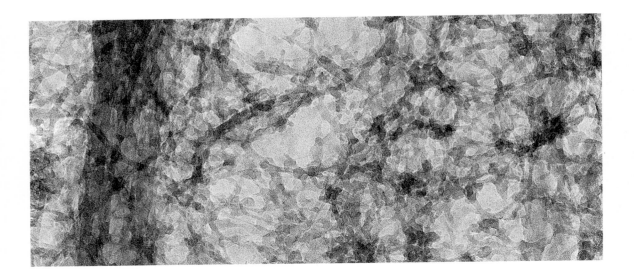

1–8 High-voltage electron micrograph. The electron beam, impelled at higher voltage, penetrates thicker sections and provides greater resolution than that in conventional transmission electron microscopes. This field includes the ground cytoplasm (hyaloplasm or cell sap). The ground substance of the cytoplasm contains a lattice of microtrabeculae. These form an irregular lattice which is continuous with the actin fibers (on the left) and support polysomes at their junction points. The microtrabeculae are about 30 to 50 Å in diameter and highly variable in length. The intertrabecular spaces provide for the rapid diffusion of water soluble metabolites. × 145,000. (Courtesy of John Wolosewick and Keith Porter.)

differences follow from the special properties of electrons. Electron beams are streams of negatively charged particles incapable of passing through glass. Hence, the lenses of an electron microscope are electromagnetic coils that surround the beam at different levels, somewhat like a set of collars. The strength of these electromagnetic lenses may be changed by varying the current passing through their coils. By varying the strength of the projector lens (the counterpart of the ocular of the light microscope), the magnification of the image formed by the objective lens is changed.

Electrons are charged particles, and because collision with charged molecules of air will absorb and deflect electrons and distort the beam, the optical system of an electron microscope must be evacuated of air. A vacuum of 10^{-4} mm Hg is commonly required. The electron stream is produced by heating a tungsten filament. The electrons are directed and impelled by moderately high voltage, usually ranging from 40,000 to 100,000 V. The higher voltages produce electron streams with shorter wavelengths, which are more penetrating and produce an image with less contrast but with higher resolution than lower voltages. Because electron beams are invisible to the eye, the images they form must be revealed by causing them to strike a fluorescent screen, and they are then recorded on a photographic plate.

Stability of the specimen is always a major consideration, and efforts must be made to protect the specimen against sublimation, distortion, and other damage by the electron beam or the vacuum. The specimen must be extremely thin for the electrons, so easily absorbed, to pass through it and create an image. Electron-microscopic sections are approximately 0.025 μm (250 Å) thick. Obtaining sections of tissues this thin has required the development of special slicing machines, *ultramicrotomes*, and a special technology of fixing and embedding tissues. Because thin sections have little intrinsic contrast, they must be stained with electron-absorbing heavy metals to provide the contrast necessary to reveal details of cell structure.

The value of the electron microscope lies in its great resolving power. Resolution of a microscope, measured as the distance between the closest two points it can distinguish as separate, depends on the wavelength of the radiation. An electron train has wave characteristics in addition to the characteristics of charge and mass. Its wavelength is small enough so that resolution of about 2 Å is possible and about 30 Å is routine. Consequently, a useful magnification of more than 500,000 is possible. The bright-field microscope, in contrast, has a resolution of approximately 0.2 μm and a useful magnification of 2,000. It has not yet proved practicable to examine living tissue by electron microscopy because of the vacuum and the damaging effects of electrons. Techniques that make it possible to obtain histochemical information at electron-microscopic resolutions have made electron microscopy increasingly productive. Moreover, quantitative analytic methods are available.

Variations on the TEM have been made. High-voltage electron microscopes capable of exceptionally high resolution exist. With accelerating voltages of a million electron-volts, they provide greater resolution and greater penetrating power of the electron beam and, therefore, the capacity to use thicker sections than is possible by conventional TEMs (Fig. 1–8).

Scanning Electron Microscopy

Scanning electron microscopy (SEM) provides a beautiful three-dimensional high-resolution image of cells and tissues (Figs. 1–9, 13–7, and 16–19). Moreover, cytochemical features can be localized on the image.

In SEM the surface of the tissue is studied. Whole mounts of tissue cultures or pieces of tissue are placed on the stage of the SEM. A slender electron beam or probe plays upon the surface, going back and forth in a regular way scanning the preparation. As the electron probe strikes the surface of the specimen, it generates several different kinds of signals. These signals include electrons (the so-called secondary electrons) and x rays. The secondary electrons may be focused on a cathode-ray tube or photographic film to form the three-dimensional image. X rays are generated when the electron probe strikes atoms having a mass greater than that of sodium. Each element is the source of x rays of distinctive wavelengths. The magnitude of the x rays generated is a function of the concentration of the element. Analysis of the x ray pattern of a tissue thus provides information on the concentration and distribution of elements.

Tissues prepared for SEM are fixed and dried. Drying at *critical point* has become the preferred method. The tissue is introduced into a suitable fluid and that fluid brought to its critical point, which is the combination of pressure and temperature at which the fluid and gaseous phases exist together without an interface or meniscus. Thus, there is no surface tension. The presence of surface tension during drying is disruptive to a tissue and causes visible distortions. After

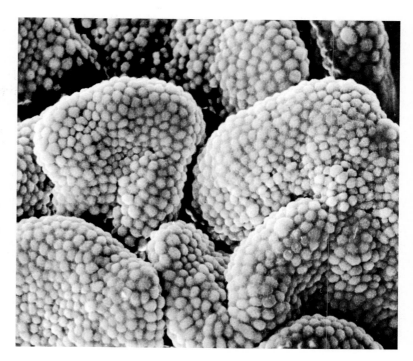

1–9 Scanning electron microscopy of the surface of the yolk sac. Note the three-dimensional character of the scanning electron micrograph. The surface is thrown up into folds, and each of the folds is beset with many cobblestonelike protuberances. The surface dips down around these protuberances. The appearance of this surface by light microscopy and transmission electron microscopy is presented in Chap. 27. (From King, B., Jr., and Enders, A. C. 1970. Am. J. Anat. 127:397.)

drying, the surface of the tissue is commonly coated in a vacuum with an electrically conductive coat of gold, gold–palladium, or carbon.

The SEM's resolution is inversely proportional to the diameter of the electron probe. Accordingly, SEMs possess very narrow, very coherent electron beams. Resolution of the SEM in the images generated by secondary electrons is 25 to 75 Å.

Biological Microscopic Preparations

Living Cells

Living cells may be maintained in tissue culture for long periods and examined by microscopy while undisturbed in culture. Tissue culture permits control of the environment and isolation of single cells or of *clones*, which are colonies derived from the proliferation of a single cell.

Maintaining cells in tissue culture requires considerable attention, involving nutritive media, control of atmospheric gases, and sterility. For short-term investigation, living cells such as leukocytes in a drop of blood may be placed on a clean slide, covered with a coverslip, sealed with petroleum jelly to prevent evaporation, placed on a warming stage, and studied under the microscope. This type of preparation is called *supravital* in distinction to more stable, longer-lasting preparations, such as whole animals or long-term tissue cultures, which are called *vital preparations*. Thus living cells may be observed with the conventional bright-field microscope or with the phase, interference, polarizing, or fluorescence microscopes. Living material may be studied unstained or it may be stained and remain alive, but such vital or supravital staining offers limited structural detail and damages the cells. Although it is valuable in special situations, as in the staining of the reticulocytes of the blood (Chap. 11), it is seldom used.

The nucleus, cytoplasm, mitochondria, Golgi apparatus, and centrioles may all be observed in the living state, as may such activities as motility of whole cells and the movement of structures within the cell.

The plasma membrane may be in active movement, associated with such processes as pinocytosis and phagocytosis (discussed under cytoplasmic vesicles, below). The study of living material offers certain satisfactions. Any scientific study induces artifacts, or departures from the natural state. A question that a scientist must always consider is whether or not the artifacts are consistent, repeatable, and significant—and therefore useful. Intuitively, one thinks that what is seen in the living cell is less apt to be an uncontrolled or misleading artifact and nearer to the typical, undisturbed life of the cell than what can be inferred from killed, sectioned, and stained tissue.

In order to obtain greater resolution and more chemical and other information about cells, it is necessary to kill them by fixation, section them into thin slices, and stain them. We shall now consider these procedures.

Fixation

Fixation is a procedure wherein a given cellular structure or activity is preserved or stabilized, often at the expense of other structures, for subsequent viewing with the microscope. Fixation is most commonly achieved by immersing the tissue in a solution of chemicals, but it may be accomplished by physical means, such as heat denaturation, freezing, or air drying. Although there are fixatives of general use, fixation may be quite selective. Thus, to study the structure of fat droplets, the tissues must be fixed in formaldehyde or other chemicals that stabilize the fat, and alcohol or other organic solvents that extract fats must be avoided. Fixatives that fix or coagulate protein are widely used because they preserve the general structure of nucleus and cytoplasm. Greater resolution and less distortion of cellular structures are obtained with a fixative that produces a fine coagulum than with one that produces a coarse one. Thus glutaraldehyde and osmium tetroxide, which cause a very fine precipitation of protein, permit high resolution without appreciable distortion of structure. They are the most widely used fixatives for electron microscopy. Phosphotungstic acid is a coarse protein precipitator that causes protoplasm to be thrown into heavy strands. For general work, therefore, it is used infrequently, but its drastic action may expose more reactive groups. More sulfhydryl groups are free to react after the coarse fixation with phosphotungstic acid than with fixatives that induce a finer coagulation of protein. For the special purpose of detecting sulfhydryl groups in tissue section, this otherwise unsatisfactory chemical may be the fixative of choice.

Fixation induces chemical change in tissue.

Thus fixatives containing heavy metals, such as Zenker's fluid, which contains mercuric chloride, may react with the carboxyl groups of tissue proteins and influence their subsequent staining. Aldehyde-containing fixatives, such as formaldehyde and gluteraldehyde, may react with amino groups in tissue and block them. Reagents such as bromine in the fixative may saturate double bonds and influence the stability and staining of lipids. Staining methods are available that detect enzyme activity. The fixative used for this purpose must be very gentle; most chemical fixatives tend to damage enzymes so much that they become inoperative and therefore undetectable.

Although fixation is commonly required in preparation for microscopic study, it must sometimes be avoided or its effects minimized because of unwanted chemical change. Some living tissues, such as a drop of blood or tissue cultures, lend themselves directly to microscopy and need not be fixed. The deleterious effects of fixation may be minimized by such maneuvers as freezing the tissue or using very dilute fixatives for very short times (see below and Chap. 2).

Embedding and Sectioning

After the tissue is fixed, it usually must be sectioned into sufficiently thin slices so that its details can be revealed by microscopy. Only in exceptional cases, as in spreading out a drop of blood on a slide, can the required thinness be obtained without slicing. The slices must be thin enough to transmit light (or electrons in electron microscopy). Moreover, since the depth of focus of microscopic objectives is shallow, clarity of detail is favored by thin sections. For light microscopy, section thickness varies from less than 1 μm to about 100 μm. Most preparations are about 5 μm thick. Slices this thin are made with an instrument known as a *microtome,* which consists of a chuck that holds the tissue, a knife, and an advance mechanism. However, tissue after fixation is often pulpy or brittle and impossible to cut into thin slices. It must be infiltrated with a stiff material that can be cut. Most of these infiltrating or embedding agents are fatty waxes, immiscible with the aqueous cytoplasm. Most fixing solutions, moreover, are aqueous. Therefore, to be embedded in the most commonly used embedding agents, which are paraffin or celloidin for light microscopy and the acrylic or epoxy resins for electron microscopy, the fixed tissues must be dehydrated. To this end the tissues are passed through a series of increasingly concentrated aqueous solutions of ethyl alcohol, acetone, or other dehydrating agents that are miscible with both water and fat. Thus the tissue may be passed through solutions of 50, 70, 80, and 95% ethanol, and then into absolute ethanol. Next, either directly or through an intermediate organic solvent like toluene, the tissue is placed in the embedding agent in a liquid phase. The embedding agent replaces the solvent and thoroughly infiltrates the tissue.

Paraffin is made fluid by temperatures above the melting point, usually about 60°C, and the dehydrated tissue is allowed to steep in molten paraffin. The preparation is then cooled. Having infiltrated the interstices of the tissue, the paraffin becomes solid, forming a block that can be cut.

In plastic embedding for electron or light microscopy, the plastic is introduced in the fluid monomeric state. With sufficient steeping, it infiltrates the tissue. Then, by means of heat or ultraviolet light, the plastic is polymerized and becomes, like paraffin, a solid in which the tissue lies thoroughly infiltrated and embedded.

However, a price must be paid to obtain such stable infiltrated blocks of tissue. The alcohols used to dehydrate tissues before infiltration extract fat, coagulate protein, and cause other chemical changes in a tissue. In order to infiltrate with paraffin, moreover, the tissue must be subjected to temperatures high enough to inactivate many enzymes. As plastic polymerizes, heat is given off and may damage the tissue. Paraffin and other embedding agents shrink and thereby distort the tissues. For these reasons, alternatives to these convenient types of embedding can be used. Water-soluble embedding agents are available that circumvent the need for dehydration so that fatty materials may be preserved.

Some enzymatic activities, however, are so fugitive that they do not withstand infiltration with an embedding agent. In such circumstances the tissue may be frozen, and the frozen block of tissue has the physical properties to permit sectioning. Freezing saves the time required for embedding. Tissues can be frozen and sections made, stained, and read in minutes, as is common practice in a surgical operating room.

Freeze-drying is a significant refinement over fixation by freezing or chemical means because it allows minimal distortion and displacement of tissues, minimal chemical extraction, and maximal preservation of enzyme activity for light microscopy. A small block of tissue is quick-frozen or quenched by immersion in isopentane in liquid nitrogen at a temperature of $-150°$ to $-160°C$. It is then placed in a vacuum and dried by sublimation of H_2O, thereby avoiding liquid H_2O, which causes displacement and extraction of cellular components. The dried tissue, while still in vacuo, may be infiltrated with molten paraffin.

In tissues that have been quenched, the sublimated water may be replaced by a chemical fixative in vapor form; this type of fixation is called *free substitution*. It offers the results of freeze-drying coupled with chemical fixation. An electron-microscopic technique, freeze-fracture-etch, has proved so valuable that it is described in detail below.

Mounting and Staining

After the tissue is sectioned for light microscopy, it is usually mounted on a glass slide and stained, although it is possible with phase-contrast or interference microscopy to study unstained tissue.

Freeze–Fracture–Etch

The technique of freeze-fracture-etch has become an invaluable method in cell biology for studying membranes (Figs. 1–10 to 1–14; Fig. 1–27). The technique avoids embedding and sectioning of tissue and may even avoid fixation. It demonstrates heterogeneity in biological membranes and illuminates the nature of cell junctions. Its applications have not been restricted to the study of membranes, however. Useful information has also been obtained on particles, filaments, ground substance within the cell, and extracellular substances. Freeze-fracture-etch depends on the rather simple fact that when a tissue is frozen and fractured, the fracture line tends to travel within membranes so as to separate them into inner and outer leaflets, thereby revealing structures previously hidden. This technique is carried out in steps (Table 1–2):

1. The tissue is removed from the body and fixed, although fixation may be eliminated.

2. After suitable rinses the tissue is transferred to glycerol. The glycerol infiltrates the tissue and protects against artifacts due to ice-crystal formation in the subsequent freezing.

3. The tissue is cut into small pieces and placed on metal (temperature conductive) discs.

4. The tissue is then plunged into a bath of isopentane, held in a temperature-conductive vessel partially immersed in liquid nitrogen. Temperature is low ($-160°C$) so that the tissue is almost immediately quenched or frozen below the eutectic point of water. This is most important because it permits freezing without ice-crystal formation in glycerated tissue. As ice crystals form, they rotate and literally cut apart the tissue, causing visible artifacts.

5. The frozen tissue is quickly transferred to the chamber of a freeze–fracture–etch machine, where a number of operations can be carried out. The chamber can be cooled to a low temperature. It contains a razor on an adjustable swinging arm that can intersect the tissue. It can be pumped out to achieve high vacuum (approximately 10^{-8} mm of mercury). Moreover, it is equipped with platinum electrodes so that platinum can be evaporated to form a film over the specimen. Within the freeze–fracture–etch machine the tissue is maintained frozen and under vacuum through the production of a platinum replica (step 8).

6. The tissue, positioned on its disc, is now fractured by the razor blade on the swinging arm. The cutting edge of the blade strikes the tissue and starts a fracture rift. The free piece of tissue above the fracture flies off and is lost. The lower part of the tissue affixed to the disc now has an exposed fracture face. The face is relatively smooth, with glasslike frozen water surrounding the tissue and filling in the spaces between membranes, particles, and other cellular and extracellular structures.

7. The freshly fractured face of tissue is kept under vacuum for a short time, usually a matter of minutes. This represents the etching phase of the process, during which some of the frozen water at the fracture face sublimates into the vacuum. As a result, membranes, granules, and other cellular structures on the fractured surface now stand out in relief, the level of the frozen water table being below them.

8. Current is passed through the platinum electrodes and a layer of platinum is evaporated over the frozen-fracture-etched surface of the tissue. This platinum layer forms a tough membranous replica of the surface. The platinum is evaporated from a point source and reaches the tissue from a given direction. The platinum covers the tissue very much as snow falling from a certain direction covers a landscape. It piles up

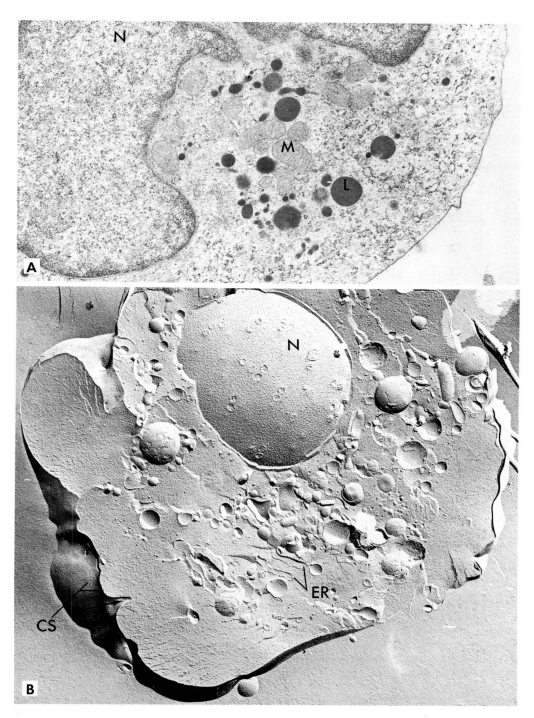

1–10 Guinea pig macrophage. **A,** A cell which has been fixed and sectioned and photographed in the electron microscope after staining with heavy metals. Nucleus **(N),** mitochondria **(M),** lysosomes **(L),** and the plasma membrane are visible by this standard technique. × 13,500. **B,** A freeze-fractured-etched macrophage, showing the nucleus **(N),** bearing nuclear pores, numerous globular profiles, two cisternae of the ER **(ER),** and an invagination **(arrow)** at the cell surface **(CS),** × 19,000. [From Daems, W. Th., and Brodero, R. *In* R. van Furth (ed.), Mononuclear Phagocytes. Philadelphia: F. A. Davis, p. 29.]

Table 1–2 Freeze–Fracture–Etch (Prepared by Dr. Maya Simionescu)

TISSUE FIXATION AND CRYOPROTECTION	FREEZING
1mm 0.5mm — 25% glycerol (diffuses into cells) 4°C	tissue — forceps — carrier freon -150°C liquid N₂ (-190°C)
FRACTURING	ETCHING (optional)
liquid N₂ knife — tissue liquid N₂ -100°C high vacuum	sublimation of ice liquid N₂ -100°C high vacuum
REPLICATION	CLEANING THE REPLICA
2 carbon backing 1 platinum shadowing liquid N₂ -100°C high vacuum	strong bleach replica to be examined by EM

on the near side of structures that rise from the surface and leaves a clear space or shadow on the far side. A carbon film is evaporated on the back of the platinum replica to strengthen it.

9. The vacuum is broken, the chamber is opened, and the disc bearing the tissue covered with a platinum replica is removed from the machine.

10. The replica is freed from the tissue by digesting the tissue away and is caught on a grid that fits into a TEM. Under the electron microscope, the grain of the platinum permits resolution to better than 30 Å.

Isolation of Whole Cells and Parts of Cells

Techniques are available for isolating cells from complex tissues and for disrupting cells to isolate their constituent parts.

A single cell type can be purified in a viable state from a complex tissue containing many cell types. For example, hepatocytes, the distinctive parenchymal cell type of liver, can be isolated from blood vessels, lymphatics, nerves, fibroblasts, macrophages, extracellular substances, and other cells and extracellular materials of the liver. The first step is to prepare a cell suspension of the tissue. In a few tissues, such as blood, this is not necessary, because the cells already are in suspension in the liquid plasma. In a solid tissue, however, such as the liver and kidney, the tissue is usually cut into pieces and subjected to enzyme digestion while it is shaken. *Trypsin*, a proteolytic enzyme produced by the pancreas, will digest virtually any protein substrate and is widely used in cell-separation procedures. With judicious application, extracellular substances will be destroyed or depolymerized and intercellular junctional complexes will be loosened without too much cell destruction. (A valuable related use of trypsin is for harvesting cells in tissue culture that are adherent to the flask walls. Brief treatment loosens the cells; overlong treatment digests and destroys them.) *Collagenase* is especially useful in freeing cells enmeshed in collagen. *Neuriminidase* can remove a sticky extrinsic carbohydrate, *sialic acid*, from the cell surface. (This example highlights a refined use of enzymes in cell biology in which certain receptors or other molecules can be specifically removed from the cell surface, such as *fucose* by *fucase*.)

After enzymatic treatment and mechanical agitation, a solid tissue is reduced to a suspension of diverse cell types and debris. A given cell type may be separated by one or more techniques. Cells will migrate differently in a countercurrent or in an electrophoretic system, and a given cell type may thereby be removed. In certain instances cells may be selectively eliminated, for example, by destroying erythrocytes with hypotonic solutions or destroying other cells with anticell antibodies. Cells may have different affinities for surfaces. If a suspension of macrophages and lymphocytes is poured through a column of glass wool, the macrophages will adhere to the glass fibers (from which they can later be removed) and the lymphocytes will go through. This technique may be refined by coating a surface with reactants that can hold certain cell types by interacting with specific cell surface receptors.

The major method for separating cells, however, is centrifugation, whereby the cells are subjected to pulls greater than gravity. (The number of gravities, or g, is a function of the speed of rotation and the distance from the center of rotation to the material in the centrifuge tube.) The rate at which a structure reaches the bottom of the centrifuge tube depends on its density and

volume. Cells or other particles may thus be separated differentially by varying the time of centrifugation, with the denser and more voluminous structures coming down first. When centrifugation is complete, moreover, the larger denser structures are on the bottom of the tube and the smaller lighter ones lie on top of them. This is the technique of *differential centrifugation*. For example, the density of red cells is approximately 1.077 and that of white cells, 1.033. As a result, on differential centrifugation, the red cells and white cells are separated so that the red cells are below and the white cells above. (The sedimentation of red cell is enhanced by their tendency to aggregate into *rouleaux*, thereby increasing their effective unit volume.) However, separation may be cleaner by interposing a density barrier. That is, a suspension of blood cells may be layered carefully over a solution of bovine albumin or sucrose whose density is between that of red and white cells. The red cells go through the density barrier and the white cells do not, and hence a better separation is achieved. This is the principle of *density-gradient* separation. The technique may be refined by using a number of layers of varying density, or going gradually from low to high density without steps, resulting in continuous, or linear, density-gradient centrifugation. If the range of densities in such multiple or continuous density barriers encompasses the densities of the cells being centrifuged into them, the cells will come to rest in the layer whose density equals its own. This technique is *isopycnic centrifugation*.

In the separation and analysis of constituent parts of a cell, the main elements of the procedure are as follow. Fresh tissue is shred into small pieces or run through a grinder. Cells are then disrupted in a blender, or with a mortar and pestle, or ground by fine sand or in a mill by a closely fitting piston riding in a test tube. The tissue is thereby reduced to a pulpy heterogenous liquid containing disrupted cells and their constitutent parts, extracellular material, and debris. This homogenate is centrifuged and its different components are isolated. The nucleus is a relatively large, heavy structure and is concentrated in fields of low gravity. Mitochondria, ribosomes, lysosomes, and other cellular elements may also be separated differentially. An isolated component may be studied by electron microscopy to confirm its nature and to determine the damage done during its concentration and the cleanness of separation.

Microchemistry and Histochemistry

Microchemical methods developed as refinements of chemical methods. With them it has become possible to take a section of a tissue, study it with the microscope, and then take the section next to it and analyze it for inorganic salts, oxidative enzymes, or other components. It is possible, moreover, to dissect sections and carry out chemical analyses on small groups of similar cells or even on single cells.

Histochemistry, the visualization of chemical reactions in microscopic preparations, is so valuable that it is accorded a full chapter (Chap. 2).

The Structure of the Cell

Biological Membranes

Membranes are essential to cells. They are metabolically active sheets that enclose the cell as the plasma membrane. They also occur within the metazoan cell as nuclear membranes, endoplasmic reticulum, Golgi membranes, and as the membranes enclosing lysosomes, pinocytotic and phagocytic vacuoles, and many other structures. Membranes thus bound the cell and compartmentalize its elements. The organization and many of the functions of the cell, such as secretion of protein, synthesis of fat, detoxification of drugs, phagocytosis, respiration, and active transport depend on membranes.

The plasma membrane is the outer limit of the living cell and its face to the environment. It controls the ease with which substances enter the cell, providing it with selective permeability. The plasma membrane contains many and diverse molecules in its surface, which confer the capacity to interact with other cells and the extracellular environment. The fluidity of the membrane is determined by its ratio of cholesterol to phospholipid. Its permeability is also dependent on its lipid content. The membrane contains enzymatic pumps that control the levels of Na^+, K^+, Ca^{++}, and other ions both in the cell and its environment. It contains the enzyme adenosine triphosphatase (ATPase), which breaks down adenosine triphosphate (ATP) to the diphosphate (ADP), thereby providing energy for active transport (pumping), endocytosis, and other energy-costing membrane functions. (See discussion under Mitochondria.)

Some of the molecules that extend from the surface of the plasma membrane are *receptors* capable of selectively linking with substances outside the cell, including receptors on other cells. Many essential cell functions are receptor-mediated, such as conduction, phagocytosis, antibody production, antigen recognition, hormone-induced activities, and other cellular interactions in embryogenesis, cell homing, and cell sorting. Some receptors are shared by many cell types, such as insulin receptors needed in carbohydrate metabolism (Chap. 22). Other receptors are quite restricted to cell type, such as the *erythropoietin receptors* on erythroblasts, needed to capture the hormone *erythropoietin*, which drives the proliferation and differentiation of red cell precursors (Chap. 12). A cell type may show a succession of receptors as it differentiates, each stage of differentiation characterized by a distinctive set of cell surface receptors or markers, well exemplified by lymphocytes (Chaps. 11 and 14).

The phenomenon of *contact inhibition* is related to properties of the cell surface. Normal cells, as can be shown in tissue culture, cease to grow or move away when they establish contact with other cells; they show contact inhibition. Malignant cells, on the other hand, are not inhibited but move over other cells.

Most cells of the body contain an array of molecules on their surfaces, distinctive to cell type, encoded by major histocompatibility complex (MHC), the "supergene" on chromosome 6 in human beings that governs many cellular interactions, including immune-related actions (Chap. 12). Although not all of these MHC-determined molecules have been characterized or their formation determined, many of them seem to possess receptor functions. Cells, particularly those that are metabolically active, must literally bristle with surface molecules, an expression of the extraordinary importance of these molecules in regulating cell function. This discussion will be carried further after the chemistry and modeling of the plasma membrane are considered.

Plasma membranes, like other membranes, are complex and diverse. Their composition and functions have been studied by a number of techniques. They can be isolated by cell disruption followed by differential centrifugation and studied by x-ray diffraction, freeze-fracture-etch, and microchemistry. The erythrocyte plasma membrane has been extensively studied because large amounts can be easily prepared. As is the case with most membranes, it is preponderantly protein (50–60% of dry weight). This composition reflects high metabolic activity and structural stability. A notable exception is the lipid-

1-11 Diagrammatic representation of the four membrane "faces" that can be studied with the freeze-fracture-etch technique as shown on an erythrocyte. Note the terms used to designate the four surfaces: **ES,** the true outside surface of the plasma membrane; **PS,** the true inside surface of the plasma membrane; **PF,** the split surface of the plasma membrane which faces away from the cytoplasm; **EF,** the split surface of the plasma membrane which faces toward the cytoplasm. Particles, representing protein molecules, are shown only on faces PF and EF. (From Weinstein, R. S. 1974. The Red Blood Cell. New York: Academic Press, Inc., p. 247.)

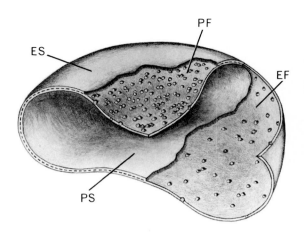

rich membrane of myelinated nerves, whose high concentration of myelin appears to serve as an insulator. Most proteins associated with cell membranes are regarded as intrinsic to the membrane because they can be removed only by drastic procedures of extraction, digestion, or denaturation. The rest of the proteins are easily removed and thus considered extrinsic. Intrinsic or extrinsic proteins include structural proteins, enzymes, and receptor substances. Many of these proteins, notably the intrinsic ones, appear to be amphipathetic, that is, asymmetric or polarized with hydrophilic groups at one pole and hydrophobic groups at the other. The implications of amphipathety are discussed below.

Lipids constitute 20 to 30% of the dry weight of erythrocyte membranes. Because lipid determines the permeability of plasma membrane, fat-soluble compounds readily enter cells, dissolving in the membrane, whereas fat-insoluble compounds enter by more complex mechanisms. The dominant lipid in the cell membrane is phospholipid, which is amphipathetic: the glycerol end is water-soluble, carrying phosphate and other ionized groups, whereas the fatty acid end is not, being lipid-soluble and hydrophobic. Other lipids include cholesterol and a minor component linked to protein or carbohydrate as lipoprotein or liposaccharide. Carbohydrate accounts for less then 10% of the weight of plasma membranes in most cells studied. It may be free as oligosaccharide or linked to protein or fat.

By TEM of sectioned tissue, the plasma membrane is approximately 75 Å in thickness with a range of about 60 to 90 Å. As with most intracellular membranes, it is seen as a trilaminar structure, termed the *unit membrane,* with outer darker lines approximately 20 Å wide and an inner lighter line, approximately 35 Å wide (Fig. 1–12). With high resolution, suggestions of bridges across the lucent central zone or of granular structures within the membrane may be present, but usually little or no specialization is evident. By negative staining some membranes, such as mitochondrial membranes, display distinctive structures (see below); but plasma membranes do not. A valuable technique in revealing structural heterogeneity in membranes is *freeze-fracture-etch* described above. By this method membranes are typically split into outer and inner leaflets, the split tending to occur in the central lucent zone (Figs. 1–11 and 1–14). As a result of this split there are four surfaces. The original surface facing to the exterior is the *E face* and the original surface facing to the interior, or protoplasm, of the cell is the *P face.* The fracture face on the exterior leaflet is the *EF* (Exterior Fracture) *face* while the fracture face on the interior leaflet is the *PF* (Protoplasmic Fracture) *face.* Particles may be seen on the split surfaces (Fig. 1–13). The number, size, and pattern of these particles differ from place to place in a given membrane and from membrane to membrane. By the use of labeled antibodies or other cytochemical procedures, it is evident that at least some of these particles are enzymes such as ATPase and adenylate cyclase.

A number of models for the organization of the plasma membrane have been put forth. That of Singer and Nicholson has received wide support (Fig. 1–14). Like other models, it postulates a lipid bilayer consisting primarily of phospholipid molecules oriented with their hydrophilic ends directed both to the outside and to the in-

1–12 Erythrocyte, peripheral cytoplasm. Note the trilaminar character of the plasmalemma, there being two dark laminae separated by a light one. This membrane is a unit membrane. × 280,000. (From the work of J. D. Robertson.)

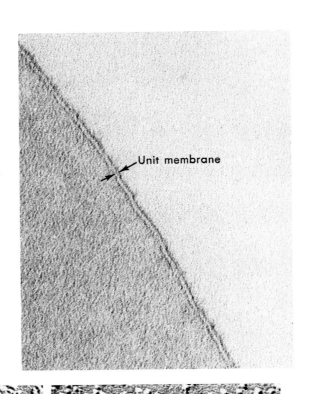

1–13 Replicas of freeze-fractured human red cell membranes. **A.** Freeze-fracture face PF originating from within the interior of the membrane shows more or less randomly distributed membrane-associated particles **(MAP),** which may represent sites of integral membrane proteins. × 120,000. **B.** Face-EF has fewer MAP than face-PF. × 140,000. **C.** Freeze-etching has exposed the true exterior surface of the red cell membrane **(*),** which appears barren and smooth. The fracture has entered the membrane **(arrows)** and exposed a PF-face for replication. × 100,000. **D.** Small fibrils **(arrows)** apparently extend from the cytoplasm of intact cells into the interior of the cell membrane. × 90,000. (From Weinstein, R. S. 1974. The Red Blood Cell. New York: Academic Press, Inc.) ▽

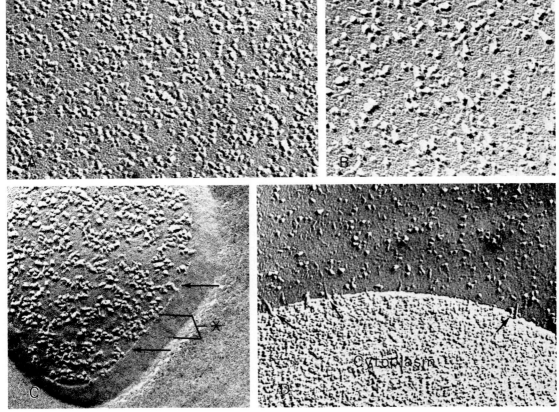

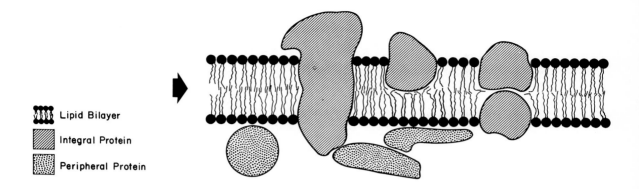

Lipid Bilayer

Integral Protein

Peripheral Protein

side surfaces. Being hydrophilic, the surfaces of the membrane interact with watery environments. Within the membrane, on the other hand, lie the long-chain nonpolar hydrocarbon portions of the fatty acid constituents of the phospholipid bilayer. The internum of the membrane is, therefore, fatty and hydrophobic. The phospholipid constituents of the outside and inside surfaces of the membrane, moreover, are somewhat different. Cholesterol molecules are dispersed throughout the membrane. Lying in the phospholipid bilayer like "icebergs in a lipid sea" are the proteins. They are most likely amphipathetic with their hydrophobic ends lying within the membrane among the hydrophobic fatty acids and hydrophilic pole protruding from the outside or inside hydrophilic surface of the membrane. Certain intrinsic proteins are longer than the width of the membrane and therefore cross it, protruding from both inside and outside surfaces. These proteins are presumably hydrophilic at the ends and hydrophobic in the center. There are places in membranes, such as in the synaptosome of nerve and junctional complexes, unusually rich in proteins, which may be linked to one another. Proteins may be fixed in the membrane or may be rather loosely attached and move about in the plane of the membrane. Such movement can be demonstrated by an experiment in which certain receptors in the plasma membrane of mouse cells are stained with a fluorescent marker of one color and those of human cells stained with a fluorescent marker of another color. The plasma membranes, and thereby the cells, are then fused by the action of sendai virus. At first the labeled receptor substances remain apart, but within 40 min they appear completely intermixed. The mixing is temperature-dependent, occurring at physiological temperature but inhibited at 4°C. This temper-

1–14 Fluid mosaic model of cell membrane. The bulk of the phospholipids (**solid circles** represent polar head groups and **wavy lines** their fatty acid chains) are organized in a discontinuous lipid bilayer. Intrinsic or integral proteins are embedded in the bilayer but can protrude from the membrane. Extrinsic or peripheral proteins may bind to phospholipid polar head groups or to the membrane via protein-protein interactions. The **arrow** shows the position of the natural cleavage plane within the center of a lipid bilayer in freeze-fracture-etch techniques. (From Weinstein, R. S. 1974. The Red Blood Cell. New York: Academic Press, Inc., p. 239.)

ature-dependence suggests simple diffusion as the basis of mixing.

In addition to proteins intrinsic to the membrane, there are peripheral proteins, the extrinsic proteins, that are linked to the membrane. The contractile protein *actin* lies directly beneath the plasma membrane in microvilli and other places and appears linked to intrinsic proteins. As a result, the plasma membrane of the microvilli is moved when actin contracts. *Spectrin* is a linear structural protein that forms a bridgework beneath the plasma membrane of erythrocytes and inserts into the underside of the membrane. This membrane-associated protein both strengthens the plasma membrane, protecting it against the shearing forces of the circulation, and anchors many of those intrinsic membrane proteins that extend into the subjacent cytoplasm. Spectrin is in the class of structural filaments known as *intermediate filaments* (page 60). A further example of membrane-associated proteins are the *cytochromes*, which are rather loosely attached to the surface of the plasma membrane. Carbohydrates are often attached to the outside of the plasma membrane. Among them are sialic acid and other glyco- or mucoproteins. The carbohydrate-rich extrinsic coat may be so heavy as to be

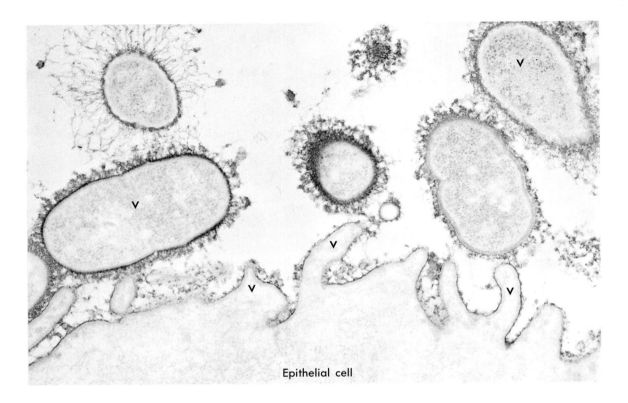

Epithelial cell

1–15 Cell surface, human buccal epithelium; electron micrograph. The free surface of an epithelial cell having large and small villi **(v)** is shown. A surface coat has been stained selectively with the dye ruthenium red. The coat, where it lies upon the plasmalemma, is relatively dense. On its free surface, on the other hand, the surface coat has a flocculent or filamentous character. × 40,000. (From Luft, John. 1971. Anat. Rec. 171:347.)

visible as a fuzzy layer called the *glycocalyx* and can be selectively stained by ruthenium red or lanthanum (Fig. 1–15). If sufficiently thick, it can be visible by light microscopy when stained by the periodic acid Schiff procedure. The sarcolemma of muscle and basal laminae in general may be regarded as sites of large-scale accumulation of proteoglycans extrinsic to the plasma membrane.

The Nucleus

The nucleus is the fundamental part of a cell that encodes the information from which the structure and function of the organism derive. The information is encoded in the genetic material DNA, complexed to simple basic proteins, histones, to form deoxyribonucleoprotein (DNP). With some exceptions, notably mitochondria, DNA lies exclusively in the nucleus. DNA is capable of replicating itself, thereby providing precise copies of the genetic code that are passed on to daughter cells by cellular division.

The nucleus also plays a central role in synthesizing proteins and polypeptides from the genetic information it carries. All the nucleated cells of the body contain the same genes, yet cells differ in their structure, function, and products. The nucleus differentially controls the use of this information from cell to cell by repressing or derepressing the action of various genes. The nucleus initiates the translation of its encoded information into the synthesis of proteins by mean of RNAs, a group of nucleic acids that differ from DNA primarily in base composition. Some RNAs are complexed to proteins to form ribonucleoprotein (RNP). The RNAs are produced in or under the control of the nucleus and are released to the cytoplasm where they engage in protein synthesis. The "machine" that assembles proteins from amino acids is a complex of RNAs and protein, the *ribosome*, whose constituents are produced in a nuclear component, the *nucleolus*. Other RNAs are *messenger RNA* (mRNA), which links ribosomes into working units called *polyribosomes*, and *transfer RNA* (tRNA), which carries amino acids to the polyribosomes to initiate protein synthesis.

A nucleus is present in virtually all differentiated metazoan cells, being absent only from mammalian erythrocytes and a few other end-stage cell types. Certain cell types have many nuclei or are polyploid (see below); the number of genes and other elements in the protein-synthesizing apparatus of a cell is thus multiplied and the cell is able to produce a greater volume of product. Hepatocytes, particularly with age, may develop two or more nuclei, and renal tubular cells may be binucleate. Osteoclasts or foreign-body giant cells may contain 25 or more nuclei. A mechanism for increasing nuclear function without increasing nuclear number is polyploidy, an increase in the number of chromosomal pairs within a single nucleus. Most somatic cells are diploid (2n), having one pair of each chromosome characterizing its species, but cells may develop two pairs (4n) or more. Hepatocytes tend to increase in ploidy with age; in old rats they are often 8n and 16n. Megakaryocytes, giant cells of the bone marrow containing a giant polymorphous nucleus may become 32n or 64n. A more restricted mechanism for increasing nuclear components is an increase in the number of nucleoli in certain oocytes, with a concomitant increase in production of ribosomal RNA.

The nucleus may occur in a dividing (mitotic or meiotic) state, during which it reproduces itself, or in a nondividing or interphase state. The interphase nucleus is most frequently encountered, because nuclear division takes approximately 1 h whereas, even in actively dividing cells, 6 h or more elapse between divisions. Many cells of the body seldom divide (e.g., hepatocytes) or never divide (e.g. nerve cells). (See section below on Life Cycle of Cells.)

In most cell types the interphase nucleus is an ovoid structure several micrometers in diameter (Figs. 1–10 and 1–16 to 1–18). In the leukocytes of blood and connective tissues, the nucleus is lobulated and hence termed polymorphous (see Chaps. 11 and 12). The nucleus is deformable and may therefore be pressed into a reniform or horseshoe shape. In contracted smooth muscle, it may be twisted like a corkscrew (Fig. 1–18).

The interphase nucleus is bounded by a nu-clear envelope and typically contains several distinctive structures. These structures include chromatin, nuclear sap or karyolymph, and one or more nucleoli. The protoplasm of the nucleus is termed *nucleoplasm* or *karyoplasm*.

Chromatin. Chromatin, by light microscopy, consists of irregular clumps or masses that, although not highly constant, tend to be characteristic in texture, quantity, and size for any given cell type. These clumps, sometimes called *karyosomes*, have an affinity for basic dye because chromatin contains DNA. DNA confers distinctive staining reactions on chromatin. Thus, chromatin is specifically stained in the Feulgen reaction. It selectively binds methyl green. In Romanovsky preparations, which are stained with methylene blue and azures, chromatin is stained violet (Chap. 11). These distinctive DNA staining reactions are abolished by pretreating the specimen with the enzyme *deoxyribonuclease*.

Chromatin is the embodiment in the interphase nucleus of the DNP of chromosomes. The chromosomes in the interphase nucleus are very slender, long, threadlike structures lying in a rather tangled mass. It is impossible to delineate individual chromosomes from this tangle. Indeed, it was at one time thought that this mass was a continuous single thread instead of individual interlaced chromosomes, and the name *spireme* was applied to it.

Chromosomes may be either coiled or uncoiled along their length. Whenever the tight coiling of the chromosome forms clumps greater than 0.2 μm in dimension, they are visible with the light microscope. Chromosomes in this form constitute the *heterochromatin*. The karyosomes are heterochromatin. In many cells, moreover, heterochromatin is also applied against the inner surface of the nuclear envelope, forming an outer rim of the nucleus interrupted only by nuclear pores (Figs. 1–10, and 1–17 to 1–19). There is also nuclear membrane–associated chromatin. Because the chromatin in uncoiled chromosomes, the *euchromatin*, is below the limit of resolution of the light microscope, euchromatin is "invisible" and cannot be differentiated from the nuclear sap. The proportions of euchromatin and heterochromatin and the distribution of heterochromatin can be quite characteristic for a given cell type. In fact, in the interphase nucleus, chromosomes may be tightly coiled in certain segments and uncoiled in other segments. Cells

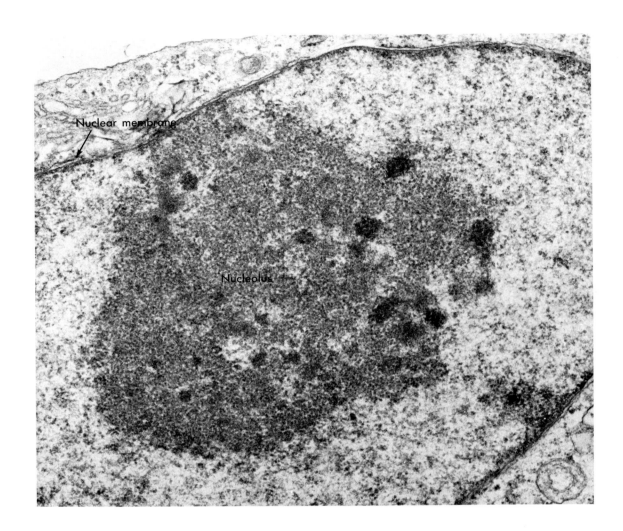

Nuclear membrane

Nucleolus

1–16 Rhesus kidney cell (strain MA 104) in culture.
The nucleolus, stained with uranyl acetate and
lead, is well developed. It touches the inside surface
of the nuclear membrane. Heterochromatin, densely
stained, is present as a rim against the inside surface
of the inner nuclear membrane. Most of the chromatin
is dispersed and presents as euchromatin. The outer
nuclear membrane (nuclear membrane) stands out
clearly. It is part of the endoplasmic reticulum and, at
places, bears ribosomes on its surface. See Fig. 1–25.
× 40,000. (From the work of A. Monneran.)

with large blocks of heterochromatin tend to be
relatively inactive in an early stage of protein
synthesis, the production of mRNA. The uncoiled chromosomes are in the functional state
that enables transcription of DNA through the
formation of mRNA. The uncoiled chromosomes

serve as a *template* for transcription of information to mRNA. This messenger leaves the nucleus and enters the cytoplasm. There, in concert
with tRNA and the ribosomal RNA (rRNA) of the
ribosomes, it synthesizes proteins whose structure was encoded in the DNA. Thus cells whose
nuclei are relatively rich in euchromatin tend to
be quite active in the transcription phase of protein synthesis. In cells of females a characteristic
mass of heterochromatin lying against the nuclear membrane represents one of the female sex
chromosomes, an X chromosome, which remains
tightly coiled through interphase. It is called *sex
chromatin* or, after its discoverer, the *Barr body*
(Fig. 1–20). It enables the genetic sex of an individual to be determined, a procedure of value in
certain endocrinopathies or congenital disturbances in which the genetic sex may not be ap-

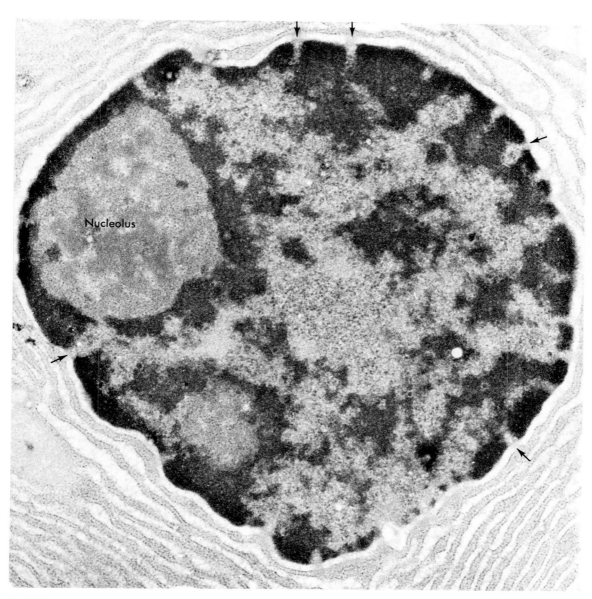

1–17 Pancreatic acinar cell. The nucleus of this cell,
which secretes digestive enzymes, has been
selectively treated to enhance the staining of DNA and
to reduce the staining of the nucleoli and other RNA-
containing structures. Chromatin is densely stained.
Much of it is marginated on the inner surface of the
nuclear membrane. Nuclear pores are prominent
(arrow), their location marked by the lightly stained
aisles between heterochromatin masses. The section
was treated with picric acid, uranyl acetate, and lead.
× 30,000. (From the work of A. Monneron.)

1–18 Contracted muscle cell. The nucleus has been
twisted into a corkscrew spiral. On relaxation,
the nucleus will untwist and be cigar-shaped.

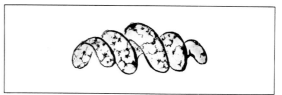

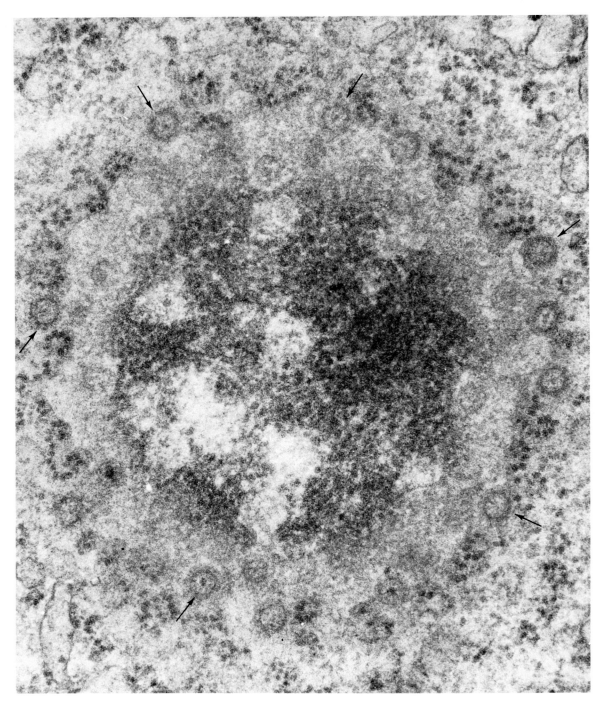

1–19 Rat hepatocyte. This is a tangential section of the nucleus, revealing nuclear pores all around **(arrow),** some with a dark central granule. Note that polyribosomes are in close association with the pores. This preparation is stained with uranyl acetate and lead. × 140,000. (From the work of A. Monneron.)

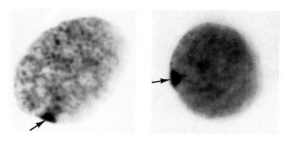

1–20 Sex chromatin of a human female. The chromatin lies against the nuclear membrane **(arrows)**. This formation of sex chromatin appears to be due to the persistent coiling in interphase in one of the X chromosomes. Human buccal mucosa. × 4000. (From the work of B. R. Migeon.)

parent. The Y (male) chromosome may be demonstrated in interphase nuclei by a special fluorescence staining method.

The elements of the interphase nucleus—namely, chromatin, nucleoli (see below), karyolymph, and nuclear membranes—are readily identified by electron microscopy. However, the correlation of electron-microscopic observations of interphase nuclei with what is inferred of the structure of chromosomes and other nuclear components from genetic and other data remains rudimentary. It is known, for example, that an uncoiled chromosome may be of the order of 10,000 times the largest dimension of the nucleus. But it is difficult to gain any appreciation from sections of nuclei of the nature of the immense folding and coiling that the chromosomes must undergo. Such inferences as electron microscopy affords come from preparations in which chromosomes are floated out of disrupted nuclei, dried down on supporting membranes, and examined whole. In these preparations high degrees of coiling and folding are evident. Pure DNA may be prepared and examined as whole, unsectioned filaments by electron microscopy. These filaments are approximately 20 Å in diameter. DNA can be identified in sectioned interphase nuclei on the basis of selective staining. It is present in filaments of varying diameter, that of the slimmest being about 100 Å. The greater thickness of DNA in sections may be due to such factors as coiling, folding, or intertwining of DNA filaments or complexing of DNA with histones or other substances.

Nucleolus. A nucleolus is a discrete intranuclear structure consisting largely of protein and

RNA, which synthesizes the major components of ribosomes. The nucleolus is well developed in cells active in protein synthesis. Such cells may contain several nucleoli. In cells synthesizing little protein, such as spermatocytes, neutrophils, and muscle cells, a nucleolus may not be evident. Nucleoli appear at certain specific sites, the *nucleolar organizing sites* in certain chromosomes (Fig. 1–21). These sites represent secondary constrictions in the chromosomes. At these sites on the chromosomes, the gene sequences *(cistrons)* are located that encode the genetic information for the synthesis of rRNA. Nucleoli remain attached to the chromosomes at nucleolar organizing sites.

Nucleoli by light microscopy are usually spherical, up to 1 μm in diameter, but may be oval or even bow-tie shaped. They are usually compact and sharply outlined, but they may be porous with fuzzy borders. Nucleoli may lie at random or against the inside of the nuclear membrane, an efficient location for discharging substances into the cytoplasm (Figs. 1–3 and 1–4).

Nucleoli are rich in RNA. Thus they absorb ultraviolet light at a wavelength of 2,600 Å, and can thereby be identified by ultraviolet microscopy. Nucleoli may be stained with pyronin in the methyl green-pyronin mixture and blue in Romanovsky blood stains. Staining of nucleoli is abolished by treating the section with *ribonu-*

1–21 Chromosomes containing nucleolar organizing sites from the clawed toad *Xenopus laevis*. They are taken from the metaphase karyotype (see text). Each of the chromosomes in the wild type contains very slender zones, the nucleolar organizing sites. In the heterozygote, on the other hand, only one pair of chromosomes contains this site. The resultant heterozygote, as discussed in the text, is nucleolar-deficient mutants. (From the work of D. D. Brown.)

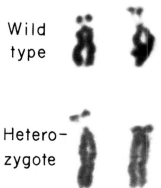

Wild type

Hetero- zygote

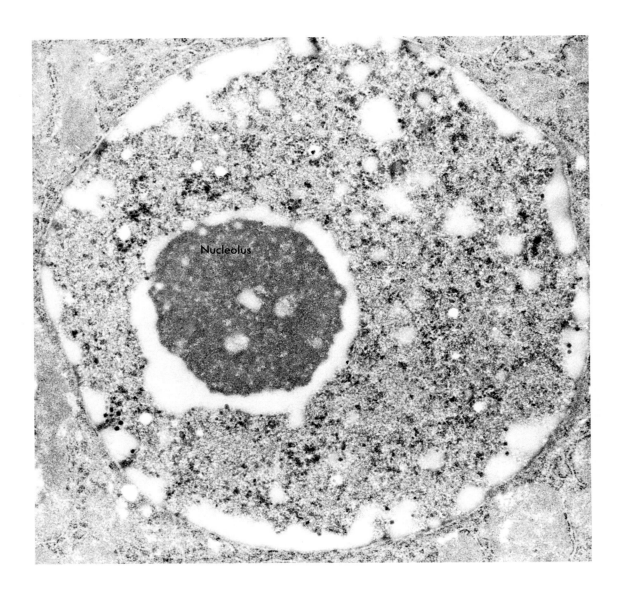

Nucleolus

1–22 Hepatocyte. In this preparation RNP is preferentially stained and chromatin is bleached. The nucleolus stands out sharply. Stained granules, presumably containing RNA, lie outside the nucleolus in association with the chromatin. There are large (400 to 500 Å) perichromatin granules and small (200 Å) interchromatin granules. × 27,000. (From the work of A. Monneron; see also Bernhard, W. 1969. J. Ultrastruct. Res. 27:250.)

clease. RNA contains the nucleotide base *uridine*. (*Thymidine* is the DNA base counterpart to uridine.) Therefore, if radioactive uridine is given to an animal, autoradiography of its cells shows positive nucleoli (Fig. 1–23).

By electron microscopy, nucleoli contain two forms of RNA (Figs. 1–16, 1–17, 1–22, and 1–23). One is granular, approximately 150 Å in diameter, and represents maturing forms of RNP particles. This is typically the dominant nucleolar structure. The second form of RNA is fibrillar, 50 to 80 Å in thickness, and is probably a precursor to the granules.

Nucleoli are not the only sites of RNP in the nucleus. Particles of different sizes and filaments of RNP lie against and between chromatin. It is likely that some of this widely dispersed nuclear RNA is mRNA (see below) produced on extended segments of DNA (euchromatin).

DNA is a component of the nucleolus, desig-

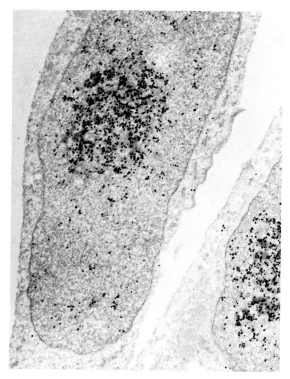

1–23 Monkey kidney cells (strain BSC). These cells, in tissue culture, were exposed to [³H] uridine (a precursor of RNA) for 30 min and then fixed and processed for EM autoradiography. The distribution of silver grains is only over the nucleus and mainly over the nucleolus. ×25,000. (From A. Monneron, J. Burglen, and W. Bernhard. 1970. J. Ultrastruct. Res. 32:370.)

nated *nucleolar chromatin* of the nucleolar organizing site of the chromosome. It occurs in twisted or single filaments 200 to 300 Å in diameter.

Poorly defined granular material, probably protein, occurs throughout nucleoli. Rarefied vacuolar zones, not membrane-bounded, may be present.

The nucleolus is a center for the synthesis of ribosomes. The size and number of nucleoli depend on the level of rRNA synthesis. In actively secretory cells (pancreatic acinar cells) nucleoli are large and multiple, whereas in cells showing a low level of protein synthesis (muscle cells, certain small lymphocytes) nucleoli may be small or absent.

Ribosomes have several subunits (see section on Ribosomes). On the basis of isolation and sedimentation analysis it appears that nucleoli

produce the subunits of ribosomes and release them to the cytoplasm. The release to the cytoplasm may be facilitated by the nucleolus moving against the nuclear membrane and discharging through nuclear pores. In the cytoplasm, the nucleolar-produced ribosomal components may mature further, perhaps by adding protein, and combine to form ribosomes.

Support for the role of nucleoli in ribosomal synthesis comes from the work of Brown and his associates on amphibian mutants lacking nucleoli. The embryo of the clawed toad *Xenopus laevis* synthesizes few ribosomes before the tail bud stage, the ribosomes from the oocyte serving until that time. A lethal anucleolate mutant of *Xenopus* may be bred from a spontaneously occurring heterozygote mutant with but one nucleolus per cell, instead of the normal two. Development of the anucleolate embryos is retarded after hatching. The embryos are microcephalic and edematous and die before feeding. The mutation that prevents the formation of a normal nucleolus also prevents synthesis of 28S and 18S rRNA, as well as high molecular-weight precursor molecules of ribosomes.

The correlation between ribosome production and nucleoli is evident in multinucleolate amphibian oocytes where the DNA specifying the sequences for 28S and 18S rRNAs is selectively replicated. As many as 1,000 autonomously functional nucleoli may occur per oocyte (Fig. 1–24).

1–24 Nucleus isolated from an oocyte of *Xenopus laevis*. The nucleus was dissected from the oocyte, flooded with cresyl violet stain, and photographed. The deeply stained spots are those of the hundreds of nucleoli which are in the plane of focus. (From Brown, D. D., and Dawid, I. B. 1968. Science 160:272.)

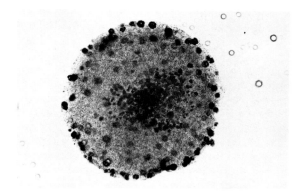

Nuclear Envelope. The nuclear envelope consists of two concentric unit membranes (Fig. 1–5). Each is approximately 70 Å in thickness, the inner one somewhat thinner. The space of the cisterna between inner and outer nuclear membranes varies in size and content. It is commonly about 150 Å wide and lucent. The outer nuclear membrane is continuous with the endoplasmic reticulum (ER), both rough and smooth. The cytoplasmic character of nuclear membrane is underscored in reformation in the telophase. The nuclear membranes are clearly formed by segments of ER, which line up around the reconstituted nuclear mass. In cells synthesizing protein, the nuclear envelope may, like the rough ER, contain the protein product. Thus, in antibody-producing cells the nuclear envelope may be distended with antibody and, indeed, is among the first places antibody accumulates. In the interphase nucleus the inner nuclear membrane is reinforced on its inner surface by a closely applied finely granular *lamina*. A subset of heterochromatin lies against the inner surface of the lamina, and, in places, penetrates it and reaches to the inner nuclear membrane (Figs. 1–25 and 1–26). This heterochromatin forms a rim around the nucleus, interrupted by nuclear pores (Figs. 1–10 and 1–16 to 1–19). During the first meiotic prophase, chromosomes may be attached to the inner surface of the inner membrane and nucleoli may lie there. Although the nuclear envelope cannot be resolved by light microscopy, its location is often revealed as a definite line representing the sum of the nuclear membranes, nuclear cisterna, and lamina.

Nuclear pore complexes represent interruptions in the nuclear membranes. At a pore complex the inner and outer nuclear membranes appear to fuse and their margins thicken to form an annulus as great as 1,000 Å in outside diameter and 600 Å inside. On surface view it is circular or octagonal in outline. By low-power electron microscopy the pore complex may appear as an aperture in the nuclear membranes with a thickened annulus, closed by a thin diaphragm that often contains a central granule. At high resolution the complex appears to be a granular and filamentous structure with eight regularly spaced granules, each about 100 Å in diameter, lying in the rim of the pore. There are, in fact, two sets of eight granules, one set lying at the outer rim associated with the outer nuclear membrane, the other at the inner rim, associated with the inner nuclear membrane (Fig. 1–25). The central gran-

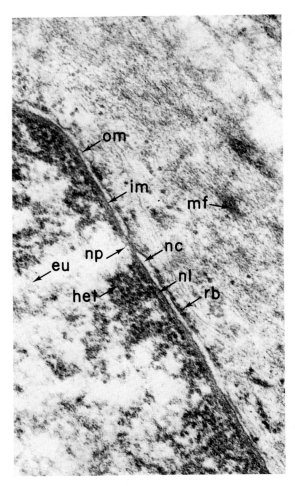

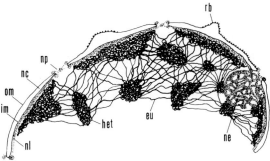

1–25 Above, an electron micrograph of a reticular cell, equine spleen, the nucleus on the left, the cytoplasm on the right. **om** outer nuclear membrane; **im** inner nuclear membrane; **nc** nuclear cisterna; **nl** nuclear lamina; **np** nuclear pore complex; **eu** euchromatin; **het** heterochromatin; **rb** ribosome; **mf** plaque of microfilaments. Courtesy of Fern Tablin. × 42,000. Below, schema of nuclear structures showing, in addition, **ne** nucleolus.

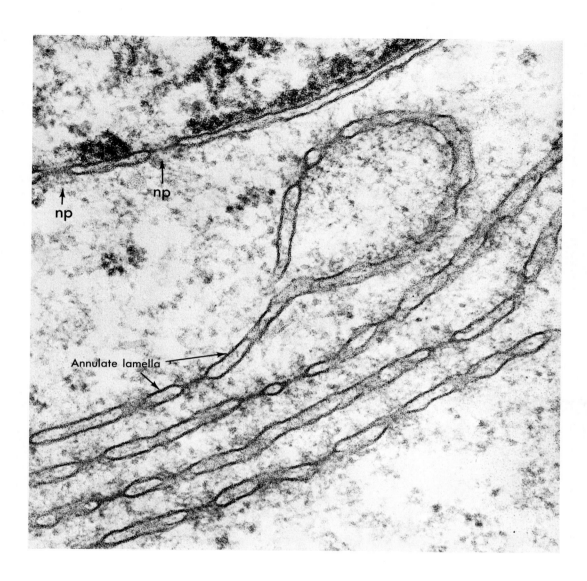

1–26 Nuclear pores and annulate lamellae. The nucleus in the left upper corner is bounded by a double membrane, each component consisting of a unit membrane (see text). Within the nucleus, densely stained chromatin is arranged against the nuclear membrane, in which two nuclear pores **(np)** are present. Within the cytoplasm, occupying much of the field, are stacks of annulate lamellae. These appear identical in structure with the nuclear membrane and, like the nuclear membrane, have frequently spaced pore complexes. × 65,000. (From Maul, G. 1970. J. Cell Biol. 46:604.)

ule is connected by filaments to the wall of the pore complex and to the annular granules. The granules and filaments may be surrounded by a particulate material. The central granule may be traversed by a slender aperture, connecting nucleoplasm with cytoplasm (Fig. 1–19).

There are very few cell types, such as the spermatozoa of bulls, that have few or even no nuclear pore complexes. In other cell types, 3 to 35% of the nuclear surface may be covered by complexes. They may be distributed over the whole nuclear surface or clustered. They may lie irregularly or regularly, falling into square or hexagonal arrays.

Nuclear pore complexes would seem to rep-

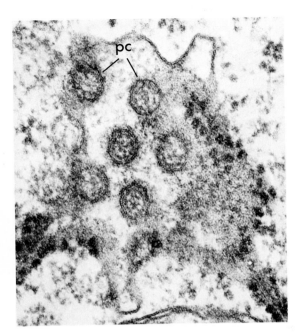

1–27 Annulate lamellae. In this face-on section, surface views of the pore complexes (**pc**) are presented. The pores appear limited by a unit membrane and have a complex, regular internal structure. × 65,000. (From Maul, G. 1970. J. Cell. Biol. 46:604.)

resent passageways, albeit restricted ones, between nucleus and cytoplasm.

Annulate Lamellae. In many cell types stacks of membranes that exactly resemble portions of nuclear membranes, pore complexes and all, may be found in the cytoplasm (Figs. 1–26 and 1–27). In germ cells they may also be present in nucleoplasm. These membranes are termed *annulate lamellae* and are especially common in germ cells and in some tumor cells. They may be continuous with ER. Their significance is not known.

The Cytoplasm

The cytoplasm surrounds the nucleus and is bounded peripherally by the plasma membrane. The cytoplasm expresses most of the functions of the cell. It is dependent on the nucleus for direction, renewal, and regeneration. Thus, isolated units of cytoplasm, exemplified by blood plate-

lets and mature erythrocytes, are capable of protein synthesis and of such specific functions as respiration and the retraction of blood clots. The cytoplasmic structures, however, such as membranes, granules, and microfilaments, which are the basis of such cytoplasmic functions, were originally synthesized and accumulated in the cytoplasm from ribosomes and other materials derived from a viable nucleus that was present at an early phase in the life cycle of these anucleate structures. The volume of cytoplasm in proportion to the nucleus, the nuclear–cytoplasmic ratio, varies considerably from cell type to cell type. In some cells, such as spermatozoa and small lymphocytes, the cytoplasm is scant. In most cells the cytoplasm is relatively abundant and exceeds the nuclear volume by a factor of 3 to 5 or more. The cytoplasm possesses distinctive organelles with specialized functions that lie in the ground substance or hyaloplasm.

Cytoplasm in the center of the cell next to the nucleus, may be gelated. It contains the centrioles and centrosphere but is usually clear of other organelles. It may be bounded by microtubules and surrounded by the Golgi apparatus. Often it pushes the nucleus aside, indenting it. This zone is called the *cell center* or *cytocentrum*. Peripheral to this zone is a solvated part of the cell containing vacuoles and granules, mitochondria, and elements of the ER. Cytoplasmic streaming occurs here, carrying the cytoplasmic organelles in rapid movement. This zone is called *endoplasm*. The peripheral cytoplasm in many cell types, particularly in free or motile cells, is gelated and often rich in microfilaments but free of other organelles. This zone is the *ectoplasm*. It is capable of rapid sol-gel transformation. Gelated ectoplasm may become liquid, particularly in motile cells or cells extending pseudopodial processes, and the already liquid endoplasm bearing organelles then flows in.

The structural protein of the hyaloplasm has a reticulated character visible in high-voltage electron micrographs (Fig. 1–8), which underscores the importance in providing the framework of the cell. Fat occurs in macromolecular micelles that may be visible. Fat sometimes coalesces to form larger fatty vacuoles, *not* bound by membrane, that are visible by electron and light microscopy (Chap. 5). Granules of glycogen may lie in the hyaloplasm, in clusters termed *alpha particles* (Fig. 1–28). However, the predominant structures carried in the hyaloplasm

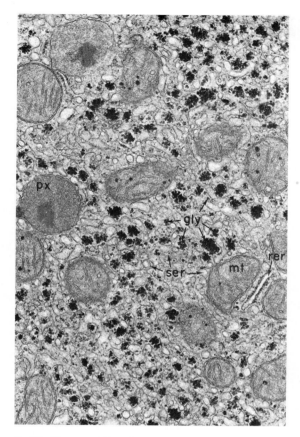

1–28 Glycogen. This electron microscopic field contains particles of glycogen **(gly).** The individual particles are termed beta particles. Ten to fifteen beta particles form an alpha particle. When glycogen is present in lysosomes, presumably to be broken down to glucose and utilized, the glycogen–lysosome structure may be termed *glycosome.* The field also contains peroxisomes **(px),** mitochondria, and endoplasmic reticulum. Most of the endoplasmic reticulum is smooth **(ser)** and contains the glycogen, a finding suggesting that smooth er has a role in glycogen synthesis. × 23,000. (From the work of Robert R. Cardell, Jr.)

are complex organelles fashioned of membranes, filaments, tubules, and granules, which we shall consider now.

Mitochondria. Mitochondria are membranous cytoplasmic organelles capable of trapping chemical energy released by oxidation of compounds derived from food. They then fix that en-

ergy in a form, *adenosine triphosphate (ATP),* that is readily utilizable by the cell. They are present as punctate or linear structures just within the resolving power of the light microscope (Figs. 1–4 and 1–29). By electron microscopy, mitochondria are tubular or spherical structures bounded by one membrane called the *outer membrane* and containing a second internal folded membrane termed the *inner membrane* (Figs. 1–30 and 1–31).

A cell obtains energy from substrates derived from food. Thus amino acids derived from protein, fatty acids from fat, and glucose from carbohydrate may be sources of energy. The major source, however, is glucose. Glucose is broken down in the cell by glycolytic enzymes to form pyruvic acid, which is then oxidized to acetyl coenzyme A. This compound then proceeds to a cycle of further oxidations, the Krebs tricarboxylic acid cycle, whose end products are carbon dioxide and water. Approximately 690,000 calories of energy per mole lie in the chemical bonds of glucose. Its breakdown to pyruvate yields approximately 40,000 calories per mole, but its complete oxidation to carbon dioxide and water through the Krebs cycle yields another 650,000 calories per mole. The energy-capturing mechanism of cells is at best only about 50% efficient, however, because half of the energy is lost as heat. Therefore, the total caloric content of glucose is never available.

Only about 350,00 calories per mole are useful to the cell. The glycolytic breakdown of glucose is anaerobic—that is, it does not use oxygen. In contrast, the mechanism of the Krebs cycle does require oxygen and is therefore respiratory in nature. The oxidation through the Krebs cycle is of the greatest importance, as indicated by its caloric yields; indeed, it is necessary to life. Blocking this system, as can be done with fluoracetate, causes death. *The Krebs cycle enzymes are present in mitochondria.*

The energy resulting from the oxidation of pyruvate to carbon dioxide and water would, by itself, yield only heat. For this energy to be of value to the metabolism of the cell, it must first be chemically fixed or stored in certain molecules and then be readily released from these molecules as needed. The cell accomplishes this by means of a distinctive enzyme system coupled into the Krebs cycle: the electron-transfer system of cytochromes. This system accepts the energy liberated in each of the steps of the Krebs

1–29 Light micrograph of a portion of the stomach lining. The preparation has been stained for NAD$^+$-dependent isocitric dehydrogenase activity (consult Chap. 2). This constitutes a selective stain for mitochondria. Nuclei are present in negative image. Two cell types are present. One, the parietal cell, is rich in granular mitochondria and carries out active transport. The second, the chief cell, has relatively few filamentous mitochondria and is concerned with the synthesis of protein. These cell types are discussed in Chap. 19. × 1,500. (From the work of D. G. Walker.)

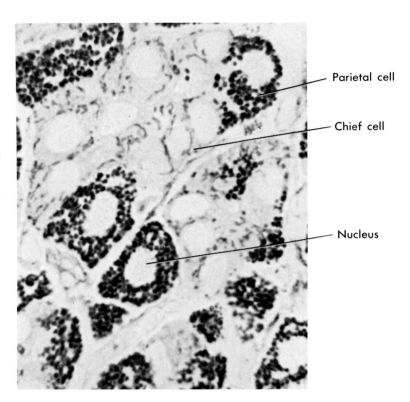

Parietal cell

Chief cell

Nucleus

cycle and incorporates it into so-called high-energy phosphate compounds, notably ATP. This is done by the conversion of *adenosine diphosphate (ADP)* to ATP. The additional phosphate bond so formed represents approximately 7,300 calories of stored energy. *The cytochrome electron-transfer system capable of fixing the energy obtained from the oxidations of the Krebs cycle into ATP lies in mitochondria.* The source of energy for virtually every energy-requiring activity of the cell is ATP. It is translocated from mitochondria into surrounding cytoplasm and its energy is released by ATPases, which lie at different locations in the cell. One depot rich in ATPase is the cell membrane. Here the energy obtained from the conversion of ATP to ADP is used in the active transport of compounds across the cell membrane.

Mitochondria may be observed in living cells by phase-contrast microscopy (Fig. 1–1). They are quite pliant and appear to be carried passively in cytoplasmic streams, twisted, bent, and changing shape. On occasion they appear contractile or motile. They are subject to swelling in certain physiological states.

Mitochondria may be vitally stained with Janus green B, pinacyanole, or other vital dyes that exist in either a colored oxidized form or a colorless reduced form. Because of their oxidative enzymes, mitochondria are able to maintain the dye in its oxidized form (a green or blue in the case of Janus green B), whereas the rest of the cytoplasm is usually unable to do so. Mitochondria stand out clearly as stained linear or punctate structures (Figure 11–5).

In fixed and stained light-microscopic preparations, mitochondria are usually demonstrated by virtue of the phospholipid contained in their membranes. Iron hematoxylin is an excellent stain for mitochondria that is used in the Regaud, Baker, and other methods, because it stains phospholipid. Sudan black B or other dyes that dissolve in lipid stain mitochondria faintly.

Mitochondria may also be demonstrated under the light microscope by cytochemical staining of the activity of their enzymes (Fig. 1–29). Thus stains that reveal the activity of succinic dehydrogenase, malic dehydrogenase, isocitrate dehydrogenase, fumaric dehydrogenase, and other oxidative enzymes effectively stain mitochondria. The cells must be carefully fixed to limit diffusion of enzymes and to retain structural clarity. Even slightly prolonged fixation destroys enzyme activity and renders the methods ineffective. Cytochemical methods provide valuable physiological information. For example, mitochondria may appear identical by methods that depend on phospholipid staining or by supravital staining or phase microscopy. Yet in such mitochondria, Krebs-cycle enzymes may have different activity, and by staining for a variety of these enzymes different functional classes of mitochondria may be recognized.

By electron microscopy, mitochondria may be recognized as distinctive tubular or, occasionally, spherical structures made of inner and outer membranes (Figs. 1–30 and 1–31). The outer membrane is unfolded. The inner membrane is folded to form *cristae*, which extend into the center of the mitochondrion. The space enclosed by the inner membrane is the *inner chamber*. It contains a finely granular material, the *matrix*. The space between outer and inner membrane is the *outer chamber*. In most mammalian cells the cristae are plates or shelves that extend partway across the inner chamber. In cardiac muscle and in kidney tubular cells there may be many cristae that reach across the mitochrondrion, whereas in macrophages there are usually few cristae, and they are short. In the testis, ovary, and adrenal gland, the mitochondria of cells secreting steroid hormones have tubular rather than shelflike cristae.

The unit membrane is modified in the cristae. The surface exposed to the inner chamber possesses knoblike repeating units attached to a basal membrane by slender stalks (Fig. 1–32). These units, called *elementary particles*, are best revealed at high magnification with negative staining after osmotic shock. Elementary particles contain a mitochondrial ATPase complex that appears to provide a channel for proton translocation. Normally the particles may be embedded in the membrane rather than project from it.

Mitochondria are subject to conformational change (Figs. 1–30 and 1–31). The *orthodox form*, described above, is typical of mitochondria in tissue section, since the methods of preparation usually result in low levels of ADP with the mitochondria inactive in oxidative phosphorylation. If, however, oxidative phosporylation is induced in isolated mitochondria by adding ADP or if measures are taken to maintain a high level of oxidative phosphorylation in tissue sections, a *condensed mitochrondrial conformation* is revealed. In this form the volume of the outer chamber is increased to approximately 50% of the organelle, and the inner chamber is reduced in volume.

Mitochondria may be isolated relatively easily by a technique that requires disruption of cells and centrifugation of the fragments. In density-gradient centrifugation, the mitochondria form a tan colored stratum lying above the nuclei and below the lysosomes and ribosomes.

Isolated mitochondria exhibit the reactions described above. In addition, they may be studied by standard chemical and microchemical methods. They may be dissociated by applying deoxycholate and other surface-active agents; in this way it has been shown that the electron-transfer system of cytochromes is firmly bound to membranes, whereas the enzymes of the Krebs tricarboxylic acid cycle are not. Electron-microscopic cytochemistry demonstrates the presence of cytochrome oxidase and other oxidative enzymes in sections of mitochondria.

Freeze-fracture-etch methods reveal particles in mitochondrial membranes (Fig. 1–33). The particles on the inner membrane are numerous and may constitute the enzymes of the electron-transfer chain of cytochrome enzymes.

The number and size of mitochondria are, in general, correlated with the level of oxidative phosphorylation. Hepatocytes may each contain about 1,000 to 1,500 mitochondria. Mature erythrocytes, totally dependent for energy on glycolysis, contain none.

Mitochondria may bear characteristic relationships to other organelles and cell structures. Their relationship is often of functional significance, as the mitochondrion is the primary source of energy. Thus in cells synthesizing protein, mitochondria may occur close to ribosomes. In cells engaged in large-scale active transport of materials across a cell membrane, such as the parietal cell of the stomach (which pumps protons across the plasma membrane in the production of hydrochloric acid), the plasma membrane dips into the cell in many folds and mitochondria are closely held in them. In striated muscle cells, which contain myofilaments that slide on one another to effect contraction, mitochondria are present close to the myofilaments. In the development of fat cells, the minute fat droplets that form and then coalesce are intimately associated with mitochondria.

38

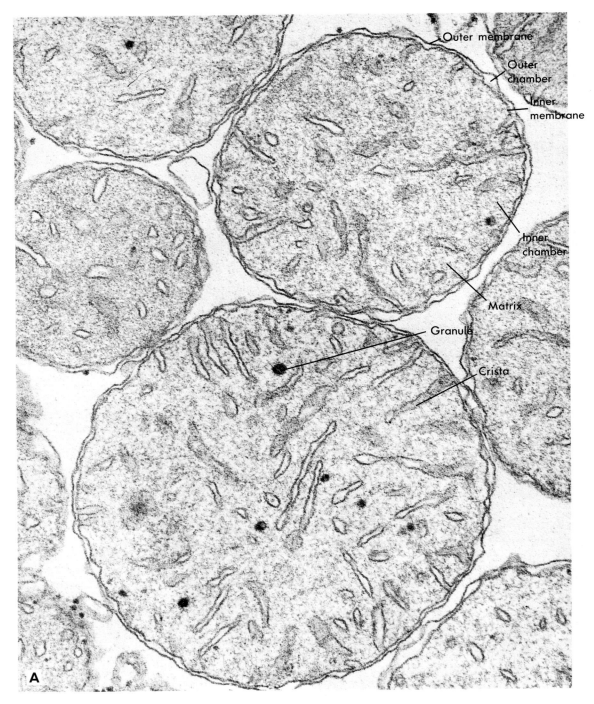

Outer membrane

Outer chamber

Inner membrane

Inner chamber

Matrix

Granule

Crista

A

1-30 Mitochondria of a rat hepatocyte. Mitochondria undergo reversible ultrastructural transformations between a condensed and an orthodox conformation in relationship to the level on oxidative phosphorylation (see text). These changes may be observed in isolated mitochondria and in tissue section. Mitochondria are isolated from disrupted hepatocytes and sectioned. **A.** The conventional

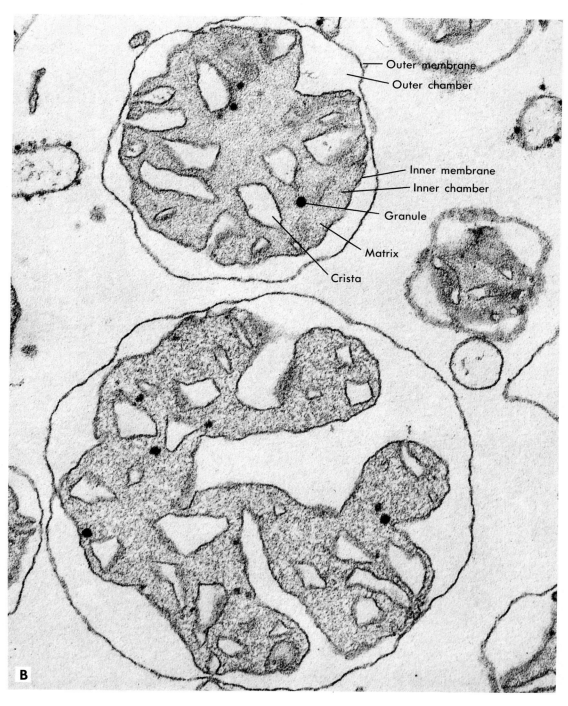

B

conformation, the outer membrane, outer chamber, inner membrane with cristae, and inner chamber containing matrix and granules may be seen. **B.** The condensed state: the outer chamber is considerably enlarged and the inner membrane and matrix thereby condensed. Each × 110,000. (From Hackenbrock, C. R., 1968. J. Cell Biol. 37:345.)

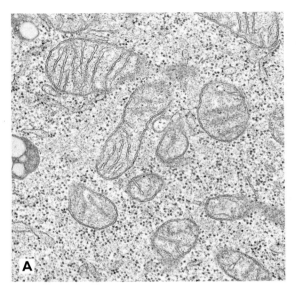

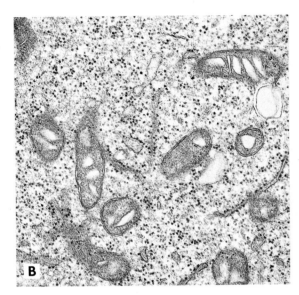

1–31 Mitochondria of an ascites tumor cell. **A.**
△ Mitochondria are present in the orthodox
conformation. A mitochondrion is enclosed in an
outer membrane. The inner membrane is folded into
cristae that extend into the matrix of inner chamber.
× 26,800. **B.** The condensed form, wherein the outer
chamber is expanded, is evident. The cytoplasm also
contains polyribosomes and rough ER. × 26,800.
(From Hackenbrock, C. R., Rehn, T. G., Weinbach,
E. C., and Lemasters, J. J. 1971. J. Cell Biol. 51:123.)

1–32 Mitochondrion from beef heart; negatively
▽ stained electron micrograph. **A.** The cristae of
the mitochondrion are outlined at a magnification of
62,000. Note that small bodies **(arrow)** appear on the
outer cristal membrane facing the interior of the
mitochondrion. **B.** Under 420,000 magnification these
small bodies, the elementary particles **(EP),** are seen
attached to the cristal membrane by a slender
stalk. (From Fernandez-Moran, H., Oda, T., Blair,
P. V., and Green, D. E. 1964. J. Cell Biol. 22:63.)

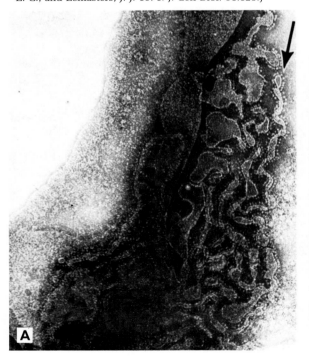

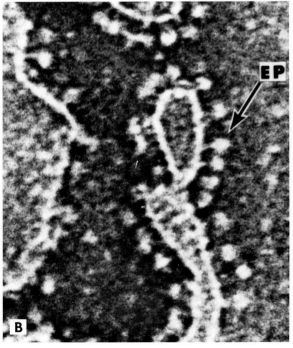

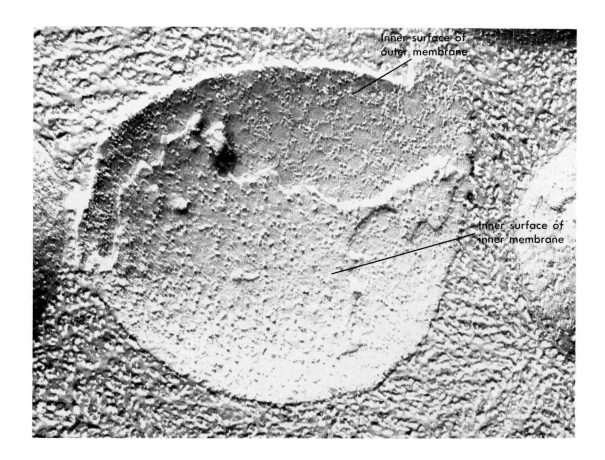

1–33 Mitochondria of a rat hepatocyte. Freeze-fracture-etch of isolated mitochondria. The fracture line exposed the inner surface of the outer membrane and the inner surface of the inner membrane. Note the rather regularly arranged system of granules on the inner surface of the outer membrane. The granules are the size of certain enzymes and may represent membrane-associated enzymes. × 110,000. (From the work of C. R. Hackenbrock.)

The primary function of mitochondria is respiratory, as has been described. They may display other activities as well, notably the concentration of cations. The dense granules of the mitochondrial matrix in the inner chamber may represent concentrations of Ca^{++}.

Mitochondria contain circular DNA typical of prokaryotes, and mitochondrial ribosomes are similar to bacterial ribosomes in several respects. There is evidence, moreover, that existing mitochondria produce new mitochondria. It is possible that in the evolution of eukaryotes, ancestral prokaryote structures established a felicitous symbiotic relationship and permitted the highly successful evolution of eukaryotes. Alternatively, the prokaryotic character of mitochondrial nucleoproteins may be the result of later eukaryotic evolution (convergent evolution) without any contribution of symbiotic prokaryotic organisms.

Endoplasmic Reticulum. The endoplasmic reticulum (ER) is a cytoplasmic system of tubules,

vesicles, and sacs or cisternae fashioned of membranes. It is continuous with the outer membrane of the nuclear envelope (Fig. 1–34). The development of ER varies with cell type and function.

The ER has been defined by electron microscopy, although it has been observed by light microscopy in some cells, notably as the sarcoplasmic reticulum, the specialized ER of striated muscle (Chap. 7). The ER was first described in fibroblasts in tissue culture examined in electron micrographs of whole mounts, i.e., without sec-

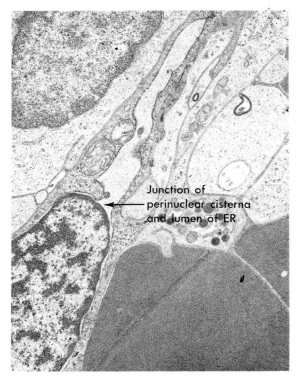

1–34 Connective tissue cell from human embryo spleen. Here the continuity of the outer nuclear membrane and the smooth ER is evident. Thus the perinuclear space and the lumen of the ER are continuous. × 12,000.

◁

Junction of perinuclear cisterna and lumen of ER

1–35 Fibroblast, tissue culture. The preparation in this electron micrograph has not been sectioned. It is a whole mount of the cell, and only the peripheral region is sufficiently thin to permit passage of the electron beam. (From the work of K. R. Porter.) ▽

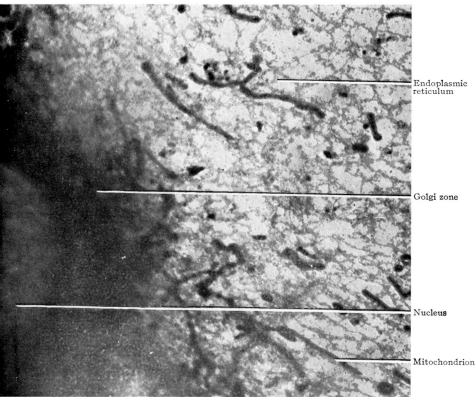

Endoplasmic reticulum

Golgi zone

Nucleus

Mitochondrion

tioning. Ordinarily, whole cells are too thick for electron-microscopic study, but cells in culture may put out cytoplasmic processes thin enough to pass an electron beam. In such preparations the ER may be seen as a cytoplasmic network (Fig. 1–35).

Two major forms of ER occur. They are *rough* or *granular* ER (Fig. 1–36), which has ribosomes on its outside surface, and *smooth* or *agranular* ER, whose surface is free of ribosomes. Ribosomes synthesize protein (see below) and need not be associated with ER. The association of ER and ribosomes occurs in cells that bind the protein they produce in membranous sacs. For example, erythroblasts synthesize the protein hemoglobin, which remains dispersed through the cytoplasm; thus, ribosomes are plentiful but little ER is present. In plasma cells, on the other hand, which synthesize large volumes of antibody, confine it by membranes, and then secrete it, rough ER is abundant. Peptide chains are synthesized in the ribosomes and sent across the ER membrane into the lumen of the ER. The ER thereby isolates synthesized material from the rest of the cytoplasm, permits further assembly of peptides into larger molecules, and conveys the material by means of *transport vesicles* to the Golgi complex where further synthesis and pro-

cessing occur. The Golgi then release the secretion enclosed in membranous sacs, the *condensing vacuoles,* which mature into secretory vacuoles. (See discussion of the Golgi complex, page 48.) Rough ER, well developed in secretory cells, is also abundant in cells that synthesize protein and hold it membrane-bounded within their cytoplasm, as in leukocytes and macrophages. These cells contain enzyme-rich membrane-bounded granules, the *lysosomes.* The formation of these granules parallels the formation of secretory vacuoles, except that the granules tend to be retained rather than released (secreted). The process of secretion is fully discussed in Chap. 21. See, particularly, Figs. 21–9 to 21–13.

In nerve cells rough ER exists as large, flattened sacs lying on one another in lamellated fashion to form masses, *Nissl bodies,* identifiable by light microscopy. Hepatic parenchymal

1–36 Hepatocyte of a rat. In this portion of the cytoplasm most of the cisternae of the rough ER were cut transversely and others tangentially. In the latter **(arrow)** the membrane of the ER and the attached polysomes are seen *en face.* A section of a mitochondrion **(mit)** is present. × 64,000. (From the work of G. E. Palade.)

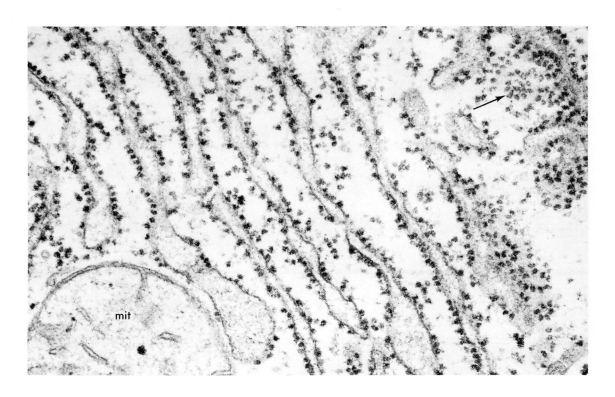

mit

cells contain smaller blocks of rough ER. In plasma cells the rough ER is rather uniformly distributed through the cytoplasm except in the region of the cytocentrum. It may be tubular, vesicular, or flattened, depending on the phase of antibody secretion. Rough ER occupies the base of the pancreatic acinar cell. This rough ER, recognizable by light microscopy as basophilic materal (because of the affinity of its ribosomes for cationic dye) is termed *ergastoplasm* (Figs. 1–3 and 1–4).

Smooth ER, free of ribosomes, occurs in a number of cell types and may have diverse functions. It has a role in the production of steroid hormones and it is abundant in such cells as the Leydig cells of the testis, which produce the steroid testosterone. Smooth ER synthesizes complex lipids from fatty acids. It also detoxifies certain drugs and becomes very prominent in hepatocytes during the inactivation of phenobarbital. In striated muscle, smooth ER is distinctly organized as the sarcoplasmic reticulum whose functions include delivering high concentrations of Ca^{++} and other ions to critical places in the sarcomere for muscular contraction and relaxation. Smooth ER in megakaryocytes delimits platelet zones in the cytoplasm and, by fusing, frees platelets from the megakaryocyte. Appropriately, this ER is termed *"demarcation membrane"*. Carbohydrate synthesis is associated with smooth ER and the Golgi apparatus. The reformation of the nuclear membrane in telophase is accomplished by smooth ER.

The membranes of the ER possess a self-healing capacity after disruption. When fractions rich in ER are recovered from disrupted ultracentrifuged cells, the ER is found as small vesicles *(microsomes)* (Fig. 1–37). Evidently the tubular system is fragmented, but the membranes reunite or "heal" to form small vesicles. After fixation with osmium tetroxide (but not gluteraldehyde) the tubular T system of sarcoplasmic reticulum is revealed as an artifactual system of vesicles— another example of the readiness with which the tubules of ER may be broken up and reformed as small vesicles.

Ribosomes. A single ribosome is below the limit of resolution of the light microscope, but in aggregate, the presence of ribosomes can be recognized. Owing, in all likelihood, to their PO_4^{3-} groups, they have a pronounced affinity for cationic or basic dyes such as methylene blue$^+$. As a result, cells rich in ribosomes are basophilic;

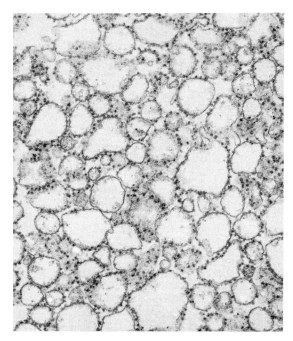

1–37 Microsomes of rat liver. The liver was disrupted and various fractions recovered by ultracentrifugation. This is the microsome fraction. It consists almost entirely of rough ER that had been disrupted and "healed" as vesicles. Ribosomes remain attached to the outer surface. × 40,000. (From the work of D. Sabatini and M. Adelman.)

this basophilia may be abolished by pretreating the tissue with ribonuclease. The intensity and disposition of the basophilia are highly characteristic of cell type. Basophilic material visualized by light microscopy has been designated *chromidial substance*. Consult the description of pancreatic islet cells (Chap. 22), lymphocytes (Chap. 11), and erythroblasts (Chap. 12) for patterns of chromidial substance.

Ribosomes are flattened, spheroidal, complex cytoplasmic particles measuring approximately 150 × 250 Å that synthesize protein (Figs. 1–38 to 1–41). They consist of RNA and protein. Their RNA is classed as rRNA, which accounts for 85% of the RNA of the cell. In addition to this form of RNA, there is mRNA and tRNA. The instruction for protein synthesis is encoded in DNA. This information is transcribed to mRNA, which is about 300 to 600 nm long, depending on the protein. Messenger RNA is produced in the nucleus, on a template of uncoiled DNA. It moves to the

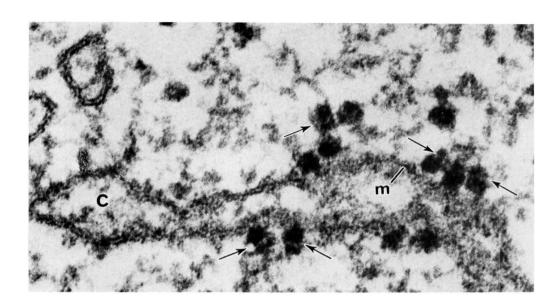

cytoplasm where it associates itself with ribosomes that lie along the mRNA like beads on a necklace. Ribosomes occurring singly in the cytoplasm are not active; only when they are linked by mRNA to form polyribosomes do they engage in protein synthesis. The ribosomes are the small machines that receive the amino acid constituents of protein, assemble them into peptide chains, and release these chains into the cytoplasm or into the lumen of the ER where they continue to aggregate to form protein. Each amino acid is brought to the ribosome by its distinctive tRNA, a low molecular-weight nucleic acid (see below) that may be produced in the nucleolar region of the nucleus (as is rRNA) and passes out of the nucleus into the cytoplasm. In protein synthesis, a ribosome moves along mRNA and reads the genetic message that has been transcribed from DNA. As the ribosome translates the message, it binds on its surface the particular activated amino acyl-tRNA specified by the codon being read and synthesizes the peptide linkage of this amino acid to the earlier ones.

The peptide chain grows larger as the ribosome moves along the mRNA, and as the ribosomes slides off the mRNA, it releases the peptide chain. As one ribosome slides off one end of the mRNA, another slides onto the other end and several ribosomes "read" or translate the mRNA at any time. The ribosomes lie on the mRNA approximately 340 Å apart (Fig. 1–40). For a poly-

1–38 Ribosomes, hepatocyte, of a guinea pig.

Ribosomes at high magnification show a larger and smaller component. When associated with the ER, the larger component lies upon the membrane. In this field a single cisterna (c) of the ER is present. The arrows indicate the position and orientation of the partitions separating the large from the small subunits of the ribosomes. Note that these partitions lie generally parallel to the surface of the membranes (m). This specimen was fixed in osmium tetroxide, embedded, sectioned, and stained with uranyl acetate. × 270,000. (From the work of D. Sabatini, Y. Toshiro, and G. E. Palade.)

peptide chain of hemoglobin 150 amino acids long, 60 to 90 sec are required for the ribosome to run the length of mRNA.

The ribosome is composed of two unequal subunits, one large and the other small (Fig. 1–42). Both are highly organized macromolecular assemblies consisting of one or more RNA molecules and numerous different proteins. In humans, as in most eukaryotes, the smaller subunit has a molecular weight of 1.5×10^6 and is composed of a single molecule of RNA with a sedimentation constant of 18S and approximately 30 different, rather small proteins (10,000 to 40,000 daltons). The small subunit functions to bind the mRNA to the ribosome and forms part of the tRNA binding site as the codon is being read by the anticodon of the tRNA. The larger subunit with a molecular weight of $3.0 \times$

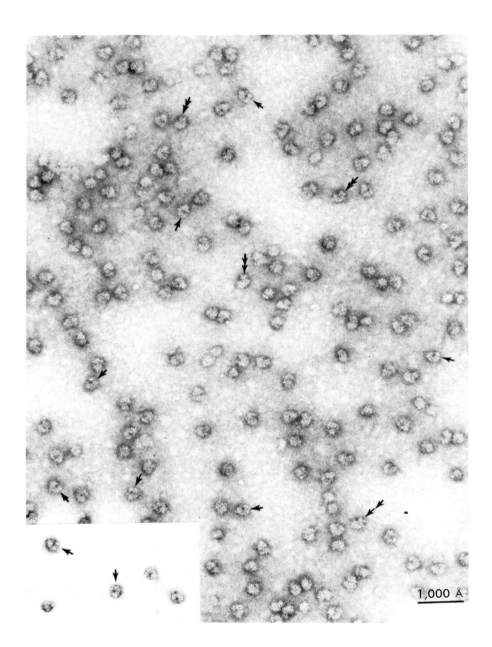

1–39 Ribosomes of a guinea pig. General view of a field of native monomeric ribosomes. Several image types are predominant. Frontal images **(arrows)** have an elongated small subunit profile and a dense spot toward the side of the separation between subunits. All frontal images in the field have this spot to the left of the observer if the particle image is oriented with the elongated small subunit horizontally and toward the top. In lateral images **(double arrows)** the small subunit produces a small rounded or rectangular profile toward one side of the large subunit profile. The inset shows images of monomeric ribosomes, reconstituted in vitro from the isolated large and small subunits. This preparation was made from ribosomes isolated by differential centrifugation of disrupted cells. The ribosomes were then floated on a membrane-covered electron-microscopic grid, dried, and negatively stained with phosphotungstic acid. × 125,000. (From the work of D. Sabatini, Y. Nonomura, and G. Blobel.)

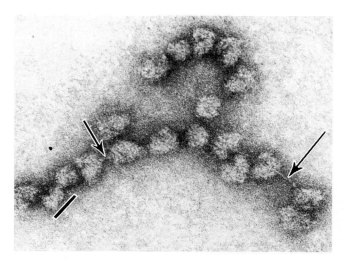

1–40 Ribosomes of a guinea pig. Here a strand of messenger RNA **(arrows)** links ribosomes into a polyribosomal unit. The mRNA runs between the small and large subunits. × 240,000. (From the work of D. Sabatini, Y. Nonomura, and G. Blobel.)

◁

1–41 An electron micrograph of *E. coli* small ribosomal subunits reacted with antibodies directed against ribosomal protein S14. The antibodies attach at only a single region in the upper one-third of the subunit, and are indicated by arrows. The centrally located pairs of subunits are connected by single IgG molecules, while the pair of subunits on the left is connected by two different IgG molecules, both attached to the same region of the subunit surface. (From the work of J. Lake, M. Pendergast, L. Kahan, and M. Nomura.)

◁

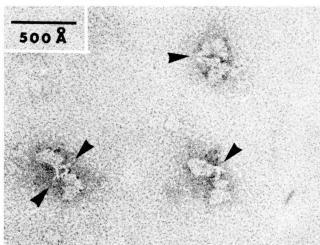

1–42 Model of the *E. coli* ribosome showing the relationship of the large and the small subunits. The view on the left shows the interface between the small subunit **(light)** and the large subunit **(dark).** This interface is an important region where the tRNAs, the mRNA, and factors involved in protein synthesis are located. In the view at the right showing the ribosome viewed from above, a prominent feature of the large subunit is the elongated projection extending from the subunit. At present, the function of this feature of the large subunit is not well understood. (From the work of J. Lake.) ▽

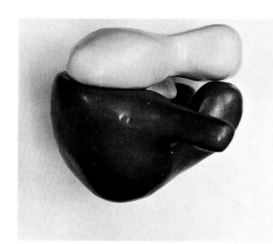

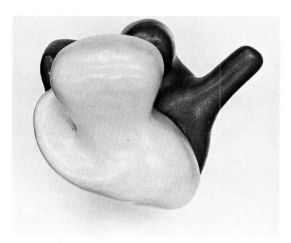

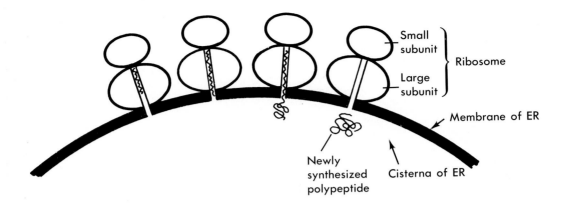

1–43 Model of the relationship between ribosomes and ER membrane. Attachment by the large subunits and orientation of the partition separating the two ribosomal subunits are strongly suggested by the evidence presented. The central channel in the large subunit and the discontinuity in the subjacent ER membrane are tentative features of the model, included only to indicate a possible pathway for the release of the newly synthesized protein in the cisternal space. (From the work of D. Sabatini and G. Blobel.)

10^6 has a sedimentation constant of 60S and contains two RNA molecules (5S and 28S) and probably a third (5.8S). The approximately 40 different proteins contained in the large subunit are on the average slightly larger than those in the small subunit. The large subunit functions in protein synthesis by forming part of the tRNA binding sites, catalyzing peptidyl transfer, and holding the growing polypeptide chain. Ribosomes bound to the rough ER are attached through the large subunit (Fig. 1–43). In bacteria, and prokaryotes in general, ribosomes (70S) and their subunits (30S and 50S) are somewhat smaller. Bacterial ribosomes differ from eukaryotic ribosomes in their responses to antibiotics affecting protein synthesis. Some antibiotics, such as puromycin, inhibit protein synthesis on both prokaryotic and eukaryotic ribosomes; others, such as cycloheximide, affect only eukaryotic ribosomes. (The ribosomes found in the mitochondria of eukaryotes differ from others in eukaryotic cytoplasm by resembling bacterial ribosomes in their responses to antibiotics.) Eukaryotic and prokaryotic ribosomes have important similarities despite their differences. The sequence of events that occur during the protein synthesis cycle is the same in both eukaryotic and prokaryotic ribosomes, and although there

are differences in size, these ribosomes greatly resemble each other in gross morphology as observed in the electron microscope.

The three-dimensional locations of specific ribosomal proteins are being mapped by using antibodies directed against individual ribosomal proteins (Figs. 1–41 and 1–44).

Polyribosomes may lie free in the cytoplasm, releasing their peptide chains into the cytoplasm for further combination and complexing. This is how hemoglobin is synthesized. Where the ribosomes attach to the outer surface of ER, the larger unit maintains attachment. The mRNA and the ER membranes are parallel. Furthermore, there may be a canal running through the larger ribosomal component at right angles to the mRNA and the ER. This canal has been postulated to run through the membranous wall of the ER, with the result that the amino acids, in peptide linkage, are "spun out" by the ribosomes directly into the lumen of the ER (Fig. 1–43). This peptide is "led" across the wall of the ER into its lumen by a signal peptide produced by the large ribosomal subunit and linked to the amino terminal of the peptide. See Chap. 21 for further discussion of secretion.

Ribosomes have a short life span. When protein synthesis ceases, they are quickly metabolized and disappear.

Golgi Complex. The Golgi apparatus or complex is a membranous system of cisternae and vesicles, usually located in or around the cytocentrum. It is involved in intracellular transport of secretory proteins, membrane proteins, and proteins that remain membrane-bounded within the cell, in distinction to proteins such as hemoglobin and keratin that lie free in the cytoplasm.

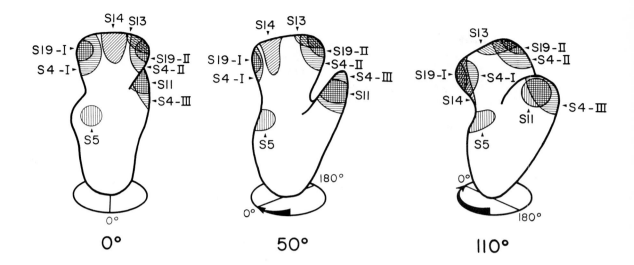

| 0° | 50° | 110° |

1–44 A diagrammatic representation of three views of the *E. coli* smaller ribosomal subunit illustrating the locations of some of the ribosomal proteins. The views from left to right represent rotations of the subunit about its long axis of 0°, 50°, and 110°, respectively. The cleft formed between the vertically oriented platform and the upper one-third of the subunit is best seen in the +50° view. The platform itself is attached to the lower two-thirds of the subunit. The vertical axis of the subunit is approximately 250 Å long. Many of the proteins are located at only a single region of the subunit but some, such as S4 and S19, are elongated and extend through the subunit. Three different regions of S4 are exposed and indicate that this protein must be at least 170 Å long. Protein S4 is required for the proper self-assembly of subunits and its extended nature may be related to its role in subunit assembly. (From the work of J. Lake, M. Nomura, and L. Kahan.)

The Golgi complex has a characteristic appearance by light microscopy. It may be a small compact structure; it may be a cluster of small structures (termed dictyosomes in earlier literature); or it may be a large netlike structure, the *internal reticular apparatus* as initially defined by C. Golgi in nerve cells. The Golgi complex is often juxtanuclear and may partially enclose the centrioles. Its size fluctuates with cell type and secretory activity. It is well developed in secretory cells, for example, in the mucus-producing intestinal epithelial cells, in plasma cells, and cells of the pituitary gland. The Golgi complex has the capacity to reduce metal salts, such as salts of osmium and of silver (Figs. 1–4 and 1–45), and may therefore be stained with these compounds. Such staining methods were responsible for the discovery of the Golgi complex.

By electron microscopy, the Golgi complex consists of 3 to 15 large flat sacs or cisternae apposed to one another. They are relatively compressed at their centers and somewhat dilated peripherally. The sacs tend to be bowed, presenting a convex *proximal face* (toward the nucleus) and concave *distal face* (away from the nucleus (Figs 1–35 to 1–37, 21–9, and 22–8). These stacked cisternae thus form bowl-shaped structures, and the Golgi complex as a whole looks like a stack of shallow bowls with the concavity directed away from the nucleus. The cisternae may communicate with one another by slender channels at places along their contiguous surfaces. The proximal membranes (those near the nucleus) are thinner than the distal membranes (facing out toward the bulk of the cytoplasm), which are more like those of plasmalemma. At the edge of the lamellated sacs, near their expanded peripheries, vesicles 400 to 800 Å in diameter are typically present. Similar vesicles may also be abundant at the distal face. The vesicles vary in size and probably fuse to form larger vesicles. They, like the lateral vesicles, may contain a dense material. The proximal face is relatively free of vesicles and has been termed the *forming face* (also known as the *cis* face). The distal face, which is typically engaged in granule formation, has been termed the *maturation face* (also known as the *trans* face) (Figs. 1–46 to 1–49).

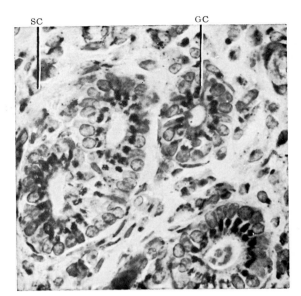

1–45 Golgi material in cells of guinea pig uterus.

The Golgi material was blackened with silver by the method of Da Fano. Large quantities of it lie above the nuclei of the glandular cells **(GC)**; smaller amounts lie next to the nuclei of the stromal cells **(SC)**. × 500.

◁

1–46 Human myelocyte. In this developing blood cell (see Chap. 11), the nucleus is lobed. Nuclear pores **(np)** are present. The cytoplasm contains granules, vesicles, rough and smooth ER, mitochondria, and free ribosomes. A Golgi apparatus is present, partially surrounding a centriole. × 26,000. (From the work of G. A. Ackerman.) ▽

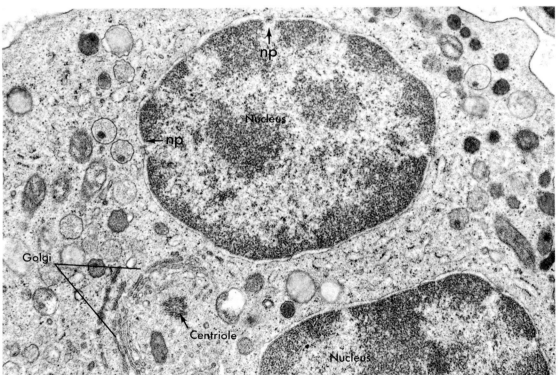

Proteins destined to be secreted or stored in lysosomes or other membrane-bounded granules are synthesized by polysomes attached to the outer surface of ER. Newly synthesized proteins collect within the lumen of the rough ER and move into contiguous ER free of ribosomes.

These elements are called "transitional elements" because they lie between the rough ER and the Golgi complex. It is thought that they bud off as *transport vesicles*, which carry quanta of ER content to the Golgi complex. The Golgi complex not only serves as a way station for pro-

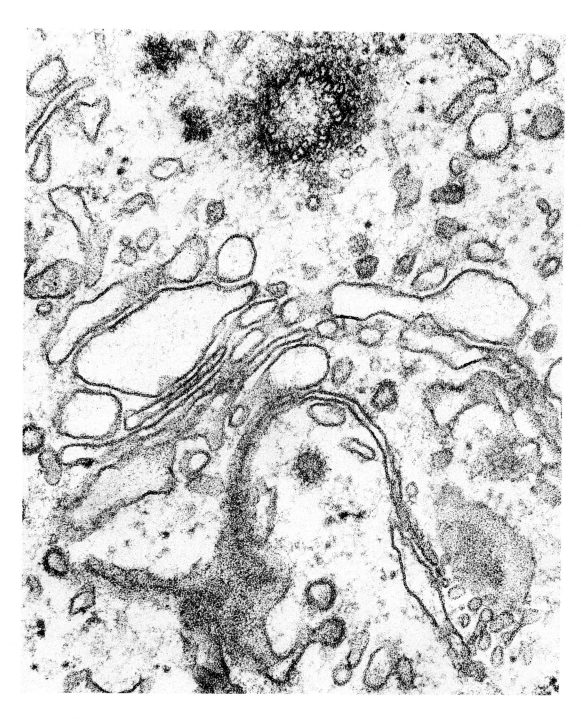

tein intracellular transport, but several covalent modifications of proteins may occur as they pass through it. For example, a portion of the carbohydrate moiety of many glycoproteins is added in the Golgi complex (e.g., immunoglobulins and pancreatic enzymes). The high concentration of

1–47 Golgi complex. It is evident, in this field, that the Golgi membranes and vesicles are made of the trilaminar unit membrane. A centriole is also present. (From the work of E. D. Hay and J. P. Revel.)

the *glycosyl transferase* enzymes on the inner surface of Golgi membranes reflects this function.

There are several patterns of secretion. In "nonregulated" secretory cells (e.g., plasma cells and fibroblasts), secretion is continuous and is effected by small Golgi-derived secretory vesicles, perhaps 50 nm in diameter. In "regulated" secretory cells (e.g., pancreatic acinar cells), on the other hand, secretion is intermittent and depends on hormonal stimuli. In this case, the secretory granules accumulate in the apical cytoplasm and may become rather large, up to 1,500 nm in diameter. In such cells, the ability of the Golgi complex to concentrate secretory protein is especially evident. Distal to the stacked cisternae are "condensing vacuoles" of irregular shape. These organelles further concentrate their content to become zymogen or storage granules. Upon hormonally triggered secretion, the granule membrane fuses with the plasma membrane. At the site of fusion the membranes break down and the contents of the secretory granule are released from the cell. See Figs. 21–9, 21–12, 21–13, and 22–8.

The Golgi complex also functions in lipoprotein synthesis. Lipids enter the Golgi cisternae from smooth ER and in the Golgi apparatus they are complexed to protein produced in rough ER. Membrane-bounded lipoprotein granules are then released from the Golgi (Figs. 1–48 and 1–49).

A major technique for delineating the sequence of protein intracellular transport is *pulse-chase electron-microscopic autoradiography*. With this method, a radioactive metabolite, such as an amino acid or sugar that will be incorporated into the macromolecular product undergoing synthesis, is injected rapidly in a single dose into an experimental animal. As a result, a short, sharply delineated "pulse" of radioactively labeled metabolite enters the synthetic process and is carried through it. By sampling tissue at appropriate times for autoradiography, the "pulse labeled" radioactive macromolecules (e.g., proteins) can be visualized at their site of synthesis and followed during transport to the site of discharge.

The Golgi complex has been isolated by differential centrifugation and has been partially characterized chemically. It consists of approximately equal parts of lipid and protein and tends to be unusually rich in nucleoside diphosphatases. These phosphatases serve as cytochemical and biochemical markers for Golgi membranes. After a short time an identical but now radioactive compound is digested rapidly. This "chases" the radioactive amino acid, diluting it out.

Smooth Vesicles and Coated Vesicles. The cytoplasm contains several kinds of membrane-bounded vesicles that enclose diverse materials and carry them from place to place within the cytoplasm and to and from the cell surfaces. These vesicles include phagosomes, macropinosomes, micropinosomes, condensing vesicles, transport vesicles and secretory vesicles. Lysosomes, peroxisomes, and microbodies may also be included and are discussed in the next section. The movement and destination of vesicles within the cell may be rather specific. For example, vesicles originating at the cell surface may selectively take in immunoglobulin, transport it across the cell using well-defined cytoplasmic streams, and release it at the lateral or basal surfaces of the cell. In addition, protein, partially synthesized in the ER, may be delivered for further synthesis to the Golgi complex by a system of transport vesicles that bud off the ER, travel to the Golgi sacs, and fuse with them.

The cytoplasm of virtually every cell contains membrane-bounded vesicles originating at the cell surface from invaginations of plasma membrane that pinch off. Because such vesicles carry material from outside into the cell, the process that results in their formation has been called *endocytosis*. In the reverse process, *exocytosis*, intracellular material is conveyed within vesicles to the cell surface where the membrane of the vesicle fuses with the plasma membrane and then breaks down, releasing the material to the extracellular compartment. In the process, the vesicle disappears and its membrane is translocated into the plasma membrane.

In endocytosis, the endocytotic vesicles may contain particulate material, such as bacteria or cell fragments. These vesicles are called *phagocytic* vesicles or *phagosomes*. Phagosomes typically flow toward lysosomes and fuse with them, forming *phagolysosomes*, *heterolysosomes*, or *secondary lysosomes* (Chap. 4). The hydrolytic enzymes of the lysosomes mix and digest the particulate material of the phagosome, and the resulting low molecular-weight compounds diffuse from the phagolysome into the hyaloplasm. Phagocytic vesicles tend to be large, visible by light microscopy. Certain cell types such as macrophages (Chap. 4) and leukocytes (Chap. 11) are

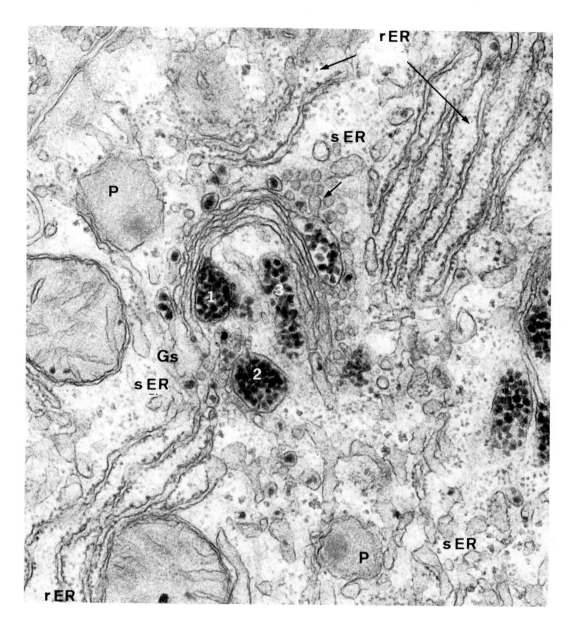

1–48 Golgi complex from a rat hepatocyte. The complex lies near the center of this field. The forming face of the Golgi, where the development of secretory product is initiated, is at the convex side of the apparatus, with extensions from the smooth ER network **(sER)** piling up from below and above, along the curved structure. This smooth ER is probably produced by the rough ER **(rER)** that surrounds the Golgi. The smooth ER may be continuous with the Golgi saccules or may break up into transport vesicles that move to the Golgi and fuse with it. A cluster of small vesicles, on top of the Golgi structure and next to a concentrating or secretory vesicle, is interpreted as representing cross sections of tubular, smooth ER extensions, with one of them **(arrow)** connecting with the concentrating vesicle. At the concave or maturing face of the Golgi three concentrating or secretory vesicles (1 to 3) are present. Each contains many small granules. At P, there are two peroxisomes (see text). Compare this process of lipoprotein granule formation with that of the formation of granules within leukocytes, described in Chap. 11. × 56,500. (From Claude, A. 1970. J. Cell Biol. 47:745.)

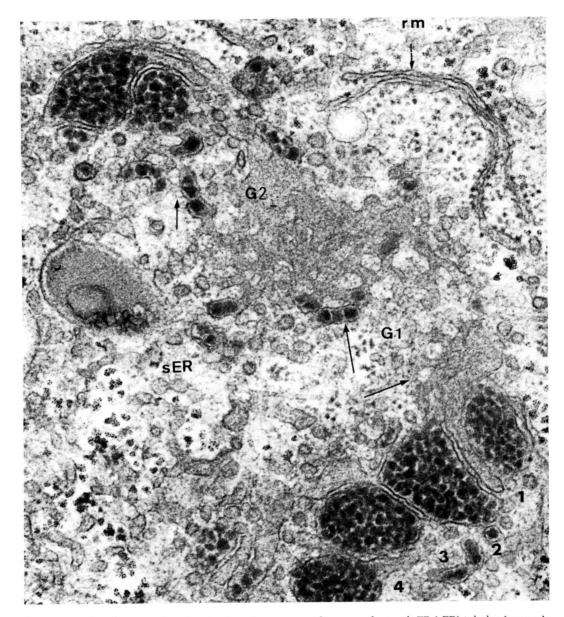

1–49 Golgi complex from a rat hepatocyte. Smooth-surfaced membranes **(rm)** similar to those in Fig. 1–48 are cut in cross section. As they are traced to the right, they are continuous with rough ER. At G2 Golgi membranes at the forming surface are cut in a plane parallel to their surface. These membranes are fenestrated and, in all probability, are formed by coalescence of smooth ER **(sER)** tubules **(arrows)** carrying rows of dense lipoprotein granules. Four large concentrating or secretory vesicles are present (numbered 1 to 4). These would develop from the maturing face of the Golgi, corresponding to the concave portion in Fig. 1–48. × 67,800. (From Claude, A. 1970. J. Cell Biol. 47:745.)

quite proficient or "professional" phagocytes. Other cell types, however, can be phagocytic, such as the endothelium of the vascular sinuses of bone marrow and spleen (Chap. 13), and phagocytosis must be regarded as a general property of cells.

Another class of endocytotic vesicles may contain fluids imbibed from the extracellular fluid at the cell surface. These are *pinocytotic vesicles* or *pinosomes* (*pino*, drinking). Pinosomes may bring fluid in unselectively or they may depend on receptors to bring material into the cell selectively, which is called *receptor mediated pinocytosis*. A type of pinosome is greater than 0.2 μm in diameter. This type is large enough to be visible by light microscopy, and in fact, was first described more than 50 years ago in living cells in tissue culture. These *macropinosomes* characteristically move in cytoplasmic streams toward the center of the cell, becoming smaller and denser as they travel, their contents presumably becoming more concentrated owing to loss of water. Macropinosomes, like phagosomes, may fuse with lysosomes.

A variety of pinocytosis undertaken by virtually every cell of the body, *micropinocytosis*, is distinguished by vesicles visible only by electron microscopy (70 to 100 nm in diameter).

The endocytic vesicular systems function to bring material into a cell, to segregate that material, and to transport it to selective destinations within the cell. In endothelium, for example, vesicles originate at the luminal surface, cross the cell and release their contents at the basal surface. Vesicles may also move in the opposite direction. This type of transit, *transcytosis*, is discussed more fully in Chap. 9. In the epithelial cells lining the gut, materials are taken up at the luminal or apical surface and transported to the lateral cell surface by vesicles and discharged into the intercellular space (Chap. 19). In addition to the discharge of immunoglobulin, the many instances of secretion are examples of exocytosis. Secretory vesicles typically derive from the Golgi complex as *condensing* or *storage vesicles*, and become secretory vesicles, which collect in the apical or secretory pole of the cell. They then move to the cell surface, fuse with the plasma membrane, open to the extracellular space, and discharge their secretion (Figs. 21–9, 21–12, 21–13, and 22–8). Secretion is discussed throughout this book, but major presentations are in the chapters on epithelium (Chap. 3), salivary glands (Chap. 7), mammary glands (Chap. 26), pancreas (Chaps. 21 and 22), and hypophysis

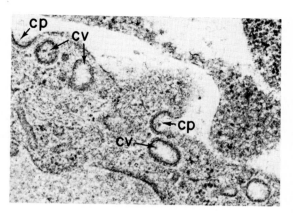

1–50 Endothelium, mouse bone marrow. Coated pits **(cp)** and coated vesicles **(cv)** are present. × 25,000. See also Figs. 3–15, and 8–36.

(Chap. 29), as well as in the earlier sections of this chapter on the endoplasmic reticulum (page 41) and the Golgi complex (page 49).

Cytoplasmic vesicles can be smooth or coated. Smooth vesicles are bounded by membrane similar to the plasma membrane. Coated vesicles are coated on their outside (cytoplasmic) surface by a protein, *clathrin*, of molecular weight 180,000. Clathrin invests the vesicle and appears in sections as radiating spikes, each about 15 nm long and about 5 nm apart, which gives the vesicle a fuzzy look. On surface view the clathrin forms a lattice of hexagons, the side of the polygons being the projections or spikes seen in sections. Coated pinosomes originate as invaginations from coated invaginations of the cell surface, *coated pits* (Figs. 1–50 and 1–51).

Coated and smooth vesicles have similar and complementary functions. Any type of vesicle may be smooth, but coated vesicles are almost always of small diameter (70–10 nm) and only in a few instances are larger. The nature and special functions of coated vesicles are being sorted out. Coated endocytotic vesicles transport immunoglobulin across the placenta from mother to fetus, thereby conferring passive immunity on the fetus. Coated vesicles also transport yolk proteins into the cytoplasm of oocytes. As the yolk-containing coated vesicles move centrally, they lose their clathrin coat and fuse with other yolk-containing vesicles to form rather large yolk vesicles. They, in turn, fuse with lysosomes, and the yolk is digested into low molecular-weight nutrients that diffuse out of the lysosome-yolk vesicle to be metabolized by the oocyte. Casein, as noted above, is carried in exocytotic coated ves-

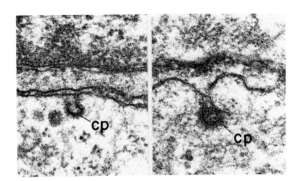

1–51 Leukocytes, mouse bone marrow. Varieties of coated pit **(cp).** left panel × 42,000, right × 70,000. See also Figs. 3–15 and 8–36. Courtesy Joyce S. Knoll

icles that may be rather large. The liver produces a very low density lipoprotein (VLDL) which it releases to the blood through exocytotic coated vesicles. VLDL is a component of blood serum that controls the dispersment of serum lipids, a factor important in the development of atherosclerosis in the walls of the blood vessels. The clathrin coat may play a distinctive role in recycling exocytic membrane. In the synaptic bulb at the end of certain nerves, a number of synaptic vesicles are present. These vesicles are bounded by smooth membrane and contain neurotransmitter substances. When the nerve is stimulated the synaptic vesicles move to the plasma membrane at the synapse, fuse with it, and discharge their contents. After discharge, the membrane of the synaptic vesicle is intercalated into the plasma membrane. It appears that this intercalated membrane may be translocated a short distance away from the synapse and then recycled into the cell where it again forms synaptic vesicles. Clathrin seems to play an essential role in this recycling by moving beneath the translocated synaptic membrane intercalated in the plasma membrane and inducing it to invaginate and pinch off in the cytoplasm as a coated vesicle. When the clathrin first moves beneath the plasma membrane, its latticework is entirely hexagonal. Then pentagons appear in the lattice, and with this change the clathrin assumes a curvilinear form, bringing in the membrane as an invaginated coated pit that proceeds to form a coated vesicle. The coated vesicle next loses its clathrin coat and becomes, once again, a smooth synaptic vesicle. Its clathrin coat appears to prevent a coated vesicle from fusing with other membranous structures. When material is endocytized by a coated vesicle, therefore, that mate-

rial remains within that vesicle as long as it remains coated. When the coat drops away, the membrane of the vesicle may fuse with similar vesicles forming larger vesicles, with lysosomes forming heterolysosomes, with plasma membrane resulting in exocytosis, or with such other membranous structures as the Golgi complex to facilitate transport and synthesis.

Lysosomes, Peroxisomes and Multivesicular Bodies. Lysosomes are membrane-bounded cytoplasmic vesicles containing 50 or more hydrolytic enzymes, virtually all of which are glycoproteins active at acid pH (Figs. 1–52 and 1–53). Lysosomes may become quite large but in their primary state usually measure 50 to 80 Å in diameter. They may be isolated by differential centrifugation of disrupted cells, where they lie centripetal to mitochondria. They may be identified

1–52 Lysosomes of the epithelioid cell of chicken. In this cell, derived from a macrophage, the cytoplasm is filled with lysosomes. They crowd out the centrosome. From the centriole, rays of gelated cytoplasm free of organelles radiate. At one place a small pocket of Golgi membranes is present. (From Sutton, J., and Weiss, L. 1966. J. Cell Biol. 28:303.)

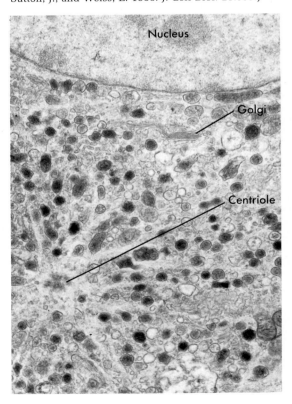

Nucleus

Golgi

Centriole

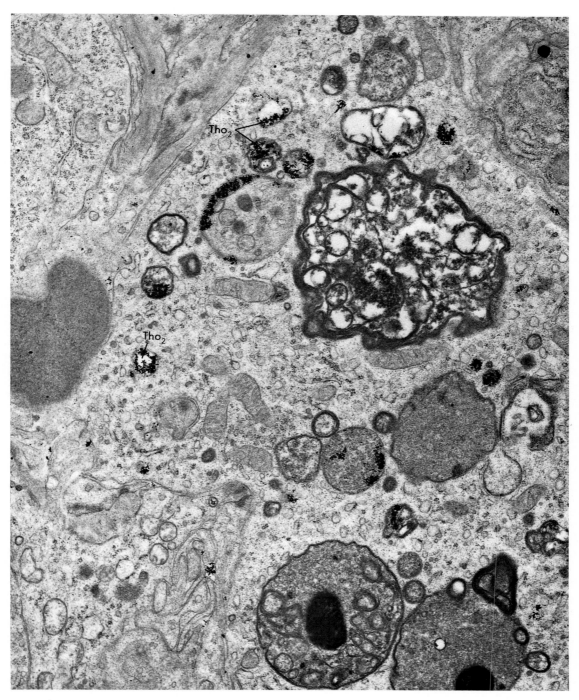

1–53 Lysosomes of a macrophage from a rabbit. This animal was given thorium dioxide (ThO_2), an electron-dense heavy metal, shortly before this cell was fixed. Heterolysosomes, considerably different in appearance, are present. Many contain some ThO_2. × 40,000. (From Weiss, L. 1964. Bull. Hopkins Hosp. 115:99.)

Table 1–3 Major Enzymatic Activities
of Lysosomes

Acid phosphatase
lipase and esterase
phospholipases
ribo- and deoxyribo-nucleases
galactos- and glucos-aminidases
fuco- and gluco-sidases
glucuronidase and hyaluronidase
aryl- and chondro-sulfatases
cathepsins and other peptidases

cytochemically by reactions for acid phosphatase, a commonly used marker, or by reactions for other enzymes they contain. In such cytochemical preparations lysosomes appear as punctate structures by light microscopy. In electron micrographs they are oval or round and contain variably dense granular material. Most cells contain lysosomes. Hepatocytes and macrophages, cell types rich in lysosomes, contain approximately 200. Their large complement of hydrolytic enzymes (Table 1–3) endows lysosomes with the capacity to hydrolyze or digest a great many substrates. The activity of these enzymes is controlled by their bounding membrane. This membrane selectively admits substrates into the lysosome and protects the cells against indiscriminate digestion by its own lysosomal enzymes.

The digestive capacities of lysosomes have been adapted to the functions of disparate cell types. In phagocytic cells, for example, lysosomes digest microbes or other phagosomal contents brought into the cell (heterophagy). In almost any cell of the body, moreover, organelles that have become worn out or exhausted and need to be replaced may be incorporated into lysosomes and digested (autophagy). Furthermore, secretory substances synthesized by endocrine cells may be digested by lysosomal enzymes and the level of secretion thereby regulated (crinophagy). In fact, lysosomes may participate in the destruction and recycling of many cell components, such as receptors and membrane.

The life cycle of lysosomes is complex and accounts for their marked structural heterogeneity (polymorphism). The primary lysosome or storage body is produced at the Golgi complex. Its genesis parallels that of secretory granules (Chaps. 3 and 21) in that its protein is synthesized in rough ER, is conveyed to the Golgi complex by transport vesicles, and in the Golgi complex it is cross-linked and aggregated, and

carbohydrate is added (see preceding section on Golgi Complex). Novikoff and his colleagues believe that lysosomes may also be produced in Golgi-associated ER, bypassing the Golgi complex proper, and they have coined the acronym "GERL complex" to encompass these cooperating structures. Primary lysosomes move to phagosomes and pinosomes and fuse with them to form secondary lysosomes, heterolysosomes, heterophagosomes, or heteropinosomes (Fig. 1–53), as described in the preceding section on smooth and coated vesicles. After fusion, the lysosomal enzymes mix with and digest the contents of the pinosomes or phagosomes. The low molecular-weight digestion products diffuse out of the lysosome into the surrounding cytoplasm where they are metabolized. Heterolysosomes may be long-lived and new endocytized material added over time. Heterolysosomes, moreover, may fuse with one another and form rather large, irregular complexes. Lysosomes finally reach a state in which the material they contain is not further degradable and their enzymatic capacity declines. They become residual bodies or telolysosomes. They may contain pigments, myelin bodies, crystals, lipids, and assorted materials. Residual bodies may be expelled from macrophages and from invertebrate cells, as amebocytes (exocytosis). Alternatively, they may accumulate in the cytoplasm as indices of "wear and tear" of aging, as exemplified by lipofuscin granules. Residual bodies, as expected, are notable in long-lived metabolically active cells, such as nerve cells and muscle cells.

Another group of secondary lysosomes consists of autophagocytic vacuoles or cytolysosomes. These vacuoles are heterolysosomes that contain some organelles of the cell such as mitochondria and ribosomes. They may originate from segments of smooth ER that curve around some cytoplasm and fuse to enclose it in a vacuole. These vacuoles may then fuse with primary lysosomes just as phagosomes do. Another mechanism accounting for their origin may be the incorporation of some cytoplasm directly into a lysosome. The formation of autophagosomes is a mechanism of "internal policing" of a cell that removes damaged or senescent cell substance. Autophagocytic vacuoles increase in starvation and aging and after tissue injury. They participate in the normal turnover of cell organelles by destroying the aged ones. Thus, mitochondria have a half-life of only 10 days in rat hepatocytes. They are removed by autophagy. Autophagocytic vacuoles form residual bodies.

Lysosomes have other metabolic functions. They may function in the degradation of glycogen. Evidence for this role comes from a type of glycogen storage disease, an illness of children characterized by a marked increase in liver size (hepatomegaly) due to the accumulation of glycogen. In this disease, lysosomes are deficient in *glycosidase*, the enzyme responsible for glycogen breakdown. Lysosomes function to regulate hormone production by *crinophagy*. The thyroid hormone *thyroxin* is produced as a conjugate of globulin. Its separation or hydrolysis from globulin seems to depend on incorporation of the thyroglobulin into lysosomes and hydrolysis by their hydrolytic enzymes. The destruction of excess mammotrophic hormone in the secretory cells of the pituitary gland and of parathyroid hormone in the secretory cells of the parathyroid gland is accomplished by autophagy of secretory granules (crinography).

Unlike secretory granules, lysosomes are typically not released but remain within the cytoplasm. Their genesis is parallel to that of secretory granules, however. In their synthesis in rough ER and Golgi complex, lysosomal enzymes retain phosphorylated mannose residues which interact with membrane receptors in the Golgi complex to induce the formation of membrane-bounded lysosomes which remain within the cytoplasm indefinitely (See discussion in Chapter 21). In the case of secretory proteins, on the other hand, the phosphorylated mannose residues are cleaved off in the ER or Golgi, leading to the formation of membrane-bounded secretory granules which do not remain within the cytoplasm but move to the cell surface and are secreted. In some instances, however, lysosomes may be secreted. Thus, transformed platelets plugging a tear in a blood vessel secrete lysosomes (lambda granules) and lysosome-related vesicles (alpha granules), which intensify blood coagulation. Osteoclasts lying on bone that is undergoing lysis seal off an area by sheetlike cytoplasmic processes whose edges attach to the bone. They then secrete their bone-dissolving lysosomal enzymes into this sealed pouch and thereby remove bone with great precision. A number of lysosome-associated diseases have been identified. The lysosomal membrane in leukocytes in Chediak-Higashi disease is abnormally resistant to fusion with phagosomes. Phagocytized bacteria are therefore not exposed to the lysosome's lytic enzymes; the cell's capacity to destroy bacteria is impaired, and affected individuals die of infection. More than 20 *storage diseases* due to deficient activity of lysosomal enzymes have been identified. In *Hurler's syndrome* connective tissue matrix accumulates because lysosomes fail to degrade acid mucopolysaccharides. The enlarged spleen (splenomegaly) and other pathology of *Gaucher's disease* seem to be due to a defect in lysosomal β-glucosidase. In glycogen-storage disease type II, α-glycosidase is absent from lysosomes so that hepatocytes (and the whole liver) become enlarged by stored glycogen-filled vesicles that cannot be metabolized. A contrasting group of lysosomal diseases is due to intracellular breakup of lysosomes. In gout, as a result of genetically induced high levels of uric acid in the body fluids, urate crystals form in the synovial cavities and other connective tissue spaces. Leukocytes engulf these crystals. As the crystals become incorporated into secondary lysosomes they disrupt the lysosomes, loosing the hydrolytic enzymes. The leukocytes are destroyed and the enzymes, released to the tissue, induce inflammation characteristic of gouty arthritis. This sequence may occur in asbestos intoxication, in experimentally induced methylcellulose disease, and in other instances in which lysosomes are confronted with irritating materials that they are unable to degrade.

Peroxisomes, or *microbodies of Rouiller* are involved in H_2O_2 metabolism. They are membrane-bounded organelles, somewhat larger than primary lysosomes (Fig. 1–48) and may be continuous with tubules of smooth ER. Peroxisomes are relatively numerous in hepatocytes (Chap. 20), in renal tubular cells (Chap. 24), and in macrophages. They contain flavin enzymes, such as *urate oxidase* and D-*amino acid oxidase*, which produce H_2O_2 by using molecular oxygen as an oxidizing agent. Peroxisomes have a variegated granular internum and, in the hepatocyte and some other cell types, contain a crystalline component that represents urate oxidase. However, H_2O_2, although necessary in a number of cellular reactions and capable of killing microorganisms, is tolerated in only low concentration by cells. In a sequential action to their generation of H_2O_2, peroxisomes, because they contain the enzyme *catalase*, convert H_2O_2 to water. Peroxisomes are also associated with α-keto acid formation and thereby participate in forming glucose from lipids and other noncarbohydrate precursors, a process termed *gluconeogenesis*.

Multivesicular bodies (MVB) are membrane-bounded vesicles 0.5 to 1.0 μm in diameter that contain a number of small vesicles with a diameter of 50 to 75 nm. They may be found in most

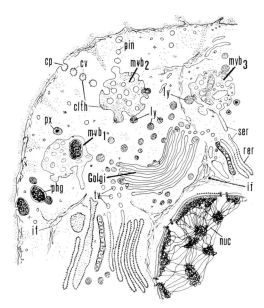

1–54 Multivesicular bodies **(mvb)** are prominent in this drawing. **mvb₁** contains a phagosome **(phg). mvb₂** receives smooth **(pin)** and coated **(cv)** pinocytotic vesicles, the latter originating as coated pits **(cp)**. Plaques of clathrin **(clth)** lie on the surface of mvb₂ and mvb₃. Lysosomes fuse with mvb. **mvb₃**, containing mitochondria and rough ER **(rer)**, is autophagocytic. It is continuous with smooth ER **(ser)**. The Golgi complex is engaged in lysosome production and receives material from the ER in transport vesicles **(tv)**. Vimentin, a class of intermediate filament **(if)** surrounds the nucleus **(nuc)** and radiates in the cytoplasm.

cell types and are more numerous in cells rich in lysosomes. The membranes bounding MVB are usually smooth, but patches of their surface may be coated (see discussion of coated vesicles above). The MVB bounding membrane itself may invaginate and form some of the smaller vesicular structures and, like peroxisomes, may be continuous with short segments of smooth ER. Multivesicular bodies appear to represent reaction vats, receiving the contents of the endocytic vesicles and lysosomes that fuse with them. As a result, MVB possess the functions of a large heterolysosome. They may also receive the contents of secretory granules by crinophagy. They incorporate peroxisomes, partaking of their functions. Indeed, peroxisomes and other cellular structures may be autophagocytized in MVB (Fig. 1–54).

Microfilaments and Intermediate (100 Å) Filaments. There are two major groups of fine fila-

ments in virtually every cell type. One group is approximately 50 Å in diameter (Fig. 1–55) and is made of *actin*. These filaments, called *microfilaments*, are contractile and are believed to underlie the locomotion of cells, the ruffling and invagination of cell membranes, contraction, and other aspects of contractility. They form the terminal web of epithelial cells and enter microvilli. They also form the contractile ring in dividing cells (Fig. 1–55). They are best developed in muscle cells (Chap. 7). A second group of fine intracellular filaments is stouter, approximately 90 to 120 Å in diameter. They represent a more diverse population of filaments than the microfilaments and are referred to as *intermediate filaments* or *100-Å filaments*. They possess mechanical functions in supporting or stiffening cells and in organizing intracellular organelles for coordinated activity.

Microfilaments are part of the actin–myosin system and become contractile by sliding over myosin filaments, as occurs in muscle cells. In nonmuscle cells actin, in the form of microfilaments, is visible by electron microscopy whereas myosin is not. Yet myosin is also present, as shown in a number of cell types by immunocytochemistry (Chap. 2). Thus, in the mitotic contractile ring in which actin microfilaments have been demonstrated by electron microscopy, the presence of myosin has been shown by fluorescence immunocytochemistry. It is likely that myosin is not visible in electron micrographs because it occurs in short segments representing oligomers, which aggregate into filaments only transiently or form filaments that our preparative methods fail to preserve. Furthermore, myosin is present in much lower concentration in most cells than actin. Its high concentration and layout in cells suggest that actin, in addition to its major contractile functions, has a cytoskeletal role. Actin can be detected by an excellent cytochemical test: its specific reaction with the S-1 subfraction of heavy meromyosin (HMM) (Fig. 1–55). The tissue is first extracted with glycerol to increase permeability and permit the penetrance of HMM. After irrigation with HMM, microfilaments become "decorated" with HMM, which gives them a characteristic fuzzy appearance resembling arrowheads. Actin may also be detected by more conventional immunocytochemical methods. Microfilaments are often concentrated at the surface of nonmuscle cells and, by high-resolution electron microscopy, appear to be attached to the cytoplasmic surface of the plasma membrane. Whether the microfilaments

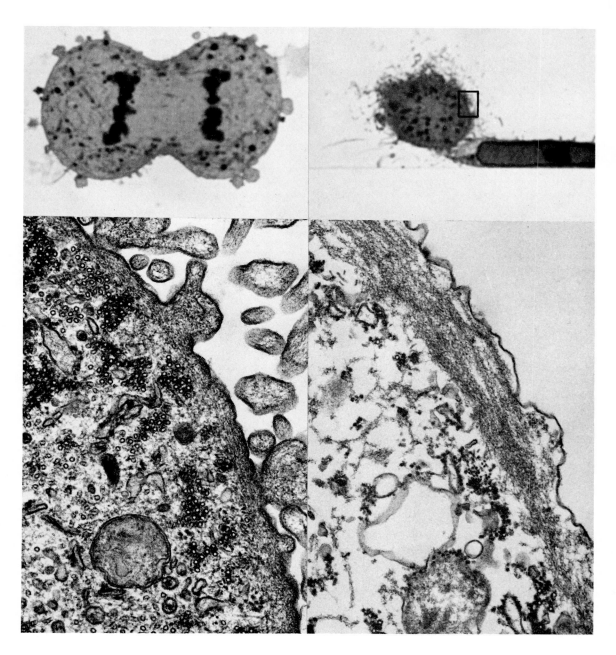

1–55 Cytoplasmic microfilaments in many cells are composed of actin. These micrographs illustrate this point for the contractile ring in dividing HeLa cells. The upper figures are light micrographs (× 2000) of 1 μm Epon sections of cells midway through cleavage: at the left parallel to the plane of the monolayer and at the right perpendicular to it at the level of the furrow constriction; hence the cell's circular profile. Electron micrographs below (× 50,000) illustrate portions of perpendicular sections, as indicated by the black rectangle. In standard preparations (lower left) the contractile ring appears as a layer of thin microfilament encircling the cell just beneath its membrane. After extraction in glycerol and irrigation with heavy meromyosin these same microfilaments appear "fuzzy" (lower right) in a way that is characteristic of actin filaments. Small circles in the electron micrographs are transverse profiles of microtubules of the mitotic apparatus. (From Shroeder, T. E. 1973. Proc. Natl. Acad. Sci. U.S.A. 20:1, 688.)

are directly linked to certain intrinsic proteins of the plasma membrane or connected through a set of anchoring proteins is not known. Microfilaments may be disaggregated and rendered functionless by the antibiotic *cytochalasin* B. (Refer to Chap. 7 for further discussion of actin and contractile filaments.)

Intermediate filaments may be divided into a number of classes, each with a distinctive cytoskeletal function. *Keratin filaments* occur in epithelial cells as *tonofilaments* and are particularly well developed in such stratified squamous epithelia as the epidermis (Chap. 17). They are tough filaments that serve to strengthen and stiffen cells, particularly at intercellular junctions, where they are closely associated with desmosomes (Chap. 3). When present in very high concentration, as in the keratinocytes of epidermis, keratin filaments laminate to form dense, strong, impermeable protective layers. Keratins are quite diverse, displaying somewhat different properties in different locations, as, for example, in the skin, snout, hoof, and feather. *Desmin filaments* hold myofibrils in place in muscle cells. In striated muscle they have distinctive locations on the myofibrils (Z, N, and M lines), and connect them to plasma membrane, mitochondria, and other elements of the cell. Desmin filaments are particularly abundant in smooth muscle cells, forming networks linking plaques of microfilaments to the cell surface. By these links desmin mechanically organizes muscle cells and coordinates the whole process of contraction. The protein *vimentin* forms intermediate filaments that enmesh the nucleus, in some cases forming a nuclear cap. They appear to control the location of the nucleus. Vimentin probably plays a role in such nuclear activities as mitosis and in maintaining nuclear–cytoplasmic passageways. *Neurofilaments* and *glial filaments* are, with microtubules, major structural elements in nervous tissue. These intermediate filaments are present in patterns and quantities distinctive to a given neural cell type. Their roles include maintaining the extraordinary asymmetry and cytoplasmic processes characteristic of neural cells (see Chap. 8). Spectrin is a tetramer found in erythrocytes where, as an intermediate filament, it forms a subplasmalemmal lattice anchored into the plasma membrane. As discussed in Chap. 11, spectrin protects the erythrocytic plasma membrane from shearing forces of flow, it stabilizes the intrinsic proteins of the cell membrane that penetrate its subplasmalemmal lattice, and it maintains the shape of the erythrocyte. Portions of the spectrin molecule occur as components of intermediate filaments in other cell types, such as macrophages and sea urchin epithelium, but the complete spectrin molecule appears restricted to erythrocytes. Spectrin, like other intermediate filaments, is conserved in evolution, being present in the red blood cells of many species with little variance in amino acids.

Microtubules. Microtubules are major structures in prokaryotic and eukaryotic cells. They function as a cytoskeleton and permit the asymmetry in shape necessary for cellular movement and differentiation. For example, the development of axons appears to depend on alignment of microtubules in the axonal processes. Dispersal of the microtubules prevents formation. Microtubules are important in intracellular transport. Particles and organelles such as mitochondria move along microtubules. The motility of cilia seems to depend on microtubules sliding upon one another.

Microtubules appear as hollow, nonbranching cylinders 210 to 240 Å in diameter and many micrometers long (Figs. 1–56 and 1–57; see also succeeding figures on centrioles and mitosis). Their dense wall is made of globular subunits 40 Å in diameter, arranged in helix with 13 subunits per turn. The center zone is lucent in most microtubules and is 160 Å in diameter. The major biochemical component of microtubules is the 110,000 dalton protein *heterodimer* tubulin, composed of α and β polypeptide subunits. Microtubules often appear in groups of 30 or 40 or more and may be connected by slender bridges.

Microtubules are the basis of such complex and well-defined structures as centrioles, cilia, and the achromatic mitotic apparatus. In addition, there are bands of microtubules in the axons of nerve cells (neurotubules), beneath the plasma membrane of many cylindrical or asymmetric cells, and within the endoplasm of such cells as macrophages. Microtubules may originate from a nucleating or initiating site in the cell. The centriole is a nucleating site for microtubular structures such as cilia and the achromatic apparatus. Most groups of microtubules are less stable than those in cilia and centrioles. They disappear with many fixatives, including osmium tetroxide, and on fixation in the cold. Microtubules are relatively easily dispersed by colchicine, vinblastine, or high hydrostatic pressure. When such dispersing factors are removed, the subunits quickly reassociate to reform microtubules.

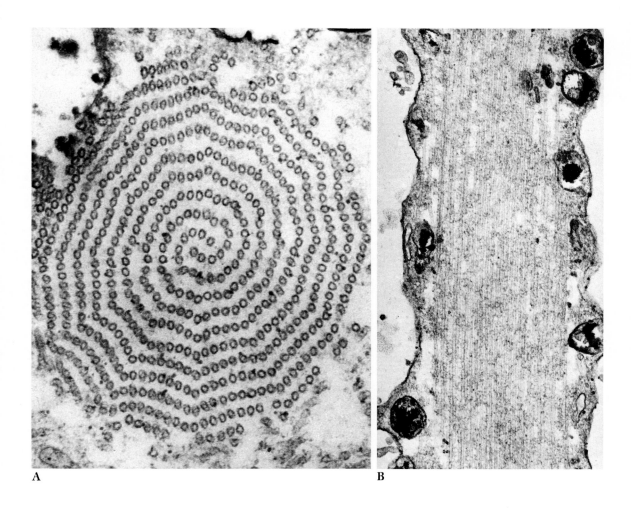

A   B

C

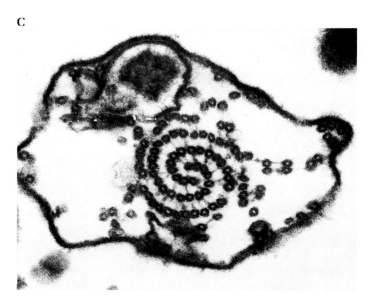

1–56 Microtubules in axoplasm of
Echinoshaerium. Much correlative
morphologic work in chemistry,
physiology, and morphology has been
done on invertebrates. **A.** Tranverse section
of an axoneme at the base of an
axopodium. There are 12 sections of
microtubules in cross section. × 70,000.
B. Longitudinal section of an axoneme.
Peripheral to the parallel array of
microtubules constituting the axoneme are
dense granules that undergo saltations.
× 40,000. **C.** Transverse section of an
axoneme heavily stained with MnO_4 to
emphasize the bridges that connect the
microtubules. × 110,000. (From Tilney,
L. G., and Porter, K. R. 1965. Protoplasma
60:317.

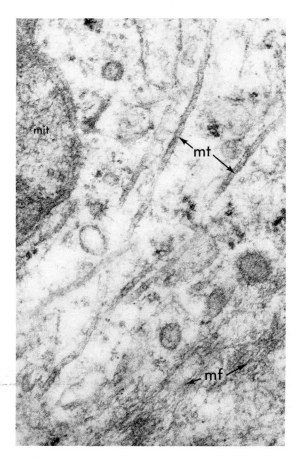

1–57 Microtubules of a human splenic reticular cell.
△   This field is from the peripheral cytoplasm and contains sections of microtubules **(mt)**, microfilaments **(mf)**, and a mitochondrion **(mit)**. × 90,000. (From Chen, L. T. and Weiss, L. 1972. Am. J. Anat. 134:425.)

Centrioles. Centrioles are cylinders, 0.25 to 2 μm in length and 0.1 to 0.2 μm in diameter, whose walls are composed primarily of microtubules. Centrioles lie in the cytocentrum and may be surrounded by microtubules radiating out into the cytoplasm. Diploid metazoan cells contain two centrioles. Multinucleate cells may contain centrioles: in osteoclasts and foreign-body giant cells, which may have 25 or more nuclei, the central regions of the cells are composed of fused cytocentra strewn with centrioles. Higher plants lack centrioles.

Centrioles function in mitosis, in the genesis of cilia, microtubules, mitochondria, and new centrioles. Unlike other cytoplasmic structures, centrioles are duplicated before mitosis.

By light microscopy, centrioles are minute rods, well stained with a number of dyes, of which iron hematoxylin is the most commonly used (Fig. 1–4).

By electron microscopy, the centriolar wall is made up of nine vanes or blades each consisting of three fused microtubules (Figs. 1–58 to 1–60). The nine blades are set next to one another, their long axes parallel; the edge of one is slightly shingled beneath the edge of its neighbor, curving around to form the cylinder that is the outer wall of the centriole. In cross section, this array resembles a pinwheel.

The fused microtubules making up each of the blades extend the length of the centriole and lie almost in a plane, with the result that the long

1–58 Centrioles of a Chinese hamster fibroblast. **A.**
▽   The centriole is cut in cross section (from an interphase cell). **B.** The centriole is cut in longitudinal section (from a metaphase cell). × 100,000. (From the work of B. R. Brinkley.)

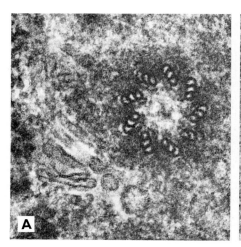

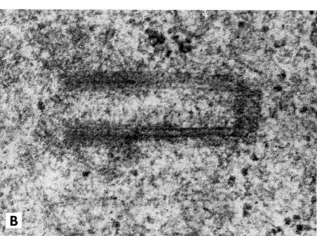

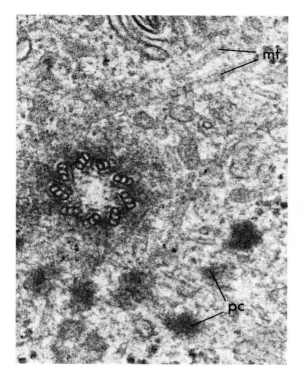

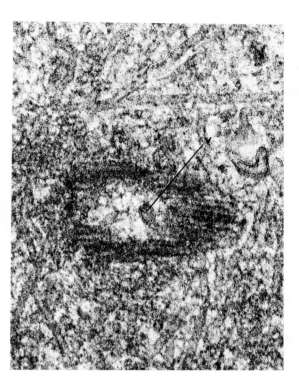

1–59 Centriole of a Chinese hamster fibroblast. The centriole is cut in cross section. Paracentriolar material **(pc)** is evident around the lower half of the centriole. Microtubules **(mt)** are also present, particularly in the upper half of the field. × 92,000. [From Brinkley, B. R., and Stubblefield, E., 1970. *In* D. M. Prescott, L. Goldstein, and E. McConkey (eds.), Advances in Cell Biology, vol. 1. New York: Appleton-Century-Crofts.]

1–60 Centriole of a melanoma cell. The centriole is cut in oblique section. It contains a small vesicle **(v).** The field surrounding the vesicle abounds in microtubules. × 120,000. (From the work of G. G. Maul.)

blades they form are slightly curved from side to side. In addition, each of the blades is subject to a slight twist about its long axis.

The principal structure within the lumen of the centriole is a 75-Å filament wound into a helix that curves against the inside surface of the wall, apparently held in place by small spurs. The lumen of the centriole may also contain a large clear vesicle. An end of the centriolar cylinder may show spokes radiating out from the wall.

Satellites are amorphous masses about 750 Å in diameter that lie close to the surface of centrioles, near an end; they may be aggregates of microtubular subunits.

A new centriole is assembled at an end of each extant centriole a few hours before DNA replication. It is oriented at right angles to the parent centriole and requires several hours to

form. A mature centriole is preceded by a *procentriole,* a cylinder 150 nm in diameter with nine single microtubules in its wall. These singlets develop into the triplets of the centriole. The procentrioles are themselves preceded by small, dense procentriolar precursor bodies, which are apparently transformed into procentrioles by the stimulation of "procentriole organizers," dense amorphous surrounding masses.

Centrioles induce microtubule formation. In mitosis they separate, move to opposite poles, and become foci for the development of the achromatic mitotic apparatus. Centrioles move beneath the cell surface and, as basal bodies, initiate the formation of cilia. Flagella are similarly related to centrioles. Basal bodies are structurally different from centrioles, primarily in possessing a basal plate that closes the end directed toward the cell membrane. The other end, directed toward the nucleus, is open and may display spokes. In spermatocytes one centriole may be associated with both the mitotic apparatus and the flagellum. Microtubular formations other

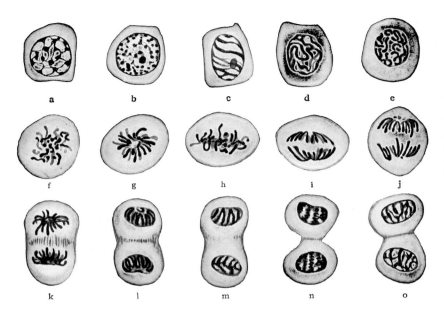

1–61 Mitosis. Epidermal cells of a mouse. These drawings are arranged in sequence from early prophase into telophase. **a** to **f**, prophase; **g** and **h**, metaphase; **i**, anaphase; **k** to **o**, telophase. Bouin fixation: iron–hematoxylin. (From the work of Ortiz-Picon.)

than those of the mitotic apparatus, cilia, and flagella may extend into the cytocentrum in characteristic alignment with centrioles.

Cell Division

The division of one cell into two is the basis of the continuity of life and underlies the complexity of metazoan organisms. The life of an individual protozoan is limited, but by cell division the line of Protozoa goes on. In Metazoa, division provides the cells that constitute these organisms and the replacement of lost cells, underlies the phenomena of cellular differentiation and specialization, and permits the continuity of the species despite the death of individuals. Several types of cell division exist. We shall consider *mitosis*, *amitosis*, and *meiosis*. Cell division may be separated into two events: *karyokinesis*, or nuclear division, and *cytokinesis*, or cytoplasmic division. As indicated above, karyokinesis may occur without cytokinesis, resulting in binucleate or multinucleate cells.

Mitosis. DNA is capable of precise replication, ensuring constancy of genetic information from generation to generation and, thereby, maintenance of the characteristics of the species. Mitosis is a complex, highly ordered process wherein the original and replicated molecules of DNA are separated from one another and distributed to two nuclei. Cytokinesis typically follows karyokinesis and two cells result. The DNA with

associated protein is organized as chromosomes, whose number is highly characteristic for a species. These chromosomes are typically matched in pairs or homologs.

The human nucleus contains 46 chromosomes, paired as 23 homologs. The partners in 22 of these pairs, the *autosomes*, are morphologically alike. The remaining two chromosomes are sex chromosomes. In the female they are matched and alike; they are the X chromosomes. In the male, however, these two chromosomes are morphologically different from one another; they are the X and Y chromosomes. Chromosomes in the interphase nucleus are so long and thin that it is not possible to recognize 46 of them.

The first phase of mitosis is *prophase* (Figs. 1–61, 1–62, 1–65, and 1–66). During prophase the extended chromosomes characteristic of the interphase become progressively thicker and

1–62 Mitosis. Human leukocytes. Only the chromosomes are stained. Each chromosome is seen to consist of two chromatids joined at the kinetochore. Note the secondary constrictions in several of the chromosomes and the presence of satellites **(arrows)**. Note, too, the coiling evident in several of the chromatids. In anaphase, two chromosomes lie near the equatorial plane, lagging behind the others in joining the two diverging masses of chromosomes. This happens frequently. Note the sharp separation furrow in telophase. Aceto-orcein stain. × 4,000. (From the work of B. Reuben Migeon.)

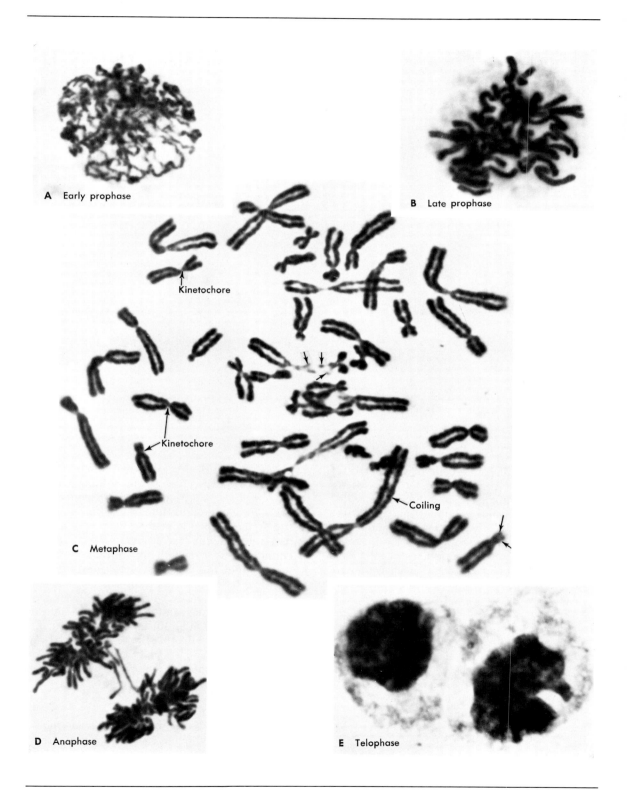

A Early prophase

B Late prophase

C Metaphase

Kinetochore

Kinetochore

Coiling

D Anaphase

E Telophase

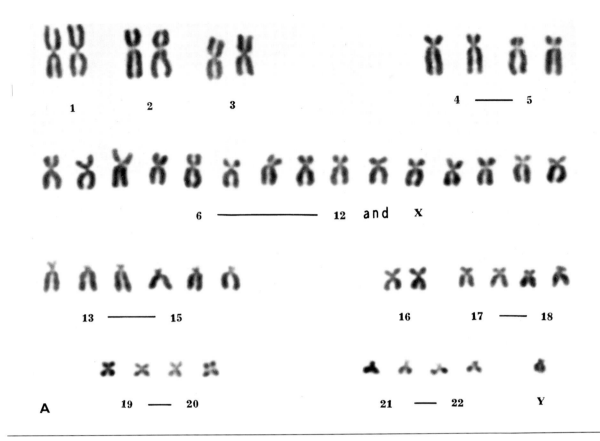

1   2   3   4 ——— 5

6 ——————— 12 and X

13 ——— 15   16   17 ——— 18

A   19 ——— 20   21 ——— 22   Y

---

more tightly coiled. The coils may undergo secondary coiling. As perceived by light microscopy, the individual chromosomes emerge from the nuclear substance as strands that appear progressively shorter, thicker, and more intensely stained. Moreover, as prophase goes on, one can see that each of the chromosomes is split longitudinally into precisely equal halves, or *chromatids*. This longitudinal splitting of the chromosome actually occurs in the S and G_2 phases just preceding mitosis but becomes apparent only in late prophase.[1] Through most of prophase the individually emerging chromosomes remain confined within the nuclear envelope and are too bunched together to be clearly characterized as to size and shape. Near the end of prophase, when the chromosomes are maximally contracted, the nuclear membrane disappears.

The centrioles diverge from one another and move to opposite poles of the cell. From the polar centrioles, radiating toward the center of the cell, into and around the mass of chromosomes, is a system of poorly stained fibers, the *spindle*. Some of them, the discontinuous fibers, attach to chromosomes. Others, the continuous fibers, pass around the chromosomes, going from one centriole to the other. In addition, a set of fibers radiates around each centriole, forming an *aster*. The fibers of the spindle and of the asters are preponderantly microtubules. They are called the *achromatic apparatus* because they lack affinity for dyes and are thus distinguished from the deeply stained ensemble of chromosomes, termed the *chromatic apparatus* (Figs. 1–61 to 1–69).

In the next phase of mitosis, *metaphase*, the chromosomes arrange themselves in an equatorial plane, forming an *equatorial plate* (Figs. 1–61, 1–62, and 1–67 to 1–69). Viewed from the side, this plate appears as a somewhat irregular,

---

[1]The centrioles duplicate in late G or early S and remain close together until prophase. See discussion of cell cycle, page 82.

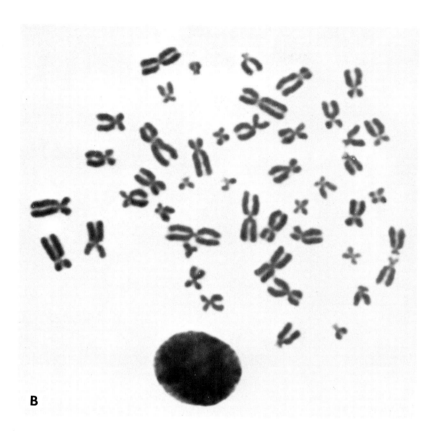

B

1–63 **A.** Human karyotype. Metaphase chromosomes have been arranged into morphologically similar groups of paired chromosomes and numbered. Pairs 1, 2, 3, and 16 can be identified as different from other chromosomes. It is impossible to separate 4 from 5, but 4 and 5 may be separated from the remainder. Similarly it is impossible to separate 6, 7, 8, 9, 10, 11, 12, and the X chromosome as different from one another, but this large group may be recognized as different from the other chromosomes. Chromosomes 13, 14, and 15, 17 and 18; 19 and 20 form similar groups. This individual is male, having an X and Y chromosome. **B.** The metaphase from which the karyotype was prepared. An interphase nucleus is present for comparison of size. Aceto-orcein stain. × 2,400. (From the work of B. Reuben Migeon.)

dense line transecting the cell. Viewed from one of the poles, the chromosomes form a circlet. Metaphase chromosomes are linear, densely stained structures. Each chromosome is constricted at one place along its length, an unstained zone called the *centromere* or *kinetochore*. The two chromatids of the chromosomes are free of one another except at the centromere, and the spindle fibers also attach there. Chromosomes may be divided into three groups, depending on the location of the centromere. If the centromere divides a chromosome into segments of equal length, the chromosome is *metacentric*. Those chromosomes separated into larger and smaller limbs by the centromere are *submedian*. Chromosomes in which the centromere is almost at the end, so that there is virtually only one limb, are *telocentric*.

The chromatic material of the chromosome may have another *secondary constriction* in one of the limbs. This constriction may have some length, and so it isolates the chromatic material

at the end of the chromosome into a *satellite*. Typically, nucleoli develop in certain zones of constriction in satellited chromosomes on reconstitution of daughter nuclei.

Metaphase chromosomes of each species may be classified on the basis of the location of the centromere, the size and shape of the limbs, and the presence of secondary constrictions and satellites. These characteristics make up the *karyotype*, or the morphology of the metaphase chromosomes. The karyotype of the human male is presented in Fig. 1–63A. The metaphase plate from which the karyotype was prepared is shown in Fig. 1–63B. The karyotype is prepared by cutting out the chromosome pairs from a photograph of a squash preparation of a metaphase cell selectively stained with a dye such as aceto-orcein. The cut-out chromosomes are then arranged in clusters of similar chromosomes. It is not possible to differentiate chromosomes occurring within a cluster by the standard aceto-orcein procedure. Thus, in the human male karyotype

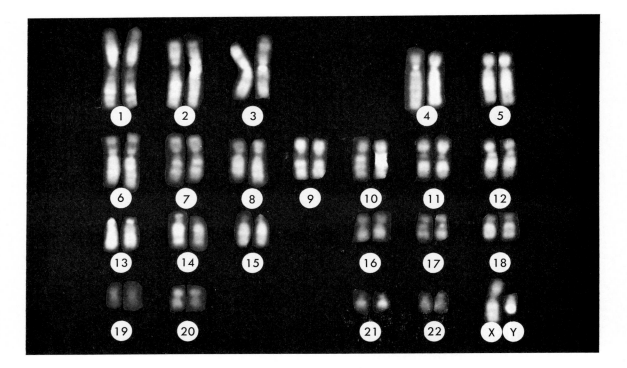

1–64 Karyotype of normal male (XY) cultured human leukocyte, showing quinacrine fluorescence patterns. Note the bandings present in each of the chromosomes. Although the significance of this banding is not understood, it has proved useful in differentiating chromosomes that are morphologically alike. Compare with the conventional karyotype in Fig. 1–63A and B. × 2,500. (From the work of W. R. Breg.) It has proved possible to obtain a similar banding pattern by staining a chromosomal preparation with a giemsa stain at a pH of about 6.8. The latter is a relatively easy procedure and may become more widely used than fluorescence staining.

one cannot separate chromosomes 6, 7, 8, 9, 10, 11, 12, and the X chromosome from one another. Certain fluorochromes produce a banded staining pattern in each of the chromosomes (Fig. 1–64). The banding pattern can also be shown in a more stable preparation by staining a squash preparation of a metaphase cell with dilute giemsa stain at pH 6.8. By this means it has proved possible to identify chromosomes not differentiable otherwise. Correlations of genetic diseases such as Down's syndrome (mongolism) and leukemia with abnormal karyotypes are being made in increasing number.

At the beginning of metaphase, the chroma-

tids of a chromosome are connected only at the centromere. At the end of metaphase the centromeres divide and each of the chromatids, now a daughter chromosome and attached to the spindle by its own centromere, moves outward from the metaphase plate toward one pole of the cell. Thus, in human somatic cells, one set of 46 chromosomes moves to one centriole and the other set to the other. This divergent movement constitutes the *anaphase* of mitosis (Figs. 1–61, 1–62, and 1–65C). The spindle fibers attached to the centromeres are responsible for the characteristic orderly diverging movement of the chromosomes in anaphase. The drug colchicine interferes with the spindle by breaking up microtubules, leaving dividing cells suspended in metaphase and unable to complete the cell division.

Anaphase is concluded when the two chromosomal masses have moved to opposite poles of the cell. There now begins the final stage of nuclear division, *telophase* (Figs. 1–61, 1–62, and 1–65), during which two daughter nuclei are formed. Nuclear membranes form around each of the chromosomal masses, nucleoli appear at the satellite-bearing chromosomes, and segments of the chromosomes uncoil to become euchromatin.

Although primary attention must be accorded

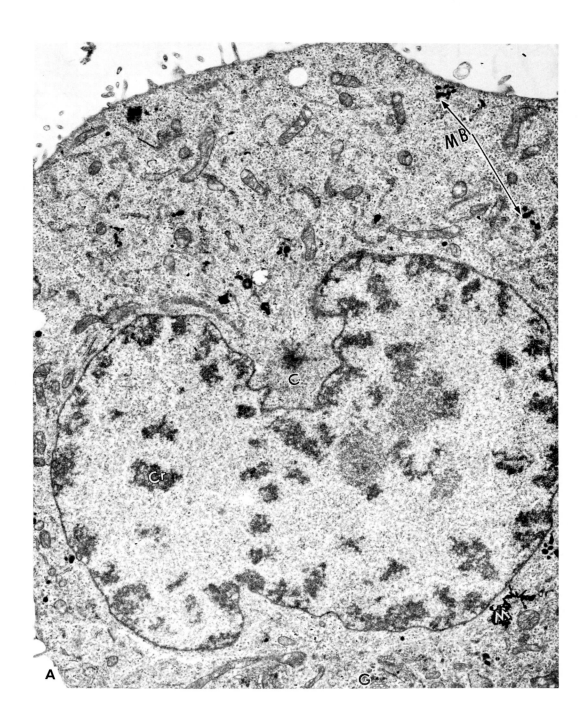

1–65 **A–D** Electron micrograph of mitosis in a human HeLa cell in tissue culture. These cells, originally derived from a carcinoma of the uterine cervix, form a strain of cells maintained in tissue culture. **A.** In early prophase, the chromatin becomes clumped because of the condensation of chromosomes **(Cr).** The nuclear membrane is still intact, and the centriole **(C)** and multivesicular bodies **(MB)** are prominent. Approximately × 3,850. (From Robbins, E., and Gonatas, N. K. 1964. J. Cell Biol. 21:429.)

(continued)

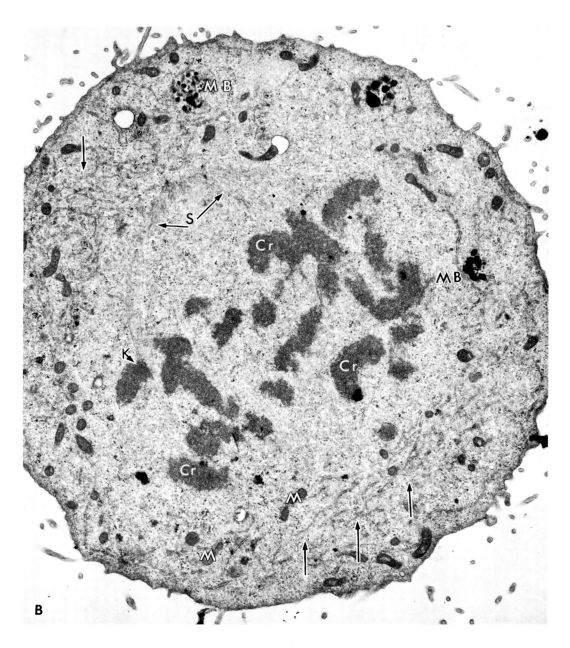

Figure 1–65 B △ and C ▷

B. In later prophase the chromosomes are close to the equatorial plate and metaphase. The spindle fibers **(S)** are seen radiating from the centriole and attached to a chromosome at the kinetochore **(K).** Approximately × 5,640. (From Robbins, E., and Gonatas, N. K. 1964. J. Cell Biol. 21:429.)

C. In late anaphase, the two chromosomal masses have moved apart. They are already surrounded by a double nuclear membrane. At the lower pole, a portion of a centriole and spindle fibers may be seen. Note how the spindle fibers are present, together with some mitochondria, in the constriction between what will be the two daughter cells. Note, too, the blebs of cytoplasm **(BL)** about the periphery of the se cells, indicating the frothing that occurs in this phase. Approximately × 5,225. (From Robbins, E., and Gonatas, N. K. 1964. J. Cell Biol. 21:429.)

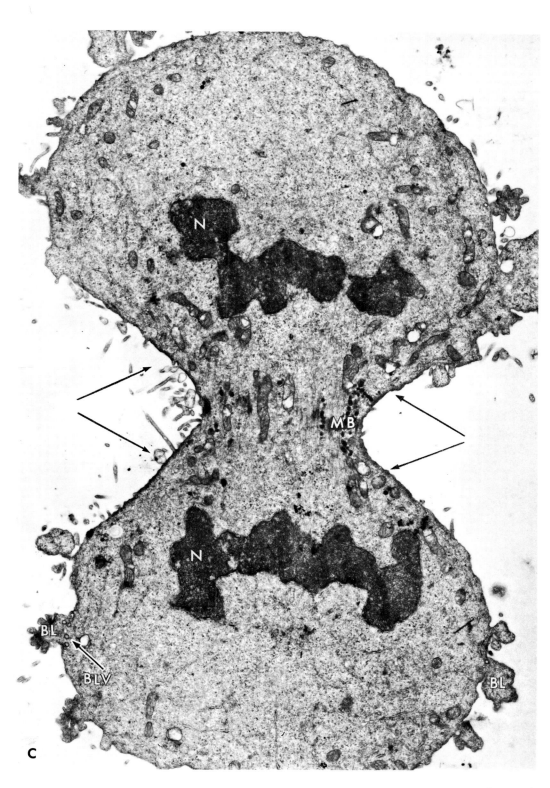

(continued)

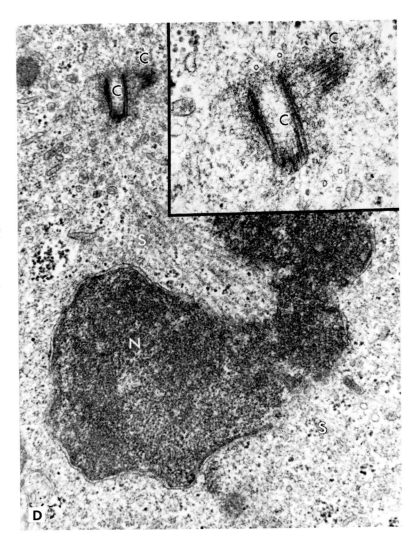

Figure 1–65D
D. Telophase. Note the presence of a double nuclear membrane about a daughter nucleus. The centriole (at higher magnification in the inset) has already been duplicated. Approximately × 13,750 (inset × 30,800). (From Robbins, E., and Gonatas, N. K. 1964. J. Cell Biol. 21:429.)

the nucleus in mitosis, characteristic changes occur in the cytoplasm. The division of the centrioles and the formation of the achromatic apparatus in prophase have already been discussed. Frothing or bubbling of the cytoplasm occurs in anaphase. During this bubbling phase, the cell surfaces are covered with microvilli. Indeed, microvilli occur throughout mitosis, being most prominent in anaphase. They also occur during G, but are usually absent or scanty in the rest of the cell cycle (Fig. 1–70). With the separation of the nuclear masses in anaphase, a partition of cytoplasmic constituents occurs. Mitochondria, lysosomes, ribosomes, and cytoplasmic membranes become distributed in

approximately equal amounts about the two newly formed nuclei. As the nuclear membrane is reconstructed, the cytoplasm becomes deeply constricted in a *constriction ring* (Figs. 1–55 and 1–65C) between the two masses of chromosomes. The cytoplasm divides, forming two equal daughter cells. For a short time, the spindle may persist as a transient bridge between daughter cells.

Amitosis. Amitosis may occur in terminal or highly transient cell types such as certain cells of the placenta or of the blood. It may also occur in some multinucleated cells, as the giant cells of the connective tissue. In amitosis the nuclear

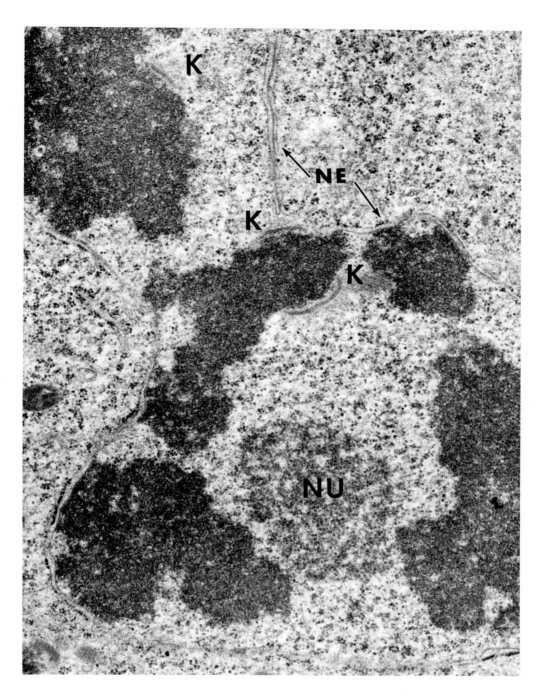

membrane appears to constrict deeply and a single nucleus becomes pinched into two. Although equal-sized daughter nuclei may sometimes result, it is impossible that a precise separation of chromosomal material can be achieved (Fig. 1–71).

1–66 Later prophase. Chinese hamster fibroblast.
Fully formed kinetochores **(K)** and a nucleus **(NU)** are present. The nuclear envelope **(NE)** is almost completely intact. [From Brinkley, B. R., and Stubblefield, E. 1970. *In* D. M. Prescott, L. Goldstein, and E. McConkey (eds.)]

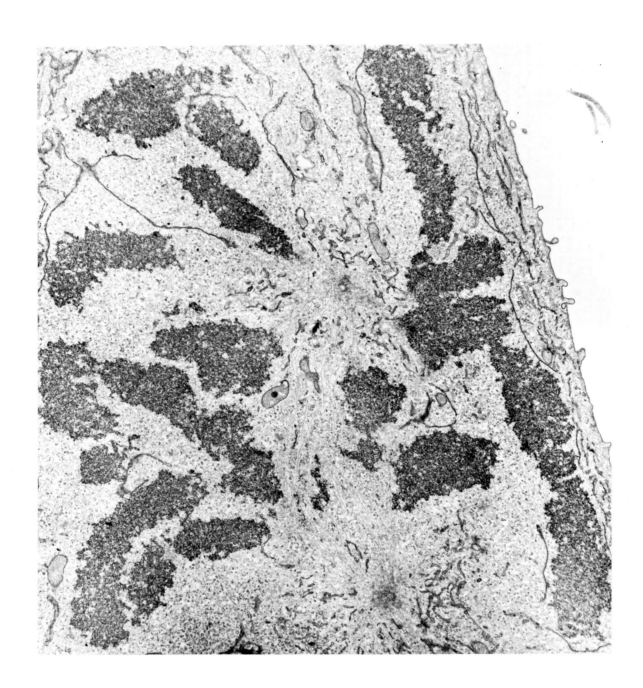

1–67 Prometaphase, rat kangaroo fibroblast. Here each of the chromosomes is tightly coiled and, although not evident, split into two chromatids. The chromosomes are moving to take positions on the metaphase plate. A centriole and microtubules are present in the cytoplasm. × 14,000. (From the work of B. R. Brinkley.)

Polyteny and Poliploidy. DNA replication may occur without nuclear division. It is characteristic of certain cell types, such as the salivary gland cells of diptera, that DNA replication occurs without subsequent chromosomal division, resulting in *polytene* chromosomes. These chromosomes replicate themselves many times over. However, the replicates remain together

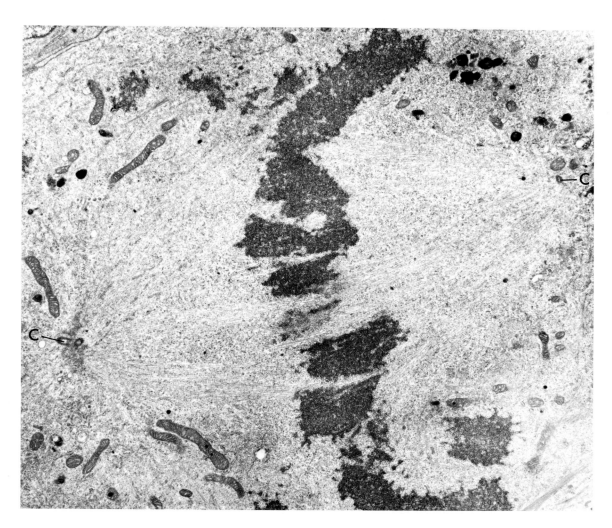

rather than move apart into separate chromosomes and thereby form giant chromosomes. Polytenic chromosomes readily show a type of banding that requires fluorochromes or special giemsa staining (Fig. 1–64) to demonstrate in other chromosomes.

DNA replication may occur with subsequent chromosomal duplication but without loss of nuclear membranes or karyokinesis, resulting in polyploid nuclei. The process has been termed *endomitosis*. Polyploid nuclei thus contain multiples of the diploid number of chromosomes. They are typically larger than diploid nuclei, as in some hepatocytes and megakaryocytes.

Meiosis. Meiosis is a type of nuclear division, restricted to gametes (i.e., spermatocytes and

1–68 Metaphase, rat kangaroo fibroblast. The metaphase plate is present in edge-on view. On the left, two centrioles **(C)** may be observed; on the right, one centriole. The microtubules of the spindle radiate from the centrioles. Both chromosomal (attached to kinetochore) and continuous (pole to pole) microtubules are present. × 10,350. (From Brinkley, B. R., and Cartwright, J., Jr. 1971. J. Cell Biol. 50:416.)

oocytes) wherein the number of chromosomes characteristic of somatic cells, the *diploid* number (2n), is halved to the *haploid* number (1n). This halving occurs because the homologs in each chromosome pair separate from one another. Each daughter nucleus in meiosis contains a set of homologs. For this reason, meiosis is called *reduction division*. The haploid nuclei of

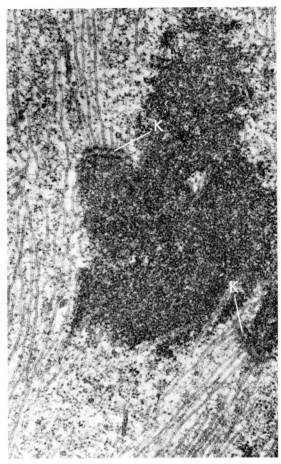

1–69 Metaphase, rat kangaroo fibroblast.
Chromosomal microtubules are inserted into kinetochores **(K).** Note the double nature of the kinetochore. Continuous microtubules pass between the chromosomes running from pole to pole without insertion into kinetochores. × 30,800. (From Brinkley, B. R., and Cartwright, J., Jr. 1971. J. Cell Biol. 50:416.)

the gametes unite and the diploid number of chromosomes is restored in the process of fertilization. The fertilized ovum and all its somatic descendants divide by mitotic division, and the diploid number is thereby maintained in somatic cells. But meiosis has the second major function of providing genetic variation by the exchange of segments between homologous chromosomes and the random selection of one of the two homologs during the reduction division into a given daughter nucleus.

Meiosis involves two successive nuclear divisions with only one division of chromosomes (Figs. 1–72 and 1–73). The first meiotic division is characterized by a prolonged prophase. In this prophase the homologous chromosomes come to lie together, closely and exactly paired in a point-for-point correspondence along their entire length *(synapsis)*. During the process the chromosomes shorten by coiling, but not as much as in the prophase of mitosis. Moreover, each of the chromosomes is observed to be longitudinally split into two chromatids. The homologous paired chromosomes, termed a *bivalent,* therefore consist of four chromatids. A spindle forms and the bivalents arrange themselves on a metaphase plate. The divergent movement of anaphase begins as the homologs, consisting of two chromatids each, move apart to opposite poles and are then separated into daughter cells at telophase. Thenceforth, after the first meiotic division, each of the daughter cells contains one of the homologous chromosomes split into two chromatids. It is of great significance that in the first meiotic division the kinetochore does not divide, as it does in mitosis, and so the chromatids remain together. A second meiotic division ensues in which the chromosomes become arranged in a metaphase plate and the kinetochores divide. The chromatids that make up each of the chromosomes are now free of one another and diverge from the metaphase plate in an anaphase movement. Later in telophase they are grouped into daughter nuclei and then daughter cells. The two meiotic divisions have thus sorted the four homologous chromatids present in prophase of the first meiotic division into four separate gametes, each of which has the haploid number of chromosomes. In a male, four functional spermatozoa will result from the two meiotic divisions. Curiously, the completion of cytokinesis in the spermatozoa is delayed so that four otherwise mature spermatozoa may remain linked in Siamese-quadruplet style. In a female four ova are produced as well, but the cytoplasmic division leaves virtually all the cytoplasm with one nucleus. The remaining nuclei, surrounded by minimal cytoplasm, cannot survive. They are called *polar bodies.* This unequal cytoplasmic division provides one nucleus with sufficient cytoplasm to support fertilization and embryogenesis. Each of the gamete nuclei contains 23 chromosomes. In female gametes one of these is an X chromosome, whereas in male ga-

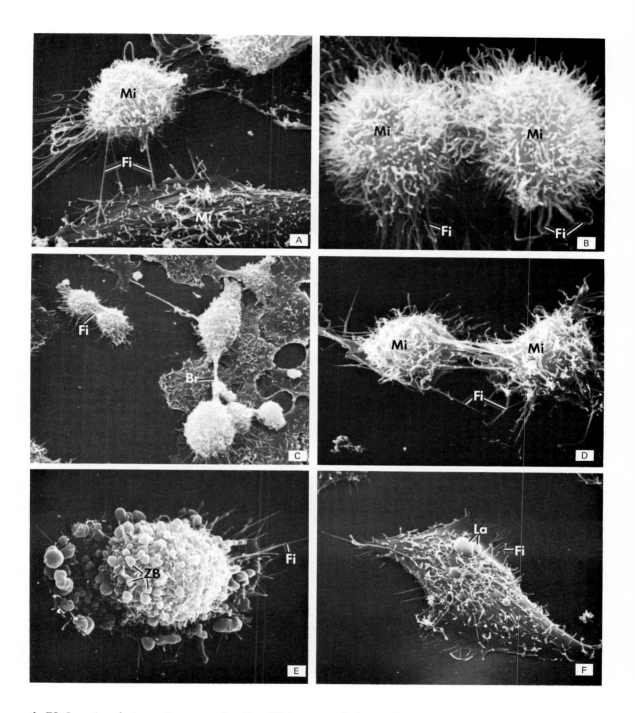

1–70 Scanning electron microscopy of cultured HeLa **(A, C, and F)** and KB cells **(B, D, and E)** in mitosis. Late stages in cell division are illustrated in B to D; interphase cells are illustrated in C, E, and F. Note the long bridge **(Br)** connecting the daughter cells in C. Other surface specializations identified are microvilli **(Mi),** filopodia **(Fi),** lamellapodia **(La),** and blebs **(ZB).** A, × 1,664; B, × 3,600; C, × 684; D, × 2,040; E, × 1,889; F, × 1,680. (From Beams, H. W., and Kessel, R. G. 1976. Am. Sci. 64:279.)

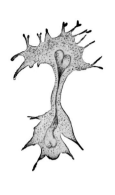
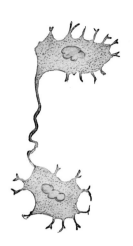
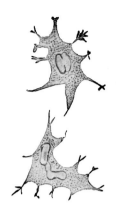

1–71 Amitosis in a histiocyte of a frog. The drawing is prepared from a cell in tissue culture. (From the work of Arnold.)

metes one is either an X or a Y. During fetal life in a human female, oocytes migrate into the ovary, proliferate by mitosis a short time, and then undergo meiosis, entering the prophase of the first meiotic division. They remain in that state until shortly before ovulation. Because a woman may ovulate until about 45 years of age, oocytes may remain in meiosis for more than 45 years. It may well be that the first meiotic prophase constitutes a particularly stable state for DNA.

Another essential function of meiosis is to provide genetic variation. It will be recalled that in diploid cells one chromosome in a homologous pair is contributed by the spermatozoon and the other by the oocyte. When the homologous chromosomes are arranged on the first meiotic metaphase plate, it is a matter of chance whether the homolog contributed by the sperm or the homolog contributed by the ovum faces a given pole. As a result, in each cell produced in the first meiotic division, the proportion of chromosomes derived from the sperm and that from

the egg are a matter of chance. This chance separation is one mechanism of genetic mixture. A second mechanism is the exchange, by homologous chromosomes, of corresponding segments. This exchange occurs when the homologs are in synapsis during the early phases of meiotic prophase I (Fig. 1–73). The extent of the exchange becomes apparent as the homologs pull away from their synaptic union. It is then seen that they frequently remain attached in one or more places. This persistent link between diverging chromosomes is termed a *chiasma*. The exchange of segments is termed *crossing over*.

The stages in meiosis are as follows (Fig. 1–72):

1. The first prophase, prophase I, is long and may be divided into five stages. In *leptotene* the chromosomes are long and thin. In *zygotene* the homologous chromosomes move toward one another and pair, lying in close touch in a point-for-point correspondence along their length (synapsis). In *pachytene* the

1–72 The stages of meiosis I and II shown schematically. A pair of homologous chromosomes, one dark and the other light, is followed through meiosis I. Then chromatids of a daughter cell are traced through meiosis II. The events are as follows:

Prophase I. Leptotene: The chromosomes become apparent as thin linear structures. Zygotene: Homologous chromosomes line up and pair with one another point to point (synapsis). Pachytene: With pairing completed, the chromosomes become shorter and thicker and each longitudinally splits into chromatids, the centromere remaining single. The four

chromatids of the two chromosomes constitute a bivalent. Chromatids from each of the homologous chromosomes may cross over one another forming a chiasma. Diplotene: The chromosomes further shorten and broaden; they also coil. Homologous chromosomes begin to move apart but are held together at the chiasma. Diakinesis: The chromosomes become broader, thicker, more tightly coiled; they move further apart.

- Metaphase I. The chromosomes are on the equatorial plate.
- Anaphase I. The chromosomes diverge, exchanging chromosomal segments at the site of the chiasma.

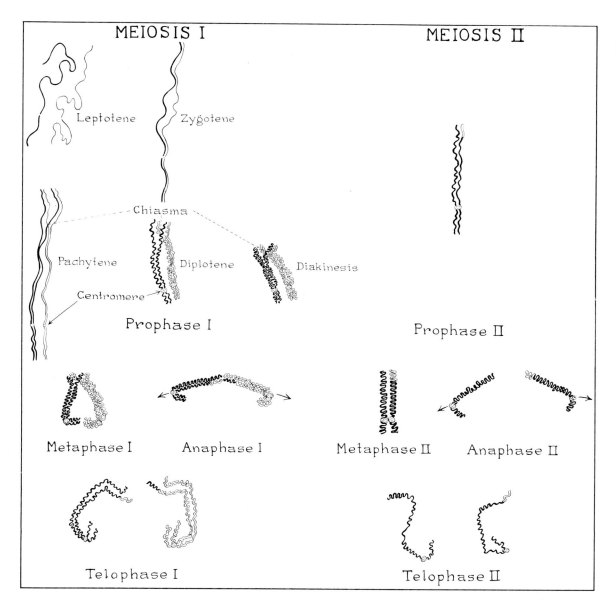

MEIOSIS I

Leptotene Zygotene

Chiasma

Pachytene Diplotene Diakinesis

Centromere

Prophase I

Metaphase I Anaphase I

Telophase I

MEIOSIS II

Prophase II

Metaphase II Anaphase II

Telophase II

- Telophase I. Each chromatid pair joined by a single centromere, lies in a daughter cell. The chromatids uncoil and lengthen to some extent.
- Chromatids in the left-hand daughter cell pass through the following stages in meiosis II.
- Prophase II. This stage is transient and possibly absent since the chromatids may move directly to metaphase II.
- Metaphase II. Chromatids become shorter, broader, and coiled. The centromere divides.
- Anaphase II. Chromatids separate and move to opposite poles.

- Telophase II. Each of the chromatids is now a daughter cell.

Thus in the course of these two divisions the four chromatids forming the bivalent of prophase I are separated, first into two daughter cells of telophase I, each containing two chromatids (4n → 2n), and then into two daughter cells again in telophase II, each containing one chromatid (2n → 1n). A total of four daughter cells is produced each having the haploid (1n) number of chromosomes. In a male individual four sperms are produced; in a female, one ovum and three polar bodies. On fertilization the diploid (2n) number is restored.

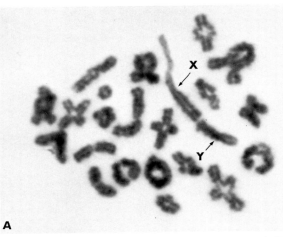

A

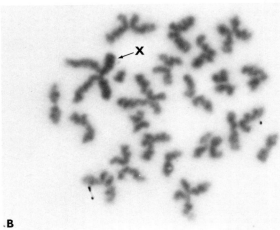

B

1–73 Meiosis in the golden hamster *Mesocricetus auratus*. **A.** Primary spermatocyte showing the 22 bivalents at the first meiotic metaphase. The X and Y chromosomes are associated terminally, the X being distinguished by its length. The autosomal bivalents demonstrate chiasmata in various stages. Note the coiling of the chromatids. **B.** Secondary spermatocyte at the second meiotic metaphase, containing the haploid number of 22 chromosomes. This cell has received the Y chromosome. At this stage, the chromosomes show "relic" spirals, which are probably remnants of coiling from the first meiotic division. Aceto-orcein stain. × 2,200. (From the work of M. Fergusen-Smith.)

chromosomes coil considerably, appearing shorter and thicker. At about this time it becomes apparent that each of the chromosomes of the bivalent contains four chromatids. The centromere does not split. In *diplotene* the chromosomes begin to separate from one an-

other, but the separation is incomplete, with chiasmata forming. The separation continues into the *diakinesis*, a stage that shows the chiasmata and the thickened, coiled, partially separated chromosomes to good advantage. The nuclear membrane disappears.

2. In metaphase I the bivalent chromosomes are arranged on an equatorial plate. There are two centromeres, one for each of the chromosomes, and the centromeres are attached to spindle fibers.
3. In anaphase I the chromosomes, each of which consists of two chromatids, move to opposite poles.
4. Telophase I follows, but the chromosomes may remain in a shortened form.

In the first meiotic division, therefore, the diploid number of chromosomes has been reduced to the haploid number; an exchange of genetic information may have occurred between the chromosomes; the distribution of chromosomes of a given bivalent to each pole has been a matter of chance, further increasing genetic variation; and each of the chromosomes is longitudinally split to form two chromatids.

5. Interphase, or *interkinesis,* is brief.
6. In prophase II a spindle forms, the nuclear membrane breaks down, and the chromosomes move equatorially.
7. In metaphase II the chromatids are arranged on an equatorial plate and their centromeres divide and become attached to spindle fibers.
8. In anaphase II the chromatids, now daughter chromosomes, move to opposite poles.
9. Telophase II is marked by the appearance of a nuclear membrane uncoiling of the chromosomes, and the development of daughter cells.

The Life Cycle of Cells

Two major types of cell may be recognized: *somatic cells,* which are the diverse cells making up the somatic structure of the body, fated to die with or before the individual they constitute; and *germ cells,* which are the gametes capable of uniting sexually with those of another individual to form a new individual.

A somatic cell begins its life span as one of the daughter cells of a mitotic division. Directly after this division the cell may undergo a period of intense protein synthesis, resulting in the emergence of the granules, filaments, or other specific structures that mark the cell as mature and specialized. As the cell matures and morphological signs of specialization occur, it is differentiated from an unspecialized, perhaps multipotential, cell into a highly specialized unit of limited cellular potency. Although a cell may appear undifferentiated, its direction of maturation may be fixed and limited genetically, only time being required to disclose the nature of the differentiation by the appearance of morphological specializations. In short, a cell that appears morphologically undifferentiated may, in fact, be quite specifically determined.

The frequency of mitotic division varies with the cell type and tissue. Tissues may be classified as showing no mitotic division, resulting in no renewal (nervous tissue); little division, resulting in slow renewal (liver and thyroid); and active division, resulting in fast renewal (gastrointestinal tract and hematopoietic tissue). Some slowly renewed tissues may be termed "conditional renewal" systems because their renewal rate can be considerably increased under certain circumstances. After partial hepatectomy, for example, the remaining hepatocytes divide very actively, providing fast renewal until the mass of the liver is restored. Even some cells showing no mitotic division may, with appropriate stimulation, proliferate and differentiate. Certain small lymphocytes (T cells) may circulate and recirculate for many years in humans without dividing, but when stimulated by the appropriate antigen, or with certain mitogens, such as phytohemagglutinin or pokeweed, they may divide rapidly, producing clones of immunologically competent cells. In neurons, mitosis occurs only prenatally and neonatally until the full number of neurons is reached. Thereafter, no replacement occurs; a cell lost diminishes the total number, and its absence may cause functional impairment. The cells in tissues undergoing slow renewal tend to be long-lived. The relatively low levels of mitotic division provide new cells to replace those dying off or to permit the growth and increased functional capacity of the tissue. Rapidly renewing tissues are characterized by short-lived cells replaced by cell division, so that a rather stable number of cells results. In the intestinal epithelium, new cells formed in the depths of the intestinal glands appear to move up the wall of the gland replacing the topmost cells, which fall into the gut lumen. As a result, the entire intestinal epithelium is renewed in a span of days. The kinetics of hematopoietic tissues, particularly of the granular leukocytes, follows this pattern.

It is possible to define a *generation time* for a population of similar cells, relating the interphase state, the period of DNA replication, and the process of mitotic division. A series of three periods follows mitosis: G_1, S, G_2, then M. G_1 is an interval or gap that follows cell division; S is the period of DNA replication; G_2 is the gap between replication of DNA and the start of mitosis; and M is mitosis.

The duration of G_1 varies greatly with cell types and mitotic turnover. In rapidly dividing cells it may be a matter of several hours. In non-renewing tissues it may last the life of the organism. Such prolonged G_1 periods may be designated G_0. S is demonstrated by autoradiography. Thymidine is a base distinctive to DNA. Therefore, replicating DNA specifically and selectively takes up thymidine. If the thymidine is radioactive, accomplished by the incorporation of tritium (^{3}H) in the molecule, and is administered during DNA replication, it is taken up by the replicating DNA and can mark it in autoradiographs. Indeed, the ability to delineate the S period by this means makes it possible to determine the entire generation time. In a rapidly renewing tissue, S is approximately 7 h. It is a matter of great interest that the DNA in a given chromosome does not all replicate at the same time. Instead, different segments of the chromosome replicate at different times in the S period, and in a characteristic sequence. G_2 is very short—about an hour—in rapidly renewing tissues. In cells destined to be polytenic, G_2 may last indefinitely. The whole of the cycle in such rapidly dividing rodent tissues as germinal centers or thymus may be about 12 h. In the epithelium of the gastrointestinal tract in humans G_2 is 1 to 7 h.; the S phase, 10 to 20 h; G_1, 10 to 20 h; and the whole of the cycle, 1 to 2 days. In rodents this cycle may take only a third of this time.

The sequences in the generation cycle may be illustrated as follows[2]:

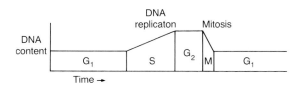

---

[2]After Lamerton, L. F., 1969, *In* Fry, R. J. M., Griem, M. L., and Kirsten, W. H. (eds.), Normal and Malignant Cell Growth. New York: Springer-Verlag.

After functioning as a mature cell for varying lengths of time, a cell dies, its death often presaged by a period of senescence. Perhaps the best-studied case is that of the erythrocyte, whose life span in the circulation of humans is approximately 120 days. Near the end of its life span, the activity of glucose-6-phosphatase and certain other enzymes declines, and the cell becomes mechanically more fragile. There are, however, no morphological concomitants of erythrocyte senescence.

In other cell types, however, morphological changes may signify senescence and coming cell death. In muscle cells, these changes include attenuation, decrease in specific functional elements such as contractile filaments, and accumulation of pigment. Other changes include diminution in mitochondria, accumulation of fat, and vacuolization of cytoplasm and nucleus. Dead cells may disappear by lysis, by phagocytosis, or by displacement from the tissue, seen in desquamated skin cells and intestinal cells.

References and Selected Bibliography

General

Baker, J. R. 1958. Principles of Biological Microtechnique: A Study of Fixation and Dyeing. New York: John Wiley and Sons, Inc.

Baker, J. R. The cell-theory: A restatement, history and critique. Q. J. Microbiol. Sci. 89:103 (1948); 90:87 (1949); 93:157 (1952).

Bensley, R. R., and Gersh I. 1933. Studies on cell structure by the freezing-drying method. I. Introduction. II. The nature of the mitochondria in the hepatic cell of amblystoma. III. The distribution in cells of the basophil substances, in particular the Nissl substance of the nerve cell. Anat. Rec. 57:205, 217, 369.

Bensley, R. R., and Hoerr, N. L. 1935. Studies on cell structure by the freezing-drying method. VI. The preparation and properties of mitochondria. Anat. Rec. 60:449.

Bodmer, W. F. 1981. The HLA system: Introduction. Brit. Med. Bull. 34:213.

Brachet, J., and Mirsky, A. E. (eds.). 1961. The cell. I. Biochemistry, physiology, morphology. II. Cells and their component parts. III. Mitosis and meiosis. IV. Specialized cells, pt. 1. V. Specialized cells, pt. 2. New York: Adademic Press, Inc.

Busch, H. B. (ed.). 1974. The Cell Nucleus. 3 vols. New York: Academic Press.

De Robertis, E. D. F., Saez, F. A., and De Robertis, E. M. F., Jr. 1975. Cell Biology, 6th ed. Philadelphia: W. B. Saunders Co.

Freeman, J. A., and Spurlock, B. O. 1962. A new epoxy embedment for electron microscopy. J. Cell Biol. 13:437.

Fuks, A., Kaufman, J. F., Orr, H. T., Parham, P., Robb, R. R., Terhorst, C., and Strominger, J. L. 1980. Structural aspects of the products of the human histocompatibility complex. Transplant. Proc. 9:1685.

Harris, H. 1974. Nucleus and Cytoplasm, 3rd ed. New York: Oxford University Press.

Karp, G. 1979. Cell Biology. New York: McGraw-Hill Book Co., Inc.

Organization of the Cytoplasm. 1982. Cold Spring Harbor Symp. Quant. Biol. Vol. 46.

Pretlow, T. G. II., Weir, E. E., and Zettergren, J. G. 1975. Problems connected with the separation of different kinds of cells. Int. Rev. Exp. Pathol. 14:91.

Siegel, B. M. (ed.). 1964. Modern developments in electron microscopy. In The Physics of the Electron Microscope: Techniques: Applications. New York: Academic Press, Inc.

Watson, D. D. 1976. Molecular Biology of the Gene, 3rd ed. New York: Benjamin.

Cell Cycle, Mitosis, and Centrioles

Ackerman, G. A. 1961. Histochemistry of the centrioles and centrosomes of the leukemic cells from human myeloblastic leukemia. J. Biophys. Biochem. Cytol. 11:717.

Bajer, A., and Mole-Bajer, 1971. Architecture and function of the mitotic spindle. Adv. Cell Mol. Biol. 1:213.

Baserga, R. (ed.). 1976. Multiplication and Division in Mammalian Cells. New York: Marcel Dekker.

Beams, W. H., and Kessel, R. G. 1976. Cytokinesis: A comparative study of cytoplasmic division in animal cells. Am. Sci. 64:279.

Brinkley, B. R., and Porter, K. R. (eds.). 1977. Symposium on "The Eukarocyte Cell Cycle." Inter. Cell Biol. New York: The Rockefeller Press, p. 409.

Brinkley, B. R., and Stubblefield, E. 1970. Ultrastructure and interaction of the kinetochore and centriole in mitosis and meiosis. In D. M. Prescott, L. Goldstein, and E. McConkey (eds.), Advances in Cell Biology, vol. I. New York: Appleton-Century-Crofts.

Bullough, W. S. 1975. Mitotic control in adult mammalian tissues. Biol. Rev. 50:99.

Edenberg, J., and Huberman, J. A. 1975. Eukaryotic chromosome replication. Ann. Rev. Genet. 9:245.

Fuge, H. 1974. Ultrastructure and function of the spindle apparatus and chromosomes during nuclear division. Protoplasm 82:299.

Gall, J. G., Porter, K. R., and Siekevitz, P. (eds.). 1981. Discovery in cell biology. J. Cell Biol. 91 (3, part 2):35.

Goss, R. T. 1970. Turnover in cells and tissues. In D. M. Prescott, L. Goldstein, and E. McConkey (eds.), Advances in Cell Biology, vol. 1. New York: Appleton-Century-Crofts, Inc.

Kornberg, A. DNA Synthesis. 1974. W. H. Freeman.

Lajtha, L. 1969. Proliferative capacity of hemopoietic stem cells. In R. J. M. Fry, M. G. Griem, and W. H. Kirsten (eds.), Normal and Malignant Cell Growth. New York: Springer-Verlag.

LeBlond, C. P., and Walker, B. E. 1956. Renewal of cell populations. Physiol. Rev. 36:255.

Lesher, S., and Bauman, J. 1969. Cell proliferation in the intestinal epithelium. *In* R. J. M. Fry, M. L. Griem, and W. H. Kirsten (eds.), Normal and Malignant Cell Growth. New York: Springer-Verlag.

Mazia, D. 1961. Mitosis and the physiology of cell division. *In* J. Brachet and A. E. Mirsky (eds.)., The Cell, vol. 3. New York: New Academic Press, Inc.

Mazia, D. 1964. The cell cycle. Sci Am. 230:54.

Mitchison, J. M. 1971. The Biology of the Cell Cycle. New York: Cambridge University Press.

Pelc, S. R. 1964. Labelling of DNA and cell division in so-called non-dividing tissues. J. Cell Biol. 22:21.

Prescott, D. M. 1970. Structure and Replication of Eukaryotic Chromosomes. 1970. *In* D. M. Prescott, L. Goldstein, and E. McConkey (eds.). Advances in Biology, vol. 1. New York: Appleton-Century-Crofts.

Prescott, D. M. 1976. The cell cycle and the control of cellular reproduction. Adv. Genet. 18:99.

Robbins, E., and Gonatas, N. K. 1964. The ultrastructures of a mammalian cell during the mitotic cycle. J. Cell Biol. 21:429.

Taylor, J. H. 1974. Units of DNA replication in chromosomes of eukaryocytes. Int. Rev. Cytol. 37:1.

Wheatley, D. N. 1982. The Centriole: A Central Enigma of Cell Biology. Amsterdam: Elsevier Biomedical Press.

Chromatin

Back, F. 1976. The variable condition of heterochromatin and euchromatin. Int. Rev. Cytol. 45:25.

Barr, M. L. 1966. The Significance of the Sex Chromatin. Int. Rev. Cytol. 19:35.

Barr, M. L. 1959. Sex chromatin and phenotype in man. Science 130:679.

Baserga, R., and Nicolina, C. 1976. Chromatin structure and function in proliferating cells. Biochem. Biophys. Acta 458:109.

Berendes, H. D. 1973. Synthetic activity of polytene chromosome. Int. Rev. Cytol. 35:61.

Elgin, S. C. R., and Weintraub, H. 1975. Chromosomal proteins and chromatin structure. Ann. Rev. Biochem. 44:725.

Fitzsimmons, D. W., and Wolstenholme, G. E. (eds.). 1975. The Structure and Function of Chromatin. Ciba Foundation Symposium 28 (new series). Amsterdam: Elsevier North-Holland.

Kornberg, R. D. 1977. Structure of chromatin. Ann. Rev. Biochem. 46:931.

Endocytosis—Cytoplasmic Vesicles

Brandt, P. W., and Pappas, G. D. 1960. An electron microscopic study of pinocytosis in ameba. I. The surface attachment phase. J. Biophys. Biochem. Cytol. 8:675.

Silverstein, S. C., Steinman, R. M., and Cohn, Z. A. 1977. Endocytosis. Ann. Rev. Biochem 46:669.

Stossel, T. P. 1974. Phagocytosis. N. Engl. J. Med. 290:717.

Straus, W. 1964. Occurrence of phagosomes and phagolysosomes in different segments of the nephron in relation to the reabsorption, transport, digestion, and extrusion of intravenously injected horseradish peroxidase. J. Cell Biol. 21:295.

Ockleford, C. D., and Whyte, A. (eds.). 1980. Coated Vesicles. Cambridge, England: Cambridge University Press.

Endoplasmic Reticulum

Brinkley, R. R., and Porter, K. R. (eds.). 1977. Symposium on "Endoplasmic Reticulum. Golgi Apparatus and Cell Secretion." Int. Cell Biol. New York: Rockefeller University Press, pp. 267-340.

Cardell, R. R., Jr. 1979. Smooth endoplasmic reticulum in rat hepatocytes during glycogen deposition and depletion. Int. Rev. Cytol. 48:221.

Depierre, J. W., and Dallner, G. 1975. Structural aspects of the membrane of the endoplasmic reticulum. Biochem. Biophys. Acta 415:411.

Porter, K. R., and Palade, G. E. 1957. Studies on the endoplasmic reticulum. V. Its form and differentiation in striated muscle cells. J. Biophys. Biochem. Cytol. 3:269.

Porter, K. R., and Yamada, E. 1960. Studies on the endoplasmic reticulum. V. Its form and differentiation in pigment epithelial cells of the frog retina. J. Biophys. Biochem. Cytol. 8:181.

Golgi Complex

Bennett, G., LeBlond, C. P., and Haddad, A. J. 1974. Migration of glycoproteins from Golgi apparatus to the surface of various cell types as shown by radioautography after labelled fucose injection into rats. J. Cell Biol. 60:258.

Dalton, E. J., and Felix, M. D. 1956. A comparative study of the Golgi complex. J. Biophys. Biochem. Cytol. 2:79.

Jamieson, J. D. 1971. Role of the Golgi complex in the intracellular transport of secretory proteins. *In* F. Clementi and B. Ceccarelli (eds.), Advances in Cytopharmacology, vol. 1. New York: Raven Books, Abelard-Schuman, Inc., p. 83.

Morre, D. J., and Oltacht, L. 1977. Dynamics of the Golgi apparatus: Membrane differentiation and membrane flow. Int. Rev. Cytol. 5:61.

Palade, G. 1975. Intracellular aspects of the process of protein synthesis. Science 189:347.

Tartakoff, A. M. 1982. Simplifying the complex Golgi. Trends Bio. Sci. 7:174.

Whaley, W. G. 1975. The Golgi Apparatus. Vienna, New York: Springer-Verlag.

Intermediate Filaments

Lazarides, E., 1980. Review Article: Intermediate filaments as mechanical integrators of cellular space. Nature 283:249.

Lysosomes

Allison, A. 1967. Lysosomes and disease. Sci. Am. 217:62.

De Duve, C. 1958. Lysosomes, a new group of cytoplasmic particles. *In* T. Hayashi (ed.), Subcellular Particles. New York: The Ronald Press.

De Duve, C. 1963. The separation and characterization of subcellular particles. Harvey Lectures 59:49.

De Duve, C. 1975. Exploring cells with a centrifuge. Science 189:186.

Holtzman, E. 1976. Lysosomes: A Survey. Vienna, New York: Springer-Verlag.

Kolodny, E. H. 1976. Lysosomal storage diseases. N. Engl. J. Med. 294:1217.

Meiosis

Comings, D. E., and Okada, T. A. 1972. Architecture of meiotic cells and mechanisms of chromosome pairing. Adv. Cell Mol. Biol. 2:309.

Moens, P. B. 1973. Mechanisms of chromosome synapsis at meiotic prophase. Int. Rev. Cytol. 35:117.

Rhoades, M. M. 1960. Meiosis. *In* J. Brachet and A. Mirsky (eds.), Cell, vol. 3, New York: Academic Press, Inc., pp. 1–75.

Stern, H., and Hotta, Y. 1972. Biochemical controls of meiosis. Ann. Rev. Genet. 9:37.

Mitochondria

Fernandez-Moran, H., Oda, T., Blair, P. V., and Green, D. E. 1964. A macromolecular repeating unit of mitochondrial structure and function: Correlated electron microscopic and biochemical studies of isolated mitochondria and submitochondrial particles of beef heart muscle. J. Cell Biol. 22:71.

Munn, E. 1975. The Structure of Mitochondria. New York: Academic Press.

Palmer, J. M., and Hall, D. O. 1972. The mitochondrial membrane system. Prog. Mol. Biol. 24:125.

Tedeschi, H. 1976. Mitochondria: Structure, Biogenesis and Transducing Function. Cell Biology Monographs, vol. 4. Vienna: Springer-Verlag.

Nuclear Envelope

Feldherr, C. M. 1962. The nuclear annuli as pathways for nucleocytoplasmic exchanges. J. Cell Biol. 14:65.

Franke, W. W. 1974. Structure, biochemistry and functions of nuclear envelope. Int. Rev. Cytol (Suppl) 4:72.

Maul, G. G. 1970. On the relationship between the Golgi apparatus and annucleate lamellae. J. Ultrastruct. Res. 30:368.

Microfilaments

LeBlond, C. P., and Clermont, Y. 1960. The cell web, a fibrillar structure found in a variety of cells in animal tissues. Anat. Rec. 136:230.

Perry, S., Margerth, A., and Adelstein, R. (eds.). 1977. Contractile Systems in Non-Muscle Tissues. Amsterdam: Elsevier North-Holland.

Pollard, T. D. 1975. Functional implications of the biochemical and structural properties. *In* S. Inoue and R. E. Stephens (eds.), Molecules and Cell Movement. New York: Raven Books, Abelard-Schuman, Ltd.

Pollard, T. D. 1976. Cytoskeletal functions of cytoplasmic contractile proteins. J. Supramol. Struct. 5:317.

Schroeder, T. E. 1973. Actin in dividing cells: Contractile ring filaments bind heavy meromyosin. Proc. Natl. Acad. Sci. U.S.A. 70:1,688.

Schroeder, T. E. 1975. Dynamics of the contractile ring. 1975 *In* S. Inoue and R. E. Stephens (eds.), Molecules and Cell Movement. New York: Raven Books, Abelard-Schuman, Ltd.

Membranes

Ash, J. F., Louvard, and Singer, S. J. 1977. Antibody-induced linkages of plasma membrane proteins to intracellular actinomyosin-containing filaments in cultured fibroblasts. Proc. Natl. Acad. Sci. U.S.A. 74:5,584.

Branton, D. 1966. Fracture faces of frozen membranes. Proc. Natl. Acad. Sci. U.S.A. 55:1,048.

Branton, D. 1971. Freeze-etching studies of membrane structure. Trans. R. Soc. Lond. (Biol.) 261:133.

Branton, D. 1966. Fracture faces of frozen membranes. Proc. Natl. Acad. Sci. U.S.A. 55:1,048.

Brinkley, B. R., and Porter, K. R. (eds.). 1977. Symposium on "Plasma Membrane Organization." *In* Int. Cell Biol. New York: Rockefeller University Press, pp. 5–28.

Cuatrecasas, P., and Greaves, M. F. 1977. Receptors and Recognition. Halsted.

Essner, E., Novikoff, A. D., and Masek, B. 1958. Adenosine triphosphatase and 5-nucleotidease activities in the plasma membrane of liver cells as revealed by electron microscopy. J. Biophys. Biochem. Cytol. 4:711.

Hughes, R. C. 1975 The complex carbohydrate of mammalian cell surfaces and their biological roles. Essays Biochem. 11:1.

Marchesi, R. T., Furthmayer, H., and Tomita, M. 1976. The red cell membrane. Ann. Rev. Biochem. 45:667.

Nicolson, G. L., Poste, G., and Ji, T. H. 1977. The dynamics of cell membrane organization. *In* G. Poste and G. L. Nicolson (eds.), Dynamic Aspects of Cell Surface Organization, vol. 3, Cell Surface Reviews. Amsterdam: Elsevier North-Holland, pp. 1–73.

Pinto da Silva, P., and Braxton, D. J. 1970. Membrane splitting in freeze-etching. Cell Biol. 45:598.

Quinn, P. J. 1976. The Molecular Biology of Cell Membranes. Baltimore: University Park Press.

Raff, M. C., and De Petris, S. 1973. Movement of lymphocyte surface antigens and receptors: The fluid nature of the lymphocyte plasma membrane and its immunological significance. Fed. Proc. 32:48.

Singer, S. J., and Nicolson, G. L. 1972. The fluid mosaic model of the structure of cell membranes. Science 175:720.

Singer, S. J. 1974. Molecular organization of membranes. Ann. Rev. Biochem. 43:805.

Microtubules

Blake, J. R., and Sleigh, M. A. 1974. Mechanics of Ciliary Locomotion. Biol. Rev. 49:85.

Borgers, M., and DeBrabander, M. 1975. Microtubules and microtubule inhibitors. New York: Elsevier North-Holland.

Olmstead, J. B., and Borisey, G. G. 1973. Microtubules. Ann. Rev. Biochem. 42:507.

Osborn, M., and Weber, K. 1977. The display of microtubules in transformed cells. Cell 12:561.

Roberts, K. 1973. Cytoplasmic microtubules and their functions. Prog. Biophys. Mol. Biol. 28:273.

Satir, P. 1974. How Cilia Move. Sci. Am. 231 (4):44.

Spooner, B. S. 1975. Microfilaments, microtubules, and extracellular materials in morphogenesis. Bioscience 25:440.

Nucleolus

Brinkley, B. R. 1965. The fine structure of the nucleolus in mitotic divisions of Chinese hamster cells in vitro. J. Cell Biol. 27:411.

Brown, D. D., and Gurdon, J. B. 1965. Absence of ribosomal RNA synthesis in the anucleate mutant of Xenopus laevis. In E. Bell (ed.), Molecular and Cellular Aspects of Development. New York: Harper & Row.

Busch, H., and Smetana, K. 1972. The Nucleolus. New York: Academic Press, Inc.

Ghosh, S. 1976. The nucleolar structure. Int. Rev. Cytol. 44:1.

Peroxisomes

DeDuve, C. 1969. The peroxisome: A new cytoplasmic organelle. Proc. R. Soc. (London) 173:71.

Novikoff, A. B., and Allen, J. M. (eds.). 1973. Symposium on "Peroxisomes." J. Histochem. Cytochem. 21:941.

Tolbert, N. E. 1971. Microbodies—peroxisomes and glycosomes. Ann. Rev. Plant. Phys. 22:45.

Ribosomes

Palade, G. E. 1975. Intracellular aspects of the process of protein synthesis. Science 189:347.

Rich, A., Warner, J. R., and Goodman, H. M. 1963. The structure and function of polyribosomes. Cold Spring Harbor Symp. Quant. Biol. 28:269.

Shore, G. C., and Tata, J. R. 1977. Functions for polyribosomes membrane interactions in protein synthesis. Biochem. Biophys. Acta 472:197.

Smith, D. W. E. 1975. Reticulocyte transfer RNA and hemoglobin synthesis. Science 190:529.

Spitnik-Elson, P., and Elson, D. 1976. Studies on the ribosome and its components. In W. E. Cohn (ed.), Progress in Nucleic Acid Research and Molecular Biology. New York: Academic Press, Inc., 17:77.

Weiss, J. M. 1953. The ergastoplasm: Its fine structure and relation to protein synthesis as studied with the electron microscope in the pancreas of the Swiss albino mouse. J. Exp. Med. 98:607.

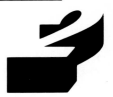

Histochemistry and Cytochemistry

Helen A. Padykula

Histochemistry–cytochemistry is a biological approach that permits a precise interpretation of the chemistry of cells and tissues in relation to structural organization. A student of histology quickly becomes aware of the intrinsic heterogeneity in the structure of multicellular organisms. Biochemical analysis alone is inadequate because homogenization of an organ obscures structural heterogeneity, which extends to the molecular level. In histochemistry–cytochemistry, by using tissue sections, morphological relationships are maintained.

The principal question asked by the cytochemist is: Where, within the organized framework of the cell, is a particular chemical component located? To identify and localize the component, a specific procedure derived from well-established reactions in inorganic or organic chemistry is used to yield a reaction product visible with microscopes. The result offers qualitative and spatial precision. For example, it has been established that glucose-6-phosphatase is localized in the rough and smooth endoplasmic reticulum as well as in the nuclear envelope of the hepatocyte and that galactose is incorporated into glycoprotein in the Golgi complex of the intestinal goblet cell. Such qualitative information is essential to an understanding of cell physiology.

Another major approach to the chemical characterization of cells and tissues is the isolation of cellular and tissue components by ultracentrifugation. Current procedures of ultracentrifugation and electron microscopy are so refined that ultra-structural entities (for example, the outer mitochondrial membrane or the Golgi complex) can be isolated, recognized, and characterized quantitatively. A limitation of this powerful methodology is that cell and tissue organization is dismantled with consequent loss of the interrelationship of component parts. Thus, the two major approaches to chemical characterization of cells are complementary in terms of the kinds of information yielded.

The potential for study of biological organization unleashed by the electron microscope's resolving power of 2 Å offers an exciting challenge to cytochemistry. Chemical localizations can be made at the ultrastructural level. The impetus provided by electron microscopy extended most of histochemistry (intratissue localizations) to cytochemistry (intracellular localizations). Much current effort centers heavily on immunocytochemistry, which has also advanced to the ultrastructural level. This powerful methodology uses the high precision of the antigen–antibody reaction to identify the location of an individual exogenous or endogenous protein or other antigen.

Significant biological concepts have emerged from the application of histochemistry and cytochemistry, only a few examples of which are cited here. Concepts of the mechanism of cellular defense have been shaped in part from information gained through the cytochemical study of phagocytosis (via identification of lysosomal derivatives by localization of acid phosphatase) and through identification of antibody-producing cells by immunocytochemistry. Interpretations related to cell differentiation, migration, and replacement have depended heavily on information gained through radioautography, which permits visualization of the location of an incorporated radioactive label. The characterization of chemical differences along the nephron is accomplished mainly through histochemistry, as the complex histological organization of the kidney makes biochemical analysis exceedingly difficult. Exploration of the heterogeneity of vertebrate skeletal muscle fibers received its direction from histochemical observations; zonation of the hepatic lobule is in part a histochemical concept. To approach problems involving multicellular systems through histochemistry, an observer must have an adequate background both in microscopic anatomy and in chemistry.

General Principles of Histochemistry

1. *The essential first step is the preservation and immobilization of the chemical substance by appropriate fixation and processing.* Cellular structure and selected chemical features must survive the procedures required to prepare a suitable tissue section for transmission microscopy. Special fixation is usually required to ensure retention of the chemical entity with its characteristic reactivity. In fixation for morphological purposes, only the macromolecular protein framework (for example, nucleoproteins, lipoproteins, glycoproteins) is retained, because the proteins are denatured and new cross-linkages are established that render them insoluble. Thus, the cytochemistry of macromolecules is more readily approached than that of small molecules, such as simple sugars, amino acids, and electrolytes, which are usually washed out of tissue sections. To preserve triglycerides and other lipids, organic solvents such as acetone, chloroform, and xylol must be avoided. The fact that glycogen is soluble in water but insoluble in concentrated ethanol should be considered in selecting an appropriate fixative. Most enzymes are inactivated to some degree by fixation, and some, in addition, are soluble. Thus, fixation preceding a cytochemical demonstration of enzymatic activitity usually represents a compromise between the quality of morphological preservation and the degree of activity.

2. *A specific chemical-identifying reaction is needed that will yield an insoluble product* composed of particles small enough to be localized among the tissue and cell components and large enough to be resolved by light and electron microscopes. In addition, the reaction product should be visible by virtue of its color (with the ordinary light microscope), by a fluorescent label (with the ultraviolet microscope), or by high electron opacity (with the electron microscope).

3. *The specificity of the histochemical test must be defined by the appropriate use of control preparations.* The importance of this principle cannot be overemphasized, as the tissue section is a heterogeneous system with highly varied chemical reactivity. Common control preparations are ones in which a significant reagent has been omitted from the reaction or ones in which the reactive substance has been removed or masked.

4. *The accuracy of the localization of the re-*

action product must be evaluated to eliminate the possibility that one of the reagents might be bound nonspecifically to a tissue component or the possibility that the reaction product might migrate or be soluble in adjacent cell inclusions, such as lipid droplets.

5. *The sensitivity of the histochemical test must be considered when evaluating results.* A negative histochemical reaction may or may not indicate the absence of a substance. Negative results may mean (1) that the material is absent or is in insufficient amount for detection, (2) that an interfering reaction is present; (3) that the substance has been chemically altered; or (4) that the substance has been lost from the tissue during preparation.

To introduce the rationale of the histochemical–cytochemical approach, these principles are illustrated in a few commonly employed procedures. For more information about these and other procedures, consult the books by Barka and Anderson and by Pearse.

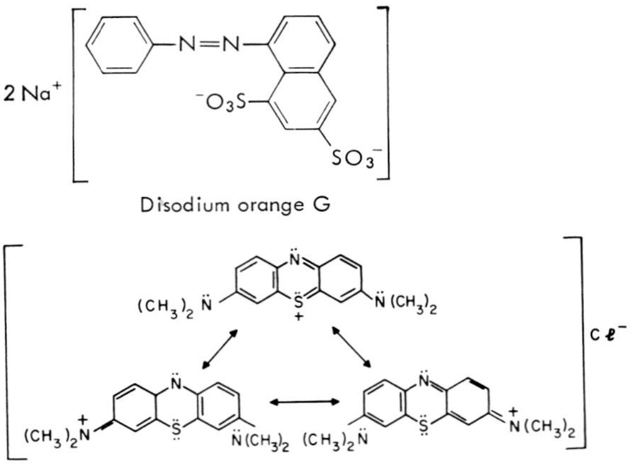

Acidophilia and Basophilia

Staining with a cationic (basic) dye and an anionic (acid) dye is the principal way of creating the color contrasts necessary for morphological study (see Chap. 1). A cellular or tissue component that binds a basic dye is termed *basophilic;* conversely, a component that binds an acid dye is *acidophilic.* The designations *acidophilia* and *basophilia* are primary and important distinctions drawn to characterize cellular and tissue components.

Here we shall consider how these cationic and anionic dyes may be used as histochemical reagents to characterize the cell. Figure 2–1 illustrates the chemical structure of a representative anionic (so-called acidic) dye, orange G, and a representative cationic (basic) dye, methylene blue.

Acidic and *basic* dyes are inherited designations that unfortunately do not conform to current definitions for an acid and a base (that is, an acid is a substance capable of donating protons and a base is capable of accepting protons). However, through long-standing usage in biological and medical sciences, an acid dye is one capable of forming a salt linkage with a positively charged tissue group; therefore, the dye molecule is negatively charged (anionic). A basic dye is positively charged (cationic) and hence forms a

Disodium orange G

METHYLENE BLUE

2–1 Formulas of a typical anionic (acid) dye, orange G, and a typical cationic (basic) dye, methylene blue. The formula for methylene blue depicts it as a resonance hybrid of three main structures (From Bergeron, J. A., and Singer, M. 1958. J. Biophys. Biochem. Cytol. 4:433.)

salt with a negatively charged tissue group. This usage is analogous to the designation of nucleic acids.

Commonly used basic dyes are methylene blue, toluidine blue, basic fuchsin, carmine, and hematoxylin. (Note below the special usage of mordants with hematoxylin.) Common acid dyes are eosin, orange G, phloxine, anilin blue, and light green. For further information on dyes, consult texts in organic chemistry.

Many substances in the protein scaffolding of the tissue section—simple proteins, nucleoproteins, glycoproteins, and lipoproteins, as well as many lipids, glycolipids, and glycosaminoglycans—have ionizable radicals that can form electrostatic (salt) linkages with these dyes. This staining capacity is more easily appreciated in relation to the chemical structure of proteins.

A protein is a polymer of a variety of amino acids; it is amphoteric because of the side groups, which impart either anionic functions (for example, phenolic hydroxyl or carboxyl groups) or cationic functions (for example, amino, imidazole, or guanidine) (Fig. 2–2). The basis of the amphoteric property is illustrated in Fig. 2–3, which indicates that the charge of an amino acid depends on the pH of the medium. Thus, the protein as a whole may act either as an anion or cation, depending on the algebraic sum of its

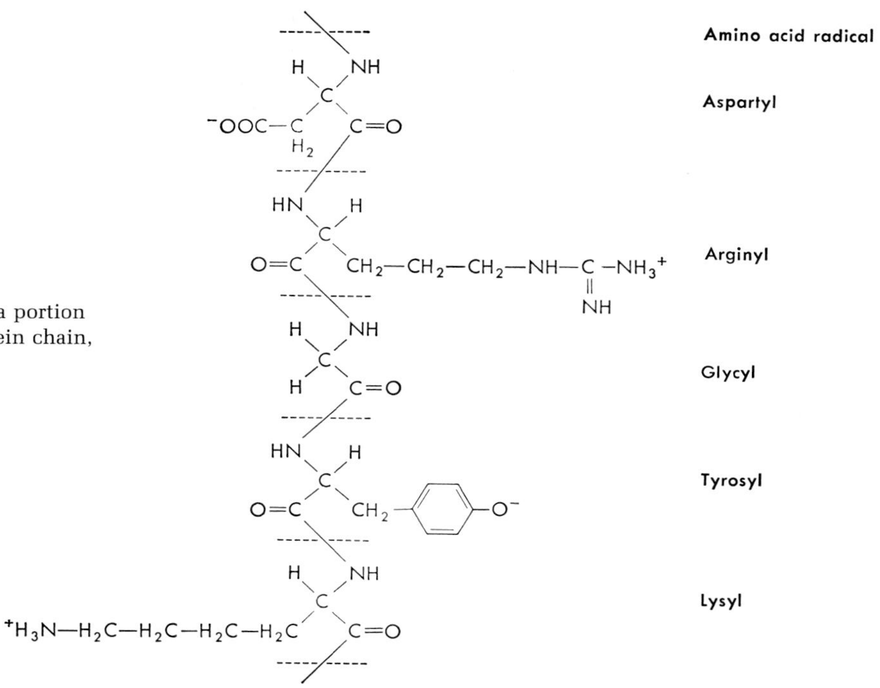

2–2 Structural formula of a portion of a hypothetical protein chain, to illustrate the presence of ionizable radicals.

positive and negative charges at the pH of its environment. The pH at which the protein approaches electrical neutrality is the *isoelectric point*.

The fixed proteins of a tissue section retain their amphoteric properties but are modified by denaturation. Actually fixation causes increased affinity for stains, because as peptide chains unfold, secondary groups become available for reaction with dye molecules. Certain fixatives (for example, those containing osmium or mercury) combine with various reactive groups in the tissue and can influence subsequent stainability considerably.

Evidence that the binding of acid (anionic) and basic (cationic) dyes by proteins is principally an electrostatic phenomenon can be obtained by experiments involving the dye-binding of a single pure protein, fibrin, at various pH levels (Fig. 2–4). The intensity of staining at each pH—that is, the amount of light absorbed—can be measured with a photometer; and when plotted against pH, curves representing the acidophilia and basophilia of the protein can be drawn. Study of Fig. 2–4 shows that the least binding of cationic and anionic dyes occurs near pH 6.0, which is near the isoelectric point of fibrin. Below its isoelectric pH, the fibrin is acidophilic (that is, it binds anionic orange G) by virtue of its overall positive charge (e.g., $—NH_2$ ionizes to $—NH_3^+$). Above the isoelectric point, the fibrin is basophilic (that is, it binds the cationic methylene blue) because of its overall negative charge (e.g., $—COOH$ ionizes to $—COO^-$).

A tissue section, however, contains a myriad of proteins that differ in their amino acid composition and, thus, in isoelectric point; at a pH that creates good color contrast for morphological study, certain tissue components will show a relative acidophilia (for example, mitochondria, collagen, and hemoglobin of red blood cells) whereas others display a relative basophilia (for example, chromatin, nucleoli, and ergastoplasm). However, the dye-binding of proteins is not only

2–3 The amino acid zwitterion: the net charge is zero at the isoelectric point. The substance is anionic above the isoelectric point and cationic below it.

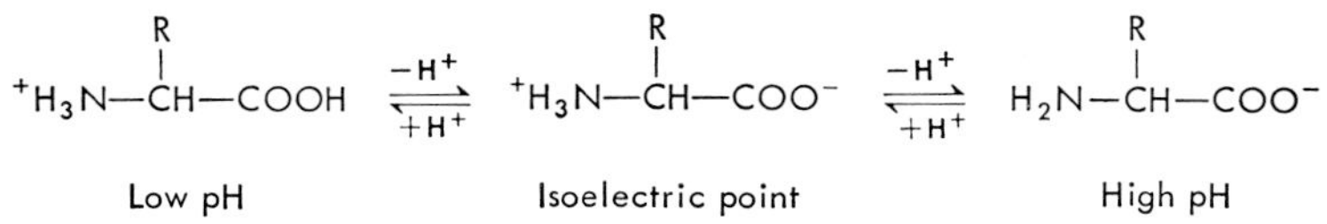

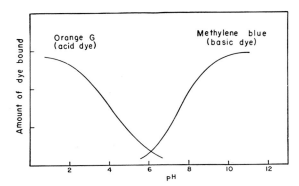

2–4 Dye-binding of a pure protein, fibrin, in solutions of constant salt and dye concentration. The amount of dye bound is calculated from the light absorption of the stained protein. For further explanation, see the text. (Courtesy of M. Singer.)

relative to their amino acid content but is also profoundly affected by the presence of associated groups, such as the phosphate groups of the nucleoproteins (Fig. 2–5). Much of the cellular basophilia commonly observed in the chromatin, nucleoli, and large aggregates of ribosomes (Fig.

2–5 Structure of a portion of DNA. The components responsible for the basophilia of chromatin are the phosphate radicals that can dissociate to form anions at the OH group. The **arrow** indicates the point between the purine and deoxyribose residues where acid hydrolysis occurs, an essential step in the Feulgen nucleal reaction.

Adenine   Deoxyribose   Phosphate

Thymine

2–6) is based on the dissociation of the phosphate groups of DNA and RNA to form negative radicals, even at relatively low pH (Fig. 2–7). Other highly basophilic structures (granules of mast cells and blood basophils) and cartilage matrix contain sulfated proteoglycans; the high electronegativity of the sulfate group causes a basophilia that persists even at pH 2 (Fig 2–7).

To identify basophilia originating from nucleoproteins, additional information derived from control preparations is required. For example, if the cytoplasm exhibits marked basophilia, a control section may be exposed to the action of the enzyme ribonuclease (RNase) before staining. Because RNase will hydrolyze and thus remove RNA present in the control, areas in the section whose dye affinity is due to RNA will not be basophilic after such treatment. Similarly, DNase can be used to remove DNA from control preparations. Also, useful information about the relative basophilia of various radicals on protein molecules can be uncovered rather simply by staining at different pH levels (Fig. 2–7). The basophilia caused by the carboxyl groups of muscle proteins will be extinguished at a higher pH than that originating from the phosphate groups of nucleoproteins. Basophilia persisting at pH 2 usually indicates the presence of the sulfate group, as in the heparin (Fig 2–8) of mast cells or chondroitin sulfate of cartilage matrix.

Intense acidophilia over a wide pH range may reflect the presence of a high concentration of proteins rich in lysine or arginine, which impart strong overall positive charge. For example, red blood cells are strongly acidophilic because they are rich in hemoglobin. The eosinophilic leukocytes obtain their name from the presence of strongly acidophilic (eosinophilic) cytoplasmic granules. We should add, however, that there are also relatively chromophobic substances, such as elastic fibers, that show little reactivity toward these aqueous dyes.

Because the dyes hematoxylin and eosin are commonly used in routine study, it should be noted that the color-bearing moiety of the hematoxylin is actually an anionic substance called hematein that is bound (or chelated) to tissue components by a multivalent metallic cation (such as aluminum or iron) known as a mordant. The hematein–mordant *complex* carries a positive charge. Although it behaves generally as a cationic dye, certain hematoxylin mixtures will stain mitochondria and other structures that are not basophilic under the conditions previously described.

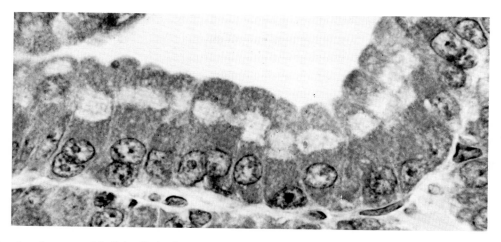

2–6 Simple columnar epithelial cells in the prostate gland of the rat. Stained with hematoxylin (basic or cationic dye) and eosin (acid or anionic dye). Dark areas represent basophilia, which is evident in the nuclei (nucleoli and heterochromatin) and in most of the cytoplasm, except for a supranuclear acidophilic region occupied by the Golgi complex.

2–7 Staining characteristics, or "signatures," of several basophilic constituents of tissues. Methylene blue staining was employed under constant conditions of salt and dye concentration. The chemical constituents responsible for the basophilia of these cells and tissue components are the sulfate groups of proteoglycan in cartilage, heparin (see Fig. 2–8) of mast cell granules; the phosphate groups of ribonucleoprotein in the Nissl bodies of neurons; and the carboxyl groups of muscle proteins. In routine preparations, most cell and tissue basophilia originates from the strongly anionic phosphate group of DNA and RNA and from the sulfate groups of certain polysaccharides. (Courtesy of M. Singer.).

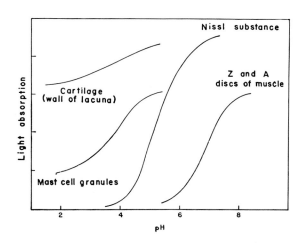

2–8 Structure of heparin hexasaccharide. This linear anionic polyelectrolyte sulfated carbohydrate molecule is a major constituent of heparin, the widely used anticoagulant. Heparin is produced in mast cells of the connective tissue. It is stored in secretory granules that are highly basophilic, metachromatic, and PAS-positive because of the strong, linear, polyanionic charge on this carbohydrate. (From Jaques, L. 1979. Science 206:528–533.)

For critical distinction between acidophilic and basophilic structures, the use of methylene blue and eosin at controlled pH levels is preferable to a hematoxylin and eosin preparation.

The semithin (or "thick") plastic section (1–2 μm), a by-product from electron microscopy, is a valuable addition to light microscopy. It offers the excellent preservation derived from the double fixation of electron microscopy (glutaraldehyde followed by osmium tetroxide) as well as thinness that facilitates intracellular distinctions. Such sections are usually stained with a single basic dye, methylene blue or toluidine blue, which are thiazine dyes that exhibit metachromasia (see below). Thus, tissue components are usually stained blue (orthochromatic) or pink-rose (metachromatic). Osmium tetroxide blocks most of the reactive groups of macromolecules, and binding of these cationic dyes can be achieved only by staining at highly alkaline pH. Thus, the terms basophilia and acidophilia are not strictly applicable. In this system, mitochondria (usually nonbasophilic structures) will bind these cationic dyes.

The "connective tissue stains" (e.g., Mallory trichrome, Masson trichrome) consist of a mixture of acid dyes, one of which (anilin blue or light green) has a distinct affinity for collagen. The color contrasts facilitate identification of the extracellular matrix of the various connective tissues.

Metachromasia

In a tissue section, *metachromasia* signals the change in the absorption spectrum of certain basic dyes when they are bound to polyanionic polymers, such as heparin (Fig. 2–8), chondromucoprotein, and nucleoprotein. Thiazine dyes (such as toluidine blue, thionine, and, to a lesser extent, methylene blue) are *orthochromatic* blue when seen in a dilute solution in a monomeric state; however, when they are concentrated in a solution, they aggregate as dimers and polymers, which absorb at a lower wave length and thus appear *metachromatic* red. Thus, different colors may be obtained from a single thiazine dye, depending on the state of aggregation of the molecules, and this state may be altered by the tissue components themselves.

For a histochemical demonstration of metachromasia, a tissue section is exposed to a dilute solution of toluidine blue. This cationic dye will bind electrostatically with anionic sites. Wherever the anionic sites are close enough, as in polyanionic polymers, the dye molecules will be aggregated by certain constituents of the tissue (Fig. 2–9A). Their interaction on the surface of the polyanion will result in a shift in absorption

2–9 A. Hypothesis concerning the basis of metachromasia in tissue sections. The polyanionic polymer on the left possesses a series of closely, uniformly spaced negative sites that react electrostatically with cationic molecules of toluidine blue. This alignment allows interaction of dye molecules that results in a metachromatic shift (red). On the right, the anionic sites are more widely and irregularly spaced; this results in an orthochromatic effect (blue). (Modified from Bradley and Wolf, 1959. Proc. Natl. Acad. Sci. 45:944.) **B.** Hypothetical representation to illustrate the alignment of two methylene blue cations with adjacent anionic groups of a phosphate polymer such as RNA or DNA. Methylene blue cations are separated by 7Å and dipolar water molecules intervene. (From Bergeron, J.A., and Singer, M. 1958. J. Biophys. Biochem. Cytol. 4:433).

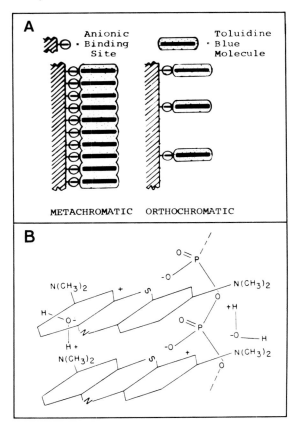

that creates the metachromatic effect. It is postulated that the distance between dye molecules should be about 5–7 Å for such interaction and that the presence of water is essential (Fig. 2–9B). Metachromasia is illustrated in Fig. 27–41, here the nuclei stain an orthochromatic blue, but the ground substance of the connective tissue is metachromatic red. Under certain conditions, nucleoproteins will also stain metachromatically but less obviously than the sulfated mucopolysaccharides. For the expression of metachromasia, the chemical nature of the binding site does not seem so important as the distribution and frequency of the negative charges (Fig. 2–9A). For a stimulating analysis of metachromasia, see Bergeron and Singer (1958).

Reactions of the Schiff Reagent with Aldehyde Groups

The Periodic Acid Schiff (PAS) Reaction for Carbohydrates

The histochemistry of carbohydrates centers around the periodic acid Schiff reaction, a procedure used routinely in most histology and pathology laboratories. It permits the localization of carbohydrate-rich macromolecules such as glycogen, glycoproteins, and proteoglycans. Glycogen is the principal storage form of carbohydrate in animals; its identification and localization is often important.

The specificity of the PAS reaction derives from the sequential use of two selective reagents, periodic acid (HIO_4) and the Schiff reagent. Periodic acid oxidizes the free hydroxyl groups on two adjacent carbon atoms, such as the 1,2-glycol linkage in hexoses or the adjacent hydroxyl and amino groups in hexosamine (Fig. 2–10). The hydroxyl groups are converted to aldehydes, the carbon-to-carbon bond is cleaved, and under the

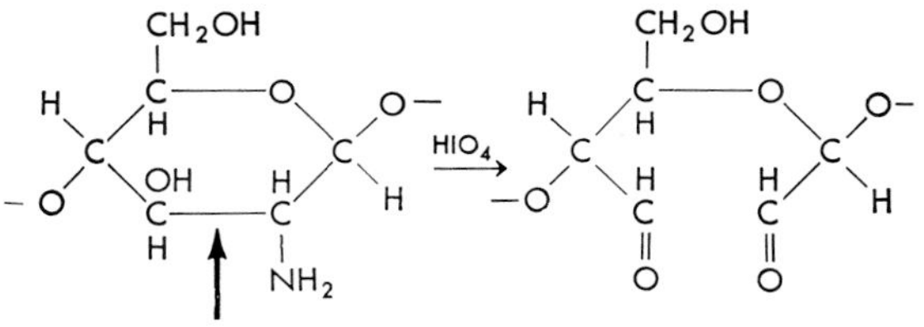

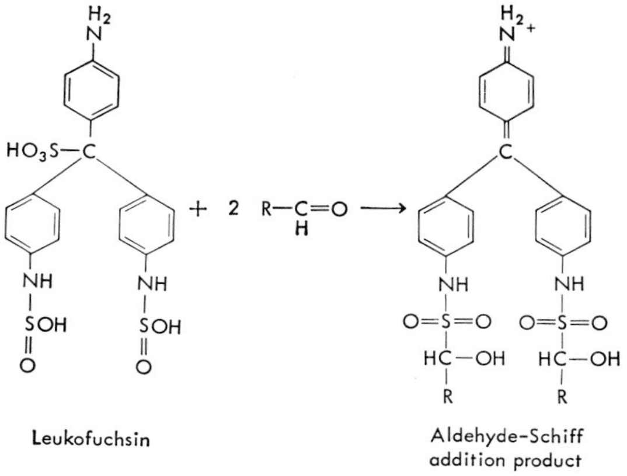

2–11 Reaction of colorless leukofuchsin with a dialdehyde to form a magenta-colored complex (see Fig. 2–12).

conditions of the PAS procedure, the oxidation does not proceed further. The resulting aldehydes react readily with the Schiff reagent to produce a stable-colored complex. The usual Schiff reagent is colorless leukofuchsin, or fuchsin–sulfurous acid, a chromogenic bisulfite compound which, when it forms an additional product with aldehydes, produces a stable red product (Fig. 2–11).

Numerous substances, especially in the epithelia and connective tissues, are reactive in the PAS method. Common reactive tissue components are glycogen, epithelial mucins, cell coats (see Fig. 2–12), basement membranes, and proteoglycans occurring in the extracellular matrix of the various connective tissues. To establish that the PAS-reactive material is glycogen, a control preparation is used that has been predigested with α-amylase, an enzyme that hydrolyzes glycogen specifically (Fig. 2–13). At the ultrastructural level, glycogen particles are recognizable as aggregates called α particles and single β particles as in muscle fibers (Fig. 7–29 and 7–31). The sorting out of the PAS-reactive substances not digested by amylase is a more difficult task, because there is considerable chemical variation among the carbohydrate polymers. Also some carbohydrate polymers are not stained by the PAS procedure, e.g., several of the hyaluronic acids and most chondroitin sulfates.

An important application of the PAS reaction will be presented in Chap. 29; this histochemical reaction facilitates the identification of the cells producing the glycoprotein hormones FSH, LH,

2–10 Oxidation of hexosamine residue of a polysaccharide by periodic acid to form dialdehydes. The point of attack is shown by the **arrow.**

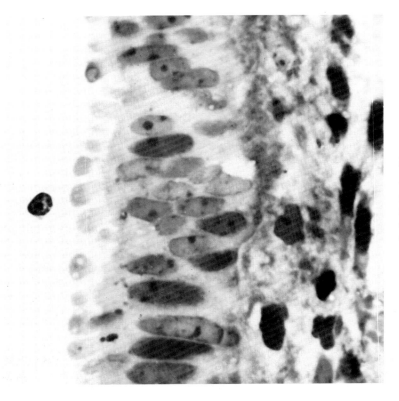

2–12 Periodic acid Schiff (PAS) reaction, rhesus monkey uterine luminal epithelium. Consult color section where this figure is shown in color and is accompanied by a more complete caption.

2–13 Glycogen synthesis in liver slices.

Radioautographs of sections stained with PAS and hematoxylin. These three sections were taken from a single liver slice (obtained from a rat fasted for 24 h) that had been incubated in a medium containing [³H] glucose for 15 min. In the control, silver grains overlay PAS-positive material, especially at the periphery of the hepatocytes. That this reactive material is glycogen is demonstrated by its complete removal by α amylase. The amylase of saliva removes the glycogen only partially. × 680. (From Coimbra and Leblond. 1966. J. Cell Biol. 30:151.)

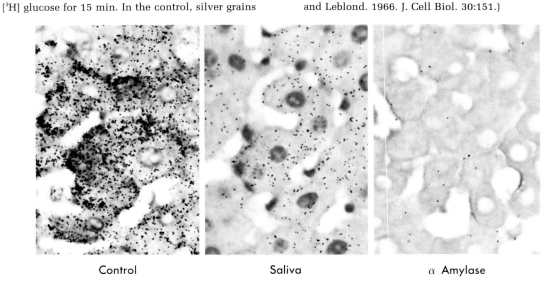

Control   Saliva   α Amylase

and TSH. At the ultrastructural level carbohydrate macromolecules may be detected by oxidation with periodic acid followed by silver methenamine as a substitute for the Schiff reagent, which yields a final reaction product of sufficient electron opacity.

A further easily-made characterization of a carbohydrate-rich substance is the determination of its degree of basophilia, such as the strong basophilia caused by the heparin (Fig. 2–7) of mast cell granules. The presence of sulfate groups or sialic acid in glycosaminoglycan confers a distinct basophilia in appropriately fixed material. Glycans with polyanionic groups can also be identified by staining with Alcian blue. Sialoglycans can be removed from the tissue section by digestion with neuraminidase.

The Feulgen Reaction for DNA

A highly specific reaction for the cytochemical localization of DNA also permits quantitative estimation by microspectrophotometry. The specificity is derived from the presence in DNA of a unique sugar, deoxyribose. The Feulgen procedure involves the hydrolytic removal of the purine groups by *mild* acid hydrolysis (Fig. 2–5). The furanose ring of deoxyribose thus opens and forms an aldehyde group that reacts with the Schiff reagent. A magenta-colored product marks the locus of DNA. One control for this test involves predigestion of the section with deoxyribonuclease; this control preparation is then stained in parallel with a standard preparation. Comparing the two preparations allows the DNA to be identified.

Usually the Feulgen-positive material is basophilic, but in some instances the high isoelectric point of the proteins (protamine) associated with the DNA competes with the cationic dye and prevents expression of basophilia. Although mitochondria contain DNA, the amount is too low for the sensitivity of these procedures.

Sudanophilia of Lipids

The most common cellular lipids are triglycerides and phospholipids. Triglycerides are metabolic reserves that occur as cytoplasmic droplets; their fluctuations within a tissue can be followed cytochemically. Phospholipids are structural

2–14 Sudan IV; representative fat-soluble dye.

components of membranes and thus are difficult to localize cytochemically. To avoid the extraction of lipids that occurs in the routine paraffin technique, lipids are often localized in frozen sections.

A widely used procedure for localizing lipids is based on the properties of the Sudan dyes. These dyes will dissolve in droplets containing triglycerides and will color them intensely. These lipid "stains" are weakly ionizable and hence can be dissolved only in nonaqueous media (Fig. 2–14). The carrier for the Sudan dye is an organic solvent in which lipids are relatively insoluble, such as 70% ethanol or propylene glycol. Because the dye is less soluble in this carrier than in lipids, "staining" occurs with substances in which the dye is partitioned, as in a separatory funnel. Stained sections are mounted in water-soluble medium (glycerol) to avoid extraction of either the dye or the lipid. Sudanophilia therefore depends on solubility rather than salt formation or the reactivity of certain end groups.

Sudan black is widely used because of its color and its ability to demonstrate lipoprotein structures such as mitochondria and myelin. Structures containing polymerized lipids (e.g., lipofuscin granules) are also stained with Sudan dyes, but crystallized lipids cannot be colored. One type of control preparation consists of lipid extraction before staining with an organic solvent such as acetone or chloroform plus methanol. Such extraction will remove triglycerides and cholesterol but not the phospholipids. Another important control is based on the extraction of the Sudan dye from the stained tissue section by excess solvent; this procedure identifies the presence of any chemical binding.

Special techniques are available for localizing cholesterol and other lipids. For a critical discussion of the cytochemistry of lipids at the light-microscopic level, see the review by Deane (1958).

Specific Proteins: Enzymes, Antigens, and Antibodies

The inherent specificity of an enzyme for its substrate or of an antibody for its antigen constitutes the basis for precise cytochemical localizations. A colored reaction product or a fluorescent or other label is needed for a light-microscopic localization. Visualization with the electron microscope, however, requires an electron-opaque product, such as one containing a heavy metal. Furthermore, the great resolving power of the electron microscope demands reaction products be composed of exceedingly fine particles, ideally as close as possible to the limit of resolution.

Enzymatic Activity

In cytochemical localizations, the enzyme itself is not directly visualized; instead a visible reaction product, which is formed as a result of catalytic activity, marks the site of activity.

Here, in simple fashion, is a typical cytochemical reaction for hydrolases and oxidoreductases: AB is the *substrate*, which undergoes an enzyme-catalyzed reaction to $A + B$. In the presence of R, a reagent capable of precipitating one of the products of the enzymatic reaction (in this case A), an insoluble complex AR is formed:

$$AB \xrightarrow[R]{\text{enzyme}} AR\downarrow + B$$

The initial insoluble complex AR may itself be colored or electron-opaque and hence may be readily visualized, or it may be insoluble but invisible and must be converted secondarily to a precipitate visible in microscopes. During incubation, conditions favorable for enzymatic activity—proper pH, ionic composition, and temperature—are maintained as closely as is compatible with the requirements for visualizing the product.

Because most fixatives inhibit enzymatic activity to some degree, the choice of fixative is critical. Enzymes vary in their sensitivity to fixation as well as in their solubility; these properties present problems to the cytochemist. To avoid denaturation and other inhibition, frozen sections of fresh tissue are prepared, usually in a cryostat (a refrigerated chamber held usually at -15 to $-20°C$ and containing a microtome). The frozen sections are incubated in an appropriate medium for demonstrating enzymatic activity. Usually the activity of fixed and unfixed sections is compared. Fixation is generally necessary, particularly at the ultrastructural level, to preserve the macromolecular structure during the subsequent cytochemical processing. Aldehydic fixatives such as formalin or glutaraldehyde are most frequently used, the latter being especially effective for dual preservation of cellular structure and protein reactivity.

As representatives of this principle of histochemistry, two examples will be cited: the Gomori procedure for phosphatases and a method for a pyridine nucleotide–dependent dehydrogenase.

Phosphatases

A versatile cytochemical approach for localizing phosphatase activity was introduced by Gomori in 1939. Phosphatases hydrolyze the ester linkages of natural organic phosphates (e.g., ATP, glucose-6-phosphate, or glycerophosphate) and liberate phosphate ions as one of the reaction products (Fig. 2–15). The released phosphate ions are then trapped, ideally at the site of the enzyme, by either lead or calcium ions to form a relatively insoluble primary reaction product, lead or calcium phosphate, that is colorless. Therefore, for light microscopy, lead phosphate is customarily converted to lead sulfide, which is black (see Fig. 2–17). However, the interference and the phase-contrast microscopes can be used to detect the primary reaction product. For electron microscopy, the second step is unnecessary because the lead phosphate itself is electron-opaque (Figs. 2–16, 2–17, and 2–18). Calcium phosphate is converted in a two-step reaction to cobalt sulfide, a brown-black precipitate for light-microscopic study. The Gomori principle is thus termed metal-salt visualization.

2–15 The Gomori acid-phosphatase reaction, pH 5.0, performed in two steps. The first yields lead phosphate, the second, lead sulfide, both of which are insoluble reaction products visible in light or electron microscopes (consult text).

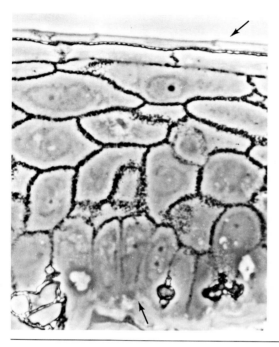

2–16 ATPase activity of the frog epidermis. In this photomicrograph, the shapes of the cells making the stratified squamous epithelium are evident because the lead sulfide reaction product, which reflects ATPase activity, is located at most cell boundaries. It is absent, however, from the free and basal surfaces of the epithelium (see **arrows**). Dendritic portions of pigment cells are also reactive in the deeper layers of the epidermis. Glutaraldehyde-fixed tissue, incubation in a Gomori-type medium for ATPase activity at pH 7.2, postfixation in OsO_4, araldite section 1 μm treated with (NH_4) S to produce PbS. $\times$ 900. (From Farquhar and Palade. 1966. J. Cell Biol.30:359.)

2–17 Radioautographic localization of the site of Na^+ $-K^+$ ATPase (N^+ pump sites) in frog epidermis. The distribution of this phosphatase activity within stratified squamous epithelium was identified by exposing fresh frog skin to a radioactive inhibitor, [^{3}H] ouabain, which binds specifically to this enzyme. Note that the silver grains occur along cell surfaces facing the intercellular compartment of this epithelium. This localization correlates well with that of epidermal ATPase activity shown in Figs. 2–16 and 2–18. **Ger,** germative layer; **Sp,** spinosal layer; **Gr,** granular layer; **MR,** macrophage. (From Mills, J. W., Ernst, S. A., and DiBona, D. R., 1977. J. Cell Biol. 73:88–110)

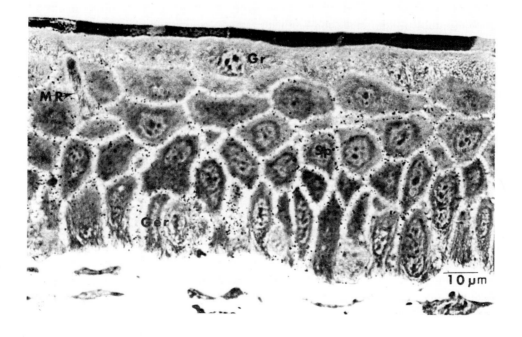

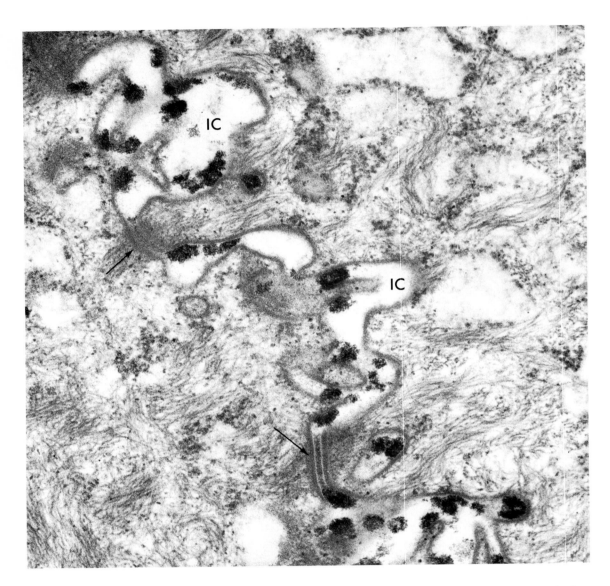

2–18 Electron micrograph of the junction of two
cells of the stratum corneum (compare with
Fig. 2–17). Lead phosphate deposits occur as
aggregates of small particles (approximately 50 Å),
which are located irregularly along the apposed
cellular surfaces as well as in the intercellular spaces
(IC). No reaction product occurs at the site of the
desmosome **(arrow).** Fixation in glutaraldehyde,
incubation in a Gomori-type medium for ATPase
activity at pH 7.2, postfixation in OsO₄, and
embedding in araldite. × 72,000. (From Farquhar and
Palade. 1966. J. Cell Biol. 30:359.)

This rationale permits localization of phosphatases over a wide range of pH. Below pH 8,
lead is the trapping ion. Although lead is useful
for both light and electron microscopy, it tends
to combine with hydroxyl ions above pH 8 and
precipitates from the medium; thus calcium is
used as the capture agent above pH 8. To localize
acid phosphatase, which has a pH optimum
near 5, the incubating medium would contain
the substrate (for example, glycerophosphate),
buffer (for example, tris maleate), and lead ion as
the capture reagent (Figs. 2–15 and 2–18). The
morphological identification of lysosomal derivatives rests heavily on this ultrastructural cytochemical demonstration of the presence of acid

phosphatase. In contrast, the muscle protein myosin has ATPase activity with an alkaline pH optimum; thus, frozen sections are incubated with ATP, barbital buffer (pH 9), and calcium ion as the capture agent. Phosphatases with a pH optimum near 7, (glucose-6-phosphatase) can be demonstrated by suitable adjustment of buffer and substrate. In addition, known activators can be incorporated to enhance catalysis and specificity.

The Gomori procedure is used widely in ultrastructural localizations because it yields an electron-opaque, lead-containing reaction product. The high resolving power of the electron microscope carries a more stringent requirement for morphological preservation than that needed at the light-microscopic level. It became apparent in initial attempts at ultrastructural cytochemistry that osmium tetroxide, although an excellent preserver of ultrastructure and a creator of contrasting densities, is a potent inhibitor of enzymes. To circumvent this problem, double fixation is employed. Initial fixation by glutaraldehyde preserves ultrastructure while retaining the reactive groups of many enzymes, antibodies, and other proteins (Sabatini et al., 1963). Then a cytochemical demonstration, such as that of the Gomori procedure, is performed, preferably on tissue slices. Such aldehyde-fixed tissues tend, however, to be too low in contrast for morphological examination; thus a second fixation with osmium tetroxide is performed to create the usual density contrasts associated with the ultrastructural image (Fig. 2–18).

Generally the specificity of enzymatic localization and identification is greatest for enzymes that are tightly bound to cellular organelles, have a high substrate specificity, or are selectively inhibited or activated by certain compounds. Controls are required to ensure that the reaction product is a result of enzymatic activity and that its location accurately reflects the site of the enzyme. The most common control preparation is one in which the substrate has been omitted; a positive reaction here would signify the presence in vivo of metallic precipitates such as calcium or iron salts or nonspecific binding of the capture reagent. Diffusion of a reaction product to another locus is also a possibility that must be considered.

Hydrolases can also be demonstrated through the so-called azo-dye procedures, which depend on a different rationale. For example, phosphatase activity can be demonstrated by using an artificial substrate, such as naphthyl phosphate.

2–19 Azo-dye procedure for localizing alkaline phosphatase activity. The enzyme hydrolyzes the substrate, naphthyl phosphate, to yield α-naphthol and phosphate ion. The diazonium salt, fast blue RR, couples with the α-naphthol to yield a bright-colored insoluble azo-dye pigment. (From Barka, T., and Anderson, P. J. 1963. Histochemistry—Theory, Practice and Bibliography. New York: Paul B. Hoeber, Inc.)

The primary reaction products are naphthol and phosphate; but in this system the naphthol instead of the phosphate is visualized by precipitation with a chromogenic diazonium compound. An azo dye is thereby formed as the final reaction product. This reaction is illustrated in Fig. 2–19.

The azo-dye principle possesses considerable versatility because the synthesis of appropriate naphthyl substrates will yield new methods. Also, the coupling of the primary reaction product, α-napthol, with the diazonium salt allows localization of various enzymes over a wide pH range. It is used to demonstrate phosphatase, esterase, sulfatase, aminopeptidase, and β-glucuronidase activities as well as the —SH, —NH$_2$, and —COOH groups of proteins. Diazonium salts exist in considerable variety and are selected in relation to both the pH of the reaction and the desired color of the final azo-dye pigment. For additional information, consult Barka and Anderson (1963), Burstone (1962), and Pearse (1968, 1972).

Representative Oxidoreductase Reactions

This class of enzymes catalyzes the transfer of hydrogen and electrons. Many biological oxidations take place with loss of hydrogen and elec-

2–20 Reduction of a soluble tetrazolium salt to its formazan, which is insoluble in aqueous solution and is colored. R is a substituted phenolic radical.

trons and without the addition of oxygen; the enzymes catalyzing such oxidations are called *dehydrogenases*. *Tetrazolium salts* provide the basis for the principal methodology for localizing dehydrogenases. Such compounds are nearly colorless, water-soluble substances that become insoluble and colored forazans upon reduction (Fig. 2–20).

The chemical reduction of tetrozoles requires quite vigorous reducing agents acting at high pH and temperature; but, in the presence of specific enzymes and substrates, the reaction proceeds at biological temperature and pH. When substrates are oxidized in vivo, hydrogen ions and electrons are transferred through a pyridine nucleotide coenzyme (NAD or NADP) to cytochrome c and from there through the electron-transport chain to oxygen. In the histochemical procedure, the tetrazolium substitutes for cytochrome c. The enzyme that transfers hydrogen ions to the tetrazolium from the reduced pyridine nucleotide is

2–21 Production of a formazan deposit as the end result of the exidation of sodium L-lactate, with nicotinamide–adenine dinucleotide (NAD) serving as the coenzyme.

called a diaphorase, or more specifically in the histochemical reaction, a tetrazolium reductase.

A representative reaction, using lactate as the initial hydrogen donor, a pyridine nucleotide coenzyme (NAD) as the initial hydrogen acceptor, and a tetrazolium salt as the final acceptor, involves a minimum of two linked enzymes, lactate–NAD oxidoreductase (lactase dehydrogenase) and $NADH_2$–tetrazolium reductase (diaphorase) (Fig. 2–21). Thus, histochemically, the activity of the second, not the primary, enzyme is being demonstrated, although the primary one is necessary for obtaining reduced coenzyme.

The reaction in which $NADH_2$ itself is supplied as substrate may be used to demonstrate the locations of the $NADH_2$–cytochrome c reductases. The insoluble dehydrogenases, those capable of being reliably visualized, reside in mitochondria and, in some cell types, also in the endoplasmic reticulum.

Control procedures to confirm the enzymatic nature of the reaction and to establish that the provided substrate is the source of the hydrogen ions include (1) inactivation by pretreatment with heat or an —SH reagent such as p-chloromercuribenzoate (since like most dehydrogenases, lactate dehydrogenase is —SH-dependent); and (2) omission of the primary substrate or of the coenzyme from the incubation medium. Control preparations to confirm the location of the enzyme are more complex, especially in this example, where the second of two enzymes is being localized.

A major problem in the use of tetrazoles in histochemistry has been the frequency of false localization of the formazans because of their solubility in lipids. This difficulty is largely overcome by substituting additional water-soluble radicals on tetrazolium salts to render their formazans virtually insoluble in lipids. Tetrazoles with highly insoluble formazans composed of fine particles are used to localize enzymatic activity with the electron microscope.

Because oxidative metabolism of nutrients provides energy, diaphorase reaction is of key importance for many biological processes. Many of the oxidative enzymes are located within mitochondria. Other methods using tetrazoles as hydrogen ion acceptors from oxidative enzymes are those for the succinate oxidase system (Fig. 2–22) and monoamine oxidase. These reactions do not require pyridine nucleotides as coenzymes. In addition, at high pH, tetrazoles can accept hydrogen ions from —SH and ketol groups.

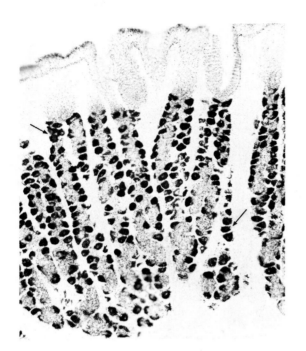

2–22 Succinic dehydrogenase activity, gastric glands
△   of the cat. This cryostat section was incubated
with succinate and neotetrazolium at pH 7.5 for 10
min. The diformazan deposits reveal various levels of
succinic dehydrogenase activity in the cells of the
gastric epithelium. The most reactive cells are the
parietal cells **(arrows)**, which have numerous
mitochondria. The mucous cells of the gastric surface
and pits are considerably less reactive. × 150.

The Visualization of Enzymatic and Nonenzymatic Hemoproteins

An important research tool in cell physiology
was introduced by Werner Straus (1957) when
he administered intravenously an exogenous enzyme, horseradish peroxidase (HRP, an oxygen
transferase that is a hemoprotein), to trace the
pathway of protein absorption in the kidney. To
identify the location of the tracer, its peroxidase
activity was demonstrated at the light-microscopic level by incubating tissue sections with
the substrate hydrogen peroxide H_2O_2 and the reagent benzidine, which upon oxidation yields a
blue color. Graham and Karnovsky (1966) provided ultrastructural visibility by substituting
benzidine with 3,3'-diaminobenzidine (DAB)
(Fig. 2–23), which upon oxidation yields an in-

2–23 The DAB procedure for demonstrating
         peroxidase activity. Hypothetical reaction for
the peroxidative or oxidative polymerization of DAB
as a consequence of the catalytic action of the
hemoprotein enzyme HRP. The oxidation of DAB
results in the formation of insoluble, colored
indamine polymers at the site of peroxidase activity.
The indamine polymer may also cyclize to form the
phenazine polymer. Visibility of these polymers with
the electron microscope is dependent on their
osmiophilia. Osmication results in the formation of
discrete, electron-opaque osmium black chelator.
(Courtesy of J. S. Hanker.) ▽

Diaminobenzidine (DAB)

Indamine polymer   Phenazine polymer

Osmium Block

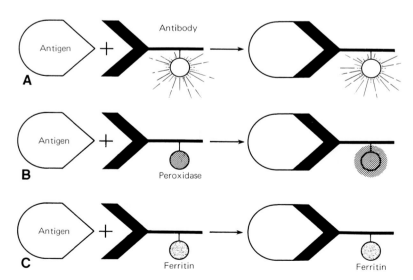

2–24 Diagram representing the reduction of a nonenzymic hemoprotein, cytochrome *c*, by DAB (top left). Oxidized polymeric products of DAB (lower left) after osmication (see Fig. 2–23) have been localized along the inner mitochondrial membrane through electron microscopy. Reduced cytochrome *c* is oxidized by O_2 through the action of cytochrome oxidase. (From Hanker, J. S. 1976. *In* Barnett, R. J. (ed.), Symposium in Electron Cytochemistry: Electron Microscopy Society of America, 32nd Annual Meeting. New York: John Wiley & Sons, Inc.)

soluble, highly colored polymeric indamine or phenazine polymers that are osmiophilic (Fig. 2–23). In the HRP reaction the DAB serves as the donor of two electrons to hydrogen peroxide. Subsequent osmication of the polymers yields a distinct electron-opaque reaction product called osmium black. Variations and limitations of the procedure are described by Essner (1974) and Hanker (1976).

The procedure involving oxidative polymerization of DAB has been used effectively to iden-

tify ultrastructurally the pathway of protein transport in a variety of cellular systems. This principle can be used to localize endogenous hemoproteins, both enzymic and nonenzymic (catelase of peroxisomes, mitochondrial cytochrome *c* and cytochrome oxidase, hemoglobin, and myoglobin). Most hemoproteins contain the iron porphyrin prosthetic group, which has peroxidatic activity, as illustrated for cytochrome *c* in Fig. 2–24.

The significance of the DAB procedure rests primarily on its effectiveness in immunocytochemical identifications of exogenous or endogenous proteins (see Fig. 2–25 and the next section).

Immunocytochemistry: Antigens and Antibodies

The high specificity within the mutual recognition between an antigen and its antibody provides potential for highly precise cytochemical identifications and localizations. *Immunocytochemistry is based on the use of specific antibodies as reagents for localizing cellular and extracellular molecular constituents.* Antibody, used as a cytochemical reagent, carries a label that can be visualized in light and electron microscopes. This powerful approach was introduced by Albert H. Coons who, in essence, adapted immunological procedures for use with tissue sections.

Initially immunocytochemistry was applied to analyses of the immune response in order to

2–25 Direct method for identifying antigens in tissue sections. An antigen can be localized by "staining" with its specific antibody labeled for visualization with light and/or electron microscopes. **A,** fluorescent dye visible in the ultraviolet microscope; **B,** enzymic label (peroxidase here) identifiable with light and electron microscopes by reaction products formed as a result of enzymic activity; **C,** electron-opaque label with distinctive ultrastructure for electron-microscopic localization. (From Junqueira, L. C., and Caneiro, J. 1980. Basic Histology. Los Altos, Calif.: Lange Medical Publications.)

identify the cells throughout the body that were involved in binding exogenous antigens or in producing antibodies to them. The significance of immunocytochemistry now extends beyond study of the immune response to the feasibility of localizing *endogenous proteins (or haptens)*. If an endogenous protein can be highly purified to serve as a valid antigen for the preparation of specific antibody, then its in situ location can be determined through immunocytochemistry. As examples, note the localization of various contractile proteins (Chapter 7), the cellular origin of the protein hormones of the anterior pituitary (Chapter 29), and maps of the antigenicity of cell surfaces.

The antigen–antibody reaction is usually performed with frozen sections in which the fixation has been modulated to precipitate the protein framework of cells and tissues without destroying antigenic determinants. Fixation changes native protein structure to a varying degree, and this creates some technical limitation.

The basic rationale for the "staining" procedure is derived from Coons's original investigation in which a fluorescent dye was conjugated in vitro with an antibody, thus labeling it without destroying the ability to form an immune complex with its antigen (Fig. 2–25). This basic procedure is widely used in cellular analysis. Fluorescent dyes, such as fluorescein and rhodamine, emit greenish or reddish color, respectively, which can be distinguished from the bluish autofluorescence of nucleic acids and certain proteins. The localization of the antigen–antibody fluorescent reaction is identified in an ultraviolet microscope. Fewer molecules of a fluorescent dye than of visible dye are required for visual detection, a property that endows immunofluorescence with greater sensitivity.

For electron microscopy, the antigen–antibody reaction is performed after the sections have been fixed with an aldehyde. Osmication occurs after the in vitro immune complex has been formed. Because electron opacity is required for visualization, antibodies are most commonly labeled with HRP or other enzymes (e.g., alkaline phosphatase) that yield electron-opaque reaction products, or with ferritin (ferric hydroxide micelles in a tetrahedral lattice create electron opacity and characteristic ultrastructure) (Fig. 2–25).

If protein *X* is to be localized within a tissue, it must first be isolated and purified to form a

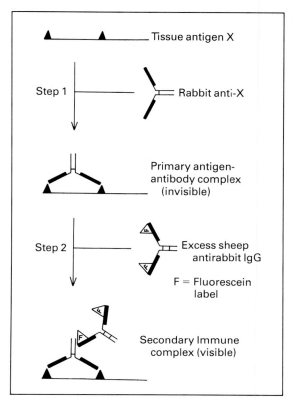

2–26 Basic principle of the indirect method for identifying antigen in tissue sections. This diagram illustrates the two-step procedure used for light-microscope identifications with ultraviolet light. See text for explanation. For electron-microscopic visualization, the labeling procedure is adapted to produce an electron-opaque reaction product. (Modified from Sternberger, L. A. 1979. Immunocytochemistry. 2nd ed. New York: John Wiley & Sons.)

suitable antigen that will stimulate synthesis of a specific antibody (usually IgG) when injected into a rabbit. In the *direct method* (Fig. 2–25), this specific antibody in rabbit antiserum is labeled with a fluorescent dye or other tag for application to sections where the antigen exists in the organized framework of the tissue.

Antigens in tissue sections are more commonly identified by an *indirect method* (Fig. 2–26) because the small amount of available specific primary antibody (antiserum) is usually a limiting factor in the "staining" procedure. The primary reaction (step 1) in the indirect method involves exposing tissue sections to *unlabeled* rabbit antibody. This exposure causes the for-

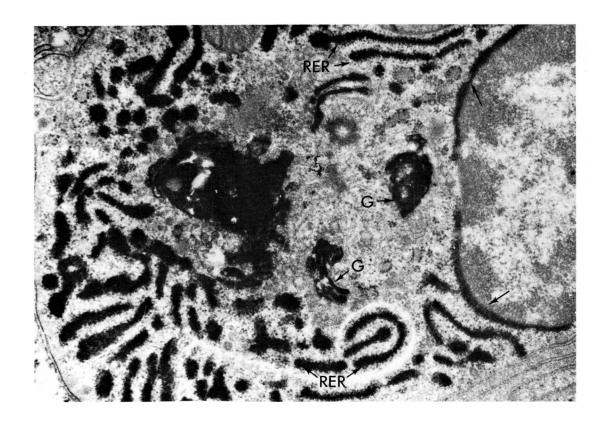

2–27 Ultrastructural localization of an antienzyme antibody produced in response to the injection of HRP, which binds specifically to its antibody. The DAB procedure of Graham and Karnovsky was used to visualize the enzymic activity of the antibody-attached HRP; the reaction product was then rendered electron-opaque by OsO_4, as shown in Fig. 2–23. In this immature plasma cell, antibody is located within the cisternae of the rough endoplasmic reticulum **(RER)** (including the perinuclear cisterna [see **arrow**], and also within the cisternae of the Golgi complex **(G).** × 23,000. (From Leduc, E. H., and Avrameas, S. 1970. Sandoz J. Med. Sci. 9:200.)

mation of an invisible antigen–antibody complex. The second step is based on the production of labeled secondary antibody to the primary antibody. An important point is that *the antibody in the primary reaction acts as an antigen in the secondary reaction.* This state is accomplished if the primary antibody is injected into another species, usually sheep, to produce a large amount of antiserum (antiimmunoglobulin G). This secondary antibody is labeled for visibility (fluorescent dye, HRP, or ferritin) and usually

can be used to detect various primary antibodies in a single species. Applied to tissue sections, it will combine with unoccupied antigenic sites in the primary immune complex and thus make it visible. This secondary reaction increases the sensitivity of the immunocytochemical demonstration considerably, probably because the secondary antiserum is richer in antibody than the primary antiserum.

From this brief account it is evident that stringent control procedures are mandatory to establish specificity of the immunocytochemical staining. For example, the immunocytochemical staining reaction should be blocked by exposure of the tissue sections to unlabeled antibody before using the labeled antibody. The specificity of the reaction depends heavily on the degree of cross-reactivity of the antibodies. Ludwig Sternberger's monograph (1979) on immunocytochemistry should be consulted for an authoritative overview of this methodology, its applications, and appropriate control experiments.

Immunocytochemical analysis of *antibody production* in vivo may be performed with antigens—such as ferritin or horseradish peroxidase

(HRP) (Fig. 2–27)—that are identifiable by microscopy. After the injection—of such an antigen into the footpad of a rabbit, specific antibody (antiferritin or antiHRP) is produced by plasma cells in the popliteal lymph node. Exposure of tissue sections of this lymph node to the appropriate antigen, ferritin or HRP, leads to the formation of an antibody–antigen immune complex. The immune complex formed by ferritin is directly visible in the electron microscope because of the characteristic tetrahedral ultrastructure of the ferritin molecule. The HRP-containing immune complex is visualized through the DAB reaction (Fig. 2–17 and 2–23) described above.

Radioautography

Radioautography (autoradiography) is a cytochemical procedure for localizing sites of radioactivity within biological specimens, usually by using tissue sections. An animal is injected with a biologically important molecule labeled with a radioactive isotope (usually tritium, (^{3}H), an isotope of hydrogen that emits particles of low energy and thus short range). For example, [^{3}H] thymidine is injected to label DNA for a study of cellular origin and turnover; to investigate protein synthesis, a tritiated amino acid is used; or for a study of glycogen synthesis, [^{3}H]·glucose serves as the precursor for this carbohydrate macromolecule (Fig. 2–13). After appropriate intervals, the animal is sacrificed and tissue sec-

tions are prepared for light and electron microscopy. Such radioactive precursors are rapidly incorporated into macromolecules that can be readily preserved in tissue sections. Then, in a darkroom, a very thin layer of photographic emulsion (suspension of silver halide crystals in gelatin) is placed on top of the tissue section (Fig. 2–28). During the subsequent period of exposure, β particles are emitted from the sites of radioactivity; some of these particles pass through the photographic emulsion and hit some of the silver halide crystals to produce a latent image (that is, small sites within a crystal where ionic silver is converted to metallic silver). After an appropriate interval of exposure, chemical development is used to convert the entire silver halide crystal that has been hit by β particles into metallic silver (true image). Finally, the unexposed crystals are dissolved out as silver thiosulfate complexes by the photographic fixer.

2–28 Diagram of a radioautographic preparation for electron microscopy. **Top:** A β particle emanating from a tritium source within a tissue section hits a silver halide crystal in the overlying gelatin photographic emulsion. This exposure creates a latent image in that crystal. **Bottom:** After photographic processing, the exposed crystal has been converted to a true image of metallic silver (developed grain) whereas the unexposed crystals have been dissolved out by the hypo solution. (Courtesy of L. G. Caro.)

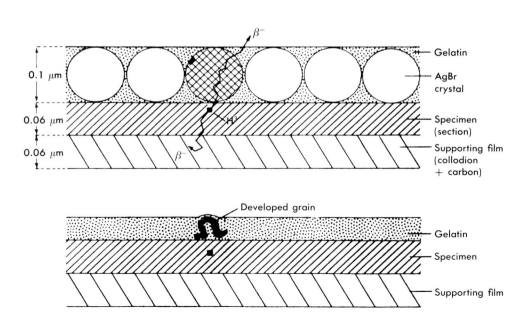

The reaction product is a pattern of metallic silver grains (Fig. 2–13) that localizes the position of the isotope. A resolution of 0.1 μm can be achieved under good conditions, and this is certainly adequate for light microscopy. In the ultrastructural image, however, precise localization requires statistical analysis, because 0.1 μm can include a variety of structures. Resolution is influenced by geometric factors such as section and emulsion thickness, and also by the size of the silver halide crystal and the resulting developed grain.

Dynamic aspects of cellular and tissue morphology can be followed through radioautography, and many important concepts have been derived from such studies, only a few of which are noted here. Concepts of of epithelial replacement, as in the gastrointestinal tract, have evolved from labeling dividing cell populations and following their subsequent migration and differentiation. The first clue that galactosyl transferase might be an enzyme of the Golgi complex was obtained from the radioautographic observation that [³H] galactose is incorporated in the Golgi region of intestinal goblet cells (Neutra and Leblond, 1966). The site of macromolecular synthesis and the subsequent path of migration can be traced by ultrastructural radioautography (for example, the synthesis, storage, and secretion of digestive enzymes by the pancreatic acinar cell) (Caro and Palade).

References and Selected Bibliography

Barka, T., and Anderson, P. J. 1963. Histochemistry—Theory, Practice, and Bibliography. New York: Paul B. Hoeber, Inc.

Bergeron, J. A., and Singer, M. 1958. Metachromasy: An experimental and theoretical reevaluation. J. Biophys. Biochem. Cytol. 4:443.

Burstone, M. S. 1962. Enzyme Histochemistry and Its Application in the Study of Neoplasms. New York: Academic Press, Inc.

Caro, L. G. 1964. High resolution autoradiography. In Prescott, D. M. (ed.), Methods in Cell Physiology, vol. 1, chap. 16. New York: Academic Press, Inc.

Caro, L. G., and Palade, G. E. 1964. Protein synthesis, storage, and discharge in the pancreatic exocrine cell. A radiographic study. J. Cell Biol. 20:473.

Conn, H. J. 1977. Biological Stains, 9th ed. Baltimore, Maryland: Williams & Wilkins.

Coons, A. H. 1959. Some reactions of lymphoid tissues to stimulation by antigens. Harvey Lectures, Series L111, p. 113.

Deane, H. W. 1958. Intracellular lipids: Their detections and significance. In Palay, S. L. (ed.), Frontiers in Cytology. New Haven, Connecticut: Yale University Press.

Essner, E. 1974. Hemoproteins. In Hayat, M. A. (ed.), Electron Microscopy of Enzymes: Princeton University Press.

Gomori, G. 1952. Microscopic Histochemistry. Chicago: University of Chicago Press.

Graham, R. C., and Karnovsky, M. H. 1966. The early stages of absorption of injected horseradish peroxidase in the proximal tubules of mouse kidney: Ultrastructural cytochemistry by a new technique. J. Histochem. Cytochem. 14:291.

Hanker, J. S. 1976. Catalytic osmiophilic polymer generation in the demonstration of membrane-bound enzymes and ultrastructural tracers in cytochemistry. In Barnett, R. J. (ed.), Symposium in Electron cytochemistry: Electron Microscopy Society of America, 32nd Annual Meeting. New York: John Wiley & Sons., Inc.

Kasten, F. H. 1960. The chemistry of Schiff's reagent. Int. Rev. Cytol. 10:1.

Leduc, E. H., Avrameas, S., and Bouteille, M. Localization of antibody in plasma cells by electron microscopy. J. Exp. Med. 127:109.

Nakane, P. K. 1970. Classifications of anterior pituitary cell types with immunoenzyme histochemistry. J. Histochem Cytochem. 18:9.

Nakane, P. K., and Pierce, G. B., Jr. 1967. Enzyme-labeled antibodies for the light and electron microscopic localization of tissue antigens. J. Cell Biol. 33:307.

Neutra, M., and Leblond, C. P. 1966. Synthesis of the carbohydrate of mucus in the Golgi complex, as shown by electron microscopic radioautography of goblet cells from rats injected with glucose·H³. J. Cell Biol. 30:119.

Pearse, A. G. E. 1968 and 1972. Histochemistry—Theoretical and Applied. 3rd ed., vols. 1 and 2. Boston: Little Brown and Company.

Sabatini, D. D., Bensch, K., and Barrnett, R. J. 1963. Cytochemistry and electron microscopy. The preservation of cellular ultrastructure and enzymatic activity by aldehyde fixation. J. Cell Biol. 17:19.

Salpeter, M. M., and Bachmann, L., and Salpeter, E. E. 1969. Resolution in electron microscope radioautography. J. Cell Biol. 41:1.

Singer, M. Factors which control the staining of tissue sections with acid and basic dyes. Int. Rev. Cytol. 1:211.

Sternberger, L. A. 1979. Immunocytochemistry, 2nd ed. New York: John Wiley & Sons.

Straus, W. 1957. Segregation of an intravenously injected protein by "droplets" of the cells of rat kidney. J. Biophys. Biochem. Cytol. 3:1037.

Swift, H. Cytochemical Techniques for nucleic acids. In Chargaff, E., and Davidson, J. N. (eds.), The Nucleic Acids, vol. 2. New York: Academic Press, Inc.

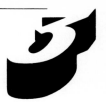

Epithelium

Eva Griepp and Edith Robbins

In multicellular organisms, individual cells are differentiated during development to perform specialized functions. Specialized cells frequently carry out their functions as multicellular aggregates of like cell types called *tissues*. Different tissues are combined in more elaborate structures called *organs*, which enable the efficient performance of complex functions.

In this chapter we shall consider *epithelium*, a tissue existing in a multiplicity of structural forms with a common role: to form continuous layers lining inner surfaces and covering outer surfaces throughout the body, or to secrete various substances, or both. Epithelial cells are held together by various membrane specializations called *junctions* and rest on an extracellular matrix called *basement membrane*; the epithelial tissues thus form a barrier between the structures underlying them and the environments confronting their free surfaces. Epithelial cells characteristically have a distinct polarity, expressed in the plasma membrane as differences in the composition of the free or *apical* surface, the *lateral* surfaces, and the *basal* surface (attached to the basement membrane), and also manifest in their internal organization, where a characteristic disposition of organelles often is found. Also, epithelial tissues lack large amounts of intercellular matrix or blood vessels between adjacent cells.

In some cases, such as in skin, the epithelial covering is mainly a protective barrier, but in many other instances, epithelial tissues serve in more complex functions, such as surface or transepithelial transport, absorption, and secretion.

Types of epithelia vary according to function: one type may have specialized structures on its free surface such as *cilia* for surface transport or *microvilli* for absorption; one may consist of a single layer of cells while another has many. The shape of the cells within different epithelia also varies, as do the characteristics and complexity of the junctions between cells. Not surprising, given the variety and ubiquity of epithelia, epithelial tissues can derive from all three embryonic germ layers: ectoderm, mesoderm, and endoderm.

Organs whose primary role is to secrete specific substances, either to a free surface *(exocrine glands)* or into the blood stream *(endocrine glands)*, are derived from and are considered epithelial tissues. Some general aspects of their organization will be considered. Only brief mention will be made of the role of epithelia in sensory perception; these specialized *neuroepithelia* such as the taste buds, olfactory epithelia, and retina are discussed in detail with their respective organs. We shall not consider the structure and function of specialized secretory cells found within epithelia but of different origins from the rest of the tissue, such as the melanocytes of the skin and the cells of the amine precursor uptake and decarboxylation (APUD) system; they are discussed elsewhere.

Epithelia are subject to stresses arising, for example, from mechanical trauma, changes in temperature, or contact with toxic substances. Therefore it is not surprising that epithelia have mechanisms for repair and renewal. The importance of understanding the mechanisms controlling the growth necessary for repair and renewal can readily be appreciated by considering that most malignant tumors—characterized by uncontrolled growth—are of epithelial origin. The means by which epithelial cells achieve and maintain polarity are also under active investigation: this is part of the more general inquiry into the mechanisms by which specialized domains of plasma membrane and specific sites of cytoplasmic localization of organelles come to exist.

Types of Epithelia

Epithelia have traditionally been classified according to two criteria: first, whether *simple*, consisting of one layer, or *stratified*, composed of several layers; and, second, whether the shape of the cells at the free surface is *squamous, cu-*

boidal, or *columnar*. Although this method of categorization is appealing, *stratified cubodial* and *stratified columnar* epithelia are rarely found (except in a few places during embryonic development, and at junctions between simple and stratified epithelia), and there are other significant epithelial types that are not easily classified according to this scheme. Three of these types are *pseudostratified columnar* epithelium, *transitional* epithelium, and *cytogenic* epithelium. Cytogenic epithelium lines the seminiferous tubules of the testis and will be considered with the male reproductive tract. Here, then, we shall consider (1) simple squamous epithelium, (2) simple cuboidal epithelium, (3) simple columnar epithelium, (4) stratified squamous epithelium, (5) pseudostratified columnar epithelium, and (6) transitional epithelium.

Simple Squamous Epithelium

Cells in simple squamous epithelium are very flat (often with the region of the nucleus creating a noticeable apical bulge), making them suitable for lining surfaces across which metabolites or gases must move rapidly (Fig. 3–1 and 3–2; see also Fig. 3–3). The *endothelium* of blood and lymphatic vessels is a simple squamous epithelium, as are the linings of the terminal air spaces, or alveoli, of the lungs (composed mostly of type I pneumocytes) and the *mesothelium* of the peritoneal cavity.

Simple Cuboidal Epithelium

Cuboidal cells, as the name suggests, are about as wide as they are tall (Fig. 3–3). They form some of the tubules and ducts of the kidney and also form ducts of other glands; they cover the choroid plexus and ciliary bodies and are active in absorption and secretion. Modified simple cuboidal epithelia are also prevalent in glands (see below). When glandular cells are grouped into small balls *(acini)* they are prismatic, or pyramidal, in appearance.

Simple Columnar Epithelium

Columnar cells are taller than they are wide and are the most strikingly polarized of the epithelia (Figs. 3–4, 3–5, and 3–6). Active in secretion, absorption or both, simple columnar epithelia form linings throughout the digestive tract, at various sites in the respiratory tract, in portions of the

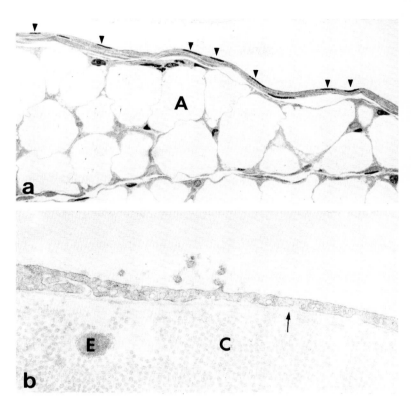

3–1 a. The simple squamous epithelium, called *mesothelium*, seen in this light micrograph covers the omentum and lines the peritoneal cavity. All that can be distinctly seen at this magnification are the nuclei of some mesothelial cells **(arrowheads).** The mesothelium rests on a basement membrane and underlying adipose tissue **(A).** × 400. **b.** Electron micrograph of a thin section of the attenuated cytoplasm of a mesothelial cell from the diaphragm of a mouse. **Arrow,** basal lamina; **E,** elastic fiber in cross section; **C,** collagen fibers in cross section. × 22,750.

female reproductive system, in the urinary system, and in the major ducts of many glands.

Stratified Squamous Epithelium

Stratified squamous epithelium is composed of a basal layer of germinative cells that are often cuboidal (Figs. 3–7 and 3–8). The basal cells give rise to several layers of more flattened cells above them, which are no longer in contact with the underlying basement membrane. Such a multilayered epithelium forms the outer layer of skin, where the most superficial cells become hard or *keratinized* (also called *cornified*) and all organelles, including nuclei, are no longer distinguishable. The family of proteins called *keratins* are present as important structural elements in most epithelial cells (Fig 3–26) and their derivatives (such as hair and sebaceous glands). However, some stratified squamous epithelia in which the surface cells remain nucleated, although also containing keratins, are called *nonkeratinized* stratified squamous epithelia. They are found in moist environments such as the mouth, esophagus, vagina, and cornea.

Pseudostratified Columnar Epithelium

Pseudostratified epithelia have nuclei situated at different levels, thus giving a multilayered impression (Fig. 3–9). But, in fact, all the cells maintain contact with the underlying basement membrane, although not all reach the free surface. Pseudostratified columnar epithelia are found in the trachea, bronchi and large bronchioles, and in parts of the male genitourinary tract. Pseudostratified epithelia are more common than truly stratified columnar epithelia, an example of which is shown in Fig. 3–10.

Transitional Epithelium

Transitional epithelium is found in the urinary tract where it lines the bladder, ureters, urethra, and the calyces of the kidney (Fig. 3–11 and 3–12). The cells of this epithelium vary dramatically in shape, from pyramidal or cuboidal to squamous, depending on how distended the structure is by the fluid it contains. In the empty bladder a stratified multilayered epithelium can be seen, but with maximal distension only two

112

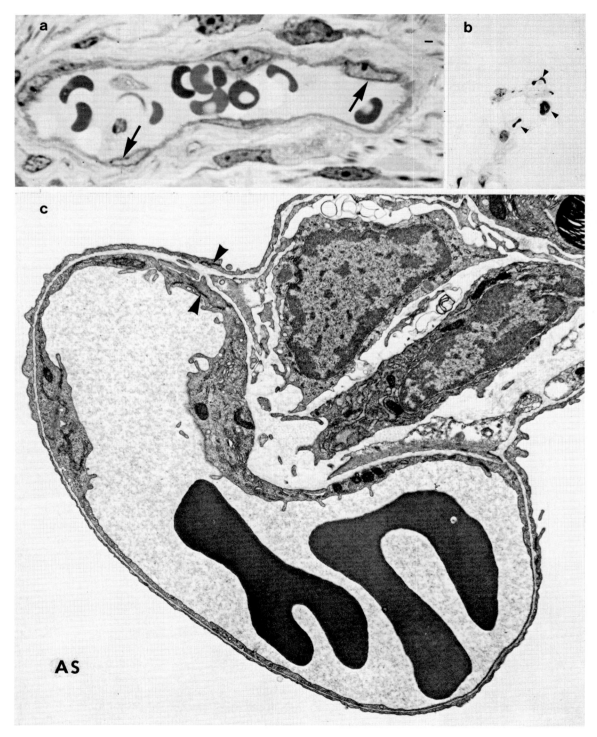

Figure 3–2

3–2 a. Light micrograph of the simple squamous epithelium, called *endothelium*, that lines all blood vessels. In this section of a small venule, **arrows** indicate the nuclei of two endothelial cells; the lumen of the vessel contains many red blood cells. × 1,600. **b.** Light micrograph of an interalveolar septum of the lung. The entire air space is covered by a simple squamous epithelium in close apposition to underlying capillaries lined by endothelium. These structures are so thin that the electron microscope is needed to show that the air–blood interface includes two cellular layers (see part c). **Arrowheads** indicate capillaries, which are identifiable because they contain dark-staining erythrocytes. × 600. **c.** Electron micrograph of a thin section of an interalveolar septum of rat lung. The endothelial cells, which form the inner lining of the capillary, and the simple squamous type I pneumocytes that line the alveolar space **(AS)** are separated from each other by a fused basement membrane. Cells of both of these simple squamous epithelia are extremely thin in the areas through which gas exchange occurs; nuclei are not included in this section (the nuclei in the upper portion of the photograph belong to connective tissue cells). The **arrowheads** indicate tight junctions, and within the lumen of the capillary are two erythrocytes. × 11,700. (From Schneeberger, E. 1978. Fed. Proc. 37:2471.)

3–3 Simple cuboidal epithelium of a bile duct **(D)** in the liver as seen in a light-microscopic section. The cells have fairly straight lateral borders, which allows the visualization of lateral cellular limits although individual plasma membranes are below the limit of resolution of the light microscope. Nuclei of endothelial cells are seen in an adjacent venule **(V).** × 400.

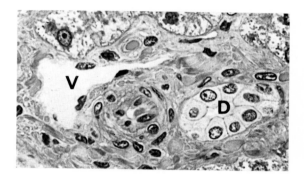

3–4 a. Cell shape is often more complex than the simple terms cuboidal or columnar imply. This diagram of a low columnar cell from the proximal convoluted tubule of the kidney illustrates the lateral and basal infoldings often seen in cells involved in water and ion transport. See Fig. 3–26 for an electron micrograph of the basal portion of such cells. (From Welling, D. J. 1979. Fed. Proc. 38.) **b.** Light micrograph of portions of cross sections of two proximal convoluted tubules in the guinea pig kidney. The lateral cell borders are indistinct because of the extensive infolding. The microvilli of the brush border **(arrow)** appear as a light zone on the apical surface of the cells. Compare with part a. × 1,480.

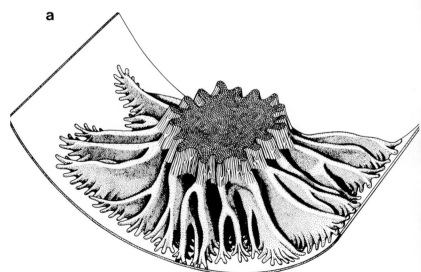

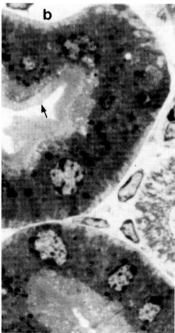

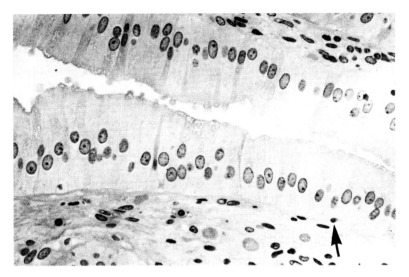

3–5 Light micrograph of simple columnar epithelium lining a monkey gallbladder. Occasional basal nuclei **(arrow)** usually belong to lymphocytes that infiltrate the epithelium. × 400.

3–6 a. A light-microscopic section of portions of two villi of monkey jejunum. The lining is composed of a simple columnar epithelium with some goblet cells. The columnar epithelial cells, but not the goblet cells, have a prominent brush (microvillous) border **(B)** and an underlying terminal web, which is visible as a dark line. Also recognizable are terminal bars and many lateral cell borders. × 400. **b** and **c.** Scanning electron micrographs of the simple columnar epithelium lining the mouse intestine. The orderly arrangement of these tall cells on the surface of the ridge and finger-like villi of this tissue makes the term "columnar" seem highly appropriate. In part b, microvilli are visualized on the free surface of the cells, and the lateral surface, which was exposed by breaking the tissue, can be seen to have multiple membrane folds. **B** indicates the basement membrane and underlying reticular extracellular matrix on which the cells rest. Part b, × 600; part c, × 6,600. (Courtesy of J. P. Revel.)

a

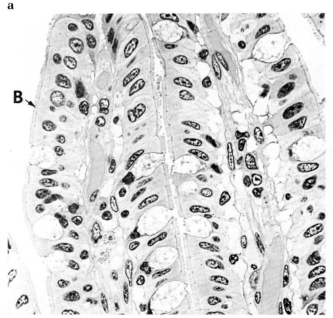

b

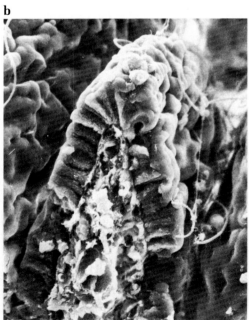

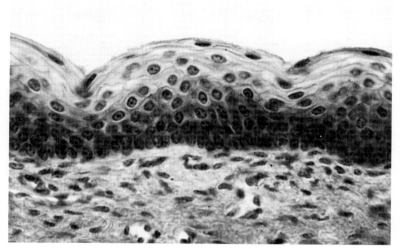

3–7 Light micrograph of nonkeratinized stratified squamous epithelium from the larynx of a rat. Note that cells retain identifiable nuclei up to the free surface. × 440.

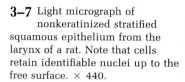

c

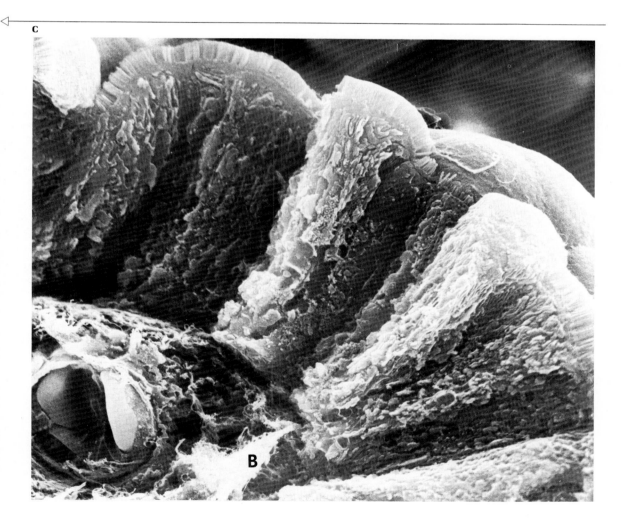

B

116

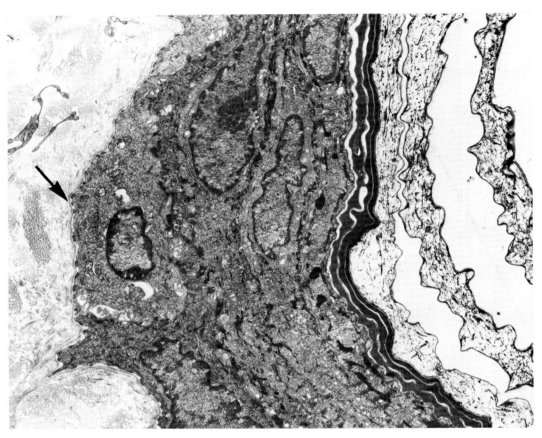

3–8 Low-power thin-section electron micrograph of stratified squamous epithelium of rat skin. Keratinized cells without nuclei are seen desquamating from the free surface. An **arrow** indicates the basal lamina. × 5,250. (Courtesy of Irene Brown.)

3–9 Light micrograph of pseudostratified ciliated columnar epithelium with goblet cells from the lining of monkey trachea. Goblet cells are not ciliated but appear so in this micrograph because of the slightly oblique sectioning. Polymorphonuclear leukocytes from the underlying connective tissue **(C.T.)** often infiltrate epithelia, and several are seen here **(arrows)**. In this epithelium all the cells contact the underlying basal lamina but their nuclei lie at different levels. This epithelium is usually composed of several different cell types as seen here. × 400.

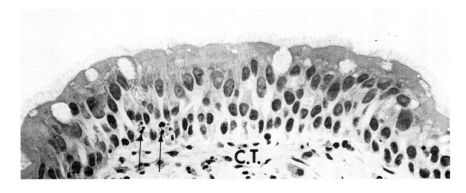

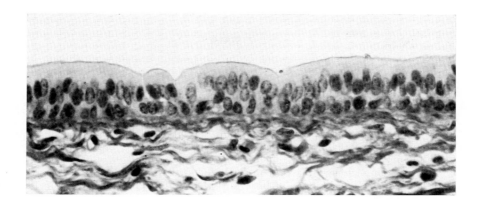

layers, a basal cuboidal and a surface squamous layer, are apparent. Study has shown that all the cells (perhaps even including those in the most superficial layer) may be anchored to the basement membrane via long, thick cytoplasmic processes (similar to the situation in pseudostratified columnar epithelia): these attachment sites allow the cells to align parallel to one another in the distended state, giving an impression of fewer layers overall. Unusual discoidal vesicles and infoldings of the plasmalemma are found in the apical cytoplasm of the most superficial cells; these differentiations of the apical membrane allow additional plasma membrane to be inserted or removed, thus allowing for the huge changes in surface area required of the epithelium during cycles of filling and emptying.

3–10 Stratified columnar epithelium of a major salivary gland duct as seen in a light-microscopic section. Stratified columnar epithelium is most often found in areas of transition between two different types of epithelium (as illustrated in Fig. 3–28). × 600.

3–11 Light micrograph of transitional epithelium lining the monkey ureter. In the relaxed state this epithelium is composed of a layer of basal cells, layers of pyriform cells, and surface cells which are often binucleate **(arrow).** The cells increase in size toward the surface, and one surface cell covers several pyriform cells. × 400.

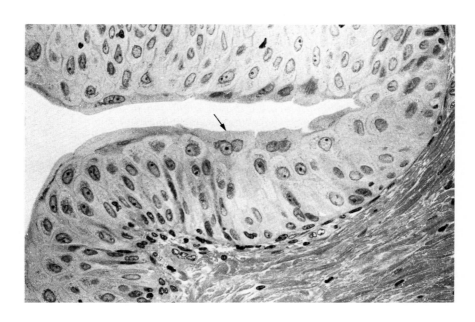

118

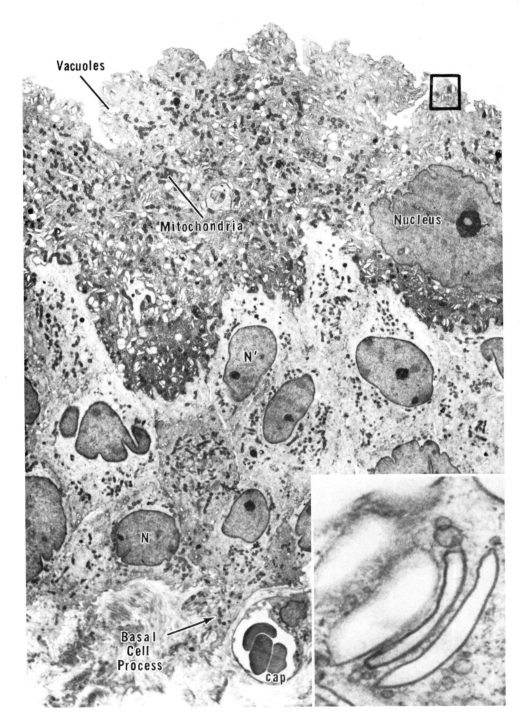

3–12 Electron micrograph of relaxed transitional epithelium lining the bladder of the mouse. The superficial cells have many mitochondria and a population of oblong vacuoles, several of which are seen at higher magnification in the **inset.** The nuclei of the pyriform **(N′)** and basal **(N)** cells are indicated. A capillary **(cap)** in the adjacent connective tissue is seen at bottom. × 1,600; inset, × 50,000. (Courtesy of J. Rhodin.)

The Polarity of Epithelial Cells

A striking and fundamental property of epithelial cells is their polarized organization, manifested not only by the characteristic locations of intracellular organelles, but also by the differential composition of the apical, lateral, and basal plasma membranes and by the special features associated with each (Fig. 3–13).

The Apical Membrane

In most epithelial cells, the membrane facing the free or luminal surface has a somewhat different complement of membrane proteins from that of the basal and lateral membranes. In the intestinal lining the apical membranes contain proteins such as *ligatin* that bind enzymes (for example, the disaccharidases, which hydrolyze sugars into absorbable monosaccharides). In kidney tubules the apical membrane is the locus of the enzymes alkaline phosphatase and leucine aminopeptidase, and the free surface plasmalemma of endothelial cells, especially in the lung, is the

site of a dipeptidase called the angiotensin converting enzyme. Many apical membrane proteins contain carbohydrate moieties that protrude from the free surface of the plasma membrane and contribute to the PAS-positive layer of apical

3–13 Surface-associated features of epithelial cells.
Not all cells have all of these structures. Some of these structures may be designated by special names, which originate from light-microscopic observations. (1) Microvilli may be irregular or regular. Regular microvilli and the glycocalyx constitute the *brush* or *striated* border. Beneath the microvilli is a region called the *terminal web*, in which microfilaments are concentrated. (2) The tight junction and subjacent zonula adherens are sometimes called the *terminal bar*. (3) The intercellular canaliculus is a space sealed by tight junctions that communicates with a free surface or lumen (see Fig. 3–19). (4) The basal lamina and subjacent reticular lamina are the *basement membrane* (see Fig. 3–23). (5) Basal infoldings and the associated mitochondria are called *basal striations*.

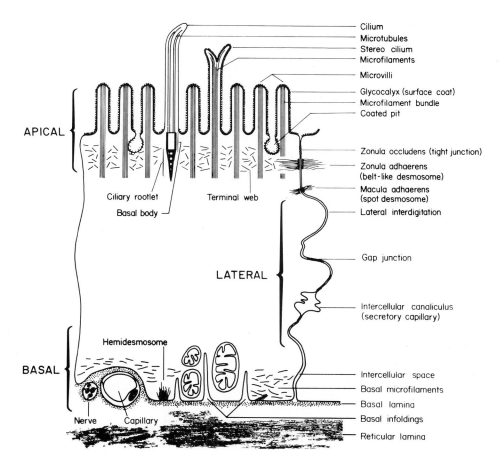

120

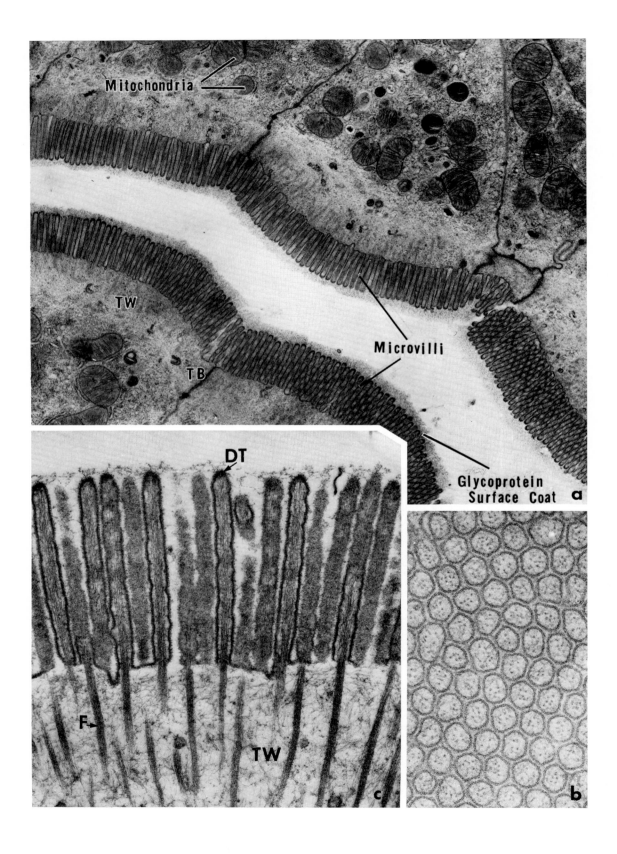

3–14 **a.** Thin section of the intestinal epithelium of the bat showing the glycoprotein coat (glycocalyx) at the apical surface of the microvillous border. **TW,** terminal web; **TB,** terminal bar. × 8,000. (Courtesy of S. Ito.) **b.** Electron-microscopic cross section of the brush border of a kidney proximal convoluted tubule cell (see Fig. 3–4). The glycocalyx is relatively thin and the cross-sectioned filamentous cores of the microvilli are clearly discernible. × 85,000. **c.** Thin section of the brush border of chicken intestinal epithelium illustrating the fine structure of microvilli. Each microvillus contains a bundle of actin filaments **(F),** which are anchored apically at the dense tip **(DT)** and basally in the terminal web region **(TW).** In some areas cross-bridges connecting the actin filaments to the membrane of the microvillus can be seen. × 52,000. (From Mooseker, M. 1975. J. Cell Biol. 67.)

⟸

membranes, also called the surface coat or *glycocalyx* (Fig. 3–14). In vascular endothelium, most apical membrane glycoproteins contain a terminal sialic acid residue that imparts a net negative charge to the luminal surface of the cells (this is true also of other epithelia). The negative charge contributes to the protective function of the endothelium by electrostatically repelling negatively charged platelets and other cells, thus preventing their attachment and the subsequent release or activation of plasma factors (such as complement) which can damage the endothelium and the underlying smooth muscle. In mucus-producing and other secretory cells like those found in the tracheobronchial tree and digestive tract (Fig. 3–6a), the release of secretory products, a process called *exocytosis*, takes place only at the apical aspect of the cell. Mucus may adhere to the epithelium, forming a thick viscous glycoprotein coat which protects against mechanical and chemical trauma, or it may be moved along the epithelial surface, trapping and removing unwanted foreign materials.

The apical membranes of some epithelial cells have unique structural features to aid in their specialized functions.

Microvilli. These small projections, found on the free surface of epithelial cells, are most numerous on those whose primary function is that of absorption or transepithelial transport. The presence of microvilli on these cells makes teleological sense, as microvilli greatly increase the surface area of membrane exposed to the lumen from which absorption is taking place. Microvilli are regular and abundant in the so-called *brush*

or *striated borders* of proximal renal tubules, the intestinal lining, and the syncytiotrophoblast of the placenta (Fig. 3–14; see also Fig. 3–20). The plasma membrane of microvilli is often associated with enzymes that facilitate absorptive functions, e.g., sugar phosphate hydrolases in the intestine, which convert disaccharides into monosaccharides.

In epithelial cells the bases of microvilli are the characteristic sites for invagination of membrane to form vesicles in which larger, nonabsorbable substances such as hemoglobin in the kidney or lipid micelles in the intestine can actively be transported into or across the epithelial layer. This process is usually called *endocytosis* (although where appropriate the term *transcytosis* can be used). It also occurs in cell types other than epithelia and often involves a protein called clathrin, which coats endocytic vesicles (Fig. 3–15). Clathrin baskets may also be involved in transport within cells, moving vesicles to the

3–15 **a.** Electron micrograph of a coated pit or developing endocytic vesicle forming from the plasma membrane of a liver cell. The cytoplasmic surface is enveloped by a "basket" composed of a protein called clathrin and possibly other proteins. × 34,000. **b.** The clathrin coat, in the form of hexagons and pentagons, can be best visualized by negative staining, as seen with these isolated vesicles from brain tissue. × ˙142,000. (Courtesy of C. DeLemos.)

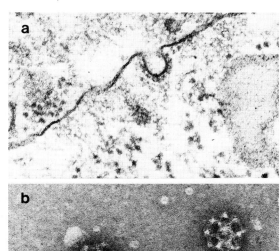

Golgi apparatus from the endoplasmic reticulum or from the Golgi to the plasmalemma.

The microvilli of the intestinal brush border have been observed to move in vivo. Although the exact nature and significance of the movement has not been determined, it is probably mediated by an interaction between actin and myosin. A bundle of actin filaments is anchored in the dense material at the tip of each microvillus. The bundle is connected by cross-bridges to the lateral plasma membrane and is also attached to the meshwork of filaments associated with the junctional region and the apical cytoplasm just below the microvilli known as the *terminal web* (Figs. 3–13 and 3–14; see also Fig. 3–18). Myosin (although not appearing as the thick filaments characteristic of muscle) and tropomyosin have also been found in association with the terminal web, but, in isolated microvilli without attached terminal web components, actin is found in association with a newly described set of proteins (villin, fimbrin, and calmodulin), some of whose functions are not yet known. In isolated demembranated brush borders, contraction of the actin filament bundles can be induced by the addition of calcium and ATP.

Stereocilia. Stereocilia are very long microvilli that sometimes branch (Figs. 3–16 and

3–17). In the epididymis and vas deferens they seem to function like ordinary microvilli; in the inner ear, they respond to mechanical displacement with alterations in membrane potential, thus mediating sensory transduction.

Cilia. In epithelia concerned with transport of substances along the epithelial surface, such as in the tracheobronchial tree, uterus, or oviduct, the free surface of epithelial cells has specialized structures called *cilia* (Fig. 3–18; see also Fig. 3–13). The core of each cilium consists of two central and nine peripheral pairs of microtubules, composed of the proteins *alpha* and *beta* *tubulin*. One tubule of each peripheral pair has crossarms composed of the protein *dynein* protruding from it; radial spokes of an unidentified additional protein are also present. By means of an energy-converting mechanism (similar to the actin–myosin interaction of muscle) involving the reversible cross-bridging of the microtubules and the ATPase activity of dynein, the cilia undergo a specific series of movements known as *beating*. Beating consists of a forward motion, the *effective stroke*, followed by a second undulation, the *recovery stroke*. The coordinated forward spreading waves of ciliary beating enable the directed propagation of mucus and particulate matter along the surface of an epithelium.

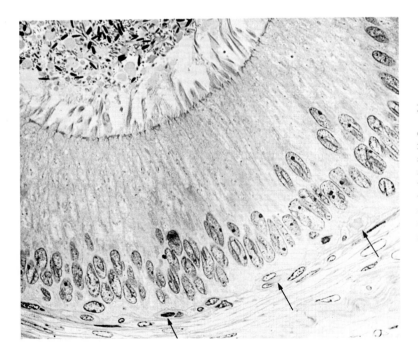

3–16 Light micrograph of pseudostratified columnar epithelium from the lining of the monkey epididymis. Stereocilia are seen clumped on the apical surface. Their obvious resemblance to cilia in the light microscope led to their inappropriate name. Small capillaries indent the basal surface of the epithelium **(arrows),** and sperm are seen in the lumen. × 400.

a

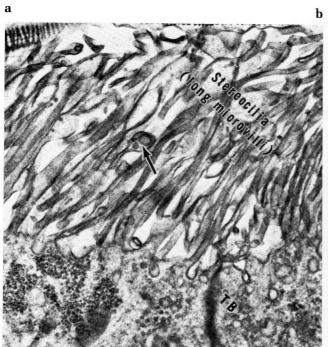

b

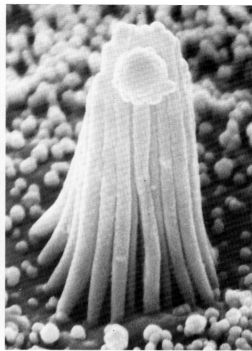

Like microvilli, cilia anchor in the terminal web region, but they attach specifically to structures called *basal bodies* containing centrioles from which the cilia arise during development.

No one yet understands fully the mechanisms by which ciliary beating is accomplished and coordinated. The cilia of individuals who suffer from a genetic defect of ciliary motion lack either the dynein arms or the radial spokes connecting the central microtuble pair to those in the periphery, thus suggesting that both are essential for proper ciliary function. The importance of normal ciliary function is dramatized by individuals with this "immotile cilia syndrome," who suffer from bronchiectasis (a kind of chronic lung infection) and sinusitis; many also have dextrocardia, a finding suggesting that ciliary motion may also play an important role in embryogenesis. Males with the immotile cilia syndrome are infertile because the movement of sperm depends on *flagella*, structures very similar to cilia which are also paralyzed by the absence of dynein or radial spokes.

In some sensory epithelia, such as the eye and the ear, cells with normal nonmotile cilia, called *kinocilia*, may function in sensory transduction. These cilia differ in structure from motile cilia.

3–17 a. Thin-section electron micrograph of the free border of the epithelium of the epididymis of bat. It can be seen that stereocilia are usually long microvilli that extend from the free surface of the epithelium into the lumen. The tips of these microvilli are often dilated **(arrow).** Endocytic vesicles forming at the bases of the microvilli (stereocilia) are particularly numerous. **TB,** terminal bar. × 12,000. (Courtesy of A. Mitchell.) **b.** Scanning electron micrograph shows stereocilia and microvilli of a hair cell from the inner ear of a bullfrog. The central kinocilium (whose substructure contains microtubules) with its bulbous tip does not taper at the base like the stereocilia. Note the length of the stereocilia compared with the surrounding, unusually rounded microvilli. × 12,000. (From Hudspeth, A. J., and Jacobs, R. 1979. Proc. Natl. Acad. Sci. U.S.A. 76:1506.)

They have nine peripheral pairs of microtubules but lack the central pair and are sometimes designated 9 + 0 to differentiate them from motile cilia with a 9 + 2 pattern.

The Lateral Membrane

The lateral membrane of epithelial cells, like the apical membrane, contains enzymes essential for

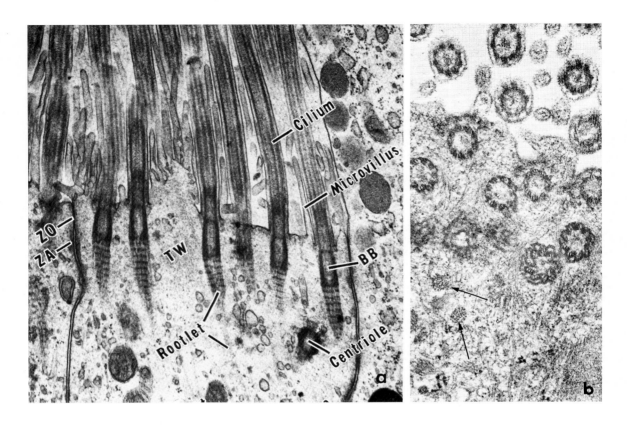

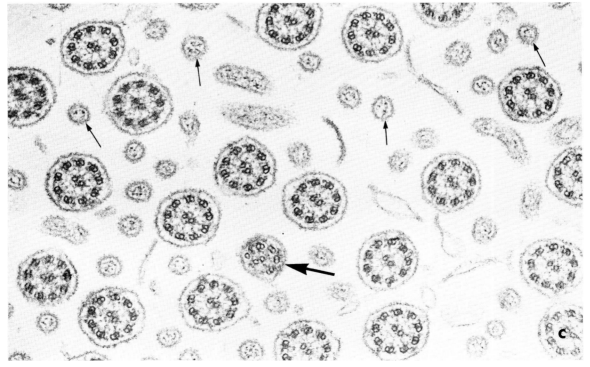

3–18 **a.** Longitudinal thin section through cilia from the lining of the human fallopian tube. Microvilli are also seen. One can distinguish several junctions between cells: the zonula occludens (**ZO**) and the zonula adherens (**ZA**). **TW**, terminal web; **BB**, basal body. × 24,000. (Courtesy of N. Bjorham and B. Fredricsson.) **b.** An electron micrograph of an oblique section of the apical surface of a ciliated bronchial cell of a monkey. Isolated oblique sections of cilia and microvilli are seen at the top of the micrograph. In the cytoplasm the triplet arrangement of the microtubules in the basal bodies can be seen especially well on the right. Also present are cross-sectioned microfilament bundles (**arrows**) of ciliary rootlets. × 44,000.
c. Electron-microscopic cross sections of normal cilia from monkey bronchial tissue similar to that of part b, showing normal central and peripheral microtubule pairs. The dynein arms, radial spokes, and nexin links are also present. The cilia are easily distinguished from cross sections of microvilli (some are indicated by **small arrows**), which contain filamentous cores. At the **large arrow** a cilium is sectioned near its tip. Because not all of its microtubules are of the same length their number appears reduced. The micrograph also has some small membrane fragments, which probably were part of the debris normally found in the mucous coat that covers the epithelial surface in vivo. × 62,500.

---

absorption and transepithelial transport. Unlike some of the apical membrane markers, however, the lateral membrane enzymes are not always unique to this membrane: enzymes such as Na^+K^+ ATPase, for example, are also present in the basal membrane.

A unique feature of the lateral surface of epithelial cells is the presence of various functionally and morphologically distinct intercellular junctions (Fig. 3–13). The *tight junction*, or *zonula occludens*, is the most apically located and serves as a permeability barrier. Below the tight junction along the lateral membrane are plaquelike zones of attachment between cells, examples of the *desmosome*, or *macula adherens*, which allow mechanical forces to be transmitted from cell to cell. Also along the lateral membrane are *gap* or *communicating junctions*, which allow ions and other small molecules to pass between adjacent cells.

Tight Junctions. In electron micrographs of thin sections of epithelial cells, *tight junctions* appear as fused regions of adjacent lateral cell membranes that are impermeable to large molecular-weight tracers (Figs. 3–19 and 3–20). The structural characteristics making this possible can better be appreciated in freeze-fracture preparations that expose the inner surfaces of the membrane. In freeze-fracture the tight junction is seen to consist of a variable number of parallel interweaving strands of intramembranous particles in the cytoplasmic (P) half of the membrane that correspond to grooves in the outer (E) half and are in register with similar structures in the adjoining cell membrane. The tight junction may be formed by fusion of integral membrane proteins of adjacent cells. However, the tight junction protein (or proteins) as well as possible associated lipids have not yet been isolated or characterized, and the process of tight junction formation is not fully understood. Freeze-fracture studies of forming tight junctions show that typical strands evolve from what are initially rows and small clusters of intramembranous particles. Physiological and morphological evidence from tissue culture systems suggests that tight junction formation requires protein synthesis and, under certain conditions, synthesis of new messenger RNA. Also, functioning microfilaments may be necessary for tight junction formation. In certain tissues, some intact tight junctions can be disrupted by ethylene glycol aminoethyl tetracetate (EGTA), a calcium chelator; tight junctions can also be destroyed by the proteolytic action of trypsin.

Physiological studies of different types of epithelia suggest that epithelia may be classified as either "tight," for example, urinary bladder, or "leaky," for example, proximal renal tubule, and that these differences in transepithelial permeability depend largely on the nature of the tight junctions between adjacent cells. In "tight" epithelia, virtually nothing can pass between adjacent cells. Consequently, the permeability of a "tight" epithelium to water and solutes is determined by the active and passive transport properties of the apical and basolateral cell membranes, i.e., *transcellular* transport. In "leaky" epithelia, the tight junctions are selectively permeable to certain substances, and the transcellular resistance to flow of water and ions is so much greater than the resistance to flow between the cells that the transepithelial resistance is considered to be determined primarily by this *paracellular* route. Attempts have been made to correlate the physiological "tightness" of the epithelium both with the number of parallel strands in the tight junction and with the integrity of individual strands (which in the P face of freeze-fracture preparations may range in appearance from individual particles to fused cords), but the relationship be-

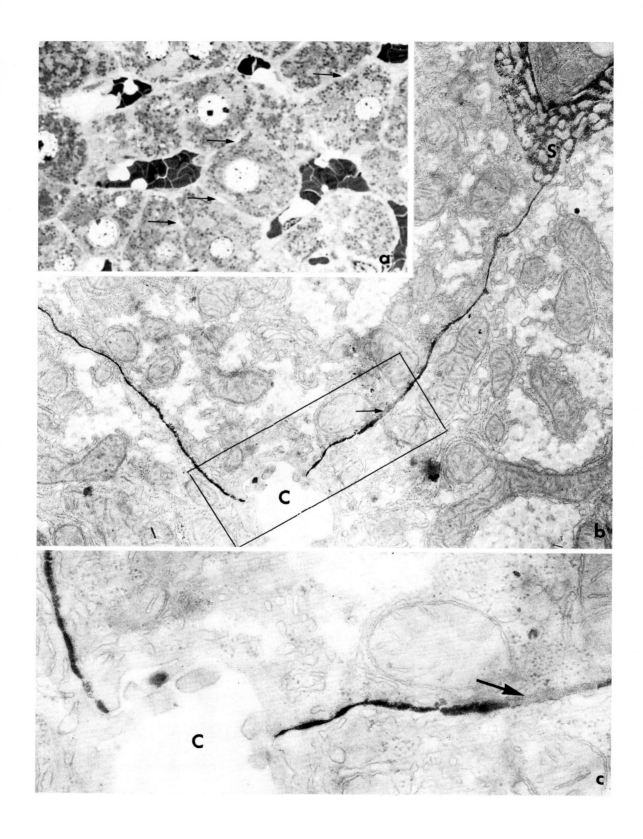

3–19 a. Light micrograph of a section of rat liver.
Hepatocytes have large, round, light-staining
nuclei. Each cell abuts a blood vessel called a
sinusoid, which can be recognized because of its
content of darkly stained red blood cells. The
hepatocyte free surface is a small region between two
cells that is sealed by tight junctions and is the
beginning of the bile duct system. It is called the *bile
canaliculus* and can just barely be visualized in the
light microscope **(arrows)**. × 1,000. **b** and **c.** Electron
micrographs of liver with the extracellular space filled
with the electron-dense marker lanthanum, which was
administered intravascularly. Note that lanthanum
entering from the sinusoid **(S)** and filling the
intercellular space cannot cross the tight junctions
near the free surface of the bile canaliculus **(C)**.
Lanthanum penetrates gap junctions, creating a
characteristic hexagonal lattice work **(arrow)**. This
section is from the liver of a starved animal; light
areas in the cytoplasm are normally filled with
glycogen. The area indicated by a **box** in part b is
enlarged in part c. b, × 18,000; c, × 50,000. (Parts b
and c courtesy of J. P. Revel.)

---

tween tight junction structure and transepithelial
permeability is not yet clear.

Other factors affecting transepithelial permeability include the shape of the cells, the ratio of
apical surface to basolateral surface, and the configuration and length of the lateral intercellular
spaces. These features may vary considerably
even within a given epithelial cell type because
of the convolutions and interdigitations of the
plasma membranes. Experimental studies in
which changing the ionic strength of bathing solutions results in altered transepithelial permeability often show more marked changes in these
other geometric factors than in the structure of
the tight junctions (see Fig. 3–24).

Desmosomes. The structure of the *desmosome* or *macula adherens*, can best be seen in
thin sections, although freeze-fracture replicas
show desmosomes as patches of large, variably
sized and irregular intramembranous particles
(Figs. 3–20 and 3–21). The desmosome consists
of a pair of dense *attachment plaques* just beneath each of the two adjacent lateral cell membranes, which are separated by a 20-nm space
that often has a central dense line. The material
filling the intercellular space in the region of the
desmosome is thought to be glycoprotein and to
attach the cells to one another. Side arms between the intermediate dense line and the outer

leaflet of each cell membrane can often be seen.
Within the cytoplasm, filaments 10 nm in diameter, called *tonofilaments*, form hairpin loops
through the dense material of the attachment
plaques. These filaments, composed of *keratins*,
are a major cytoskeletal element within most epithelial cells (see Fig. 3–22). The network of desmosomes and tonofilaments is thought to enable
an epithelial sheet to distribute its mechanical
stress and retain its functional integrity.

The process of desmosome formation is only
beginning to be studied. Although the molecular
components of the desmosome have not been
identified, indirect evidence suggests that desmosomes are probably somewhat heterogeneous
in structure and function. Studies show, for example, that epithelia with more stable intercellular associations, such as stratified squamous
and some glandular epithelia, require proteolytic
agents or detergents to dissociate their desmosomes. However, desmosomes from some simple
columnar epithelia, characterized by cell migration and relatively rapid turnover, can be disrupted simply by chelation of extracellular calcium.

In addition to the usual *spot* (macular) desmosomes, a more extensive structure resembling
a desmosome is found between columnar epithelial cells. Called an *intermediate junction, belt
desmosome,* or *zonula adherens,* this structure
surrounds the cell just basal to the zonula occludens. The function of the zonula adherens, like
that of the macula, is thought to be adhesion, but
the filaments attaching to the dense plaque are
somewhat smaller (7 nm) and are composed of
actin rather than keratin; these filaments are primary components of the *terminal web*. The *fascia adherens* of the intercalated disc (which
holds cardiac muscle cells together) resembles
the zonula adherens.

Gap Junctions. *Gap junctions*, like tight
junctions, are appreciated best in freeze-fracture
preparations, but they can also be recognized in
electron-microscopic thin sections (Figs. 3–19 to
3–23). In the region of a gap junction the adjacent cell membranes, although closely apposed,
are separated by a 2-nm space (the "gap"), which
distinguishes the appearance of gap junctions
from tight junctions in thin sections. This gap or
space is bridged by connecting structures. These
connecting structures are clearly recognizable after special preparative procedures such as permeation of the extracellular space with an elec-

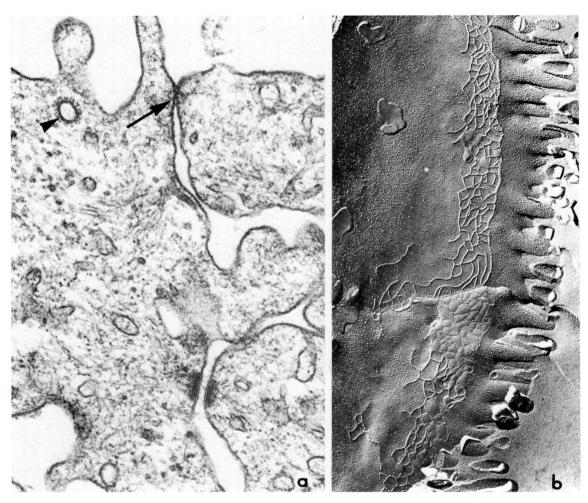

3–20 a. Thin-section electron micrograph showing
        the tight junction region (and a desmosome) of
the lateral surface of two epithelial cells. Note that at
the tight junction the adjacent plasma membranes
appear to fuse **(arrow).** The desmosome lacks some of
the intercellular material sometimes seen. (Compare
with Fig. 3–21a.) The **arrowhead** indicates a coated
vesicle (see Fig. 3–15). × 66,000. **b.** Freeze-fracture

appearance of a tight junction in mouse intestinal
epithelium. The tight junction is characterized by
interweaving strands on the **P** (cytoplasmic) face and
grooves on the **E** (extracellular) face. To the right are
microvilli, showing the localization of the tight
junction near the apical surface of the cell. × 30,000.
(Courtesy of J. P. Revel.)

tron-dense substance like lanthanum (Fig. 3–19).
In freeze-fracture preparations, gap junctions
consist of a variable number of 9- to 11-nm intramembranous particles on the cytoplasmic (P)
fracture face; these particles are packed together
more closely than the somewhat smaller particles in the rest of the membrane and are surrounded by a relatively particle-free halo. The
extracellular (E) face of the gap junction looks

like a collection of pits corresponding to the particle array on the cytoplasmic (P) face.

  In molecular and functional terms, the gap
junction is the best characterized of all the intercellular junctions. It is generally agreed that its
function is to provide a low-resistance channel
between adjacent cells for the passage of ions
and other small molecules (molecular weight
less than 800 daltons). Gap junctions are not

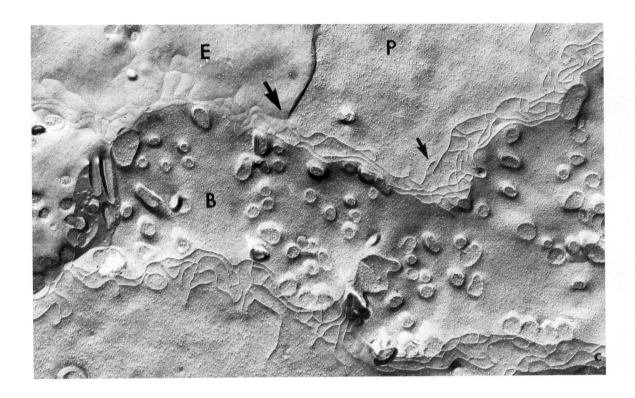

Figure 3–20 c. Freeze-fracture view of the tight junction surrounding the bile canalicular (free) surface of a rat hepatocyte. Both the P and E faces of the tight junction are shown. **B** indicates bile canalicular plasmalemma with cross-fractured microvilli. The fracture plane jumps from the P face of one cell to the E face of the adjacent cell at the level of the tight junction and the intercellular space can be seen to be obliterated **(large arrow).** Small arrays of intramembranous particles resembling gap junctions are occasionally seen among tight junction strands **(small arrow).**

× 45,000. (Courtesy of A. Yee.)

only present in epithelial tissues; they are almost ubiquitous, being absent only in mature skeletal muscle and isolated cells such as blood cells and spermatozoa. The importance of gap junctions in a tissue such as a cardiac muscle is well understood: it is clear that the almost unrestricted passage of ions between cells—ionic coupling—is required for coordinated and synchronous contraction of adjacent muscle cells. In other tissues, such as epithelia, it is not as certain why gap junctions are present. By use of radioactively labeled compounds it has been shown that cells linked by gap junctions can transfer essential nutrients such as nucleotide precursors to one another, a function that has been termed *metabolic cooperation*. It has also been demonstrated that gap junctions may be capable of allowing transfer of mediators of hormonal stimulation such as cyclic AMP between cells. Although it is quite conceivable that gap junctions enable the passage of signals, for example, allowing cilia to beat in a coordinated fashion, or directing cells to migrate to sites of injury, or stimulating or arresting growth, the evidence for such functions is as yet only suggestive.

The proteins comprising the gap junction have been isolated from the plasmalemma of liver cells in a number of species and also from heart tissue. It is generally agreed that a major component has a molecular weight of about 26,000. A partial amino acid sequence of liver gap junction protein has recently been published. The currently accepted model of gap junction structure, based on x-ray diffraction studies, postulates an aligned hexagonal grouping of subunits in the

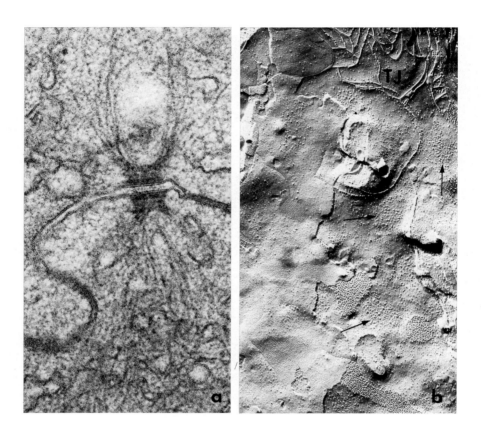

3–21 a. Thin section of the lateral membranes of two cells at the site of a desmosome from mouse stomach. This micrograph shows clearly the space between adjacent cell membranes, the dense plaque just beneath each membrane, and the insertion of tonofilaments into the plaques. × 50,000. (Courtesy of J. P. Revel.) **b.** Freeze-fracture appearance of desmosomes **(arrows)** as well as tight and gap junctions from the epithelial lining of mouse stomach. The **P**-face intramembranous particles of the desmosomes are irregular and of several sizes in comparison with the much more uniform size and packing of those in the extensive areas of gap junctions present. The desmosomal areas are also less well demarcated than the gap junctions (also see Fig. 3–22b). Note that the tight junction **(TJ)** is toward the apical surface. × 42,000. (Courtesy of J. P. Revel.)

adjacent membranes of coupled cells, with each subunit containing a central hydrophilic channel or pore approximately 1.5 nm in diameter. The idea that a single intramembranous particle may suffice for ionic coupling is supported by studies demonstrating some coupling in the absence of recognizable gap junction particle arrays; the characteristic morphological picture of clusters of particles would then reflect the convenience of gathering junctional elements in an area of close membrane apposition. However, changes detected in the packing of particles within junction arrays when cells are known to be functionally uncoupled (as in hypoxia) have been used as evidence against the single-particle hypothesis.

Intercellular permeability, determined principally by gap junctions, can be studied by using intracellular microelectrodes not only to record the transmission of current between cells, but also to inject compounds of different molecular weights whose distribution it is possible to monitor visually. The questions remain, however, whether gap junction permeability differs in different cell types, and whether permeability through a junction is equal in both directions. Some evidence suggests that permeability can be regulated physiologically, perhaps by changes in intracellular calcium concentration.

The formation and turnover of gap junctions have been studied morphologically and physiologically in several experimental systems, with conflicting results, especially with regard to how

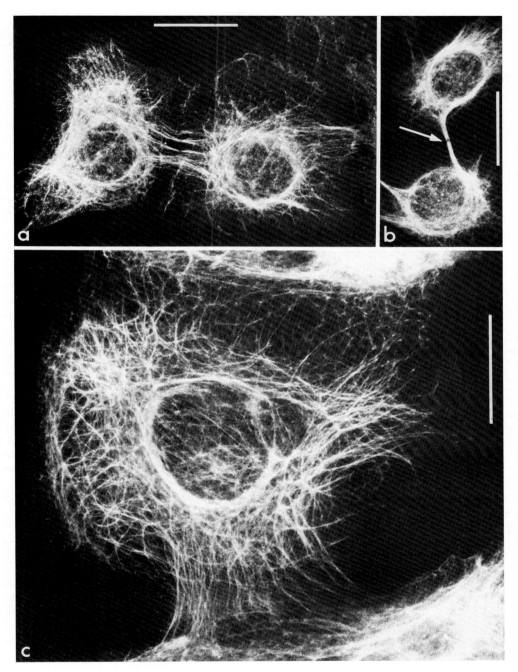

3–22 Cytoplasmic keratin networks of mammary epithelial cells in tissue culture visualized by a fluorescent antibody. Such cytoskeletal substructures of keratin can be found in most epithelial cells along with other major cytoskeletal networks composed of actin, tubulin, and desmin, which are found in many other cell types as well. Part **a** shows the keratin filaments of desmosomes and part **b** illustrates their absence **(arrow)** in the midbody of the telophase spindle. **Bars** = 20 μm. Approx. mag.: a, × 1,000; b, × 1,100; c, × 1,500. (From Franke, W., et al. 1978. Exp. Cell Res. 116:429.)

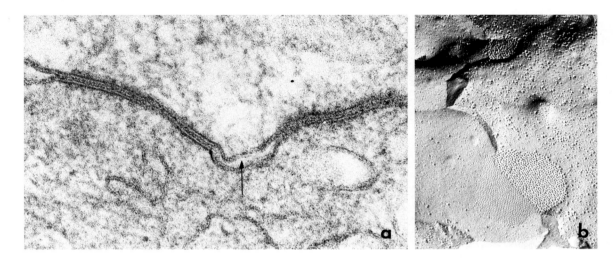

3–23 a. Thin section of two gap junctions between lining cells of mouse stomach. Although the membranes are in close apposition, a characteristic gap of 2 nm, which distinguishes gap from tight junctions, can be seen. An **arrow** indicates the widened intercellular space between the two junctions. ×115,000. (Courtesy of J. P. Revel.) **b.** Freeze-fracture appearance of a gap junction from mouse gallbladder. Note that the intramembranous particles comprising the gap junction are slightly larger and more densely packed than those on the P face of the membrane. On the E face of the membrane of the adjacent cell, a regular array of pits defines the gap junction. × 50,000. (Courtesy of J. P. Revel.)

the protein is destroyed: by internalization into vesicles or by morphologically undetectable dispersal of the components within the plane of the membrane. Little is known about how the process of junction formation is regulated. There is some evidence that gap junction formation requires protein synthesis; it can be triggered in vitro by contact between cells and in vivo by certain hormonal stimuli. Recent studies in rat liver suggest that turnover of gap junctions normally is more rapid than some other membrane proteins; the rate of turnover can be increased by physiological stress, as in partial hepatectomy.

The Basal Surface

The membrane of the basal surface of an epithelial cell (See Fig. 3–13) contains proteins that always differ from those in the apical membrane, but not always from those of the lateral membrane. The most widely studied basolaterally lo-

cated enzyme is Na^+K^+ ATPase, which transports sodium out of the cell and potassium inward. This ATPase can be localized histochemically or by using radioactive ouabain, a digitalis glycoside that binds to the enzyme and inhibits its function. The basal membrane of many secretory cells is also thought to contain the receptors for various hormones. Endocytosis at the basal membrane may be important in the transepithelial transport (transcytosis) of immunoglobins in such organs as the neonatal intestine and the placenta. In stratified squamous epithelia, so-called *hemidesmosomes* are present on the basal membrane and are thought to function in anchoring the cell to the extracellular matrix.

Epithelial cells elaborate and secrete through the basal membrane some of the constituents of *basement membrane,* an extracellular layer that is a matrix composed of collagen (often of two or more different types), other glycoproteins and mucopolysaccharides, and sometimes elastic fibers. The basement membrane varies in its composition and appearance according to location, but some form of it underlies all epithelia (Figs. 3–24, 3–25, and 3–26; see also Figs. 3–1, 3–6, 3–8, and 3–13). Although epithelial cells make some components of their own basement membrane, some interaction with underlying mesenchymal cells or connective tissue may be required. The *basal lamina* (sometimes called basement lamina) is a thin amorphous sheet closely applied to the cells, which contains a particular type (IV) of collagen. It is the component of basement membrane common to all epithelial tissues; it cannot usually be seen with the

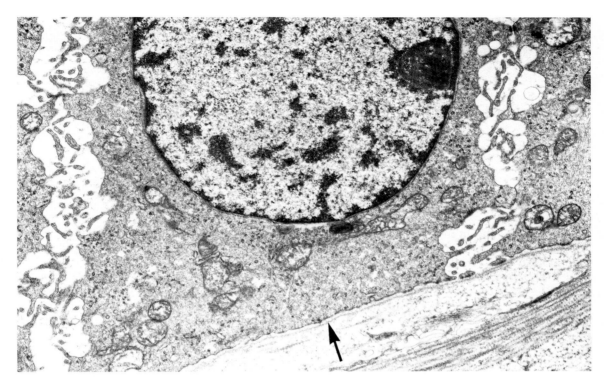

3–24 Electron micrograph of the basal portion of the simple columnar epithelium of the human gallbladder (see Fig. 3–5) showing dilated lateral spaces as well as the basal **(arrow)** and reticular laminas. × 14,200.

3–25 Thin-section electron micrograph of the special basement membrane of the kidney glomerulus, which acts as a filter for blood. (For views of other less specialized basement membranes see Figs. 3–23 and 3–26.) On one side of the basement membrane is the capillary **(C)** lined by a fenestrated **(arrow)** endothelium. The glomerular epithelium is composed of special cells called podocytes. The foot processes that give this cell type its name are seen on the other (urinary) surface of the basement membrane. **N,** podocyte nucleus. × 48,000.

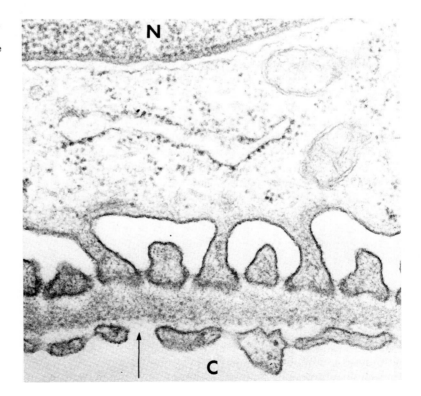

light microscope. Below the basal lamina, in some tissues, is the *reticular lamina*, which varies in its composition and remains poorly characterized. It can be visualized by light microscopy if PAS or silver stains are used to stain its carbohydrate components or reticular fibers.

The function of the basement membrane is not well understood. It probably serves as a substrate for migration of epithelial cells, such as those in the intestinal lining. It may have a role in stabilizing tissue shapes, since its removal during embryogenesis causes developing salivary glands to lose their characteristic structure. In the kidney, the special basement membrane of the glomerulus (Fig. 3–25) is thought to function as a selective permeability barrier, contributing to the process of ultrafiltration of plasma to form urine. The absence of basement membrane in certain malignant tumors suggests that it may be important in growth control; metastasis of cancer cells is considered to begin when the basement membrane is breached.

Intracellular Polarity

Especially in actively secretory epithelia, polarity is reflected both by the characteristics of the plasma membrane and by the pattern of intracellular organization. For example, in glandular cells the rough endoplasmic reticulum is often found near the base of the cell, the Golgi apparatus above the nucleus toward the middle of the cell, and the secretory and condensing vacuoles near the apical surface. By use of radioactively labeled amino acids or monosaccharides or both, progression of synthesis of a glycoprotein product after stimulation (generally via receptors at the basal surface) can be followed. First, the radioactive substances are incorporated into polymers in the rough endoplasmic reticulum; next they are seen in the Golgi apparatus; then in the vesicles; and finally, one can trace the substances in the discharge of secretory contents into the lumen by exocytosis at the apical surface. The process of secretion thus demonstrates the utility of the observed intracellular polarity.

The localization of the mitochondria within epithelial cells may also reflect function. In absorptive cells, mitochondria are usually near the apical surface. In secretory cells and cells resorbing ions and H_2O they are found basally, often in close association with basal infoldings, which increase basal surface area (Fig. 3–26).

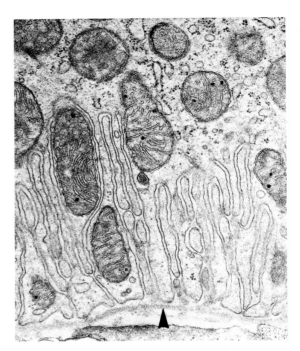

3–26 Thin-section electron micrograph of the basal portion of a kidney tubule cell from guinea pig. Note the basal infoldings, which include interdigitated processes from an adjacent cell and are associated with mitochondria. An **arrowhead** indicates the basal lamina. × 19,000. (Courtesy of V. Black.)

Experimental Studies of Polarity

How is membrane polarity achieved and maintained? This question is now of great interest because its answer may elucidate the general mechanisms by which membrane proteins find their appropriate destinations. It has been observed that certain classes of infective viruses will bud only from the apical surface of epithelial cells, whereas others bud exclusively from the basolateral membrane. Further investigation has shown that glycosylation of the viral proteins is not required for polarized viral budding, thus suggesting that, in general, the carbohydrate portion of glycoproteins may not be required for their transport to and insertion at their proper membrane destinations. Other studies monitoring the distribution of intramembranous particles (presumably complexes of integral membrane proteins) in relation to tight junction formation suggest that the tight junction may be essential for establishing and maintaining epithelial membrane polarity.

Renewal and Turnover of Epithelial Cells

An essential feature of many epithelia is a constant cycle of renewal and shedding. This cycle can be a direct consequence of function, as in *holocrine* glands, where the entire cell becomes the secretion, or it can occur where the outermost cells are constantly exposed to various kinds of trauma, as is true for epidermis, mucous membranes, and intestinal linings. Autoradiographic studies have demonstrated that within most epithelia only certain cells, called *stem cells,* are normally responsible for the steady supply of new cells. However, under unusual circumstances other cells may demonstrate some regenerative potential (reserve stem cells). Experiments involving extensive acute injury (i.e., irradiation of intestine or sudden bladder distension) have shown that most of the new cells are provided by an accelerated rate of turnover of the usual stem cells, with some contribution from the first generation of daughter cells (secondary stem cells).

In general, stem cells are relatively undifferentiated, they lie at the base of the epithelium, and although they give rise to a few stem cells to perpetuate the pool, they principally give rise to more differentiated daughter cells that migrate to exposed regions and are eventually shed. The small, relatively quiescent population of stem cells from which the rest of the epithelium derives possibly represents a mechanism for guarding against the extensive mutagenesis that might occur if all cells were turning over rapidly. The conservation of the original genetic material might be further assured if, as some evidence suggests, the same strand of DNA were retained by some of the original stem cells after each successive division. This mechanism adds to other safeguards of genetic integrity that may be present, such as the ultraviolet-absorbing pigment melanin of skin.

Rates of cellular renewal in epithelia vary widely, from a few days in the intestinal linings to months or years in epithelia less subject to abrasion such as in the vas deferens. In relatively stable populations of simple epithelia—for example, vascular endothelium or the epithelium of the cornea—as the initial response to injury,

cells will migrate to cover a wounded or denuded area, following which there is gradual proliferation from the edge of the damaged region.

Glands

Glandular tissues have traditionally been classified as epithelial, even though *endocrine glands,* which produce hormones entering the bloodstream, often differ in appearance from typical epithelial tissues. In *exocrine glands,* which secrete substances onto a free surface, the similarity to other epithelial tissues is more obvious.

Exocrine glands are classified both according to their structure and the type of secretion they produce (Figs. 3–27, 3–28, and 3–29). Glands are called *holocrine* if whole cells are secreted, as is the case in sebaceous glands. If only a part of the apical cytoplasm of the cell is lost, as in the secretion of lipids by the mammary glands, the glands are called *apocrine.* In most exocrine and endocrine glands, only the secretory product itself is released: these glands are called *merocrine.* Merocrine glands are further categorized by the type of secretory product: *mucous cells* make a viscous, carbohydrate-rich secretion; *serous cells* produce a more watery, protein-rich secretion, often high in enzyme activity. Viewed through the light microscope, mucus-producing cells look empty because the nuclei and endoplasmic reticulum of these cells are pushed toward the basal surface, and the mucus that fills the apical cytoplasm in vivo is not well preserved or stained by routine methods. Serous cells, often quite basophilic because they have more abundant endoplasmic reticulum, are not distended by as large a volume of secretion as

3–27 Diagrams of simple and compound forms of glands. Secretory portions of the gland are stippled. Sometimes alveoli are called acini. (Courtesy of E. Hay.)

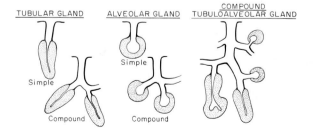

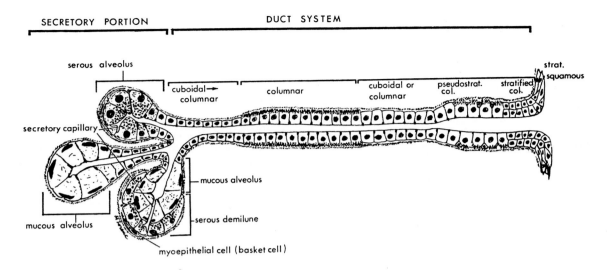

3–28 Diagram of an idealized exocrine gland with both serous and mucous secretory elements and a simplified duct system. Note that mucous alveoli in some glands have caps or demilunes of serous cells, which empty their secretory products into *secretory capillaries* (also called *intercellular canaliculi*). *Myoepithelial cells* are found within the basal lamina around the alveoli of some glands and help propel secretory products. Some parts of duct systems transport ions and water; the cells of these regions often have basal infoldings with associated mitochondria, as illustrated in the columnar portion of the duct system of this diagram. (Modified from an original of M. Lorenc; courtesy of V. Black and Department of Cell Biology, N.Y.U. School of Medicine.)

mucous cells. With good preservation, the secretory granules of serous cells can be seen with the light microscope (Fig. 3–30).

Exocrine glands are also classified by their organization (Fig. 3–27). Single secretory cells, often found scattered among nonsecretory cells within an epithelium (in the tracheobronchial tree, for example), are called, logically, *unicellular*. Unicellular mucus-producing gland cells, most often found between columnar cells, have constricted basal regions and are called *goblet cells* (Figs. 3–6 and 3–10). In multicellular glands the secretory cells may form along ducts *(tubules)* or terminal sacs *(alveoli)*. If more than

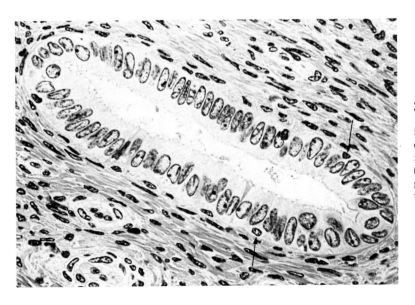

3–29 This simple tubular gland of the uterine endometrium is composed of simple columnar epithelium and has occasional intraepithelial lymphocytes **(arrows)**. Intracellular secretory granules are not recognizable in this light micrograph. × 360.

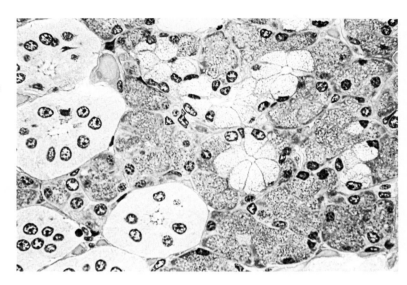

3–30 Light micrograph of a submandibular gland of the monkey, which has both serous and mucous acini. The mucous acini are distinguished by their empty-appearing cytoplasm from the serous cells, which contain recognizable secretory granules. Cross sections of ducts composed of simple columnar epithelium are also present (left side of micrograph). × 400.

one tubule or alveolus connects to a duct leading to the surface, the glands are called *compound tubular, compound alveolar,* or *compound tubuloalveolar.*

Endocrine glands are ductless, having lost their original embryonic connections to the surface from which they invaginated. Cells of some endocrine glands, like the thyroid, closely resemble other epithelial cells in structure. Others have quite various appearances, lacking a true free surface, but sharing such characteristics of epithelial cells as the presence of junctions and evidence of polarity. The endocrine glands will be considered in detail in subsequent chapters.

References and Selected Bibliography

Transitional Epithelium

Petry, G., and Amon, H. 1966. Licht und electronmikroskopische Studien über Struktur and Dynamik des Übergangsepithels. Z. Zellforsch. 69:587.

Severs, N. J., and Hicks, R. M. 1979. Analysis of membrane structure in transitional epithelium of rat urinary bladder. J. Ultrastruct. Res. 69:279.

Cilia and Stereocilia

Afzelius, B. A. 1976. A human syndrome caused by immotile cilia. Science 193:317.

Hudspeth, A. J., and Jacobs, R. 1979. Stereocilia mediate transduction in vertebrate haircells. Proc. Nat. Acad. Sci. USA. 76:1506.

Sturgess, J. M., Chao, J. Wong, J., Aspin, N., and Turner, J. A. P. 1979. Cilia with defective radial spokes. A cause of human respiratory disease. N. Engl. J. Med. 300:53.

Zanetti, N. C., Mitchell, D. R. and Warner, F. 1979. Effects of divalent cations on dynein cross bridging and ciliary microtubule sliding. J. Cell Biol. 80:573.

Cytoskeleton

Bretscher, A., and Weber, K. 1980. Fimbrin, a new microfilament-associated protein present in microvilli and other cell surface structures. J. Cell Biol. 86:335.

Drenckhahn, D., and Groschel-Stewart, U. 1980. Localization of myosin, actin, and tropomyosin in rat intestinal epithelium: Immunohistochemical studies at the light and electron microscope level. J. Cell Biol. 86:475.

Franke, W. W., Weber, K., Osborn, M., Schmid, E. and Freudenstein, C. 1978. Antibody to prekeratin. Exp. Cell Res. 116:429.

Geiger, B., Tokuyasu, K. T., Dutton, A. H., and Singer, S. J. 1980. Vinculin, an intracellular protein localized at specialized sites where microfilament bundles terminate at cell membranes. Proc. Nat. Acad. Sci. U.S.A. 77:4127.

Mooseker, M. S. 1976. Actin filament-membrane attachment in the microvilli of intestinal cells. *In* Cell Motility, Book B, Goldman, R., Pollard, T., and Rosenbaum, J. (eds.). Cold Spring Harbor, New York: p. 631.

Sun, T-T, Shih, C., and Green, H. 1979. Keratin cytoskeletons in epithelial cells of internal organs. Proc. Nat. Acad. Sci. U.S.A. 76:2813.

Weihling, R. R. 1979. The cytoskeleton and the plasma membrane. Meth. Archiev. exp. Pathol. 8:42.

Junctions

Borysenko, J. Z., and Revel, J. P. 1973. Experimental manipulation of desmosome structure. Am. J. Anat. 137:403.

Bullivant, S. 1978. The structure of tight junctions. *In* Ninth International Congress on Electron Microscopy, Toronto, III:659.

Claude, P. 1978. Morphological factors influencing transepithelial permeability: A model for the resistance of the zonula occludens. J. Membrane Biol. 39:219.

Dragsten, P. R., Blumenthal, R., and Handler, J. S. 1981. Membrane asymmetry in epithelia: Is the tight junction a barrier to diffusion in the plasma membrane? Nature 294:718.

Nicholson, B. J., Hunkapiller, M. W., Grim, L. B., Hood, L. E., and Revel, J. P. 1981. Rat liver gap junction protein: Properties and partial sequence. Proc. Nat. Acad. Sci. U.S.A. 78:7594.

Staehelin, A. L. 1974. Structure and function of intercellular junctions. Int. Rev. Cytol. 39:191.

Symposium. Molecular and morphological aspects of cell-cell communication. In vitro 16(12):1007 (7 papers).

Yancey, S. B., Nicholson, B. J. and J. P. Revel. 1981. The dynamic state of liver gap junctions. 1981. J. Supramolec. Struct. Cell. Biochem. 16:221.

Permeability and Transport

Diamond, J. M. 1979. Osmotic water flow in leaky epithelia. J. Membrane Biol. 51:195.

Kraehenbuhl, J. P., and Kuhn, L. 1978. Transport of immunoglobulins across epithelia. *In* Transport of Macromolecules in Cellular Systems, Silverstein, S. C. (ed.). Berlin: 1979, p. 213.

Reuss, L. (chairman). 1979. Symposium: Electrophysiology of epithelial transport. Six papers by many authors. Fed. Proc. 38:2750.

Schneeberger, E. 1978. Structural basis for some permeability properties of the air-blood barrier. Fed. Proc. 37:2471.

Basement Membrane

Huang, T. W. 1978. Composite epithelial and endothelial basal laminas in human lungs. Am. J. Pathol. 93:681.

Kefalides, N. A., Alper, R., and Clarke, C. C. 1979. Biochemistry and metabolism of basement membranes. Int. Rev. Cytol. 61:167.

Thaslaff, I., Barrach, H. J., Foidart, J.-M., Vaheri, A., Pratt, R. H., and Martin, G. R. 1981. Changes in the distribution of laminin, type IV collagen, B.M.−1 proteoglycan and fibronectin during mouse tooth development. Dev. Biol. 81:182.

Connective Tissue

Burton Goldberg and Michel Rabinovitch

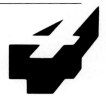

The connective tissues are defined as the complex of cells and extracellular materials that provides the supporting and connecting framework for all the other tissues of the body. Thus, epithelia, endothelia, mesothelia, nerves, and muscle rest on or are ensheathed by connective tissues.

The connective tissues consist of extracellular *fibers*, amorphous *ground substance*, and a population of connective tissue cells. The fibers are assembled mainly from the proteins *collagen* and *elastin*. The ground substance, which fills the spaces between cells and fibers, contains soluble precursors of the fibrous proteins, proteoglycans, glycoproteins, other molecules secreted from the cells, and molecules passed by the vascular filters.

Mesenchyme is a loose connective tissue network formed early in embryonic development from mesoderm and neuroectoderm. Mesenchyme contains stellate-shaped cells dispersed in a viscid ground substance. The mesenchymal cell is the ancestor of most of the indigenous cells of adult connective tissues, including the fibroblast, chondroblast, osteoblast, odontoblast, reticular cell, and adipocyte. The macrophage and mast cell are classified as indigenous cells of connective tissues but they originate from bone marrow precursors. We classify all these cell types as *resident cells* because they are constantly present in relatively fixed numbers and characteristic distributions in the various types of normal adult connective tissues. The resident cells produce the bulk of the intercellular materials in connective tissues, but epithelia and endothelia may also form some of these molecules.

The smooth muscle cell, which can be classified as a resident connective tissue cell in blood vessels and other organs, is also a source of matrix materials.

The resident cells contrast with *immigrant cells*, which appear transitorily in connective tissues as part of the inflammatory reaction to cell injury. During the inflammatory reaction, neutrophils, eosinophils, basophils, cells of lymphocytic lineage, and monocytes pass in large numbers from blood vessels into the surrounding connective tissues. These hematogenous cells tend to disappear from the tissues as the inflammatory reaction subsides. In certain connective tissues one may observe a few lymphoid cells, neutrophils, and eosinophils in the absence of documented injury. In the course of tissue injury, inflammation, and repair, increased numbers of fibroblasts appear within the connective tissues. According to one view, this expanded population of fibroblasts is derived from primordial mesenchymal cells that have persisted in adult tissues. Another view holds that the pericyte of capillaries and venules (see Chap. 9) is stimulated to divide, migrate, and undergo fibroblastic differentiation after tissue injury. However, well-differentiated adult fibroblasts can also undergo rapid serial divisions in vivo and in vitro, so there is no compelling need to postulate that fibroblasts at sites of tissue injury and repair necessarily originate from another cell type.

Comparison of connective tissues from different organ systems reveals considerable morphological diversity. The proportion of cells to fibers and ground substance, and the amounts, kinds, and organization of the extracellular materials may vary greatly from tissue to tissue. Table 4–1 classifies connective tissues and indicates their range of morphological diversity.

Loose (areolar) connective tissue, widely and abundantly distributed in the body, is characterized by a relative predominance of resident cells (e.g., fibroblasts, adipocytes, macrophages, and mast cells) over fibrous elements (Fig. 4–1). Loose connective tissue is typically interposed between tissues that can move somewhat with respect to one another, such as the mucosa and submucosa of the intestine. Areolar tissue also ensheaths blood vessels, nerves, and muscles, and it establishes the fascial planes exploited by the anatomist and surgeon. The fat-laden adipocyte characterizes *adipose tissue*, which can be considered a special category of loose connective tissue.

Table 4–1 Classification of Connective Tissues

I. Embryonic: mesenchyme

II. Adult

  A. Connective tissues proper
    1. General
      Loose (areolar)
        As in subcutis, mesentery, omentum, lamina propria of tubular epithelial organs
      Dense
        Irregular: as in periosteum, dermis, organ capsules
        Regular: as in tendons, ligaments, cornea
    2. Special
      Adipose
      Reticular
  B. Cartilage
  C. Bone

In *dense* connective tissue collagen fibers predominate over cells. The fibers are not preferentially oriented in dense irregular connective tissue (for example, in the dermis), but they are oriented preferentially in such dense regular tissues as tendons, ligaments, and the substantia propria of the cornea.

The term *reticular tissue* is applied to the delicate network of branched fibers (reticulum, reticulin) that support epithelia and endothelia and form a meshwork between the cells of the spleen, lymph nodes, and bone marrow.

Cartilage and bone are traditionally placed in separate categories because of their special architecture; however, they clearly can be considered as very dense connective tissues in which the predominant extracellular materials fulfill important weight-bearing and mechanical functions.

The cells and extracellular materials of connective tissue make up a functional complex determining the structural integrity of tissues and organs. In addition to their mechanical functions, the fibrous proteins and ground substance influence the transport of molecules across extracellular compartments. The cells of the connective tissues also have important roles in the storage of vital metabolites, in immune and inflammatory responses, and in tissue repair after injury. In this chapter we shall discuss the structure and functions of the fibroblast, the macrophage, and the mast cell. The chemistry of the fibrous proteins, proteoglycans, and glycoproteins will be described in sufficient detail to

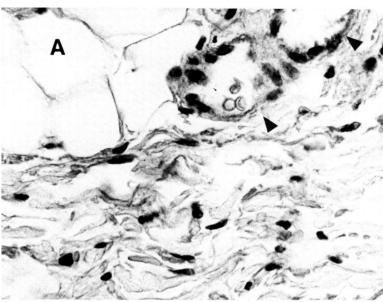

4–1 Loose connective tissue. The field shows collagen fibers adjacent to blood vessels **(arrowheads)** and fat **(A).** The collagen fibers are not oriented or tightly packed, and most cells between the fibers are presumed to be fibroblasts. × 550.

provide some understanding of how these molecules are assembled into functional units in tissues.

The Fibroblast

In conventional sections of connective tissue the fibroblast is a spindle-shaped cell with tapering eosinophilic cytoplasmic extensions (Fig. 4–2). Its nucleus generally has a regular elliptical contour, contains two to four nucleoli, and has sparse and scattered chromatin. In very dense

4–2 General appearance of fibroblasts in moderately dense connective tissue. The nuclei are regularly elliptical and the cytoplasmic borders are not well resolved from the adjacent collagen fibers. × 1,500.

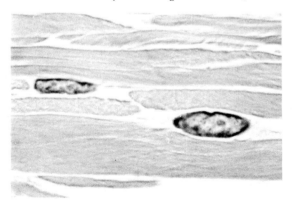

connective tissue, fibroblasts appear to be compressed between the thick bundles of collagen, for their nuclei are more elongated and darkly stained, and their cell borders usually cannot be resolved in routine preparations.

The shape of the fibroblast can vary from the simple elongated spindle; it is influenced by the nature of the substrate to which the cell attaches, the space available for movement over the substrate, and by stimulation for division. Consider, for example, fibroblasts inoculated at low cell-density into culture plates: in this setting they flatten onto the surface, send out cytoplasmic extensions with ruffled borders, and move about assuming many irregular shapes (Fig. 4–3). The fibroblast is capable of serial replication in vivo and in vitro; when the cell enters the mitotic phase, it loosens its attachment to a surface and becomes spherical. After telophase, the daughter cells flatten onto available surfaces and once again assume extended forms.

The ultrastructural organization of the differentiated fibroblast reflects the commitment of that cell type to the synthesis of molecules destined for secretion into the extracellular space. Thus, the typical fibroblast has a well-developed granular endoplasmic reticulum on which the precursor polypeptides of collagen, elastin, proteoglycans, and glycoproteins are synthesized (Fig. 4–4). The cisternae of the rough-surfaced endoplasmic reticulum contain finely granular or filamentous material, which presumably repre-

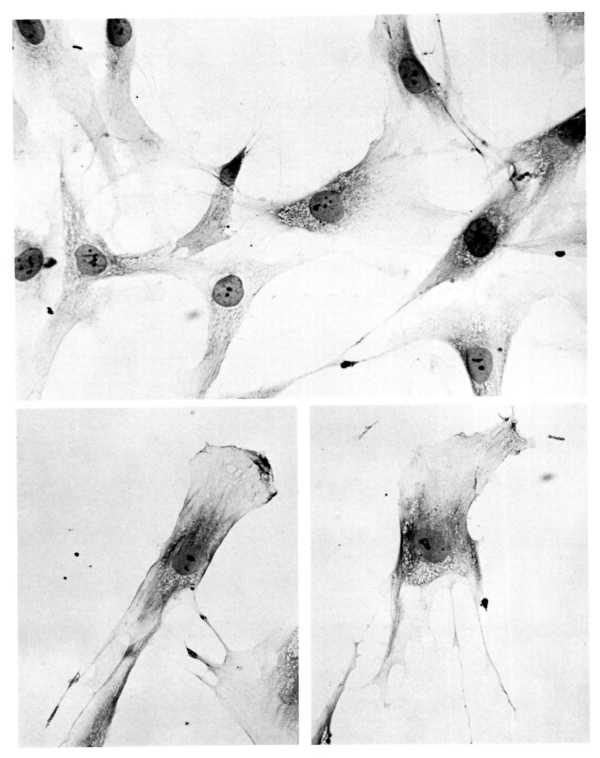

4–3 Cultured fibroblasts from human skin. Photomicrographs illustrate some of the shapes fibroblasts may take when their movement is not restricted by adjacent cells or fibrous elements. × 1,200.

4–4 Electron micrograph of cytoplasm of a fibroblast shows a tangential section through the granular endoplasmic reticulum (**E_g**). The polysomes are seen as curved chains; the cisterna contains granular material. **Arrows** indicate profiles of agranular ergastoplasm in continuity with granular reticulum. Smooth vesicles could represent transitional vesicles moving to the Golgi zone. × 74,000. (From Goldberg, B. and Green, H., 1964. J. Cell Biol. 22:227.)

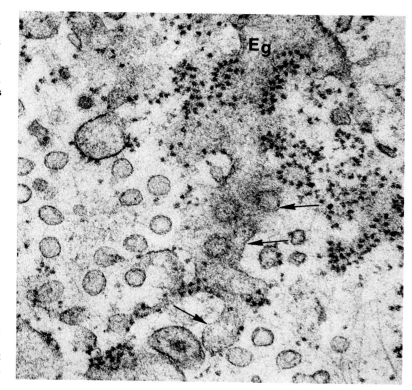

4–5 Electron micrograph shows surfaces of two fibroblasts. Smooth vesicles (**V_s**) appear to be fusing with the plasma membranes and discharging their contents into the extracellular space (**ECS**). A banded collagen fiber (**C**) is present between the cells. × 74,000. (From Goldberg, B., and Green, H. 1964. J. Cell Biol. 22:227.) ▽

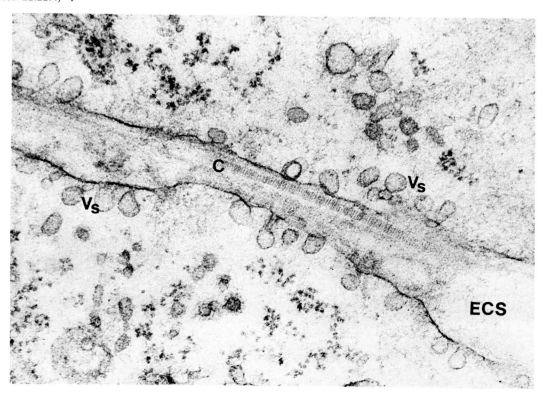

sents the soluble precursor molecules that have been precipitated during fixation and staining. The molecules in the cisternae are transported to a well-defined Golgi zone by transitional vesicular elements. Although the molecules are chemically modified in the Golgi zone, they do not generally appear to be subject to concentration and storage in condensing vacuoles. Accordingly, smooth-surfaced secretory vesicles that move from the Golgi zone to the plasma membrane do not usually contain greater concentrations of material than the cisternae of the granular endoplasmic reticulum. The secretory vesicles fuse with the plasma membrane to release their soluble contents into the extracellular space (Fig. 4–5). Further biochemical modifications of the secreted molecules may follow, and insoluble collagen and elastic fibers are deposited in the extracellular space close to the cell surface.

The fibroblast contains the usual complement of cytoplasmic organelles and inclusions. The mitochondria tend to be long and slender, and fat droplets and primary and secondary lysosomes are occasionally prominent. Microtubules are present and appear to be required for the translocation of secretory vesicular elements. Additionally, bundles of actin microfilaments are prominent; they are implicated in general cellular motility. Fibroblasts in healing wounds frequently have deeply indented nuclei and cytoplasmic bundles of microfilaments with dense bodies, which make them resemble smooth muscle cells. Such "myofibroblasts" are thought to play a role in the contraction of wounds.

The cells with a fibroblastic structure that form the fine collagenous reticulum in lymph nodes, spleen, and bone marrow are called reticular cells. Unfortunately, other cell types in lymphoid tissues have also been called reticular cells, but the term is best reserved for cells that share fibroblastic structure and function. The osteoblast, chondroblast, odontoblast, and smooth muscle cell are the mesenchymally derived cells that form the matrix materials in specialized connective tissues.

Extracellular Components of Connective Tissue

Collagen

Collagen is a protein that forms extracellular fibers or networks of basement membrane in practically every tissue of the body. Depending on the structural and functional requirements of a particular tissue, the fibers may be abundant (dense connective tissue) or sparse (loose connective tissue) and may be arranged in distinctive patterns. For example, in tendons and ligaments, the collagen fibers are thick and long and are grouped into large parallel bundles to provide the required tensile strength. In contrast, collagen fibers tend to be wrapped helically around the long axes of tubular expansile structures such as blood vessels, intestine, and glandular ducts. In cartilage and bone, calcium phosphate crystals are deposited on collagen fibers, contributing to the mechanical properties of the skeleton. In the cornea the collagen fibers form alternating orthogonal lamellae, which by their spacing and angular orientation permit the cornea to function as a refractive element of the eye. Although the cornea is continuous with the sclera, collagen fibers are not arranged orthogonally in the scleral coat. In the transparent vitreous humor, the collagen fibrils are thin, sparse, randomly oriented, and embedded in a gel of hyaluronic acid.

For most of the examples cited, the collagenous units are in the form of fibers; by electron microscopy such fibers usually display a characteristic "native" pattern of transverse bands (Fig. 4–6).

Collagen molecules are also components of basement membranes, structures that characteristically lie beneath epithelia, endothelia, and mesothelia and that stain strongly with PAS. By light microscopy basement membranes appear as a single layer of variable thickness, but with the electron microscope their components can be resolved. Just beneath the epithelium is an unstained layer containing proteoglycans and glycoproteins (the lamina rara), followed by a distinct and constant layer, the basal lamina, composed of a stained feltwork of nonbanded collagenous fibrils (Fig. 4–7). Beneath the basal lamina another space is often interposed, below which thin fibers of banded collagen (reticular fibers or reticulin) may be present. As will be discussed, the basal lamina and reticulin are formed from different molecular types of collagen. In certain tissues the basement membranes may vary both in thickness and in the prominence of the component layers. For example, the capsule of the lens of the eye is an epithelial basement membrane about 12 μm thick. In contrast, the capillaries of the renal glomerulus have a basement membrane with a thickness of 0.3 μm (300 nm), consisting of a basal lamina (called the lam-

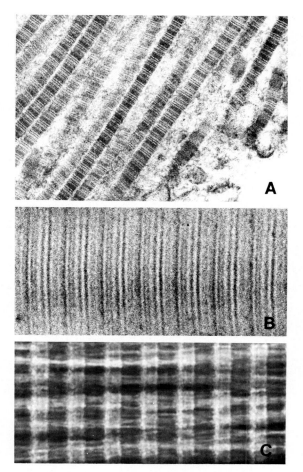

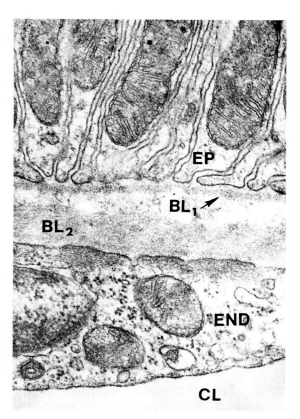

4–7 Electron micrograph of basal laminae of proximal convoluted tubule of kidney **(BL₁)** and capillary **(BL₂)**. Note lack of banding in the laminae. **EP,** epithelium of renal tubule; **END,** endothelial cell of capillary; **CL,** capillary lumen. Molecules exchanged between the renal tubule and the capillary must traverse the collagenous basal laminae. × 41,000. (Courtesy of Edith Robbins.)

4–6 Electron micrographs of native collagen fibers. **A.** Positively stained collagen fibers with characteristic cross-striations and periodicity. × 59,000. (Courtesy of Edith Robbins.) **B.** Positively stained rat tail tendon. Higher magnification emphasizes regularity of bands across the fiber and the repeat period of 670 Å. × 149,000. **C.** Negatively stained collagen fiber formed by warming a neutral salt solution of human collagen to 37° C. The repeat period is 670 Å, but only two major intraperiod bands are present. × 149,000.

ina densa) and two distinct unstained layers called the internal and external lamina rara. Figure 4–7 illustrates the basement membranes of a capillary and an adjacent renal tubule; in this instance the individual basal laminae are of different thickness, and reticulin fibers are not interposed between the basement membranes.

Collagen thus serves a wide variety of structural and mechanical functions, and as a component of basement membranes it helps to deter-mine vascular and epithelial permeability. Conventional histological stains for light microscopy aid in identifying the various fibrous forms of collagen in different tissues, but they are not specific for the protein. Collagen fibers can be identified specifically by their banding pattern in the electron microscope, their wide-angle x-ray diffraction pattern, their amino acid composition, or by immune staining.

Molecular Structure. We must know the general structure of the collagen molecule to understand the biosynthesis of the protein and how the molecules aggregate to form the characteristic fibers in the extracellular space. Cold neutral salt or acidic solutions will extract the collagen molecule from the banded collagen fibers of growing

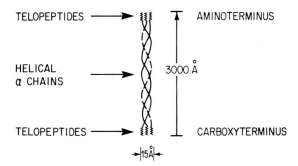

TELOPEPTIDES ——————→ AMINOTERMINUS

HELICAL
α CHAINS ——————→ 3000 Å

TELOPEPTIDES ——————→ CARBOXYTERMINUS

←15Å→

4–8 Schematic diagram of the triple helical collagen molecule. The three chains are helical except for the short terminal segments (the telopeptides). The aminotermini of all three chains are at the same end of the molecule. The **dotted line** indicates that one chain may differ in primary structure from the other two chains, as is the case for type I collagen. Triple helical molecules containing only one chain class are known (see Table 4–2).

animals. Analysis has shown the collagen molecule to consist of three polypeptide chains (α chains) of equal length, each with a molecular weight of approximately 95,000 (Fig. 4–8). The aminotermini of the three chains are at the same end of the molecule. The individual chains form a left-handed helix, but the three chains are coiled around the central axis to form a right-handed major helix. The molecule overall has the shape of a rod, about 3,000 Å long and 15 Å in diameter. The molecular structure is determined by its unique amino acid composition: every third residue in the helical chains is glycine, and the imino acids proline and 4-hydroxyproline together account for another 23% of the residues. The imino acids direct the helical conformation by their rotational restrictions, and hydroxyproline also helps to stabilize the triple helix by contributing to interchain hydrogen bonds. The other amino acids of the chains are not critical for the general helical structure, but their polar and nonpolar side chains are directed out from the central axis and thus are available to interact with other collagen molecules or noncollagenous components of the connective tissues. Such interactions contribute to the assembly of collagen molecules into fibers.

Hydroxyproline is a convenient analytical marker for collagen because it occurs in only one other structural protein (elastin) and then in much lesser amounts. The amino acid 5-hydrox-

ylysine is unique for collagen, but it is much less abundant than hydroxyproline. Galactose, or the disaccharide galactose–glucose, is covalently linked to the hydroxyl group of some of the hydroxylysine residues. The function of these sugars is unknown. At both the amino- and carboxytermini of each α chain are 16 to 25 residues that are nonhelical because of their low content of glycine and imino acids. These abbreviated nonhelical extensions are called telopeptides and are represented by the pleated lines in Fig. 4–8. Lysine and hydroxylysine residues in the telopeptides participate in covalent cross-linking of collagen molecules after the molecules aggregate to form fibers. The telopeptides are remnants of much larger extensions originally present in procollagen, the precursor form of collagen.

There are at least five genetically distinct molecular types of collagen in tissues. All have the triple helical structure described above and depicted in Fig. 4–8, but they differ from each other in the primary structure of their constituent α chains. Table 4–2 gives the current nomenclature, chain compositions, tissue distributions, and some distinctive features of the collagen types.

Type I, the most abundant of the collagens, was the first to be isolated and extensively analyzed, and so is considered to be prototypic. Type I molecules contain two α-chain classes, each determined by a different gene and hence differing in primary structure. Type I molecules typically assemble to form the very thick, distinctly cross-banded collagen fibers of connective tissues. A trimer of type I α1 chains has been found in small amounts in fetal and pathological tissues and in certain culture systems; its tissue form and physiological significance are not known. Collagen types II and III each contain only one chain class and tend to form thin crossbanded fibers. It is not known whether fiber size is determined only by the structure of the constituent collagen molecules or whether interactions with proteoglycans and glycoproteins also play a role. To this point, the thin fibers of type II collagen are characteristically embedded in the dense proteoglycan matrix of cartilage, and type III fibers are typically stained by reduced silver salts, a reaction ascribed to a coating of glycoproteins or proteoglycans on the fibers. Collagen types I to III are the best characterized with respect to molecular structure and tissue distribution and they are referred to collectively as the *interstitial collagens*.

Table 4–2 Collagen Types

Type	Molecular form	Tissue distributions	Features
I	$[\alpha 1(I)]_2\alpha 2(I)$	Ubiquitous. Majority of collagen in bone, tendon, dentine, and adult skin	Relatively low content of Hyl and glycosylated Hyl. Forms banded fibers of large diameter in vivo
I (trimer)	$[\alpha 1(I)]_3$	Fetal, neoplastic, and inflamed tissues. Certain culture systems	In vivo fiber form unknown
II	$[\alpha 1(II)]_3$	Characteristic of hyaline cartilage. Also in nucleus pulposus, vitreous of eye, and cultured embryonic cornea and neural retina	Intermediate content of Hyl and glycosylated Hyl. Forms banded fibers of small diameter in vivo
III	$[\alpha 1(III)]_3$	Same as type I but almost absent in bone and very low in tendon. Most prominent in fetal skin, healing wounds, and tissues with major smooth muscle component	Chains cross-linked by carboxyterminal disulfide bonds. Greater than $^1/_3$ glycine. High 4-Hyp. Low content of Hyl and glycosylated Hyl. Forms banded fibers of small diameter (argyrophilic reticulin) in vivo
IV	? $[\alpha 1(IV)]_2\alpha 2(IV)$ $[\alpha 1(IV)]_3$ $[\alpha 2(IV)]_3$	Basal laminae (e.g., lens capsule, parietal yolk sac, glomerular basement membrane)	High 3-Hyp. Richest in Hyl and glycosylated Hyl. Relatively rich in larger hydrophobic residues. Chains have helical and nonhelical domains and are cross-linked by disulfide. bonds. Forms feltwork of nonbanded fibrils in vivo
V	? $[\alpha l(V)]_2\alpha 2(V)$ $[\alpha l(V)]_3$ $[\alpha 2(V)]_3$ $[\alpha 3(V)]_3$	Almost ubiquitous: relatively prominent in amnion, chorion, muscle, and tendon sheaths	High Hyl and glycosylated Hyl; low alanine. Form thin, nonbanded pericellular laminae

[a]Hyl; hydroxylysine. Hyp; hydroxyproline.

Collagen chains isolated from extracts of basement membranes (e.g., lens capsule and glomerular basement membrane) represent a fourth type of collagen. Such chains are distinguished by size, enrichment in hydrophobic amino acids, and content of 3-hydroxyproline, half-cystine, and glycosylated hydroxylysine. Recent evidence indicates that these extracts contain two classes of chains, but it is not known whether the chains are constituents of one heteropolymeric molecule or whether they each form different molecules containing only one chain class. The fibrillar, nonbanded basal laminar layer of basement membranes is formed mostly by type IV collagen.

A fifth collagen type was designated when three additional collagen chains, αA, αB, and αC, were discovered in extracts of placental tissues. These chains have been renamed α2(V), α1(V), and α3(V), respectively. Type V chains have now been isolated from various tissues, and it is by no means clear if the three chain classes always coexist in given tissues, whether they form heteropolymeric or homopolymeric molecules in vivo, and if they should be exclusively classified as basement membrane collagens. A current view is that these collagens can form thin, nonbanded pericellular laminae around smooth and skeletal muscle cells and fibroblasts.

At least two additional collagen isotypes have been recently isolated from cartilage; most probably other genetic types of collagen will be discovered. It is presumed that each genetic type of collagen represents an evolutionary selection for a molecular form better suited for certain functions. Thus, it appears that type III collagen is better suited than type I for particular functions in fetal skin, healing wounds, and distensible tissues. To define these unique functions and to re-

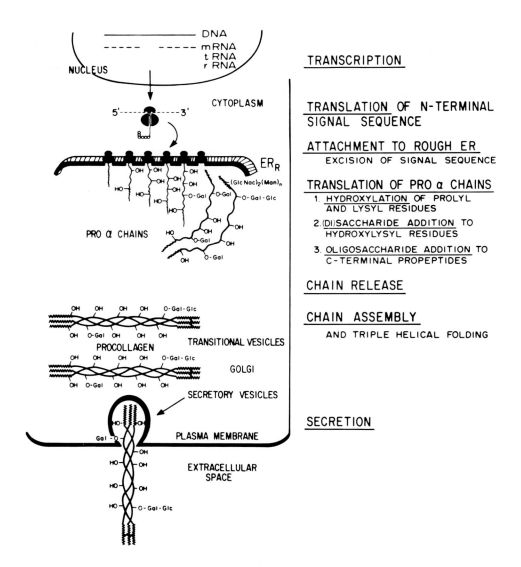

4–9 Collagen biosynthesis: intracellular events and secretion.

late them to the molecular differences among the collagen types remain important tasks.

The fibroblast is responsible for synthesizing the bulk of type I collagen, and its counterpart, the osteoblast, synthesizes the type I collagen of bone. Cartilage collagen (II) is synthesized by the chondroblast. Type III collagen of skin is synthesized by the fibroblast. Apparently, a skin fibroblast may simultaneously synthesize types I and III collagen. The type III collagen found in the muscularis of arteries, intestine, and uterus is synthesized by smooth muscle cells. Smooth

muscle cells also synthesize type I collagen. Basement membrane collagen (IV) is synthesized by endothelial cells of vessels and by various types of surface epithelia. Evidence suggests that type V chains may be synthesized by smooth and skeletal muscle cells, fibroblasts, and some epithelia such as hepatocytes.

Biosynthesis. Most of what we know about collagen biosynthesis has been learned from studying fibroblast systems synthesizing type I collagen, but the mechanisms to be described are probably generally valid for other cell types that synthesize other molecular forms of collagen. The biosynthetic steps are shown schematically in Figs. 4–9 and 4–10.

4–10 Collagen biosynthesis: extracellular events. The propeptides are enzymatically cleaved from the ends of the procollagen molecule, leaving the abbreviated telopeptides of collagen. Collagen molecules aggregate to form fibers. Enzymatic oxidative deamination **(1)** of lysyl or hydroxylysyl residues in the telopeptides introduces reactive aldehydic groups. These aldehydic groups react with the ε-amino groups of lysine or hydroxylysine in adjacent molecules **(2)** to form Schiff bases **(3)**.

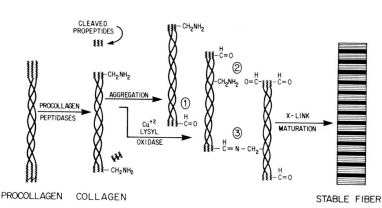

Translation of collagen chains may begin on free polysomes, but aminoterminal "signal" sequences on the nascent polypeptides direct the attachment of the polysomes to the endoplasmic reticulum. The "signal" sequences are excised by proteases, and translation of the chains proceeds with the nascent chains vectorially oriented into the cisternae. The translated chains are precursor forms (pro α chains), having nonhelical polypeptide extensions (propeptides) at the amino- and carboxytermini that are much larger than the telopeptides of the collagen molecule extracted from fibers. Amino acids are incorporated into the nascent chains via transfer RNAs by the usual mechanisms except for hydroxyproline and hydroxylysine. These residues arise from the enzymatic hydroxylation of specific prolyl and lysyl residues in peptide linkage in the growing nascent chains. The two hydroxylating enzymes (prolyl and lysyl hydroxylase) are contained within the granular endoplasmic reticulum; atmospheric O_2, α-ketoglutarate, ferrous ions, and ascorbate function as substrates or cofactors for both of the hydroxylations.

Certain hydroxylysyl residues in the nascent chains become O-glycosidically linked to galactose, and then a glucose residue may be linked to the galactose. These glycosylations require the respective uridine diphosphate sugars and specific galactosyl and glucosyl transferases. Glycosylations involving the carboxyterminal propeptides utilize different mechanisms. In this case, an oligosaccharide unit of N-acetylglucosamine and mannose residues is preassembled on a lipid carrier (dolichol phosphate) and then transferred to an asparaginyl residue in the propeptide chain.

Pro α chains released from polysomes pass into the cisternae of the rough endoplasmic retic-

ulum where some of the hydroxylations and glycosylations described above might be completed. Three pro α chains are covalently assembled by the formation of interchain disulfide bonds between carboxyterminal propeptides. Then noncovalent interactions in the helical collagen domains of the chains stabilize triple helical folding. In addition to their role in chain assembly, the propeptides may serve to keep the assembled procollagen molecule in solution and to aid in its subsequent transcellular movement through membrane-bounded compartments. Assembly of procollagen probably begins in the cisternae, and the molecule is then transported to the Golgi complex via transitional elements of the rough endoplasmic reticulum. Procollagen is transported from the Golgi complex to the cell surface via secretory vesicles, which then fuse with the plasma membrane to discharge the soluble precursor molecules. The transcellular movement and secretion of procollagen require energy, and the microtubular system is necessary to translocate the vacuolar elements. Once secreted from the cell, procollagen is enzymatically converted to collagen (Fig. 4–10). The fibroblast secretes amino and carboxyl procollagen peptidases that excise the respective propeptides from the ends of the precursor, leaving the nonhelical telopeptides as remnants of the original precursor sequences. The collagen molecule that is generated now aggregates in a specific manner to form collagen fibers.

Some elements of the general biosynthetic scheme presented in Figs. 4–9 and 4–10 are provisional. For example, some of the registration peptides of procollagen may be enzymatically excised just before secretion occurs, which may explain the fibrous aggregates observed in secretory vesicles of the odontoblast. Another possibility is that the excision of propeptides may occur after the molecules have polymerized to form thin fibrils in the extracellular space.

The biosynthesis of collagen is evidently complex, for it involves the balanced synthesis of pro α chain classes, posttranslational hydroxylations and glycosylations of specific residues, and extracellular modifications of the precursor so that the final molecule can be incorporated into a type of fiber appropriate to the tissue. If a cell synthesizes two molecular forms of collagen simultaneously, the complexities are increased. Controls clearly must operate at the level of genomic transcription so that the proper kinds and amounts of messenger RNA are released to the cytoplasm. Translational controls may further modulate the balanced synthesis of different chain classes. Presumably the hydroxylations, glycosylations, assembly, and extracellular processing of the precursors are critically determined by the primary structure of the pro α chains, but controls affecting the activities of the various enzymes could also be superimposed.

The biosynthesis of types II and IV collagen illustrates some of the variations that may be imposed on the general scheme. In chondroblasts, type II pro α chains are released into the cisternae of the rough-surfaced endoplasmic reticulum, but they are assembled into a three-chain molecule in this compartment more slowly than type I pro α chains. Assembly of type II pro α chains may not be completed until the chains are transported to smooth-surfaced compartments, and this delay may allow for the more extensive glycosylation of the hydroxylysine residues in this type of collagen. It has been shown for type IV procollagen that the propeptides of the secreted molecule are not subject to extensive excision by peptidases, and the relatively intact procollagen molecule is incorporated into the structure of basal laminae.

Fibrillogenesis. Most collagen in the body is in the form of fibers that display a characteristic "native" pattern of cross-banding when positively or negatively stained with heavy metal ions and examined by electron microscopy (Fig. 4–6). The native pattern is characterized by a major axial repeat period of 670 Å within which 12 dark bands may be resolved under optimal conditions of positive staining. A negatively stained native fiber shows the same repeat period, but within it are only two major bands: a dark zone where the stain penetrates, and a light zone where the stain is excluded.

When neutral salt solutions of pure collagen

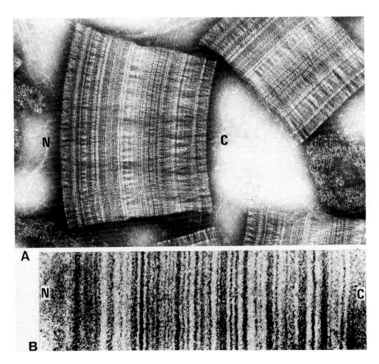

4–11 Electron micrographs of SLS aggregates of collagen. Aggregates are formed by in-register, side-to-side packing of identically polarized molecules. Thus, the length of the aggregate is that of the collagen molecule (3,000 Å) and the aggregates have amino- and carboxyterminal ends (labeled **N** and **C**, respectively). **A.** SLS aggregates of type II collagen, negatively stained. × 133,000. **B.** SLS aggregate of type I collagen, positively stained. The vertical dark bands are formed by binding of stain to charged residues in register across the aggregate. × 280,000. (Courtesy of Romaine R. Bruns.)

are warmed to 37° C the protein precipitates in the form of native fibers. Thus, the native fiber can be considered to be a polymer of collagen molecules and its ultrastructure to result from a specific mode of molecular packing. The nature of that molecular packing was suggested by analysis of another form of aggregated collagen, the segment long spacing (SLS) form (Fig. 4–11). SLS forms precipitate when ATP is added to an acidic solution of collagen; in this instance the aggregates are 3,000 Å in length because they are formed by side-to-side packing of the molecules with their ends in register. Additionally, the molecules have the same polarity so that like residues are in register across the SLS aggregate. Because heavy metal stains used for electron microscopy bind to polar residues, the observed cross-bands represent a map of the distribution of polar side chains along the length of the collagen molecule. Fibrils are formed when molecules are aligned end to end, or when they are overlapped along their long axis. Accordingly, it was found that when SLS forms were overlapped by approximately one quarter of their length, the band pattern of the native fiber could be reconstructed. Therefore a two-dimensional quarter-stagger model of molecular packing for the native fiber was proposed (Fig. 4–12). There are five essential elements of the model: (1) The collagen molecule has a length of 4.4 D; D equals 670 Å. (2) The molecules in the fiber have the same polarity. (3) Axial displacement of adjacent molecules by a distance D produces fibers with a repeat period of D. (4) There is a gap of 0.6 D between the carboxy- and aminotermini of successive molecules lying in the same plane. (5) Mass per unit length alternates within the period, corresponding to an overlap zone of 0.4 D and a hole (gap) zone of 0.6 D. The model accounts for the banding pattern of positively and negatively stained native fibers. In the latter case, the stain penetrates maximally into the hole zone to produce the dark band. The model is also in accord with currently available sequence data for type I collagen chains.

We are still uncertain about how collagen molecules are packed in three dimensions in the native fiber. All of the proposed three-dimensional models incorporate the axial stagger principle described above, but they differ with respect to the symmetry of the lateral spacing of the molecules. A five-stranded rope model has a limiting microfibrillary unit composed of five axially staggered molecules in cylindrical array.

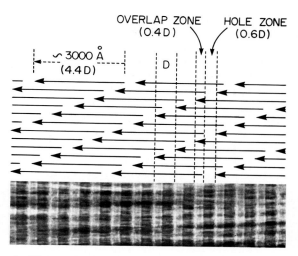

4–12 Two-dimensional model for packing of collagen molecules **(arrows)** in the native-type fiber. **Arrowheads** indicate aminoterminal ends. Adjacent molecules are longitudinally displaced by a distance D (approximately 670 Å) to form a fiber of repeating period D. The electron micrograph of a negatively stained fiber **(below)** shows that each period consists of light overlap zone (0.4 D) from which the stain is mostly excluded, and a dark hole zone (0.6 D) into which the stain penetrates. (Adapted from the model of Hodge, A. J., Petruska, J. A., and Bailey, A. J. 1965. Structure and Function of Connective and Skeletal Tissue. London: Butterworths & Co., Ltd., p. 31.)

The native fibril and the SLS form are only two of many possible periodic structures that can result from electrostatic and hydrophobic interactions between collagen molecules. Moreover, if collagen molecules precipitate without statistical symmetry, nonperiodic aggregates will be generated. Fundamentally, the specificity for all the possible forms of aggregation resides in the primary structure of collagen, but pH, temperature, ionic environment, and noncovalent interactions with noncollagenous molecules can favor one form of collagen packing over another. The essential point is that the chemical environment in vivo is controlled so that collagen types I, II, and III generally pack as native fibrils. Type IV collagen is an exception, for basal laminae are characterized by a feltwork of nonperiodic fibrils. It has been suggested that the galactose-glucose disaccharide or the bulky heteropolysaccharide groups that are covalently linked to type IV collagen molecules prevent native fibrillar packing. Although lacking periodicity, the fibrillar networks of basal laminae have a structural order that determines their capacity to function as molecular sieves.

When loose connective tissues are stained with alkaline solutions of silver salts, a delicate network of very thin silver-stained fibers can be seen by light microscopy. These reticular fibers (reticulin) often underlie basal laminae of various types and contribute to the supporting stroma of epithelial and hematopoietic tissues. Because thick collagenous fibers do not stain intensely with the silver stain, reticulin and collagen were once assumed to be different fibrous proteins. We now believe, however, that most reticulin is collagen, because electron microscopy shows that argyrophilic reticular fibers may have the characteristic periodicity of collagen. We also believe that most reticulin is formed from type III collagen and that its argyrophilia is best ascribed to a coating of proteoglycans and glycoproteins on these thin collagen fibers. In some tissues argyrophilic reticulin may fail to show collagen periodicity. In these instances the collagen may have aggregated randomly or be of the basal laminar type, or the observed materials might be composed almost entirely of proteoglycans and glycoproteins.

We have emphasized that collagen fibers in particular tissues are distinctive in their numbers, length, thickness, and spatial orientation. We do not yet understand how these particular arrangements are achieved. It has been suggested that the initial assembly of the fibril may be critically influenced by interactions between the collagen molecules and cellular surfaces, such interactions occuring either within secretory vesicles or on the plasma membrane of the secreting cell. Fibril growth away from the cell might also be influenced by interactions with negatively charged proteoglycans and glycoproteins; such interactions might determine the rate of polymerization and the ultimate size and orientation of the collagen fiber generated. Directional forces produced by musculoskeletal activity could also serve to orient formed collagen fibers. A better understanding of fibrillogenesis awaits a more detailed knowledge of the interactions between the collagens, the cells, and the noncollagenous molecules of the connective tissue matrix.

Cross-Linking of Collagen Fibers. Noncovalent interactions between collagen molecules are mainly responsible for the assembly of the collagen fiber; once formed, however, the fiber becomes stabilized by covalent intermolecular cross-links. These cross-links are initiated when a specific copper-dependent amine oxidase (lysyl oxidase) secreted by the fibroblast converts certain lysyl and hydroxylysyl ε-amino groups to aldehydes. Most of these converted residues are at the ends of the α chains, i.e., in the telopeptides. Intra- and intermolecular cross-links between α chains can now form by the reaction of two aldehydic groups (an aldol condensation product) or by the formation of an aldimine bond (a Schiff base) between an aldehyde and the ε-amino group of an unmodified lysyl or hydrosylysyl residue. The latter type of adduct is shown in the scheme of Fig. 4–10.

The cross-linking process is an extracellular event and it is suspected that oxidative deamination of the lysyl and hydroxylysyl residues occurs after procollagen peptidases have removed the propeptides from procollagen. Noncovalent associations bring the molecules into the staggered array of the native fibril, and where aldehydic and ε-amino groups are apposed cross-links are formed nonenzymatically.

A more complete description of the chemistry of the collagen cross-links is beyond our scope, but we emphasize the functional importance of these bonds. Introduction of covalent cross-links into the fiber increases its tensile strength by preventing slippage between molecules, renders the fiber less soluble, and decreases the fiber's susceptibility to proteolytic turnover. The cross-linking process is finely controlled: collagen fibers from particular tissues have characteristic kinds and amounts of cross-links, which largely determine the mechanical properties of the fibers. For example, a more chemically stable intermolecular cross-link is achieved when an aldimine bond is made between two hydroxylysyl residues. Such cross-links are characteristically abundant in cartilage and bone.

When normal collagen cross-linking is disturbed, as may occur in certain inherited and acquired diseases (see below), the consequences can be dramatic. For example, the skin may become hyperextensible; ligaments, tendons, and fasciae may weaken, bones may grow improperly; wounds may heal poorly; and blood vessels can dilate and rupture.

Degradation (Turnover) of Collagen. Under physiological conditions of pH and temperature the collagen molecule retains its triple helical structure, thus remaining resistant to digestion by most tissue proteases. Yet collagen molecules and fibers undergo significant degradation during growth, remodeling, involution, and inflammation and repair of tissues. Collagen turnover in these instances is initiated by the action of enzymes with specific affinities for native interstitial collagens (types I, II, and III). These enzymes are called the animal collagenases to distinguish them from collagenases synthesized by bacteria. Cell types that synthesize animal collagenases include fibroblasts, synovial cells, polymorphonuclear leucocytes, macrophages, and epithelia of skin and cornea.

Although the collagenases from the different cell types may differ in their affinities for collagen types I, II, and III, they all appear to cleave the molecules in the same manner: the three helical chains of the native molecule are cleaved at a single site 750 Å in from the carboxylterminus, thus generating two triple helical fragments that represent, respectively, 75% and 25% of the original molecule. Occasionally a collagenase may make secondary clips through the three chains of the larger cleavage product. If the fragments are not bound by intermolecular cross-links to other molecules of a fiber, they can go into solution and diffuse away. The triple helical fragments have lower melting points than the parent molecule and so are denatured to random coils at body temperature. Denatured, they are susceptible to further digestion by the collagenases or by other neutral proteases in the extracellular space. Additionally, the molecular fragments, or partially digested fibrils, may be phagocytized by macrophages and degraded within secondary lysosomes by proteases with acid pH optima.

The purified collagenases that digest the interstitial collagens do not degrade collagen types IV and V, but there is evidence that certain tumor cells, activated macrophages, and polymorphonuclear leucocytes can synthesize enzymes that attack these collagens.

For the normal remodeling of connective tissues during growth or after injury and repair, there must be a proper balance between the formation and resorption of collagen fibers. How this linkage between collagen synthesis and turnover is achieved is not known in detail, but there are clues about how collagenase activity is modulated. Synthesis of collagenases by various cell types can be stimulated by hormones, prostaglandins, and substances secreted from lymphocytes (lymphokines) and macrophages. Some

collagenases are synthesized and secreted as inactive precursors (zymogens) that must be modified by proteases before they can digest collagen. Finally, inhibitory molecules that complex with activated collagenases have been identified in a variety of tissues.

Collagen and Disease. The pathogenesis of certain inherited and acquired diseases of connective tissue is now understood in terms of disturbances in the intracellular and extracellular steps of collagen biosynthesis and turnover.

Molecular defects in collagen can arise from mutations in the genes coding for the structural and enzymatic proteins of the biosynthetic pathways. The diseases or syndromes caused by such mutant genes are defined by their patterns of inheritance, their clinical manifestations, and the gene product that is defective. The Ehlers-Danlos syndromes, for example, represent several categories of patients with inherited defects in the formation or stability of collagen fibers. The symptom complexes in such patients include hyperextensible skin, hypermobile joints, hernias, poor wound healing, skeletal deformities, and ocular fragility. Some of these syndromes are due to a lack of lysyl hydroxylase or lysyl oxidase activities or are caused by a mutation affecting the propeptide sequence in the region subject to cleavage by an aminoterminal procollagen peptidase. Although different gene products are affected in these syndromes, the clinical manifestations in all of them are ascribed to inadequate cross-linking of collagen fibers. The enzymic defects prevent the formation of stable hydroxylysyl-derived cross-links or reduce cross-linking in general. The retention of aminoterminal propeptides is assumed to disturb molecular packing and subsequent cross-linking of fibers.

Included in the Ehlers-Danlos syndromes are other patients with fragile, easily bruised, translucent skin, who are prone to rupture of the intestine or large blood vessels. In these patients, synthesis or secretion of type III collagen is reduced.

Scurvy is an acquired disease of collagen metabolism caused by a lack of dietary vitamin C (ascorbic acid). In scurvy, collagen fibers are not formed and consequently bone growth and dentition are abnormal, wounds and fractures do not heal, and capillaries are susceptible to rupture. This disease complex is related to the requirement for vitamin C in the enzymatic hydroxylation of the prolyl and lysyl residues of collagen.

A procollagen molecule lacking hydroxyproline residues has an unstable triple helix and is prone, therefore, to denaturation and proteolytic turnover. Moreover, such underhydroxylated procollagen molecules are secreted at an abnormally slow rate from the fibroblast. The few collagen fibers that may be assembled extracellularly will not be adequately cross-linked because they lack the stable hydroxylysine-derived bonds. Such fibers will be mechanically deficient and subject to degradation.

There are many other acquired diseases in which the metabolism of collagen is altered significantly. In rheumatoid arthritis the destruction of the articular cartilage is due to the release of specific collagenases and proteases from the inflamed synovial membrane. Alterations in vascular basal laminae characterize much of the pathology of diabetes mellitus. In atherosclerosis and hypertensive vascular disease some of the changes in the blood vessels are due to the secretion of increased amounts of collagen by smooth muscle cells.

Diseases with an inflammatory component, whether of infectious, metabolic, or autoimmune origin, inevitably affect collagenous structures, and new collagen fibers are deposited as part of the reparative response to tissue damage. The resulting collagen scars can further limit function and contribute to the morbidity of disease. This brief overview shows that the prevention and rational treatment of many diseases will require an understanding of collagen structure, function, and metabolism.

Elastic Fibers

Elastic fibers stretch easily and return to their original length when the deforming force is removed. They are found in tissues normally subject to stretching and expansile forces, such as arteries, the vocal cords, pleura, trachea, bronchi, pulmonary alveolar septa, certain ligaments (ligamenta flava of humans, ligamentum nuchae of ruminants), auricular cartilage, Scarpa's fascia of the anterior abdominal wall, and the skin. Special stains (Verhoeff's stain, Weigert's resorcin-fuchsin) are required to identify elastic fibers in histological preparations for light microscopy (Fig. 4–13). The thickness, length, and disposition of the fibers differ in different tissues. In arteries, elastic fibers form two thick concentric lamellae, the elastica interna and externa, and elastic fibers are also dispersed through the me-

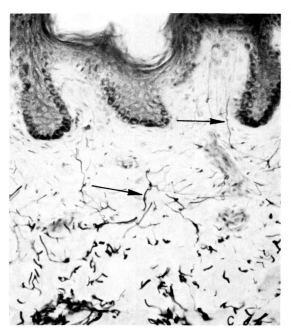

4–13 Elastic fibers **(arrows)** in dermis of skin are stained black with Verhoeff's stain. × 600.

dia of the artery as a concentric, highly fenestrated network. In mesentery, fasciae, and skin, the thin and scattered fibers form networks between bundles of collagen. In the peripheral portions of the respiratory tree, very thin elastic fibers follow the course of the bronchioles, alveolar ducts, and sacs.

By electron microscopy most of an elastic fiber appears to be composed of material whose structure is neither fibrillar nor periodic and that has little affinity for the standard staining reagents (Fig. 4–14). However, at the periphery of the amorphous component, the stains define microfibrils approximately 110 Å in diameter. When elastic fibers are forming, the microfibrillar component appears first and then the amorphous component accumulates to form the bulk of the fiber.

The chemical compositions of the amorphous and microfibrillar components of the fiber differ from each other. *Elastin*, the insoluble protein that remains after connective tissues are digested with dilute alkali, is derived from the amorphous component of the elastic fiber. Like collagen, about one-third of the residues of elastin are glycine, about 11% are proline. Unlike collagen, elastin is composed mostly of nonpolar hydro-

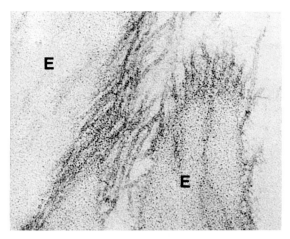

4–14 Electron micrograph of elastic fibers. The fibers are composed of amorphous elastin **(E)** and a peripheral microfibrillar protein. × 84,400. (Courtesy of Russell Ross.)

phobic amino acids, and it has little hydroxyproline and no hydroxylysine. Also and uniquely, elastin contains desmosine and isodesmosine (Fig. 4–15), which function as covalent cross-links in and between the polypeptide chains. Elastin stains poorly with ionic dyes because it

4–15 The structure of desmosine **(A)** and isodesmosine **(B)**. The isomers function as cross-links in elastin.

contains relatively few charged amino acids; the preponderance of hydrophobic residues and the presence of cross-links account for elastin's insolubility.

The microfibrillar protein is composed mainly of hydrophilic amino acids. It contains much less glycine than elastin and has no hydroxyproline, desmosine, or isodesmosine. It contains a relatively large number of half-cystine residues, which are absent from elastin. Accordingly, when elastic fibers are treated with chemical agents that break disulfide bonds, the microfibrils are solubilized and the elastin is left as an insoluble residue. Neutral sugars represent about 5% of the weight of the microfibrillar protein.

Fibroblasts and smooth muscle cells synthesize the molecules that form the elastic fiber. The microfibrillar protein and elastin are synthesized on the rough endoplasmic reticulum and reach the cell surface by the same organellar pathways used for other secretory proteins. Little is known about the detailed structure of the microfibrillar protein and how its synthesis, secretion, and extracellular assembly are coordinated with elastin biosynthesis. As for elastin, the best evidence favors its synthesis and secretion as a single, soluble polypeptide chain of about 70,000 daltons ("tropoelastin"). Assembly and cross-linking of individual tropoelastin chains to form the amorphous component of the elastic fiber occur in the extracellular space. The desmosine and isodesmosine cross-links of elastin are initiated by an enzymatic reaction like that described for the cross-linking of collagen. A copper-dependent lysyl oxidase catalyzes the oxidative deamination of the ε-amino groups of specific lysyl residues in the polypeptide chains of elastin. Three aldelydic residues ("allysyl" residues) formed by this reaction condense with a fourth intact lysyl residue to give the carbon and nitrogen ring structure of the desmosines (Fig. 4–16). Thus, the desmosines have the potential of cross-linking four tropoelastin chains. The formation of the cross-links could be the nucleation step for the aggregation of elastic fibers, could add soluble tropoelastin chains to an insoluble fiber matrix, or could occur with time in a preassembled elastic fiber.

Available data suggest various structural models for elastin. One model, derived from the structure of rubber, posits a three-dimensional network of randomly coiled chains joined by covalent cross-links. The noncovalent interchain forces are considered to be weak and the cova-

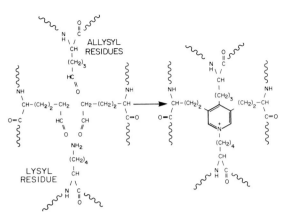

4–16 Schematic diagram showing how four lysine residues form the desmosines and how the latter may potentially link four elastin chains.

lent cross-links to be widely spaced. Thus, minimal unidirectional forces would produce extensive slippage of chains (stretching) before the cross-links restricted their movement. Because the thermodynamics of stretching of elastin does not fit that of rubber, other models have been proposed that depict elastin as a syncytium of easily deformable globular or fibrillar corpuscles behaving as an array of interconnected springs.

Elastic fibers may be altered by disease. In severe atherosclerosis the elastic laminae and networks in arteries are subject to thinning and fragmentation, and lipids and calcium are deposited upon the fibers. Such arteries lose their normal elastic recoil and can become dilated. In pulmonary emphysema there is abnormal enlargement of air spaces distal to terminal bronchioles, associated with destruction of alveolar septa and diminished elastic recoil of the lung. Patients with pulmonary emphysema are short of breath and display an increased expiratory effort. Some forms of pulmonary emphysema are thought to follow the destruction of elastic and collagen fibers by lysosomal elastases released from neutrophils and macrophages.

The Ground Substance

The cellular and fibrous components of connective tissues are surrounded by materials collectively called the *ground substance*. The ground substance is poorly stained and appears amorphous in conventional preparations, but we know that proteoglycans and glycoproteins form most of the interstitial ground substance.

Proteins with covalently attached carbohydrate units are called proteoglycans or glycoproteins. The general characteristics of these two classes of glycoconjugates are compared in Table 4–3. Within each class are molecules that do not fulfill all criteria, and some of these exceptions will be noted.

Proteoglycans

The proteoglycans are secreted products of resident cells of the connective tissues. The proteoglycans are polyanions and hence, when present in sufficient concentrations (for example, in cartilage), they stain with conventional basic dyes such as hematoxylin. In lower concentrations, they may be detected with special cationic dyes (for example, colloidal iron, alcian blue), which have a high affinity for the anionic groups of the macromolecules. Toluidine blue and crystal vi-

Table 4–3 Characteristics of Proteoglycans and Glycoproteins

PROTEOGLYCANS	GLYCOPROTEINS
1. High relative content of carbohydrate	1. Low relative content of carbohydrate
2. Carbohydrate chains longer and linear	2. Carbohydrate chains shorter and branched
3. Carbohydrate chains composed of repeating disaccharide units (a) Repeating units consist of hexosamines (D-glucosamine or D-galactosamine) and uronic acids (D-glucuronic or L-iduronic)	3. Carbohydrate chains not composed of repeating disaccharide units (a) Uronic acids absent
4. Fucose, sialic acid, and mannose residues uncommon	4. Fucose, sialic acid, and mannose residues common
5. High content of ester sulfate groups	5. Absence of ester sulfate groups
6. Unique xylose to serine linkage in some proteoglycans	6. Other types of carbohydrate–protein linkage

olet are cationic dyes that undergo characteristic spectral shifts (metachromasia) when reacting with the anionic groups of the proteoglycans. The proteoglycans are grouped according to the composition of the polysaccharide chains (glycosaminoglycans) attached to the protein core.

Hyaluronic Acid. We are not certain if hyaluronic acid is a true proteoglycan because we do not have firm evidence that its polysaccharide chains are covalently linked to protein. Its carbohydrate chains are formed from repeating units of N-acetylglucosamine and D-glucuronic acid, and it is estimated that about 2,500 such units form chains of approximately 10^6 daltons. In contrast to the other glycosaminoglycans, hyaluronic acid is not sulfated. Hyaluronic acid is widely distributed in loose connective tissues. It is a major component of synovial fluid and the vitreous body of the eye, and it has been extracted in significant amounts from cartilage, blood vessels, skin, and umbilical cord.

Chondroitin Sulfate. The repeating unit is N-acetylgalactosamine and D-glucuronic acid, and the hexosamine is variously sulfated at carbons 4 or 6. Approximately 60 repeating units contribute to an estimated molecular weight of about 30,000. This molecule predominates in cartilage, bone, and blood vessels, but it has also been identified in skin, cornea, and other connective tissues.

Dermatan Sulfate. The repeating unit is N-acetylgalactosamine-4-sulfate and L-iduronic acid. This is a stereoisomer of chondroitin 4-sulfate in which L-iduronic acid has generally replaced D-glucuronic acid, although a few of the latter groups may still occur in each polysaccharide chain. Its molecular weight is comparable to that of chondroitin sulfate. Dermatan sulfate is found mostly in the skin, but is has also been demonstrated in blood vessels, heart valves, tendons, and the connective tissues of the lung.

Keratan Sulfate. The repeating unit is N-acetylglucosamine-6-sulfate and galactose. In this structure the degree of sulfation of the hexosamine group can vary considerably. Moreover, the galactose residues may be sulfated in position 6, and galactosamine may also be present. Two keratan sulfate types have been identified: Type I, located exclusively in the cornea; type II, found in association with chondroitin sulfate in skeletal tissues such as cartilage and the nucleus pulposus. The keratan sulfates have characteristics of both proteoglycans and glycoproteins. Although composed of repeating disaccharide units, the keratans lack uronic acid residues. Their carbohydrate chains tend to be short, and they contain fucose, sialic acid, and mannose residues. Type I keratan sulfate is unique among the proteoglycans for having an N-glycosidic bond between an N-acetylglucosaminyl residue and the amido nitrogen of an aspariginyl residue in the polypeptide chain. This type of linkage group is commonly found in glycoproteins.

Heparan Sulfate. The repeating unit is N-acetylglucosamine and D-glucuronic acid, but some iduronic acid residues are also present. Sulfate esters are formed with the nitrogen group of deacetylated glucosamine and with oxygens of the hexosamine and iduronic acid residues. Heparan sulfate appears to be a ubiquitous surface component of many cell types; one form of this proteoglycan may be localized in the lamina lucida zone of basement membranes.

Heparin, the anticoagulant and antilipemic agent, is related structurally to heparan sulfate. In contrast to the latter, however, it has a higher content of N-sulfated glucosamine and O-sulfated iduronic acid residues. Heparin is characteristically synthesized and stored within mast cells.

The proteoglycans are thus classified according to the nature of their repeating disaccharide units but considerable molecular heterogeneity can exist within each group. For example, keratan sulfate from the cornea is not the same molecule as keratan sulfate from cartilage, and there may be a unique heparan sulfate-containing proteoglycan in basement membranes. Even when a given proteoglycan is carefully isolated from a single tissue or cell type, the molecules are often polydisperse in size. This heterogeneity can be due to differences in lengths of the protein cores or to variations in the number, size, or degree of sulfation of the glycosaminoglycan chains. For example, the size polydispersity of rat mast cell heparin has been ascribed to attachment of varying numbers of glycosaminoglycan chains of constant size and sulfation to a constant core protein.

The complex organization of the proteoglycans is illustrated by the model proposed for the proteoglycans of cartilage (Fig. 4–17). The fundamental structural unit is called the *proteogly-*

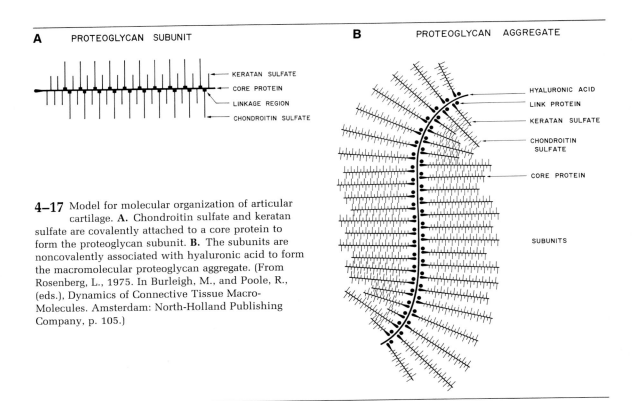

A   PROTEOGLYCAN   SUBUNIT

← KERATAN SULFATE
← CORE PROTEIN
← LINKAGE REGION
← CHONDROITIN SULFATE

B   PROTEOGLYCAN   AGGREGATE

← HYALURONIC ACID
← LINK PROTEIN
← KERATAN SULFATE
← CHONDROITIN SULFATE
← CORE PROTEIN

SUBUNITS

4-17 Model for molecular organization of articular cartilage. **A.** Chondroitin sulfate and keratan sulfate are covalently attached to a core protein to form the proteoglycan subunit. **B.** The subunits are noncovalently associated with hyaluronic acid to form the macromolecular proteoglycan aggregate. (From Rosenberg, L., 1975. In Burleigh, M., and Poole, R., (eds.), Dynamics of Connective Tissue Macro-Molecules. Amsterdam: North-Holland Publishing Company, p. 105.)

can subunit; it appears to consist of a core protein of variable length, to which are covalently linked chondroitin sulfate and keratan sulfate chains. The length of the core protein appears to determine the number of polysaccharide chains attached. The proteoglycan subunits in turn form a *proteoglycan aggregate* by noncovalent attachments to a hyaluronic acid backbone. Subunits are associated with hyaluronic acid through an invariant region of the core protein and an additional link protein.

Biosynthesis and Catabolism. Generally the proteoglycans are synthesized and secreted by cells derived from the primitive mesenchyme, for example, fibroblasts, chondroblasts, osteoblasts, synovial cells, and smooth muscle cells. Translation of the protein moiety of these molecules is restricted to the rough-surfaced endoplasmic reticulum, and the addition of the carbohydrate residues probably begins before the polypeptide is released from the ribosome. The polysaccharide chains are assembled by catalyzed stepwise transfers of monosaccharides from nucleotide sugar donors. This is the mechanism except when the linkage to protein is

made through an N-glycosidic bond between *N*-acetylglucosamine and an asparagine residue in the nascent peptide chain (as in keratan sulfate I). In this instance a core oligosaccharide is preassembled on a lipid carrier, dolichol phosphate, and the oligosaccharide is then transferred to the nascent peptide.

The polysaccharide chains are subject to such modifications as trimming by glycosidases, addition of new terminal sugars, deacetylation, introduction of sulfate groups, and epimerization of D-glucuronyl residues to L-iduronosyl residues. These reactions can begin in the rough endoplasmic reticulum and be completed in the Golgi zone. Secretion of the molecules occurs by transport to the plasma membrane via smooth-surfaced vesicles. Assembly of proteoglycan subunits into larger aggregates probably occurs after secretion from the cell.

The proteoglycans turn over more rapidly than collagen in both growing and adult individuals. The catabolic turnover of the polysaccharide components of the proteoglycans is accomplished by a series of exoglycosidases, sugar sulfatases, and some endoglycosidases acting sequentially. These enzymes are contained within lysosomes of the cellular elements of the connective tissues. Much of our knowledge of these degradative pathways has come from studying patients with inherited deficiencies in these enzymes. In these diseases, the "mucopolysaccharidoses," partially digested proteoglycans accumulate in the tissues, causing characteristic clinical and biochemical disturbances. Less is known about the turnover of the protein cores of the proteoglycans, but we assume it is accomplished by a variety of intracellular and extracellular proteases.

Structure and Function. The polysaccharide chains of proteoglycans are thought to be generally unbranched. The sulfate and carboxyl groups in the repeating disaccharide units of the chains provide a high density of anionic charges that promote an elongated chain configuration. The protein moieties of the molecules may also impose configurational restraints. The proteoglycans thus extend through a larger volume of solution ("domain") than do uncharged, highly folded molecules with similar molecular weights. The elongated proteoglycans tend to become entangled and form three-dimensional nets with themselves and other polymeric molecules in the connective tissue spaces.

Most of the functions of the proteoglycans can be related to the chemical and physical properties mentioned above. We have noted the affinity of cationic dyes for the anionic groups of the polysaccharide chains. In vivo, the proteoglycans presumably interact electrostatically with a variety of cationic molecules and, through such binding, play a significant role in the transport of electrolytes and water. We have said that proteoglycans might interact with positively charged collagen molecules to affect collagen fiber formation. The permeability, transport, and osmotic functions of interstitial fluid can also be modified by the entangled proteoglycans acting as molecular sieves to exclude or entrap molecules of different sizes. Such networks increase the viscosity of interstitial fluids and can thus contribute to their lubricative and mechanical functions. Because of its high molecular weight, hyaluronic acid contributes importantly to the viscosity of interstitial fluids. The viscous or gel-like nature of tissue fluids may also help to limit the spread of bacteria. Additionally, special antilipemic and anticoagulant functions are recognized for heparin and dermatan sulfate.

In summary, the proteoglycans help to maintain the proper homeostatic environment for cells and fibrous elements. Their diversity and heterogeneity reflect their adaptation for different functions in different types of tissue.

Structural Glycoproteins of Connective Tissues

Procollagens, collagens, and the microfibrillar protein of elastic fibers all have covalently attached carbohydrate residues and thus are properly classified as glycoproteins. Recently, two additional glycoproteins, *fibronectin* and *laminin*, have been identified as structural elements of the connective tissue matrix.

Fibronectin is a major surface glycoprotein of the fibroblast but it is also synthesized by other mesenchymally-derived cells, by epithelia and endothelia, and by some marrow-derived cell types. The protein is synthesized as a 220,000-dalton monomer with complex oligosaccharide chains linked to asparaginyl residues. Fibronectin appears at the cell surface as a disulfide-linked dimer and, with time, disulfide-linked multimers are formed. Fibronectin is readily shed into the extracellular space and appears in the blood plasma; in this plasma form, fibronectin is also called cold insoluble globulin.

Interest in the fibronectin molecule as a component of the structural matrix of connective tissues was generated by the observation that fibronectin mediates the attachment of fibroblasts to collagen gels in vitro. Also, immunofluorescent staining demonstrates fibronectin in most connective tissues, where it is generally associated with the interstitial collagens. It has been proposed that collagen and fibronectin form an integrated fibrillary network in vivo that influences the adhesion, motility, growth, and differentiation of cells. Fibronectin also has been shown to bind to proteoglycans, fibrinogen, and fibrin, to mediate platelet–collagen interactions, and to function as a chemotactic agent and opsonin.

Laminin is a recently discovered noncollagenous glycoprotein; it is a constituent of basement membranes. Laminin is composed of at least two large polypeptide chains (mol wts 220,000 and 440,000) joined by disulfide bonds. Immunofluorescence studies with antibodies against laminin show that it is produced by a variety of cultured cells and that basement membranes in normal tissues contain laminin or an immunologically related protein. Purified antibodies to laminin do not react with fibronectin or with type IV collagen. Evidence suggests that within normal basement membranes laminin is a component of the amorphous unstained layers (the laminae rarae).

Macrophages

Macrophages are long-lived, actively phagocytic cells that are widely distributed throughout the body. They share both a common origin, the bone marrow, and common biological properties, including the secretion of a variety of important molecules. Their very effective phagocytosis subserves a crucial role in the clearance and disposal of microorganisms, damaged body constituents, and particulate pollutants. Macrophages and their precursors are classed within the "mononuclear phagocyte system" (MPS). Significantly, the MPS can respond to appropriate stimulation, often mediated by products of activated lymphocytes, with both quantitative (numerical) and qualitative (cellular) changes. The cellular changes include enhanced microbicidal ability and growth-inhibitory or lytic effects on tumor cells. Besides these direct roles, macrophages participate in the immune responses in various other ways.

The importance of phagocytic cells in antibacterial defense was first delineated in 1882 by Elie Metchnikoff. Starting with observations of transparent starfish larvae, Metchnikoff examined phagocytosis in the various animal phyla. He found that vertebrates characteristically possessed two types of cells able to fight invading microorganisms. The cell types were the microphages (small eaters), now known as polymorphonuclear leukocytes (PMN), and the macrophages (big eaters). The latter included the monocytes of the blood and the phagocytic cells found in many tissues and organs. Early in the twentieth century, other investigators showed that acid disazo dyes (trypan blue, for example) injected into animals accumulated in certain cells in different tissues and organs. This collection of cells was named by Aschoff the "reticuloendothelial system" (RES), a term which unfortunately persists in the literature. Aschoff proposed that the RES was not only involved in defense but had other functions such as hematopoiesis, blood destruction, and metabolism of iron, bilirubin, and fat. Several of the cells included in the RES (Table 4–4) belong to the original macrophage population described by Metchnikoff. It is now known that the disazo dyes are bound to plasma albumin and taken into cells by pinocytosis. Indeed, as the dyes administered in vivo are also captured by other cells such as kid-

Table 4–4 Components of the Reticuloendothelial System

Sinus lining macrophages
Lymph sinuses
Blood sinuses
Liver (Kupffer cells)
Spleen
Bone marrow
Adrenal cortex
Anterior pituitary
Microglia (central nervous system)
Reticular cells of lymphatic tissues
Tissue macrophages (histiocytes)
Blood macrophages (monocytes)

Source: Lord Florey. 1970. General Pathology, 4th ed. London: Lloyd-Luke (Medical Books) Ltd., p. 156.

ney tubular epithelia, dye uptake alone cannot be used to define the macrophage system. Several cells included in the RES, such as those lining the sinusoids of the spleen, or the fibroblastic reticular cells of hematopoietic tissues, are only weakly phagocytic and differ from monocytes and macrophages in their recognition of particulate matter.

In recent years the RES has been reexamined and a new concept, the mononuclear phagocyte system (MPS), has been proposed in its stead. As shown in Table 4–5, the MPS excludes some of the cells of the RES and adds others. Minimal criteria for inclusion of cell types in the MPS are (1) derivation from bone marrow precursor cells, (2) characteristic cell structure, and (3) high level of phagocytic activity mediated by immunoglobulin and components of the serum complement system. Other cell types, such as fibroblasts, thyroid epithelium, or pigmented retinal cells, can ingest certain particulate materials, but such uptake is not increased by immunoglobulins and complement. PMNs are arbitrarily excluded from the MPS classification, even though they share many properties with the cells of the MPS.

Origin, Fate, and Life Span of Macrophages

In rodents, macrophages of inflammatory exudates as well as resident macrophages from the peritoneal cavity and the parenchyma of the liver and lung are derived from circulating monocytes. Macrophages are now thought to originate in the following way (see Fig. 4–18). A stem cell for the monocyte is derived from a pluripotential bone marrow cell. Such stem cells, which have not been identified morphologically, are also found

Table 4–5 The Mononuclear Phagocyte System

Cells	Localization
Stem cell (committed) ↓	Bone marrow
Monoblasts ↓	Bone marrow
Promonocytes ↓	Bone marrow
Monocytes ↓	Bone marrow Peripheral blood
Macrophages	Tissues
	Connective tissue (histiocytes)
	Liver (Kupffer cells)
	Lung (alveolar macrophages)
	Lymph nodes (free and fixed macrophages)
	Spleen (free and fixed macrophages)
	Bone marrow (macrophages)
	Serous cavities (pleural and peritoneal macrophages)
	Bone tissue (osteoclasts [?])
	Nervous system (microglial cells)

Source: van Furth, R. (ed.). 1975. Mononuclear Phagocytes in Immunity, Infection and Pathology. Oxford: Blackwell Scientific Publications, Ltd. (Reproduced by permission of the author and publisher.)

in the yolk sac and in the liver in embryonic and fetal life. Postnatally, maturation occurs in the bone marrow, and mature monocytes are released into the circulation. Release must occur steadily and rapidly because there is only a small pool of monocytes in the marrow. Monocytes remain in circulation for about 40 h, enter the connective tissues, and increase in size, lysosomal enzyme content, and endocytic activity; they are thus operationally recognized as macrophages. Under experimental or pathological conditions macrophages can show replicative activity. Their

life span varies in different tissues but may be several months or more, which agrees with the extended longevity of macrophages maintained in tissue culture. There is also in vivo evidence for macrophage translocation within the body; for example, labeled macrophages transferred to the peritoneal cavity can later be found in the liver, spleen, and thymus.

In response to foreign bodies and to certain infections (for example, tuberculosis and leprosy), macrophages can fuse to form giant cells that can have 20 or more nuclei. Alternatively, in chronic granulomas, macrophages may establish tight junctions, become less phagocytic, and show fewer lysosomes. Because of their resemblance to epithelia, these modified macrophages are called *epithelioid cells*. Epithelioid cells seem to wall off inflammatory sites.

In vitro studies have strengthened this concept of the origin and fate of mononuclear phagocytes. Colonies of murine macrophages have been shown to arise when marrow cell suspensions or cell suspensions from peripheral tissues (lung, spleen, or thymus) are cultivated in

4–18 Cell lineage of mononuculear phagocytes. The pluripotent stem cell (CFU-S) can differentiate into stem cells of more restricted potential. These include CFU-Meg (that differentiate into megakaryocytes), BFU-E (that differentiate into erythrocytes), CFU-Ly (that differentiate into lymphocytes), CFU-Eo (that differentiate into eosinophils), CFU-Bas (that differentiate into basophils), and CFU-GM (that differentiate into both neutrophils and monocytes). The evidence for the presence of CFU-Ly and CFU-Bas is less secure than for the other stem cells. See discussion of hematopoietic stem cells. (Adapted from R. van Furth "Mononuclear Phagocytes in Immunity, Infection and Pathology" page 162. Blackwell Scientific Publications, Ltd. Oxford, 1975.)

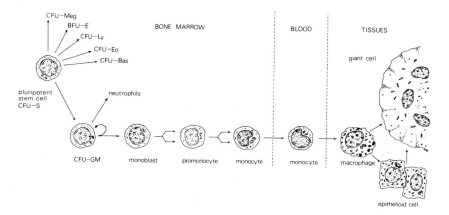

the presence of required growth factors. One of these factors—the "granulocyte-macrophage colony stimulating factor," produced by mouse fibroblasts—has been characterized, isolated, and purified to homogeneity. Transformation of human blood monocytes into macrophages in culture is also readily accomplished. Finally, a variety of rodent and human macrophage-like cell lines have been developed. These lines allow the production of large numbers of cells for biochemical studies and provide the opportunity to select for variants defective in certain phagocytic and metabolic functions.

Structure of Macrophages

With the light microscope and the usual tissue sections stained with hematoxylin and eosin, it is difficult to identify quiescent macrophages with any certainty. An irregularly shaped nucleus and abundant and eosinophilic cytoplasm may help in the identification, but fibroblasts, lymphoid cells, or pericytes may have similar features. In sections or imprints, macrophages may be better identified by cytochemical methods for lysosomal enzymes, such as acid phosphatase, glucuronidase, or fluoride-resistant esterases. Monocytes and macrophages are well stained by these techniques. The recent availability of monoclonal antibodies to immunoglobulin receptors (Fc receptors) on the macrophage plasma membrane may permit cells of the monocyte–macrophage series to be identified more precisely by immunofluorescence and immune electron microscopy.

Unequivocal identification of macrophages by ultrastructure alone is often impossible. By electron microscopy the macrophage surface is thrown into numerous folds or fingerlike processes (Figs. 4–19 and 4–20). The surface processes participate in spreading, phagocytosis, and cell movement and essentially provide reserve plasma membrane. The cell nucleus is often indented and the cytoplasm typically contains abundant endocytic vacuoles, lysosomes, and phagolysosomes (Fig. 4–21). Mitochondria and the cytoskeletal elements—microtubules, microfilaments, and intermediate filaments—are present. Bundles of actin-rich microfilaments are often arranged under the plasma membrane and are prominent at sites where the membrane adheres to substrates or to phagocytized particles. Microfilaments appear to be involved in adhesion, endocytosis, and movement, but they may also inhibit the fusion of lysosomes with the

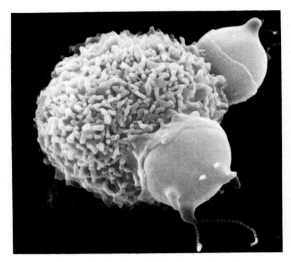

4–19 Scanning electron micrograph of freshly explanted mouse macrophage in the process of ingesting aldehyde-treated erythrocytes. Small fingerlike processes decorate the surface of the phagocyte. The macrophage periphery extends as a collar over the erythrocytes. × 4,600. (Courtesy of J. P. Revel, M. Rabinovitch, and M. J. DeStefano.)

plasma membrane. A relatively large Golgi region participates in the maturation of the lysosomes and in membrane recirculation. Smooth and rough endoplasmic reticulum are prominent, and the latter is the site of synthesis of lysosomal hydrolases as well as of many macromolecules secreted by macrophages. Mature and functionally activated macrophages have more complex and numerous surface folds and increased numbers of vacuoles, lysosomes, phagosomes, and endoplasmic reticular elements.

Biological Properties of Macrophages

Endocytosis. Macrophages are very active in pinocytosis and phagocytosis, processes collectively known as endocytosis. In pinocytosis, droplets of fluid are taken up, together with dissolved solute and macromolecules or small particles (Fig. 4–19 and 4–21). The efficiency and selectivity of this form of uptake are often increased by binding of the material to the cell surface (adsorptive pinocytosis). Pinocytic vesicles can be seen with the light microscope (macropinocytosis), but often they can be resolved only with the electron microscope (micropinocytosis). The vesicles (pinosomes), which are formed by invagination at the plasma membrane, pinch off from the membrane, fuse with other pinosomes,

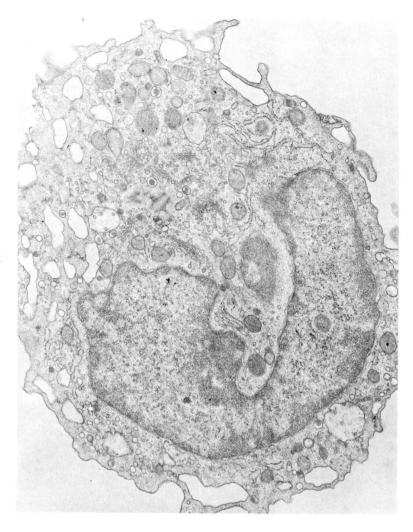

4–20 Transmission electron micrograph of normal mouse macrophage. Notice the pinocytic vacuoles, lysosomes, and abundance of Golgi elements. × 16,000. (From van Furth, R., Hirsch, J. G., and Fedorko, M. 1970. J. Exp. Med. 132:794.)

and are translocated toward the Golgi region. Possibly, the intracellular movement of pinosomes is guided by microtubular arrays. In the juxtanuclear region, pinosomes fuse with primary lysosomes to form secondary lysosomes in which ingested material can be stored and enzymatically degraded.

In contrast to pinocytosis, phagocytosis generally allows the uptake of particles 0.5 μm or more in diameter, but the distinction between pinocytic and phagocytic uptake is not always clear. Phagocytosis requires that the particle be attached to the surface of the macrophage before it is taken up (Fig. 4–22). In pinocytosis such interaction may not always occur. For this reason, pinocytic uptake is of lower specificity than phagocytic uptake. Some particles, as well as cells (e.g., lymphocytes), can attach to the mac-

rophage surface without significant incorporation. Because binding is not necessarily followed by the ingestion step, only the latter is the hallmark of phagocytosis.

Particle attachment is not an energy-dependent process, but particle ingestion is blocked by low temperature or by metabolic inhibitors. Ingestion is accomplished by progressive spreading of the phagocyte plasma membrane and underlying cell cortex over the surface of the attached particle (Figs. 4–19 and 4–22). The membrane motility required for particle ingestion is assumed to utilize forces generated by the submembranous actin-rich bundles of microfilaments. The formation of the phagocytic vacuole or pouch requires resealing of the plasma membrane and of the membrane surrounding the particle. Like the pinosome, the phagocytic vacuole

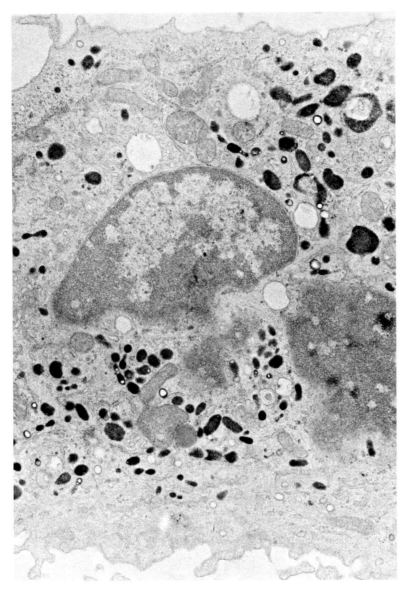

4-21 Normal macrophage incubated with horseradish peroxidase for 1 h, washed, and left in peroxidase-free medium before fixation and staining with the diaminobenzidine method for peroxidase activity. Intensely stained lysosomes indicate uptake and accumulation of peroxidase by pinocytosis. × 20,000. (Courtesy of Ralph Steinman.)

is transported toward the cell center. In this process of engulfment only a small amount of medium is trapped in the phagocytic vacuole (phagosome).

Endocytosis can lead to extensive interiorization of the plasma membrane of macrophages and other cells. Macrophages in culture can take in by pincocytosis the equivalent of their total surface area every 30 min. An important question relates to the fate of the interiorized membrane constituents. Although some may be degraded within the lysosomes, most of the membrane components are reused without significant degradation. Interiorized membrane is probably recycled in the form of tiny vesicles, which appear to transit through in the Golgi region, move to the cell periphery, and fuse with the plasma membrane.

Phagocytic Recognition. The process by which phagocytes select the particles to be taken up is called "phagocytic recognition." Phagocytosis is one of the ways the organism distinguishes "self" from "nonself" or from "altered

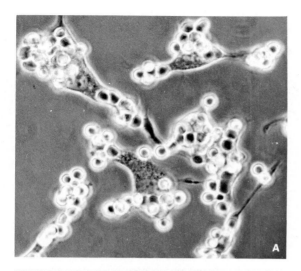

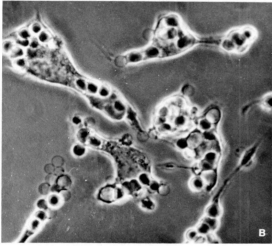

4-22 Cultivated macrophages, phase contrast.

Macrophages were incubated with erythrocytes coated with immunoglobulin G antibody. The cells were rinsed to remove free erythrocytes, photographed **(A)**, incubated in medium of lower osmolarity, fixed, and photographed again **(B)**. In part A, refractile erythrocytes are attached to the macrophages. These erythrocytes are lysed by the low-osmolarity medium and thus ingested red cells (which escape lysis) are clearly seen in part B. Some erythrocyte ghosts remained attached to the macrophages. × 500.

self." Some inert materials and certain bacteria may be ingested in the absence of specific recognition factors from the serum. The interaction of such particles with phagocytes may be due to nonspecific electrostatic or hydrophobic forces. This "nonimmunological" phagocytosis is partic-

ularly relevant to the function of lung (alveolar) macrophages, which must clear the airways of such materials as carbon, silica, berylium, asbestos, cellulose, cotton fibers, and other particulate industrial pollutants. Phagocytosis of microorganisms may involve more specific interactions, for example, the recognition by macrophage receptors of mannose and glucose residues of peptidoglycans on the microbial surface.

Many pathogenic microorganisms or intact cells cannot be ingested without first being coated with certain serum proteins termed "opsonins" which "butter" the particles for phagocytosis. The main recognition factors in serum are certain immunoglobulins (IgG, IgM), and molecules derived from the third component of complement (C3). Complement is a system of proteins in serum that interact both with each other and with antibody and other molecules to kill cells or bacteria by lysis. Antibody and complement provide a finer degree of selectivity than nonimmunological, nonspecific forms of phagocytosis. In essence, the phagocytes recognize not the particle surface proper but the antibody (usually of the IgG class) or complement bound to the particle. The particle-bound recognition factors interact with specific receptors on the phagocyte surface to trigger particle attachment and ingestion. Because macrophages (and also PMNs) interact with a segment of the heavy chains of the IgG molecules (the Fc domain), the macrophage receptors for IgG are called Fc receptors. Similarly, complement receptors are present; they are designated C3 receptors.

IgG induces both particle attachment and ingestion, whereas certain split products of C3 mostly induce the binding of the particles to unstimulated phagocytes. C3 fragments will, however, induce ingestion by inflammatory or activated macrophages in contrast to "resting" cells. Phagocytosis is most efficient when both IgG and C3 are present on the particles. For instance, very low concentrations of IgG antibody are needed to promote incorporation of particles bound via the C3 receptors.

Monoclonal antibodies specific for Fc receptors have been prepared and functional Fc receptors from mouse and human phagocytes have been immunoprecipitated and their constituent glycoproteins isolated and characterized. Thus, the function of Fc receptors can now be analyzed in molecular terms. There appears to be a family of related Fc receptor glycoproteins present on the surface of macrophages, granulocytes, and B lymphocytes and on a subset of T lymphocytes.

Three different receptors have been characterized in mouse macrophages and two in human macrophages and monocytes. The receptors differ as to their specificity for IgGs of different subclasses, their sensitivity to proteolytic enzymes, and their recognition by specific antibodies. Fc receptors are also expressed on neonatal intestinal epithelial cells, syncytial trophoblasts of the placenta, and yolk sac epithelium of certain species. In all these examples the Fc receptors are involved in the transport of IgG across epithelia. It is not known whether these Fc receptors are structurally related to those of phagocytic cells.

The interaction between IgG molecules and phagocyte Fc receptors has two important features. First, the receptors can freely move in the plane of the plasma membrane, allowing their distribution to "adapt" to that of particle-bound IgG. Second, particle interiorization requires that a critical number of Fc receptors be occupied, and it is probable that approximation or "cross-linking" of vicinal receptors is a necessary step for phagocytosis. Dimers or higher aggregates of IgG have a higher affinity for the phagocytes than monomeric IgG and are rapidly taken up. Thus, ingestion is related to the density of IgG molecules expressed on the surface of the particles to be taken up. It is also possible that a change in the conformation of the Fc portion of the IgG occurs when antibody molecules bind antigen and that this change in conformation is "recognized" by the Fc receptor. As the IgG interacts with the receptors, membrane and subjacent cytoplasm spread over the particle by a zippering-like mechanism. After the Fc receptors are engaged, microfilament function is activated in a process requiring divalent ion fluxes. Phagocytosis is then completed.

Two separate complement receptors are also found on the macrophage surface. These receptors bind two sequential products of C3, namely C3b and C3d. Functionally similar receptors for C3b have been demonstrated on the surface of human erythrocytes, PMNs, B lymphocytes, mast cells, and the visceral epithelial cells of the kidney glomerulus. From several of these cells a C3b-binding glycoprotein has been isolated by immunoprecipitation and characterized. Antibodies to this glycoprotein block the binding of C3b-coated particles to monocytes, PMNs, and B lymphocytes.

The presence of phagocytic receptors for IgG and complement on the surface of macrophages and PMNs distinguishes these cells ("professional phagocytes") from other phagocytic cells (epithelial cells and fibroblasts, for example). The latter, "nonprofessional" phagocytes, will not specifically ingest particles coated with antibody or complement. Damaged cells and extracellular materials are also avidly phagocytized by macrophages. This recognition may be mediated by the ubiquitous glycoprotein fibronectin (see above), which is found both in the plasma and in the tissues. Fibronectin has high avidity for materials found in damaged tissues, such as fibrin, denatured collagen, actin, and DNA. Complexes of these materials with fibronectin lead to binding and possibly to ingestion and degradation by macrophages. Apparently, then, fibronectin functions as a relatively nonspecific opsonin involved in recognition of such tissue damage as may arise during the course of normal morphogenesis or the inflammatory process. The postulated receptors for fibronectin may not be present on PMNs.

Postengulfment Events. Pinocytic and phagocytic vacuoles fuse with lysosomes, membrane-bounded vesicles containing a battery of hydrolytic enzymes. This fusion results in the formation of phagolysosomes or secondary lysosomes. The pH within these organelles is approximately 5, close to the optimum pH of the lysosomal hydrolases. The hydrolases digest macromolecules, and digestion intermediates of molecular weights below 300 daltons may diffuse out of the lysosomes. Materials that cannot be digested may be stored in lysosomes for long periods. Genetically determined defects of lysosomal hydrolases can lead to a variety of "storage diseases" in which undigested materials accumulate within macrophages and other cells.

Microbicidal Mechanisms. Many kinds of bacteria are killed within phagosomes of the macrophages but the mechanisms involved are not entirely understood. By itself, the low pH inside the phagosomes may reduce the viability of microorganisms. Lung macrophages contain the polysaccharidase lysozyme, which digests the walls of many bacteria. A peroxidase is involved in the bactericidal activity of monocytes, but the enzyme is absent in tissue macrophages. Importantly, monocytes, macrophages, and polymorphonuclear granulocytes, when triggered by particles or other membrane stimuli, rapidly increase their oxygen consumption and generate the superoxide anion (O_2^-). The superoxide anion spontaneously or enzymatically dismutates into hydrogen peroxide (H_2O_2). Highly reactive and short-lived hydroxyl radicals and possibly singlet oxygen are also formed. These molecules appear to be involved in the microbicidal and cytostatic–cytotoxic activities of the phagocytes. A plasma membrane NADH (or according to others, NADPH) –dependent oxidase is involved in the production of the oxygen reduction species. Particle attachment to the phagocytes is sufficient to trigger the initial generation of O_2^-. Thus, as a consequence of particle–phagocyte interactions, the oxygen metabolites are released into the surrounding medium as well as within the phagocytic vacuoles. When the trigger is soluble, as is the case with the complement split product C5a and other chemotactic factors, or when phagocytosis is inhibited or impossible (e.g., macrophages on insolubilized immune complexes or antibody on a large target cell), the oxygen radicals are released extracellularly. This has implications for the damage of cells or other tissue components by phagocyte-produced oxygen radicals.

Certain microorganisms thrive and multiply within macrophages. Examples are the leprosy and tubercle bacilli and protozoa such as *Toxoplasma*, *Trypanosoma cruzi*, or *Leishmania*. These organisms escape destruction in mononuclear phagocytes by a variety of mechanisms. Thus, *Toxoplasma* and *Leishmania* seem to trigger only minimal formation of oxygen radicals at the time of phagocytosis by macrophages. Phagocytic vacuoles containing *Toxoplasma* or tubercle bacilli do not fuse efficiently with primary lysosomes; this finding may explain the survival of these parasites within phagocytes. In other instances, phagolysosomal fusion does occur, but the organisms are resistant to both the lysosomal hydrolases and the low intravacuolar pH. Finally, organisms such as *Trypanosoma cruzi* escape from phagocytic vacuoles and then lodge and multiply within the cytosolic compartment. Thus, a variety of ingenious escape mechanisms—besides others involving the immune responses of the host—permit the establishment of intracellular infection.

Exocytosis. When macrophages bind to particles or to immune complexes, particularly when ingestion is inhibited or when the phagocytes interact with certain complement fragments (C5a), lysosomal enzymes are released into the extracellular space. This release occurs by fusion of lysosomes with the phagocytic pouch or with the plasma membrane. The enzymes released, together with the oxygen reduction species which are also generated, can increase tissue damage in several forms of inflammation. Experimentally, release can be obtained easily by incubation of cells with particles (for instance, yeast cell walls or opsonized erythrocytes) in the presence of the fungal metabolite cytochalasin B, which interferes with the assembly of actin-rich microfilaments and inhibits particle ingestion. Alternatively, lysosomal enzyme release can be induced by plating the phagocytes over substrate-bound immune complexes. Macrophages spread over the immobilized complexes and their frustrated attempt at phagocytosis causes lysosomes to fuse with the adherent surface of the plasma membrane.

Exocytosis in toto of undigestible materials, as found in some free-living amoebae, has not been demonstrated in macrophages. However, release has been reported of small amounts of semidigested or "processed" macromolecules such as hemocyanin previously fed to the phagocytes.

Chemotaxis. Monocytes and macrophages are attracted toward certain substances termed chemotactic factors; that is, they move directionally against concentration gradients of these factors. Chemotactic factors for monocytes include C5a, a product of the activation of the complement cascade; N-formyl-methionyl peptides; and hydroxylated derivatives of arachidonic acid. One product of stimulated lymphocytes is also chemotactic for monocytes and may account for the accumulation of macrophages in inflammatory lesions infiltrated by lymphocytes. Chemotaxis is often assayed by placing cells on top of a filter with pores of sufficient diameter to admit the cells (about 5 μm). Solutions of chemotactic factors are placed in the bottom of the chamber (with an appropriate control medium in the upper compartment), and thus a concentration gradient of the chemotactic factor is built across the membrane. Chemotactic activity is measured by counting cells that migrate into or through the porous membrane over time. Usually, the chemotactic factors also increase the rate of random movement of the monocytes when applied in the absence of a gradient (chemokinesis). Therefore, adequate controls are needed to distinguish chemotactic (directional) from chemokinetic (in-

Table 4–6 Secretory Products of Macrophages

Enzymes
  Lysosomal hydrolases
  Neutral proteinases: plasminogen activator, collagenase, elastase, proteoglycan degrading enzymes. These enzymes participate in tissue remodeling and damage.
  Lysozyme (a carbohydrase that digests the cell walls of many microorganisms)
  Arginase
Proteins of the complement system: C1q, C2, C3, C4, C5, factors B and D. These proteins are involved in the classic and the alternative pathways of complement activation.
Molecules that regulate cell activities and cell proliferation:
  Interferon: macrophages may be an important source of this antiviral factor, which can also be produced by many other cell types.
  Granulocyte and macrophage colony stimulating factors (CSFs)
  Mitogenic protein (for T cells), formerly termed lymphocyte activating factor (LAF), now called "interleukin 1"
  Immunosuppressive factors
  Factors that enhance the growth of fibroblasts
  Factors that enhance the growth of endothelial cells
  A macromolecular factor chemotactic for polymorphonuclear neutrophils
Other macromolecules
  Endogenous pyrogen: this molecule, perhaps identical to the mitogenic protein, is a mediator of fever.
  Alpha-2-macroglobulin: inhibits a variety of proteolytic enzymes
  "Tissue factor" or thromboplastin-like procoagulant factor(s)
Arachidonic acid derivatives
  Leukotriene C (slow reacting substance of anaphylaxis)
  Prostaglandins: E_2 is the major compound; PGI_2; thromboxane A_2; $PGF_2\alpha$.
  These are important mediators of inflammation and of platelet and leukocyte function.
Other small molecules
  Cyclic AMP, nucleosides
  Superoxide and hydroxyl radicals; H_2O_2: relevant to the microbicidal and cytocidal properties of macrophages

Source: Modified from Davies, P., and Bonney, R. J. 1979. J. Reticuloendothol. Soc. 26:37–47.

creased random movement) effects of chemotactic factors.

Macrophages as Secretory Cells. Table 4–6 lists the impressive range of molecules synthesized and secreted by macrophages. Several products are of critical importance in the defense against microorganisms, viruses, and tumor cells. Examples are lysozyme, an enzyme that degrades the components of the cell wall of many bacteria; components of the complement system, involved in the lysis of bacteria and cells as well as in opsonization; the antiviral glycoprotein interferon; and hydrogen peroxide and free radicals of oxygen, which, as discussed above, play a major role in microbicidal and cytocidal activities of macrophages. Other macrophage products, such as the neutral proteases, participate in extracellular degradation of connective tissue con-

stituents and are thus relevant to tissue remodeling as well as to tissue damage. The proteases can also trigger the clotting, complement, and kinin cascades and lead to the generation of important inflammatory mediators such as bradykinin and the chemotactic factor C5a. Additionally, a family of derivatives of arachidonic acid, including prostaglandins, hydroxylated derivatives of arachidonic acid and the more complex lipids known as leukotrienes, act as mediators of inflammation, and affect the functions of granulocytes, platelets, endothelia, smooth muscle and other cell types. Other factors, such as "interleukin 1," affect the function of lymphocytes and help regulate the immune responses (see below). Other, as yet poorly characterized factors, enhance the growth of fibroblasts and of capillary endothelial cells, cell types also involved in inflammation and repair. Several directly or indirectly generated macrophage products are chemotactic for PMNs and fibroblasts, and at least one factor, "endogenous pyrogen," is an important mediator of fever.

Macrophage secretory activity can be regulated by diverse membrane stimuli. The secretion of lysosomal enzymes, prostaglandins, hydrogen peroxide, or superoxide anion, for example, is clearly enhanced by phagocytosis and interaction with immune complexes. Nanogram amounts of microbial constituents known as lipopolysaccharides effectively stimulate the secretion of a variety of macrophage products such as neutral proteinases, pyrogen, procoagulant factor, colony stimulating factor, and interleukin 1. Experimentally, the production of neutral proteinases, hydrogen peroxide, or free radicals of oxygen can be enhanced by the tumor promoter phorbol myristate acetate, by certain lectins, or, importantly, by preliminary exposure to products of activated lymphocytes (lymphokines). Finally, the secretion of lysozyme appears "constitutive," as it is not influenced by phagocytic or other membrane stimuli.

Participation in the Immune Response. Macrophages are involved both in the production of antibody and in cell-mediated immune responses. Examples of the latter are delayed hypersensitivity reactions, transplant rejections, and the control of intracellular infections. Macrophages ingest and degrade particulate antigens or aggregated proteins and, at a simple level, help prevent the inhibition of the immune response by antigen overload. However, macrophages participate in the immune responses in other, "positive," ways. Indeed, the most immunogenic antigens are those avidly captured by macrophages. Molecules that bypass macrophages, such as monomeric serum albumin or globulin, not only are weak antigens but also easily induce immunological tolerance. When such molecules are aggregated, and thus made palatable to macrophages, their immunogenicity is markedly enhanced and tolerance becomes difficult to obtain.

Positive participation of macrophages in the immune responses involves processing and presentation of antigen to lymphocytes and the production of immunoregulatory molecules by macrophages. Macrophages may "present" or display antigens on their surface and the macrophage-bound antigen can trigger the proliferation or activation of T and B lymphocytes. Experimentally,

antigens associated with macrophages appear to be more immunogenic in vivo and in vitro than equivalent amounts of free antigens. Such antigens may be simply bound to the macrophage surface, on the way to interiorization, or they may be ingested, partially digested, or processed, and then reappear on the macrophage surface in a more immunogenic form. The triggering or activation of lymphocytes by macrophage-bound antigen requires physical contact between the two cell types and, in the case of the T cells, the interaction also depends on precise genetic restrictions. A proportion of macrophages (varying with the source of the phagocytes) express a histocompatibility (transplantation) antigen coded for by a chromosomal locus called Ia. Ia antigens of macrophages and T cells must match for successful antigen presentation.

A series of immunoregulatory soluble molecules is also produced by macrophages. The best known is the mitogenic protein (interleukin 1), which is required for the proliferation and survival of T and B lymphocytes. Proliferating T cells can then reciprocate by producing macrophage-activating factors. Macrophages also produce other factors that cause the differentiation of B lymphocytes into plasma cells, affect the differentiation of T lymphocytes, or inhibit lymphocyte proliferation and function (immunosuppressive factors).

Other Ia-positive cells derived from bone marrow may be involved in antigen presentation to the lymphocytes. These cells are the poorly phagocytic dendritic cells present in some lymphoid tissues, and the possibly related Langerhans cells of the dermis. Dendritic and Langerhans cells are apparently not of monocyte–macrophage lineage.

Macrophage Activation. In vitro and in vivo experiments demonstrate that macrophages subjected to appropriate stimuli undergo morphological, biochemical, and functional changes consistent with enhanced activity. Examples of such stimuli are systemic infections with obligatory or facultative intracellular microorganisms, such as the agents of tuberculosis, listeriosis, toxoplasmosis, or leishmaniasis. Macrophages can also be activated by administering certain killed microorganisms (e.g., *Corynebacterium parvum*) or cell wall components from bacteria (peptidoglycans, muramyldipeptides). However, the most common mechanism that underlies macrophage activation is exposure of macrophages to lymphocyte products (lymphokines). Activated macrophages are characterized by increased size, adhesiveness, expression of plasma membrane Ia antigens, and production of enzymes such as collagenase or plasminogen activator. Importantly, activated macrophages triggered by phagocytosis, immune complexes, chemotactic factors, tumor promoters, or other stimuli generate larger quantities of oxygen reduction products (O_2^-, H_2O_2, OH·) than do the corresponding resting, nonactivated phagocytes. The two most important features of macrophage activation are enhanced microbicidal activity and enhanced cytotoxicity toward tumor target cells. Microbicidal activity is conveniently tested with parasites adapted to intracellular life such as *Toxoplasma* or *Leishmania*. The cellular changes that characterize activated macrophages are most often correlated with increased numbers of macrophages at the sites of infection, either by recruitment from circulating moncytes or by proliferation of pre-existing macrophages.

Lymphokines are released into culture media when sensitized lymphocytes are incubated with the immunogen or when normal lymphocytes are incubated with plant lectins such as phytohemagglutinin or concanavalin A. Macrophages from normal animals acquire enhanced microbicidal or cytotoxic activity when incubated with such lymphokine preparations in vitro, and this effect is potentiated by lipopolysaccharides. The activation is reduced when the lymphokines are removed from the macrophage cultures. The macrophage-activating lymphokine(s) have so far resisted adequate purification and characterization.

There is considerable in vivo evidence that successful host defense against obligatory or facultative intracellular organisms requires interactions between macrophages and T lymphocytes. The macrophages, having phagocytized the organisms, present the antigens of the organism to T lymphocytes. The T-lymphocyte population in turn expands and secretes lymphokines, which affect the macrophages by (1) increasing their numbers; (2) causing chemotactic recruitment, and (3) activating them to kill the phagocytosed organisms. The activation is nonspecific in the sense that macrophages activated during the course of infection with one microorganism are also better able to kill other infectious agents or tumor cells.

Growth of certain tumors can be inhibited by the local or systemic administration of bacterial products to animals or humans (e.g., *C. parvum*; muramyldipeptides; lipopolysaccharides), but it remains to be shown that this form of immunotherapy is mediated primarily by macrophage activation. To best exploit the cytotoxic capacity of macrophages in tumor therapy, methods to direct monocytes into the tumors and to activate the phagocytes locally must be developed.

Mast Cells

Mast cells were discovered by Paul Ehrlich in 1877 when he was a medical student. He showed that certain cells in connective tissues contained granules that stained characteristically with basic aniline dyes. He presumed that the granules represented stored nutrients and hence named the cells "mast cells," in a reference to "feeding" in German. The granules were "metachromatic"; that is, the color they acquired differed from that of the dye in solution. It is now known that mast cells stain with basic and metachromatic dyes such as toluidine blue or thionine because the cells contain a high concentration of the sulfated proteoglycan heparin.

Mast cells are best identified by their numerous basophilic and metachromatic granules. Rat mast cells are easily seen with conventional fixation, but staining human mast cell granules requires special fixatives and stains. Thus, although mast cells are widely distributed in human tissues, they are not observed in routinely fixed and stained specimens.

Mast cells are ubiquitous in connective tissues and are most often observed adjacent to blood vessels (Figs. 4–23 and 4–24). They are particularly numerous at sites where the body meets the outside environment, such as in the skin (where there are about 10,000 mast cells per cubic millimeter of dermis) and in the lining of the respiratory and digestive tracts. Rat mast cells found in the mesentery or in the peritoneal fluid have been a favorite subject for experimental studies, but there are morphological, compositional, and pharmacological differences between the human and rodent cells.

By light microscopy, in appropriately prepared material, mast cells are relatively large (20–30 μm) and filled with characteristic basophilic and metachromatic granules that often obscure the cell nucleus. Electron microscopy shows that mast cell granules are bound by a unit membrane. Human granules are heterogeneous and contain lamellar bodies, whorls, or

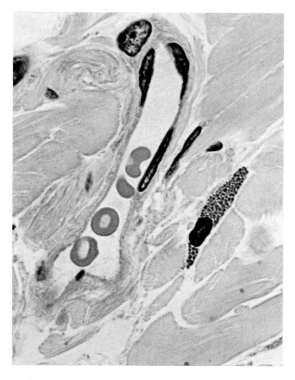

4–23 Human mast cell between collagen bundles in thin section of skin. A venule is also shown. × 800. (Courtesy of Edith Robbins.)

paracrystalline structures (Fig. 4–25), whereas the granules are more homogeneous in the rat mast cells (Fig. 4–26). Besides the specific granules, mast cells contain the usual cytoplasmic organelles such as mitochondria, Golgi, endoplasmic reticulum, microtubules, and microfilaments.

Mast cells are long lived. Recently, pure populations of mouse mast cells were obtained from cultures of fetal liver or adult bone marrow enriched with lymphocyte culture supernatants. The mast cells divided continuously and the growth factor was shown to derive from T lymphocytes and was partially purified.

Mast cells should be distinguished from polymorphonuclear basophils. Basophils are also marrow-derived but belong to the granulocytic series. They are found in small numbers in the circulating blood but can accumulate in tissues at sites of delayed hypersensitivity reactions. Basophils are smaller than mast cells and contain a multilobed nucleus, whereas the nucleus of the mast cells is unilobed. The granules of basophils are less numerous than those of mast cells but they are alike with respect to basophilia and metachromasia, and similar but not identical in appearance in the electron microscope. Instead of heparin, basophil granules contain chondroitin sulfate, dermatan sulfate, and small quanti-

4–24 Electron micrograph of human mast cell from a biopsy of the rectal submucosa. The mast cell is situated between two small blood vessels. × 7,500. (From Lagunoff, D. 1972. J. Invest. Dermatol. 58:296.)

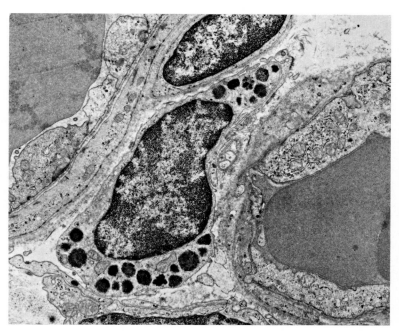

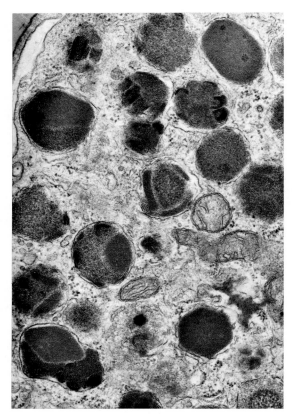

4–25 Portion of cytoplasm of human mast cell showing granules with denser cores or with lamellar or paracrystalline arrays. × 25,800. (From Lagunoff, D. 1972. J. Invest. Dermatol. 58:296.)

ties of heparin sulfate. Otherwise mast cells and basophils contain and secrete similar substances. Mast cells and basophils are derived from different bone marrow precursors, so mast cells are not basophils that have migrated into the tissues.

Mast cells and basophils, like macrophages, polymorphonuclear neutrophils, eosinophils, and platelets, secrete pharmacologically potent mediators upon appropriate stimulation. These mediators can elicit such phenomena as edema, pain, shock, hypercoagulation, and fever. In humans, mast cell mediators are usually released in "immediate hypersensitivity" reactions, which occur shortly after a sensitized individual is challenged with the antigen. Thus, mast cells participate in conditions such as asthma, hay fever, urticaria, drug reactions, and anaphylactic shock. All of these conditions involve the participation of a special class of immunoglobulin

called immunoglobulin E (IgE). In addition, mast cells and basophils have receptors for the complement split products C3a and C5a and thus participate in reactions that involve the activation of the complement cascade.

Table 4–7 lists the mediators produced by human mast cells and basophils. Here we shall present some relevant properties of the primary (stored) and secondary (nonstored) mediators. Histamine increases the permeability of small venules by inducing the formation of gaps between endothelial cells. Leakage of plasma protein and fluid accounts for edema (swelling), one of the features of inflammation. Histamine also induces the contraction of smooth muscle. Slower contraction of smooth muscle is induced by leukotriene C, a mediator previously called "slow reactive substance of anaphylaxis," which does not exist preformed as does histamine. Leukotriene C is also produced in relatively large quantities by mononuclear phagocytes and is a derivative of arachidonic acid. Another mediator, platelet-activating factor (PAF), is also formed upon stimulation of mast cells and basophils. Platelet-activating factor is a lipid derivative that releases serotonin from platelets at very low concentrations. Release of eosinophil chemotactic factors stored in the mast cells possibly accounts for the accumulation of eosinophils at sites of allergic reactions, such as the nasal mucosa in hay fever, the bronchial mucosa in asthma, or the gut mucosa in parasitic infestations. In the human, heparin may not be released together with the other mediators. Heparin is not only involved in lipid metabolism but inhibits the Hageman factor–dependent induction of coagulation as well.

Mediator release from human mast cells and basophils mainly involves IgE. IgEs are preferentially synthesized after exposure to certain antigens such as those present in ragweed or pollen or in many metazoan parasites, particularly worms. IgE is found in serum at very low concentrations (less than 300 ng/ml), but its Fc domain (located in the heavy chains) has a very high avidity for specific receptors on the surfaces of mast cells and basophils. These receptors are termed IgE receptors. Consequently, most of the IgE in the body is fixed to the surface of these cells. Because there is a slow exchange or equilibration of IgE antibodies on the cells with those of the plasma, specific IgE antibodies can remain cell-bound for several weeks after passive antibody administration to animals or man. When sensitized hosts or the isolated mast cells or ba-

Table 4–7 Mediators Produced by Human Mast Cells and Basophils

I. Primary: Granule-associated

Mediator	Function
Histamine (Beta imidazolyl ethylamine)	Increases vascular permeability and contracts smooth muscle
Heparin[a] (Sulfated proteoglycan)	Anticoagulant and activates lipoprotein lipase
Chymase (Chymotrypsin-like neutral protease)	Degrades connective tissue constituents and may activate the kinin and clotting cascades
Eosinophil chemotactic factors (Tetrapeptides and larger peptides)	Attract eosinophils and neutrophils
N-acetyl beta glucosaminidase and Beta glucuronidase	Contribute to degradation of connective-tissue glycosaminoglycans

II. Secondary: Unstored

Arachidonic acid derivatives[b]	
Leukotriene C (Hydroxy-cysteinyl-eicosatetraenoic acid)	Increases vascular permeability and induces slow contraction of smooth muscle
Prostaglandins 5-membered carbon ring with two (7- and 8-membered) carbon side chains	Stimulate adenyl cyclase with numerous vascular, smooth-muscle, platelet, and cellular actions
Hydroxyarachidonates	Powerful chemotactic factors for neutrophils
Platelet activating factor (PAF)[b] (a glyceryl ether phosphoglyceride)	Aggregates platelets and induces release of serotonin
Products of oxygen metabolism[b] Hydrogen peroxide; superoxide radical; singlet oxygen; hydroxyl radical	Cause tissue damage

Source: Modified from Austen, K. F. 1979. Harvey Lect. 73:93.

[a]Basophils contain other sulfated glycosaminoglycans.
[b]Several derivatives also produced by macrophages, granulocytes, and platelets.

sophils are reexposed to minute amounts of antigen (e.g., micromicrograms of ragweed pollen antigen), the antigen molecules interact with the mast cell–bound antibody, triggering the release of mediators over a period of minutes. Release from basophils may take longer. Crucial to the release is the requirement that vicinal cell-bound IgE molecules are "cross-linked" or clustered by the binding to a single antigen molecule. This requirement leads to the approximation of the IgE receptors, which are independently mobile in the plane of the membrane and which probably then interact with submembranous cytoskeletal components.

The analogy with the function of the Fc receptor in macrophages should be evident. It is probably the close approximation of at least two receptors that triggers the release of mediators. Indeed, it has been shown that release can be induced by (1) dimers of IgE applied in the absence of antigen, (2) IgG antibodies against IgE class immunoglobulins, or (3) certain anti-IgE receptor antibodies. In all of these situations clustering of

receptors occurs. Recently the receptors for IgE have been purified and their glycoprotein components isolated and characterized. The interaction of IgE molecules with IgE receptors should soon be understood at the molecular level.

Mediator release dependent on IgE is inhibited by agents that increase the levels of cyclic AMP (cAMP) in the mast cells and basophils. Drugs such as isoproterenol act on beta-adrenergic receptors of mast cells and increase the synthesis of cAMP. Other agents such as theophylline (a methylxanthine) increase cAMP levels by inhibiting a diesterase that degrades cAMP. In both instances mast cell release is inhibited. On the other hand, agents that lower the cAMP content of mast cells (or increase cyclic GMP) increase mediator release and can induce asthmatic attacks. These responses are relevant to the pathogenesis and management of allergic conditions. A rare disease called diffuse urticaria pigmentosa is associated with increased numbers of mast cells. The mast cells in patients with this disease are also abnormally fragile, and simply

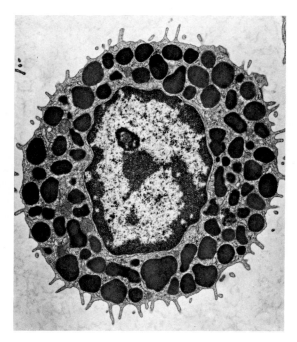

4–26 Electron micrograph of peritoneal mast cell from a rat. Note relative uniformity in granule densities. × 6,200. (From Lagunoff, D. 1972. J. Invest. Dermatol. 58:296.)

stroking the skin results in mediator release and the formation of wheals (dermographism).

Mediator release can be demonstrated with suspensions of mast cells or basophils or with slices of tissues (such as lung) that are rich in mast cells. These preparations have provided important information about the mechanisms of release of the mediators and have helped in the development of drugs that inhibit or facilitate the release reaction.

Ultrastructural studies of the release reaction (Figs. 4–26 and 4–27) show that the peripheral granules fuse with the plasma membrane to discharge their contents. The membranes of granules toward the center of the cell may fuse with each other, creating channels that connect with the cell surface (Fig. 4–27). The process of mediator release or secretion is energy-dependent, requires Ca^{++}, and seems to involve microfilaments.

Connective Tissues in Inflammation and Repair

The inflammatory reaction encompasses neural, vascular, cellular, and humoral responses to tissue injury. Examples of such injury are mechan-

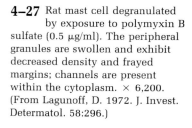

4–27 Rat mast cell degranulated by exposure to polymyxin B sulfate (0.5 μg/ml). The peripheral granules are swollen and exhibit decreased density and frayed margins; channels are present within the cytoplasm. × 6,200. (From Lagunoff, D. 1972. J. Invest. Determatol. 58:296.)

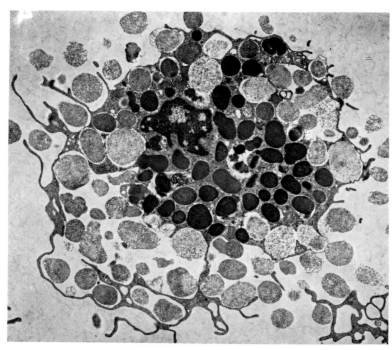

ical trauma, burns, or invasion of tissue by microorganisms. The initial reaction to injury is probably a transient vasoconstriction, but it is followed rapidly by vasodilation involving arterioles and venules. The dilated vessels leak increased amounts of fluid and plasma proteins into the supporting connective tissues. Local hemoconcentration increases the viscosity of the blood, and the flow of blood slows in the venules. Because of an undefined alteration of either the endothelial cells or leukocyte surfaces, or both, circulating white blood cells adhere to the lining of the venules. First, polymorphonuclear neutrophils and then monocytes move between the loosened endothelial cell junctions, penetrate the layers of the basement membrane, and reach the supporting connective tissues. This movement of the leukocytes represents a crucial event in the development of the inflammatory response and is presumably enhanced and directed by the release of chemotactic factors in the tissues.

The PMNs and the newly arrived or resident macrophages phagocytize microbial agents, damaged cells, and extracellular materials, and release products that further amplify the inflammatory reaction. Polymorphonuclear neutrophils, monocytes, and macrophages are not the only cells involved in inflammation. In varying degrees, depending on the nature of the injury and its temporal development, mast cells, eosinophils and basophils, lymphocytes, and platelets may also play a role. In addition, endothelial cells and fibroblasts participate in the repair of damaged tissues.

The vascular and cellular phases of inflammation are orchestrated by a large number of pharmacologically active molecules called mediators. Some of these molecules are released by the resident or immigrant cells of connective tissue. Mediators can also be generated by the action of cell-derived proteolytic enzymes on precursor proteins of plasma. These plasma-derived mediators can also be generated without the intervention of cellular proteases.

The actions of cell and plasma-derived mediators include vasodilation and increased permeability of venules; chemotaxis of leukocytes; and activation of clotting factors and fibrinolytic enzymes. Tables 4–6 and 4–7 include mediators of inflammation produced by macrophages and mast cells. A variety of effector molecules with roughly similar actions can be released at sites of inflammation. It is thus difficult to ascribe any of the features of inflammation to the release of a single mediator. For example, vasodilation and increased vascular permeability can arise from the release of histamine contained in the granules of mast cells and basophils, from the synthesis of leukotriene C by these and other cells, and from the generation of the nonapeptide bradykinin from plasma precursors. Similarly, the influx of PMNs and monocytes in inflammation can be related to the release of various cellular or plasma-derived chemotactic factors. The chemotactic factors include hydroxyarachidonates released from leucocytes, C5a generated from the complement cascade, and cleavage products of fibrinogen.

Enzymes able to degrade most biological macromolecules are contained within and released from inflammatory cells, particularly the PMNs and macrophages. These enzymes help degrade cells and matrix materials damaged by injury and may, in certain circumstances, further extend the zone of tissue damage. Another class of potentially damaging molecules released from inflammatory cells are the oxygen-derived free radicals.

Repair of irreversibly damaged cells and connective tissue matrixes begins while inflammation is still present. Because most cells of the body are capable of replication, surface and glandular epithelia and endothelia, hematopoietic cells, and fibroblasts lost in the course of injury and inflammation can be replaced by the replication and differentiation of undamaged progenitors. Stromal (matrix) repair is marked by the proliferation of fibroblasts and vascular endothelial buds, which move into the injured site. The endothelial buds come to line new capillary channels and they and the fibroblasts secrete new matrix materials, notably fibronectin, collagens, and proteoglycans. Fibronectin can bind to fibrinogen and fibrin at the site of injury, and the fibrillary network so formed can serve as a scaffold for migrating cells. The collagen deposited is largely responsible for restoring the tensile strength of the damaged tissue. The developing collagen scar is subject to remodeling by a process of enzymatic turnover and deposition of new fibers. In the initial stages of repair, type III collagen fibers are more numerous than type I fibers, but later type I fibers predominate.

The entire complex of inflammatory cells, proliferating fibroblasts, endothelia, new capillaries, and secreted glycoproteins and proteoglycans is called *granulation tissue*. In time, the cellular content of the granulation tissue diminishes, the capillary channels collapse, and a relatively avascular collagen scar marks the site of previous injury. Ideally, the repair reactions should restore normal form and function. In cases of limited injury where only surface epithelia are lost and damage to supportive basement membranes and stroma is minimal, normal function and form can be restored. Often regeneration of parenchymatous epithelia is imperfect and the resultant increase in collagen content and distortion of epithelial–stromal relationships produce functional deficits. Reactive fibrosis can also cause narrowing of tubular organs and the formation of adhesions between mesothelial surfaces.

The repair reaction requires, at a minimum, signals for cell replication and differentiation, chemotactic factors, and controlled synthesis and turnover of matrix proteins. Some of these signals or mediators are generated by elements of the earlier-occurring inflammatory reaction. For example, factors released from platelets, macrophages, and lymphocytes can stimulate fibroblasts to divide and synthesize matrix proteins. Collagenases released from neutrophils and macrophages digest collagen; and collagenous fragments have been shown to be chemotactic for fibroblasts. Thus, tissue injury is followed by a complex set of interrelated cellular and humoral reactions that remove or neutralize injurious agents, eliminate the damaged tissue, and promote healing. Most of these reactions occur in the connective tissues and most healing depends on the deposition of collagen.

References and Selected Bibliography

The Fibroblast

Gabbiani, G., Majno, G., and Ryan, G. B. 1973. The fibroblast as a contractile cell: The myofibroblast. In Kulonen, E., and Pikkarainen, J. (eds.), Biology of the Fibroblast. New York: Academic Press, Inc., p. 139.

Goldberg, B., and Green H. 1964. An analysis of collagen secretion by established mouse fibroblast lines. J. Cell Biol. 22:227.

Weinstock, M., and Leblond, C. P. 1974. Formation of collagen. Fed. Proc. 33:1205.

Collagen: Structure and Metabolism

Bornstein, P., and Byers, P. H. 1980. Disorders of Collagen Metabolism. In Metabolic Control and Disease, 8th ed., Bondy, P. K., and Rosenberg, L. E. (eds.). Philadelphia: W. B. Saunders Co., p. 1089.

Bornstein, P., and Sage, H. 1980. Structurally distinct collagen types. Ann. Rev. Biochem. 49:957.

Bornstein, P., and Traub, W. 1979. The Chemistry and Biology of Collagen. In The Proteins, vol. 4, Neurath, H., and Hill, R. L. (eds.). New York: Academic Press, Inc., p. 412.

Fessler, J. H., and Fessler, L. I. 1978. Biosynthesis of procollagen. Ann. Rev. Biochem. 47:129.

Gross, J. 1974. Collagen biology: Structure, degradation, and disease. Harvey Lect. 68:351.

Harris, E. D., Jr., and Krane, S. M. 1974. Collagenases. N. Engl. J. Med. 291:605, 652.

Kefalides, N. A. (ed.). 1978. Biology and Chemistry of Basement Membranes. New York: Academic Press, Inc.

McKusick, V. A. 1972 Heritable Disorders of Connective Tissues. St. Louis: C. V. Mosby Co.

Miller, E. J. 1976. Biochemical Characteristics and Biological Significance of the Genetically Distinct Collagens. Mol. Cell. Biochem. 13:165.

Ramachandran, G. N., and Reddi, A. H. (eds.). 1976. Biochemistry of Collagen. New York/London: Plenum Press.

Elastic Fibers

Franzblau, C. 1971. Elastin. In Comprehensive Biochemistry, Florkin, M., and Stotz, E. H. (eds.), vol. 26C. Amsterdam: Elsevier, p. 659.

Ross, R., and Bornstein, P. 1971. Elastic fibers in the body. Sci. Am. 224:44.

Sandberg, L. B., Soskel, N. T., and Leslie, J. G. 1981. Elastin structure, biosynthesis, and relation to disease states. N. Engl. J. Med. 304:566.

Proteoglycans and Structural Glycoproteins

Lennarz, W. J. (ed.). 1980. The Biochemistry of Glycoproteins and Proteoglycans. New York/London: Plenum Press.

Pearlstein, E., Gold, L. I., and Garcia-Pardo, A. 1980. Fibronectin: A review of its structure and biological activity. Mol. Cell. Biochem. 29:103.

Ruoslahti, E., Engvall, E., and Hayman, E. G. 1981. Fibronectin: Current concepts of its structure and functions. Collagen Rel. Res. 1:95.

Timpl, R., Rohde, H., Robey, P. G., Rennard, S. I., Foidart, J.-M., and Martin, G. R. 1979. Laminin—a glycoprotein from basement membranes. J. Biol. Chem. 254:9933.

Macrophages

Books (see also references in 4th ed.)

Metchnikoff, E. 1968. Immunity in Infective Diseases. Binnie, F. G. (Transl). New York: Johnson Reprint Corporation.

Nelson, D. S. (ed.). 1976. Immunobiology of the Macrophage. New York: Academic Press, Inc.

Pick, E., and Landy, M. (eds.). 1981. Lymphokines and Macrophage activation. Vol. III of Lymphokines. New York: Academic Press, Inc.

Sbarra, A. J., and Strauss, R. R. (eds). The Reticuloendothelial System. 1980. *In* Biochemistry and Metabolism, vol. 2. New York: Plenum Press.

Van Furth, R. (ed.). 1980. Mononuclear Phagocytes. Functional Aspects. 2 vols. The Hague, Netherlands: Martinus Nijhoff Publishers.

Articles and Reviews

Badway, J. A., and Karnovsky, M. L. 1980. Active oxygen species and the functions of phagocytic leukocytes. Ann. Rev. Biochem. 49:695.

Davies, P., and Bonney, R. J. 1979. Secretory products of mononuclear phagocytes. A brief review. J. Reticuloendoth. Soc. 26:37.

Fearon, D. T. 1980. Identification of a membrane glycoprotein that is the C3b receptor of the human erythrocyte, polymorphonuclear leukocyte, B lymphocyte and monocyte. J. Exp. Med. 152:20.

Hart, P. D. 1979. Phagosome-lysosome fusion in macrophages: Hinge in the fate of ingested microorganisms? *In* Lysosomes in Applied Biology and Therapeutics, Dingle, J. T., Jacques, P. J., and Shaw, I. H. (eds.), vol. 6. Amsterdam: North Holland Co., p. 409.

Horwitz, M. A., and Silverstein, S. C. 1981. Activated human monocytes inhibit the intracellular multiplication of legionnaires' disease bacteria. J. Exp. Med. 154:1618.

Johnston, R. B., Chadwick, D. A., and Cohn, Z. A. 1981. Priming of macrophages for enhanced oxidative metabolism by exposure to proteolytic enzymes. J. Exp. Med. 153:1678.

Nathan, C. F., and Cohn, Z. A. 1981. Cellular components of inflammation: monocytes and macrophages. *In* Textbook of Rheumatology, Kelley, W. N., Harris, E. D., Ruddy, S., and Sledge, C. B. (eds.), vol. 1. Philadelphia: W. B. Saunders, p. 136.

North, R. J. 1978. The concept of the activated macrophage. J. Immunol. 121:806.

Silverstein, S. C., Steinman, R. M., and Cohn, Z. A. Endocytosis. Ann. Rev. Biochem. 46:669.

Unanue, E. R. 1978. The regulation of lymphocyte functions by the macrophage. Immunol. Rev. 40:227.

Unkeless, J. C., Fleit, H., and Mellman, I. S. 1981. Structural aspects and heterogeneity of immunoglobulin Fc receptors. Adv. Immunol. 31:247.

Zuckerman, S. H., and Douglas, S. D. 1979. Dynamics of the macrophage plasma membrane. Ann. Rev. Microbiol. 33:267.

Mast Cells (see also references in 4th ed.)

Austen, K. F. 1979. Biologic implications of the structural and functional characteristics of the chemical mediators of immediate-type hypersensitivity. Harvey Lectures 73:93.

Kitamura, Y., Matsuda, H., and Hatanaka, K. 1979. Clonal nature of mast cell clusters formed in W/W^v mice after bone marrow transplantation. Nature 281:154.

Kitamura, Y., Yokoyama, M., Matsuda, H., and Ohno, T. 1981. Spleen colony-forming cell as common precursor for tissue mast cells and granulocytes. Nature 291:159.

Lagunoff, D. 1978. Mast cell secretion: Membrane events. J. Invest. Dermatol. 71:81.

Metzger, H. 1978. The IgE-mast cell system as a paradigm for the study of antibody mechanisms. Immunol. Rev. 41:186.

Nabel, G., Galli, S. J., Dvorak, A. M., Dvorak, H. F., and Cantor, H. 1981. Inducer T lymphocytes synthesize a factor that stimulates proliferation of cloned mast cells. Nature 291:332.

Razin, E., Cordon-Cardo, C., and Good, R. A. 1981. Growth of a pure population of mouse mast cells in vitro with conditional medium derived fom concanavalin A-stimulated splenocytes. Proc. Nat. Acad. Sci. U.S.A. 78:2559.

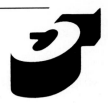

The Adipose Tissue

M. R. C. Greenwood and Patricia R. Johnson

Adipose tissue, commonly called fat, occurs in virtually every mammalian organism. It has long been considered a type of connective tissue and can be described as a loose association of lipid-filled cells *(adipocytes)* and associated stromal vascular cells held in a matrix of collagen fibers. Adipocytes occur in two major forms: unilocular, with a single large inclusion of lipid, and multilocular, with many smaller lipid inclusions. The unilocular adipocyte is the characteristic cell type of white adipose tissue, the primary energy-storage compartment of the mammal. The multilocular adipocyte is characteristic of brown adipose tissue, which functions as a heat-production organ in the mammal.

In humans, roughly 15% of the body weight in a normal man is adipose tissue; fat accounts for approximately 22% of body weight in women. Although normally the percent of body weight that is fat appears to remain fairly constant throughout the adult life span, in pathological conditions such as obesity and anorexia nervosa adipose tissue has a remarkable capacity to change its size. In obesity, the total weight of adipose tissue may increase by more than 100%; in anorexia nervosa, its weight may decrease to 3% of normal.

This unique property of the tissue reflects the function of the unilocular white adipocyte itself. Although adipose tissue of the adult mammal contains many cell types in addition to the adipocyte, most of the physiological functions of the tissue are thought to result from changes in lipid storage and mobilization by the adipocyte. The other cell types in the tissue accounting possibly for as much as 80% of tissue DNA are cells in the vascular bed, fibroblastic connective tissue cells, leukocytes, and macrophages. Although these cells are obviously necessary for tissue integrity, support, and nutrition, they have no known specialized role in adipose tissue function per se.

Distribution of Adipose Tissue

In mammals, white and brown adipose tissues serve different functions, occur in different amounts, and are distributed differently in the body. Until the recent comprehensive report of Pond (1978) few systematic data existed on the relative distribution of fat among the various vertebrate species. Heat generation and mechanical protection of organs have been considered as determinants of the distribution of body fat. Pond's findings suggest that factors such as buoyancy, locomotor mechanics, and the modification of body contours for social and sexual signaling are also important determinants. In some higher primates and marine mammals, certain fat masses appear in only one sex and age group, suggesting that social and sexual factors are the major selective forces leading to their development. Fat distribution in humans is relatively atypical among mammals in respect to its quantity, its location, and its very marked capacity to vary with age, sex, and race.

White adipose tissue is characterized by a white or yellow color, is less well vascularized and innervated than brown adipose tissue, and the fat cells are unilocular. In the rat, major deposits of white adipose tissue occur (1) subcutaneously, as a sheath around the scapular, axillary, and cervical regions and in the inguinal area with minor amounts around the buttocks; (2) intraabdominally in retroperitoneal, mesenteric, and omental regions; and (3) in association with the gonads—the intraabdominal parametrial pad in the female and the well-known epididymal pad that lines the epididymis and testis of the male and normally lies at least partially in the scrotal sac. In the human, the more or less continuous subcutaneous layer shows sexual dimorphism, being better developed, particularly in abdominal and buttocks regions, in women than in men. This difference in the subcutaneous adipose depot between men and women accounts, in large measure, for the difference in total body fat seen in the two sexes. The retroperi-

toneal, mesenteric, and omental depots are well developed in both sexes; and, unlike the rat, the human male has no epididymal fat pad.

Brown adipose tissue, whose only known function is heat production, has been found in newborn mammals of nearly all examined species (Fig. 5–1). In nonhibernators, the relative weight of the tissue declines during the course of maturation. However, in rats it may increase again during prolonged exposure to cold.

In the adult rat, brown adipose tissue occurs mainly in the interscapular region and the axillae. Some minor deposits exist adjacent to the thymus and in the dorsal midline region of the thorax and abdomen. In the adult human, brown adipose tissue deposits are essentially absent, but tissue closely resembling the brown adipose tissue of rodents does occur in human fetuses and newborns. According to Merklin, the major deposits of brown fat in the human fetus are located in the posterior cervical, axillary, suprailiac, and perirenal regions (Fig. 5–1). Lesser deposits exist in the interscapular, anterior mediastinal, intercostal, anterior abdominal, and retropubic areas. As the individual ages, a gradual and selective replacement of these brown fat deposits by white adipose tissue takes place.

Morphology of White Adipose Tissue

Light Microscopy

The cells of white adipose tissue are characterized by one large lipid inclusion resulting from distension of the cytoplasm and apposition of the nucleus to the plasmalemma, and giving the cell a signet-ring shape. In tissue sections these cells are typically polygonal and range in size from 25 to 200 μm. By light microscopy, the cytoplasm is a thin rim surrounding the bulk lipid droplet. Cytoplasmic organelles are difficult to decipher, but mitochondra may be demonstrated by the use of vital dyes such as Janus green. Mitochondria are generally noted in the thicker part of the cytoplasmic rim near the nucleus. The nucleus is flattened against the plasma membrane by the large central lipid inclusion.

Between 60 and 85% of the weight of white adipose tissue is lipid, 5 to 30% water, and 2 to 3% protein. The lipid is 90 to 99% triglyceride. Thin-layer chromatographic analysis has demonstrated that small amounts of free fatty acid, diglyceride, cholesterol, and phospholipid, and trace quantities of cholesterol ester and mono-

180

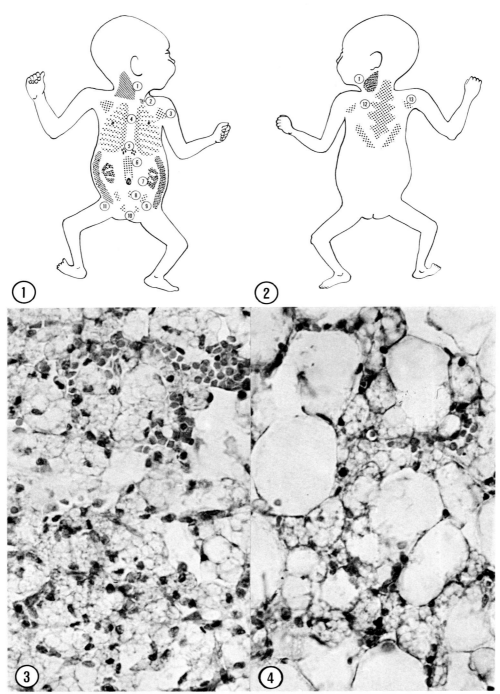

5–1 **1** and **2.** Anterior and posterior views of the fetus illustrating the position of brown fat bodies and fat cell composition. (1) Posterior cervical, (2) axillary, (3) intercostal, (4) anterior mediastinal, (5) anterior abdominal, (6) perirenal, (7) urachal, (8) inferior epigastic, (9) retropubic, (10), suprailiac, (11) interscapular, (12) deltoid, (13) lateral trapezial. Dense dot pattern represents predominantly multilocular fat cells; light dot pattern depresents mixed multilocular and unilocular fat cells. **3.** Suprailiac brown fat body of a 7-month fetus. Multilocular cells predominate. H & E × 250. **4.** Axillary brown fat body of a 7-month fetus. There is a mixture of unilocular and multilocular fat cells. × 250. (From Merklin, R. 1973. Anat. Rec. 178:637.)

glyceride are present. The fatty acid composition of the triglyceride component is a complex array reflecting the influence of dietary fat as well as patterns of synthesis from carbohydrate. Six fatty acids contribute more than 90% of the total mixture: myristic, palmitic, palmitoleic, stearic, oleic, and linoleic.

Electron Microscopy

Until recently, the electron microscope has not been used extensively in studies of adipose tissue. This is probably because of preparation difficulties encountered in dealing with the large amounts of lipid present in adipose cells. The early investigations of Chase showed that adipose cells had a peculiarly filamentous structure, either closely applied to the plasmalemma or as an integral part of the cell membrane. Wasserman and MacDonald (1960) noted that, rather than having such a closely applied extracellular collagenous structure, the fat cell was enveloped by a structure similar to, probably identical to, basement membrane complex. However, Chase's suggestion that a filamentous collagenous structure is in immediate contact with the adipocyte plasmalemma has been confirmed recently by scanning electron-microscopic studies of adipo-

cytes from rat bone marrow (Fig. 5–2). More recent studies, which meet current standards for well-fixed material, have all demonstrated that properly fixed adipose cells show normal cell membranes: Golgi, endoplasmic reticulum, a basement membrane complex, and pleomorphic mitochondria (Fig. 5–3 and 5–6). These intracellular structures are present in adipocytes from chick bone marrow tissue and adipocyte cell culture, in isolated adipocyte preparations, as well as in mammalian whole-tissue preparations. All the intracellular organelles are present in the cytoplasmic rim of the adipocyte (Fig. 5–3). The predominant morphological characteristic of the adipocyte is, of course, the large lipid inclusion. The lipid inclusion itself seems devoid of any inclusions or intracellular organelles. It is not entirely clear how the lipid inclusion enlarges. However, time-lapse photography has demonstrated that viable cells in culture show coalescence of lipid droplets after a few days. Pinocytotic vesicles were observed in cells from both in vivo and in vitro studies. Cushman reported that mature adipocytes pinocytose and remove serum albumin from media. It has been suggested that the pinocytotic vesicles deliver their contents directly to the large lipid inclusions.

Although no one has suggested that the mul-

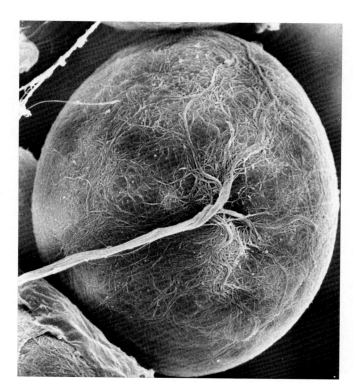

5–2 Scanning electron micrograph of adipocyte from rat thymus held by reticular fibers. ×2,750. (Courtesy of L. Weiss.)

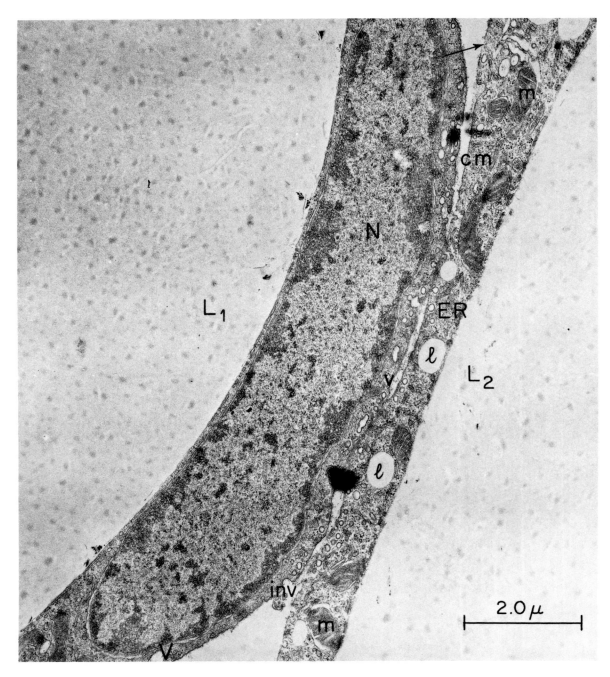

5–3 Isolated adipose cells incubated 60 min in KRB–albumin buffer in the presence of 1.0 μg epinephrine per ml. **L₁** and **L₂**, large, central lipid droplets; **l**, cytoplasmic lipid droplet; **cm**, cell membrane; **m**, mitochondrion; **N**, nucleus; **V**, vacuole; **v**, vesicle; **inv**, invagination; **ER**, endoplasmic reticulum; **arrows,** break in cell membrane. × 15,000. (From Cushman, S. W. 1970. J. Cell Biol. 46:326.)

tilocular droplets in fat cells are membrane-bound, the central lipid inclusion of the unilocular adipocyte may be membrane-bound. Some investigators have reported an electron-dense region at the edge of the lipid droplet, whereas others have found fine filaments (80–100 Å in diameter) arranged in an orderly array and proximate to the lipid droplet. It seems reasonable to conclude that some specialized structures may be associated with the large lipid droplet but that a true membrane boundary does not exist.

Innervation and Vascularization of White Adipose Tissue

According to Ballantyne and Rafferty, the sole innervation of rat epididymal adipose tissue is postganglionic sympathetic and noradrenergic and is arranged as periarteriolar plexuses. Adipocytes are not directly in contact with nerve terminals (Fig. 5–4). Innervation of white adipose tissue appears to be vasoconstrictor in nature, because neural stimulation causes a reduction in the volume of the tissue. However, stimulation also causes an increase in lipolysis, the breakdown of triglyceride in the central droplet, and the release of free fatty acids and glycerol from adipose tissue. The explanation for this finding, in view of the lack of direct innervation to the adipocyte, is that adrenergic-stimulated lipolysis is the result of release of norepinephrine from the perivascular plexuses and its transport through the plasma to adipocyte membrane receptors. The lipolytic response is mediated by beta adrenoreceptors. However, the vasoconstrictor response of the vascular system to neural stimulation is mediated by alpha adrenoreceptors, and intravascular norepinephrine causes vasodilation that is mediated by alpha adrenoreceptors of the vascular system itself (Belfrage, 1978). Thus, the tissue response to catecholamines depends on whether their route of arrival is via the neural or the humoral pathway, on fine tuning of responses by the adipocyte itself, and on the vascular system, which ultimately carries away the products of lipolysis.

Although white adipose tissue has been considered to be poorly vascularized, each adipocyte

5–4 **(Top, left)** Formaldehyde-induced fluorescence in nerve fibers around a blood vessel in rat epididymal adipose tissue. Technique of El-Badawi and Schenk; section thickness 20 μm. × 72. **(Top, right)** Silver-impregnated nerve fiber around an arteriole in rat epididymal adipose tissue. Technique of Holmes; section thickness 12 μm. × 350. **(Bottom, left)** Silver-impregnated nerve fiber around an arteriole in a section of rat epididymal adipose tissue previously incubated in a solution of collagenase to digest connective tissue fibers. Incubated in 0.1% collagenase for 5 h; silver impregnation by the technique of Holmes; section thickness 12 μm. × 350. **(Bottom, right)** Section of rat epididymis impregnated with silver after treatment with collagenase. Bundles of nerve fibers are readily demonstrated after such treatment. Incubated in 0.1% collagenase for 5 h; silver impregnation by the technique of Holmes; section thickness 12 μm. × 240. (From Ballantyne, B., and Rafferty, A. T. 1974. Cytobios. 10:187.)

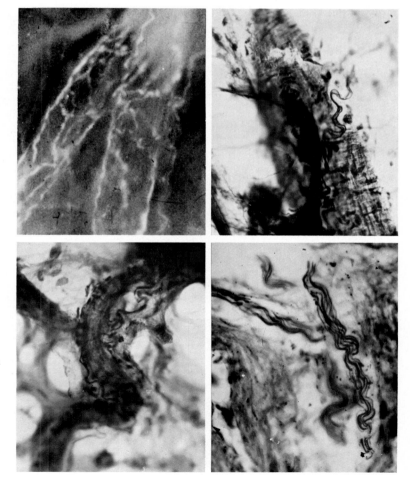

is actually in contact with at least one capillary. The blood supply is adequate to support the very active metabolism of the thin rim of cytoplasm that surrounds the large lipid inclusion. Moreover, adipose tissue blood flow has been measured as varying with the nutritional state and body weight of the animal. For example, blood flow per gram of tissue increases during fasting in rats, dogs, and humans.

Morphology of Brown Adipose Tissue

Light Microscopy

The tissue is composed of loosely arranged lobules that become more compact with aging. The multilocular adipocytes vary in shape from round to polygonal or elongated. The most common state is polygonal, and the cells may reach 60 μm in diameter. The characteristic brown color of the tissue derives from its rich vascularization and the numerous mitochondria present in individual cells (Fig. 5–11).

Electron Microscopy

By electron microscopy, the plasmalemma of brown adipocytes is relatively free of pinocytotic invaginations. A fine fibrillar network fills the narrow intercellular spaces. The mitochondria vary greatly in size and in shape, being round, oval, or filamentous. Lipid droplets within each cell may reach 25 μm in diameter, but they, too, show considerable size variation. Golgi structures are apparent, but rough endoplasmic reticulum and glycogen deposits are sparse (Fig. 5–5).

Innervation and Vascularization of Brown Adipose Tissue

Brown fat differs from white fat in that the adipocytes themselves, in addition to being richly supplied by blood vessels, are directly innervated by sympathetic adrenergic neurons. Bargmann et al. have demonstrated by electron microscopy that paravascular nerves originating from the sympathetic nervous system innervate the interscapular brown fat of the rat. These neurons are nonmyelinated fibers, containing many microtubules with a central filament and some small mitochondria. In addition, their unmyelinated axons are found closely attached to adipocytes, frequently embedded in invaginations of the adipocyte plasma membrane. These terminal axons often contain synaptic vesicles, and it is proposed that these synaptic terminations on adipocyte membranes are the site of release of catecholamines. The existence of these "short adrenergic neurons" that directly innervate brown fat adipocytes has been confirmed by fluorescent histochemical studies of interscapular brown fat from immunosympathectomized rats (Derry et al., 1969). Presumably, it is the short adrenergic neurons that provide the rapid thermogenic response of brown adipose tissue to cold stress.

Origin, Development, and Growth of Adipose Tissue

Nature of the Precursor Cell

Unlike hematopoietic, muscle, or pancreatic beta cells for which functional correlates can be measured before the cells assume their characteristic morphology, the precusor adipose cell possesses no morphological or enzymatic marker. Most of the morphological criteria for identifying or counting adipocytes depend on the presence of accumulated lipid within the cell after proliferation has ceased and cell DNA content is diploid. The earliest investigations into the development of adipose tissue were conducted by Fleming in 1871. He carried out extensive observations of adipose tissue and suggested that adipocytes were derived from mesenchymal cells. During the same period, Toldt (1870) hypothesized that adipocytes were specific cell types of nonmesenchymal origin. His hypothesis was based on the observation that developing fat globules had their own vascular system and were separate from surrounding connective tissue.

Controversy continued into the 1920s and 1930s. Evidence for the idea that adipocytes were modified fibroblasts was strengthened by the investigations of Clark and Clark using rabbit-ear windows. They showed the appearance and apparent differentiation of fibroblasts into a lipid-laden adipose cell shaped like the face of a signet ring. When the cell was depleted of lipid, it returned to fibroblast type. Such studies tended to give strong support to the theory of the adipose cell as a modified fibroblast. Evidence supporting Toldt's concept of adipose tissue as a distinct organ was presented by Wasserman and Hausberger. Wasserman (1926) demonstrated that distinct primitive organs of white adipose tissue existed in human embryos and were derived from reticuloendothelial tissue. Wasserman contended that fat tissue consisted of fat organs,

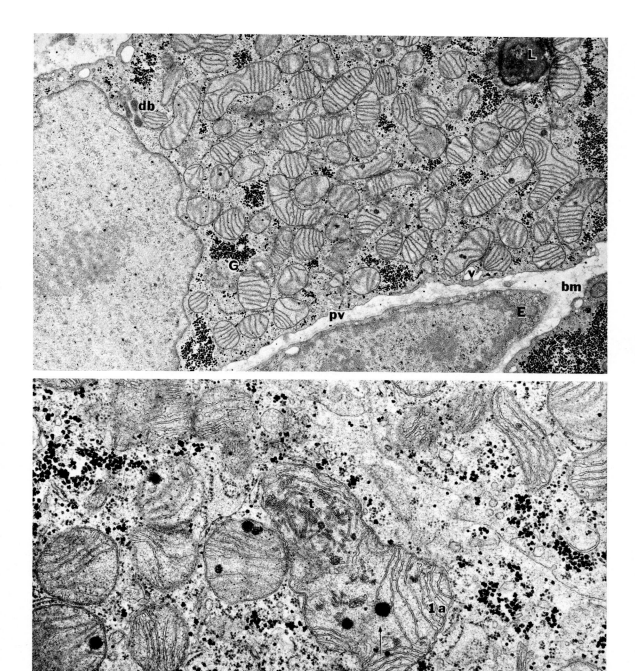

5–5 Top: Parts of adipocytes from a 20-day fetus. Compared with an 18-day fetus, the cells have more cytoplasm and mitochondria are closer together. Their cristae are lamellar, the matrix is denser, and inclusions are more numerous and larger. Masses of glycogen particles **(G)** have accumulated. The cytoplasmic matrix contains fewer ribosomes. Pinocytotic vesicles **(pv)** and vacuoles **(v)** are more frequent. Lipid droplets **(L)** are larger. An endothelial cell **(E)** of a tangentially sectioned capillary is rich in ribosomes. A thin basement membrane **(bm)** envelops it. **db,** dense bodies. × 13,000. **Bottom:** A large mitochondrion in an adipocyte from a 20-day fetus. Its complex inner structure comprises lamellar cristae **(la),** several material inclusions **(arrow)** of various sizes and densities, and a multitude of tubular elements **(t).** (From Suter, E. R. 1969. Res. Lab. Plasma 21:3.)

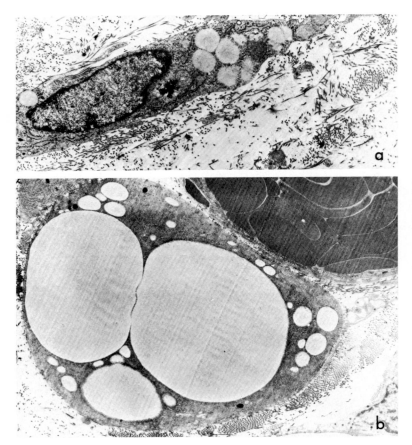

5–6 Developing inguinal adipose tissue in the rat. Cells that are putative preadipoblasts have typical fibroblastic morphology before lipid accumulates **(a).** Lipids first accumulate as small intracellular droplets **(b),** which later coalesce forming the single large lipid droplet characteristic of the white adipocyte shaped like a signet ring. (Courtesy of J. Roth and P. R. Johnson.)

each of which derived from a single primordial cell. His theory was substantially strengthened by Hausberger's finding in 1938 that tissue taken from presumptive adipose tissue sites and transplanted to nonadipose tissue sites did differentiate into fat tissue and *not* into connective or other tissue types. The transplantation studies combined with the observation that adipose tissue arises in well-defined rather than random areas in normal organisms still constitute some of the most convincing evidence that adipose tissue can be considered an organ.

Results from our laboratory on developing inguinal adipose tissue in the rat and from the work of Slavin (1979) on developing inguinal, epididymal, and mesenteric tissue in the mouse suggest that adipocyte precursors appear in loose connective tissue between 17 days prenatal and 3 days postnatal. Electron micrographs show cells that have typically fibroblastic structure before lipid accumulates (Fig. 5–6a). Lipids first accumulate as small intracellular droplets (Fig. 5–6b), which later coalesce to form the single

large lipid droplet characteristic of the signet-ring-shaped white adipocyte.

The concept that adipocytes originate from a specific precursor cell in defined anatomical locations has found recent support in studies of cells cultured from mouse embryonic tissue (the 3T3-L1 cell line) and from rat and human adipose tissue. Cells derived from the stromal–vascular fraction of collagenase-digested adipose tissue, when grown in cultures enriched with insulin, sera, and various lipid components, have been shown to accumulate large amounts of lipid and to exhibit adipocyte-specific enzyme activity (Fig. 5–7). These studies lend credence to the concept that "preadipocytes" exist in adipose tissue, which, under appropriate stimulation, will differentiate into fat cells. Rat or human skin fibroblasts do not differentiate in this fashion under similar culture conditions (Fig. 5–7). Recent studies by Faust et al. (1977a) using lipectomy in the rat also point to the existence of precursor adipocytes. Subcutaneous inguinal fat depots were surgically removed from adult rats; the de-

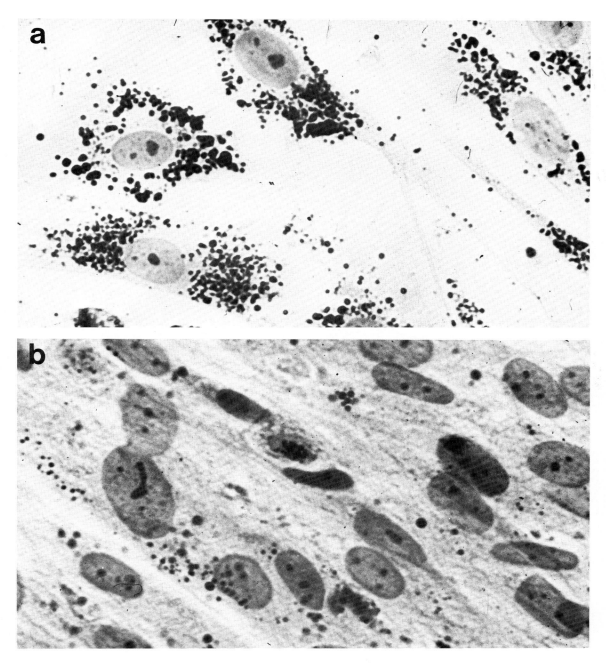

pots eventually regrew, regenerating precisely
the same number of adipocytes that were present
in control sham-operated animals of the same
age and body weight. The fact that these new
cells matched control values not only in number
but also in size is presumptive evidence for precise regulation of adipose tissue cellularity.

Electron-microscopic studies have now provided well-fixed samples of mature adipocytes, yet

5–7 a. Morphology of differentiating precursors of
adult human omental adipocytes in culture.
Early monolayer confluency. **b.** Morphology of human
abdominal skin fibroblasts at monolayer confluency.
× 400. (From Van, R. L. R., and Roncari, D. A. K.,
1978. Cell and Tissue Res. 195:317.)

they have not elucidated a structural–functional relationship that could be used to follow, or to identify precisely, the preadipocyte or adipogenic cells. At present, the clearest demonstrations of a functional marker for the preadipocyte have come from the work of Mohr and Beneke (1969) and Pilgrim (1971). Mohr and Beneke demonstrated the presence of an α-naphthyl acetate esterase in fibrocytic cells that did not yet have lipid accumulations. Because similar-appearing cells were also gylcogen-positive, they suggested that these cells were precursors to cells that later became osmophilic and still later, assumed the appearance of mature adipocytes. The accumulation of glycogen has been shown to precede fat deposition in starved and refed rats and presumably occurs in the normal development and differentiation of adipose tissue. Pilgrim, using these reactions to study the development of adipose tissue in pre- and early postnatal rat epididymal fat pads, found that the proliferative index measured by tritiated thymidine autoradiography was highest in esterase- and glycogen-positive cells lacking lipid vacuoles. He suggested that these cells were preadipocytes. Nonetheless, there is still no clear-cut morphological or cytochemical marker that can be used to distinguish fibroblast-like cells that will become adipocytes from fibroblast-like cells that will not differentiate into adipocytes.

There is disagreement among investigators about the relationship of brown to white adipose tissue. During normal adipocyte development, cells are multilocular before the numerous small lipid inclusions coalesce into a single large droplet of triglyceride. Starvation and refeeding studies have also indicated that when white adipocytes deplete lipid, they become miltilocular and look much like brown adipocytes. Although it may be true that in some specific anatomical locations white adipose tissue appears where brown adipose tissue had previously existed, the reverse is not true; brown adipose tissue does not occur in all the anatomical locations that contain white adipose tissue. It seems likely, therefore, on both anatomical and functional bases that brown and white fat are fundamentally different.

Postnatal Growth

The postnatal growth of adipose tissue has been thoroughly studied in the rat. We know that the size of the adipose tissue mass is a function of both the number and size of adipocytes. During growth of the tissue mass, well-defined stages occur that are characterized either by changes in the number of adipocytes (brought about primarily by mitotic activity in precursor cells, that is, *hyperplastic* growth) or by a change in the size of adipocytes (brought about primarily by intracellular lipid accumulation, that is, *hypertrophic* growth). In the rat epididymal fat pad, from birth until the fourth postnatal week growth of adipose tissue is hyperplastic. From the fourth to the fourteenth week, both hyperplasia and hypertrophy contribute to the enlargement of the adipose tissue mass; from 14 weeks until senescence, hypertrophic growth predominates. Therefore, influences early in postnatal life may produce long-lasting effects on the number of fat cells, whereas influences later in life are more likely to change cell size only. However, it has recently been shown that when rats are fed highly palatable diets they consume a large excess of calories (Faust et al., 1977b). Their fat cells greatly enlarge to what may be considered a maximum size of approximately 1.6 µg of lipid per cell. When this maximum cell size has been reached, the number of cells begins to increase in the adipose depots. If such overfed rats return to a diet of the less palatable laboratory chow, fat cells shrink back to the more usual size of 0.6 µg of lipid per cell, but the number remains elevated. Clearly, after fat cells are formed, at whatever stage in the animal's development, they remain throughout its life.

Abnormal Growth: Obesity

The major pathological condition of adipose tissue, obesity, can also be described on the basis of cellularity changes. The classification of obesity on these grounds has become a common practice. Both in humans and in rodents at least two forms of obesity based on adipose depot morphology have been proposed: (1) hyperplastic–hypertrophic and (2) hypertrophic. Furthermore, some researchers suggest that the hyperplastic–hypertrophic type occurs primarily in early-onset obesities. In children, the hyperplastic–hypertrophic form of obesity has been reported as early as 2 years of age. In hyperplastic obesity, the total number of fat cells may exceed by three- to fourfold the number found in the normal-weight adult. The exact developmental sequence of cellularity characteristics in the human is not yet known. However, it has been suggested that the human, unlike the rat, has both an early postnatal proliferative period and a pre-

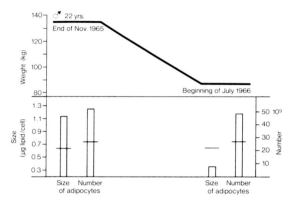

5–8 Adipose cell size and total adipose cell number before and after weight reduction. (From Knittle, J. L. 1974. Sandoz J. Med. Sci. 13:3, 57.)

pubertal proliferative period. Whatever the developmental pattern, investigators agree that once formed, fat cells remain in the tissue throughout life with little or no removal or replacement. The adipocyte lipid is in a constant state of dynamic equilibrium, with lipogenesis and lipolysis being controlled by numerous stimuli, as will be discussed below. Weight reduction in humans and in the rat comes about when caloric restriction limits substrate availability to the adipocyte, inhibiting lipogenesis and enhancing lipolysis (fat mobilization). The morphological result of caloric restriction is a reduction in the size of individual fat cells with no reduction in their number (Fig. 5–8).

Structural–Functional Relationships in the White Adipocyte

In white adipose tissue, the major biochemical functions are associated with the deposition and mobilization of triglyceride lipid in response to caloric demands. The structural–functional correlates of lipid deposition and mobilization are not well understood, but the mechanisms for controlling the balance between the two are related to neuroendocrine secretions and to the nutritional status of the individual. In fact, the white adipocyte has become a favorite subject for study by endocrinologists who wish to unravel mechanisms of hormone action because it is exquisitely sensitive to a number of hormones—for example, insulin, catecholamines, glucagon, ACTH, thyroxine, TSH, and somatotropin, all of which are essentially lipolytic, except insulin which inhibits lipolysis and promotes lipogenesis. The development by Rodbell (1964) of a tech-

nique for isolating intact white adipocytes stimulated the use of these cells for investigation of hormone binding and metabolic regulation. Most attempts to document the cytological and morphological changes in the white adipocyte that are related to biochemical function have been done in cells or tissues derived from animals that were starved, or starved and refed, or that had received injections of hormones, hormone agonists, or hormone antagonists.

Morphological Correlates of Fasting

The original light-microscopic observations of changes brought on by fasting were made by Clark and Clark in 1940 when they observed subcutaneous fat transplanted to a transparent rabbit-ear preparation. They observed that the unilocular signet-ring white adipocytes became multilocular and decreased in diameter when the cells mobilized lipid. This transition from a unilocular to multilocular conformation by cells undergoing lipolysis has been repeatedly confirmed in other tissue sites at the light-microscopic level by other investigators.

In intact white adipose tissue of rats, morphological correlates of the fasting state can be detected after 24 h. At this time, the number of micropinocytotic invaginations increases and pseudopod-like evaginations of cytoplasm appear. However, there are no detectable changes in the size or the appearance of the unilocular fat droplets. After the 48 h of fasting, the size of the unilocular lipid droplet decreases, and some of the cells begin to assume a multilocular appearance. After 72 h of fasting, adipocyte morphology is distinctly altered (Fig. 5–9). Adipose cells are reduced in size and contain many and smaller lipid droplets. The plasmalemma surface becomes very irregular. In addition, the smooth endoplasmic reticulum appears to be proliferating and becomes more obvious than that seen in normal adipose tissue (Fig. 5–9). Some investigators have reported that fenestrated double-membrane envelopes are in close apposition to the lipid droplets and are more visible during fasting. Mitochondrial size and shape do not appear to be affected during fasting.

With continued fasting, white adipocytes may become spindle-like and appear more like fibroblasts, containing few, if any, fat droplets. They may show further indentations of the cell surface, and the size of the micropinocytotic vesicles may be enlarged, reaching 600 to 1,000 Å. Some investigators have demonstrated that the

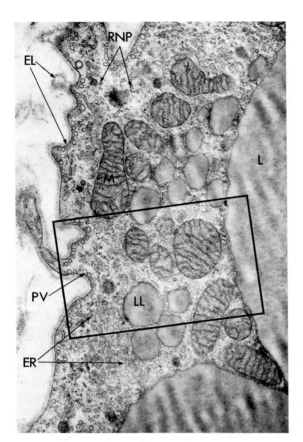

5—9 Portion of a mesenteric adipose cell from a 3-day starved rat. Smaller lipid droplets **(LL)** are seen near the large central lipid droplet **(L)**. Note the abundance of micropinocytotic vesicles **(PV)** and endoplasmic reticulum **(ER)**. The external lamina **(EL)** is clearly visible, especially where it juts out beyond the plasma membrane. **RNP,** ribonucleoprotein particles. × 32,000. (From Slavin, B. G. 1972. Rev. Cytol. 33:297.)

smooth endoplasmic reticulum abundant in adipocytes from starved rats appears to be continuous with the micropinocytotic invaginations at the surface of the cell. However, other investigators, although finding proliferation of smooth endoplasmic reticulum, have not been able to document the continuity between the smooth endoplasmic reticulum and the micropinocytotic invaginations. Jarett and Smith have suggested that the observed pinocytotic microvesicles are part of an alveolar-like interconnecting system with the cell surface, which functions to increase surface area and thus facilitate cytoplasm—surface interaction.

The freeze-fracture studies of Carpentier and co-workers (1977) have produced a quantitative estimate of these membrane changes during lipolysis. The data show that the total number of invaginations of the cell surface does not change during fasting, but rather that the number per unit surface area in local areas increases (Fig. 5–10). This finding, interpreted to mean that a localized clustering of invaginations occurs during lipolysis, tends to support the hypothesis of Jarett and Smith that these finger-like processes are constantly open to the extracellular space. Likewise, the intramembraneous particles seen in the freeze-fracture replicas (Fig. 5–10) remain constant in number, but show local increases. Because these particles are protein in nature, the results imply that the rapid changes in cell size that occur during lipolysis are due to alteration of the lipid content of the membrane, but not of the total protein content. Such changes would likely alter topography in the protein—lipid bilayer.

Other, and much less understood, cellular inclusions that have been reported by various investigators are the complex vesiculated bodies and pentalaminar membranous structures described by Napolitano and Gagne (1963). These structures are spherical in shape, usually membrane-bound, and slightly larger than mitochondria. Within these vesiculated structures are a variety of granules and vesicles of differing size and electron opacity. In the white adipose cell there seems to be no morphological change in the nucleus or the nucleolus except for, perhaps, the increased number of nuclear pores occasionally seen during fasts.

Morphological Correlates of Fat Deposition

During the postulated development of an adipocyte, the cell goes from a fibroblast spindle-shape with small lipid inclusions to a multilocular stage with larger but numerous lipid inclusions to a state of a single, large lipid inclusion. This progression from multilocular to unilocular is thought to be associated with the normal process of lipogenesis and development. During development and during refeeding after a fast, it has been reported that glycogen is deposited in the cytoplasm prior to lipid filling. Hietanen and Greenwood (1977) have recently shown that increased lipoprotein lipase activity in adipose tissue precedes lipid deposition during early development; they have suggested that the onset of

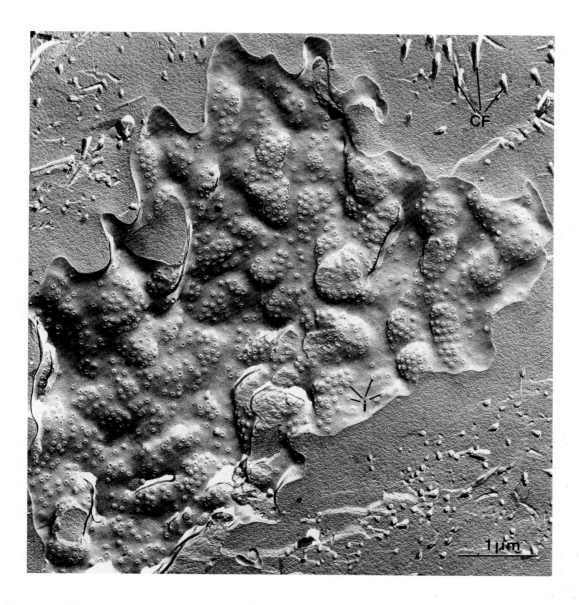

lipoprotein lipase activity is related to preadipocyte differentiation. Napolitano has described
the morphological changes that occur during development, and presumably, during refeeding after a fast. This description has been modified in
the light of more recent work (Fig. 5–11).

As the cell accumulates lipid, the following
morphological changes have been noted. In fi-
broblast-type cells, visible osmophilic lipid
droplets are first noted at one pole of the cell.
The lipid droplets tend to coalesce at one pole
and become pregressively multilocular and then
unilocular. At first, lipid droplets are found free

5–10 B face of an adipose cell plasma membrane of a
9-day starved rat. (Note that according to new
nomenclature the B face is now called the E face.)
Clusters of invaginations **(i)** are seen on protruding
areas of the outer leaflet of the membrane. **CF,**
collagen fibers. × 21,000. (From Carpentier, J. L.,
Perrelet, A., and Orci, L. 1977. Morphological changes
of the adipose cell plasma membrane during lipolysis,
J. Cell Biol. 72:104.)

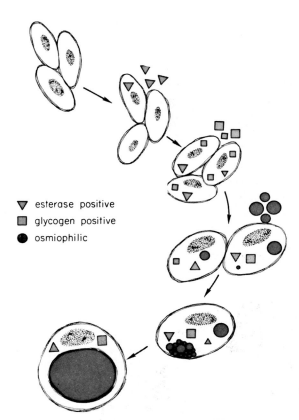

▽ esterase positive

☐ glycogen positive

● osmiophilic

5–11 A generalized schema for the development of an adipose cell. The sequential acquisition of esterase activity, glycogen deposition, and lipid accumulation is depicted as described in the text.

in the cytoplasm, apparently morphologically unrelated to the organelles. As lipid accumulates, the plasma membrane shows several micropinocytotic vesicular areas, and the external lamina elaborates. There is also a gradual reduction in the amount of endoplasmic reticulum, and smooth-surfaced vesicles appear in abundance. Their origin is unclear. The amount of Golgi apparatus diminishes. At no time during the process does any specific organelle show intimate association with lipid droplets.

Biochemical Correlates of Ultrastructure

Attempts to correlate biochemical function with ultrastructural changes have met with varying success. Hollenberg et al. studied the subcellular distribution and composition of exogenously synthesized lipids in isolated white adipocytes.

Their results indicate that after a brief incubation of isolated fat cells with labeled glucose, acetate, or palmitic acid, more than 90% of the newly synthesized triglyceride is stored in the bulk lipid or unilocular lipid inclusion, indicating rapid intracellular transport and storage. However, when the relative specific activity of the organelles was monitored after cell fractionation, the order of highest specific activity of the organelle triglyceride was mitochondria, microsome, liposomes,[1] soluble supernatant, and bulk lipid. They believe that these experiments establish the structural correlates of the intracellular pools of lipid known to exist in adipose tissue, that is, a rapidly exchanging pool and a large-storage, slowly exchanging pool with lipids that are less active metabolically (Fig. 5–12).

Using isolated fat cells, Cushman (1970) has been able to demonstrate the uptake by micropinocytotic vesicles of radioactive colloidal gold and radiolabeled glucose (Fig. 5–3). The function of these micropinocytotic vesicles is yet to be established physiologically, but presumably they represent a mechanism for transport of large molecules.

Although few morphological correlates of changes in the cytophysiology of the white fat cell have been reported to date, numerous reports relate to the hormonal binding sites associated with the fat cell plasmalemma. Both lipolysis and lipogenesis are regulated by hormones, and both lipolytic and antilipolytic hormones are believed to initiate their action by first binding with the adipocyte plasma membrane. Hormone-specific receptor proteins in the adipocyte plasma membrane bind with the hormone. The binding is generally followed by an activation or inhibition of the adenylate cyclase enzyme system in the membrane. Activation of adenylate cyclase results in an increase in the intracellular concentration of cyclic adenosine 3′,5′-monophosphate (cyclic AMP), which mediates the intracellular action of the hormone according to the "second messenger" hypothesis of Sutherland and Rall.

Cyclic AMP achieves its effects by interacting

---

[1]Liposomes are isolated as a floating fraction from adipose cell homogenates. They vary in diameter from 0.5 to 2 μm and contain neutral lipids. Each is surrounded by a single layer of electron dense membrane; dense osmophilic aggregates are associated wih the limiting material. Some liposomes have a granular-appearing membrane. There are some structural similarities between liposomes and the morphology of chylomicra." (Hollenberg et al., 1970.)

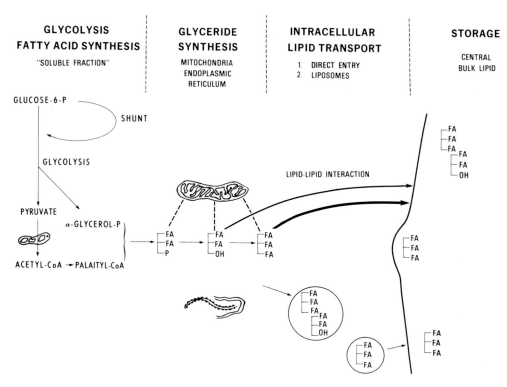

GLYCOLYSIS
FATTY ACID SYNTHESIS
"SOLUBLE FRACTION"

GLYCERIDE
SYNTHESIS
MITOCHONDRIA
ENDOPLASMIC
RETICULUM

INTRACELLULAR
LIPID TRANSPORT
1. DIRECT ENTRY
2. LIPOSOMES

STORAGE
CENTRAL
BULK LIPID

GLUCOSE-6-P

SHUNT

GLYCOLYSIS

LIPID-LIPID INTERACTION

PYRUVATE

α-GLYCEROL-P

ACETYL-CoA → PALAITYL-CoA

5–12 Glyceride synthesis and storage in the adipose cell; structure-function correlation. (From Hollenberg, C. H., Angel, A., and Steiner, G. 1980. Can. Med. Assoc. J. 103:843.)

with the regulatory subunit of specific enzymes known as protein kinases. When cyclic AMP binds to the regulatory subunit of the enzyme, it alters the enzymic conformation so that the catalytic subunit is free to perform its function. Protein kinases catalyze the transfer of terminal phosphate groups from ATP to a variety of intracellular enzymes whose activity depends on their state of phosphorylation or dephosphorylation. For example, the enzyme, hormone-sensitive lipase, which catalyzes the hydrolysis of triglyceride during lipolysis, is inactive in its dephosphorylated form. It is activated by phosphorylation catalyzed by a cyclic AMP–dependent protein kinase. Thus, when physiological concentrations of the catecholamines bind at beta-adrenergic receptor sites in the adipocyte membrane, adenylate cyclase activity is stimulated, intracellular cyclic AMP concentration rises, protein kinase and then hormone-sensitive lipase are activated, and lipolysis proceeds at an elevated rate. Kinetic studies comparing the rate of cyclic AMP formation and the rate of lipolysis, as well as studies using agonists and antagonists to various lipolytic hormones, suggest that cyclic AMP may be compartmentalized within the cell relative to concentrations of intra-

cellular enzymes and the location of cell-surface hormone receptors. As yet, no morphological evidence to confirm such compartmentalization has been presented.

Although it is clear that insulin binds to fat cell membranes and that the effect of insulin on the fat cell is to stimulate lipogenesis and to inhibit lipolysis, the number, nature, and binding affinity of insulin receptors are all matters of great controversy. It has been variously reported that there are high-affinity binding sites ($K_D = 5 \times 10^{-11}M$), low-affinity binding sites ($K_D = 5 \times 10^{-9} M$), and as many as 30,000 and as few as 3,000 insulin receptor sites per fat cell. Furthermore, it has been suggested that insulin inhibits cyclic AMP production by binding at an adrenergic receptor site as well as at its own specific receptor and that it can stimulate cyclic AMP accumulation under conditions of accelerated lipolysis. Regardless of what the specific kinetics of binding are and of what the interaction with

194

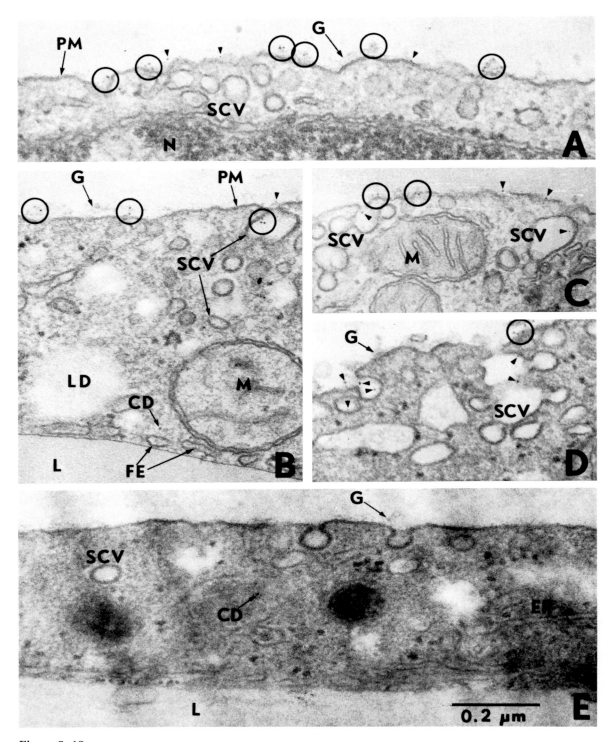

Figure 5–13

5–13 Intact adipocytes were isolated, incubated, and prepared for electron microscopy. In order to allow better visualization of ferritin–insulin molecules, sections were examined without staining. All micrographs were oriented with the plasma membrane toward the top of the figure and the central lipid depot to the bottom. Micrographs × 100,000

PM, plasma membrane; **G**, glycocalyx; **SCV**, surface connected vesicles; **N**, nucleus; **LD**, cytoplasmic lipid droplet; **CD**, cytoplasmic density; **M**, mitochondria; **FE**, fenestrated envelope; **L**, central lipid depot; **ER**, endoplasmic reticulum. (From Jarett, L., and Smith, E. M. 1975. Proc. Natl. Acad. Sci. U.S.A. 72:3526.)

5–14 Sections of adipocytes fixed after incubation with 10 microunits of insulin per milliliter without glucose for 10 min. **S**, extracellular space; **L**, lipid drop within the fat cell. **a.** Section through the central part of an adipocyte showing cytoplasmic envelope that surrounds lipid. Two microtubules **(mt₁)** lie nearly in the plane of the section; another **(mt₂)** is transverse to it (× 18,000). **b.** Fairly thick section near one pole of a cell. Plane of section nearly tangent to lipid droplet. Arrows indicate some of the many microtubules in this section. The tubules appear to form a network tangent to the fat droplet (× 18,000). **c.** Enlargement of region of adipocyte outline in part b. Note electron-lucent region around each tubule (× 30,000). (From Soifer, D., Braun, T., and Hechter, O. 1971. Science [Wash. D.C.] 179:269.)

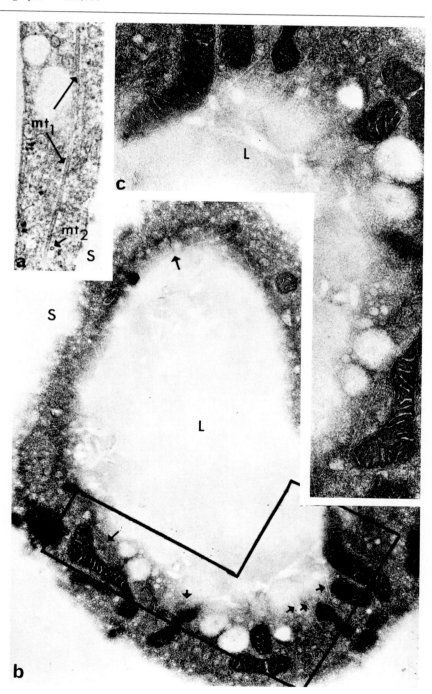

the adenylate cyclase system is, that insulin does bind to the surface of the adipocyte has been elegantly demonstrated by Jarett and Smith (1975) using covalently linked ferritin–insulin complexes. The ferritin–insulin complex provides an electron-microscopic marker for the insulin receptor and reveals that the receptor exists in association with the glycocalyx coating in the external surface of the intact adipocyte plasma membrane (Fig. 5–13). The fact that the insulin receptor is associated with the surface coat of the fat cell supports other studies which suggest that the insulin receptor may be glycoprotein in nature.

It has been demonstrated recently that, in addition to binding to cell-membrane receptor sites, insulin promotes microtubule assembly in isolated rat adipocytes (Fig. 5–14). Other stimuli, such as oxytocin and high concentrations of glucose, do not promote the assembly of microtubules. Because colchicine inhibits the insulin stimulation of lipid and glycogen synthesis in the fat cell but does not influence insulin stimulation of glucose oxidation, it was suggested that

microtubule assembly may be important as part of the direct effect of insulin in inhibiting lipolysis and promoting lipogenesis. Nonetheless, with the possible exception of this microtubule assembly study and the freeze-etched preparations, the internal morphological correlations associated with hormone binding to the fat cell surface have never been documented systematically.

A quantitative study of changes in the adipocyte plasma membrane under the influence of a lipogenic stimulus (insulin) or a lipolytic stimulus (glucagon or epinephrine) has been conducted using the freeze-fracture technique. Carpentier et al. (1976) reported that the number of intramembranous particles seen in the fractured faces of plasma membrane increased in membranes from white adipose cells that had been incubated with insulin, but decreased in preparations from cells that had been incubated with either glucagon or epinephrine. Because these intramembranous particles, which may be seen in both the P and E faces of a fractured plasma membrane (Fig. 5–15) are believed to be membrane proteins (possibly hormonal receptors, membrane-bound enzymes, or both), these data may be the first quantifiable morphological evidence of the modulation of membrane and, thus, of cellular function by a hormone. In these same preparations, the number of membrane invaginations was increased by all three hormones as compared with untreated material, but the size and shape of all membrane structural components remained unaltered regardless of treatment.

5–15 Details of both A and B faces seen at high magnification. The reverse appearance of the membrane invaginations as well as the unequal number of intramembranous particles are clearly evidenced. × 126,000. [Note that according to the new freeze-etching nomenclature (Branton, D., et al. 1975. Science [Wash., D.C.] 190:54]), the A face is now called the P face, and the B face is called the E face.] (From Carpentier, J. L., Perrelet, A., and Orci, L. 1976. J. Lipid Res. 17:335.)

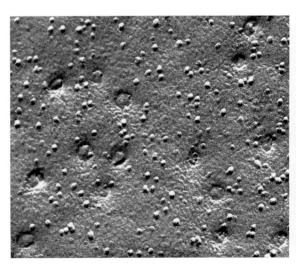
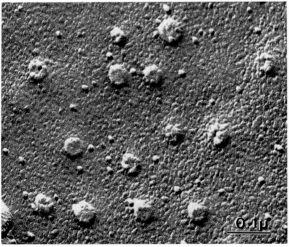

Structural–Functional Relationships in the Brown Adipose Tissue

There are several known functional differences between brown and white adipose tissue. Some of them have been reviewed by Hull and Segall (1966). Perhaps the most striking physiological difference is that brown fat mobilizes little, if any, triglyceride in response to dietary restriction and increases triglyceride deposition very little in response to overfeeding; however, brown fat stores do respond dramatically, both during development and in mature mammals (especially hibernators), to the demands of cold stress.

5–16 **A.** Brown adipocyte from a newborn rat. Several mitochondria contain large matrix inclusions. In most of them a tubular substructure is visible. In filamentous mitochondrial profiles the cristae are oriented lengthwise. Two kinds of particles occur in the cytoplasmic matrix; the smaller less dense ones are ribosomes, and the larger black-appearing ones are glycogen granules. × 24,500.
B. Brown adipocyte from a 17-h-old rat. The mitochondrial matrix inclusions have disappeared, and in their place much smaller granular elements are visible. The mitochondria are somewhat larger and more nearly round. The cytoplasm contains only ribosomes, and no glycogen remains. × 24,500. (From Suter, E. R. 1969. Specialia, 15:3.)

A

B

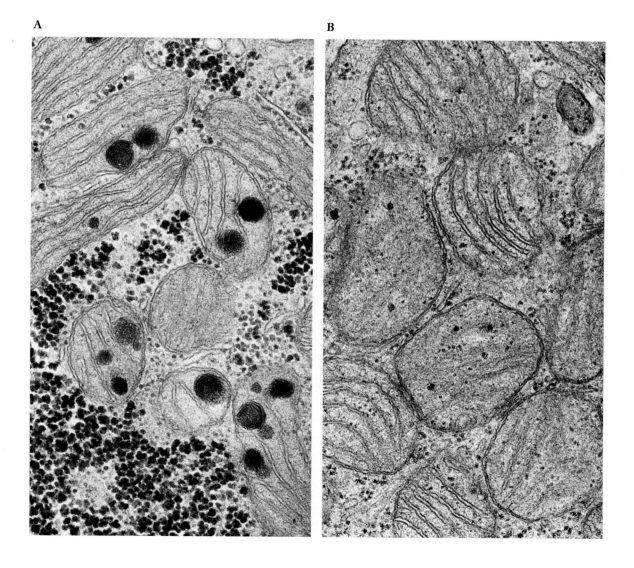

White adipose tissue undergoes lipolysis and becomes depleted during a fast even at higher-than-normal environmental temperature. Brown adipose tissue, in contrast, rapidly mobilizes lipid when the animal is cold-stressed, but brown adipocytes may remain lipid-filled even when the animal is starved to death in a thermoneutral environment. The thermogenic properties of brown adipose tissue are thought to result from cyclic AMP modulation of norepinephrine stimulation. The noradrenergic stimulation results from neural innervation of individual fat cells and the subsequent activation of adenylate cyclase through adrenergic receptors in brown adipose tissue cell membranes.

It has recently been suggested by investigators in the United Kingdom and Canada that brown fat may be involved in a diet-induced thermogenic response, similar to the response induced by cold stress. Thus when an animal or human increases food intake, brown fat cell mitochondria may increase the degree to which they are "loosely coupled," i.e., oxidize substrate without subsequent ATP formation, thereby using up excess substrate and preventing its storage in white adipose tissue. This mechanism has been advanced as a possible means by which mammals regulate body weight, and it has been reported that the obese hyperglycemic mouse has a deficit in brown fat.

Structural—functional relationships in brown adipose tissue both during development and in response to stimuli are much more clearly documented than those in white adipose tissue. During the first few days of rat postnatal development, brown adipose tissue progressively loses cellular glycogen deposits, the diameter of the multilocular lipid droplet decreases, and dense bodies and cytolysosomes become more prominent. Major changes in mitochondrial ultrastructure are also noted. Principally, the mitochondria swell and cristae are reoriented to a transverse configuration. Inclusions that are typically noted in the internal mitochondrial matrix in prenatal development and under thermoneutral conditions are decreased in number (Fig. 5—16). The ultrastructural changes presumably associated with lipid mobilization in cold stress can be produced both in vivo and in vitro by norepinephrine administration. The ultrastructural effects are blocked by the use of Trasicor (a beta-adrenergic blocking agent) and mimicked by theophylline. Presumably, the effect of theophylline is to inhibit the intracellular phosphodiesterase, leading to decreased degradation of cyclic AMP and to consequently higher intracellular cyclic AMP levels. Therefore, theophylline administration leads to higher cellular lipolytic activity. Although many points about structural correlates of brown adipose tissue must still be established, the process of neural integration and substrate mobilization reflected in the ultrastructural changes described above is most probably correct.

References and Selected Bibliography

General

Cushman, S. W. 1970. Structure–function relationships in the adipose cell. I. Ultrastructure of the isolated adipose cell. J. Cell Biol. 46:326.

Cushman, S. W. 1970. Structure–function relationships in the adipose cell. II. Pinocytosis and factors influencing its activity in the isolated adipose cell. J. Cell Biol. 46:342.

Greenwood, M. R. C., and Hirsch, J. 1974. Postnatal development of adipocyte cellularity in the normal rat. J. Lipid Res. 15:474.

Heitanen, E., and Greenwood, M. R. C. 1977. A comparison of lipoprotein lipase activity and adipocyte differentiation in growing male rats. J. Lipid Res. 18:480.

Hollenberg, C. H., Angel, A., and Steiner, G. 1970. The metabolism of white and brown adipose tissue. Can. Med. Assoc. J. 103:843.

Mohr, W., and Beneke, G. 1969. Histochemische Untersuchungen de Enstehung von Fettzellen. Virchows Arch. B 3:13.

Napolitano, L. 1963. The differentiation of white adipose cells. An electron microscopic study. J. Cell. Biol. 18:663.

Pond, C. M. 1978. Morphological aspects and the ecological consequences of fat deposition in wild vertebrates. Am. Rev. Ecol. Syst. 9:519.

Renold, A. E., and Cahill, G. F. 1965. Adipose tissue. In Handbook of Physiology, Sect. 5. Washington, D.C.: American Physiological Society.

Slavin, B. G. 1972. The cytophysiology of mammalian adipose cells. Int. Rev. Cytol. 33:297.

Brown Adipose Tissue

Bargmann, W., Hehn, G. V., and Linder, E. 1968. Über die Zellen des braunen Fettgewebes und ihre Innervation. Z. Zellforsch. Mikrosk. Anat. 85:601.

Derry, D. M., Schonbaum, E., and Steiner, G. 1969. Two sympathetic nerve supplies to brown adipose tissue of the rat. Can. J. Physiol. Pharmacol. 47:57.

Hull, D., and Segall, M. M. 1966. Distinction of brown from white adipose tissue. Nature (Lond.) 212:469.

Merklin, R. 1973. Growth and distribution of human fetal brown fat. Anat. Rec. 178:637.

Suter, E. 1969. The fine structure of brown adipose tissue. Lab. Invest. 21:246.

Suter E. R. 1969. The fine structure of brown adipose tissue. I. Cold-induced changes in the rat. J. Ultrastruct. Res. 26:216.

Suter, E. R., and Staubli, W.. 1970. An ultrastructural histochemical study of brown adipose tissue from prenatal rats. J. Histochem. Cytochem. 18:100.

Development and Regeneration

Faust, I. M., Johnson, P. R., and Hirsch, J. 1977a. Adipose tissue regeneration following lipectomy. Science (Wash., D.C.) 197:391.

Pilgrim, C. 1971. DNA synthesis and differentiation in developing white adipose tissue. Dev. Biol. 26:69.

Slavin, B. G. 1979. Fine structural studies on white adipocyte differentiation. Anat. Rec. 195:63.

Van, R. L. R., and Roncari, D. A. K. 1978. Complete differentiation of adipocyte precursors. Cell Tissue Res. 195:317.

Endocrine Control and Metabolism

Belfrage, E. 1978. Vasodilation and modulation of vasoconstriction in canine subcutaneous adipose tissue caused by activation of β-adrenoreceptors. Acta. Physiol. Scan. 102:459.

Carpentier, J. L., Perrelet, A., and Orci, L. 1976. Effects of insulin, glucagon and epinephrine on the plasma membrane of the white adipose cell: A freeze-fracture study. J. Lipid Res. 17:335.

Carpentier, J. L., Perrelet, A., and Orci, L. 1977. Morphological changes of the adipose cell plasma membrane during lipolysis. J. Cell Biol. 72:104.

Cuatrecasas, P. 1971. Insulin—receptor interactions in adipose tissue cells: Direct measurement and properties. Proc. Natl. Acad. Sci. U.S.A. 68:1264.

Fain, J. N. 1975. Insulin as an activator of cyclic AMP accumulation in rat fat cells. J. Cyclic Nucleotide Res. 1:359.

Gliemann, J., Gammeltoft, S., and Vinten, J. 1975. Insulin receptors in fat cells. Relationship between binding and activation. Isr. J. Med. Sci. 2:656.

Jarett, L., and Smith, R. M. 1975. Ultrastructural localization of insulin receptors on adipocytes. Proc. Natl. Acad. Sci. U.S.A. 72:3526.

Kono, T., and Barham, F. W. 1971. The relationship between the insulin-binding capacity of fat cells and the cellular response to insulin. J. Biol. Chem. 246:6210.

Napolitano, L., and Gagne, H. 1963. Lipid-depleted white adipose cells: An electron microscope study. Anat. Rec. 147:273.

Robinson, G. A., Butcher, R. W., and Sutherland, E. W. 1971. Cyclic AMP. New York: Academic Press, Inc.

Rodbell, M. 1964. Metabolism of isolated fat cells. I. Effects of hormones on glucose metabolism and lipolysis. J. Biol. Chem. 239:375.

Soifer, D., Braun, T., and Hechter, O. 1971. Insulin and microtubules in rat adipocytes. Science (Wash., D.C.) 179:269.

Wasserman, F., and MacDonald, T. F. 1960. Electron microscopic investigation of the surface membrane structures of the fat cell and of their changes during depletion of the cell. Z. Zellforsch. Mikrosk. 52:778.

Innervation

Ballantyne, B., and Raftery, A. T. 1974. The intrinsic autonomic innervation of white adipose tissue. Cytobios 10:187.

Obesity

Faust, I. M., Johnson, P. R., and Hirsch, J. 1977b. Diet-induced adipocyte number increase in adult rats: A new model for obesity. Am. J. Physiol. 235:E279.

Hirsch, J., and Knittle, J. L. 1970. Cellularity of obese and non-obese human adipose tissue. Fed. Proc. 29:1516.

Johnson, P. R., and Hirsch, J. 1972. The cellularity of adipose depots in six strains of genetically obese mice. J. Lipid Res. 13:2.

The Skeletal Tissues

Webster S. S. Jee

The skeletal tissues, cartilage and bone, are a highly specialized type of connective tissue that forms the skeletal framework of most vertebrates. They are distinguished from other types of connective tissue by the preponderance of solid intercellular material. Cartilage has a firm gel, whereas bone, because of the calcified matrix, is hard. The complex mineral substance within the organic matrix of bone is composed chiefly of calcium, phosphate, and carbonate.

Cartilage and bone serve as a permanent and temporary skeletal tissue throughout the vertebrates. They form the endoskeleton, the supporting structure, and the levers of the locomotion system to which are attached muscles and ligaments of the vertebrate body. Lower vertebrates have a permanent cartilaginous skeleton. In humans most of the embryonic skeleton is initially cartilaginous but is eventually replaced by bone. However, some cartilage does persist as the articular surfaces of movable joints, as the walls of the respiratory tract, and as parts of the base of the skull.

The distinctive properties of cartilage include its low metabolic rate, avascularity, capacity for continued growth, and high tensile strength coupled with resilience and elasticity. In contrast, bone is harder, much more vascular, more complex in structure, and constantly renews itself to meet both mechanical and metabolic demands. The bony skeleton contains approximately 99% of the calcium in the body and also serves as a major storehouse for calcium.

Cartilage

Cartilage is a specialized form of supporting connective tissue composed of cells, fibrous macromolecules, and ground substance. The cartilage cells (chondrocytes) synthesize matrix and encase themselves within cavities (lacunae). The matrix, primarily responsible for the physicochemical properties of cartilage, is composed of fibers embedded in a ground substance.

The toughness and rigidity of cartilage enable it to withstand shearing and contribute to a "friction-free" surface at the articular surfaces of bones. Cartilage provides a resilient form of support and has a crucial role as a precursor or "model" for the embryonic development and subsequent growth of many bones.

There are only three types of mature cartilaginous tissue: hyaline, elastic, and fibrocartilage. They differ in the distribution and quantity of fibers and chondrocytes within the matrix. Of the three, hyaline cartilage is most prevalent.

Hyaline Cartilage

In adults, hyaline cartilage is present in the walls of the major respiratory passages (nose, larynx, trachea, and bronchi), on the ventral ends of ribs, and on the bone surfaces of joints (articular cartilage). In the fetal and postnatal growing human, it is also found at the core of developing long bones, thus providing a temporary skeleton for the embryo and a model for the growth in length of bone. Fresh hyaline cartilage is grossly structured as plates, columns, or irregular masses and is translucent bluish-white.

Development. All cartilage develops from mesenchymal tissue (Fig. 6–1). At the site of chondrogenesis, mesenchymal cells round out and proliferate to form closely packed agglomerations. At this stage of differentiation the cells have transformed into chondroblasts, and the tissue is called precartilage. Subsequently, the chondroblasts begin to synthesize and secrete matrix into the extracellular space, entrapping themselves within lacunae, which become further separated by the formation of additional matrix. The cells completing this sequence have been transformed into mature cartilage cells, or chondrocytes.

At the same time, the outermost region of mesenchyme surrounding the precartilage condenses to form a fibrous sheath around the newly formed cartilage. This fibrous covering, the perichondrium, is composed of an outer fibrous layer of dense connective tissue and an inner or chondrogenic layer of flattened cells having the potential to differentiate into chondrocytes.

Growth. Many of the individual chondrocytes within lacunae divide and may create lacunae packed with a mass of cells called an isogenous group or cell nest (Figs. 6–1 to 6–3). Each cell in the cell nest is a clone of the first chondrocyte within that lacuna. The progeny eventually become partitioned by the secretion of matrix, resulting in the expansion of the cartilage from within, a process known as interstitial growth.

As the matrix ages, it becomes increasingly rigid. Interstitial growth declines rapidly with age because the matrix is no longer able to expand. Further growth proceeds by the addition of cartilage on the existing outer surfaces beneath

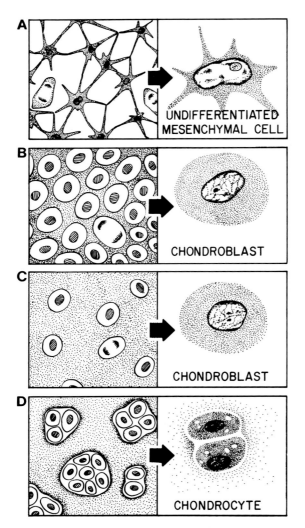

6–1 The origin and development of hyaline cartilage.
A. The mesenchyme; precursor of all types of cartilage. **B.** The precartilage; the mesenchymal cells contract their processes, proliferate, and differentiate into chondroblasts. **C.** The secretion of new matrix; chondroblasts are entrapped in lacunae and separated from each other by the formation of new extracellular matrix. **D.** The isogenous group; chondrocytes within lacunae divide to create isogenous groups. Lacunae are surrounded by a condensation of the matrix called territorial matrix; the remaining matrix is called interterritorial matrix.

the perichondrium in a sequence referred to as appositional growth. Appositional growth occurs when the undifferentiated cells of the inner chondrogenic layer of perichondrium proliferate and differentiate into chondroblasts that deposit matrix around themselves.

In early embryonic development, appositional and interstitial cartilage growth occur in concert. Later growth is primarily appositional. At maturity, the chondrogenic activity of the perichondrium becomes dormant and is stimulated only after cartilage injury.

Chondrocytes. Chondrocytes change cytologically with age. Young cells are flattened or elliptical with their long axis oriented parallel to the surface. In contrast, older cells are round or hypertrophied (having a diameter up to 40 μm) and lie within cell nests (Figs. 6–1 to 6–3). The nucleus is ovoid and contains one or two nucleoli. The cytoplasmic organelles of chondrocytes are similar to those found in fibroblasts, which also synthesize extracellular matrix. In actively growing cartilage, there is an abundance of granular endoplasmic reticulum and a prominent Golgi zone. Secretory vesicles are associated with the Golgi region and secrete material into the surrounding matrix. In mature chondrocytes the endoplasmic reticulum is less abundant, the Golgi region less extensive, and large accumulations of cytoplasmic glycogen are frequently present.

In many histological preparations, chondrocytes may appear stellate and detached from the lacunar wall (Figs. 6–2 and 6–3). This appearance is due to shrinkage during the fixation, dehydration, and staining.

Matrix. Unstained, hyaline cartilage matrix appears homogeneous. The collagen fibers are not visible because (1) most of the collagen is in the form of submicroscopic fibrils and (2) the refractive index of collagen is very close to that of the surrounding ground substance. However, these fibers may be readily visualized by polarized light microscopy.

Actually, the matrix of hyaline and of the other cartilage types shows considerable biochemical and ultrastructural variability. For example, the matrix nearest the chondrocytes contains few or no collagenous fibrils and fibers and shows an intense basophilia and a strong periodic acid Schiff reaction. The basophilic rims of matrix around lacunae collectively form the capsular or territorial matrix, whereas the less basophilic matrix located between lacunae is known as interterritorial matrix (Fig. 6–3).

The physical and chemical properties of hyaline cartilage result directly from the matrix synthesized and secreted by the chondroblasts and chondrocytes. Hyaline cartilage matrix contains

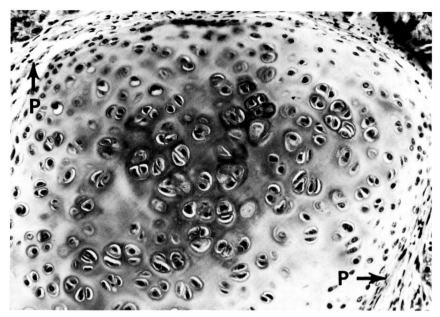

6–2 Photomicrograph of hyaline cartilage, a part of
△   the nasal choanae of a young cat. The cells
immediately beneath the perichondrium (**P**) are single
and elongated. The central located chondrocytes are
larger, are distributed as isogenous groups, and have a
more intense staining of the capsular matrix.
Hematoxylin–phloxine–orange stain. ×240.

6–3 A high magnification of a portion of the hyaline
▽   cartilage seen in Fig. 6–2. Interterritorial matrix
(**B**); intense staining of the territorial matrix (**C**)
immediately surrounding the groups of isogenous
cells. Hematoxylin–phloxine–orange stain. ×370.

collagen and proteoglycans. The proteoglycans
have a protein core with covalently bound chondroitin sulfate and keratan sulfate side chains.
Seventy-five percent of the wet weight of cartilage matrix represents tissue fluids held in place
by these macromolecules. The proteoglycans are
believed to bind cations by weak chemical bonds
and thereby to play an important role in the
transport of water and electrolytes within the
matrix. Proteoglycans also bind to collagen fibers
and fibrils, forming a network that contributes to
the gel-like qualities of the ground substance and
acts as a molecular sieve to limit the free movement of large macromolecules. Similar to other
secretory products, the protein component of
proteoglycans is synthesized on granular endoplasmic reticulum. After protein synthesis, polysaccharides synthesized within the Golgi region
are added, and sulfation and packaging within
secretory vesicles follow. The specific proteoglycans found in all cartilage are chondroitin 4- and
6-sulfates, keratan sulfate, and some hyaluronic
acid. The proportion of each varies with the anatomic site, source, and age.

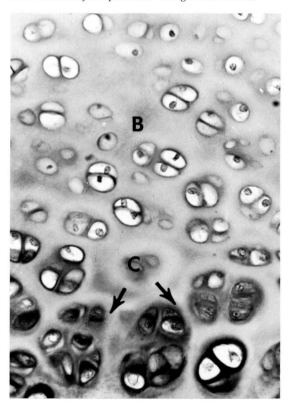

The collagen content of hyaline cartilage matrix varies between 50% and 70% of the dry weight. Cartilage is unique in containing only type II collagen. Chondroblasts and chondrocytes secrete collagen as tropocollagen molecules consisting of triple helixes of three α1 (II) proteins. In the extracellular fluid, the tropocollagen is then enzymatically linked into stable collagen fibers and fibrils. Electron micrographs reveal that the fibers and fibrils of cartilage matrix are finer than those in fibrous or dense connective tissue. Most of these fibers have a variable periodicity and fail to show the characteristic 640 Å banding seen in connective tissue and bone. In fact, some extremely fine fibrils have no periodicity. Bundles of collagen have been seen only in articular hyaline cartilage. This evidence probably indicates that the collagen is less polymerized in most hyaline cartilage than other types of connective tissue.

Elastic Cartilage

Elastic cartilage is typically found in regions requiring a flexible form of support: the auricle of the ear, the walls of the external auditory canals and Eustachian tubes, the epiglottis, and parts of the corniculate and cuneiform cartilages of the larynx. Because of a preponderance of elastic fibers, fresh elastic cartilage appears yellow and more opaque than hyaline cartilage.

The histogenesis of elastic cartilage differs slightly from that of hyaline cartilage. Elastic cartilage first appears as fibroblasts and as numerous fibril bundles, which are not characteristic of either elastin or collagen. The fibroblasts are transformed to chondroblasts that secrete matrix around themselves and, by some unknown mechanism, the previously undifferentiated fibrillar bundles are transformed into elastic fibers. The elastic fibers are highly branched and are more dense in the central region of the cartilage, often obscuring the ground substance (Fig. 6–4). At the periphery, a perichondrium is formed as in hyaline cartilage. The elastic fibers are less dense near the perichondrium and gradually blend into the fibrous layer.

The chondrocytes of elastic cartilage are identical in appearance with those of hyaline cartilage, occurring within lacunae either singly or in cell nests (Fig. 6–4). The growth of elastic cartilage is also essentially the same as that of hyaline cartilage.

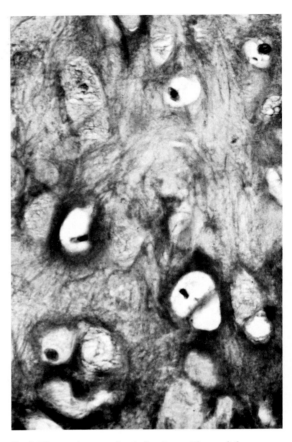

6–4 Photomicrograph of elastic cartilage of the epiglottis of an adult man. The dark staining elastic fibers are seen in the matrix between cell groups. Hematoxylin and eosin stain. ×370.

Fibrocartilage

Fibrocartilage is located in a few regions where firm support and tensile strength are necessary: the intervertebral discs, the pubic symphysis, the linings of tendon grooves, the attachments of tendons and ligaments, and the rims of certain articular cartilage; it is also the type of cartilage formed after injury. Fresh samples have a firm fibrous texture that macroscopically resembles dense connective tissue.

Fibrocartilage differs dramatically from hyaline cartilage (Fig. 6–5). The ground substance is sparse, and numerous collagenous fibers are visible as large irregular bundles between groups of chondrocytes. Occasionally, the chondrocytes are aligned in rows parallel to the collagen bun-

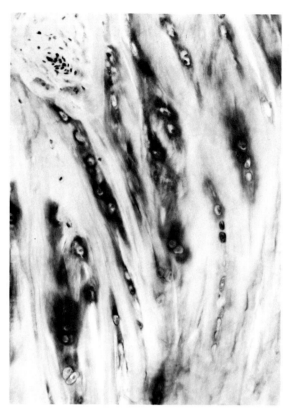

6–5 Photomicrograph of fibrocartilage of the knee joint of a young chick. The rows of chondrocytes are surrounded by deeply staining matrix. Wright's stain. ×240.

dles. However, more often they are distributed individually or in pairs. Fibrocartilage further differs from hyaline and elastic cartilage by its acidophilic staining quality owing to the preponderance of cationic collagenous fibers.

The development of fibrocartilage reflects its intermediate nature between dense connective tissue and hyaline cartilage. Fibrocartilage never occurs alone, but merges with neighboring hyaline cartilage, ligaments, or tendons. Fibrocartilage arises initially as ordinary connective tissue in which fibroblasts gradually transform into chondroblasts and secrete a thin layer of matrix around themselves. The secretion by the chondroblasts and chondrocytes is limited, and the collagenous bundles fail to become infiltrated by the sparse matrix. In contrast to other types of cartilage, a perichondrium fails to form in fibrocartilage.

Nutrition

Because it is a nonvascular tissue, cartilage has a slow turnover and an inherent stability during weight bearing. Early embryonic cartilage is filled with blood vessels. Only later does it become avascular. The chondrocytes receive nutrients and rid waste products via diffusion. The great fluid content of the matrix permits dissolved gases, nutrients, and waste products to diffuse readily to and from capillaries located outside the perichondrium. This limited diffusion is adequate for cartilage because chondrocytes function predominantly by glycolytic metabolism as an adaptation to their slightly anaerobic environment. Consequently, cartilage has an extremely high lactate content. When cartilage acquires blood vessels, it becomes converted into either bone or other types of connective tissue. Furthermore, if the cartilage becomes too thick, the diffusion distances become too great and the chondrocytes become necrotic.

Regressive Changes

Both elastic and fibrocartilage are fairly resistant to damage and aging. However, hyaline cartilage frequently undergoes numerous degenerative changes. As hyaline cartilage ages, a decline in matrix basophilia and a gradual loss of chondrocytes occur. Subsequently, the matrix becomes opaque, hard, and brittle because of calcium carbonate deposits. This impregnation of the matrix interferes with the diffusion of nutrients and wastes, leading to cell death and dissolution of the matrix.

This kind of regressive change occurs normally in a type of bone formation known as endochondral ossification. In this process the hyaline cartilage undergoes a sequence of cell proliferation, maturation, hypertrophy, and finally cell death concurrent with the calcification of its matrix. These transforming chondrocytes form a plate called the growth plate, and the cytological changes are localized into specific zones (Fig. 6–6). The sequential degenerative changes eventually result in the calcification of the matrix and the enlargement of lacunae that, in turn, provide a calcified cartilage substrate or "scaffolding" for the formation of bone. Little was known about the mechanism of matrix calcification until recently, when a variety of electron-micrographic and biochemical studies indicated that chondrocytes play a major role in

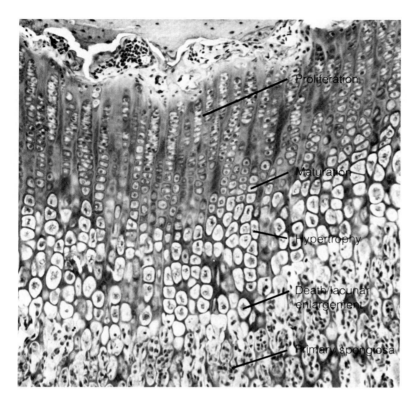

6–6 Photomicrograph of endochondral ossification in decalcified longitudinal sections through growth plate of proximal end of the tibia of a rat. Sequential degenerative changes of chondrocytes result in the production of calcified cartilage cores to serve as scaffolding for bone formation. The sequence involves cartilage proliferation, maturation, hypertrophy, death and lacunar enlargement, and calcification of matrix. Mineralization is not apparent in this decalcified section. Hematoxylin and eosin stain. ×104.

the mineralization of intercellular matrix. Matrix vesicles containing calcium and phosphate are probably derived from the cytoplasmic membrane of chondrocytes and are left behind by contraction of cell membrane to form initial sites of cartilage mineralization. Amorphous calcium phosphate occurs first, and hydroxyapatite then forms within the vesicles. Needle-like structures believed to be crystals of bone mineral (hydroxyapatite) lie within the vesicles. It has been postulated that the hydroxyapatite crystals burst through the vesicle membrane to be deposited into the matrix.

A rare pathological condition occurs within hyaline cartilage. It is characterized by the presence of silky, lustrous parallel fibers inappropriately called asbestos fibers. These fibers may soften and cavities develop.

Regeneration

Except in young children, human cartilage has a limited capacity to regenerate. When cartilage is damaged in adults, the injured region becomes necrotic. The area is then filled with newly formed connective tissue from the perichondrium and nearby fascia. Some of the connective tissue slowly differentiates into cartilage cells and lays down fibrocartilage. However, most of it remains as a scar of dense connective tissue. Fractured mature cartilage, on the other hand, is usually united by a permanent fibrous tissue that may eventually be replaced by bone.

Transplantation of Cartilage

Because extraskeletal sources available for autografts are limited, damaged or missing hyaline cartilage is frequently replaced by transplantation using homografts from people who have recently died. These homografts have been successful because the matrix acts as a barrier that permits only limited diffusion of high-molecular-weight substances and contains an antiangiogenesis factor against the invasion of host blood vessels and fibroblasts. Thus, exposure to the immunologically reactive cells is restricted. The success of the transplant further depends on the quantity and distribution of nearby vessels for nutrient diffusion.

Bone

Bone differs from other connective tissue by its rigidity and hardness owing to the inorganic salts impregnated in the matrix. Bone enables the skeleton to maintain the shape of the body and to protect the soft tissues of the cranial and thoracic cavities. It provides the framework for the bone marrow and transmits the force of muscular contraction from one part of the body to another during movement. The skeleton is also important metabolically for the regulation of fluids in the body. The mineral content of bone serves as a reservoir for ions, particularly calcium.

Macroscopic Structure of Bone

On a gross level, all bones are composed of two basic architectural structures: cortical or compact and trabecular or cancellous bone. With the exception of microscopic channels, cortical bone is a dense solid mass. Trabecular bone, in contrast, appears as a lattice of rods, plates, and arches individually known as trabeculae (Figs. 6–7, 6–8, and 6–12). The two bone structures differ radically in their bone marrow or soft tissue content. The soft tissue content of cortical bone is usually less than 10% by volume, whereas it is 75% by volume in trabecular bone.

The mass of an adult human skeleton is composed primarily of compact bone: approximately 80% of the skeletal mass is cortical bone. Cortical bone forms the outer wall or "shell" of all bones. The remaining 20% of the mass is trabecular bone. It is primarily limited to the central region of bones and contains marrow.

The long bones (e.g., humerus, femur, and tibia) provide an excellent descriptive model for the macroscopic structures of bone. A typical adult long bone consists of a central cylindrical shaft, or diaphysis, and two roughly spherical ends, the epiphyses (Fig. 6–9). Connecting the diaphysis with each epiphysis is a cone-shaped region, the metaphysis. Whereas the diaphysis is primarily compact in structure, the epiphysis and metaphysis are mainly composed of interior trabecular bone with a shell of compact bone. In the growing animal, the epiphysis is separated from the metaphysis by a thick plate of hyaline

6–7 Bone section and radiograph of dried proximal end of femur. × 0.5. **A.** Photograph of 8-mm-thick proximal femur cut in a frontal plane. The head and greater trochanter are covered by a thin shell of cortical (compact) bone, whereas the shaft is covered by a thick cylinder of cortical (compact) bone. Note the arching pattern of trabeculae (**double arrow**). **B.** Radiograph of same bone section.

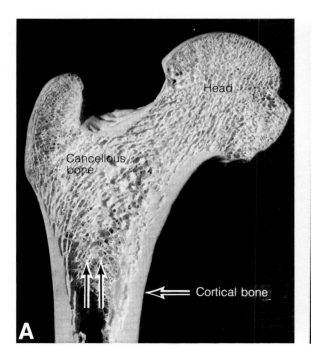

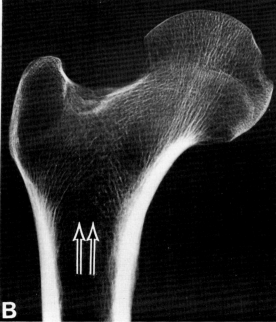

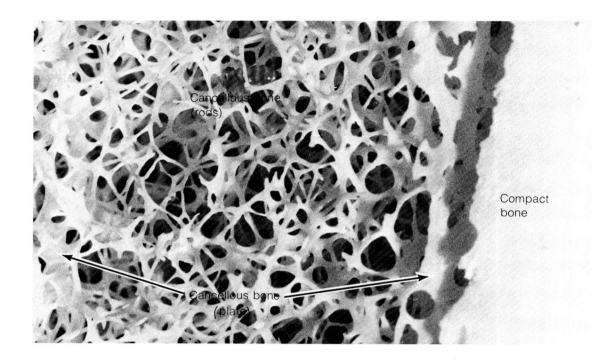

Cancellous bone
(rods)

Cancellous bone
(plate)

Compact
bone

6–8 Photograph of a thick ground section of part of the proximal tibia showing the cortical (compact) bone and the trabecular (cancellous) bone. The trabecular bone consists of vertical trabecular plates with perforations and a network of trabecular rods or bars. In living specimens, bone marrow occupies the intertrabecular spaces. ×4.

cartilage known as the epiphyseal–metaphyseal complex or growth plate. The growth plate and the adjacent cancellous bone of the metaphysis constitute a region where cancellous bone production and bone elongation occur. In the adult, the cartilaginous growth plate has been replaced by trabecular bone formed at the adjacent epiphysis and metaphysis. Obliteration of the cartilage by fusion of the two cancellous bone masses is called the "closure of the epiphysis" and "synostosis." On the articulating (joint) surface at the ends of long bones, the cortical shell of compact bone (subchondral bone) is covered by a thin layer of specialized hyaline cartilage, the articular cartilage.

The outer surfaces of most bones are covered by a sheath of fibrous connective tissue and an inner cellular, or cambian, layer of undifferentiated cells, the periosteum. The periosteum has the potential to form bone during growth and fracture healing. It is not present in areas where tendons and ligaments insert on bones, on bone ends that are lined with articular cartilage, on surfaces of the sesamoid bones, or in subscapular areas and the neck of the femur. The marrow cavity of the diaphysis and the cavities of cancellous bone are lined by a thin cellular layer, the endosteum, which also has osteogenic properties.

Microscopic Structure of Bone

Adult mammalian bone, whether compact or cancellous, is lamellated. The lamellations appear as stacks of parallel or concentrically curved sheets or lamellae and resemble the multiple layers of plywood. Each lamella is approximately 3 to 7 μm thick and its collagen fibers are oriented parallel to each other. In histological preparations, the lamellations are best seen by polarized light. The successive lamellations appear as alternating bright and dark layers, a result of the differing orientation of collagen fibers within adjacent lamellae (Fig. 6–10). By scanning electron microscopy these lamellae are seen as fibrous plates separated by bands of interlamellar cement (0.1 μm thick).

Regularly spaced throughout lamellar compact and cancellous bone are small cavities, or lacunae, connected by thin tubular channels

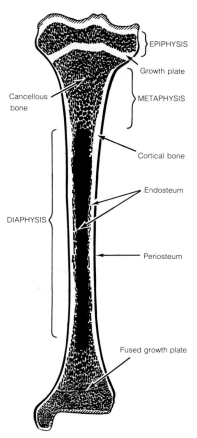

EPIPHYSIS

Growth plate

Cancellous
bone

METAPHYSIS

Cortical bone

Endosteum

DIAPHYSIS

Periosteum

Fused growth plate

6–9 Schematic diagram of a tibia. The interior of a
typical long bone showing the growing proximal
end with a growth plate and a distal end with the
epiphysis fused to the metaphysis.

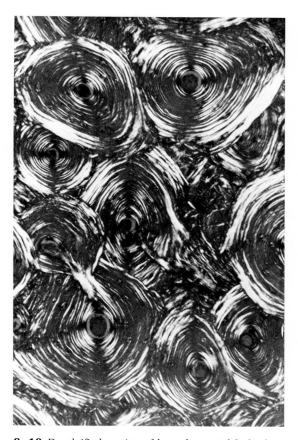

6–10 Decalcified section of bone from midshaft of a
horse humerus photographed in polarized
light. The complete and partial osteons possess
alternating bright and light concentric layers that
result from differing orientation of collagen fibers in
the successive lamellae. Note the interstitial lamellae
between completed osteons and Volkmann's Canal
between osteons at center of print. ×130. (Courtesy of
L. Krook.)

called canaliculi. Entrapped bone cells, or osteocytes, and their long cytoplasmic processes occupy the lacunae and canaliculi, respectively
(Figs. 6–11 and 6–12). These cell processes
within canaliculi communicate by gap junctions
with processes of osteocytes lying in adjacent lacunae. Canaliculi open to extracellular fluid at
bone surfaces, thus forming an anastomosing
network for the nutrition and metabolic activities
of the osteocytes.

The lamellae of compact bone have three major patterns:

1. Circular rings of lamellae can be arranged
   concentrically around a longitudinal vascular
   channel. These concentric lamellae vary in
   size and have from four to 20 layers. Collectively, the vascular channel and the surrounding concentric lamellae form a structure
   called an osteon or Haversian system (Figs.
   6–10 to 6–13).
2. Several layers of lamellae can extend uninterrupted around the circumference of the shaft.
   They are located on the external surfaces of
   cortical bone immediately underneath the
   periosteum, and on the internal surface, adjacent to the endosteum. These lamellae are collectively called surface or circumferential lamellae (Figs. 6–12 and 6–13).
3. Angular fragments of previous concentric and
   circumferential lamellae can fill the gaps be-

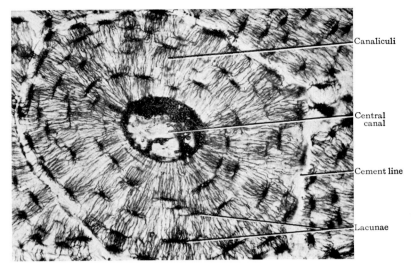

6–11 Ground cross section of a typical osteon of human femur. The lacunae, canaliculi, Haversian or central canal, and cement line are clearly evident. ×225.

Canaliculi

Central canal

Cement line

Lacunae

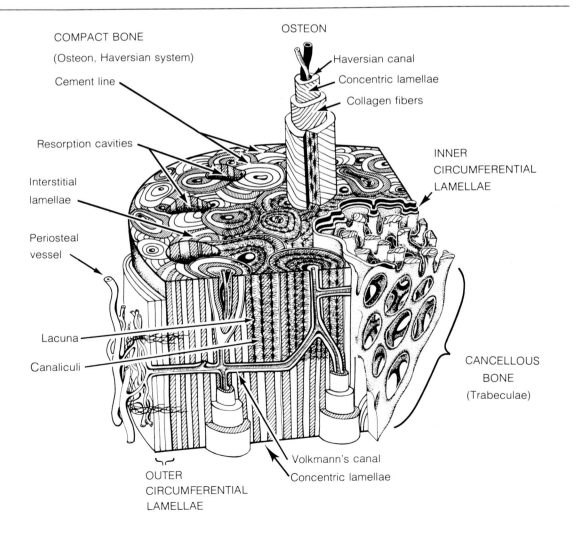

COMPACT BONE

(Osteon, Haversian system)

Cement line

Resorption cavities

Interstitial lamellae

Periosteal vessel

Lacuna

Canaliculi

OSTEON

Haversian canal

Concentric lamellae

Collagen fibers

INNER CIRCUMFERENTIAL LAMELLAE

CANCELLOUS BONE

(Trabeculae)

OUTER CIRCUMFERENTIAL LAMELLAE

Volkmann's canal

Concentric lamellae

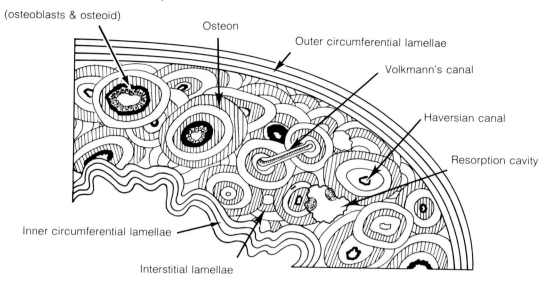

Forming osteon or Haversian system

(osteoblasts & osteoid)

Osteon

Outer circumferential lamellae

Volkmann's canal

Haversian canal

Resorption cavity

Inner circumferential lamellae

Interstitial lamellae

tween Haversian systems. They are called interstitial lamellae (Figs. 6–12 to 6–14).

Because most human compact bone is in the form of an osteon, morphologists have classified the osteon as the main bone structural unit of cortical bone. A typical osteon consists of a central or Haversian canal surrounded by concentric lamellae (Figs. 6–11 and 6–12). Each canal is 30 to 70 μm in diameter and contains nutrient vessels, nerves, and connective tissue. The Haversian canals communicate with the periosteum, bone marrow, and each other through transverse or oblique channels called Volkmann's canals

6–12 Schematic view of a part of the proximal shaft of a long bone containing cortical **(left)** and trabecular **(right)** bone. The cortical bone is composed mainly of Haversian systems or osteons of concentric lamellae with inner and outer circumferential lamellae at the periphery. Many completed osteons can be seen, each with its central Haversian canal, cement line, concentric lamellae, canaliculi, and lacunae. Note the orientation of the collagen fibers in successive lamellae in the protruding osteon. Cross connections between osteons are established by Volkmann's canals. Volkmann's canals connect with periosteal vessels and the marrow cavity and, unlike the Haversian canals, lack a covering of concentric lamellae. Interstitial lamellae are seen between completed Haversian systems. Three resorption cavities are also depicted.

6–13 Schematic diagram of a portion of a ground cross section of a typical adult cortical bone.

(Figs. 6–10, 6–12, and 6–13). Volkmann's canals can be differentiated from Haversian canals by their lack of concentric lamellae.

Surrounding the outer border of each osteon is a "cement line," a 1- to 2-μm-thick layer of mineralized matrix deficient in collagen fibers (Fig. 6–11). Two types of cement lines have been observed: arrest lines and reversal lines. Reversal lines are irregular or scalloped; arrest lines have a smooth and even contour. The arrest lines result when bone formation resumes after an interruption. In contrast, reversal lines occur when bone formation follows a phase of bone removal, or resorption. These lines provide histological evidence of the history of a specific region of bone.

Adult cancellous bone consists of a network of anastomosing trabeculae with intertrabecular spaces containing bone marrow (Figs. 6–7, 6–8, and 6–12). Most trabeculae are less than 0.2 mm in thickness and contain no blood vessels. The osteocytes are nourished by diffusion from the trabecular surface by the canaliculi extending to the surface. A few trabeculae are thicker than 0.2 mm and their central portion generally contains an osteon-like structure (i.e., concentric lamellae surrounding a blood vessel) (Fig. 6–14).

Each trabecula is composed of a mosaic of angular segments, each segment formed by parallel

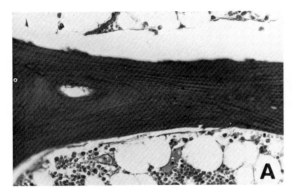

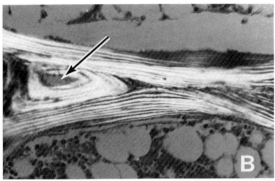

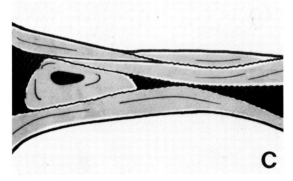

6–14 Photomicrograph showing several trabecular packets. ×130. **A.** Ordinary bright field micrograph of a portion of trabecula from human iliac biopsy specimen. **B.** The same area photographed through the polarizing microscope. Note the alternating bright and dark layers of lamellar bone in the trabecular packet. The packets are delineated by scalloped cement lines. The packet designated by the arrow shows concentric lamella forming an osteon-like structure within the trabecula. This osteon-like structure permits nutrients to reach interior osteocytes within the trabecula. **C.** Schematic diagram of the same area outlining possible trabecular packets or fragments of packets (interstitial lamellae). (Courtesy of P. Meunier.)

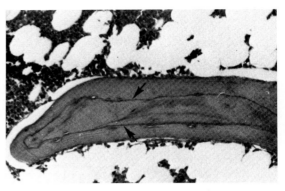

6–15 A portion of trabecula stained to show the cement lines **(arrows).** × 130 (Courtesy of P. Meunier.)

sheets of lamellae (Fig. 6–14). These segments of lamellar bone are called trabecular packets and are functionally analogous to the osteon, the bone strucutural unit of compact bone. The trabecular packet is the bone structural unit of cancellous bone (see Table 6–7). An idealized trabecular packet is shaped like a shallow crescent with a radius of 600 μm and is about 50 μm thick and 1 mm long. As with compact bone, cement lines hold the trabecular packets together (Fig. 6–15).

Composition of Bone Matrix

The two major components of mineralized bone are organic matrix and inorganic salts. Inorganic material makes up 76% of cortical bone and organic matrix, 24%.

Organic Matrix. The organic matrix is defined as the extracellular organic phase, composed primarily of protein, glycoprotein, and polysaccharide, which is secreted by and surrounds the osteogenic cell. It consists predominantly of collagenous fibers embedded in an amorphous ground substance. Collagen constitutes 90% of the organic matrix.

Amorphous Ground Substance. The amorphous ground substance is a noncollagenous cementing substance in which collagen fibers and crystals are embedded. It is what remains after the fibers and crystal have been removed. Although not fully characterized, bone ground substance is known to contain sialoproteins, phosphoproteins, glycoproteins, γ-carboxyglutamic acid–containing proteins, and small amounts of proteoglycans, lipids, and peptides. These components are characterized by their highly acidic nature, high aggregation tendencies, and rather peculiar calcium-binding properties. Complexes of these proteins with collagen have been reported.

Mineralization may be affected by glycoproteins, phosphoproteins, proteoglycans, and lipids present in unmineralized matrix. These substances may act to carry calcium and phosphate as bound ions or as crystal nucleators and may affect collagen spacing and cross-linking.

Bone Collagen. Bone collagen, like the collagen of tendons, skin, dentin, and fascia, is composed exclusively of type I collagen. Its helix consists of two α_1 chains of identical amino acid sequence and a single α_2 chain. The α_2 chain shows considerable homology with the α_1 chain but has a different amino acid sequence. Bone collagen also has the characteristic "native" pattern of cross-striations seen in other collagens. These striations represent changes in density resulting from the staggered arrangement of collagen molecules into fibrils. The staggering is due to the overlapping of neighboring collagen molecules by one-quarter of their length. This results in a gap known as a hole zone or pore of approximately 400 Å between the end of one molecule and the beginning of the next. Such holes are the site of 50% of the hydroxyapatite crystals deposited in bone. In addition, the holes in mineralized collagen of bone and dentin are larger than those in unmineralized collagen of tendon.

Collagen in bone and dentin calcifies, whereas the type I collagen found in skin and tendon does not. This difference may be due not to specific properties of the collagen alone, but to the interaction of the collagen fibrils with macromolecules within the extracellular matrix. Recently, phosphoproteins and proteins containing γ-carboxyglutamate have been proposed as possible regulators of mineral deposition.

Several biochemical differences exist between the collagen of bone and dentin and that of tendon and skin. These differences involve the posttranslational modification of the collagen and the distribution of intermolecular cross-links. The most striking modification is the ratio of diglycosylated to monoglycosylated hydroxylysine, which is 2.06 in skin in contrast to 0.47 in bone. Bone and skin collagen also differ in the relative proportion of specific cross-links. For example,

bone has more cross-links formed by two hydroxylysyl residues.

In summary, both the posttranslational and intermolecular modifications may be important in determining some of the physical properties of type I collagen found in bone and dentin. Bone and dentin collagen is less soluble, more densely packed, and less hydrated than type I collagen of skin. It differs from both tendon and skin collagen by not swelling when exposed to dilute acids. However, how and to what extent these biochemical differences contribute to the capacity to mineralize remain unknown.

Bone Mineral. Mineral constitutes 75% of bone weight. By volume, the mineral content of bone is 50%, in a form similar to hydroxyapatite $(Ca_{10}(PO_4)_6(OH)_2)$. In mature bone, the hydroxyapatite is present as needles, thin plates, or leaves 15 to 30 Å in thickness and 100 Å long. A crystal is believed to have three zones: (1) crystal interior, (2) crystal surface, and (3) hydration shell. The hydration layer facilitates the exchange of ions between hydroxyapatite and the body fluid. These bone crystals are minute and impure, containing many ions other than calcium, phosphate, and the hydroxyl ions found in pure synthetic hydroxyapatite. Furthermore, there are substanital quantities of carbonate, citrate, sodium, and magnesium in bone mineral. The magnesium and citrate are surface-bound. The quantity of fluoride is variable. Trace amounts of iron, zinc, copper, lead, manganese, tin, aluminum, strontium, boron, and silicon have also been reported.

The hydroxyapatite crystals are regularly distributed at intervals of 600 or 700 Å along the length of the collagen fibers. Ground substance surrounds and stabilizes these crystals. This interaction of hydroxyapatite with collagenous fibers and noncollagenous proteins brings about the hardness and rigidity of bone.

During growth, the amount of organic material per unit volume remains relatively constant, but the amount of water decreases and the proportion of bone mineral increases, attaining a maximum of about 65% of the fat-free dry weight of the tissue in adults.

Bone Cells

Five kinds of bone cells can usually be recognized in the growing and adult skeleton: osteoprogenitor cells, osteoblasts, osteocytes, osteoclasts, and bone-lining cells.

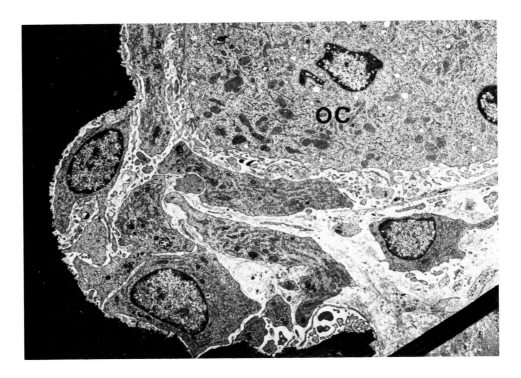

6–16 Electron micrograph of a typical reversal zone of a bone remodeling unit. At the upper right corner is an inactive osteoclast **(OC)** off bone surface. Within the well-defined Howship's lacuna, adjacent to bone that appears black, are mononuclear cells with numerous cytoplasmic extensions and lysosomes. ×3000. (From Baron, R., and Vignery, A. 1981. Bone Histomorphometry, W. S. S. Jee and A. M. Parfitt (Eds.), S.N.M.P.D., Paris, Courtesy of authors and Société Nouvelle de Publications Medicales and Dentaires)

Osteoprogenitor Cells. Osteoprogenitor cells have the capacity for mitosis and further differentiation and specialization into mature bone cells. There are two types of osteoprogenitor cells; one type (preosteoblasts) gives rise to bone-forming osteoblasts, and the other type (preosteoclasts) gives rise to bone resorbing osteoclasts.

Osteoprogenitor cells are spindle-shaped with oval or elongated nuclei and inconspicuous cytoplasm. They are commonly found near bone surfaces and other bone cells. The two types of osteoprogenitor cells can be recognized by electron microscopy. One type, the osteoblast precursor, has some endoplasmic reticulum and a poorly developed Golgi region. The other type, the osteoclast precursor, has more mitochondria and free ribosomes (see Fig. 6–16).

Osteoblasts. Osteoblasts are bone-forming cells. They synthesize and secrete unmineralized bone matrix, the osteoid (Figs. 6–17 to 6–19). Osteoblasts also appear to participate in the calcification of bone, and they seem to regulate the flux of calcium and phosphate in and out of bone.

Active osteoblasts are plump cells, usually cuboidal or polygonal, and rarely undergo mitosis. They are found in sheets on bone surfaces where bone is actively formed (Fig. 6–18). The nucleus has a single nucleolus usually lying in the cytoplasm farthest from the bone. The cytoplasm is deeply basophilic, owing to the large content of ribonucleoprotein, except in the center of the cell where a well-developed Golgi apparatus lies. Active osteoblasts give a strong histochemical reaction for alkaline phosphatase that disappears when the cells cease their synthetic activity. This enzyme is believed to play a role in calcification, perhaps by breaking down local inhibitors of calcification in the matrix, by releasing phosphate ions from substrates, or both. These actions would increase the calcium and phosphate ion products and encourage mineral precipitation and crystallization.

Osteoblasts have a fine structure expected of cells engaged in protein synthesis and secretion. There is an extensive rough endoplasmic reticu-

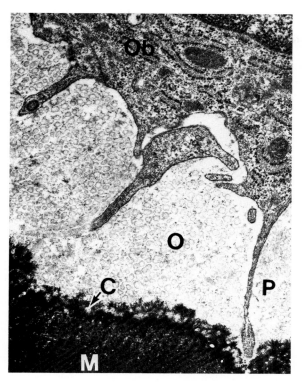

6–17 Electron micrograph of an osteoid seam. A region of osteoid **(O)** between edge of an osteoblast **(Ob)** and mineralizd matrix **(M)**. The osteoblast contains mitochondria and rough endoplasmic reticulum with three cytoplasmic processes **(P)** protruding into the osteoid. Note cement line **(C)** separating old bone from new bone. ×3,000. (Courtesy of R. Baron and A. Vignery.) ◁

6–18 Electron micrograph of osteoblasts. Notice the prominent Golgi complex **(GC)** and extensive rough endoplasmic reticulum **(rER)**. Adjacent to the osteoblasts are the unmineralized matrix or osteoid seam **(O)** and the mineralized matrix. The mineralized matrix is black because of the electron scattering of the hydroxyapatite crystals. ×5,500. (Preparation by S. C. Miller.) ▽

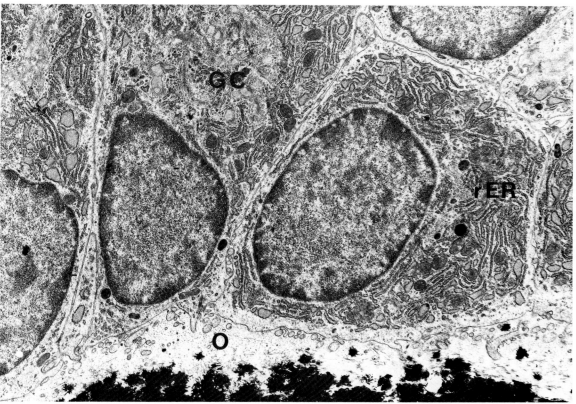

lum often in parallel array. The Golgi membranes are well developed with numerous saccules containing collagen precursors. Many secretory vacuoles are associated with the Golgi apparatus (Fig. 6–18). Osteoblasts have many microfilament-rich, finger-like processes that extend into the developing bone matrix and contact cell processes from osteocytes embedded in it.

Osteocytes. Osteocytes, the principal cells of fully formed bones, are housed in lacunae (Figs. 6–19 and 6–20). Osteocytes derive from osteob-

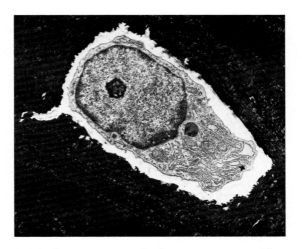

6–20 Electron micrograph of a young osteocyte. The cell still has some Golgi membrane and numerous rough endoplasmic reticulum. Notice that it does not completely fill its lacuna. The clear space around the cell is occupied by an unmineralized matrix in which collagen fibers are partially visible. At the left, a cell process is seen entering into a canaliculus. ×4,000. (Courtesy of S. C. Miller.)

6–19 Decalcified section of the trabecular bone from the secondary spongiosa of a growing rat tibia. Osteoblasts **(OB)** with prominent Golgi complex line most of the bone surfaces. A few osteoclasts can be seen **(arrows)**. Osteocytes are seen in their lacunae in bone near island of acellular calcified cartilage cores **(c)**. The bone marrow **(BM)** fills the spaces between trabeculae. ×300. (From the work of Miller, S. C., and Jee, W. S. S. 1979. Anat. Rec. 193:439. By permission of authors and Alan R. Liss, Inc., Publisher.)

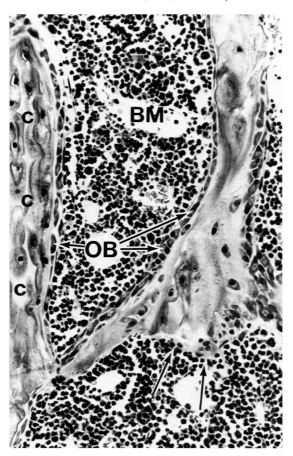

lasts that have secreted bone around themselves. The younger osteocytes, found near bone surfaces, are in rounder lacunae; the older cells are in oval or lenticular lacunae. As osteocytes become older and occupy less space in the lacunae, the amounts of rough endoplasmic reticulum and Golgi membranes decrease. Osteocytes do not divide; only one cell is ever found in a lacuna.

Osteocytes have many slender cell processes that can extend for considerable distances in canaliculi. These cell processes contain extensive microfilaments and often contact cell processes of other osteocytes and bone surface cells. At points of contact between osteocytes or between osteocytes and bone surface cells, gap junctions are present. This finding explains how the cells can survive in such an isolated environment. Nutrients may pass into and waste products out of the osteocytes by several possible pathways. Ions and small molecules might pass through the gap junctions of adjoining cell processes; another possibility is that fluids percolate through the space between the cells and their processes and the canalicular and lacunar walls. (See section on Role of Bone in Calcium Homeostasis).

Some morphologists believe that the osteocyte

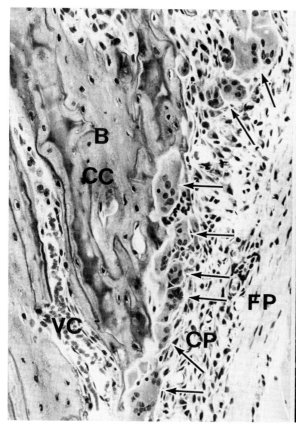

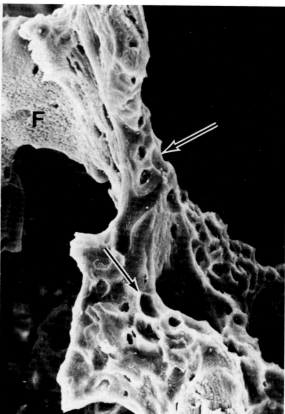

6–21 Light micrograph of osteoclasts. Osteoclasts **(arrows)** containing many nuclei on metaphyseal periosteal surfaces of growing rat tibia. The cellular **(CP)** and fibrous **(FP)** periosteum, longitudinally oriented vascular canals **(VC)** coursing through bone **(B)**, and dark staining calcified cartilage cores **(CC)** are evident. Decalcified, hematoxylin and eosin stain. ×250. (From the work of Miller, S. C., and Jee, W. S. S. 1979. Anat. Rec. 193:439. By permission of authors and Alan R. Liss, Inc., Publisher.)

6–22 Scanning electron micrograph of trabecular bone. Well-defined osteoclastic resorption pits (Howship's lacunae; **arrows**) and rough surfaces suggestive of active bone formation **(F)** are seen on trabecular bone surface. ×300. (From Miller, S. C., and Jee, W. S. S. 1979. Anat. Rec. 193:439. By permission of authors and Alan R. Liss, Inc., Publisher.)

can periodically remove and replace perilacunar bone, a unique form of bone surrounding the osteocyte to a depth of about 1 μm. The evidence for removal and replacement is (1) the variation in the size of the lacunae; (2) the presence of osmophilic laminae that resemble reversal lines in perilacunar bone; (3) the incorporation of a fluorescent bone marker, tetracycline, in perilacunar bone; and (4) the ultrastructural morphology reflecting bone-forming and resorbing clastic activities. An argument against osteocytic resorption, or osteocytic osteolysis, is that periosteolytic osteolysis has never been seen with scanning

electron microscopy. Further studies are necessary to resolve this controversy.

Osteoclasts. Osteoclasts are multinucleated giant cells responsible for the resorption of bone (Fig. 6–21). The cells range from 20 to over 100 μm in diameter and contain from two to 50 nuclei. Actively resorbing osteoclasts are usually found in or near cavities on bone surfaces called resorption pits or Howship's lacunae (Fig. 6–22). The cytoplasm of the osteoclast is often foamy in appearance and has acidophilic staining characteristics. In the light microscope, the surface of the osteoclast adjacent to the bone often has a striated appearance corresponding to an area of extensive membrane infoldings termed the "ruf-

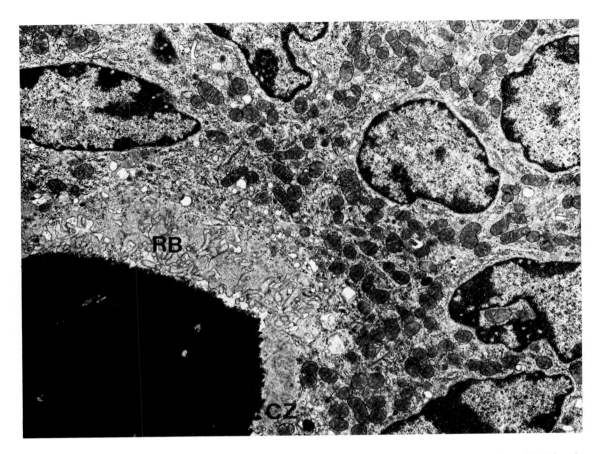

6–23 Electron micrograph of a part of an osteoclast. The osteoclast has multiple nuclei, numerous mitochondria, ruffled border **(RB)**, and clear zone area **(CZ)**. ×6,500. (From Miller, S. C., and Jee, W. S. S. 1979. Anat. Rec. 193:439. By permission of authors and Alan R. Liss, Inc., Publisher.)

fled border." The ruffled border, best observed by electron microscopy, is a unique surface modification of the osteoclast that apparently facilitates bone resorption (Fig. 6–23). The plasma membrane of the ruffled border appears to be coated with small 15-nm bristle-like structures that may contribute to the transport of materials across the membrane. Cinematographic studies of living osteoclasts in culture demonstrate that the ruffled border is highly motile. Bone can be seen dissolving beneath it.

The ruffled border is surrounded by an ectoplasmic-like zone devoid of organelles yet containing many actin filaments. This area is commonly called the clear or filamentous zone (Fig. 6–23). This clear zone around the ruffled border seems to be a site of adhesion of the cell to the bone surface and may also act as permeability seal to maintain a microenvironment conducive to bone resorption. Osteoclasts that lack ruffled borders are not capable of resorbing bone. This is the situation in osteopetrosis, a genetic disease characterized by defective bone resorption.

Dispersed throughout the cytoplasm are abundant mitochondria and small amounts of rough endoplasmic reticulum. Multiple Golgi complexes are found, usually around the multiple nuclei. Pairs of centrioles corresponding to the number of nuclei are gathered together in a region called the centrosome. The numerous granules and vacuoles in osteoclasts stain with acid phosphatase, the marker enzyme for lysosomes. The larger vacuoles are usually near the ruffled border region of the cells where they apparently form. Some of the vacuoles appear to contain breakdown products of the bone.

Osteoclasts can respond rapidly to calcium-regulating hormones by changing their cell specialization and functions. For example, parathyroid hormone (PTH) causes the rapid mobilization of calcium from bone, resulting in increased serum calcium levels. After the administration of exogenous PTH, osteoclasts quickly develop ruffled borders or enlarge existing ruffled borders, suggesting an increase in bone resorption. On the other hand, calcitonin (CT), which acts to suppress the release of calcium from bone and leads to lower serum calcium levels, causes the rapid disappearance of ruffled borders on osteoclasts.

Bone-Lining Cells. Most bone surfaces in the adult skeleton are covered by very flat and elongated cells with spindle-shaped nuclei commonly called bone-lining cells, although they are known by other names including surface osteocytes and resting osteoblasts (Fig. 6–24). We know very little about these cells and only in recent years have they been studied, even though they are the most common bone surface cells in the adult human skeleton.

Bone-lining cells are believed to be derived from osteoblasts that have ceased their activity and flattened out on the bone surface. They contain few organelles, and the nuclei are often less than 1 μm thick in the adult skeleton. The bone-lining cells are commonly joined to their neighbors by gap junctions and send cell processes into canaliculi to join the cell processes of osteocytes (Figs. 6–25 and 6–26).

Bone-lining cells may have several functions. They may serve as inducible osteogenic cells that could divide and differentiate into osteoblasts. They may also serve as an ion barrier separating the fluids percolating through the osteocyte and lacunar canalicular systems from the interstitial fluids. This membrane barrier around bone may contribute to mineral homeostasis by regulating the fluxes of calcium and phosphate in and out of bone fluids; it may also control the growth of bone crystals by maintaining a suitable microenvironment.

The Origin of Bone Cells. For many years it was thought that osteoblasts, osteocytes, and osteoclasts were simply different functional expressions of the same cells. The intermediate of all the mature bone cells was thought to be the osteoprogenitor cell, which presumably could differentiate into osteoblasts and osteoclasts depending on the immediate need. During the past decade, however, much experimental evidence has demonstrated that osteoblasts and osteoclasts derive from distinct cell lines. The osteoblast arises from fibroblast-like cells; the osteoclasts

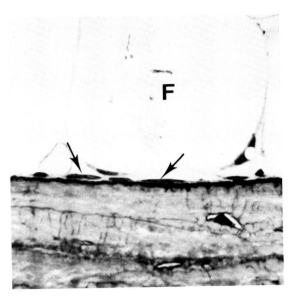

6–24 Bone lining cells on surface of bone spicule. The nuclei of bone lining cells **(arrows)** are usually flat and their cytoplasm is difficult to see under light microscopy. The surrounding fat cells **(F)** are apparent. Methylene blue, azure II, and basic fuschin stain of 1-μm-thick Epon section. ×700. (Courtesy of S. C. Miller.)

6–25 Electron micrograph of cytoplasmic processes joined by a gap junction **(arrow)** from two neighboring lining cells. ×57,400. (From Miller, S. C. and Jee, W. S. S. 1980. Anat. Rec. 198:163. By permission of authors and Alan R. Liss, Inc., Publisher.)

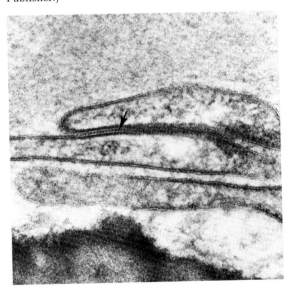

release of lysosomal enzymes and other protein-

Table 6–2 Comparison of Cortical and Trabecular Bone

	Cortical	Trabecular
Fractional volume (mm³/mm³)	0.95	0.20
Surface/bone volume (mm²/mm³)	2.5	20
Total bone volume (mm³)	1.4 × 10⁶	0.35 × 10⁶
Total internal bone surface (mm²)	3.5 × 10⁶	7.0 × 10⁶

ᵃThe whole skeleton contains 11.5 × 10⁶ mm² of surface, which includes 0.5 × 10⁶ for cortical endosteal surface.

and the vitamin D metabolites, the exact physiological role of these stimulatory and inhibitory agents is unknown.

Some investigators believe that the osteocytes both form and resorb bone. Osteocytes enlarge their lacunar cavities by removing perilacunar bone through a process known as osteocytic osteolysis. In contrast, young osteocytes may also add small amounts of bone onto the lacunar walls. This bone differs from that formed by osteoblasts by having a lower mineral content. It has been proposed that this "low-density bone" is more soluble and, therefore, capable of exchanging mineral with the surrounding extracellular fluid. Hence, the perilacunar bone may serve as a mineral reservoir rather than contrib-

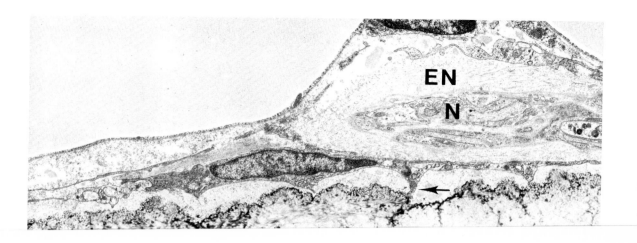

Table 6–4 Activators and Inhibitors of Bone Resorption

Activators	Inhibitors
Parathyroid hormone	Calcitonin
1.25(OH)$_2$ vitamin D$_3$	Diphosphonates
Osteoclast activating factor(s)	Phosphate
Prostanoids	Mithramycin
Vitamin A	Colchicine
Thyroxine	Glucocorticoids
Complement	Estrogen (high doses only)
Endotoxin	Glucagon
Lipopolysaccharides	
Ionophores	Membrane-stabilizing drugs
Epidermal growth factor inhibitors	Carbonic anhydrase
Cyclic nucleotides (DBcAMP, cAMP)	Anticonvulsants
Heparin	Glucagon
Mechanical stimulation	Collagen fragments
Serum albumin components	Nerve growth factor
Collagenase	Cartilage inhibitor

Source: From Ibbotson, K. J., D'Souza, S. M., Kanis, J. A., Douglas, D. L., and Russell, R. G. G. 1980. Metab. Bone Dis. Relat. Res. 2:177. (Permission of authors and Société Nouvelle de Publications Médicales et Dentaires.)

ute to the bone's structural integrity under normal conditions.

The extent to which osteocytic osteolysis occurs is controversial. Some researchers propose that the relative increases in lacunar size are not due to osteocytic resorption, but to decreased rates of bone formation.

Bone Formation. The formation of bone occurs in two phases: matrix formation and mineralization. Matrix formation precedes mineralization and occurs at the interface between osteoblasts and existing osteoid. Mineralization occurs at the junction of osteoid and newly mineralized bone, a region known as the mineralization front. This front advances as the osteoid becomes mineralized. Chemically it is characterized by a high concentration of phospholipid, zinc, and silicon, which appear histologically as a line of confluent toludine-blue stained granules.

Because mineralization lags behind matrix production, there remains a layer of unmineralized matrix called the osteoid seam (Figs. 6–17 and 6–18). The "mineralization lag time" is normally 10 days in the adult and results in an osteoid seam width of 8 to 10 μm. In contrast to adult bone, embryonic bone formation has a very short mineralization lag time, resulting in a thin osteoid seam and more rapid mineralization.

Before mineralization, the matrix undergoes a series of events: (1) an increase in the cross-linking of collagen fibers; (2) binding of phospholipids to collagen fibers; (3) an increase in the concentration of noncollagenous matrix proteins, especially γ-carboxyglutamic acid–containing protein; (4) binding of calcium to these matrix proteins; (5) the accumulation of silicon and zinc; and (6) an early increase followed by (7) a later decline in glycosaminoglycans. The importance of each of these steps in preparing the matrix for mineralization is unclear.

The mechanism that initiates bone mineralization is unknown. However, recent studies have proposed numerous factors controlling the deposition of mineral into bone matrix. Both osteoblasts and osteocytes are believed to somehow regulate local concentrations of calcium and phosphate, thus promoting a phase of mineralization. The presence of "holes" or nucleation sites created by the packing arrangement of collagen may stimulate mineralization, and it is likely that modifications in the collagen organization may regulate the site of formation, type of mineral, and amount of mineral deposited. Recent studies show that the collagen-associated mineral may be in ribbon form rather than crystalites; these studies thus question the role of "holes" as representing crystal limits or templates. Noncollagenous proteins, such as γ-carboxyglutamic acid–containing proteins, have also been suggested as inhibitors of mineral deposition. These proteins readily bind calcium and phosphate and may help regulate the matrix microenvironment with these ions. The presence of the enzyme alkaline phosphatase within osteoblasts and other cells in bone may also control mineralization. The enzyme catalyzes the degradation of inorganic pyrophosphate, a potent inhibitor of mineralization. In addition, the presence of specific components of ground substance such as glycosaminoglycans may limit the degree and rate of mineralization.

Many investigators believe that the matrix vesicle mechanisms of cartilage calcification may also apply to the mineralization of bone. However, to date, matrix vesicles have been found only in sites of rapid calcification (e.g., embryonic bone, calcifying epiphyseal growth carti-

6–27 Microradiograph of a 200-μm-thick cross section of cortical bone from a 19-year-old. The different shades of gray represent different degrees of mineralization (concentrations of hydroxyapatite). In resorption cavities **(RC)** and Haversian canals **(HC)**, there has been no absorption of x-rays; the black film shows a lack of calcification. Recently formed Haversian systems or osteons **(O)** are incompletely calcified (low-density bone) and appear dark gray, whereas older Haversian systems **(HS)** are more calcified (higher density bone) and appear light gray. The interstitial lamellae **(IL)**, being the oldest and fully calcified (high-density bone), appear near white. The resorption cavities near the periosteum **(upper)** are resorbing non-Haversian bone and will be replaced by secondary Haversian bone. Several osteons have a layer of high-density bone **(HD)** outlining the Haversian canal. ×57. (Courtesy of J. Jowsey.)

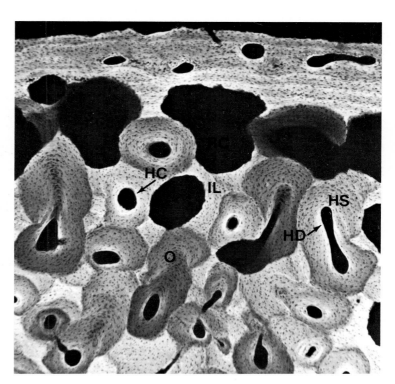

lage, fracture healing, and growing antlers). Matrix vesicles have not been observed in mature bone. Probably the noncollagenous proteins or mechanisms other than the matrix vesicles, or both, have a more important role in the calcification of adult bone.

Although a continuous process, mineralization has been divided into primary and secondary phases. Primary mineralization lasts several days and is responsible for 70% of total mineralization. This initial phase has been postulated to be under the control of the osteoblast on the osteoid surface and the osteocyte within a lacuna of osteoid. Secondary mineralization occurs over the next several months and results in an additional 20 to 25% of total mineralization. It is most likely governed by both the chemical composition of the fluid surrounding the matrix and the accessibility of the mineral to the matrix. By some unknown mechanism, osteocytes prevent the continued calcification of matrix. Good examples of osteons with varying degrees of mineralization can be seen in the long bone midshaft of a young adult (Fig. 6–27).

The rate of bone formation can be determined in humans and experimental animals by administering tetracycline or other fluorescent bone markers. Tetracycline is an antibiotic that is incorporated at the mineralization front, thus resulting in bands of tetracycline-labeled bone. The labeled bone fluoresces under ultraviolet light and provides a marker of the location and rate of bone formation (Figs. 6–28 to 6–30).

Vascular and Nervous Supply of Bone

The routing of blood is closely related to patterns of growth, modeling, and remodeling. Most of the blood supply to the cortex of the long bone shaft comes by way of medullary vessels (Figs. 6–31 and 6–32), which consist of the nutrient artery and the metaphyseal and epiphyseal arteries after the epiphyseal–metaphyseal growth plate has closed. Periosteal vessels probably contribute little. In childhood, before the epiphyses have closed, the terminal branches of the nutrient arteries and metaphyseal arteries at the growth plate loop back toward the venous circulation and do not anastomose with the epiphyseal vessels. Arterial pressure drives blood from the endosteum to the periosteum. Cortical bone is supplied exclusively with cortical branches of marrow arteries that flow into fenestrated capillaries in Haversian and Volkmann's canals to en-

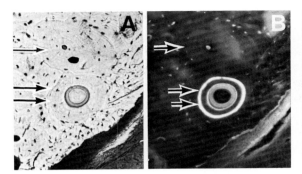

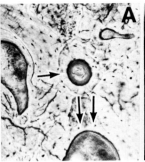
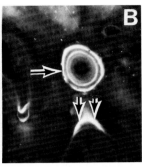

6–28 Two Haversian systems from the midshaft of the rib of an 18-month-old dog. The dog was injected with a 2-day course of tetracycline followed by a 2-day course of (2,4-bis)-N-N¹-di(carboxymethyl) aminomethyl fluorescein[B] (DCAF) 12 days later, immediately followed by rib biopsy. **A.** Ordinary light micrograph showing forming **(double arrows)** and completed **(single arrow)** osteons. Ground section, 100 μm thick, stained with Villanueva's bone stain. **B.** Fluorescent micrograph showing a double labeled Haversian system. This particular osteon was forming bone during the two fluorescent labeling periods. Note the difference in thickness between the two concentric labels. The outer band, corresponding to the first period of tetracycline labeling, is thicker than the inner label, which shows a deceleration of bone apposition as the formation of the osteon nears completion. Note third fluorescent ring caused by the autofluorescence of osteoid. ×250. (Courtesy of L. Flora.)

6–29 Ordinary light and fluorescent microscopy of a ground cross section of rib bone from the same dog as in Fig. 6–28. **A.** Ordinary light micrograph showing two forming osteons and part of the endosteal bone surface **(lower right; double arrows).** Note dark staining osteoid on the inner surface of the forming osteon (arrow). Ground section, 100 μm thick, section stained with Villanueva's bone stain. **B.** Fluorescent micrograph of three labeled bone formation sites showing a double concentric **(single arrow)** and partial labeling of the forming osteons. A portion of the endosteal surface is also labeled **(double arrows).** ×250. (Courtesy of L. Flora.)

sure circulatory exchange for all the osteocytes. These vessels drain centrifugally into the periosteal plexus. The marrow arteries also give off branches that flow into a large marrow sinusoidal system and into the central venous sinus and nutrient veins. The sinusoid and capillary network both in marrow and in cancellous bone is called the functional vascular lattice.

We know little of the hemodynamics of the circulation in bone. It has been estimated from studies in laboratory animals that the rate of cortical blood flow is 18 ml per 100 g bone per min and the rate for the diaphyseal marrow is 21 ml per 100 g per min. The intravascular pressure is high at the endosteal surface, about 60 mm Hg, and low at the periosteal surface, about 15 mm Hg.

Haversian canals, periosteum, and medullary vessels are innervated. Poorly myelinated nerve fibers are present in Haversian canals. Lymphatic channels are present in periosteum, but not in bone cortex or marrow.

6–30 Double tetracycline-labeled trabecula. A buried double-tetracycline label **(A)** spanning the upper bone surface and a short double label **(B)** near the lower bone surface of part of a trabecula from an human iliac biopsy sample. Note also thin tetracycline labels outlining the trabecular surfaces **(C).** Microphotograph under ultraviolet light. ×130. (Courtesy of P. Meunier.)

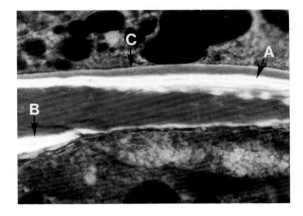

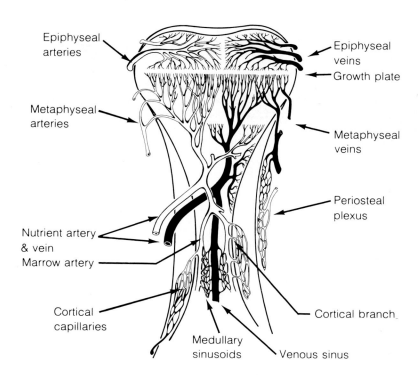

6–31 Diagram of longitudinal section of proximal portion of growing long bone illustrating bone vascularization. Several discrete points of arterial inflow (nutrient, metaphyseal, and epiphyseal arteries) supply regional sinusoidal networks within the bone and marrow. These drain into venous channels that exit at the bone surface. When growth is complete, the growth plate disappears and the trabecular bone circulation of the epiphysis and metaphysis join together.

Histogenesis

In the histogenesis of bone, the first bone tissue formed is an immature type known as primary or woven bone. The primary bone is a temporary material that is either replaced by secondary (lamellar) bone or removed to form the bone marrow cavity. Woven bone is characterized by the random orientation of its collagen fibers. On a microscopic level, the osteocytes embedded within primary bone are fewer and less uniformly distributed than those of secondary or lamellar bone. Woven bone further differs from secondary bone in that its matrix is lower in mineral content. Primary bone is formed in regions of initial bone formation within the embryo and in select sites later (e.g., fracture healing, ectopic ossification, and bone tumor formations). Like lamellar bone, woven bone may be either compact or cancellous. Lamellar bone replaces primary bone, except for a few locations (e.g., tooth sockets and sutures of the cranial bones).

In contrast to the microstructure of primary bone, the collagen fibers of secondary bone are

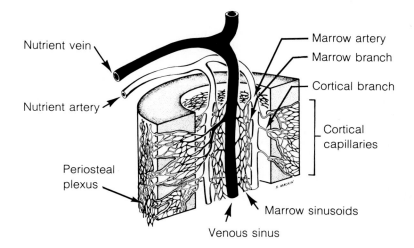

6–32 Diagram of blood supply of a long bone shaft. Blood flows from the nutrient artery to marrow arteries, and then flows into smaller marrow and cortical branches. Cortical branches supply the cortical bone through cortical capillaries that drain into the periosteal plexus. Marrow branches supply the marrow sinusoids that drain into the venous sinus.

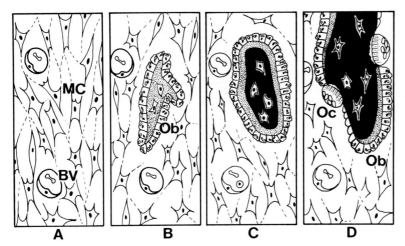

6–33 Diagram of stages of intramembranous ossification.
A. The mesenchyme (**MC**), which is the precursor of membrane bone. Blood vessel (**BV**). **B.** The initial step is the differentiation of mesenchymal cells into osteoblasts (**Ob**) and the secretion of osteoid (**stippled**). **C.** Osteoid (**stippled**) synthesis and mineralization entrap more osteocytes in lacunae (mineralized bone is black). **D.** Synthesis and calcification of matrix by osteoblast (**Ob**) to form bone spicule. Osteoclasts (**Oc**) are modeling spicules. Several such sites arise simultaneously at an ossification center so that the fusion of the growing spicules form the primary spongiosa. (See Fig. 6–34.)

regularly arranged as ordered sheets within individual lamellae. These lamellae are arranged either as parallel sheets or concentrically around a vascular channel. In both forms, lamellae differ from primary bone by having their respective collagen fibers oriented perpendicular (90°) to the collagen bundles of adjacent lamellae; thus successive lamellae appear as alternating light and dark bands by polarized light microscopy (Figs. 6–10 and 6–14). Secondary bone also differs from woven bone by the presence of a higher density of osteocytes, which are more uniformly distributed.

As discussed, histogenesis proceeds by the initial formation of primary (woven) bone, which is later replaced by secondary (lamellar) bone or bone marrow. This sequence of formation occurs via two major modes of osteogenesis: intramembranous and endochondral ossification. The two processes differ by the initial material on which the woven bone is formed. When formation takes place within primitive connective tissue (mesenchyme), the process is called intramembranous ossification. When formation occurs in preexisting calcified cartilage, it is called endochondral or intracartilaginous ossification.

The actual processes of bone tissue formation are essentially the same in both modes of ossification and proceed by the following sequence: (1) osteoblasts differentiate from mesenchymal cells; (2) osteoblasts deposit matrix that is subsequently mineralized; (3) bone is initially laid down as a network of immature (woven) trabeculae, the primary spongiosa; (4) the primary spongiosa is replaced by secondary bone, or removed to form bone marrow, or converted into primary cortical bone by the filling of spaces between the trabeculae ("compaction").

Intramembranous Ossification. The frontal and parietal bones, as well as parts of the occipital and temporal bones and the mandible and maxilla develop by intramembranous ossification. For this reason they are often referred to as membrane bones. The process of intramembranous ossification occurs within an area of well-vascularized primitive connective tissue (mature mesenchymal and epithelial tissue). Direct bone formation occurs without prior formation of cartilage, although an epithelial–mesenchymal interaction appears to be necessary. During the eighth week of human fetal life, a cluster of mesenchymal cells differentiates into osteoid-secreting osteoblasts (Fig. 6–33). This stage appears as thin bars of eosinophilic osteoid covered with basophilic osteoblasts within a mass of primitive connective tissue.

As the bars of osteoid thicken and mineralize, increasing amounts of osteoid are deposited by osteoblasts. The process results in numerous osteoblasts becoming entrapped within the newly formed bone and transformed into osteocytes. These osteocytes remain connected to each other and surface osteoblasts by their cytoplasmic processes. The deposition of bone around the osteoblasts and their processes creates the lacunae and canaliculi, completing the formation of a primitive lacunar–canalicular system.

At this stage of ossification, the trabeculae are thin and needle-like. These fine trabeculae of woven bone are lengthened and thickened by continual osteoblastic apposition. They form a

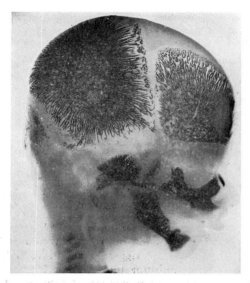

6–34 Head of a human embryo at 3.5 months gestation, stained with alizarin and cleared to reveal the primary spongiosa radiating from the centers of intramembranous ossification in the frontal and parietal bones. ×1.5. (Courtesy of L. Bélanger.)

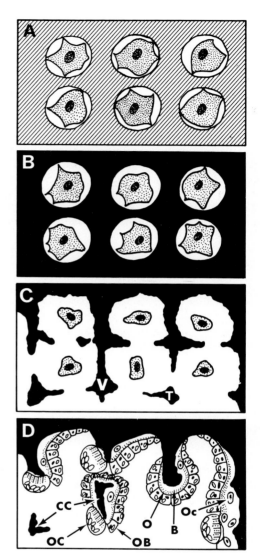

6–35 Diagram of early stages in endochondral bone formation (ossification). **A.** Hypertrophy of chondrocytes and lacunae. **B.** Mineralization of cartilaginous matrix (calcified cartilage matrix is black). **C.** Death of chondrocytes and resorption of transverse septa **(T)**, leaving behind vertical septa **(V)** of calcified cartilage. **D.** Invasion of the area by bone and bone marrow progenitor cells, and the deposition of osteoid **(O) (stippled area)** by osteoblasts **(OB)** on fragments of calcified cartilage cores **(CC)** to form the primary spicules or trabeculae. These trabeculae are composed of primary bone **(B)**, and calcified cartilage cores lined with a thin layer of osteoid, osteoclasts **(OC)**, and osteocytes **(Oc)**.

network of trabecular bone known as the primary spongiosa (Fig. 6–34).

In areas of primary spongiosa destined to become compact bone, the continued deposition of bone on existing trabecular surfaces results in the filling of the intertrabecular spaces (Fig. 6–43). In such compaction, layers of woven bone are formed onto the existing trabecular surface as irregular concentric layers to produce primary Haversian systems. They differ from secondary Haversian systems or osteons in their irregular shape, uneven distribution of osteocytes, and random orientation of collagen fibers.

Other regions of the primary spongiosa are destined to persist as cancellous bone. In these areas the thickening of the trabeculae ceases and the connective tissue between the trabeculae differentiates into the hematopoietic tissue of bone marrow. At the same time both the osteoblasts that have finished forming bone and the mesenchymal cells located near the endosteal surface transform into an endosteum. The remaining envelope of connective tissue at the periosteal surface condenses, forming a periosteum.

Endochondral Ossification. The bones of the base of the skull, the vertebral column, the pelvis, and the extremities develop by endochondral ossification. They are called cartilage bones because they are initially formed within hyaline cartilage (Fig. 6–35). The center of ossification begins with the maturation and eventual hypertrophy of chondrocytes within lacunae. This is followed by the calcification of the hyaline matrix between the enlarged chondrocyte lacunae, resulting in the eventual death of the chondrocytes. Some vertical cartilage septa and all the horizontal septae are resorbed by chondroclasts. The surrounding calcified cartilage matrix, known as calcified cartilage cores, provides a scaffolding for the formation of primary trabeculae. The onset of bone formation may be promoted by some signal passing from the hypertrophic cells to the adjacent perichondral cells. Precursor cells within the periosteum differentiate into osteoblasts and, along with periosteal vessels, invade the resorbed cartilaginous space to appose bone on the calcified cartilage cores. The bone-lined calcified cartilage cores form a latticework of primary trabeculae called the primary spongiosa.

Most of the primary spongiosa is converted into secondary (lamellar) spongiosa by the simultaneous removal of regions of calcified cartilage cores and woven bone and addition of newly formed secondary trabeculae. Concurrently, a bone marrow forms within the perivascular space from mesenchymal connective tissue.

Organogenesis

The construction of a bone as a functional organ is a complex process. Bone constantly enlarges and renews itself during development and, at the same time, adapts to support, protection, mechanical strength, and numerous metabolic and hematopoietic activities. Therefore, the formation of a functionally competent bone is the culmination of several closely integrated processes: (1) intramembranous ossification, (2) endochondral ossification, (3) growth, (4) the molding or "modeling" of bone into its desired shape, and (5) the constant replacement of relatively old bone by "remodeling." Organogenesis can best be demonstrated by following the histological changes in the development of a typical long bone from an extremity.

Development of a Long Bone from a Cartilaginous Model. At sites of future bone formation in the embryo, the mesenchymal tissue condenses to form a rough outline of the future bone (Fig.

6–36). Subsequently, the cells enlarge, differentiate, and secrete a hyaline matrix around themselves, resulting in the formation of a hyaline cartilage model. At the same time, the outer mesenchymal tissue condenses to form a perichondrium. The perichondrium is composed of an outer fibrous layer and an inner chondrogenic layer. The cartilage model continues to grow in size. Longitudinal growth occurs by the division and enlargement of chondrocytes within lacunae (interstitial growth), whereas growth in width occurs primarily by the differentiation of new chondroblasts within the chondrogenic layer (appositional growth).

The Primary Ossification Center. With growth of the cartilage model, the perichondrium is invaded by capillaries, triggering the transformation of the perichondrium into a periosteum. The chondrogenic layer is converted into an osteogenic layer that forms osteoblasts. Subsequently, the osteoblasts form bone on the inner aspect of the periosteum. Thus, by continuing intramembranous ossification at the periosteum, a hollow cylinder of trabecular bone called the periosteal bone collar is formed (Fig. 6–36).

Concurrently the hyaline cartilage within the middle of the diaphysis becomes calcified and primary spongiosa develops by endochondral ossification (Fig. 6–36). Here is the sequence of events: As chondrocytes swell and matrix becomes calcified, the chondrocytes die (because of limited nutrient diffusion) and some of the calcified matrix is removed by lytic action of chondroclasts. This results in the initiation and growth of a primary bone marrow cavity. A "periosteal bud" of blood vessels and perivascular tissue grows into the shaft, invading this cavity. Next, pluripotential cells within the perivascular tissue differentiate into bone marrow cells and osteoblasts. The osteoblasts migrate toward the remaining calcified cartilage cores and, by apposing bone onto the cores, form primary trabeculae. In contrast to the totally woven trabeculae formed by intramembranous ossification, the trabeculae formed by endochondral ossification consist of a calcified core encased by woven bone.

The changes that occur in the interior of the cartilage model and under the periosteum result in the "primary center of ossification." However, in a technical sense this term is misleading because there are actually two separate centers, one at the periosteal collar (by intramembranous os-

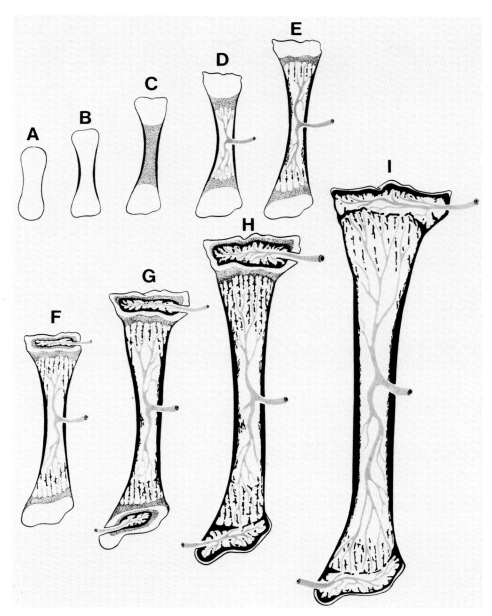

6–36 Diagram of the development of a typical long bone made of cartilage. The hyaline cartilage is clear, the calcified cartilage is stippled, and bone tissues are black. **A.** Cartilage model. **B.** Periosteal bone collar forms before cartilage calcification. **C.** Cartilage begins to calcify. **D.** Periosteal bud (blood vessels and perivascular mesenchyme) enters the calcified cartilage. The formation of the periosteal bone collar and the endochondral ossification at the center of the cartilage model is known collectively as the primary center of ossification. **E.** Blood vessels and vascular mesenchyme divide into two zones of ossification (growth plates). **F.** Blood vessels and perivascular mesenchyme invade upper epiphyseal cartilage (secondary center of ossification) to form the epiphyseal ossification center and growth plate. **G.** Later, lower epiphyseal ossification develops. **H.** As the bone slows down growing in length, the lower growth plate disappears and their epiphyseal and metaphyseal trabeculae fuse (closure of epiphyses). **I.** The same events happen with the upper growth plate. The bone marrow cavity, blood vessels of the diaphysis, metaphyses, and epiphyses now intercommunicate throughout the length of the bone.

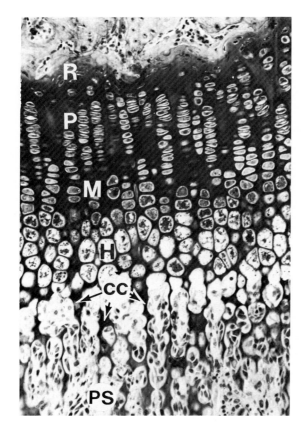

6–37 Endochondral ossification in longitudinal section through the zone of epiphyseal–metaphyseal growth plate and portion of primary spongiosa of the proximal end of the tibia of a rat. Resting **(R)**, proliferating **(P)**, maturing **(M)**, hypertrophic **(H)** cartilage zones, calcified cartilage cores **(cc)**, and primary spongiosa **(PS)** are evident. Decalcified H & E stain. ×125. (Courtesy of T. Wronski.)

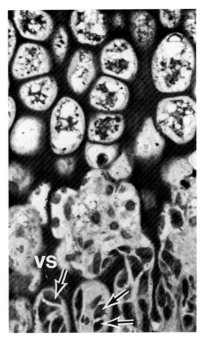

6–38 Enlarged photomicrograph of the hypertrophic, provisional calcification zones of the growth plate and adjacent primary spongiosa seen in Fig. 6–37. Note the loss of calcified horizontal septa, the persistence of vertical calcified cores **(VS)**, and the deposition of bone upon calcified cartilage core by osteoblasts **(arrows)** to form primary spicules in the primary spongiosa. ×330. (Courtesy of T. Wronski.)

sification) and one at the center of the cartilage model (by endochondral ossification).

Expansion of the Primary Ossification Center. As endochondral ossification progresses from the diaphysis toward each end of the cartilage model, the mass of hyaline cartilage thins and becomes oriented into two growth plates. The chondrocytes within the plates are arbitrarily separated into five transversely oriented zones to be described in detail below. These zones and the primary and secondary spongiosae collectively form the epiphyseal–metaphyseal complex. The expansion of each metaphysis dur-

ing the longitudinal growth of bone is accompanied by the simultaneous circumferential expansion of the periosteal bone collar, which also grows in the direction of the epiphyses. The details of this process will also be discussed below.

Appearance of the Secondary Ossification Center. In addition to the primary or diaphyseal center of ossification, most long bones contain two secondary or epiphyseal centers of ossification (Fig. 6–36). Ossification here forms the epiphyses and closely approximates the sequence of endochondral ossification seen at the primary ossification center. The cartilage at the end of bone represents a growth zone similar to the growth plate. However, it differs by expanding predominantly by radial rather than longitudinal growth. Furthermore, because most of the cartilage of the epiphysis lacks a perichondrium, there is no counterpart to a periosteal bone collar; only a thin shell of compact bone is formed.

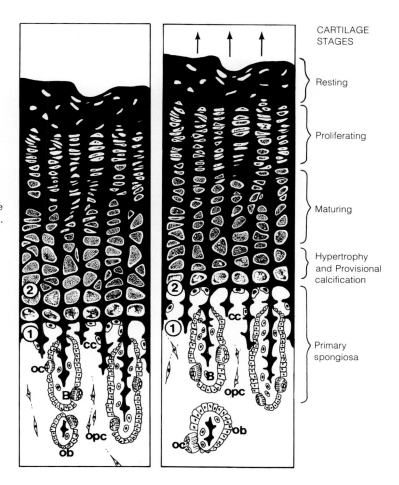

6–39 Diagrams of two longitudinal sections through the same growth plate and portion of primary spongiosa showing the movement of the bony epiphysis away from any given fixed position in the growth plate during growth. The diagram on the right shows the changes that have occurred during a short period of time after that represented in the left panel. The changes include hypertrophy, death of two horizontal rows of chondrocytes, apposition of bone on calcified cartilage cores, and the advancement of the bony epiphysis for the same distance. Points **1** and **2** are fixed points, which remain at the same level in both diagrams, but the bony epiphysis and the growth plate have moved upward in the diagram on the right. Bone **(B)**; osteoblast **(ob)**; calcified cartilage core **(cc)**; osteoclast **(oc)**; osteoprogenitor cell **(opc)**.

CARTILAGE STAGES

Resting

Proliferating

Maturing

Hypertrophy and Provisional calcification

Primary spongiosa

The Epiphyseal–Metaphyseal Complex (the Growth Plate). The growth plate is a transverse disc that separates epiphyseal from diaphyseal bone. Its overall function is twofold: (1) it drives the process of bone elongation and (2) it provides a scaffolding for the construction of cancellous bone within the metaphysis. Together with the metaphyses, the growth plates constitute the longitudinal growth zone of bones. Essentially all increases in length occur at the growth plate, and approximately 90% of all trabecular bone is initially generated there.

Five zones within the growth plate are distinguished on the basis of the cellular (chondrocytic) changes in the hyaline cartilage (Figs. 6–37 and 6–39). From the epiphyseal end they are: (1) the zone of resting cells, (2) the zone of cell proliferation, (3) the zone of cell maturation, (4) the zone of cell hypertrophy, and (5) the zone of provisional calcification. Cells in the last four zones are reasonably well organized into columns parallel to the long axis of the bone. This gives the faulty impression that the chondrocytes are moving toward the metaphysis within the columnar pathways. Actually the chondrocytes go through a normal progression of proliferation, maturation, hypertrophy, and death while remaining stationary with respect to the bone structure (Fig. 6–39). The deception is created by the addition of newly formed chondrocytes at one end while chondrocytic death at the opposite end is constantly removing mature chondrocytes and calcified matrix. This process results in the maintenance of a growth plate with a fairly constant thickness throughout longitudinal growth. Because of the critical importance of the growth plate in the process of prenatal, infant, and adolescent skeletal growth, we shall expand on the features discussed above.

The uppermost region of growth cartilage, the

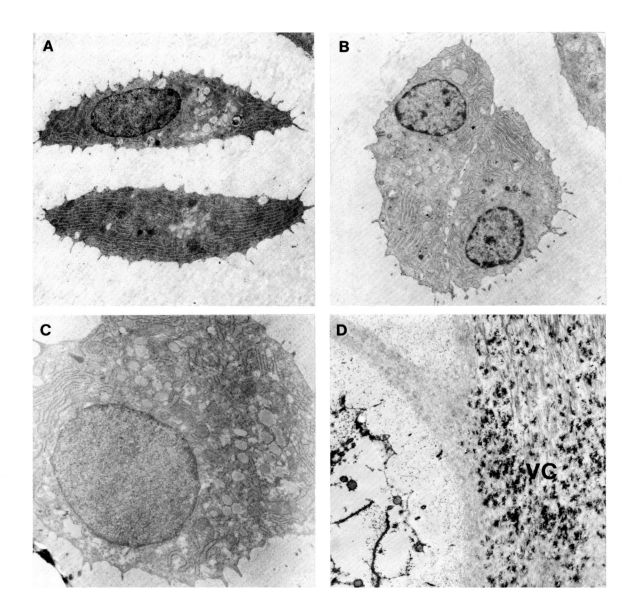

6–40 Electron micrographs of parts of the growth plate. **A.** Proliferating chondrocyte. ×3,250. **B.** Maturing chondrocyte. ×4,950. **C.** Hypertrophic chondrocyte. ×6,300. **D.** Part of degenerating and dying chondrocyte and the mineralization of the vertical cartilage septum **(VC).** ×4,000. (Courtesy of J. Yee.)

zone of resting cells (Figs. 6–37 and 6–39), is the smallest area and is composed of only a few chondrocytes. Although its function is not known, this zone may serve as a source of cells.

The next region is the zone of proliferation. It is characterized by many mitotic figures, flattened chondrocytes, and synthesis and secretion of matrix. This zone is the driving force behind bone elongation. After several mitoses, the chondrocytes become ovoid and constitute the zone of cell maturation.

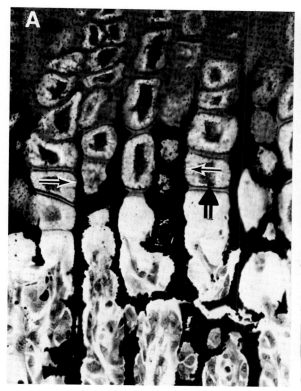
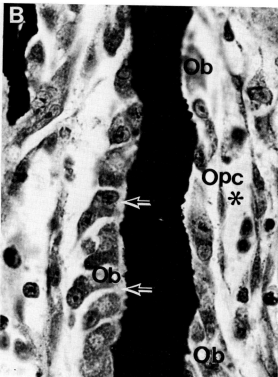

The chondrocytes of the zone of maturation function almost exclusively in the synthesis of matrix and the preparation of the matrix for calcification (Fig. 6–40). The maturing chondrocytes become larger and accumulate glycogen within their cytoplasm. At this stage they constitute the zone of cell hypertrophy. These "hypertrophic" chondrocytes are very large vacuolated cells with swollen and pyknotic nuclei. The matrix of this area become reduced to thin longitudinal and transverse septae because of the enlargement of the lacunar spaces (Fig. 6–41). As the hypertrophic cells merge into the final zone, the hyaline matrix becomes increasingly calcified, resulting in the restricted diffusion of nutrients and the ensuing death of the hypertrophic chondrocytes. Between the columns of cells, the vertically oriented matrix becomes fully calcified, whereas the septae between lacunae fail to calcify (Fig. 6–40).

The uncalcified transverse septae are removed at the junction of the growth plate and the metaphysis by the lytic action of the dying chondrocytes and by chondroclasts. In contrast, approximately one-third of the calcified longitudinal

6–41 A. Section through the lower growth plate and upper metaphyseal portion of the epiphyseal–metaphyseal growth complex **(open arrow)**. Note the mineralization **(closed arrow)** of horizontal and vertical septa in the zone of provisional calcification and the preponderance of vertically oriented calcified cores and bone spicules. **B.** Enlargement of bone spicules shown in the lower right corner of **A.** Spicule of calcified cartilage core and bone lined by osteoblasts **(Ob).**) Calcified cartilage and bone are not distinguishable by this staining method. Note thin osteoid seam **(arrows)** between osteoblast and bone **(black).** An osteoprogenitor cell **(Opc)** is located between osteoblast and blood vessel **(*). A,** ×225; **B,** ×600. Von Kossa–methyl green–pyronine stain. (From Schenk, R., et al. 1973. Calc. Tiss. Res. 11:196. By permission of authors and Springer-Verlag, Publisher.)

septae persist. They become the scaffolding for the formation of primary trabeculae.

Metaphysis. The spongiosa of the metaphysis consists of two parts, primary and secondary. The primary spongiosa slowly replaces the regions previously occupied by the growth plate as

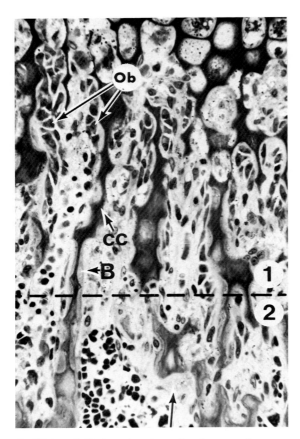

6–42 Decalcified section through primary and secondary spongiosa of a growing rat tibia. In the primary spongiosa **(1)**, plump osteoblasts **(Ob)** are apposing bone **(B)** on dark-staining, calcified cartilage core **(cc)** to form primary spicules. The bone stains poorly in these decalcified sections, but calcified cartilage and bone are distinguishable by this technique. In the secondary spongiosa **(2)**, numerous osteoblasts and occasional osteoclast **(arrow)** line bone surfaces of thicker trabeculae. The calcified cartilage cores persist in secondary spongiosa of rapidly growing bones. In more slowly elongating bones, the calcified cartilage cores are replaced by secondary bone. × 200. (Courtesy of T. Wronski.)

the bone elongates (Figs. 6–37 to 6–39, 6–41 and 6–42). At the front of the advancing metaphysis are capillary loops and perivascular connective tissue that carries osteoprogenitor cells into the newly formed osteogenic area. The preosteoblastic progenitor cells differentiate into osteoblasts that rapidly apply woven bone onto the surfaces of the longitudinal calcified septae, thus creating the trabeculae of the primary spongiosa. Osteoclasts also differentiate from specific osteoprogenitors (preosteoclasts). They resorb some of the calcified septae to make room for the forming trabeculae and marrow cavity. In regions where the primary trabeculae are formed, the osteoclasts are outnumbered by osteoblasts 10 to one within the primary spongiosa.

Eventually, most of the primary spongiosa is converted into secondary (lamellar) spongiosa by the simultaneous removal of woven bone and calcified cartilage cores and addition of secondary (lamellar) bone.

Circumferential Growth of the Bone Shaft. It must be stressed that the transformation of the cancellous periosteal bone collar into a compact bone shaft occurs simultaneously with the initiation of embryonic endochondral ossification at the epiphyseal–metaphyseal complex. In this sequence, the hollow cylinder of primary spongiosa is converted into compact bone by the previously detailed process of compaction, resulting in temporary trabeculae and a primary Haversian system. As the fetus grows, woven trabecular bone is rapidly formed on the periosteal surface of the shaft (fast periosteal bone formation) by osteoblasts arising from the periosteum. These segments of woven trabecular bone are not laid down in sheets, but form first as perpendicular columns and later as horizontal bars across the tops of these columns (Fig. 6–43). This process results in the formation of numerous **T**-shaped trabeculae lined up longitudinally on the outer surface of the shaft. Three-dimensionally, a peri-

6–43 Diagram of the cross section from the mid-shaft of a long bone as a function of age. The evolution of the cortical mid-shaft involves the compaction of the primary spongiosa, rapid periosteal bone formation coupled with enlargement of the marrow cavity, and replacement of primary bone with secondary osteons, slow surface bone formation, replacement of old osteons with new ones and slower periosteal bone formation coupled with more rapid cortical–endosteal bone resorption. **A.** Formation of periosteal bone collar of primary spongiosa. Spicules

of primary bone **(stippled area)** lined by osteoblasts **(Ob)**. Some osteoclasts **(Oc)** are seen at the cortical–bone marrow **(BM)** interface. Cellular **(CP)** and fibrous periosteum **(FP)**. **B.** Formation of primitive cortex by filling of trabecular space by compaction, and rapid periosteal bone formation by laying down T-shaped spicules leading to longitudinally disposed grooves. The groves become roofed over to form tunnels and are then filled in by forming primary osteons **(PHS)**. Compaction also occurs simultaneously as the trabecular spaces are filled with primary osteons

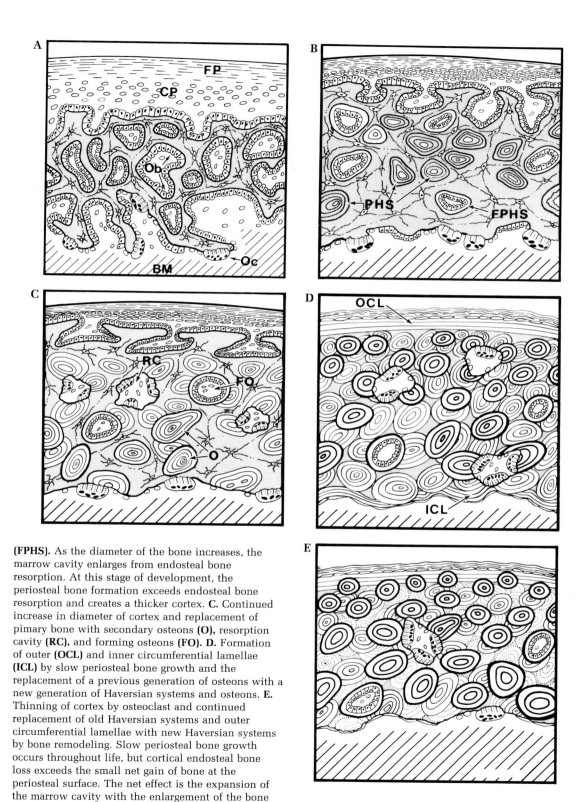

(FPHS). As the diameter of the bone increases, the marrow cavity enlarges from endosteal bone resorption. At this stage of development, the periosteal bone formation exceeds endosteal bone resorption and creates a thicker cortex. **C.** Continued increase in diameter of cortex and replacement of pimary bone with secondary osteons **(O)**, resorption cavity **(RC)**, and forming osteons **(FO). D.** Formation of outer **(OCL)** and inner circumferential lamellae **(ICL)** by slow periosteal bone growth and the replacement of a previous generation of osteons with a new generation of Haversian systems and osteons. **E.** Thinning of cortex by osteoclast and continued replacement of old Haversian systems and outer circumferential lamellae with new Haversian systems by bone remodeling. Slow periosteal bone growth occurs throughout life, but cortical endosteal bone loss exceeds the small net gain of bone at the periosteal surface. The net effect is the expansion of the marrow cavity with the enlargement of the bone circumference.

osteal surface stripped of its periosteal covering would theoretically appear as longitudinal furrows between trabecular projections. Periosteal vessels and undifferentiated connective tissue migrate into the furrows and are then "roofed" by the continued osteoblastic apposition onto the horizontal bars. This structure forms a longitudinal tunnel that becomes the site of a new primary Haversian system.

The continual rapid periosteal formation of primary trabeculae and osteons buries the earlier-formed osteons, but these early osteons remain connected to a nutrient supply by the original vessel on the periosteal surface. The subsequent apposition of bone around these vessels results in the formation of Volkmann's canals coursing obliquely from Haversian canals to the bone exterior.

In concert with the addition of periosteal bone, bone is resorbed at the endosteal surface of the bone shaft. In other words, new bone is being added to the outside of the hollow bone cylinder while a lesser amount is being removed from the inside. The net result is enlargement of the cylindrical marrow cavity, increase of the outer diameter, and a slow increase in the thickness of the shaft wall. To illustrate the importance of this process, if for some reason endosteal resorption were absent, the shaft wall would become extremely thick and the marrow cavity would remain no wider than the original primitive marrow cavity of the fetus.

Another process occurs within the bone shaft during development and maturation. It involves the gradual replacement of the primary Haversian systems with secondary Haversian systems composed of lamellar bone. The replacement originates within Volkmann's and Haversian canals when localized masses of progenitor cells and vascular buds branch off, differentiate into osteoclasts, and excavate new tunnels within the primary osteons. Subsequently, osteoblasts differentiate from preosteoblasts to lay down lamellar bone and form a secondary Haversian system (see section below on bone remodeling for details of this process). This ultimately results in the total replacement of woven bone with lamellar bone, which forms a structurally sounder shaft.

As the bone approaches its full width and length, both the fast periosteal formation of primary trabeculae and osteons and the endosteal resorption slow and finally stop. Next, the shaft is finished off by the slow addition of layers of lamellar bone on both endosteal and periosteal

Table 6–5 Some Factors Affecting Cortical Envelope Sizes

Factors	Effect on envelopes[a]		
	Periosteal	Haversian	Endosteal
Accelerated longitudinal growth	I	0	I
Decreased longitudinal growth	D	0	D
Aging	I	I	I
Growth hormone	I	0	D
Adrenal corticosteroid	0	± I	I
Estrogens	0	0	0
Androgens	0	0	0
Muscular exercise	I	0	D
Thyroxine	?	I	I

[a]I, increase; 0, no effect; D, decrease.

Source: Modified from Frost, H. M. 1973. Bone Remodeling and Its Relationship to Metabolic Bone Diseases. Springfield, Ill: C. C. Thomas. (Courtesy of H. M. Frost and C. C. Thomas, Publisher.)

surfaces. This surface lamellar bone constitutes the inner and outer circumferential lamellae. They function as protective layers and as structural reinforcement for the osteons within the walls of the shaft. Thus, the midshaft of a typical long bone from a young adult may be seen in a cross section, from outside inward with (1) periosteum, (2) outer circumferential lamellae, (3) mature osteons, (4) actively forming osteons, (5) resorption cavities, (6) interstitial lamellae, (7) inner circumferential lamellae, and (8) endosteum.

Factors affecting cortical envelope sizes during growth and development and aging are summarized in Table 6–5.

Modeling

The alteration of the size and shape of bones by bone formation and resorption at different surfaces and rates during the growth process is known as modeling. Modeling serves primarily to alter the amount of bone that is present and to determine its form. The sequence differs from the replacement process of remodeling, which limits the formation and resorption to the same site. Because bone is simply replaced by new bone in remodeling, moreover, there is no change in shape. Further differences between

Table 6–6 Comparison of Modeling and Remodeling

	Remodeling	Modeling
Location	Spatially related	Different surfaces
Coupling	A → R → F	A → F; A → R
Timing	Cyclical	Continuous
Extent	Small (< 20%)[a]	Large (> 90%)
Apposition rate	Slow (0.3–1.0 μm/d)	Fast (2–10 μm/d)
Balance	No change or net loss	Net gain

[a]Of available surface.

Source: From Parfitt, A. M. 1982. The physiologic and clinical significance of bone histomorphometric data. *In* R. R. Recker (ed.), Bone Histomorphometry: Techniques and Interpretation. Boca Raton, Fla.: CRC Press. (Courtesy of A. M. Parfitt and CRC Press, Publisher.)

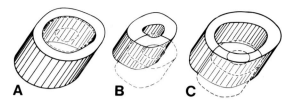

6–44 Diagram of the growth and modeling of the mid-shaft of a long bone. The growth process causes uniform enlargement **(A)**. The modeling process shifts bone surface in tissue space **(B)**. Some anatomists call the shift of any individual surface *drift*, the sum of drifts within a bone is termed modeling. Growth and drift acting together enlarge the bone shaft and change its shape **(C)**.

bone modeling and remodeling are listed in Table 6–6. Modeling occurs continually throughout the growth period and occurs at all bone surfaces. The rate of modeling varies in proportion to the growth rate. For example, in 4-week-old rats the rate is as high as 10 μm/day compared to 2 μm/day in 14-week-old rats; in children the modeling rate is approximately 2 to 3 μm/day.

Classic examples of the modeling process include: (1) the drifting of the midshaft during growth, (2) the shaping of the ends (flaring) of long bones during growth, and (3) the enlargement of the cranial vault and the modification of the cranial curvature.

Normally, during growth the rates of external apposition of new bone and internal resorption are regulated so that the cylindrical shaft expands markedly in diameter, whereas the thickness of its wall and the marrow cavity increase slowly. Bone surfaces can be moved to fulfill biomechanical demands. For example, a coordinated action of bone resorption and formation of one side of the periosteal and endosteal surfaces will move the entire shaft to the right or left, thus allowing some bones to grow eccentrically rather than concentrically (Fig. 6–44). Morphologists call the motion of any individual surface a drift. Drift is another term for modeling. Such behavior is seen in human ribs, femur, tibiae, and radii.

Flaring of the Ends of Long Bones. The diaphysis of most long bones flares outward as it approaches the epiphysis. As a result, the cortex surrounding the metaphysis is much greater in diameter than the shaft of the diaphysis, creating

what is known as the metaphyseal funnel. As longitudinal bone growth occurs, one can see that the wide metaphyseal funnel, a product of the growth plate, is later occupied by a narrower shaft. Such a dramatic change in shape is accomplished as the simultaneous resorption of the funnel region periosteally (the "cut-back zone") and the formation of bone on the opposing endosteal (inner) surface occur while bone is being formed at the adjacent periosteal surface (toward the midshaft) and resorbed at the endosteal surface (Fig. 6–45). Consequently, the diverging walls of the metaphyseal funnel are being straightened and are contributing to the lengthening of the shaft as the shaft is expanding radially and its marrow cavity is being enlarged. This pattern may be modified by drugs (Fig. 6–46).

Alteration of the Curvature of the Cranial Vault. As the cranium enlarges, the curvature of its bones must decrease. This change in curvature involves the apposition of new bone and the resorption at different localized sites (Fig. 6–47). This process is complicated by additional bone formation at the sutures.

Remodeling

Bone formed at infancy is structurally inferior, and the quality of bone in the adult tends to diminish with time. Therefore, like many other tissues, bone must replace or renew itself. This replacement of immature and old bone occurs by a sequence of resorption and production of new lamellar bone. The result is remodeling, necessary to produce and maintain biomechanically and metabolically competent bone.

In humans after 1 year of age, the primary

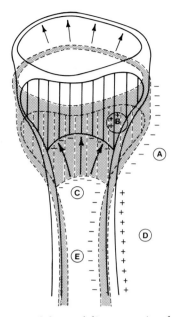

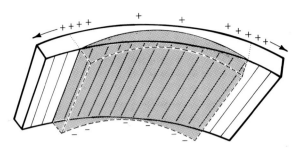

6–47 Enlargement of cranial vault. The cranial vault becomes less convex to accommodate the growing brain through differing rates of bone deposition and resorption from the center or periphery. At the periphery, both bone formation (+) and resorption (−) exceed that at the center. Simultaneously, additional bone is added laterally at the sutures **(arrows).**

6–45 Diagram of the modeling occurring during growth of proximal end of tibia. Frontal section of original proximal tibia is indicated as stippled area. The situation after a growth period of 21 days is superimposed. **A.** Reduction of metaphyseal funnel into a narrower shaft by osteoclastic resorption along periosteal surface of metaphysis (−). **B.** Thickening of cortex by osteoblastic bone formation along cortical endosteal surface of metaphysis (+). **C.** Enlargement of marrow cavity by osteoclastic resorption of metaphyseal trabecular bone (−). **D.** Increase of the diameter of the shaft by periosteal bone formation (+). **E.** Enlargement of the marrow cavity by cortical endosteal bone resorption (−).

6–46 Microradiograph of proximal tibia from control and diphosphonate (a bone resorption depressor agent) treated growing rats. **A.** Control rat with concave-shaped periosteal metaphysis **(arrow).** **B.** Treated rat with convex shaped periosteal metaphysis **(arrow)** and increased metaphyseal and epiphyseal bone mass due to inhibition of bone resorption. ×4. (From the work of Miller, S. C., and Jee, W. S. S. 1979. Anat. Rec. 193:439. By permission of authors and Alan R. Liss, Inc., Publisher.)

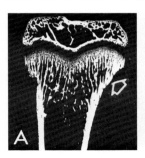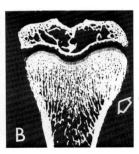

compact and cancellous bone formed during infancy is resorbed and replaced by secondary osteons and trabecular packets. (Quantitative data on structural units of cortical and trabecular bone are listed in Table 6–7). The remodeling does not end with the replacement of primary bone by secondary bone, but continues throughout life. Secondary bone is continually destroyed and replaced (Fig. 6–43). Another product of bone remodeling is the interstitial lamellae of adult bone. They are persisting fragments of large bone units that were partially resorbed by continual bone remodeling.

The remodeling occurs at scattered locations, or foci, on bone surfaces. On each focus are specialized groups of cells with a finite life span that

Table 6–7 Comparison of Adult Cortical and Trabecular Bone Structural Units

Bone structural units[a]	Cortical	Trabecular
Length (mm)	2.5	1.0
Circumference (mm)	0.6	0.6
Wall thickness (mm)	0.075	0.040
Number/mm³ bone volume	15	40
Total number in skeleton	21×10^6	14×10^6

[a]Cortical bone values derived from rib; trabecular bone data derived from ilium; cortical bone structural units (Haversian systems or osteons) are assumed to have a mean cement line diameter of 0.19 mm and mean haversian canal diameter of 0.04 mm.

Source: After Parfitt, A. M. 1982. The physiologic and clinical significance of bone histomorphometric data. In R. R. Recker (ed), Bone Histomorphometry: Techniques and Interpretation, Boca Raton, Fla.: CRC Press. (Courtesy of A. M. Parfitt and CRC Press, Publisher.)

accomplish one "quantum of turnover" (i.e., the erosion and refilling of one quantum of bone). Such a group of cells, along with the quantum of bone remodeled, is referred to as a bone remodeling unit or bone multicellular unit.

Bone remodeling units travel through the cortex or across the trabecular surface, each bone remodeling unit replacing approximately the same volume of old bone by new. At each remodeling focus, the bone remodeling unit undergoes a series of cellular events that follow a coordinated and predictable sequence (Fig. 6–48). This sequence begins with activation of progenitor cells, probably both local and blood-borne which proliferate into a group of newly formed osteoclasts. These osteoclasts excavate a volume of old bone to make way for the formation of a new bone structural unit. When they have completed their task the osteoclasts disappear. There is then produced a reversal zone in which the irregular surface of the resorption space is smoothed off and

6–48 A bone remodeling unit, a portion of rat alveolar bone showing the bone remodeling sequence. Undecalcified section, 4μm thick. ×550. **A.** Resorption phase. An active osteoclast **(OC)** creating a Howship's lacuna. The two lacunae to the left may possibly contain parts of osteoclasts. Note clear zone **(arrows)** and intervening brush border of osteoclast. Osteocyte **(Oc)** and bone **(B).** Toluidine blue stain. **B.** Reversal phase. Howship's lacunae containing partially liberated osteocyte **(white arrow),** mononucleated precursor cells and osteoblasts with prominent Golgi complex **(black arrow).** Masson-Goldner trichrome stain. **C.** Formation phase. Beginning bone formation with osteoblasts in Howship's lacunae. Note distinct cement line **(white arrows),** denoting the boundary between new and old bone. Masson-Goldner trichrome stain. **D.** Active formation phase. Palisades of osteoblasts **(OB)** apposing osteoid **(O)** to fill in previously formed Howship's lacunae. Note recently formed osteocyte **(Oc).** Masson-Goldner trichrome stain. (From Vignery, A., and Baron, R. 1980. Anat. Rec. 196:191. By permission of authors and Alan R. Liss, Inc., Publisher.)

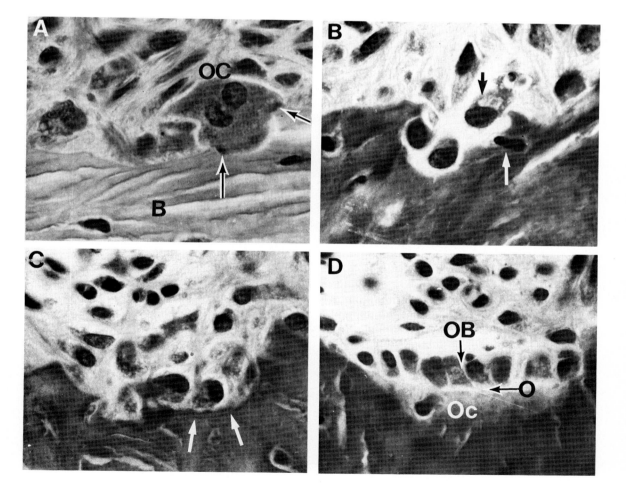

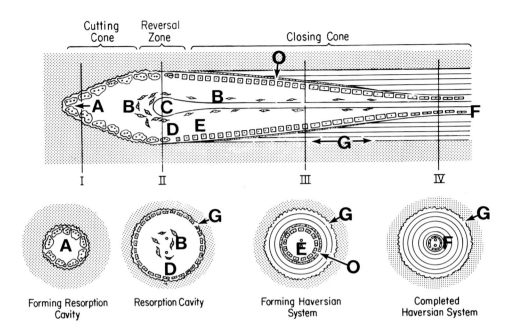

6–49 Diagram showing a longitudinal section through a cortical remodeling unit with corresponding transverse sections below. **A.** Multinucleated osteoclasts in Howship's lacunae advancing longitudinally from right to left and radially to enlarge a resorption cavity. **B.** Perivascular spindle-shaped precursor cells. **C.** Capillary loop. **D.** Mononuclear cells lining reversal zone. **E.** Osteoblasts apposing bone centripetally in radial closure and its perivascular precursor cells. **F.** Flattened cells lining Haversian canal of completed Haversian system. Transverse sections at different stages of development: **(I)** resorption cavities lined with osteoclasts; **(II)** completed resorption cavties lined by mononuclear cells, the reversal zone; **(III)** forming Haversian system or osteons lined with osteoblasts that had recently apposed three lamellae; and **(IV)** completed Haversian system with flattened bone cells lining canal. Cement line **(G)**; osteoid **(stippled)** between osteoblast **(O)** and mineralized bone. (From Parfitt, A. M. 1976. The action of parathyroid hormone on bone. Relation of bone remodeling and turnover, calcium homeostasis, and metabolic bone disease. I. Metabolism 25: 809–844. By permission of author and Grune and Stratton, Inc., Publisher.)

a cement line laid down. Next appears a group of newly formed osteoblasts, which produce new bone structural units.

The above sequence is tightly controlled. Each bone remodeling unit is activiated by one of many stimuli (e.g., PTH) of the precursor cells of osteoclasts (A), osteoclastic resorption (R) of preexisting bones, and osteoblastic formation (F) to replace the bone resorbed, in an unvarying succession symbolized by Frost as A → R → F (ARF). In a normal adult, the time scale for one bone remodeling cycle (sigma) is about 4 months.

Haversian or Cortical Remodeling. Cortical remodeling is the destruction of compact bone followed by the construction of a new Haversian system (Fig. 6–49). The osteoclasts of the bone remodeling unit form a resorption tunnel within the bone, which is refilled centripetally by the osteoblastic apposition of concentric lamellae to form a secondary Haversian system or osteon. Viewed longitudinally, a mature cortical remodeling unit consists of a cutting cone, a reversal zone, and a closing cone. In cross section they are called forming resorption cavities, resorption cavities, and forming Haversian systems and they form the Haversian systems or osteons. The cutting cone creates a space for the future osteon. In humans, the cutting cone is burr-shaped, about 400 μm long and 200 μm wide at its base. Most of the cutting cone is lined by osteoclasts. Behind the cutting cone is a reversal zone, or mature resorption cavity, where resorption has been completed but formation has not begun. The reversal zone is of variable length and is mostly lined by osteoprogenitor cells (Fig. 6–49). Both mononuclear phagocytes and preosteoblasts are

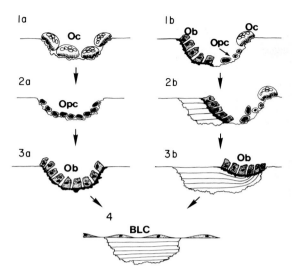

6–50 Diagram of two types of trabecular bone remodeling units. **Oc** = osteoclast, **Opc** = Osteoprogenitor cells, **Ob** = osteoblast, **BLC** = bone lining cell. **a.** Resorption completed before formation begins. The middle panel shows resorption cavities or space equal to that of a future trabecular packet lined with mononuclear cells typical for a reversal zone. **b.** Resorption followed closely by formation, as illustrated for cortical bone in Fig. 6–48.

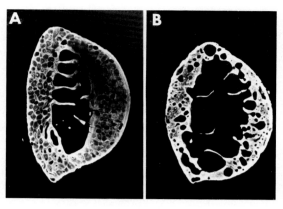

6–51 **A.** Changes in cortical bone as a function of age as seen in microradiograph of 100-μm-thick midshaft of rib from a 1.5-year-old female beagle dog. **B.** A 15-year-old female beagle dog. The thinning of the cortex and trabeculae and the increase in cortical porosity with advancing age is apparent. Bone loss predominately from the cortical–endosteal surface. × 8.

present. Behind the reversal zone is an elongated cavity lined by osteoblasts covering an osteoid seam known as the closing cone. Here, the resorption tunnel is being refilled from the cement line inwards by the formation of concentric lamellae by osteoblastic apposition. Concentric lamellae are laid down until a normal Haversian canal diameter has been attained, resulting in the completion of a new secondary Haversian system or osteon.

Trabecular Bone Remodeling. Unlike cortical remodeling, which proceeds by the tunneling activity of the cutting cone osteoclasts, trabecular remodeling occurs on a bone surface, the trabecular–endosteal surface (Fig. 6–50). However, in most other aspects, a trabecular remodeling unit is very similar to a cortical remodeling unit. Parfitt has proposed one type of trabecular remodeling in which resorption is completed before new bone formation begins and another type in which new bone formation occurs while resorption is still active (Fig. 6–50). Comparisons of bone structural units, bone dynamics, and turnover in adult cortical, trabecular, and whole skel-

eton and factors affecting the bone remodeling sequence are summarized in Tables 6–7 and 6–9.

Age-Related Bone Loss and Osteoporosis

The loss of bone is a universal component of aging. Reviews of the subject in humans suggest:

1. With advancing age, bone is lost from all parts of the skeleton, but not in equal amounts.
2. The loss of bone begins approximately 10 years earlier and proceeds approximately twice as fast in women as in men.
3. Both cortical and trabecular bone are thinned primarily by the removal of bone at the endosteal surfaces.
4. Cortical bone loss occurs predominantly at the cortical–endosteal surface and to a small degree from the enlargement of the Haversian canals (Figs. 6–51A and B). A small net gain of bone at the periosteal surface partially offsets this loss. The net effect is an expansion of the marrow cavity with enlargement of the bone circumference to a lesser degree.
5. Age-related cancellous bone loss is due to the imbalance of excess resorption relative to formation in bone remodeling; the amount of bone replaced at the trabecular–endosteal remodeling sites appears to decrease with advancing age. The sequence of A → R → F is often uncoupled because trabecular plates are perforated or lost, thus reducing the available

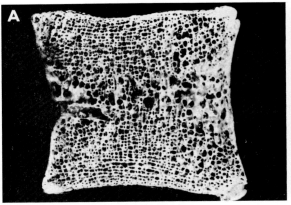

6–52 Photograph of a 2–3 mm thick sagittal sections of part of the lumbar vertebral bodies from an 18-year-old male **(A)** and 80-year-old female **(B). A.** Horizontal elements consisting of perforated transverse plates (seen on edge) stabilize the closely spaced broad flat vertical plates. Note the broad plate-like structure surrounding the basivertebral vein on the left and the plate-like structures on the right which form a fuzzy triangle. The penetrated plates in the end zones are seen as continuous long transverse trabeculae. **B.** An 80-year-old female with age-related bone loss. Note the thinned plates and rods, reduced number of horizontal intercommunicating elements, and the enlarged spacing between the vertical and horizontal elements. ×2. (Courtesy of J. S. Arnold.)

bone surface for bone formation (Figs. 6–52A and B.

6. Bone resorption remains unchanged or is decreased, whereas bone formation decreases with age.

In many cases the reduction of bone mass in specific parts of the skeleton progresses to levels that are no longer sufficient to maintain mechanical support. This results in a condition called "osteoporosis." Osteoporosis is not a single disease, but rather a group of diseases of varied causes that are characterized by osteopenia (reduced bone volume), fracture, backache, and vertebral deformities. The condition is virtually asymptomatic except for backache and associated fractures that occur after minimal trauma. Epidemiological studies have shown osteoporosis to be the principal cause of fractures in the elderly; it afflicts almost 25% of all postmenopausal women in North America and northern Europe.

Osteoporotics are characterized by osteopenia,

a reduction in bone volume compared to others of matched age, sex and race. Most believe that the reduction in the quantity of bone is the primary contributor to the fractures. It is possible that a reduction in the quality of bone with age is an additonal factor, but present techniques have failed to verify this.

The principal question in the etiology of osteoporosis is whether persons have attained osteopenia from a faster rate of age-related bone

6–53 Diagram illustrating the course of bone gain and loss throughout life. Horizontal dotted line represents level below which structural failures of fractures are likely to occur. This level is reached earlier in women (♀) than in men (♂) because of the differences in the magnitude of the age-related bone loss. In both sexes, level is reached earlier in those who accumulate less bone during growth **(lower set of curves)** than those who accumulate more bone **(upper set of curves).** (Legend and figure from Parfitt, A. M., and Duncan, H. 1975. *In* R. H. Rothman and F. A. Simeone (eds.), The Spine, vol. II. Philadelphia: W. B. Saunders, p. 648. By permission of the authors and W. B. Saunders, Publisher.)

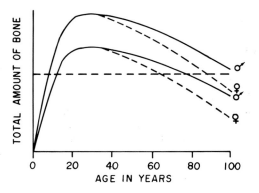

loss, or the accumulation of less than normal quantities of bone during growth and development (Fig. 6–53). Current evidence indicates that osteopenia leading to osteoporosis may be caused either by one of these phenomena, or by a combination of both, and that at any age the trabecular bone volume is less in osteoporotics than in controls. Additional studies measuring the rate of bone remodeling in osteoporotic patients have shown that 60% of the subjects exhibit normal bone remodeling (normal resorption and formation surfaces), while 30% had a normal remodeling rate coupled with a decrease in their formation rate. Only 10% of the sample had an elevated remodeling rate. In light of this evidence, it appears probable that a large number of osteoporotics show normal bone turnover and that the decreased bone volume seen in these osteoporotics is probably due to the presence of a low volume of bone formed during development and growth. therefore, individuals who have attained a large skeletal mass prior to the onset of age-related bone loss will have a sufficient amount of structural bone thoughout their lifespan. This hypothesis is circumstantially supported by limited epidemiological evidence; both white males and black Americans have significantly greater peak skeletal masses than do white females. Correspondingly, they also exhibit a much lower incidence of osteoporosis. Furthermore, obese people also appear to be resistant to osteoporosis, as the increased amount of chronic mechanical strain tends to stimulate increases in skeletal mass.

Osteopenia may also result from an episode of bone loss. If the bone loss occurs at an early age, the skeleton may make it up by bone formation (Fig. 6–54). However, if such an event occurs during adulthood, the potential to regain bone is lost and permanent skeletal deficit results. For example, a common form of osteoporosis is known as postmenopausal osteoporosis. This affliction, characterized by rapid bone loss in postmenopausal women, is believed to be caused by the sudden decreases in estrogens that accompany menopause. Estrogen supplements prevent further bone loss but fail to regain any substantial quantities of bone.

Repair

Repair of bone serves to heal injuries from traumatic causes and walls off harmful processes such as infection, neoplasm, or physicochemical irritants. Repair usually responds rapidly regard-

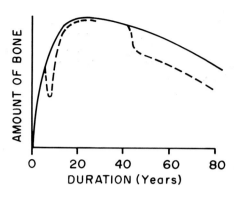

6–54 Diagrammatic illustration of bone loss in idiopathic osteoporosis and recovery during growth and aging. Solid line represents normal gain and loss throughout life. If onset is before skeletal maturity (left-hand dotted line), almost complete recovery is possible. If onset is in adult life (right-hand dotted line), the same degree of bone loss leaves a permanent deficit even when the disease becomes inactive. (From Parfitt, A. M. and Duncan, H. 1975. *In* R. H. Rothman and F. A. Simeone (eds.), The Spine, vol. II. Philadelphia: W. B. Saunders, p. 665. By permission of authors and W. B. Saunders, Publisher.)

less of the condition of the skeleton. Repair occurs in two major stages: the initial repair and the remodeling stage. The classic example of repair is fracture healing.

When a bone is fractured, hemorrhage occurs between the broken ends and the adjacent torn periosteum and muscle. Fracture healing begins with the clotting of extravasated blood. Organization of the hemorrhage follows and is accomplished by ingrowth of granulation tissue from the adjacent bone marrow, periosteum, and muscles within a few days. The torn ends of the periosteum and endosteum, and the bone marrow adjoining the fracture supply cells that proliferate and differentiate into fibrous tissue, fibrocartilage, and hyaline cartilage to form a callus. The appearance of cartilage in the callus is most prominent in fracture of long bones with displacements or large defects. Long bones formed by endochondral ossification invariably produce cartilaginous callus, whereas flat bones formed by intramembranous ossification heal without the appearance of cartilage. The callus provides a provisional scaffold that eventually will be replaced by bone. New woven bone is formed at the periosteal and endosteal surfaces and replaces the callus. The speed of these events depends on local and systemic factors. Local factors include the magnitude of the defect and its immobilization. Rigid fixation favors the formation of bone. The damaged tissue also seems to introduce local factors that stimulate osteogenesis. Systemic factors include the age and the nutritional state of the individual. Repair is rapid in young people, in whom bone formation occurs as early as 48 h. Bony union of the fracture occurs when the new spongy bone units are formed across the fracture line. Subsequently, there is compaction, modeling (resorption of excess bone), and remodeling (formation of lamellar bone). Lastly, nonunion of fractures is rare.

Thus far nothing specific, except electricity and bone morphogenic protein (BMP), has been found to stimulate bone formation. It has been postulated that electrical sources (piezoelectric, solid-state, and streaming potentials) from extracellular matrix of bone and from activated mesenchymal cells in adjacent tissue are needed in bone regeneration. Bone morphogenic protein, a bone growth factor derived from decalcified bone matrix, also causes new bone formation when implanted into fracture sites.

Histophysiology

Bone, as the principal tissue of the skeletal system, has a dual function: it acts as structural support and as a reservoir for calcium and phosphorus. Four functional cell systems are involved with the accumulation and maintenance of structural bone: (1) the endochondral ossification system, which regulates growth in length and generates cancellous bone; (2) the intramembranous ossification system, which regulates growth in width and generates cortical and cancellous bone; (3) the modeling system, which regulates size and shape; and (4) the remodeling system, which regulates bone turnover (Table 6–8).

There are two functional cell systems involved with calcium levels: (1) the osteocyte–bone-lining cell system, which regulates plasma calcium homeostasis, and (2) the osteoclast–osteocyte system, which rapidly corrects errors in steady-state calcium levels (Table 6–12).

Factors Affecting Endochondral Ossification. Longitudinal bone growth and the accumulation of trabecular bone depend on cartilage growth and endochondral ossification at the epiphyseal–metaphyseal growth complex. These processes are subject to at least four kinds of regulations: (1) genetics, (2) mechanical stresses, (3) hormones, and (4) nutrition. Genetic determinants control the appearance of osteogenesis (the timing and order of ossification) and regulate the fusion of epiphyses, whereas mechanical stresses participate in determining bone shape and internal structure. Hormones can affect growth and maintenance of bone; vitamins are important in conditioning normal ossification.

Growth hormone, thyroxine, adrenal cortical hormones, vitamin D, and vitamins A and C are important in skeletal maturation (Table 6–10). Growth hormone and thyroxine stimulate the proliferative stage of the endochondral ossification process. Growth hormone stimulates cell division and protein, deoxyribonucleic and ribonucleic acid, and mucopolysaccharide synthesis in cartilage. These effects are mediated by somatomedin, a polypeptide growth factor produced by liver and possibly by the kidney in response to growth hormone. The oversecretion and undersecretion of growth hormone lead to gigantism and dwarfism, respectively.

Thyroxine makes its essential contribution to bone growth and development by promoting cartilage cell maturation and, to a lesser extent, car-

Table 6–8 Comparison of Bone Dynamics and Turnover in Cortical, Trabecular, and Whole Skeleton

Factor	Cortical	Trabecular	Whole skeleton
Mineral apposition rate (μm/d)[a]	0.8	0.6	0.67
Duration of BRU resorption (days)	24	21	21
Duration of BRU formation (days)	124	91	101
Duration of remodeling period (days)	147	112	122
Total birth rate (per h) [b]	180	720	900
Bone turnover rate (%/yr)	3	26	7.6
Total turnover (mg Ca/day)	70	158	220

[a]Corrected for orientation.
[b]Activation of new bone remodeling unit (BRU).

Table 6–9 Factors Affecting the Bone Remodeling Sequence

Stages	Factors accelerating	Factors decelerating
Activation	Acromegaly Thyrotoxicosis Postinjury Osteoporosis Hyperparathyroidism	Hypothyroid Hypoparathyroid Estrogen Ionization Irradiation
Resorption	Hypercortisonism Hypogonadism Hyperparathyroidism Age-related expansion of marrow cavity Thyrotoxicosis Immobilization	Calcitonin Diphosphonate
Formation	Sodium fluoride Phosphate Mechanical exercise	Immobilization Hypercortisonism Age
Uncoupling		Excessive exogenous glucocorticoids Cushing's syndrome Hyperparathyroidism

tilage growth. The mode of action of thyroxine is not understood. Undersecretion of thyroxine (e.g., hypothyroidism) is associated with decreased synthesis and release of the growth hormone, which leads to cretinism, a form of dwarfism and mental deficiency. An excess of thyroid hormone (e.g., hyperthyroidism) is rare in children, and it is associated with an acceleration of both growth and osseous development.

Male and female sex hormones regulate growth rates by controlling the appearance of ossification centers and the rate of maturation. The closure of epiphyses is correlated with the rate of development of the gonads. For example, the adolescent growth spurt is associated with increased secretion of sex hormones. In cartilage, estrogens reduce mucopolysaccharide content and increase calcium content; both of these ac-

Table 6–10 Factors Influencing Endochondral Ossification

Stages in the endochondral ossification process	Factors accelerating the stage	Factor decelerating the stage
1. Proliferative stage	GH, T_4	Estrogens, ACH, mechanical compression, excessive androgens, removal of GH and/or T_4
2. Sequence of differentiation		
a. Cartilage matrix synthesis and lacunar hypertrophy	GH, T_4	Vitamin D and C deficiencies (?), anything retarding stage 1, excess Vitamin A
b. Mineralization of the matrix	Vitamin D, GH, T_4	Vitamin D deficiency, PTH, anything retarding stage 1, hypophosphatemia (?)
3. Production of primary spongiosa	None known other than GH, T_4	Vitamin C and D deficiencies, anything retarding stage 1
4. Replacement by secondary spongiosa	GH, T_4	Vitamin C deficiency, anything retarding stage 1

Abbreviations: ACH, adrenocortical hormone; GH, growth hormone; T_4, thyroxine.

Source: Modified from Frost, H. M. 1972. The Physiology of Cartilaginous, Fibrous and Bony Tissue. Springfield, Ill.: C. C. Thomas. (Courtesy of H. M. Frost and C. C. Thomas, Publisher.)

tions promote skeletal maturation. When testosterone is administered to rats, glycogen reserves are increased and the calcifying zone of the epiphyseal plate widens; these events are related to accelerated cartilage maturation.

Growth retardation of children who were given glucocorticoids has been attributed to the inhibitory effects of glucocorticoids on cartilage and bone. Overdose or excessive secretion of glucocorticoids slows or depresses the growth of the epiphyseal plate and leads to a change of osteoblasts to a resting state. The result is that the epiphyseal plate is thinned and the metaphyseal spongy bone is reduced in mass, density, and turnover. These steroids can inhibit the proliferation of cartilage cells directly or indirectly by depressing the release of growth hormone, which would account for the reduction in cell division and the thinning of the growth plates.

Some adrenocortical hormones are needed to support bodily functions essential to growth. Untreated adrenalectomized animals do not grow normally, but growth resumes with replacement therapy.

Vitamin D deficiency leads to a widening of the epiphyseal growth plate, increased numbers of hypertrophic cartilage cells, wide osteoid seams, and decreased linear growth. This pathological condition appears to be related more to defects in mineralization and the subsequent failure to resorb the growth plate. The condition is called rickets; in an adult, it is called adult rickets or osteomalacia. Osteomalacia is caused by a retarded synthesis rate and the failure of osteoid to mineralize.

Vitamin A deficiency results in decreases in bone resorption, collagen synthesis, and mineral accretion, and thus alters bone modeling. It leads to an enlarged bone, which causes compression of the nerves leaving the skull or spinal canal. Excessive intake of vitamin A stimulates bone resorption and results in irregularities in the columnar architecture of the growth plate. The vitamin first activates the existing osteoclasts and then stimulates the differentiation of monocytic osteoprogenitor cells so that the number of osteoclasts is increased.

In vitamin C deficiency (scurvy), bone formation is impaired because of decreased synthesis of collagen and of glycosaminoglycans. In scorbutic children, the growth cartilage cells continue to multiply in columns, and the matrix calcifies to form a fragile brittle network. This lesion can be seen radiographically and is known as a scorbutic band or Trummerfeld. Formation of osteoid ceases, osteoblasts are scarce, and fibroblasts of connective tissue predominate. The osteoclasts are less affected. This condition is a direct consequence of the impaired hydroxylation of collagen proline and lysine, in which ascorbic acid is required as a reducing cofactor.

Role of Bone in Calcium Homeostasis. Because the skeleton contains 99% of the total body calcium, it is not surprising that bone tissue acts as a calcium reservoir. Skeletal calcium has a key role in calcium homeostasis by maintaining levels of plasma calcium essential for the stability of a wide variety of biological processes. The function of neural, muscular, and secretory tissue is extremely sensitive to even minor changes in plasma calcium. For example, small decreases in plasma calcium concentration cause both a dramatic increase in neuromuscular excitability and the syndrome of tetany. Moreover, calcium ion must be present for cell cohesion and in numerous enzymatic reactions.

In humans, the normal plasma calcium concentration is approximately 10 mg per dl plasma and normally ranges within 1 mg per dl of this value. Kinetic studies show that a large part of the plasma calcium (approximately 7 mg/dl) is maintained by a continuous exchange of calcium ion between bone tissue and extracellular fluid. The interchange occurs between the hydroxyapatite crystals of all bone surfaces and proceeds independently of any changes in bone volume (i.e., formation and resorption). For example, under conditions of low plasma calcium (hypocalcemia), there is an increase in the outward flux of calcium ions from bone mineral into the surrounding extracellular fluid. In contrast, when plasma calcium is abnormally high (hypercalcemia), there is an increase in the inward flux of calcium ions from the extracellular fluid into bone mineral.

This process of calcium exchange is called the blood–bone transfer or disequilibrium. The transfer of calcium ions occurs between the bone and the plasma fluid compartments. The bone fluid compartment is a continuous narrow tissue-fluid space surrounding available bone surfaces (Fig. 6–55). It is located between the bone-lining cells and/or osteoblasts and the endosteal bone surfaces, and between the osteocytes and their lacunar and canalicular walls. Immediately out-

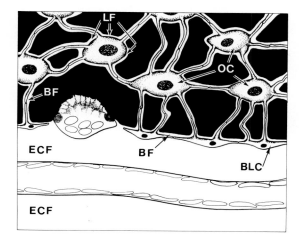

6–55 A diagrammatic representation of the role of bone fluid compartment in the postulated control of plasma calcium. It is now postulated the bone fluid is continuously circulated through each subcompartment: extracellular fluid **(ECF)**; bone-lining cell **(BLC)**; bone fluid **(BF)**; bone **(black)**; lacuna fluid **(LF)**; and osteocyte **(OC)**. Calcium ions enter the bone fluid compartment through channels between cells that line the bone surface and are actively returned to extracellular fluid through lining cells on the surface of bone. The activity of parathyroid hormone increases the entry of calcium ion into bone lining cells, which increases transcellular transport unidirectionally toward the extracellular fluid.

side the bone fluid compartment is a perivascular fluid compartment consisting of regions surrounding the vascular tissue within the Haversian canals, Volkmann's canals, bone marrow, and other vascular spaces.

Because the skeletal response to acute hypocalcemia is much too fast to involve bone resorption, investigators generally agree that plasma calcium homeostasis is governed by the blood–bone disequilibrium at quiescent bone surfaces rather than by bone resorption sites. Some authors have proposed that the blood–bone transfer is driven by an active pumping of calcium ions from the bone fluid compartment into the perivascular compartment by the bone-lining cells and osteocytes (Fig. 6–55). Other proposed mechanisms are membrane compartmentalization, pinocytic calcium transfers, localized acid production, local solubizers, and a stabilized regulator phase. Microelectrode measurements have shown that the bone fluid compartment contains lower concentrations of calcium, magnesium, and sodium while having relatively higher potassium than plasma fluids, a disequilibrium suggestive of a pumping mechanism. Such a transport system may greatly aid the movement of calcium ion out of the microenvironment of the bone surface. Once in the perivascular space, the ions move freely in and out of capillaries, governed by the concentration gradient.

The process of calcium exchange discussed above accounts only for 7 mg/dl of the 10 mg/dl found in plasma. The remainder of the calcium may be mediated by the actions of PTH and by a group of recently discovered hormones that are metabolites of vitamin D. Both are believed to cooperate in the following manner. In response to hypocalcemia, the parathyroid gland secretes PTH, which subsequently binds to membrane receptors on bone and renal tissue. In the kidney, PTH stimulates the production of a vitamin D metabolite, $1,25(OH)_2D_3$. The $1,25(OH)_2D_3$ acts on the intestine to stimulate intestinal absorption of dietary calcium and, together with PTH, promotes the mobilization of calcium ion from bone. At the same time, PTH and possibly $1,25(OH)_2D_3$ conserve calcium by stimulating the renal reabsorption of calcium ion. The resultant rise in plasma calcium to normal levels (normocalcemia) inhibits the secretion of PTH through a negative feedback loop (Fig. 6–56).

The mechanism by which PTH and $1,25(OH)_2D_3$ mobilize calcium from bone is still unknown. Possible mechanisms for calcium mobilization by PTH and $1,25(OH)_2D_3$ involve the previously discussed process of acute increase in osteoclastic and osteocytic resorption (osteocytic osteolysis) and stimulation of the calcium pump of the bone-lining cells and osteoblasts. Bélanger has proposed that physiological levels of PTH stimulate the osteocytic resorption of perilacunar bone and thereby liberate calcium. However, such changes in lacunar size have been documented only with pharmacological doses of PTH and in various pathological disorders and have not been seen during normal homeostasis. The osteoclastic and osteocytic resorption system can best be regarded as a system for correcting errors in steady-state calcium levels by acute changes in resorptive activity of osteoclasts and osteocytes.

The second hypothetical mechanism involves an increase in the pumping of calcium out of the bone fluid compartment. Such stimulation

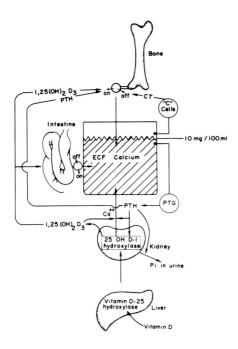

6–56 A diagrammatic representation of the calcium
homeostatic mechanism involving the vitamin
D–endocrine system. In response to hypocalcemia, the
parathyroid glands secrete parathyroid hormone. The
parathyroid hormone in turn binds to the kidney and
bone. In the kidney it stimulates production of 1,25-
$(OH)_2D_3$. The 1,25-$(OH)_2D_3$ then stimulates intestinal
absorption of calcium and together with the
parathyroid hormone stimulates the mobilization of
calcium from bone and renal reabsorption of calcium.
The resultant rise in plasma (**ECF**) calcium shuts off
secretion of the parathyroid hormone. (From DeLuca,
H. F. 1980. Nutrition Rev. 38:171. Courtesy of the
author.)

would thereby push calcium toward the plasma. Recent morphological evidence leaves no doubt that bone-lining cells do respond to PTH, but the chemical and biochemical processes remain obscure.

In summary, two functional cell systems in bone participate in calcium homeostasis: (1) the osteocyte–bone–lining cell system, which in collaboration with the kidney regulates plasma calcium homeostasis, and (2) the osteoclast–osteocytic system, which rapidly corrects errors in steady-state calcium levels (Table 6–12). The error-correcting system acts in minutes and hours whereas the blood–bone equilibrium system acts in days. The remaining cell system in bone is the osteoclast–osteoblast system, which regulates bone remodeling, turnover, and balance of structural bone. Note that all these systems are stimulated by PTH (Table 6–11).

It should be reemphasized that PTH, the most important hormone affecting the skeletal system, has two functions: (1) to stimulate and control the rate of bone remodeling, and (2) to stimulate mechanisms for the control of plasma calcium level. Parathyroid hormone immediately affects the osteocyte–bone-lining cell and the osteoclastic and osteocytic resorption systems active in calcium homeostasis; it has a prolonged effect on osteoclast formation and accelerated bone remodeling involved in the maintenance of structural bone. At low levels of PTH secretion, bone formation equals or exceeds bone resorption; at higher levels of PTH, resorption exceeds formation and results in bone loss during remodeling.

Even less is known about the regulatory response to high levels of plasma calcium (hypercalcemia). Entry of calcium ion into existing surface mineral probably partially lowers plasma calcium toward the normal value of 10 mg/dl.

Table 6–11 Comparison of Functional Systems in Structural Bone

	Systems			
	Endochondral ossification	Intramembranous ossification	Modeling	Remodeling
Function	Longitudinal growth Production of cancellous bone mainly	Growth in width Production of cortical bone mainly	Shape Size	Turnover of bone
Cells	Chondroblasts Chondroclasts Osteoblasts Osteoclasts	Osteoclasts Osteoblasts	Osteoclasts Osteoblasts	Osteoclasts Osteoblasts

Table 6–12 Comparison of Two Functional Systems in Bone Calcium Homeostasis

	Systems	
	Error-correcting	Blood–bone equilibrium
Function	Restore baseline plasma Ca	Determine steady-state level of Ca
Cells	Osteocytes Osteoclasts	Bone-lining cells Osteocytes
Affected by PTH	Yes	Yes
Time scale[a]	Minutes–hours	Days

[a]Reaction time to PTH.

Source: Modified from Parfitt, A. M. 1979. Metab. Bone Dis. Relat. Res. 1:279; courtesy of A. M. Parfitt and Société Nouvelle de Publications Médicales et Dentaires, Publisher.

However, the mechanism of further lowering is the subject of controversy. In many mammals, the hormone calcitonin acts to lower both blood calcium and phosphate in response to hypercalcemia. However, its role in normal adult humans is unknown because changes in calcium metabolism are not associated with extremes in hormone production. For example, normal plasma calcium is seen in cases of both calcitonin deficiency (thyroidectomy) and calcitonin excess (medullary carcinoma of the thyroid). The only action now attributable to calcitonin is the depression of osteoclastic resorption and an inhibition of the activation of remodeling and modeling.

Joints

All bones are interconnected by articulations or joints to form the skeleton. These joints are composed of a wide variety of connective tissue structures that permit varying amounts of movement between adjacent bones. If the connection permits very little or no bone movement, it is called a *synarthrosis*. Slightly movable joints are *amphiarthroses*, and those that contain a fluid-filled cavity and are freely movable are referred to as *diarthroses*. The amphiarthroses and diarthroses bear most of the skeletal load. They may be involved in musculoskeletal diseases.

Synarthroses

Synarthrotic joints are either nonmovable or show very limited movement. They may be fur-

ther differentiated into three subclasses by the type of tissue involved in the union. When the articulation is via connective tissue, it is termed a *syndesmosis*; when the linkage is through cartilage, a *synchondrosis*; and if the connection is bone, a *synostosis*.

Syndesmosis. Both the tibiofibular joints and the numerous sutures of the cranial bones constitute the syndesmotic joints. The syndesmotic joints are remnants of the mesenchymal tissue mass that forms the adjacent bones. For example, in the cranial bones, the centers of ossification slowly transform the mass of undifferentiated connective tissue into bone. Eventually, all that remains of these masses is a thin band of connective tissue at the bone junctions, or sutures. This undifferentiated connective tissue contains osteogenic precursors that can subsequently add bone to the free edges by appositional bone growth, resulting in the enlargement of the cranial cavity. Upon maturity, the skull stops growing and the connective tissue suture may be slowly replaced by bone, transforming the syndesmotic joint into a synostosis.

Synchondrosis. In synchondroses, bones are joined by hyaline cartilage. In most cases, these joints are present only during development and growth and show only limited mobility. The junction of the ribs and the sternum is such a joint. The growth plate in the growing mammal is also a synchondrotic joint. It connects the epiphyses and metaphyses of the long bones. Like the syndesmotic joints, the major function of synchondroses is to permit continued bone growth and expansion. This is accomplished by the process of endochondral ossification discussed above. Synchondroses are also similar to syndesmoses in their frequent conversion to synostoses after the suspension of bone growth.

Synostosis. These joints are formed from bone arising within either connective tissue or cartilage joints. Because most synostotic joints occur in adults, they are believed to function in stabilizing parts of the skeleton after the bones have stopped growing.

Amphiarthroses

These articulations are made up of numerous intervertebral discs situated between the vertebral bodies and joined together by ligaments. Each disc is constructed like a car tire and is composed of a soft gelatinous inner tube or core known as the nucleus pulposus surrounded by a fibrous outer casing, the annulus fibrosus (Fig. 6–57). The annulus is composed of concentrically arranged fibrocartilage encased within a sheath of dense connective tissue all derived from mesenchymal tissue. The arrangement of these concentric fibrous rings is shown in Fig. 6–57. In contrast, the nucleus pulposus arises from the notochord and is composed of a few round mesenchymal cells embedded in a mucoid semifluid gel. Functionally, it is the nucleus that attenuates and dissipates the forces on the spine. Unfortunately, the nucleus undergoes chondroid metaplasia, making it brittle and inelastic with age, and the annulus becomes less absorbent because of increased collagen content, loss of moisture, and a decrease in sulfated glycosaminoglycans.

6–57 Schematic representation of parts of two vertebral bodies and the intervertebral disc.
A. Horizontal section through disc. The disc consists of an *annulus fibrosus* composed of concentric fibrous rings surrounding the *nucleus pulposus*.
B. The nucleus pulposus abuts against the hyaline cartilaginous plate of the vertebral bodies.
C. Ligaments reinforce the anterior and posterior fibers of the annulus.

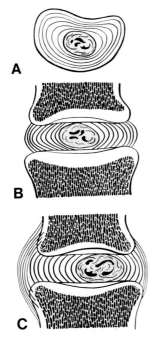

The fibers of the annulus are firmly attached to the vertebral bodies and are arranged in lamellae with fibers of one layer running at an angle to those of the deeper layer. This arrangement with the investing vertebral ligaments permits limited vertebral movements.

Diarthroses

General Structure. In diarthroidal joints, a capsule joins the ends of the bones. This capsule is lined with a synovial membrane and encloses a fluid-filled cavity (the articular or synovial cavity). The synovial fluid is critical in reducing the friction between the hyaline cartilage covering the opposing articular surfaces. The major structures of the diarthroidal joint are summarized in Fig. 6–58.

Development. The cartilage model of bone expands before the primary center of ossification appears. As the cartilage expands lengthwise, the two ends of adjacent bones approach each other and initiate the formation of a diarthroses. The development begins with the condensation of mesenchyme between the future bones into a primitive joint plate known as the interzonal mesenchyme (Fig. 6–58).

Concurrently, the outermost ring of mesenchyme condenses to form an outer sheath, which is the counterpart of the primitive perichondrium on the adjacent bones. This membrane is a primitive joint capsule. It envelopes the interzonal mesenchyme like a sleeve and is continuous with the perichondrium of both adjacent bones. As development proceeds, an amorphous intercellular gel and tissue fluid appear between the mesenchymal cells of the interzonal region. These fluid spaces coalesce to form cavities. Eventually a large continuous synovial cavity occupies the site formerly occupied by the mesenchymal plate. The formation of the cavity allows the cartilage caps to meet and articulate. Subsequently, the cavity further extends along the sides of the cartilaginous ends to overlap and create numerous folds.

After the cavitation of the synovial cavity, the primitive joint capsule completes its differentiation into two layers. The outer layer of mesenchyme is converted into a dense fibrous tissue that constitutes the joint capsule proper, and the inner layer differentiates into a cellular layer. This inner layer is the synovial membrane or synovium.

6–58 Schematic representation of the major stages in the development of a diarthroidal joint. **A.** Early limb bud showing the *blastema*. The condensation of mesenchyme. **B.** Cartilage model of bone, primitive joint capsule, and interzonal mesenchyme **(IM)** of joint with the cellular material already loosely arranged. **C.** Cleft **(C)** formation, the early development of the joint cavity. **D.** Mature synovial or diarthroidal joint. The opposing articular surfaces are covered by articular cartilage; synovial lining covers the joint capsule.

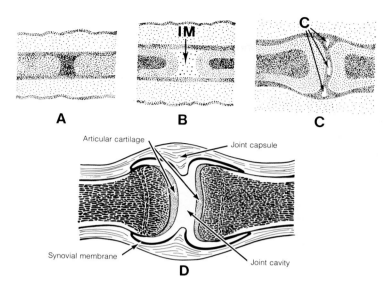

A   B   C

Articular cartilage   Joint capsule

Synovial membrane   Joint cavity

D

The initial configuration of a joint is governed genetically. However, the final phase of the development of diarthroses in utero depends on the intrauterine mechanical forces arising from newly formed skeletal muscle. When the fetal joints are unable to move, the synovial cavities and the adjacent structures either fail to develop completely or become fused.

Articular Cartilage. The articular cartilage found in the diarthroidal joints is, in most respects, typical of hyaline cartilage. However, articular cartilage does differ from hyaline in lacking a perichondrium and having a unique collagen organization. This structural modification of the cartilage matrix may be discussed as three arbitrary zones (Fig. 6–59): a tangential layer with the fibers oriented parallel to the surface, a deep radial zone with fibers at right angles to the surface, and a transitional zone uniting these two zones. The network closely resembles numerous overlapping arches, which are called Benninghof arcades. Such an orientation creates a densely packed network of collagen immediately beneath the articular surface, resulting in an ideal structure for sustaining the constantly changing stresses on the joint surface.

Within this collagenous framework are proteoglycans together with large amounts of water and cartilage cells between the collagen. The chondrocytes can be divided into layers or zones. At the surface is a narrow layer of flattened chondrocytes called the gliding layer or

6–59 Schematic drawing depicting the four zones and the arrangement of the collagen fibers in the articular cartilage. At the surface is the gliding layer or tangential zone **(TA)**, followed by transitional **(TR)**, radial **(R)**, and calcified **(CC)** zones of cartilage. The tidemark **(T)** separates the radial and calcified cartilage zones and represents the superficial edge of the calcified cartilage. The cartilage is anchored on subchondral bone **(black)**. The articular surface is devoid of perichondrium and synovial membrane. Collagen fibers are first parallel and then perpendicular to the cartilage surface. The deeper layers form Benninghof arcades **(B)**.

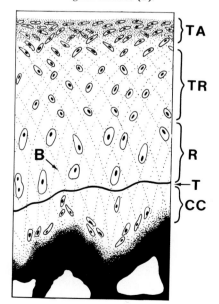

tangential zone. Beneath this zone is the transitional zone in which the ovoid-to-rounded chondrocytes are distributed randomly. The transitional zone overlies a radial zone, below which is the zone of calcified cartilage. Between the last two zones is the "tidemark," a thin wavy basophilic line representing the superficial edge of the layer of calcified cartilage; this structure appears as the "joint surface" in x-ray films. Lastly, the layer of calcified cartilage fuses with the subchondral bone, a mature type of cortical bone with Haversian systems. During the growth of the epiphyses of the long bones, the chondrocytes in the deeper (but not the deepest) layers undergo the same sequence of proliferation, maturation, hypertrophy, and calcification as those of the growth plate. In fact, this region should not be considered articular cartilage but the growth zone for subchondral bone. After epiphyseal growth is complete, the lower zones of chondrocytes become converted into compact bone and the more superficial layers remain as the articular covering.

As stated above, the ground substance of both hyaline and articular cartilage is composed of the proteoglycans chondroitin sulfate, keratan sulfate, and a small amount of hyaluronic acid. These proteoglycans avidly bind water, causing the ground substance to swell and, consequently, to inflate the collagen matrix into a taut network. When a load is placed on the surface, this fluid is readily extruded, lubricating the joint space ("weeping lubrication"). In turn, removing the load results in the reabsorption of the fluid by the matrix. The net effect of these two activities is functionally the same as a pumping mechanism for the transport of nutrients and wastes through the avascular cartilage.

Joint Capsule and Synovial Membrane. The joint capsule consists of an outer layer of dense fibrous tissue lined by an inner, loosely constructed synovial membrane. The joint capsule is continuous with the outer layer of adjacent periosteum and is attached to the margins of the articular cartilage. The layer is relatively inelastic and therefore contributes to the stability of the diarthroidal joint. Regions of the capsule are thickened to form ligaments, and occasionally gaps may be found within the capsule. Where these gaps occur, the synovial membrane forms outpouchings called bursae. The bursae separate the main body of the joint from the muscle or tendon and hence act to reduce the friction on

these structures. They are formed over pressure points after birth.

The synovial membrane is a loosely textured sheet of vascular connective tissue, similar to pericardium, peritoneum, and pleura in structure, which lines the joint capsule but not the articular cartilage surfaces. Its free surface facing the joint cavity consists of one or three cell layers of synovial cells overlying a loosely textured fibrous connective tissue layer. This fibrous connective tissue layer contains numerous capillary vessels, which merge into a deeper portion adjacent to the capsule that is made up of more densely compact fibrous tissue. The synovial stroma consists of a loose network of collagen fibers and ground substance (Fig. 6–60) well supplied with capillaries, lymphatics, and nerves. An important characteristic is the absence of any basement membrane in the synovial membrane, which means that capillary walls have no barrier to separate them from the joint cavity. Thus, the

6–60 Drawing of the synovial membrane. Two to three layers of synovial cells **(SC)** lining small villi. The more superficial portion of the membrane beneath the lining cells consists of loose fibrous connective tissue **(LCT)** with numerous capillaries; the deeper portion approaching the capsule is formed by more dense fibrous tissue **(DCT).** Basement membrane is lacking throughout the synovial membrane; thus the joint cavity can be considered an intercellular space.

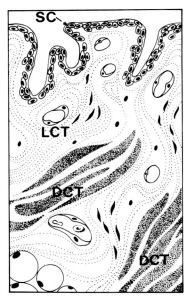

joint cavity can be considered an intercellular space. This way of seeing the joint cavity is important for understanding the process of exudate formation in inflammatory joint diseases.

The synovial membrane or synovium lies adherent to adipose tissue, areolar tissue, or the inner surface of the synovium is smooth, glistening, and commonly thrown into folds of villi. The synovium is also highly vascularized; it contains a larger caliber of capillary than most regions of the body, and many of these capillaries are fenestrated and coiled into a glomeruloid arrangement. In addition, these vessels frequently course extremely close to the inner surface of the membrane. These special features result in the rapid exchange of fluid and small molecules in the blood and the synovial fluid.

Synovial membranes may be distinguished morphologically by the type of underlying tissue: areolar, adipose, or fibrous. The areolar form overlies, as the name implies, loose connective tissue. It is found in joints or parts of joints not subjected to pressure or strain such as the suprapatellar pouch of the knee. The surface layer consists of two or three rows of rounded fibroblasts or fibroblasts with extensive processes embedded in a layer of collagenous fibers. Commonly, there is an elastic lamina located at the base that prevents the membrane from being pinched between opposing articular surfaces. In addition to the fibroblasts, there are a few leukocytes, macrophages, and lymphoid wandering cells.

The fibrous form is found overlying ligaments, tendons, and other regions frequently subjected to tension. The underlying dense connective tissue contains sparsely distributed fibroblasts often within matrix capsules. The surface layers are somewhat more cellular than the deep tissue. In regions subjected to extremely high forces, fibrocartilage develops.

Adipose synovial membrane lines the intraarticular fat pads of diarthroidal joints. The membrane is composed of a single layer of surface cells anchored on a thin layer of collagenous connective tissue.

Two cell types line the synovium. Some of the cells resemble macrophages, having a cell surface with many filopodia and a cytoplasm with a large Golgi apparatus, numerous lysosomes, and scanty rough endoplasmic reticulum. They are collectively called histocytic type A cell (or M—macrophage—like). The second cell type resembles fibroblasts and is characterized by a smoother cell surface and an abundance of granular endoplasmic reticulum. These cells are more electron-dense than A cells and are called B cells (or F—fibroblast—like). This classification is not rigid, and the two cell types may represent different functional stages of the same cell, since intermediate forms have been observed. Functionally, these cells secrete the synovial mucin and are phagocytic.

Synovial Fluid. Synovial fluid is produced from the combination of the ultrafiltrate from the synovial capillaries with the mucin produced by the type B synovial cells. The fluid portion differs from blood serum by containing only one-third of the protein content. The proteins are principally albumin, although enzymatic proteins and complement system proteins are also present. The synovial mucin secreted by the type B lining cells contributes to the viscosity of the synovial fluid. The mucin consists of hyaluronic acid and covalently bound proteins. Hyaluronic acid is highly polymerized and is responsible for the viscous properties of the synovial fluid. However, the lubricating qualities of the fluid are probably derived from a glycoprotein constituent and not hyaluronate.

Microscopic examination of synovial fluid is an invaluable tool for the diagnosis of numerous joint disorders. In normal synovial samples, there are fewer than 300 leukocytes per mm^3 and no more than 25% of them are polymorphonuclear leukocytes. Fibrinogen and larger protein molecules are normally absent or are present only in relatively small amounts compared with plasma values.

Repair of Articular Cartilage

Repair is limited to the periphery of the joint, where the cartilage is immediately adjacent to the synovial membrane. In these regions, the lining cells proliferate and produce a form of fibrocartilage rather than normal articular cartilage. If damage occurs outside this area, the cartilage fails to repair because of the inability of mature cartilage to mitose.

Aging

After the third decade, the intervertebral disc shows a decrease in water and a progressive degeneration of the nucleus pulposus. The number of cells decreases and a loss of metachromatic material occurs accompanied by a loss of turgor. These changes, together with the age-related osteopenia, result in an increased incidence in pathology of the disc and vertebra.

Articular cartilage exhibits progressive changes with age. By age 30, tears are seen. They lead to fibrillation of the surface, tangential cracks, or deep vertical fissures. Chondrocytes cluster in larger numbers of individual lacunae in the transitional and radial zones. Progressive cell death occurs and the depth of the cartilage layers decreases to a point where the calcified zone is exposed or removed. Often subchondral bone becomes highly polished to an ivory-like finish (eburnation). New bone forms at the joint margins and the subchondral bone marrow becomes hyperemic and fibrotic.

Cartilage cell number decreases with advancing age. Dying cells are commonly observed, and microscars are seen as replacement of disintegrated cartilage. The total uptake, rates of uptake, and turnover of ^{3}H-histidine, glycine, and proline diminish with age. The changes in cartilage matrix are interesting. The glycosaminoglycan content of costal cartilage decreases with age, primarily owing to a loss in chondrotin-4-sulfate (chondrotin-6-sulfate decreases only slightly). Keratosulfate content increases to a plateau from birth to old age and constitutes 50% of the total glycosaminoglycans in the aged. Whether or not these changes occur in articular cartilage is disputed.

Articular cartilage exhibits the lowest proliferative activity of all skeletal tissue. The uptake of ^{3}H-thymidine cannot be detected in mature animals.

Synovial membrane shows age-related changes in fibrosis, in formation of villous membrane, in focal accumulation of mononuclear cells, and in the viscosity of synovial fluid. After the fourth decade, the synovial fluid becomes more viscous as the levels of hyaluronate decrease.

References and Selected Bibliography

General

Bourne, G. H. (ed.). 1972. The Biochemistry and Physiology of Bone, 2nd ed., vol. I–IV. New York: Academic Press, Inc.

Frost, H. M. (ed.). 1964. Bone Biodynamics. Boston: Little Brown.

Hancox, N. M. 1972. The Biology of Bone. Cambridge: Cambridge University Press.

Johnson, L. C. 1964. Morphologic analysis in pathology: The kinetics of disease and general biology of bone. In Bone Biodynamics, Frost, H. M. (ed.). Boston: Little Brown, p. 543.

Lacroix, P. 1949. L' Organisation des Os. Paris: Masson et Cie.

McLean, F. C., and Urist, M. R. 1968. Bone, An Introduction to the Physiology of Skeletal Tissue, 3rd ed. Chicago: The University of Chicago Press.

Rasmussen, H., and Bordier, P. 1974. The Physiological and Cellular Basis of Metabolic Bone Disease. Baltimore: Williams & Wilkins.

Simmons, D. J., and Kunin, A. S. 1979. Skeletal Research: An Experimental Approach. New York: Academic Press.

Sokoloff, L., and Bland, J. H. 1975. The Musculoskeletal System. Baltimore: Williams & Wilkins Co.

Vaughan, J. M. 1981. The Physiology of Bone. Oxford: Clarendon Press.

Origin of Bone Cells

Fischman, D. A., and Hay, E. D. 1962. Origin of osteoclast from mononuclear leucocytes in regenerating new limbs. Anat. Rec. 143:329.

Friedenstein, A. J. 1973. Determined and inducable osteogenic precursor cells. In Hard Tissue, Growth, Repair, and Remineralization, Ciba Foundation Symposium II (New Series). Amsterdam: Excerpta Medica, p. 169.

Jee, W. S. S., and Nolan, P. N. 1963. Origin of osteoclasts from fusion of phagocytes. Nature 200:225.

Kimmel, D. B., and Jee, W. S. S. 1980. Bone cell kinetics during longitudinal bone growth in the rat. Calcif. Tis. Int. 32:123.

Owen, M. 1978. Histogenesis of bone cells. Calcif. Tis. Res. 25:205.

Scott, B. L. 1967. Thymidine-^{3}H electron microscope radioautography of osteogenic cells in the fetal rat. J. Cell Biol. 35:115.

Walker, D. G. 1973. Osteopetrosis cured by temporary parabiosis. Science 180:875.

Young, R. W. 1962. Cell proliferation and specialization during endochondral osteogenesis in young rats. J. Cell Biol. 14:357.

Growth and Development

Arnold, J. S., and Jee, W. S. S. 1957. Bone growth and osteoclastic activity as indicated by radioautographic distribution of plutonium. Am. J. Anat. 101:367.

Frost, H. M. 1972. The Physiology of Cartilaginous, Fibrous and Bony Tissue. Orthopaedic Lectures, vol. II. Springfield, Ill.: C. C. Thomas.

Frost, H. M. 1973. Bone Modeling and Skeletal Modeling Errors. Springfield, Ill.: C. C. Thomas.

Hall, B. K. 1978. Developmental and Cellular Skeletal Biology. New York: Academic Press, Inc.

Johnson, L. C. 1966. The kinetics of skeletal remodeling. In The Structural Organization of the Skeletal, Birth Defects, original article series, Milch, R. A.

(ed.). New York: The National Foundation March of Dimes, p. 66.

Bone Remodeling

Frost, H. M. 1973. Bone Remodeling and Its Relationship to Metabolic Bone Diseases. Springfield, Ill.: C. C. Thomas.

Parfitt, A. M. 1979. Quantum concept of bone remodeling and turnover: Implications for the pathogenesis of osteoporosis. Calcif. Tis. Res. 28:1.

Histomorphometry

Frost, H. M. 1969. Tetracycline-based histological analysis of bone remodeling. Calcif. Tis. Res. 3:211.

Jaworski, Z. F. G. (ed.) 1976. Bone Morphometry. Ottawa, Canada: University of Ottawa Press.

Jee, W. S. S., and Parfitt, A. M. (eds.). 1981. Bone Histomorphometry. Paris: Société Nouvelle de Publications Médicales et Dentaires.

Kimmel, D. B., and Jee, W. S. S. 1980. A quantative histologic analysis of growing long bone metaphysis. Calcif. Tis. Int. 32:113.

Merz, W. A., and Schenk, R. K. 1970. Quantitative structural analysis of human cancellous bone. Acta Anat. 75:54.

Meunier, P. J. (ed.). 1979. Bone Histomorphometry. Paris, France: Societé Nouvelle de Publications Medicales et Dentaires.

Parfitt, A. M. 1982. The physiologic and clinical significance of bone histomorphometric data. In Bone Histomorphometry Techniques and Interpretation, Recker, R. R. (ed.). Boca Raton, Florida: CRC Press, Inc.

Physiology

Aurbach, G. D. (ed.). 1976. Parathyroid Gland. Handbook of Physiology, vol. 7, Am. Phys. Soc. Baltimore: Williams & Wilkins.

Ibbotson, K. J., D'Souza, S., M., Kanis, J.A, Douglas, D. L., and Russell, R. G. G. 1980. Physiological and pharmacological regulation of bone resorption. Metab. Bone Dis. Rel. Res. 2:177.

Marshall, J. H., Lloyd, E. L., Rundo, J., Liniecki, J., Marotti, G., Mays, C. W., Sissons, H. A., and Snyder, W. S. 1973. Alkaline earth metabolism in adult man. Health Phys. 24:125.

Neuman, W. F., and Neuman, M. W. 1958. The Chemical Dynamics of Bone Mineral. Chicago: University of Chicago Press.

Parfitt, A. M. 1976. The actions of parathyroid hormone on bone. Relation to bone remodeling and turnover, calcium homeostasis and metabolic bone disease. I–IV. Metabolism 25:809, 909, 1033, and 1157.

Rasmussen, H., and Bordier, P. 1978. Vitamin D and bone. Metab. Bone Dis. Rel. Res. 1:7.

Talmage, R. V. 1970. Morphological and physiological considerations in a new concept of calcium transport of bone. Am. J. Anat. 129:467.

Osteoporosis

DeLuca, H. F., Frost, H. M., Jee, W. S. S., Johnston, C. C., and Parfitt, A. M. (eds.). 1981. Osteoporosis: Advances in Pathogenesis and Treatment. Baltimore: University Park Press.

Frost, H. M. 1979. Treatment of osteoporoses by manipulation of coherent bone cell populations. Clin. Orthop. 143:277.

Metabolic Bone Diseases

Avioli, L. V., and Krane, S. M. 1977, 1978. Metabolic Bone Disease, vols. I and II. New York: Academic Press, Inc.

Frame, B., Parfitt, A. M., and Duncan, H. (eds.). 1973. Clinical Aspects of Metabolic Bone Diseases. Amsterdam: Excerpta Medica.

Harris, W. H., and Heaney, R. P. 1969. Skeletal renewal and metabolic bone disease. N. Engl. J. Med. 28:253.

Jowsey, J. 1977. Metabolic Disease of Bone. Philadelphia: W. B. Saunders.

Nordin, B. E. C. 1973. Metabolic Bone and Stone Disease. Baltimore: Williams and Wilkins.

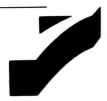

The Muscular Tissue

Geraldine F. Gauthier

The function of movement in multicellular organisms is usually assumed by specialized cells, called muscle fibers, which contract on appropriate stimulation. This property is also seen in other structures such as cilia and flagella. These various motile systems have in common the ability to transform chemical into mechanical energy by enzymatically splitting ATP, and each possesses precisely arranged filamentous proteins. Comparable proteins have now been implicated in motility in a wide variety of cell systems. In muscle cells, filaments are oriented parallel to the direction of movement and, because of their precise arrangement, constitute the actual contractile machinery of the cell. In the vertebrate body, three types of muscle are distinguished on the basis of the appearance and location of their constituent cells: smooth, skeletal, and cardiac. All three types are composed of asymmetric cells, or fibers, with the long axis arranged in the direction of movement.

Smooth muscle, which is the simplest in appearance of the three types, consists of narrow and relatively short tapering cells, each with a single centrally located nucleus. This type of muscle occurs in the walls of the viscera and hence is often called *visceral* or *involuntary* muscle. Skeletal muscle is associated, as the name implies, with the body skeleton. The cells are greatly elongated, and each contains many peripheral nuclei. Because of the conspicuous transverse striations of the individual cells, skeletal muscle is also referred to as *striated* muscle. It is controlled by the somatic nervous system and hence is often called *voluntary* muscle. Car-

diac muscle is a highly specialized form of *involuntary striated* muscle found only in the heart and, in some species, in the walls of the pulmonary vein. It is similar to skeletal muscle in that the cells are transversely striated and multinuclear but, as in smooth muscle, the nuclei are centrally located.

The descriptions that follow, emphasize the appearance of muscle as it occurs in the mammal. Reference will be made to other vertebrate classes, however, particularly where information is otherwise limited. Skeletal muscle will be considered in particular detail, since it has been the primary source of data on relationships between structure and function. Cardiac muscle will be considered in a separate chapter.

Skeletal Muscle

General Features

Skeletal muscle (Fig. 7–1) consists of long bundles of more or less parallel cells called *muscle fibers.* Cross-sectional dimensions (see Fig. 7–7) vary from about 10 to 100 μm. In longitudinal section, these cells are clearly marked by transverse striations (Figs. 7–2 and 7–3), and nuclei are located just beneath the cell membrane, or

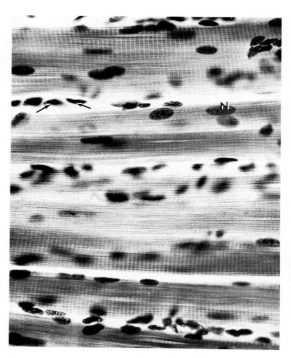

7–2 Longitudinal section of several skeletal muscle fibers (cat tongue). Each fiber is characterized by a transverse pattern of alternating dark A bands and light I bands, repeated along the length of the fiber. In certain areas, individual myofibrils can be recognized by their longitudinal orientation. Nuclei **(N)** are located at the periphery of the fibers. Angular structures **(arrows)** between fibers are distorted red blood cells present within capillaries, which closely invest individual muscle fibers. Iron-hematoxylin. × 560.

7–1 Longitudinal organization of skeletal muscle. Dimensions are based on rabbit psoas muscle. (From Huxley, H. E. 1960. *In* Brachet, J., and Mirsky, A. E. (eds.), The Cell, vol. 4. New York: Academic Press, Inc.)

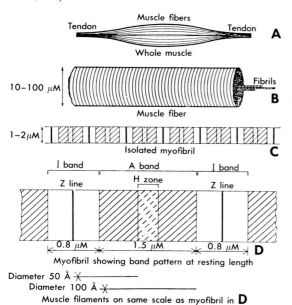

sarcolemma. The fibers contain smaller parallel units about 1 to 3 μm in diameter, the *myofibrils,* which are also transversely striated (Fig. 7–1 and 7–4) and are composed, in turn, of *myofilaments* visible only with the electron microscope (Fig. 7–5). The myofilaments are not transversely striated but are responsible for the striations because of their arrangement within the myofibril (Fig. 7–6).

Skeletal muscles are attached to bony structures by tendons, which are continuous with a covering of connective tissue over the entire muscle, the *epimysium.* This outermost connective tissue extends into the muscle and surrounds bundles, or *fascicles,* of muscle fibers, forming the *perimysium,* which eventually divides into a delicate sheath of reticular fibers around each muscle fiber called the *endomysium.* Blood vessels and nerves follow these

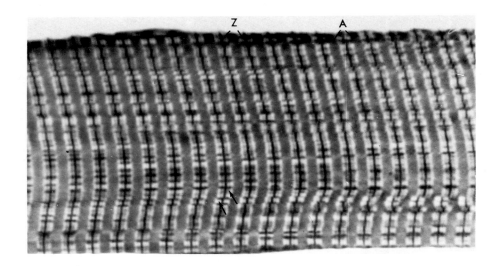

7–3 Longitudinal section of a single muscle fiber
△ (guinea pig plantaris). The transverse banding
pattern is clearly resolved, and part of a peripheral
nucleus is visible at the upper left of the fiber. A
bands are dark; I bands are light and are bisected by a
very dark, narrow Z line. The precise alignment of
paired mitochondria **(arrows)** in transverse rows over
the I bands, on either side of each Z line, creates the
impression of an additional interrupted dark band in
this position. Toluidine blue. × 1,900.

7–4 Electron micrograph of a portion of a fiber (rat
▽ semitendinosus). Several myofibrils are present
in this longitudinal section, and at least two
sarcomeres are included in each myofibril. The regular
arrangement of transverse bands in each myofibril
gives rise to the banding pattern of the whole fiber
seen with the light microscope (Fig. 7–3). Profiles of
paired mitochondria **(arrows)** are present on either
side of the electron-opaque Z line (see also Fig. 7–5).
× 17,500.

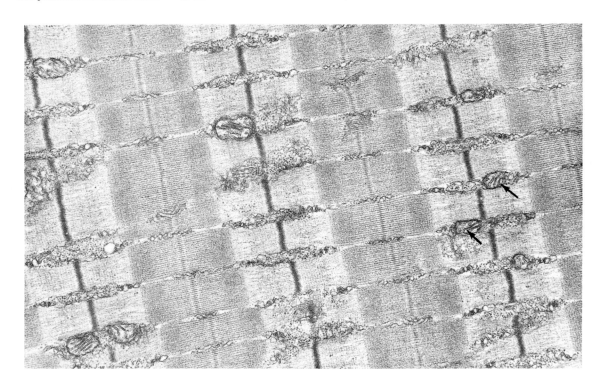

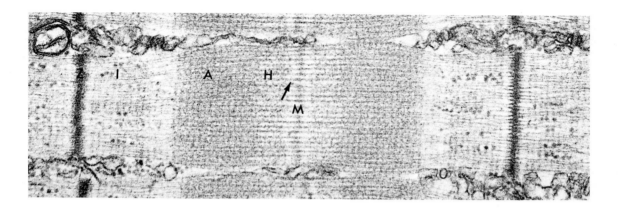

7–5 Single sarcomere from a preparation similar to that in Fig. 7–4. The conspicuous Z line marks the longitudinal extent of this structural and functional unit. The myofilaments, which compose the myofibrils, are visible, but their arrangement is more readily apparent in Fig. 7–6. All the major transverse bands can be seen in this micrograph, including the pseudo H band **(arrow)**, which is often confused with the H band. Glycogen particles occur among the filaments of the I-band region. × 48,000.

sheaths into the interior of the muscle, and a rich capillary network closely invests each muscle fiber.

Skeletal muscle fibers also contain a cytoplasm, or *sarcoplasm*, which occupies the limited space between the abundant myofibrils. Muscle fibers are conventionally depicted in longitudinal section, and emphasis is usually placed on the myofibrillar component. However, mitochondria are usually conspicuous components of

7–6 Sarcomere from rabbit psoas muscle that has been glycerinated, removing soluble components of the sarcoplasm. In this type of preparation, it is possible to discern the organization of myofilaments, which constitutes the ultrastructural basis of transverse banding in the myofibril. In the A band, there is a simple alternation of thick and thin filaments in this particular plane of section, and in the I band there are only thin filaments. The thick filaments

extend to the limits of the A band, where their ends become tapered **(arrow)**. The thin filaments extend from each Z line through both the I band and A band, but terminate at the H band. Bridgelike structures (myosin cross-bridges) extend radially from the surfaces of the thick filaments. Six such structures are arranged in a helical pattern that is repeated every 400 Å along the thick filament (see Fig. 7–19). × 128,000. (From Huxley, H. E. 1957. J. Biophys. Biochem. Cytol. 3:631.)

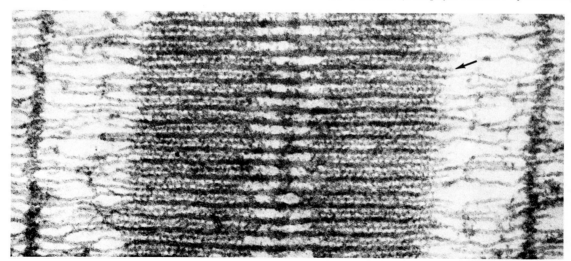

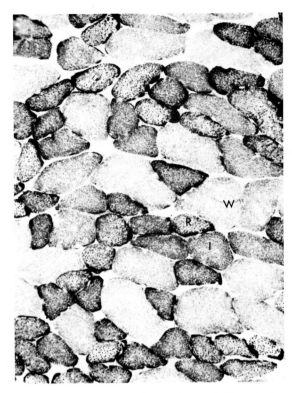

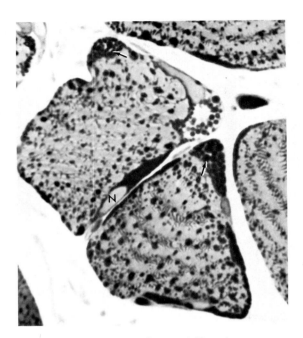

7–7 Transverse section of several muscle fibers (rat diaphragm), showing the localization of succinic dehydrogenase activity. Reaction product reflects the location of mitochondria. Small (red) fibers **(R)** are rich in mitochondria, especially along the periphery; large (white) fibers **(W)** have a low mitochondrial content; and intermediate fibers **(I)** have characteristics between the two. × 200.

7–8 Transverse section of two red fibers (rat diaphragm), illustrating the distribution of mitochondria, which are stained darkly with toluidine blue. The myofibrils appear relatively unstained. Large circular profiles of mitochondria form conspicuous peripheral aggregations **(arrows)** at sites where enzymatic activity is demonstrated (Fig. 7–7) and are also abundant in the interior of the fibers. Nuclei (N) appear in negative image. × 1,200. (From Gauthier, G. F. 1970. *In* E. J. Briskey, Cassens, R. G., and Marsh, B. B. [eds.]. The Physiology and Biochemistry of Muscle as a Food, Vol. 2. Madison: The University of Wisconsin Press, p. 103.)

the sarcoplasm (Figs. 7–7 and 7–8). Interfibrillar mitochondria are arranged in pairs at regular intervals in relation to the banding pattern of the myofibrils (Figs. 7–3 and 7–4). These paired mitochondria, characteristic of mammalian skeletal muscle fibers in general, encircle the myofibrils at the level of the I bands (see Fig. 7–28B). Their arrangement is readily visible in transverse sections of the muscle fibers (Fig. 7–9), where they appear as filamentous profiles. In longitudinal sections of the fibers (Figs. 7–3 and 7–4), these mitochondria are usually sectioned transversely and thus appear as elliptical profiles on either side of the Z line. In a tangential section through a myofibril, mitochondrial profiles extend transversely across the I bands (see Fig. 7–29). In certain types of fibers, mitochondria also form more continuous longitudinal rows and subsarcolemmal aggregations (see Fig. 7–36), which are apparent in transverse as well as in longitudinal sections (Figs. 7–7 and 7–8).

The sarcoplasm also contains an elaborate membrane system, the *sarcoplasmic reticulum*, which surrounds individual myofibrils (Figs. 7–9 and 7–10). This system will be discussed in a later section. In addition, a Golgi apparatus is present in the perinuclear sarcoplasm. Glycogen, in the form of β particles, is abundant between myofibrils, particularly in the region of the I bands, and it occurs within the myofibrils as well (Figs. 7–5, 7–9, and 7–10). Lipid droplets are frequently closely associated with large mi-

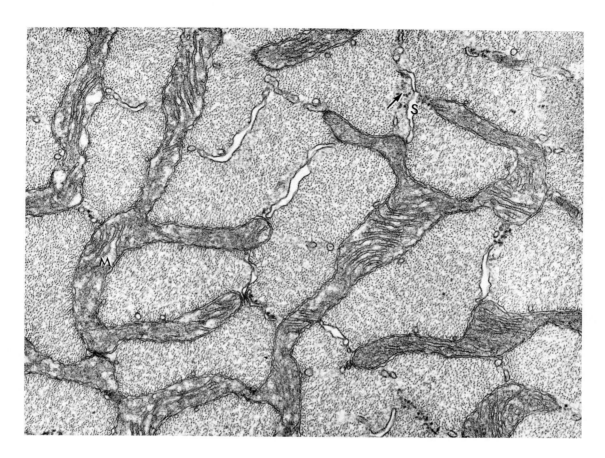

tochondria (see Fig. 7–36). Both lipid and glycogen provide metabolic fuel for the contractile machinery.

Composition of the Myofibril

The banding pattern of the skeletal muscle fiber reflects the ultrastructural organization of each myofibril. Knowledge of this pattern is fundamental to understanding the mechanism of contraction. *The two largest bands are named according to their appearance in polarized light* (Figs. 7–11 and 7–12). Certain bands exhibit positive birefringence, which reflects a parallel arrangement of asymmetric subunits. These birefringent or anisotropic bands are called *A bands* and are bright when viewed with a polarizing microscope (Fig. 7–12). They alternate with dark isotropic *I bands*, and the pattern is repeated along the length of the myofibril. Each A band has a less birefringent central zone called the *H band*, and each I band is bisected by a distinct

7–9 Electron micrograph of a transverse section (rat semitendinosus). The section passes through the I band and, therefore, through only the thin filaments that compose this part of the sarcomere. Bracelet-like mitochondria (**M**) encircle individual myofibrils; these mitochondria appear as paired elliptical profiles on either side of the Z line in longitudinal sections of a muscle fiber (Figs. 7–3 and 7–4). In addition, profiles of the sarcoplasmic membrane systems (**S**) surround individual myofibrils, and clusters of glycogen particles (**arrow**) occur close to them. × 42,000.

Z line. The M line marks the center of the H band, and in some instances (in insect muscle, for example), an N line is apparent on either side of the Z line. When viewed with phase-contrast optics (Fig. 7–11) or with ordinary light after staining with a cationic dye (Figs. 7–2 and 7–3), the banding pattern appears reversed. That is, the A band and Z line are basophilic or dark and the I and H bands are light. The various bands

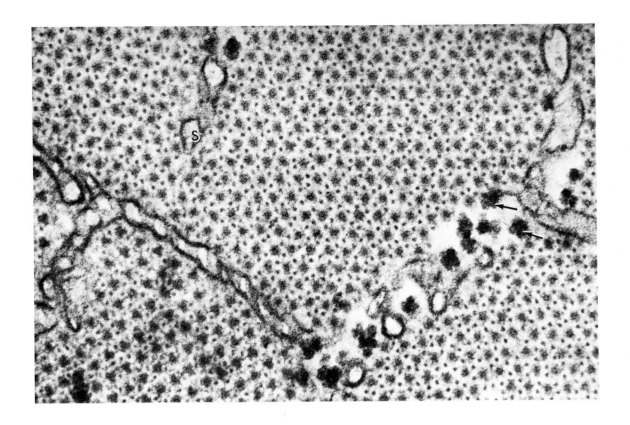

7–10 Transverse section through the A-band region
△ (frog sartorius). Both thick and thin filaments
are present, and each thick filament is surrounded by
six thin filaments, giving rise to a precise hexagonal
array. The presence of cross-bridges imparts a rough
surface to the thick filaments. Myofibrillar boundaries
are marked by profiles of the sarcoplasmic reticulum
(S) and by glycogen particles **(arrows).** × 150,000.
(From Huxley, H. E. 1968. J. Mol. Biol. 37:507.)

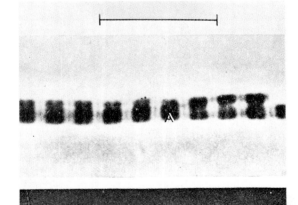

7–11 (upper) A single isolated myofibril (glycerinated
7–12 (lower) rabbit psoas), illustrating the banding
pattern with phase-contrast optics and
with polarized light. In the phase-contrast image (Fig.
7–11), the A band and Z line are dark and the I band
is light. When viewed with polarized light (Fig. 7–12),
the A band and Z line are bright and the I band is
dark. (From Hanson, J., and Huxley, H. E. 1955. *In*
Fibrous Proteins and Their Biological Significance,
No. 9, Symposia of the Society for Experimental
Biology. New York: Academic Press, Inc.) ▷

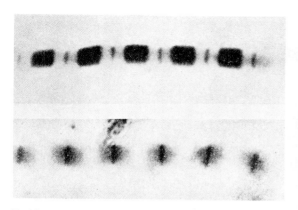

7–13 (upper) Single myofibril (glycerinated rabbit
7–14 (lower) psoas) photographed with phase-contrast
optics showing the appearance before
(Fig. 7–13) and after (Fig. 7–14) extraction of myosin.
Following removal of myosin, the density of the A
band is decreased but that of the I band and the Z line
remains. (From Hanson, J., and Huxley, H. E. 1955. *In*
Fibrous Proteins and Their Biological Significance,
No. 9, Symposia of the Society for Experimental
Biology. New York: Academic Press, Inc.)

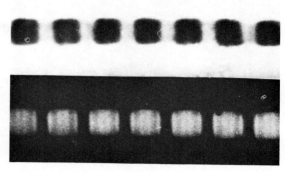

7–15 (upper) Myofibril (chicken breast muscle) treated
7–16 (lower) with a fluorescent antibody to myosin
and photographed using phase-contrast
(Fig. 7–15) and fluorescence (Fig. 7–16) microscopy.
The site of fluorescence (antimyosin) in Fig. 7–16
corresponds to the dark (A band) in Fig. 7–15. (From
Pepe, F. A. 1966. J. Cell Biol. 28:505.)

also usually appear this way in electron micrographs (Figs. 7–4 and 7–5), but the appearance with polarized light is the basis for the more widely used nomenclature. The segment between two successive Z lines is called a *sarcomere* (Fig. 7–5) and is approximately 2 to 3 μm long, with the A band contributing 1.5 μm and each full I band, about 0.8 μm. This structural and functional unit is repeated along the length of the myofibril.

Biochemical analysis shows that the myofibril consists of a number of proteins. Two of these, *myosin* and *actin*, account for most of the dry weight of the myofibril. Their interaction to form *actomyosin* is fundamental to myofibrillar contraction. Two other proteins, *tropomyosin* and *troponin*, have a regulatory role in the contractile process. Troponin, in particular, inhibits the formation of actomyosin when the calcium level is low (see Cohen, 1975). It is also possible to localize some of these proteins within the sarcomere. If, for example, myosin is extracted from a preparation of myofibrils, the density of the A band is diminished (Figs. 7–13 and 7–14), indicating that myosin is located in this region. The fluorescent antibody technique has become an increasingly useful tool for localizing muscle

proteins. An antibody to myosin, for example, is conjugated with a fluorescent dye, and this complex is allowed to interact with a preparation of myofibrils. The complex becomes bound to the site where myosin is located, and the fluorescence serves as a visual marker. The site of fluorescence, and therefore of myosin, is the A-band region of the myofibril (Figs. 7–15 and 7–16). With similar procedures, actin can be demonstrated in the I band along with troponin and tropomyosin.

Ultrastructurally, the myofibril is composed of two major types of filaments, one thicker than the other (Figs. 7–6 and 7–10). When extracted myofibrils are examined with the electron microscope, loss of myosin is associated with loss of the thick filaments, which indicates that the thick filaments are composed largely of myosin. The thin filaments, on the other hand, are composed primarily of actin. In 1957, H. E. Huxley demonstrated the exact arrangement of these filaments, which established the ultrastructural basis of the banding pattern and of the contractile mechanism as well. In the A band, thick (approximately 150 Å) filaments alternate with thin (50 Å) filaments (Figs. 7–6 and 7–10). The thick filaments are 1.5 μm long and extend only to the limits of the A band, where their ends become tapered. The thin filaments, however, extend from each Z line for a distance of 1 μm through the I band and into the A band. They are

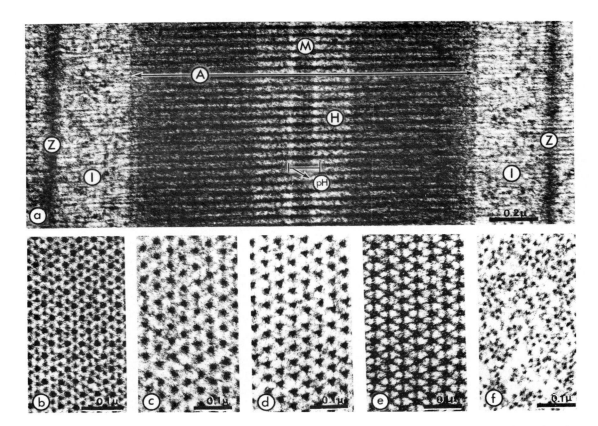

7–17 Single sarcomere (fish muscle) in longitudinal section **(a),** showing transverse banding pattern together with corresponding transverse sections through each of the bands. The A band **(A)** consists of both thick and thin filaments **(b),** the H band **(H)** and the bridge-free pseudo H band **(pH),** only of thick filaments (**c** and **d,** respectively). The M band **(M)** also contains thick filaments, but conspicuous transverse extensions (M bridges) are present as well **(e).** In the I band **(I)** only thin filaments are present **(f).** (From Pepe, F. A. 1976. *In* Timasheff, B. N., and Fasman, G. D. (eds.), Biological Macromolecules Series, vol. 5, part A. New York: Marcel Dekker, Inc., chap. 7.)

absent from the H band. The banding pattern therefore results from the presence or absence of overlap between the two sets of filaments (Figs. 7–6, 7–17, and 7–18). The A band, relatively dense when viewed with the light microscope, consists of both thick and thin filaments (Figs. 7–6 and 7–10). The less dense I band consists only of thin filaments (Figs. 7–6 and 7–9), and the H band, only of thick filaments (Fig. 7–17a and c). In transverse section, the filaments appear as more or less circular profiles in a remark-

ably precise hexagonal pattern. In the A-band region, where the two sets of filaments overlap, each thick (myosin) filament is surrounded by six thin (actin) filaments (Figs. 7–10, 7–17b, and 7–18). In addition, a series of bridgelike structures extends radially from the thick filaments toward the thin filaments (Figs. 7–6, 7–10, 7–17b, and 7–18). Six of these bridges are arranged around each thick filament in a helical pattern that is repeated about every 400 Å along the length of the thick filament (Fig. 7–19). The absence of bridges from the center of the H band produces an area of lower density often confused with the H band itself; this is called the *pseudo H band* (Fig. 7–17a and d). The bridges, which are part of the myosin molecule, possess ATPase activity, and play a major role in the interaction of actin and myosin during contraction (see below).

The M line reflects a structural modification at the center of the thick filament. Six radially arranged extensions are connected with six adjacent thick filaments in a transverse plane (Fig. 7–17e). It is likely that additional elements link these components together, but the structural

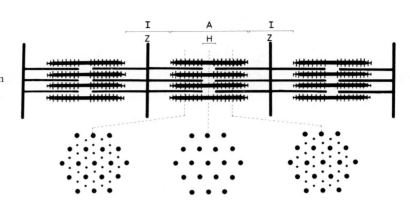

7–18 Diagrammatic interpretation of the organization of filaments giving rise to the transverse banding pattern. (From Huxley, H. E. 1969. Science (Washington, D. C.) 164:1356.)

configuration is not certain (see Luther and Squire, 1978). The precise register of this pattern across the myofibril gives rise to a narrow, relatively electron-opaque band at the center of each sarcomere when viewed in longitudinal section (Figs. 7–5 and 7–17a). These so-called M bridges are not composed of myosin and should not be confused with the cross-bridges located in the A band proper (see below). The function of the M line is not clear, but it may contribute to the ordered arrangement of thick filaments within the sarcomere.

Perhaps the least understood structural component of the myofibril is the Z line. The thin filaments composing the I band are arranged so

7–19 Diagram illustrating the helical organization of cross-bridges along the thick filament. The arrangement of six successive bridges corresponds to the 400-Å intervals observed in electron micrographs of sectioned muscle fibers. (From Huxley, H. E., and Brown, W. 1967. J. Mol. Biol. 30:383.)

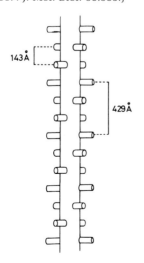

143Å

429Å

that, in longitudinal sections of the myofibril, each thin filament on one side of the Z line faces the space between two thin filaments on the opposite side, and connecting elements appear to run obliquely across the Z line, creating a zigzag appearance (Fig. 7–20). In myofibrils sectioned

7–20 Appearance of the Z line in a longitudinal section of a myofibril (rat semitendinosus). Each I-band filament on one side of the Z line faces the space between two filaments on the opposite side, and there appear to be filamentous structures connecting these filaments obliquely within the Z line itself. × 117,000.

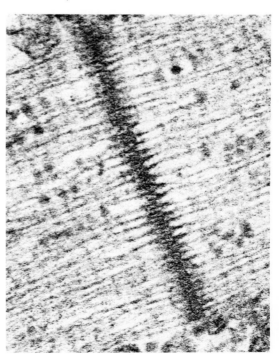

transversely, filamentous components in the region of the Z line form a tetragonal pattern. On the basis of studies of amphibian muscle, it appears that each terminating I-band filament forms the apex of a pyramid whose base is a square formed by four I-band filaments from the opposite side of the Z line. The sides of the pyramid are formed by the oblique structures composing the Z line itself. The arrangement in mammalian muscle is even more complex. A number of models have been proposed, but none has been fully satisfactory. Actin, tropomyosin, and α-actinin appear to be the major proteins of the Z line, but otherwise the chemical and structural composition remains puzzling.

The Ultrastructural Basis of Contraction

Early observation with the light microscope showed that during contraction the sarcomere becomes shorter. The I band in particular decreases in length, but the length of the A band does not change. The mechanism by which this occurs can be explained by the ultrastructure of the sarcomere. The extent to which the thick and thin filaments overlap accounts for the change observed with the light microscope. X-ray diffraction data and direct observation with the elctron microscope have established that as the sarcomere shortens, the thin filaments of adjacent I bands are pulled toward the center of the A band, thereby obliterating the H band and decreasing the width of the I band (Fig. 7–21). According to this so-called *sliding filament hypothesis* (Hanson and Huxley, 1955), the A band maintains its original length because the thick and thin filaments themselves do not shorten. The detailed events that take place as actin and myosin combine and chemical energy is converted to mechanical energy are not fully understood, but recent studies of the molecular basis of contraction are rapidly adding new information. The evidence suggests that the bridges move toward the actin filaments, engage them, and cause them to move along the myosin filament (see Huxley, 1969.)

The Molecular Configuration of the Myofilaments

Myosin can be enzymatically cleaved into two fragments, called light meromyosin (LMM) and heavy meromyosin (HMM). The former provides

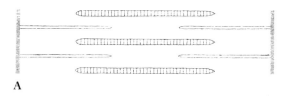

A

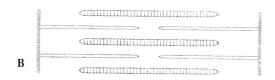

B

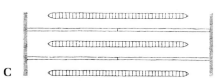

C

7–21 Diagram illustrating how the thin filaments of the I band may be pulled progressively toward the center of the A band during contraction, thereby decreasing the width of the I band (**B** and **C**) and eventually obliterating the H band (**C**). The sarcomere in **B** is at resting length; in **A** it is stretched; and in **C**, contracted. (From Huxley, H. E. 1958. Sci. Am. 199[5]:66.)

the linear "backbone" of the myosin molecule, whereas part of the latter projects outward from this backbone at regular intervals. Arrangement of LMM units parallel to one another but in a slightly staggered fashion (Fig. 7–23A) would permit the HMM units to occur at intervals of about 400 Å, thereby accounting for the spacing of bridges seen with the electron microscope and the periodicity of skeletal muscle observed by x-ray diffraction (429 Å). Each visible bridge, therefore, reflects a portion of a single HMM unit. Electron micrographs of synthetic filaments prepared form purified myosin confirm this arrangement. Such preparations consist of tapered filaments, approximately 150 Å in diameter and 1.5 μm long, each resembling intact A-band filaments with their bridgelike projections (Figs. 7–22 and 7–23A). Under appropriate conditions, the molecules are aligned with their HMM portions polarized toward either end of the filament, leaving a bare zone that is equivalent to

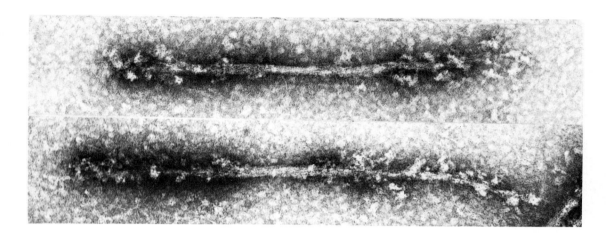

the bridge-free zone in the intact sarcomere. The HMM fragment of myosin can be further cleaved into two proteolytic subfragments (see Lowey, 1971). One of these, HMM S-2, is attached in series with the LMM "backbone," forming the so-called rod portion of the molecule. The other subfragment, HMM S-1, represents the two "heads" that extend at an angle from the rod (Fig. 7–23B). There are, in addition, low-molecular-weight subunits, or "light chains" that are non-covalently bound to the head region, each head having two moles of light chain. Their role in

7–22 Purified myosin, showing two examples of synthetic filaments aggregated at low ionic strength. Projections correspond to bridgelike structures seen in intact myofibrils (Fig. 7–6), and the bare central zone corresponds to the bridge-free pseudo H band. × 145,000. (From Huxley, H. E. 1963. J. Mol. Biol. 7:281.)

vertebrate skeletal muscle is not clear but, in certain invertebrate muscles and in vertebrate smooth muscle, light chains are involved in regulating contractile activity, which is dependent on calcium concentration.

Preparations of pure actin can form thin filaments whose dimensions are comparable to intact I-band filaments. Each filament consists of a two-stranded helix with a turn approximately every 360 Å. The periodicity of actin is therefore close but not equal to that of myosin. The individual strands (F-actin) composing the helix are actually a linear array of globular units called G-actin (Fig. 7–24). Although the periodicity of actin is 360 Å, that of the I band itself is actually greater, approximately 400 Å. This most likely reflects the arrangement of troponin and tropomyosin in the I band. The regulatory proteins are closely associated with actin in the thin filament. Tropomyosin occupies the groove formed by the twisted double strands of actin, and troponin is confined to more circumscribed sites along the filament (Fig. 7–25). These proteins prevent contraction in the absence of calcium. When the level of calcium is low, tropomyosin is situated more peripherally along the thin filament and thus blocks G-actin monomers from interacting with myosin. When the level of calcium is suffi-

7–23 **A.** Diagrammatic interpretation of the arrangement of myosin molecules giving rise to the myosin filament, based on images such as those seen in Fig. 7–22. LMM units are parallel to the longitudinal axis of the filament, and HMM units extend at right angles from them. (From Huxley, H. E. 1963. J. Mol. Biol. 7:281.) **B.** Schematic representation of the myosin molecule. (From Lowey, S., et al. 1969. J. Mol. Biol. 42:1.)

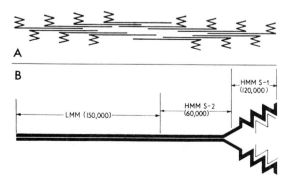

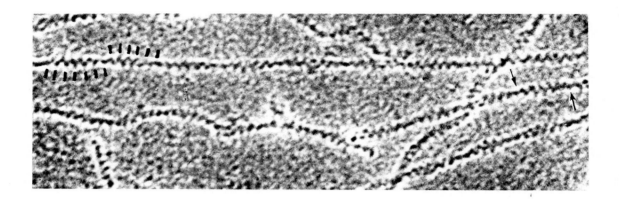

7–24 Purified F-actin showing the beaded appearance **(arrows)** of several filaments and the helical arrangement of strands of G-actin monomers. × 525,000. (From Hanson, J., and Lowy, J. 1963. J. Mol. Biol. 6:46.)

ciently high, calcium binds to troponin, which causes the tropomyosin molecule to move into the groove, occupying the position shown in Fig. 7–25. Previously blocked sites on the actin filament are thus made available for eventual contact with myosin heads (see below).

When pure HMM or HMM S-1 is added to a preparation of F-actin, the fragments attach precisely to the F-actin filaments (Fig. 7–26), and the complex has a 360-Å periodicity, which is characteristic of actin. This molecular interaction suggests that in whole muscle, the HMM or bridge portion of the thick filament makes physical contact with the thin filament at the start of contraction. The polarity of the attachment, moreover, is consistent with the ability of the filaments to slide in one specific direction. It is postulated that the HMM or bridge portion

7–25 Diagrammatic interpretation of the organization of actin, troponin, and tropomyosin to form the I-band filament. Globular monomers of G-actin are arranged in rows forming a two-stranded helix, which corresponds to the structures visible in Fig. 7–24. (From Ebashi, S., et al. 1969. Q. Rev. Biophys. 2:351.)

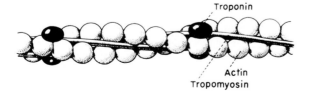

swings out radially toward an adjacent thin filament while maintaining its base in the myosin filament (Fig. 7–27).

The Sarcoplasmic Membrane Systems

Each myofibril is surrounded by an elaborate system of membranes aligned precisely with respect to the banding pattern of the myofibrils (Figs. 7–28A and B and 7–29). It is apparent that a relationship exists between the sarcoplasmic membranes and the conduction of the impulse leading to contraction. The complex arrangement of tubules and cisternae that compose this system is best understood in the relatively simple form that exists in certain amphibian muscles (Fig. 7–28A). A parallel array of tubules is oriented along the long axis of the myofibril. They extend along the full length of the A band and most of the I-band region of each sarcomere and fuse in the region of the H band to form a fenestrated cisterna. As the tubules approach the Z lines at each end of the sarcomere, they join to form greatly expanded *terminal cisternae,* which run parallel to each Z line. Each terminal cisterna is faced by an equivalent structure on the opposite side of the Z line. This membrane complex is referred to collectively as the *sarcoplasmic reticulum.* It is associated with a transverse membrane system that originates at the cell surface. Between two terminal cisternae a tubular element runs transversely at the Z line. It extends through the sarcoplasm and is continuous with comparable tubules at the same level of adjacent myofibrils. These transverse tubules compose the *T system,* which is separate from the sarcoplasmic reticulum. Two adjacent cisternae plus the intervening T tubule are called a *triad* (Fig. 7–30).

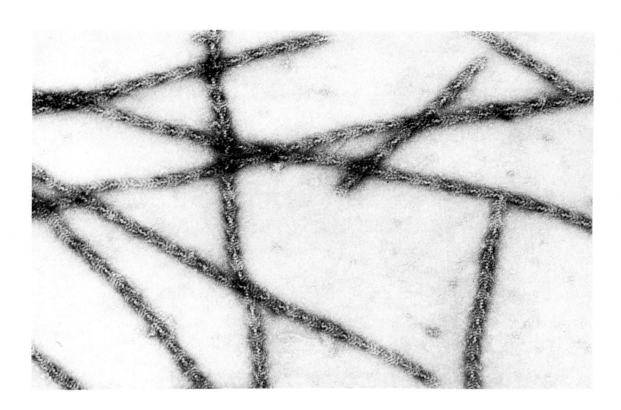

7–26 Isolated thin filaments treated with S-1
△ subfragments of HMM. The bridgelike units
have become attached to the thin filaments at regular
intervals, reflecting the periodicity of F-actin. Note
that the subunits project at an angle from the
filaments and have a definite polarity, which is the
same along the entire length of a given filament.
× 180,000. (From Huxley, H. E., and DeRosier, D. J.
1970. J. Mol. Biol. 50:279.)

7–27 Diagram illustrating a possible mechanism
▽ whereby a HMM bridge can make contact with
a nearby thin filament to bring about a sliding of the
filaments with respect to each other. The LMM unit
remains as part of the thick filament itself, whereas
the HMM portion swings out radially. The S-1
subfragment of the latter is thus brought into contact
with the thin filament. For simplicity, only one
"head" (**S-1**) is depicted but, in fact, each molecule
has two heads. (From Huxley, H. E. 1969. Science
[Wash., D. C.] 164:1356.)

In mammalian skeletal muscle, the general arrangement of these two systems is similar except
that triads are located not at the Z line, but at the
junction of the A and I bands (Fig. 7–28B). An
additional network of tubules connects the terminal cisternae over the intervening I-band and
Z-line regions (Fig. 7–29). In addition, the fused
portion of the system over the H-band region
may be either cisternal or tubular.

Although terminal cisternae and T tubules are
separated from each other, the intervening space
is occupied by regularly spaced densities or
"feet," which are closely associated with the
membranes of both systems. The membrane of
the terminal cisterna may, in some preparations,
be invaginated at regular intervals along the sur-

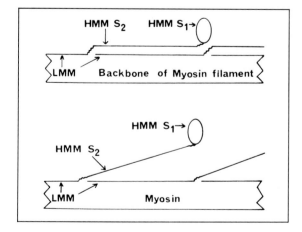

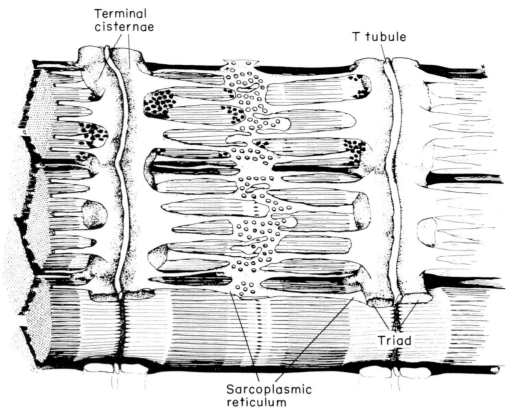

Terminal cisternae

T tubule

Triad

Sarcoplasmic reticulum

7–28 A. Three-dimensional model of the sarcoplasmic membrane systems and their relationship to myofibrils in the frog sartorius muscle. Note that triads (terminal cisternae of the sarcoplasmic reticulum plus the intervening T tubule) in this amphibian muscle are aligned with the Z lines of the myofibrils. Compare with Fig. 7–28B. (From Peachey, L. D.. 1965. J. Cell Biol. 25:209.)

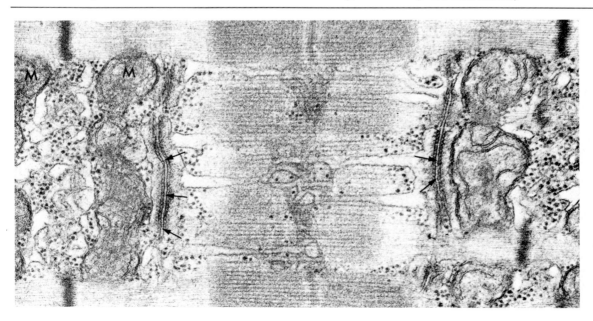

T tubule

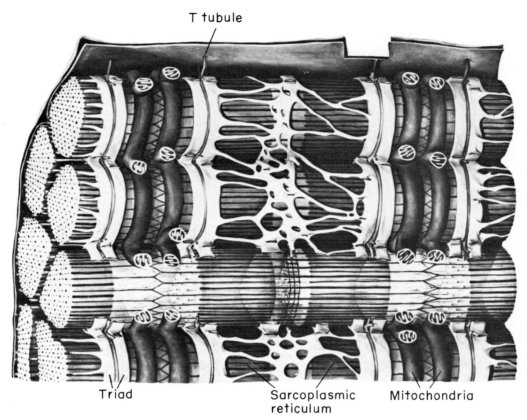

Triad   Sarcoplasmic   Mitochondria
reticulum

7–28 **B.** Three-dimensional model of the sarcoplasmic membrane systems in the rat diaphragm. Note that triads in this *mammalian* muscle are aligned with the A–I junctions in close association with I-band mitochondria. (From Schmalbruch, H. 1970. Advances in Anatomy, Embryology and Cell Biology, Ergeb. Anat. Entwicklungsgesch. 43(1):3. Berlin: Springer-Verlag.)

7–29 Electron micrograph showing tangential section of a single sarcomere (rat diaphragm). The sarcoplasmic reticulum extends over the A band and into the I band and forms a tubular network in the region of the H band. Longitudinal tubules give rise to terminal cisternae closely associated with the transversely oriented T tubule **(arrows).** The triads, in this *mammalian* muscle, are located near the junction of the A and I bands. The part of the sarcoplasmic reticulum that connects with that of the succeeding sarcomere is not fully included in this plane of section. Portions of it are visible between paired I-band mitochondria **(M),** which are closely aligned with the triads. See also Fig. 7–30. × 42,500. (Courtesy of H. A. Padykula.)

face facing the T tubule, and the resulting "scalloped" profile (Fig. 7–30) corresponds to sites where the feet are located.

Various kinds of evidence indicate that the T system is continuous with the plasmalemma of the muscle cell. Electron micrographs of certain fish muscles reveal a direct continuity between the T tubule and the sarcolemma (Fig. 7–31). In addition, when frog muscle fibers are immersed in a solution of ferritin, this electron-opaque protein is subsequently seen within the T tubule, which suggests a functional continuity as well. The form and distribution of the T system would thus permit a wave of depolarization to be rapidly distributed from the cell surface deep into the interior of the fiber to each myofibril. Comparative physiological studies have shown, in fact, that muscle fibers whose triads are located at the Z line can be made to contract when a stimulating electrode is placed at the Z line,

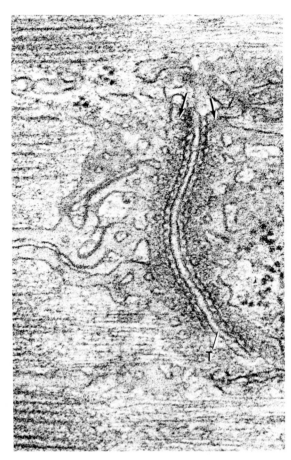

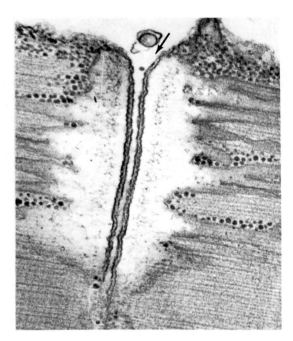

7–31 Single triad (fish muscle) illustrating the direct continuity between the membrane of the T system and the sarcolemma at the upper surface of the fiber **(arrow).** × 60,000. (From Franzini-Armstrong, C., and Porter, K. R. 1964. J. Cell Biol. 22:674.)

7–30 Single triad (rat semitendinosus). The membranes of both terminal cisternae **(arrows)** appear to be "scalloped" along the surface that faces the T tubule **(T)** (see text). At the left, longitudinal tubules of the sarcoplasmic reticulum from the A-band region connect with one of the terminal cisternae. × 94,500.

leads to the interaction of actin and myosin, and thus excitation and contraction are said to be "coupled."

The Neuromuscular Junction

The plasma membrane of the muscle cell, or sarcolemma, is structurally equivelent to the plasma membrane of other cell types, and a typical basal lamina is applied to its outer surface. It is electrically polarized; appropriate stimulation, usually by a nerve fiber, depolarizes the membrane and leads to contraction of the muscle fiber. Branches of each motor nerve fiber terminate at specific sites along the muscle fiber called *neuromuscular junctions*. The relationship between nerve fiber and muscle fiber is intimate and complex (Figs. 7–32 and 7–33). At all points, the plasmalemmae of the two cells remain separate, but the surface of the muscle fiber invaginates to form a shallow trough, the *primary synaptic cleft*, which receives the nerve terminal, or *axonal ending*. The sarcolemma invaginates further

whereas fibers whose triads are located at the A–I junction can be made to contract only if the same electrode is placed at the A–I junction. The manner in which information is transmitted from the T system along the length of the myofibril is less clear, but structural relationships between the T system and the terminal cisternae suggest that there is some form of communication between them (see Franzini-Armstrong, 1980). Ultimately, calcium is released from binding sites in the sarcoplasmic reticulum, probably at the terminal cisternae. Subsequent binding of calcium to the regulatory proteins (see above)

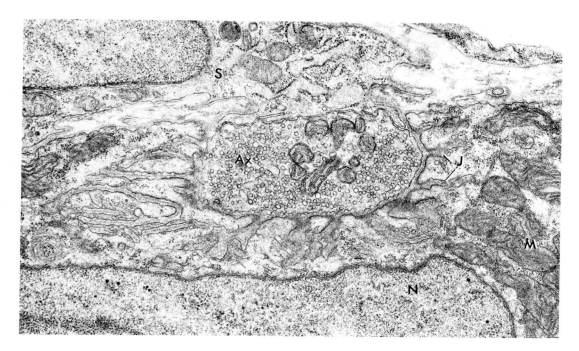

to form numerous deep *secondary synaptic clefts*, or *junctional folds*, which greatly increase the surface area of the muscle fiber (Fig. 7–33). The axon loses its myelin sheath as it approaches the neuromuscular junction, and its basal lamina, together with that of the Schwann cell (see Chap. 8), fuses with that of the muscle fiber. This cell coat extends into the primary synaptic cleft as a single layer, separating nerve fiber from muscle fiber. It enters each junctional fold and forms a coating over its inner surface. The portion of the muscle fiber that contributes to the neuromuscular relationship is called the *muscle sole plate*, or *motor end plate*. Nuclei and mitochondria are particularly abundant in this socalled junctional sarcoplasm. Cisternae of roughsurfaced endoplasmic reticulum and free ribosomes occur in this region also, perhaps in relation to synthesis of a receptor protein. The axonal ending is typically filled with vesicles called *synaptic vesicles*. Mitochondria are present, but filaments and microtubules, characteristic of the more proximal part of the axon, are not. Although myelin is absent from the axon at the neuromuscular juction, a Schwann cell remains closely associated with the axon and forms a covering over the junctional complex (Fig. 7–32). In this way, the axonal ending is enclosed by the Schwann cell on one surface and by the muscle fiber on the other. Processes of the Schwann cell

7–32 Neuromuscular junction of a red fiber (rat diaphragm). The axonal ending **(Ax)** is located in a depression of the surface of the muscle fiber (primary synaptic cleft), and the surface is further invaginated to form junctional folds or secondary synaptic clefts **(J)**. Axonal vesicles and mitochondria are present in the axon. Part of a Schwann cell **(S)** covers the upper surface of the axon, and a nucleus **(N)** and mitochondria **(M)** are present in the sarcoplasm below the axonal ending. Structural organization is more readily apparent in the diagram in Fig. 7–35A. × 22,500. (From Gauthier, G. F. 1970. *In* Briskey, E. J., Cassens, R. G. and Marsh, B. B. [eds.], The Physiology and Biochemistry of Muscle as Food, vol. 2. Madison: University of Wisconsin Press, p. 103.)

may, in addition, be interposed between the axonal ending and basal lamina (Fig. 7–35A).

The neurotransmitter acetylcholine is presumably stored in the numerous synaptic vesicles in the axonal ending. The vesicles tend to be clustered close to dense cytoplasmic bands that occur at intervals along the prejunctional plasma membrane. These so-called active zones are located opposite the openings of the junctional folds in the muscle fiber, and they correspond to sites where acetylcholine is released by exocytosis (Fig. 7–34; see also Figs. 8–76 and 8–78). Substantial evidence suggests that after acetylcholine is released, new synaptic vesicles are

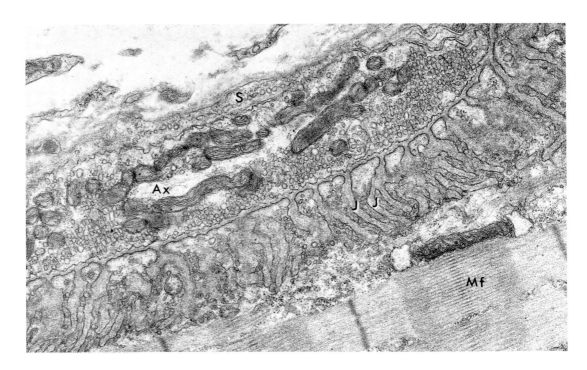

7–33 Neuromuscular junction of a white fiber (rat diaphragm). Junctional folds (**J**) are longer and more closely spaced than in the red fiber (Fig. 7–32), and axonal vesicles are more closely packed. **Ax,** axonal ending; **S,** Schwann cell; **Mf,** myofilaments. ×24,000. (From Padykula, H. A., and Gauthier, G. F. 1970. J. Cell Biol. 46:27.)

formed by a process of "recycling" (see Heuser, 1976). The vesicle membranes become confluent with the presynaptic membrane, and subsequently the membrane is returned by endocytosis to the axonal ending. A major structural element in this process is a system of coated vesicles (Fig. 7–35B). Released neurotransmitter is transported across the synaptic cleft where it interacts with receptor molecules in the postsynaptic membrane, principally near the entrance to the junctional folds. Recent experiments using freeze-fracture techniques have revealed that specific particles, believed to be the receptors for acetylcholine, occur on the outermost surface of certain types of postsynaptic membranes; the number and distribution of particles closely approximate the receptor density predicted by chemical and physiological measurements.

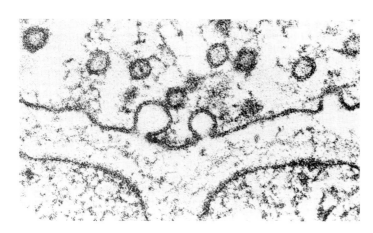

7–34 High-resolution electron micrograph of a portion of a neuromuscular junction that was stimulated and then quick-frozen so that synaptic vesicles were "caught" in the process of exocytosis. (See Fig. 7–35B.) An "active zone" (center) is located at the axonal ending, opposite the opening of a junctional fold. A dense cytoplasmic band occurs on the inner surface of the axonal plasmalemma, and two vesicles on either side of this band are apparently in the process of fusing with the plasmalemma. (From Heuser, J. E. 1977. *In* W. M. Cowan and J. A. Ferrendelli [eds.], Neuroscience Symposia, vol. 2. Bethesda, Md: Society for Neuroscience.)

7–35 **A.** Generalized diagrammatic interpretation of the neuromuscular relationship. A Schwann cell **(S)** forms a covering over the axonal ending **(Ax)**, and its basal lamina becomes fused with that of the muscle fiber, forming a coating that extends along the primary synaptic cleft and into each secondary synaptic cleft or junctional fold **(J)**. Nuclei, mitochondria, free ribosomes, and rough endoplasmic reticulum occur characteristically in the junctional sarcoplasm. Myofilaments are present at the bottom of the diagram. **B.** Diagram illustrating the process of acetylcholine release and membrane recycling in the frog neuromuscular junction. Synaptic vesicle membrane **(left)** fuses with the axonal plasmalemma as acetylcholine is released from the nerve terminal (see Fig. 7–34). The vesicle membrane becomes confluent with the axonal plasmalemma and then membrane is returned, by a system of coated vesicles **(right)**, to the interior of the axonal ending. (From Heuser, J. 1976. *In* Thesleff, S. [ed.], The Motor Innervation of Muscle. London: Academic Press, p. 51.)

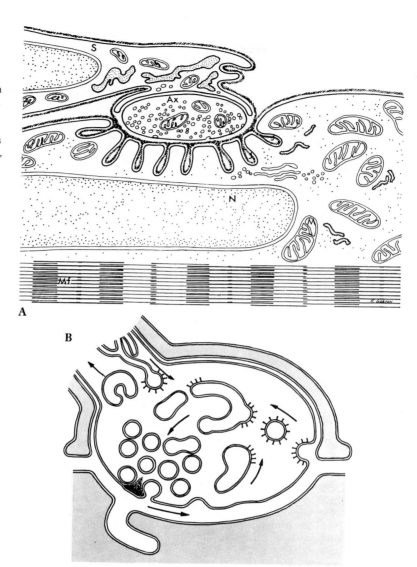

The Heterogeneity of Skeletal Muscle Fibers

It has long been known that skeletal muscles differ in their color, certain muscles being redder than others when viewed grossly. The fibers composing an individual muscle differ also, and the resulting heterogeneity is especially conspicuous after histochemical procedures to localize enzymatic activity (See Gauthier, 1971). Fibers differ, for example, in mitochondrial enzymatic activity, and this activity is, for the most part, inversely proportional to the cross-sectional dimensions of the fibers (Fig. 7–7). In the mammal, small fibers, which are rich in mitochondria, are prevalent in red muscles and are thus called *red fibers.* Large fibers with a low mitochondrial content predominate in white muscles and are called *white fibers.* Fibers with characteristics between the two, but that superficially resemble red fibers, are also prevalent in red muscles and are called *intermediate fibers.* It is also possible to distinguish these three types of fibers by their ultrastructural features. In the red fiber (Fig. 7–36), numerous large mitochondria with closely packed cristae form conspicuous aggregations beneath the sarcolemma and longitudinal rows between myofibrils. The intermediate fiber

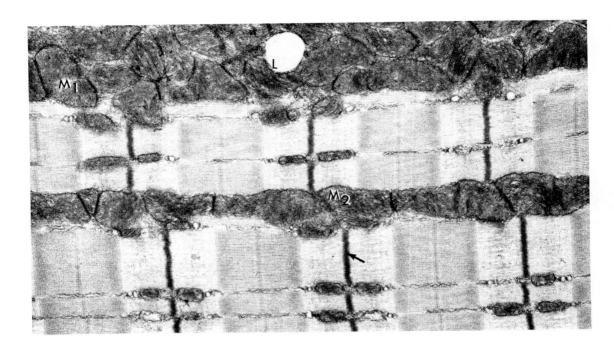

7–36 Longitudinal section of a typical red fiber (rat semitendinosus). Large mitochondria (**M₁**) with closely packed cristae are aggregated just beneath the sarcolemma and in longitudinal interfibrillar rows (**M₂**). The Z line **(arrow)** is relatively wide. Compare with Fig. 7–37, which is at the same magnification. × 16,500. (From Gauthier, G. F. 1970. *In* Briskey, E. J., Cassens, R. G., and Marsh, B. B. [eds.], The Physiology and Biochemistry of Muscle as Food, vol. 2. Madison: University of Wisconsin Press, p. 113.)

is similar except that mitochondria tend to be smaller and their cristae less abundant than in the red fiber. Also, the Z line is noticeably thinner in the intermediate fiber. In the white fiber (Fig. 7–37), subsarcolemmal and interfibrillar mitochondria are sparse, and paired elliptical profiles at the I bands, which are present in all three fiber types, are the major form. The Z line in the white fiber is about half as wide as that of the red fiber. Interestingly, the red fiber, which is the smallest fiber, has the highest concentration of mitochondria, particularly at the cell surface. These features are consistent with a high rate of metabolic exchange.

Ultrastructural features of the neuromuscular junctions of red and white fibers indicate that differences exist also in the motoneurons serving these fibers. The number of synaptic vesicles and the number and complexity of junctional folds are greatest in white fibers (Fig. 7–33) and least in red fibers (Fig. 7–32). Experiments with cross-innervation have shown that the microscopic distribution of fiber types as well as physiological and biochemical properties of the muscles are altered when the nerve supplies are switched. It has been demonstrated also that stimulating a particular motor neuron can cause a single type of muscle fiber to change cytochemically. It is evident, therefore, that the pattern of distribution of fiber types is influenced by the nervous system, and these findings are consistent with the distinctive ultrastructural features of the muscle fibers and their neuromuscular junctions.

Physiological data indicate that red muscles contract more slowly than white muscles, so it has been assumed that the red fiber is a slow fiber. However, physiological properties attributed to individual fibers have been derived largely from the measurements on whole muscles. The functional significance of individual fiber types is now beginning to be understood. The physiological properties of individual motor units (see Chap. 8) vary within a muscle, and there is also significant chemical heterogeneity among the myofibrillar proteins. For example, different isozymes of myosin exist within individual muscles, and they can be localized directly with respect to individual fibers, even within a mixed

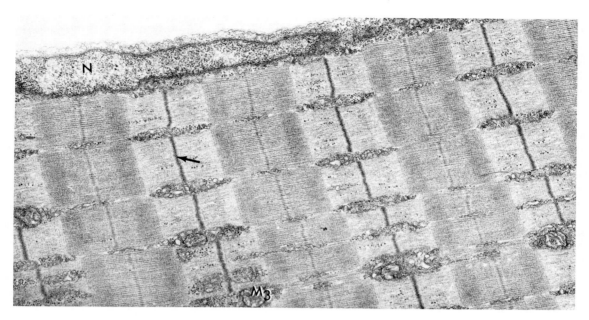

7–37 Typical white fiber (rat semitendinosus). The
△ nucleus **(N)** is included. Subsarcolemmal and
interfibrillar mitochondria are small and sparse.
Paired mitochondria **(M₃)** at the I bands, which are
characteristic of mammalian skeletal muscle in
general, are the predominate form in the white fiber.
The Z line **(arrow)** is about half as wide as the red
fiber (Fig. 7–36). × 16,500. (From Gauthier, G. F.
1969. Z. Zellforsch. 95:462.)

7–38 Serial transverse sections of several skeletal
▽ muscle fibers (rat diaphragm) showing the
reciprocal response to fluorescein-labeled antibodies
specific for "fast" **(left)** and "slow" myosin **(right).** In
the left panel all white **(W)**, intermediate **(I)**, and some
red **(black R)** fibers react with anti-"fast" myosin, and
thus they appear bright with the fluorescence
microscope. All other red fibers **(white R)** are
unreactive, but they react strongly with anti-"slow"
myosin **(black R** in the right panel). (From Gauthier,
G. F., and Lowey, S. 1979. J. Cell Biol. 81:10.)

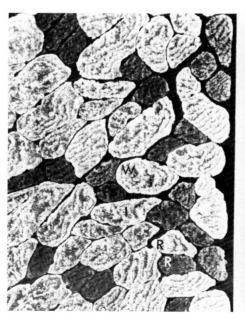

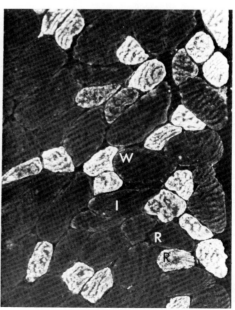

population, by using the procedures of immuno-cytochemistry (see Chap. 2). In this way, chemical properties can be correlated with microscopic characteristics of the fibers. As expected, all white and intermediate fibers react with anitbodies specific for "fast" (white) myosin. In contrast, certain red fibers react with antibodies against "slow" myosin. However, a significant number of red fibers (about 40%) react with antibodies against "fast" myosin (Fig. 7–38). Hence there are two categories of red fibers, and the characteristics usually associated with red fibers (wide Z line, for example) do not necessarily imply a slow speed of contraction. Evidence suggests that the four types of muscle fibers that can be identified in a fast-twitch muscle correspond to four types of motor units with different contraction times.

7–39 Transverse section of frog intestine showing the typical appearance of the circular layer of smooth muscle adjacent to connective tissue **(CT)** of the submucosa. The fibers are arranged circumferentially with their narrow tapered ends adjacent to the wider central regions of nearby fibers. Nuclei are centrally located. Cell boundaries are somewhat difficult to distinguish. (H&E) × 500.

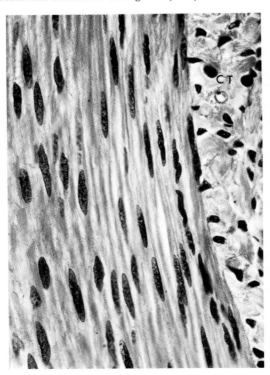

Smooth Muscle

General Features

Smooth muscle plays a critical role in maintaining the caliber of the lumens of the viscera and certain blood vessels. By contraction or relaxation of the component fibers, physiological processes such as digestion, respiration, and blood flow can be regulated. Accordingly, the fibers are arranged in characteristic directions, reflecting the functional activity of the organ (Fig. 7–39). Connective tissue, carrying blood vessels and autonomic nerve fibers, penetrates among individual fibers, but the amount of stroma varies across species and among the organ systems of a given species (for example, compare Figs. 7–39 and 7–40).

Smooth muscle fibers are narrow and tapering, and their length varies from about 20 μm in certain small blood vessels to 500 μm or more in the gestational uterus. The nucleus is centrally located, and there are no transverse striations (Fig. 7–40). A typical basal lamina is applied to

7–40 Longitudinal sections of several smooth muscle fibers (lateral vaginal canal of the opossum). Because of the relative abundance of connective tissue in this bundle of smooth muscle, the cellular outlines are clearly distinguished. Nuclei occupy the broad central regions of these tapering fibers. (H&E) × 760.

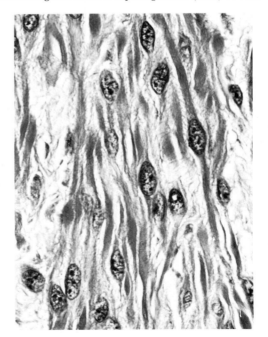

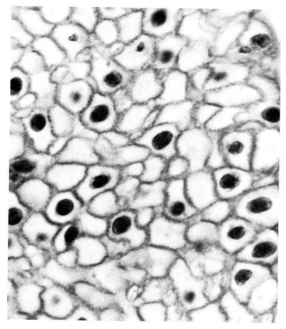

the outer surface of the sarcolemma. In fact stained basal laminae aid in visualizing individual fibers (Fig. 7–41).

The arrangement of fibers is staggered so that the broad nuclear region of one fiber lies opposite the narrow tapered end of an adjacent fiber (Fig. 7–39). A transverse section would therefore pass through the nuclear level of only certain fibers and through the tapered ends of those that intervene (Fig. 7–41). At various points, adjacent fibers form an intimate association, called a nexus, or gap junction, where electrical coupling is believed to be facilitated.

The cytoplasmic organelles, which include mitochondria, Golgi apparatus, scattered profiles of rough endoplasmic reticulum, and free ribosomes, are mostly confined to a conical region at each pole of the nucleus (Fig. 7–42). The rest of the sarcoplasm is occupied primarily by thin filaments. Characteristic dense bodies, into which the thin filaments appear to insert, are distributed throughout the sarcoplasm (Fig. 7–42).

7–41 Transverse section of smooth muscle fibers △ (stomach of the grasshopper mouse), which has been stained by the periodic acid–Schiff reaction and with hematoxylin. The carbohydrate component of the conspicuous basal lamina is stained, which facilitates visualization of individual fibers. Note that the plane of section passes through the broad nuclear regions of only certain fibers and through the broad nuclear regions of only certain fibers and through the narrow tapered ends of others. × 1,200.

7–42 Electron micrograph of a longitudinal section ▽ of a smooth muscle fiber (ileum of a 13-day-old rat). Part of the centrally located nucleus (**N**) is included at the left. Mitochondria, a Golgi apparatus, and ribosomes are particularly abundant in the conical perinuclear region. The remainder of the fiber is occupied by thin filaments and by dense bodies **(arrows)** into which the filaments appear to insert. There are no transverse striations. × 17,220.

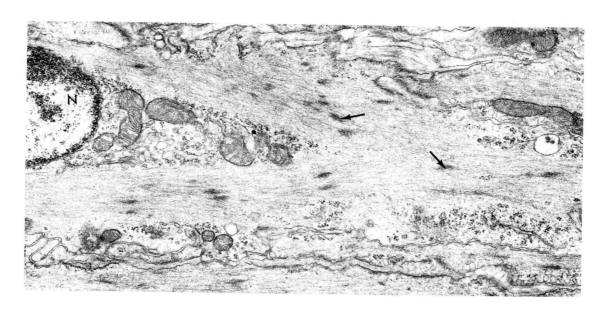

The Ultrastructural Basis of Contraction

Much less is known about the mechanism of contraction in smooth muscle than in striated muscle. Because transverse banding is lacking the sliding filament hypothesis initially seemed inappropriate. Both myosin and actin can be demonstrated by chemical procedures, but conventional ultrastructural preparations ordinarily reveal only a homogeneous population of thin filaments.

Under appropriate conditions, thick filaments can be demonstrated in smooth muscle, although the ratio of thick to thin filaments is low (Fig.

7–43 Transverse section of smooth muscle from rabbit portal-anterior mesenteric vein. Both thick and thin filaments are evident in this preparation, although the spatial arrangement is different from that of striated muscle (Fig. 7–10). × 153,000. (From Somlyo, A. P., et al. 1973. Philos. Trans. R. Soc. Lond. 265:223.)

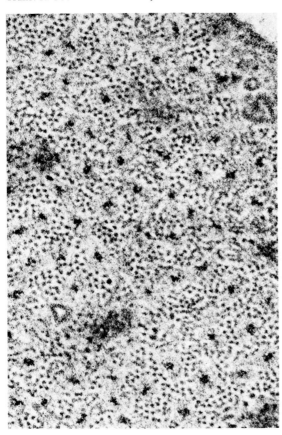

7–43). Also, synthetic myosin filaments can be prepared. They closely resemble the filaments prepared from skeletal muscle myosin, but there are important differences (see Hinssen et al., 1978). The assembly of myosin molecules is not usually bipolar as it is in skeletal muscle. The myosin cross-bridges extend the entire length of the filament; they are polarized in a single direction along one side of the filament and in the opposite direction along the other. In this "side-polar" configuration there is no central bridge-free zone, such as that seen in the skeletal thick filament. This arrangement has the advantage that actin and myosin could interact without interruption for the entire length of a thick filament. The sliding filament hypothesis may therefore be applicable, with some modification, to smooth as well as skeletal muscle.

References and Selected Bibliography

Cohen, C. 1975. The protein switch of muscle contraction. Sci. Am. 233–5:36.

Franzini-Armstrong, C. 1980. Structure of sarcoplasmic reticulum. Fed. Proc. 39–7:2403.

Gauthier, G. F. 1971. The structural and cytochemical heterogeneity of mammalian skeletal muscle fibers. In Podolsky, R. J. (ed.), The Contractility of Muscle Cells and Related Processes. Englewood Cliffs, N.J.: Prentice-Hall, Inc., p. 131.

Gauthier, G. F. 1976. The motor end-plate. In Landon, D. N. (ed.), The Peripheral Nerve. London: Chapman and Hall Ltd., p. 464.

Gauthier, G. F. 1980. Distribution of myosin isozymes in adult and developing muscle fibers. In Pette, D. (ed.), Plasticity of Muscle. Berlin: Walter de Gruyter, p. 83.

Hanson, J., and Huxley, H. E. 1955. The structural basis of contraction in striated muscle. In Fibrous Proteins and Their Biological Significance. No. 9. New York: Academic Press, Inc.

Hanson, J., and Lowy, J. 1963. The structure of F-actin and of actin filaments isolated from muscle. J. Mol. Biol. 6:46.

Heuser, J. 1976. Morphology of synaptic vesicle discharge and reformation at frog neuromuscular junction. In Thesleff, S. (ed.), The Motor Innervation of Muscle. London: Academic Press, p. 51.

Heuser, J. E., and Salpeter, S. R. 1979. Organization of acetylcholine receptors in quick-frozen, deep-etched, and rotary-replicated Torpedo postsynaptic membrane. J. Cell Biol. 82:150.

Hinssen, H., 'Haese, J. D., Small, J. V., and Sobieszek, A. 1978. Mode of filament assembly of myosins from muscle and nonmuscle cells. J. Ultrastruct. Res. 64:282.

Huxley, H. E. 1957. The double array of filaments in cross-striated muscle. J. Biophys. Biochem. Cytol. 3:631.

Huxley, H. E. 1963. Electron microscope studies on the structure of natural and synthetic protein filaments from striated muscle. J. Mol. Biol. 7:281.

Huxley, H. E. 1969. The mechanisms of muscular contraction. Science 164:1356.

Knappeis, G. G., and Carlsen, F. 1962. The ultrastructure of the Z disc in skeletal muscle. J. Cell Biol. 13:323.

Lowey, S. 1971. Myosin: Molecule and filament. In Timasheff, S. N., and Fasman, G. D. (eds.), Biological Macromolecules Series, vol. 5, pt. A. New York: Marcel Dekker Inc., chap. 5.

Luther, P., and Squire, J. 1978. Three-dimensional structure of the vertebrate muscle M-region. J. Mol. Biol. 125:313.

MacLennan, D. H., and Campbell, K. P. 1979. Structure, function and biosynthesis of sarcoplasmic reticulum proteins. Trends in Biochem. Sci. 4:148.

Moore, P. B., Huxley, H., and DeRosier, D. J. 1970. Three-dimensional reconstruction of F-actin, thin filaments and decorated thin filaments. J. Mol. Biol. 50:279.

Peachey, L. D. 1965. The sarcoplasmic reticulum and transverse tubules of the frog's sartorius. J. Cell Biol. 25:209.

Pepe, F. A. 1971. The structural components of the striated muscle fibril. In Timasheff, S. N., and Fasman, G. D. (eds.), Biological Macromolecules Series, vol. 5, pt. A. New York: Marcel Dekker, Inc., chap. 7.

Porter, K. R., and Palade, G. E. 1957. Studies on the endoplasmic reticulum. III. Its form and distribution in striated muscle cells. J. Biophys. Biochem. Cytol. 3:269.

Robertson, J. D. 1956. The ultrastructure of a reptilian myoneural junction. J. Biophys. Biochem. Cytol. 2:381.

Somlyo, A. P., Somlyo, A. V., Ashton, F. T., and Vallieres, J. 1976. Vertebrate Smooth Muscle: Ultrastructure and Function. In Goldman, R., Pollard, T., Rosenbaum, J. (eds.), Cell Motility. Cold Spring Harbor Laboratory, p. 165.

The Nervous Tissue

Edward G. Jones and W. Maxwell Cowan

Development of Nervous Tissue

Neural Induction and the Formation of the Neural Tube

Except for the sensory epithelia and the associated ganglion cells of certain of the cranial nerves, all elements of the central and peripheral nervous systems are derived from a specialized region of ectoderm along the dorsal midline of the embryo. Initially, this zone is indistinguishable from the rest of the ectoderm, but under the inductive influence of the underlying notochord and the adjoining mesoderm, its cells become elongated and appear to be irreversibly determined to form neural tissue. In the human embryo, at about the 18-day stage, this specialized zone forms a slipper-shaped area immediately rostral to the *primitive knot*, or *Hensen's node*, and in transverse sections appears as a thickened and slightly depressed region dorsal to the notochord (Fig. 8–1). The central portion of this region is called the *neurectoderm*. Interposed between it and the nonspecialized or *somatic* ectoderm is a second specialized zone, the *neurosomatic junctional region*. The neurectoderm will form the *neural* (or *medullary*) plate from which the entire central nervous system is derived; the neurosomatic junctional region will give rise to the cells of the *neural crest* from which much of the peripheral nervous system (and a number of other tissues) will be formed.

As the epithelium of the neurectoderm thickens, the lateral edges of the neural plate become increasingly elevated to form a *neural groove* bounded on either side by raised *neural folds* (Fig. 8–1). Toward the end of the third embryonic week the lips of the neural groove fuse together in the upper cervical region. From this region the process of fusion extends rostrally and caudally, converting the original neural plate into a *neural tube* (Fig. 8–1). For a time, the tube remains open at its rostral and caudal ends (the openings are called the *anterior* and *posterior neuropores*), but with the closure of the neuropores (during the fourth embryonic week), it becomes completely closed. When the folds of the neural groove fuse, the cells of the neurosomatic junctional region are separated from both the somatic ectoderm and the neurectoderm and come to occupy a position along the dorsolateral aspect of the neural tube. This initially more or less continuous column of cells constitutes the *neural crest*. Subsequently, three vesicular swellings—called the *prosencephalic*, *mesencephalic*, and *rhombencephalic vesicles*—appear in the rostral part of the neural tube; respectively, they give rise to the forebrain, midbrain and hindbrain. The more caudal, unexpanded portion of the neural tube forms the spinal cord.

Histogenesis in the Neural Tube

Until shortly after its closure, the neural tube consists of a simple, columnar epithelium. However, as cell proliferation proceeds, the wall of the tube soon becomes converted into a *pseudostratified* epithelium, with nuclei at several levels but with each cell retaining a basal cytoplasmic process in contact with the *basement membrane*, or *basal lamina*, which surrounds the neural tube and separates it from the adjoining mesodermal tissues. The luminal processes of the cells are ciliated and joined to each other by a series of *junctional complexes* (or *terminal bars*). The epithelium as a whole is variously

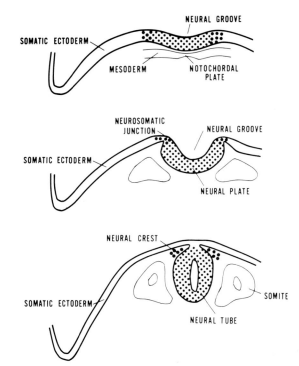

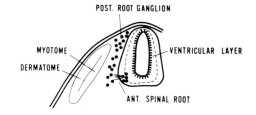

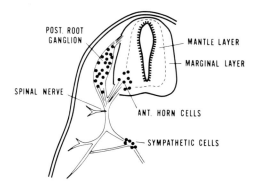

8–1 The sequence of changes that lead to the formation of the spinal cord and the associated nerve roots from the neural plate and the adjoining neurosomatic junctional region.

named the *germinal epithelium,* the *neuroepithelium,* and the *matrix* or *ventricular layer;* from it derive both the neuronal and supporting elements of the central nervous system.

As Figs. 8–2 and 8–3A show, all the readily identifiable mitotic figures in the neuroepithelium are found along its ventricular or luminal border. This unusual appearance results from the fact that although all the cells of the neuroepithelium are of the same type, their nuclei take different positions according to their stage in the cell cycle. This idea was initially formulated on cytological grounds in 1931 by Sauer, but it has been experimentally confirmed in several ways. Of these, the most convincing has been the analysis of cell proliferation in the neuroepithelium by tritiated [³H]thymidine autoradiography.

In autoradiographs of the neural tube taken within an hour or two after the administration of a small dose of [³H]thymidine to an animal, the label can be seen to have been incorporated into the DNA of cells whose nuclei lie in the basal or middle thirds of the neuroepithelium (Fig. 8–3B). At this time all other nuclei in the epithelium appear unlabeled. However, if the autoradiographs are prepared at a later time, say 8 to 12 h after administering the isotope, *most* of the nuclei in the epithelium (including those in the later stages of mitosis—metaphase, anaphase, and telophase) will be labeled. This type of experiment not only demonstrates that *all* the cells in the neuroepithelium are capable of DNA synthesis (and hence, of mitosis) but also suggests that cell proliferation in the epithelium proceeds in the following characteristic sequence. Interphase cells in the neuroepithelium (that is, those in the G_1 *phase* of the cell cycle—see Chap. 1) are elongated and their nuclei are in the upper or middle thirds of the epithelium (Fig. 8–2). As they enter the S *phase* of the next cycle, their nuclei first come to lie deeper within the epithelium; progressively later in this phase (which generally lasts about 8 to 12 h), the nuclei begin to migrate toward the luminal pole of the cell (Fig. 8–2). By the time the cell enters the G_2 *phase* of the cycle, its nucleus is close to the luminal margin, and the cell as a whole is beginning to round up by withdrawing its basal process from the basal lamina (Fig. 8–2). The G_2 phase lasts no more than 1 to 2 h and leads directly into the *M phase,* or mid- and late-mitotic phase of the cell cycle. Immediately before cytokinesis, the now more-or-less spherical cells appear to lose parts of their junctional complexes;

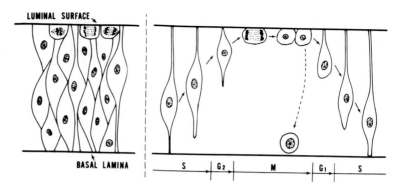

8–2 The pseudostratified character of the neuroepithelium and the pattern of interkinetic nuclear migration during the major phases of the cell cycle in the neuroepithelium.

this must be an extremely rapid process, because shortly after cytokinesis the two daughter cells resulting from telophase appear to have reconstituted the junctional complexes. The entire M phase lasts about 1 h and leads directly into the G_1 phase (which is of variable duration). During the G_1 phase the cells again become elongated, their nuclei descend, and their abluminal processes reestablish an association with the basal lamina (Fig. 8–2) before the next round of DNA synthesis. The changes in the structure of the cells at different phases of the cell cycle are

strikingly demonstrated in scanning electron micrographs (Fig. 8–4).

The duration of each phase of the mitotic cycle varies somewhat from region to region in the neural tube and with the age of the embryo. (At late embryonic stages the G_1 phase becomes progressively longer and the entire cycle may take as long as 48 to 96 h.) However, the pattern of DNA synthesis and the interkinetic migration of the nuclei of the neuroepithelial cells remain the same. The process of cell proliferation continues in this manner for a variable period of time in

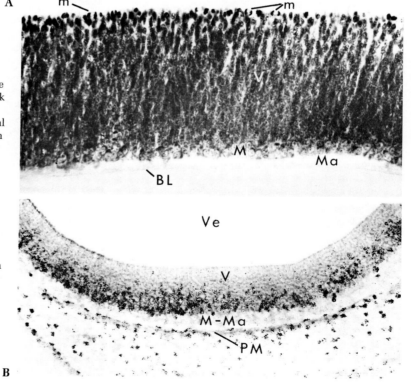

8–3 **A.** A photomicrograph of the neuroepithelium of the chick optic tectum with the mitotic figures **(m)** confined to the luminal surface. Postmitotic cells **(M)** form a mantle or intermediate zone immediately above the marginal zone **(Ma)**. **BL**, basal lamina. Thionin stain. × 450.
B. An autoradiograph of the neuroepithelium a short time after the administration of [³H]thymidine. Only the nuclei in the deeper part of the ventricular zone **(V)** are labeled, together with cells in the surrounding pia mater **(PM)**. **Ve**, ventricle. × 90.

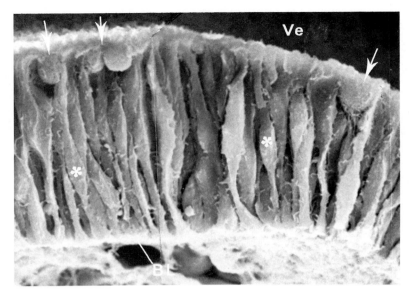

8–4 A scanning electron micrograph of the neuroepithelium to show the form of the interkinetic cells (marked by **asterisks**) and the dividing cells at the ventricular surface **(Ve)** marked by **arrows. BL:** basal lamina. × 1,300. (From Seymour, R. M., and Berry, M. 1976. J. Comp. Neurol. 160:5. Courtesy of Dr. M. Berry.)

different regions of the neural tube. However, at some point DNA synthesis ceases in certain of the neuroepithelial cells. The time at which the first postmitotic cells appear can also be readily determined by [³H]thymidine autoradiography, which has been used experimentally to establish the "dates of birth" of various classes of neurons. On completing their last mitotic division, one or both of the daughter cells become arrested in the G₁ phase of the cell cycle, and, in this state, the cells migrate out of the neuroepithelium and come to lie in a layer deep to the nuclei of the neuroepithelial cells. This newly formed layer of postmitotic cells is known as the *mantle* or *intermediate zone* (Fig. 8–3A and B); it is the growth of this layer that leads to the progressive expansion of the walls of the brain and spinal cord. The region of the neural tube between the developing mantle zone and the basal lamina is called the *marginal zone*. Initially this zone contains only the basal processes of the neuroepithelial cells, but it is soon invaded by the processes of the postmitotic cells in the mantle zone of the same area and by processes entering it from other parts of the nervous system.

We do not know what factor, or factors, bring about the cessation of DNA synthesis in certain cells while permitting it to continue for several further cell cycles in others. Nor is it known whether the two daughter cells of a terminal mitosis are both determined to form either nerve cells (or *neurons*) or supporting cells (*neuroglial*

cells), or if one cell may later differentiate into a neuron and the other into a glial cell. At present only three generalizations seem justifiable. First, in most regions of the nervous system the first neurons and the first glial cells *seem* to be formed at the same time. Second, glial cell proliferation generally continues for some time after all the neurons are formed, and indeed most glial cells retain the capacity for further division throughout the life of the organism. Third, the larger nerve cells are generated earlier than the smaller neurons in the same region. There is also some evidence that the positional information that determines where the larger (projection) neurons will send their axons becomes fixed at the time of the last mitotic division. In view of the importance of the changes that occur in the neuroepithelial cells when they become postmitotic, it is somewhat surprising that they show so little morphological evidence that the differentiated state has been established. In the light microscope, the only indications that the cells have made this transition are (1) their location in the mantle zone, and (2) the fact that they appear more rounded and have rather more cytoplasm. In the electron microscope they can be seen to have lost their junctional complexes, but otherwise they display the same cytoplasmic organelles as the neuroepithelial cells.

The cells of the mantle zone are customarily called *neuroblasts* (if they give rise to mature neurons) or *glioblasts* (if they form neuroglial

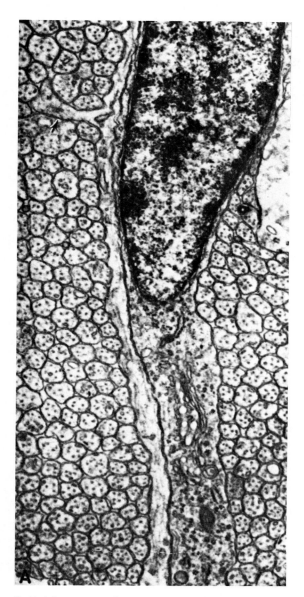

changes that they undergo (including the growth and elaboration of their various processes and appendages) simply reflect their prior commitment to the neuronal or glial cell line.

The subsequent fate of these cells and their mature morphological appearance will be considered in a later section. With the notable exception of the last remaining neuroepithelial cells, which persist in the mature nervous system as the *ependymal cells* lining the ventricular system of the brain and spinal cord, all cells in the nervous system migrate, at least once, from the region in which they are generated to their definitive location. The details of the migratory process remain to be determined (at present it is thought to be similar to the migration of ameboid cells elsewhere), but one intriguing suggestion is that migrating neurons may be directed toward their terminal loci by the neighboring preformed neuroglial cell processes. Certainly, in many parts of the nervous system, the glial cells have long radially oriented processes (which may extend across most of the thickness of the expanding neural tube, or its derivatives), and the migrating neurons are nearly always found in close association with such processes (Fig. 8–5). In certain genetic disorders characterized by early degeneration or incomplete development of the glial cells, the neurons in the affected regions fail to migrate in the normal manner.

Some Less Common Histogenetic Patterns

The pattern of cell proliferation, differentiation, and migration just described is typical of most regions of the central nervous system, but in certain regions a different sequence of events occurs. In the cerebral hemispheres, a second proliferative zone appears immediately deep to the neuroepithelium. In this *subependymal* or *subventricular* layer (Fig. 8–6), cellular proliferation leading to the production of neurons and glial cells persists for some time after mitosis in the neuroepithelium has ceased. In the cerebellum, there is an early migration of a population of precursor cells (that is, true neuroblasts) from the neuroepithelium to form a second proliferative zone on the outer surface of the cerebellar cortex. In this layer (known as the *external granular layer*), cell proliferation continues for several weeks, the precursor cells giving rise to at least four different classes of neuron, including the enormous population of small granule cells whose later migration is illustrated in Fig. 8–6.

8–5 A low-power electron micrograph of a migrating granule cell (right) associated with a glial process (left) in the developing cerebellar cortex. × 21,300. (From Rakic, P. 1971. J. Comp. Neurol. 141:253. Courtesy of P. Rakic.)

cells). However, because the neuroblasts can no longer divide, the suffix *blast* (often used in cytology for a precursor cell) is inappropriate; *neuroblast* should be replaced by *young neuron*. In sum: the newly formed neurons and neuroglial cells are differentiated cells, and the further

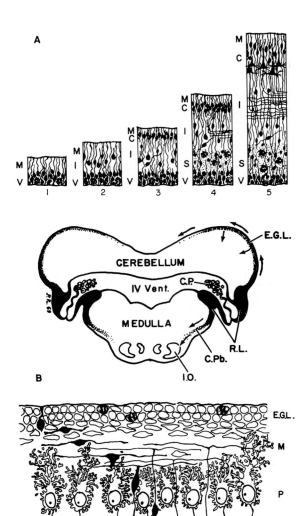

8–6 **A.** The progressive enlargement of the marginal and mantle or intermediate **(I)** zones of the neural tube at the expense of the neuroepithelial or ventricular **(V)** and subventricular **(S)** zones. **B.** The formation of the proliferative external granular layer **(EGL)** of the cerebellum from the rhombic lip **(RL)** of the developing brainstem. Several of the nuclei of the brainstem are also formed from the rhombic lip **(arrows). C.** Proliferation in the external granular layer and the migration of the granule cells **(G)** of the cerebellar cortex. (Drawings by P. Rakic to illustrate various of his publications, from Sidman, R. L. 1970. *In* The Neurosciences, Second Study Program. New York: Rockefeller University Press; courtesy of R. L. Sidman and P. Rakic.)

As they migrate from the neuroepithelium, or from one of the secondary proliferative zones in the central nervous system, the differentiated neuronal and glial cell precursors either are ellipsoidal in shape or have a single leading process. Such cells are said to be *apolar* and *unipolar*, respectively. A few neurons in the vertebrate central nervous system persist into adult life as *unipolar neurons*, but most pass through a *bipolar phase*. Several different classes of bipolar neurons are seen in the mature nervous system (Fig. 8–7), but the great majority develop a number of processes and are collectively called *multipolar neurons*. The development of the glioblasts is less well documented, and although it is formally convenient to divide them into two classes—astroblasts and oligodendroblasts (for the precursors of astrocytes and oligodendrocytes, which are the two main categories of supporting cell in the central nervous system)—there is little cytological distinction between them.

The Neural Crest and Its Derivatives

Whereas the neuroepithelium gives rise only to neurons, glial cells, and the modified columnar epithelium that forms the ependymal lining of the ventricles and the choroid plexuses (*see* below), the *neural crest* gives rise to an extremely diverse range of cells and tissues. Most of the nonneural derivatives are dealt with elsewhere in the appropriate chapters of this volume; they include:

1. The cells of the pia mater and arachnoid mater
2. Certain of the branchial cartilages and odontoblasts, and some of the cranial mesenchyme
3. Pigment-producing cells of the skin and subcutaneous tissues
4. Chromaffin tissue, including the chromaffin cells of the adrenal medulla

The neural derivatives include most of the sensory neurons of the cranial and spinal sensory ganglia, the postganglionic neurons of the sympathetic and parasympathetic ganglia, and the Schwann cells of the peripheral nervous system, including the sheath or satellite cells of the ganglia. At present we know little about the factors responsible for this morphogenetic diversity, but it is clear that many of the cells of the neural crest are determined, at a very early stage in development, to follow one or another line of dif-

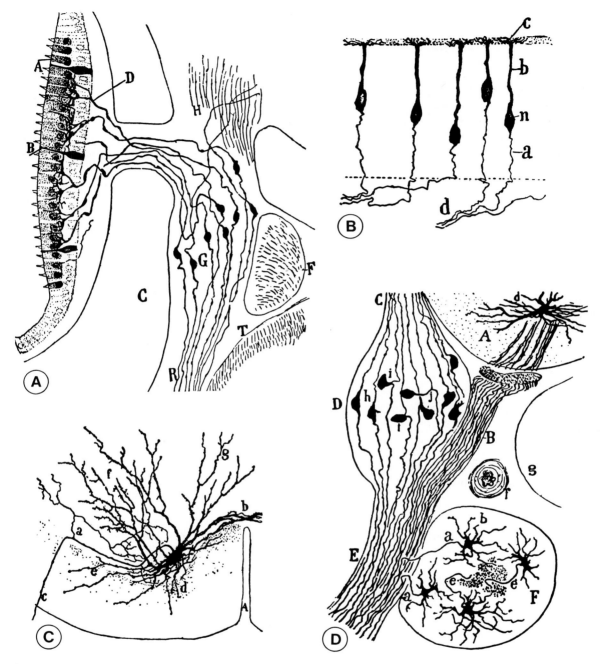

8–7 A variety of neurons stained by the Golgi method. **A.** Bipolar cells **(G)** of the vestibular ganglion in the mouse. Peripheral branches **(D)** innervate vestibular hair cells; central branches **(R)** pass to brain. **B.** Bipolar neurons in the olfactory mucosa with peripheral processes **(b)** and centrally projecting axons **(a)**. **C.** A large multipolar neuron in the anterior horn of the spinal cord. **D.** Spinal ganglion cells at different stages in development from their early bipolar form **(h)** to the mature pseudounipolar form **(i)**. (**A,** spinal cord; **B,** ventral root; **F,** sympathetic ganglion.) (From Cajal, S. Ramón y. 1909. Histologie du Système Nerveux de l'Homme et des Vertébrés, vol. 1. Republished 1952. Madrid: Consejo Superior de Investigaciones Cientificas.)

ferentiation. The neuronal derivatives of the crest show almost the same range of morphological specializations as do the cells in the central nervous system. Most of the cells begin as *apolar* neuroblasts; those in the sensory ganglia associated with cranial nerves V, VII, IX, X, and XI and with the dorsal roots of spinal nerves become *bipolar* and then, because the two processes come together and fuse, become *secondarily unipolar* (and for this reason are sometimes referred to as *pseudounipolar* neurons) (Fig. 8–7). The sympathetic and parasympathetic neuroblasts generally grow many processes and become *multipolar*.

Other Neural Derivatives

The sensory epithelia of certain of the cranial nerves, and the associated sensory ganglion cells, derive either wholly or in part from specialized ectodermal thickenings, or *placodes*. The first of these is the nasal placode, which gives rise to the olfactory epithelium in the upper part of the nose, including the olfactory receptors. The latter are modified bipolar neurons, with a shorter peripheral process or dendrite being specifically adapted to respond to the presence of odoriferous molecules in the overlying mucous layer, and with a longer central process (or axon) passing into the olfactory bulb. Parts of the trigeminal (Vth), facial (VIIth), glossopharyngeal (IXth), and vagal (Xth) ganglia are also formed from placodes. The thickened epithelial cells sink beneath the rest of the ectoderm and then proliferate and migrate toward clusters of neural crest cells that form the remaining parts of the ganglia. The *acousticovestibular placode* gives rise to the sensory epithelia of the internal ear and to the bipolar ganglion cells of the *acoustic* (or *spiral*) ganglion and on the *vestibular ganglion*. It is not known if the sheath cells in the trigeminal, facial, glossopharyngeal, or vagal ganglia are derived from the placodes or from the neural crest, but in the case of the acoustic and vestibular ganglia, it is quite clear that the placodal epithelium can form both neurons and sheath cells.

The Structure of Neurons and Neuroglial Cells

The result of the histogenetic sequence outlined above is the production of two classes of cells that together constitute the nervous tissue. They are the nerve cells, or *neurons*, and the supporting or *neuroglial* cells.

Neurons

Functionally, the most significant single feature of neurons is that they are surrounded by an *excitable membrane* which, under normal resting conditions, is capable of maintaining a differential distribution of ions on either side of it. This membrane in turn gives rise to the so-called resting membrane potential of about 90 mV (inside negative), which may be either partially or wholly depolarized or hyperpolarized by influences from other nerve cells. In addition, each neuron has a characteristic morphological structure. Different classes of neuron may have radically different appearances (see Figs. 8–7 to 8–9), but all neurons have an underlying similarity in form. The expanded part of the cell containing the nucleus is the *cell soma*; in certain types of preparations, this is the only part of the neuron stained (see Fig. 8–10). However, when the cell is stained in its entirety (for example, by means of the Golgi method; see Figs. 8–11 and 8–12), one or more slender processes, which may be of considerable length and highly branched, can be seen extending from the soma. All the neurons illustrated in Fig. 8–8 have two distinct types of processes: a number of *dendrites* and a single *axon*. The *dendrites* are drawn out of the soma in such a way that it is often difficult to define their exact point of origin; and they usually undergo several generations of branching that become progressively narrower in diameter. Together with the soma, the dendrites provide the main recipient surface of the nerve cell, and the processes of other nerve cells terminate on them at specialized regions of contact called *synapses*. The sum of the influences (excitatory and inhibitory) exerted by other nerve cells at any instant determines the state of excitability of the neuron, and the soma–dendritic membrane can be regarded as an integrating mechanism that adds these influences together.

Also arising from the soma (or less commonly from one of the dendrites) is a single process, the *axon*. The axon is usually thinner than the dendrites, and when it arises from the soma, it usually does so at a clearly recognizable elevation, the *axon hillock*. Just beyond this elevation, the axon narrows over a length of a few microns, forming what is known as the *initial segment* of the axon. Beyond the initial segment it may at first increase in diameter somewhat, but as it passes to its destination, its diameter tends to re-

8–8 **A.** A pyramidal neuron from the cerebral cortex with a prominent apical dendrite **(b)**, several basal dendrites **(a)**, and a lengthy axon **(e)** which gives off a number of collateral branches **(c)** and enters the subcortical white matter. **B.** A variety of short-axon (Golgi type II) cells in the cerebral cortex. **a,** stellate; **b,** "spider-web"; **d,** "double bouquet." **C.** A cerebellar Purkinje cell with its extensive planar-arranged dendritic tree, axon **(a)** and recurrent axon collaterals **(b).** (From Cajal, S. Ramón y. 1911. Histologie du Système Nerveux de l'Homme et des Vertébrés, vol. 2. Republished 1952. Madrid: Consejo Superior de Investigaciones Cientificas.)

main relatively uniform until it reaches its terminal arborizations. Although usually longer than the dendrites, the axon is of variable length and may terminate close to or at considerable distance from the soma. Along its course it may give off branches, the largest of which are termed *axon collaterals.* They may accompany the main axonal trunk or they may reenter the area containing the parent cell, in which case they are called *recurrent collaterals.* The axon and its branches are the main transmitting channels through which the neuron affects other nerve cells and other tissues such as muscles and glands, usually by the rapid conduction of nervous impulses.

The Shapes of Neurons. From the above it is apparent that neurons exhibit what has sometimes been called *dynamic polarization;* that is, they have a receiving surface—the synaptic sites on the dendrites and soma; an integrating mechanism—the somatic and dendritic membrane; an

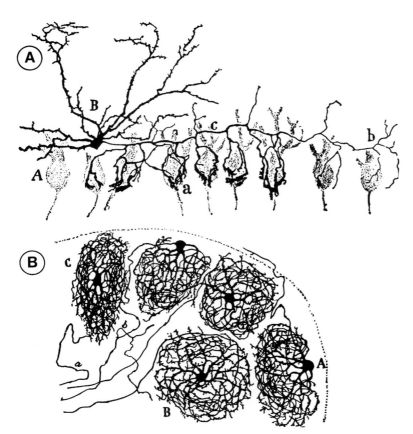

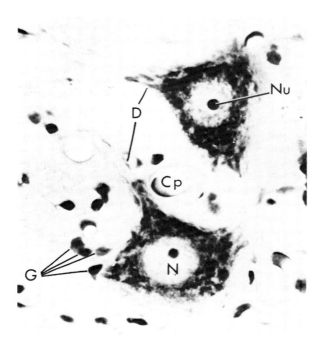

8–9 A. A basket neuron from the cerebellum with its axon **(c)** giving off characteristic axonal baskets **(a)** surrounding adjoining Purkinje cells **(A).**
B. Multipolar neurons with complex dendritic arborizations in the inferior olivary nucleus. (From Cajal, S. Ramón y. 1909. Histologie de Système Nerveux de l'Homme et des Vertébrés, vol. 1. Republished 1952. Madrid: Consejo Superior de Investigacions Cientificas.)

8–10 Two motoneurons from a Nissl-stained preparation of the spinal cord of a cat. Note the large, angular Nissl bodies in the cytoplasm, the pale nuclei **(N)**, the prominent nucleolus **(Nu)**, and the extension of the Nissl material into the large dendrites **(D)**. Several small glial cells **(G)** are also shown, and a small capillary **(Cp)**. × 480.

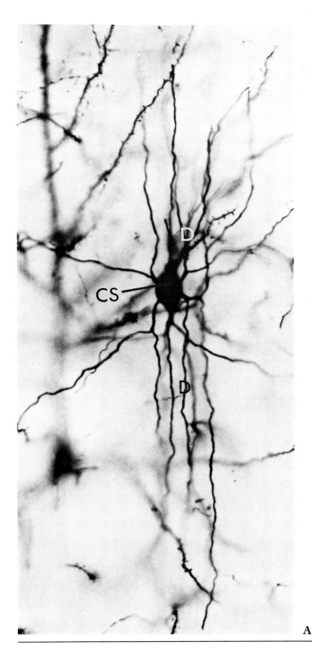

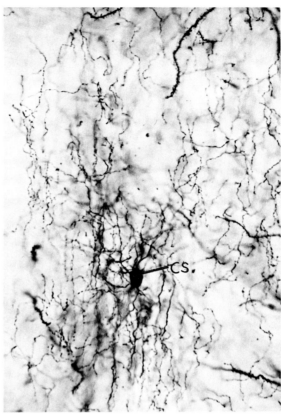

8-11 Photomicrographs of Golgi-impregnated cells from the cerebral cortex of a monkey. Note that the dendrites **(D)** ramify in all directions and that the cell on the right has an extensive locally ramifying axonal plexus. **CS,** cell soma. **A,** × 300; **B,** × 330. (From Jones, E. G. 1975. J. Comp. Neurol. 160:205.)

impulse initiating mechanism—the initial segment of the axon; and an impulse conducting process—the axon itself. Most neurons conform to this basic pattern of organization, although the overall shape of different nerve cells may vary considerably.

Perhaps the simplest class of neuron is that in which only a single process arises from the soma; such cells are commonly called *unipo-*

lar neurons. From the single process, several branches are usually given off, some of which are mainly receptive and function as dendrites; others are effectors and together they represent the branching axonal plexus of the cell. Unipolar neurons are particularly common in invertebrates. In vertebrates, true unipolar neurons are rare.

A second class of neuron that is also relatively

294

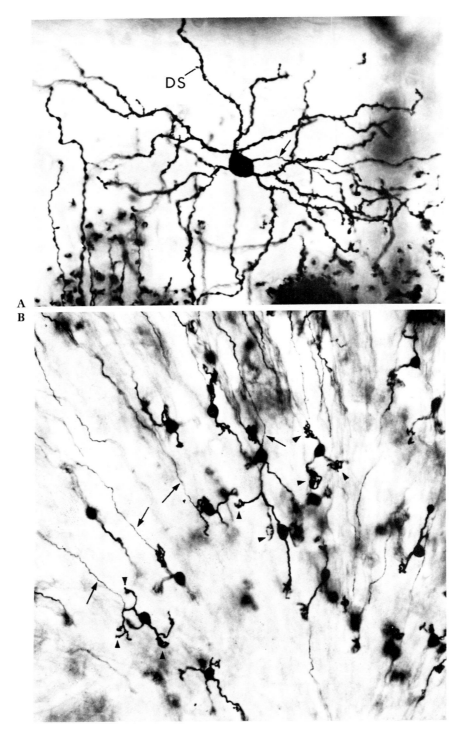

8–12 Photomicrographs of a stellate cell **(A)** and several granule cells **(B)** in Golgi-stained preparations of the cerebellar cortex of a monkey. **Arrows** indicate axons. **Arrowheads** in **B** indicate the terminal claws on the dendrites of the granule cells. Some of the axons of these cells arise from the dendrites. **DS,** dendritic spine. × 500.

uncommon in vertebrates, being found primarily in the retina and in the vestibular and acoustic ganglia, is the *bipolar neuron* (Fig. 8–7). Such neurons are relatively symmetrical, with the axon (or central process) and a single dendritic (or peripheral) process arising from opposite poles of the ovoid or elongated soma. The dendrite may or may not branch profusely, and the axon may be short (as in the retinal bipolar cells) or long (as in the vestibular and acoustic ganglion cells). A unique type of unipolar cell is found in the dorsal root ganglia of the spinal nerves and in the sensory ganglia of certain of the cranial nerves (Fig. 8–7). These cells, referred to above as *pseudounipolar neurons*, give rise to a single process that bifurcates into a peripheral process directed toward the skin and underlying tissues and a central process that enters the spinal cord or brainstem. It should be noted, however, that both the central and peripheral processes resemble axons in their structure and in their ability to conduct nerve impulses.

All other classes of neuron in the adult nervous system are *multipolar neurons*. That is, the parent soma gives rise to more than one dendritic trunk. Most neurons have only a single axon, although rare cases with multiple axons have been described. In a few special cases to be described later, the cell may lack an axon altogether. Within the general category of multipolar neurons, many types have characteristic shapes that are surprisingly constant from species to species and, within any one species, from individual to individual. These types have generally been given special names that either describe some aspect of their morphology or record the name of the investigator who first described them.

Perhaps the most typical multipolar neurons (Fig. 8–7) are the *motor cells*, or *motoneurons*, of the ventral horn of the spinal cord. The large somata of these cells customarily give rise to six or more large dendritic trunks that radiate in all directions from the perikaryon and branch into secondary and tertiary dendrites. The length of the primary dendrites is fairly uniform, so that the total *dendritic field*, (that is, the spatial volume occupied by all the dendrites together) is nearly symmetrical and, when viewed three-dimensionally, forms a round or ovoid figure enclosing the perikaryon.

In some cases the dendritic fields are particularly symmetrical, and because the dendrites radiate more or less uniformly in all directions, these cells are called *stellate neurons*. However,

few of the cells that are commonly termed stellate, such as those in the fourth layer of the cerebral cortex, have uniform dendrites or dendritic fields. More often, the field tends to be eccentric or flattened in one dimension, and then the cells are described as *spindle-shaped* or *fusiform*, for example.

Several types of multipolar neurons that have been given special names are shown in Figs. 8–8 and 8–9. Some of these neurons have long axons that leave the territory of the cell soma, and each has a highly characteristic dendritic field. The *Purkinje cells* of the cerebellar cortex have only ascending dendrites directed toward the surface of the cerebellum, but these dendrites and their branches are all oriented in the plane at right angles to the long axis of the cerebellar folia so that the dendritic field has a very narrow profile when viewed from the side. The *pyramidal cells* of the cerebral cortex are so named because of the pyramidal shape of their somata. From the base of the perikaryon, four or more branching *basal dendrites* extend laterally and downward; from its apex, an *apical dendrite* ascends toward the surface of the cortex giving off side branches along its course and commonly ending in a small spray of laterally directed branches. Another class of cells has a dendritic field in the shape of an inverted cone; these are the *mitral cells* of the olfactory bulb, so named because the shape of the cell soma was thought to resemble a bishop's miter.

In an unusual class of small multipolar cell, an axon is lacking altogether. These cells are most common in the retina, where they are called *amacrine cells* and in the olfactory bulb, where they are called *granule cells*. Although these cells lack an axon, they can influence the activity of other nerve cells by means of unusual specializations of their processes, which seem to have some of the characteristics of axons and dendrites (see Fig. 8–38).

In some instances the name given to a neuron is determined by the nature of its axonal ramifications. This is especially true of neurons with relatively short axons that break up into their terminal branches close to the parent cell soma. A well-known example is the *basket cell* of the cerebellar cortex, whose axons give sprays of small branches that enclose the somata of adjoining Purkinje cells as though in a series of baskets (Fig. 8–9 and 8–25). The small cell from the cerebral cortex illustrated in Figs. 8–7 and 8–11B with its highly branched and intensely intertwined axon, was called a spider-web cell by the

Spanish histologist Ramón y Cajal. Cajal referred to other cells of the type illustrated in Fig. 8–7 as double bouquet cells because of their long ascending and descending axonal systems. These latter two examples are of interest because they show that cells with essentially the same type of dendritic field (both would be called stellate cells) may give rise to quite different systems of axon branches.

The three examples given above show that the nature of a cell's axonal plexus may be just as characteristic as the shape of its dendritic field. And, as in the case of dendritic fields, certain basic types can be recognized. Very shortly after introducing the stain upon which so much of our knowledge of the shapes of nerve cells depends, the Italian histologist Camillo Golgi pointed out that most nerve cells fall into one of two classes. These two classes have come to be called Golgi type I and Golgi type II neurons. Golgi type I neurons have long axons that pass out of the region in which the parent cell soma is situated and terminate at some distance, either in some other part of the nervous system or in another tissue such as skin or muscle. The motoneurons of the spinal cord, the pyramidal cells of the cerebral cortex, and the Purkinje cells of the cerebellar cortex are all examples of Golgi type I cells. Golgi type II neurons, on the other hand, have short axons that ramify locally in the region of the parent cell soma and may not even extend much beyond the confines of its dendritic field (like the spider-web cell shown in Fig. 8–11B).

To get an idea of the significance of the Golgi classification, consider, for example, any of the ascending sensory pathways of the nervous system. The cells with long axons are the main transmission lines conveying information from the periphery through various synaptic relay centers (nuclei) to the cerebral cortex. Cells with short axons are situated at each synaptic station; they may influence cells with long axons that project up to the next level. The Golgi type II cells thus serve as modulators of synaptic transmission in the long pathways of the nervous system. A common alternative term for these cells is, therefore, *interneurons*, since they are, in a sense, intercalated between any two links in a long pathway.

The name applied to a particular type of nerve cell may vary depending on the nature of the histological preparation in which it is observed. The names of the examples cited above were derived from the *total* appearance of the nerve cell—soma, dendrites, and axon—as seen in the silver impregnation method of Golgi. Unfortunately, some names are based on the appearance of the cells when stained by more routine histological techniques that show only the cell somata. For example, the small stellate neurons of the cerebral cortex (Fig. 8–8) have been called granule cells, but the same term has also been applied to quite different cells in the cerebellar cortex (Fig. 8–12B), the dentate gyrus, the olfactory bulb, and certain other sites, even though their dendritic and axonal configurations are not at all comparable.

Factors Governing the Size and Shape of Neurons. Neurons differ greatly both in size and shape. Possibly the smallest neurons in the mammalian central nervous system are found in parts of the hypothalamus. Such neurons have somata measuring little more than 3 to 4 μm in diameter, and their axons and dendritic fields are comparably small. Among the largest cells are the giant pyramidal cells of the motor area of the cerebral cortex whose somata may measure as much as 120 μm in their largest dimension; and, in addition to giving rise to a long, thick apical dendrite, they have axons that may be 50 cm or more in length. Between these two extremes, all sizes can be found.

Two factors appear to determine the size of a cell: (1) the number, length, and diameter of its processes, and (2) the number of synapses that it receives on its surface. It is a useful generalization that neurons with the longest and thickest axons have the largest somata. In the case of one of the larger motoneurons in the lumbar or sacral parts of the spinal cord, for example, the axon may be almost a meter in length and 15 to 20 μm in diameter. Clearly, most of the volume of the cell is in the axon. As the axon itself appears to be incapable of synthesizing proteins and most other structural or functional constituents, the cell soma must maintain the appropriate amount of metabolic machinery to support the axon. Similarly, cells with long, thick, profusely branching dendrites also have large somata, and even though the dendrites have certain synthetic capabilities, there is evidence that they, too, are partly maintained by the soma.

The number and length of the dendrites possessed by a particular cell seem to be related to the number of synaptic contacts that it receives from the axons of other cells. The large motoneurons of the spinal cord, which integrate activity from many diverse sources, have been estimated to receive as many as 10,000 synaptic contacts, and the large Purkinje cells of the cerebellum may receive as many as 200,000. Small interneurons, on the other hand, have not only short axons of small diameter but also relatively few dendrites and ultimately few synaptic contacts.

The Structure of Nerve Cell Somata

Along with providing a large surface area of membrane that may receive synaptic contacts from other neurons, the cell soma, which contains the nucleus, is the trophic or nourishing center of the nerve cell. Chief among the functional characteristics of the nerve cell other than those concerned with the integration and transmission of nervous activity is the need to maintain itself and to supply various organelles and macromolecules to the terminals of its axon. This is achieved by the active synthesis in the soma of large amounts of proteins, lipids, etc., and a highly efficient somatofugal transport system that delivers these metabolic products and organelles to the cell's processes.

The Nucleus. The *nucleus* of most nerve cells is either spherical or ovoid, and is large relative to the size of the perikaryon.[1] Because a substantial part of the genome is continually being transcribed in keeping with the active synthetic state of the cell, it is euchromatic; that is, the nuclear chromatin is generally dispersed when seen with the electron microscope and the nucleus usually has a vesicular appearance when viewed with the light microscope (Fig. 8–10). The nuclear envelope, with its nuclear pores, is typical of that of all eukaryotic cells (Fig. 8–13). One, and sometimes two or even three prominent nucleoli are present within the nucleus; their fine structure is also typical of that in other protein-synthesizing cells. Associated with the nucleoli may be one or more "satellites," of which the female sex chromatin (corresponding to the heterochromatic X chromosome) is the best known (Fig. 8–14); this satellite was first described in neurons by Barr. These so-called Barr bodies may be attached to the nucleolus, to the inner face of the

nuclear membrane, or to both. Other nucleolar satellites and crystalline or filamentous intranuclear particles are occasionally seen, but they are uncommon and of uncertain significance.

The Perikaryon. Perhaps the most striking feature of the perikarya of neurons is the large amount of ribosomal material that they contain, a material that indicates the high rate of protein synthesis in these cells. As seen in the electron microscope, the ribosomal material is mainly in the form of multiple stacks of rough endoplasmic reticulum, but a great many free ribosomes and polyribosomal rosettes are also present. These clustered masses of free and attached ribosomes are strongly basophilic, and when nervous tissue is stained with basic dyes and viewed in the light microscope, many neurons are seen to contain irregularly shaped clumps of intensely stained cytoplasmic inclusions. These inclusions are customarily called *Nissl bodies* after the German neurologist F. Nissl, who first used aniline dyes to study the nervous system. Although the cytoplasm of all neurons is basophilic because of their rich content of RNA, not all neurons have distinct Nissl bodies. Such bodies can be seen particularly well in the large motoneurons of the spinal cord (Figs. 8–10 and 8–13) and in large dorsal root ganglion cells; the cytoplasm of smaller neurons merely shows a diffuse, dustlike basophilia.

The *Golgi complex* is also prominent in all neurons; at the electron-microscopic level, it is commonly seen as several groups of flattened and dilated smooth-walled sacs and vesicles of variable size, usually near the nucleus but sometimes extending into the bases of the larger dendrites (Figs. 8–13 and 8–15). The reason for this well-developed Golgi complex is incompletely understood; but by analogy with its appearance in other secretory cells it probably is engaged in both the glycosylation of proteins and the packaging of secretory products within membrane-bound vesicles. The most common vesicles found in neurons are the *synaptic vesicles*, which are present in large numbers in axon terminals and appear to contain the neurochemical transmitter agents that mediate synaptic function (see p. 309). We do not know to what extent these vesicles are produced in the perikaryon or in axon terminals. However, the cell bodies of some types of neuron contain variable numbers of membrane-bound dense vesicles that represent their main neurosecretory product or en-

---

[1]At one time it was thought that the nuclei of many large neurons (for example, those of the pyramidal cells of the hippocampus and the Purkinje cells of the cerebellum) were tetraploid, but this appears to have been due to a technical error in measuring the cells' DNA content.

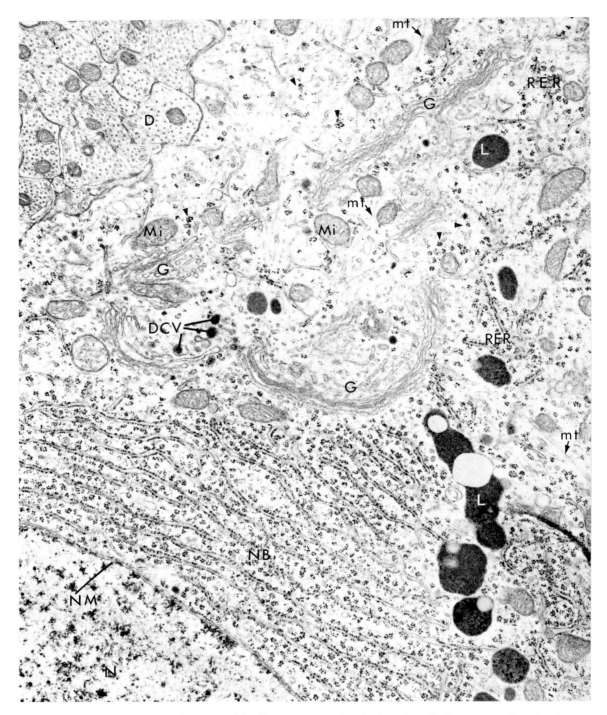

8–13 An electron micrograph of a pyramidal cell from the cerebral cortex showing the nucleus **(N)** with its surrounding envelope **(NM)**, a prominent Nissl body **(NB)**, several lysosomes **(L)**, mitochondria **(Mi)**, dense-core vesicles **(DCV)**, and microtubules **(mt)**. The cell has an extensive Golgi complex **(G)**, a good deal of rough endoplasmic reticulum **(RER)**, and free ribosomes **(arrowheads)** outside the obvious Nissl body. In the upper left corner there are several transversely sectioned dendrites **(D)** containing microtubules cut in transverse section. × 25,000.

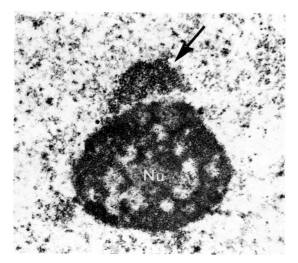

8–14 Nucleolus **(Nu)** and nucleolar satellite **(arrow)** from cortical neuron of a female rat. × 29,000.

zymes involved in its synthesis. In certain small neurons of the autonomic nervous system, for example, many dense-core vesicles about 600 to 800 Å in diameter are present in the perikaryon as well as in the axons and their terminals. These vesicles contain catecholamines which, when condensed with formaldehyde, cause the neurons to be intensely fluorescent under ultraviolet light (Fig. 8–16).

Neurosecretory products that do not act as chemical transmitter agents at synapses but are released into the general circulation are such

polypeptide hormones as oxytocin and vasopressin, and the various hypothalamic-releasing hormones. These hormones are produced by the neurons in the hypothalamus and are transported in membrane-bound vesicles down their axons for release near the blood vessels of the neurohypophysis or the median eminence. The neurosecretory material is synthesized in the endoplasmic reticulum, packaged in the Golgi complex, and transported in large (approximately 2,000 Å) membrane-bound, dense-core vesicles. Aggregations of these vesicles in the axons and their terminals may be selectively stained by means of the Gomori technique, and in the light microscope they appear as large granular masses called *Herring bodies.*

As might be expected in metabolically active cells, *mitochondria* are also present in very large numbers in neuronal perikarya (Fig. 8–13). They vary a great deal in size, density, and general configuration, but probably not more so in these than in other cells.

Some of the most ubiquitous elements in neuronal perikarya are the large numbers of *microtubules* and *neurofilaments.* Aside from the fact that they are found in all parts of the perikaryon, the microtubules (which have a diameter of about 250 Å) appear to be identical to those in

8–15 An osmic-acid-stained preparation of a spinal ganglion to show the reticular appearance of the Golgi apparatus. × 500.

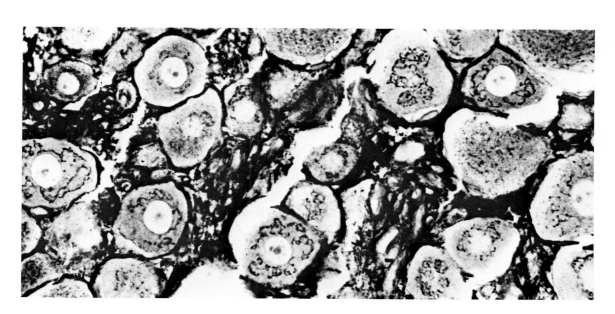

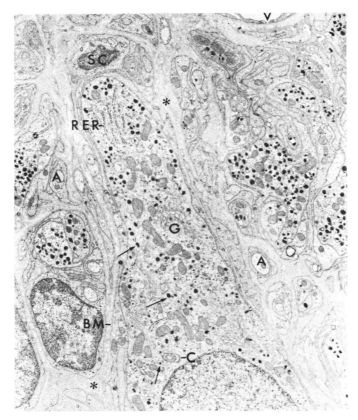

8–16 Electron micrograph of a catecholamine-synthesizing neuron from the nodose ganglion of a cat. Note the dense-core vesicles in the cytoplasm **(arrows)**. **RER,** rough endoplasmic reticulum; **G,** Golgi region; **C,** cilium; **V,** blood vessel. × 13,500. (From Grillo, M. A., Jacobs, L., and Comroe, J. H., Jr. 1974. J. Comp. Neurol. 153:1; courtesy of M. A. Grillo.)
◁

8–17 Lipofuscin granules **(arrows)** in the cytoplasm of neurons in the human superior cervical ganglion. **C,** satellite Schwann cells. × 300.   ▽

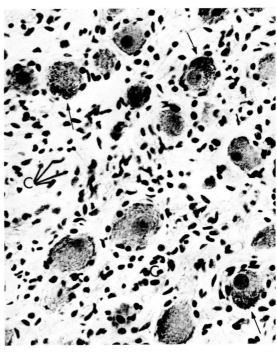

other cells (Figs. 8–13 and 8–19). At present it is not known if neurofilaments (which have a diameter of about 100 Å) are identical to the intermediate filaments (Fig. 8–19B) seen in other cells, and until their substructure and chemical composition have been adequately characterized, this will remain unsolved. Of course, both microtubules and neurofilaments are visible only at the electron-microscopic level. However, when neurons are stained with certain heavy metals (especially silver salts), thick, intertwined fibrillar strings up to 2 or 3 μm in diameter can be seen; they are known as *neurofibrils* (Fig. 8–24). It is thought that they represent metallic silver deposited on bundles of neurofilaments; but in some cases, at least, the silver deposits may be around microtubules as well. As in the case of Nissl bodies, neurofibrils appear most distinctly in large neurons; in smaller cells the neurofibrillar methods give a more diffuse staining of the cytoplasm, although the staining is probably still associated with neurofilaments.

Lysosomes of various kinds are also found in neurons. They appear as dense, or multivesicular, bodies exhibiting positive acid phosphatase activity. Their number varies from neuron to neuron and seems to increase with the age of the individual. The yellowish pigment *lipofuscin*, which accumulates in neurons with advancing age, probably represents insoluble residues remaining from lysosomal activity. In the human brain, the yellowish lipofuscin pigment may build up with age to the extent that it may occupy more than half the cross-sectional area of the somata of certain cells (Fig. 8–17). Its ultrastructural counterpart is a heterogeneous membrane-bound body composed of dense particles and lipid-filled vacuoles (Fig. 8–13). Other pigments occur naturally in certain groups of neurons. Perhaps the best known is the melanin of the nerve cells in the substantia nigra of the midbrain. The pigment seems to be absent in human infants, but by puberty it has reached its maximal development. This pigment is also enclosed in membrane-bound structures resembling lysosomes.

Neurons also frequently contain one or two typical centrioles, usually associated with a cilium that may protrude for some distance from the cell surface. Their significance is quite obscure; possibly they simply reflect the epithelial origin of the nerve cells.

The Structure of Dendrites

In some respects, dendrites can be regarded as extensions of the cell soma. For example, at both the light- and electron-microscopic levels it is difficult to define the point at which the soma ends and a dendrite begins. The dendrites appear as though they were "drawn out" from the soma, and most of the organelles typical of the perikaryon extend for considerable distances into the dendrites. The main-stem dendrites of larger neurons can usually be seen in material stained with routine neurohistological stains, because they often contain Nissl bodies or dispersed Nissl substance as distinct as that found in the soma (Figs. 8–10 and 8–22A). By electron microscopy, considerable amounts of rough-surfaced endoplasmic reticulum, free ribosomes, and components of the Golgi complex are often seen in the proximal portions of dendrites (Fig. 8–18).

As they extend away from the soma, the dendrites taper and the successive generations of branches to which they give rise are always of smaller diameter than the parent trunk. In some

neurons the dendrites appear to be beaded with irregular dilatations and constrictions. In some instances, this appearance may be artifactual; but in others, the beading clearly reflects the natural state of the dendrites.

As the dendrites extend away from the soma, the rough endoplasmic reticulum and other organelles become progressively diminished; and in the more peripheral dendrites, rough endoplasmic reticulum and free ribosomes are sparse or lacking entirely. The presence of ribosomal material is important, however, because at the electron-microscopic level it serves to distinguish dendrites from axons. But the most striking feature of dendrites is the presence of many microtubules and neurofilaments (Figs. 8–18 and 8–19). In general, they are much more conspicuous than in the soma and are more regularly aligned along the axis of the dendrite. The number of filaments and tubules seems to vary with the diameter of the dendrite and the distance from the soma. Some microtubules and neurofilaments may extend from the soma almost to the tips of the dendrites; as the dendrites branch, bundles of filaments and tubules diverge into the branches. The microtubules are thought to be involved in the transport of various materials, including proteins and such organelles as mitochondria, from the perikaryon to the distal portions of the dendrites. By tracing the movement of labeled proteins after injecting radioactive precursors into the soma, it has been possible to demonstrate "dendritic transport" with a rate of about 3mm/h, a rate comparable to that at which certain materials move down the axon. This transport is inhibited by drugs, such as colchicine and vinblastine, which cause a breakdown of microtubules. The role of the neurofilaments is unknown.

One of the most distinctive features of dendrites is the presence on their surfaces of synaptic contacts made by the axon terminals of other neurons. The structure and general distribution of synapses will be discussed elsewhere. Here we need only note that all dendrites receive synaptic contacts at various points along their length. In addition, the dendrites of many (but by no means all) classes of neurons have multiple small protrusions (dendritic spines) that are specialized to receive synaptic contacts.

As seen in Golgi preparations, a typical dendritic spine is a pedunculated structure with an expanded tip measuring 0.5 to 2 μm in diameter, and a narrow stalk 0.5 to 1 μm long (Fig. 8–20).

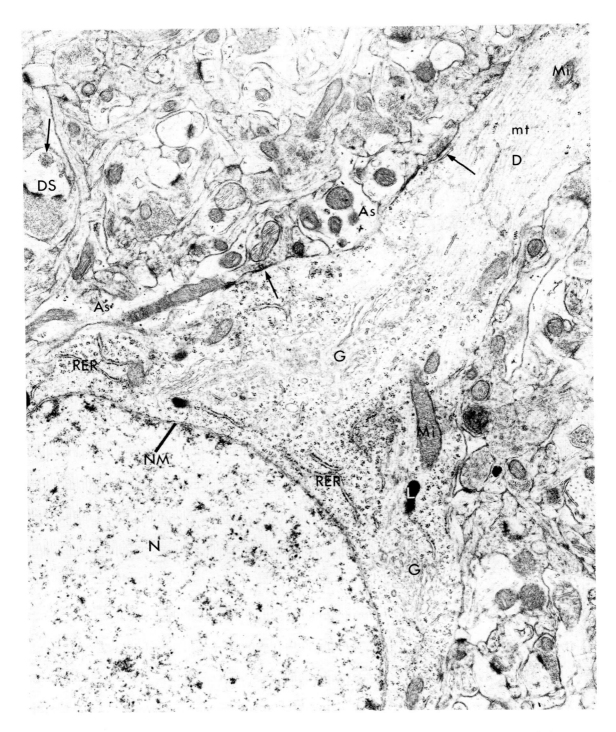

8–18 An electron micrograph of the apical portion of a pyramidal neuron from the cerebral cortex, with its apical dendrite extending toward the upper right corner. **N,** nucleus; **NM,** nuclear envelope; **RER,** rough endoplasmic reticulum; **G,** Golgi complex; **L,** lysosome; **Mi,** mitochondrion; **mt,** microtubules; **D,** dendrite; **As,** astrocytic processes; **DS,** dendritic spine with spine apparatus **(arrow).** The **arrows** in the cell soma mark the sites of two synapses on the surface of the neuron. × 15,000.

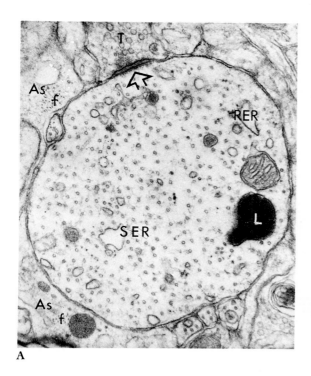

A

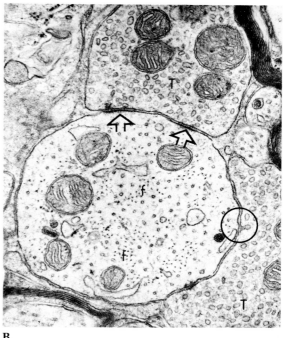

B

By electron microscopy the stalk can often be seen to contain one or more microtubules; but the expanded tip usually appears as an amorphous matrix (Fig. 8–21), except at the point of synaptic contact where a considerable amount of electron-dense material is attached to the postsynaptic membrane. In many spines, one or more smooth-walled vesicular or saclike structures are seen, often alternating with bands of electron-dense material; they constitute a special organelle of unknown function called the spine apparatus.

On any given neuron, the spines may vary considerably in shape and size. Generally, those situated most distally are the longest and may even be bifid, and those near the soma are the smallest and are often simple, sessile protrusions of the dendritic surface, usually without a spine apparatus. There is also a fairly consistent relationship between the number of dendritic spines and the distance from the soma. Generally, there are few or no spines on the proximal portions of the stem dendrites but their amount quickly increases to a maximum, maintained over the middle portion of the dendritic system, and then declines again toward the distal portions of the dendrites (Fig. 8–37). Although the significance of this characteristic spine distribution is difficult to assess, it is clear that, when present, the

8–19 Electron micrographs of two transversely sectioned dendrites that contain saccules of smooth endoplasmic reticulum **(SER)**, many microtubules, and neurofilaments **(f)**. The dendrites are contacted by axon terminals **(T)**, which form distinct synapses at the points marked by the large **open arrows.** The dendrites are surrounded by astrocytic processes **(As)**, which also contain filaments **(f)**. **L,** lysosome. The circled area in **B** shows an endocytotic vesicle thought to indicate retrieval of synaptic vesicle membrane from membrane of terminal. **A,** ×38,500; **B,** ×29,000 (From Rockel, A. J., and Jones, E. G., 1973. J. Comp. Neurol., 147:61.)

spines represent the principal synaptic surface on the dendrites. The dendritic spines may also be labile structures in the sense that they may disappear after deafferentation or sensory deprivation and possibly with increasing age.

Structure and Function of Axons

Unlike dendrites, the axon usually appears as a unique and sharply defined process. It usually arises from the soma as a conspicuous conical elevation called the axon hillock (Figs. 8–22 to 8–24), but it may also arise from the basal portion of a stem dendrite. The *initial segment* of the axon is commonly the narrowest portion of

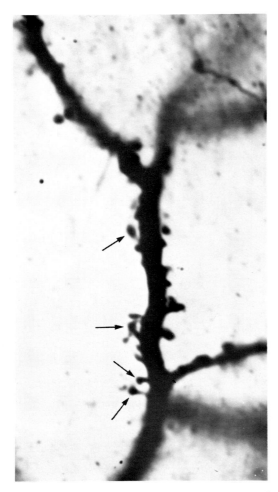

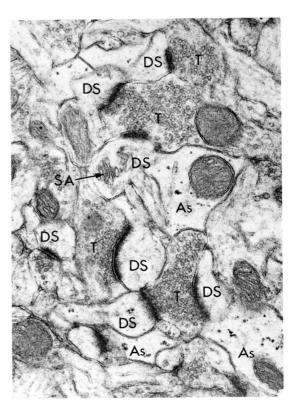

8–21 Electron micrograph of a series of dendritic spines **(DS)**, each contacted by an axon terminal **(T)**. One spine contains a spine apparatus **(SA). As,** astrocytic cytoplasm. Cerebral cortex of rat. × 28,000.

8–20 A high-power light micrograph of a portion of a dendrite of a cell in the inferior colliculus of a cat, stained by the Golgi method, to show the appearance of the dendritic spines **(arrows).** × 1,800. (From Rockel, A. J., and Jones, E. G. 1973. J. Comp. Neurol. 147:11.)

the process, and, like the axon hillock, has a number of distinctive morphological features. The most obvious feature of the axon hillock is the relative absence of free ribosomes and rough-surfaced endoplasmic reticulum, so that in Nissl-stained preparations it appears as a palely stained, triangular or fan-shaped area free of Nissl granules. In electron micrographs, the most obvious ultrastructural feature of the axon hillock is the presence of many microtubules and neurofilaments streaming from the perikaryon into the initial segment. The extent of the initial

segment is easiest to define in cells whose axons subsequently acquire a *myelin sheath;* in them the segment reaches from the apex of the axon hillock to the beginning of the myelin sheath. It is characterized by the absence of ribosomes and rough-surfaced endoplasmic reticulum and by two special features (Fig. 8–22B). The first feature is the presence of an electron-dense "under-coating" beneath the plasma membrane (or *axolemma*). The undercoat measures about 200 Å in thickness and is deficient only beneath the regions of synaptic contact that are sometimes made by the terminals of other axons on the initial segment. The membrane of the initial segment generally has the lowest threshold of excitability, and is therefore commonly the site of initiation of the nervous impulse. To what extent the dense membrane undercoat facilitates this is not known, but it is noteworthy that a similar

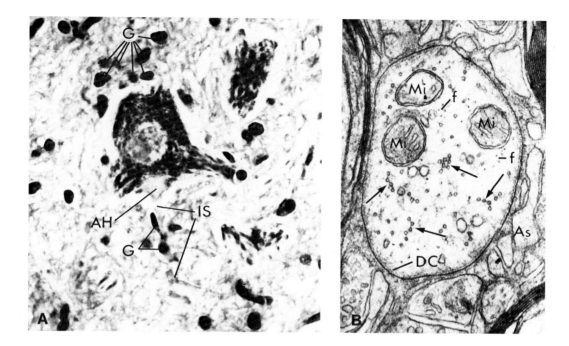

dense undercoat is found at the nodes of Ranvier in myelinated axons (see below).

The second distinguishing feature of the initial segment is the fact that the microtubules passing through it are collected into small bundles. In these bundles the individual microtubules are linked at intervals to one or more of their neighbors by multiple small cross-bridges best seen in cross sections of the initial segment (Fig. 8–22B). When seen in longitudinal sections, the electron-dense cross-bridges resemble the rungs on a ladder, which in myelinated axons can be followed to the point where the myelin sheath is acquired. In axons that do not acquire a myelin sheath, the fasciculation of the microtubules and the dense membrane undercoat cease at a comparable distance from the soma. These two features of the initial segment seem to be peculiar to the central nervous system; they have not been found in neurons of the dorsal root ganglia or autonomic nervous system.

In addition to the microtubules, the axon contains a variable number of neurofilaments of unknown function (Fig. 8–53). They are commonly regarded as semirigid structures that provide a skeletal framework for the axon, but this has not been proved; other suggestions—for example, that they guide the axon toward its destination during development—are dubious. We do know,

8–22 In a Nissl-stained preparation the axon hillock **(AH)** and initial axonal segment **(IS)** appear essentially unstained. An electron micrograph of a tranversely sectioned initial segment shows a characteristic electron-dense undercoating beneath the axolemma **(DC)**, and fasciculated clusters of microtubules **(arrows). Mi,** mitochondria; **f,** neurofilaments; **G,** glial cells; **As,** astrocytic cytoplasm. **A,** motoneuron of cat, thionin stain, × 650. **B,** electron micrograph from cat inferior colliculus, × 40,000.

however, that in cold-blooded animals the number of neurofilaments increases during cold adaptation, and in all animals their number increases after injury to the axon.

The Terminations of Axons

Axons end by forming functional contacts with other nerve cells, muscle fibers, or gland cells. In the central nervous system the axon of a neuron terminates on other nerve cells in the specialized junctions already referred to as synapses. As an axon approaches the region of the nervous system in which it terminates, it generally branches repeatedly; if it has a myelin sheath, the initial branches are myelinated, but as they approach the neurons with which they are destined to

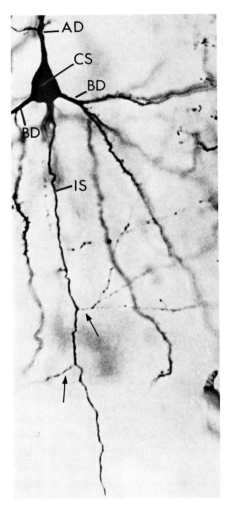

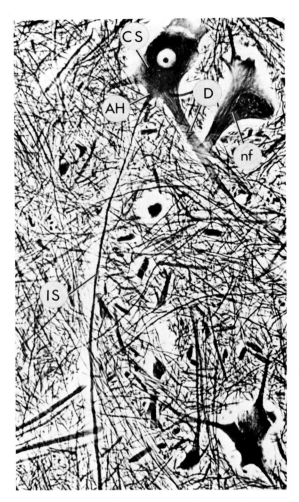

8–23 Pyramidal cell from the cerebral cortex of a monkey showing collateral branches **(arrows)** arising from initial segment of axon **(IS). BD,** basal dendrites; **CS,** cell soma; **AD,** apical dendrite. Golgi stain. × 700.

8–24 Motoneuron from spinal cord of a cat showing axon hillock **(AH)** and initial segment **(IS).** Dendrites **(D)** and cell soma **(CS)** contain neurofibrils **(nf)** best seen in part of second cell to right. Bodian stain. × 850.

make synaptic contact, they usually branch again (Figs. 8–25 and 8–26), and the final branches are unmyelinated.[2]

The appearance of the endings in silver-stained preparations is variable, but because they

---

[2]The individual branches making up the terminal spray engendered by a long axon are commonly called *telodendria* (singular, telodendron). This term, which means "branches at a distance," is often inappropriate if applied to the branches of a short, unmyelinated axon belonging to a Golgi type II neuron, for in the highly branched axonal plexus commonly engendered by such a cell, it is not possible to distinguish a major parent trunk much beyond the initial segment.

are usually in the form of tiny swellings on the axon branches, they are customarily called synaptic *boutons* (or buttons) (Figs. 8–26 to 8–28). A synapse is formed where a synaptic bouton becomes closely associated with a portion of the membrane of another nerve cell (commonly its soma or dendrites) and where, by means of a series of morphological specializations to be described below, the release of a neurochemical transmitter agent from the axon terminal can influence the conductance of the recipient (or *postsynaptic*) cell. Synaptic boutons may occur as swellings at the very ends of the terminal branches of an axon, in which case they are

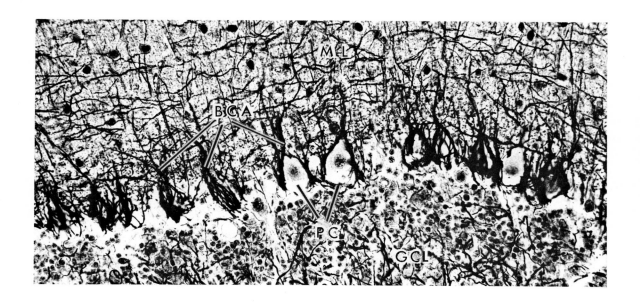

8–25 Basket cell axons **(BCA)** traversing molecular layer **(ML)** of cat cerebellum and descending to form terminal baskets over somata of Purkinje cells **(PC). GCL,** granule cell layer. Reduced silver stain. × 500.

8–26 Terminal axon **(open arrow)** branching **(arrow)** and terminating as a series of terminal boutons **(arrow heads)** on soma **(CS)** and axon initial segment **(IS)** of a pyramidal cell in the cerebral cortex of a monkey. **AD,** apical dendrite; **DS,** dendritic spines. Golgi stain. × 500. (From Jones, E. G. 1975. J. Comp. Neurol. 160:205.)

called *boutons terminaux.* Some axon terminals are exceedingly large and may cover a great deal of the surface of the postsynaptic cell, in which case they may be called *calyces,* or *baskets* (Figs. 8–9 and 8–25). Other synaptic contacts may occur at intervals along a terminal segment of an axon or, in the case of a short axon, along most of its length. In this situation, they are usually called *boutons en passant* (or *boutons de passage*) (Figs. 8–26 and 8–27). The term synapse was introduced by Sherrington in 1897, and even at that time there was good physiological evidence (based on the direction of transmission of nervous impulses from cell to cell and the differential sensitivity of the junctional region to pharmacological agents such as nicotine) that this was a functionally specialized part of the nervous system. Morphological evidence about the nature of the synapse rested solely on the knowledge that axonal boutons terminaux could be seen making contact with the somata and dendrites of nerve cells. Only since electron microscopy has been used to study the nervous system have the structural correlates of synaptic activity become fully understood.

A typical synapse in the central nervous system consists of a presynaptic element and a post-

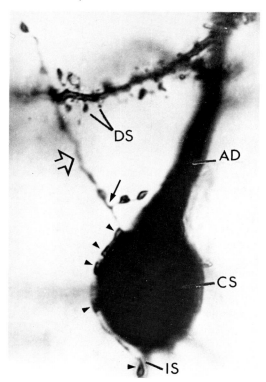

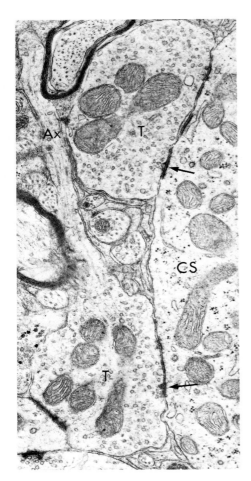

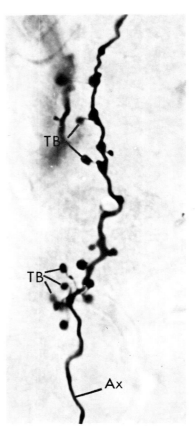

8–27 Electron micrograph showing preterminal axon **(AX)** and two terminal boutons **(T)** making synaptic contact **(arrows)** on cell soma **(CS)** of a neuron in inferior colliculus of a cat. × 18,000. (From Rockel, A. J. and Jones, E. G. 1973. J. Comp. Neurol. 147:61.)

8–28 Terminal portion of an axon **(Ax)** in inferior colliculus of cat showing terminal boutons **(TB)**. Golgi stain. × 1350. (From Rockel, A. J., and Jones, E. G. 1973. J. Comp. Neurol. 147:11.)

synaptic element in close association with one another at a region of membrane specialization and separated only by a narrow extracellular cleft (Figs. 8–27 and 8–29). The commonest form of synapse in the central nervous system is one in which the presynaptic element is a synaptic bouton and the postsynaptic element a dendrite. This type of synapse will be used to illustrate the general form (Fig. 8–30). The membranes of the pre- and postsynaptic elements are aligned to one another with a gap of only 200 to 300 Å between them and without any intervening tissue elements. The region of apposition between the axon terminal and the dendrite is usually some-

what more extensive than the region of membrane specializations that seems to constitute the active zone of the synapse. At the apparently active zone, the gap between the pre- and postsynaptic profiles, usually called the *synaptic cleft*, often becomes slightly wider than the 150- to 200-Å gap that separates other contiguous profiles in the nervous system, and it may contain fine filaments or dense material derived from the outer leaflets of the opposed pre- and postsynaptic membranes, which are much more electron-dense than elsewhere. In addition to being denser, the membrane specializations appear thicker than the rest of the dendritic or axonal membrane, because attached to them is electron-dense material that extends for a variable distance into the pre- and postsynaptic cytoplasm (Figs. 8–30 and 8–31). On the presynaptic side

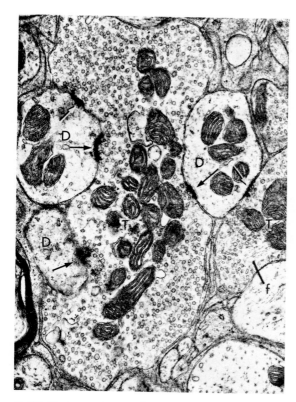

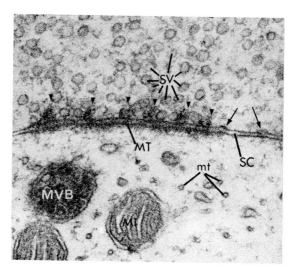

8–30 Electron micrograph of a synapse, showing synaptic vesicles **(SV)**, presynaptic dense projections **(arrowheads)**, and possible sites **(arrows)** of incorporation of synaptic vesicle membrane into membrane of terminal. **MT**, membrane thickening; **SC**, synaptic cleft. Postsynaptic dendrite contains mitochondria **(Mi)**, a multivesicular body **(MVB)**, and microtubules **(mt)**. × 57,000. (From Rockel, A. J., and Jones, E. G. 1973. J. Comp. Neurol. 147:61.)

8–29 Electron micrograph from inferior colliculus showing two terminal boutons **(T)** of the type illustrated in Fig. 8–28. They make synaptic contacts **(arrows)** with small dendrites **(D)**. One terminal contains a small cluster of neurofilaments **(f)**. × 27,000 (From Rockel, A. J., and Jones E. G. 1973. J. Comp. Neurol. 147:61.)

the material appears as a series of conical protrusions from the membrane. On the postsynaptic side, there is often a greater amount of dense material attached to the inner surface of the postsynaptic membrane; it is more homogeneous than on the presynaptic side and can extend for a considerable distance into the dendritic cytoplasm. The membrane thus appears "thicker" than that on the presynaptic side. In other words, the synaptic membrane specializations are asymmetrical. The pre- and postsynaptic membranes and their associated dense material most probably have a different protein composition from the rest of the nerve cell membrane. One clear manifestation of this is the fact that they may be selectively stained in electron-microscopic preparations with phosphotungstic acid.

The second distinguishing feature of a syn-

apse is the presence in the presynaptic element of large numbers of clear-centered vesicles (*synaptic vesicles*) with diameters ranging from 400 to 600 Å. These vesicles contain neurotransmitter substances that are the basis of chemical synaptic action. The concentration of the vesicles is usually greatest near the presynaptic membrane specialization, and many lie between the presynaptic dense projections of the membrane. As an action potential invades the axon terminal, synaptic vesicles fuse with special "release sites" in the presynaptic membrane between the dense projections and there discharge their content of transmitter into the synaptic cleft. The transmitter then diffuses to the postsynaptic membrane where it interacts with special receptor molecules in the postsynaptic membrane; this leads to a change in the membrane conductance of the postsynaptic neuron.

The only other consistent components of every synapse are mitochondria in the presynaptic process, their number varying with the size of the terminal (Figs. 8–27 and 8–29). In addition, a few sacs or tubules of agranular endoplasmic reticulum may be present and in some

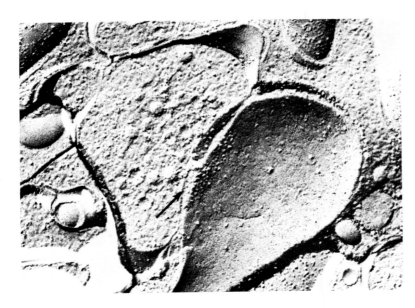

8–31 Freeze-etch preparation of a synaptic contact in cerebellum. **Arrow** indicates synaptic cleft. Note synaptic vesicles in terminal **(left)** and particles in postsynaptic membrane of Purkinje cell dendritic spine **(right).** × 79,000. (From Landis, D. M., and Reese, T. S. 1974. J. Comp. Neurol. 155:93; courtesy of Dr. T. S. Reese.)

cases microtubules and neurofilaments also extend into the axon terminal. The neurofilaments, if found in the presynaptic process, are either diffusely scattered or occasionally aggregated in a single bundle that forms a loop or ring around a central cluster of mitochondria. In the latter case, neurofibrillar stains often show the axon terminals as ringlike boutons (Fig. 8–75B).

From electrophysiological studies, we know that synapses may be either *excitatory* or *inhibitory* depending on whether their activation drives the membrane potential of the postsynaptic neuron toward or away from its threshold level for firing nerve impulses. In chemical synapses these effects are usually mediated by different neurotransmitter agents because, as a general rule, an individual nerve cell releases only one kind of transmitter agent from its axon terminals. Certain transmitters that have differing actions at different postsynaptic sites presumably do so because of differences in the postsynaptic receptors or in the properties of the postsynaptic membranes.

In parts of the vertebrate central nervous system, inhibition has often been found to involve Golgi type II neurons. Such neurons are, therefore, often termed *inhibitory interneurons*. Examples of such inhibitory interneurons are the basket cells of the cerebellum and the Renshaw cells of the spinal cord. However, not all inhibitory neurons are of the Golgi type II variety; the Purkinje cells of the cerebellum have relatively long axons, but we now know that they act to inhibit the cells of the deep cerebellar nuclei. Conversely, not all neurons with short axons are inhibitory; some (for example, the granule cells of the cerebellum) are clearly excitatory.

Synapses in the central nervous system vary in their morphology. The earliest indication of this came from the work of E. G. Gray, who noted in 1959 that synapses could be divided into two categories on the basis of differences in the width of the synaptic cleft and in the extent of the postsynaptic membrane thickenings. The typical axodendritic synapse described on page 306 is an example of what Gray referred to as a *type I synapse* (Fig. 8–32). The two characteristics of this type of synapse are a widening of the intercellular gap at the synaptic cleft to approximately 300 Å and a pronounced accumulation of dense material beneath the postsynaptic membrane. The most striking feature of these synapses is the asymmetry in the pre- and postsynaptic membrane specializations; thus they are now referred to as *asymmetrical synapses*. In Gray's second type of synapse (type II synapses, Fig. 8–33) the synaptic cleft is only slightly wider than the normal intercellular gap (approximately 200 Å) and the postsynaptic membrane specialization is less marked. Little or no dense material is seen attached to the deep surface of the postsynaptic membrane, and because the two apposed membranes appear equally "thick," such synapses are now usually called *symmetrical synapses*.

Although the pre- and postsynaptic mem-

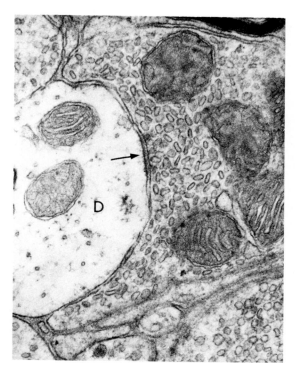

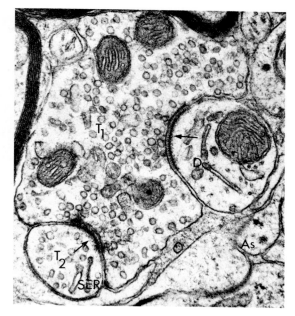

8–32 Flattened vesicle-containing axon terminal making symmetrical synaptic contact **(arrow)** with a dendrite **(D)** in inferior colliculus of cat. × 36,000. (From Rockel, A. J., and Jones, E. G. 1973. J. Comp. Neurol. 147:61.)

8–33 Spherical vesicle-containing terminal **(T₁)** making asymmetrical synaptic contacts **(arrows)** with a dendrite **(D)** and another axon terminal **(T₂)**. Thalamus of cat. **SER,** smooth endoplasmic reticulum; **As,** astrocytic processes. × 35,000.

brane specializations appear in single electron micrographs as linear structures, they are, in fact, fairly extensive plaquelike structures that may measure as much as 1×1 μm. The postsynaptic plaques of asymmetrical synapses are frequently perforated in one or more places, so that in a section passing perpendicularly through the plaque, the axon terminal appears to be associated with two or more postsynaptic "thickenings" (Fig. 8–29). Perforation of the postsynaptic plaques seems to be uncommon in symmetrical synapses.

Although to some extent the asymmetrical and the symmetrical synapses represent the extremes of a continuum, most synapses encountered can be placed readily in one or the other class. The significance of this is emphasized by the observation that the synaptic vesicles in the presynaptic processes associated with the two classes may also differ. If nervous tissue is fixed in aldehyde-containing solutions with buffers of relatively high osmolality, the synaptic vesicles in some axon terminals become "flattened,"

ovoid, or disc-shaped (Fig. 8–32), whereas those of other terminals retain the spherical form commonly seen after osmium tetroxide fixation alone (Fig. 8–33). Uchizono first noted that in the cerebellar cortex, where the functions of most synaptic contacts are known, this flattening of the synaptic vesicles occurs only in the terminals of known inhibitory neurons. Furthermore, because the synaptic vesicles in the terminals of the granule cell axons (which are known to be excitatory) remain spherical (S vesicles) under the same conditions of fixation, it was suggested that the presence of flattened (or F) vesicles in aldehyde-fixed material might serve as an identifying marker for inhibitory synapses and that spherical vesicles might always be associated with excitatory synapses. The subsequent association of flattenable synaptic vesicles with symmetrical membrane specializations and spherical vesicles with asymmetrical membrane thickenings, made first by Colonnier for synapses in the cerebral cortex, strengthened the idea that there was a close relationship between vesicle morphology and functional synaptic type. The flattening of the synaptic vesicles is clearly an artifact in-

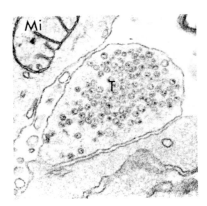

8–34 Noradrenergic terminal **(T)** from tissue culture of rat superior cervical ganglion. Note large proportion of dense-core vesicles demonstrated by soaking tissue 10^{-5}M norepinephrine before fixation. **Mi,** mitochondrion. × 40,000. (Courtesy of Dr. M. I. Johnson.)

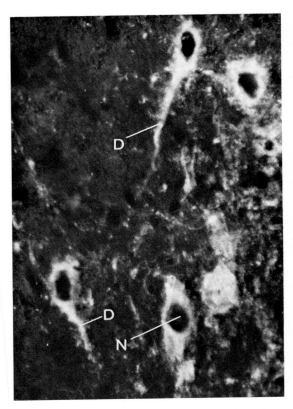

8–35 Noradrenergic neurons in locus coeruleus of a rat demonstrated by binding of a fluorescent-labeled antibody to enzyme dopamine-β-hydroxylase. **D,** dendrites; **N,** nucleus × 950. (Courtesy of B. K. Hartman and L. W. Swanson.)

duced by the high osmolality of the aldehyde fixative solutions, but in many parts of the brain and spinal cord, the flattening is sufficiently consistent to provide a useful basis for classifying synapses. However, it has become clear that the association of flattened synaptic vesicles and the presence of an inhibitory synaptic transmitter is not universal. Several instances are now known in which the presynaptic process exerts an inhibitory influence but contains spherical vesicles. The mechanism responsible for the flattening of certain synaptic vesicles is not clear, but it presumably reflects some basic differences either in the vesicle membrane or possibly in its content of synaptic transmitter. In some situations the vesicles that become flattened in aldehyde-fixed material are clearly of the same size as those that remain spherical, but others that become irregular in shape (or pleomorphic) are distinctly smaller in diameter.

A third distinct class of synaptic vesicle has been recognized in axons that are known to release catecholamines or indoleamines. This will be considered in greater detail in the section on the autonomic nervous system, but we shall note here that the terminals of certain classes of aminergic neurons in the central nervous system contain small, spherical vesicles with electron-dense "cores" identical to those found in sympathetic nerve terminals (Fig. 8–34). These vesicles have diameters of 400 to 600 Å, with dense cores approximately 250 Å in diameter. In routinely fixed material the granular vesicles of

these "G synapses" are not particularly prominent, because the material in the dense cores is not well retained. However, if the tissue is fixed in potassium permanganate or presoaked in the appropriate biogenic amine, the cores are seen to be present in most of the vesicles.

Such small dense-core vesicles are to be distinguished from a larger type that is found in small numbers in virtually every type of axon terminal in the nervous system. The larger vesicle has a diameter of approximately 1,000 Å and a core diameter of approximately 500 Å. One or more of them may be found in terminals containing small dense-core vesicles or clear vesicles, either spherical or flattened, and occasionally they are even found in the neuron soma. Their significance is unknown.

Other, even larger dense-core vesicles (up to 2,000 Å in diameter) are associated with the transport and release of various hormones by the neurosecretory neurons of the hypothalamus (*see* p. 131 and Chap. 29).

The site of formation of the clear and smaller dense-core vesicles is not certain. Some evidence suggests that they may be formed in the Golgi complex of the neuronal soma and that they are transported down to the terminals as part of the general "axoplasmic flow." This view is based partly on the known functions of the Golgi complex and partly on the fact that the neuronal soma usually contains considerable amounts of the appropriate neurotransmitter substance and of the enzymes involved in its synthesis. For example, the somata of neurons that release norepinephrine at their axon terminals contain norepinephrine and the enzyme dopamine-β-hydroxylase (which produces norepinephrine from dopamine—the amine of dihydroxyphenylalanine) (Fig. 8–35). On the other hand, smooth-walled, clear-centered vesicles are rarely seen in axons or in the somata of neurons, and since it is known that substantial amounts of most neurotransmitters can be synthesized in axon terminals, it is evident that many vesicles must be formed locally within nerve endings, possibly from the smooth endoplasmic reticulum. Direct evidence for this comes from studies on the uptake of exogenous proteins by axon terminals (Fig. 8–36). If a histochemically identifiable marker such as the enzyme horseradish peroxidase is present in the extracellular space surrounding the terminals of an axon, it is rapidly taken up by the terminals in coated vesicles. At a slightly later stage, peroxidase-laden coated vesicles can be seen to fuse with the cisternae of smooth endoplasmic reticulum in the terminal and to lose their coats or shells, which appear to remain free in the terminal. Synaptic vesicles, containing horseradish peroxidase, then bud off from the cisternae and are free to pass toward the presynaptic membrane, to fuse with it, and in the process to release the enzyme (and whatever transmitter may have been incorporated into the vesicles) into the synaptic cleft. If the terminal is subjected to repetitive stimulation, it can also be shown that as it becomes depleted of synaptic vesicles, its circumference is progressively enlarged. These experimental observations suggest a continuous recycling of the synaptic vesicle membrane, with the vesicular membrane first becoming incorporated into the presynaptic membrane, then moving to one side of the presynaptic specialization, and finally being returned to the interior of the axon terminal in the form of a coated vesicle.

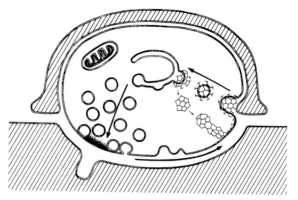

8–36 Postulated mechanism for recycling of synaptic vesicle membrane at neuromuscular junction. Vesicles discharge contents by exocytosis and membranes are incorporated into membrane of terminal; moving away from synaptic region, incorporated membrane is taken up as coated vesicle by endocytosis; joining smooth endoplasmic reticulum, it loses dense coat and is pinched off as new synaptic vesicle. (From Heuser, J. S., and Reese, T. S. 1973. Evidence for recycling of synaptic vesicle membrane during transmitter release at the frog neuromuscular junction. J. Cell Biol. 57:315; courtesy of T. S. Reese.)

The Distribution of Synapses. Axon terminals may make synaptic contacts with any portion of the surface of another neuron (Fig. 8–37). Although the majority occur on dendrites and perikarya, the axon terminals of one neuron may also contact the axon of another; the only parts of nerve cells that have never been seen to receive a synapse are those segments of an axon covered by a myelin sheath.

Synapses on dendritic spines are usually termed *axospinous synapses*. They are usually found on the expanded tips of spines, and each spine receives at least one. Because not all neurons have spines on their dendrites, axospinous synapses are not always present; however, when they are present, they tend to be of the asymmetrical type, and the weight of evidence points to their being excitatory in function. Synapses on the shafts of dendrites are called *axodendritic synapses*. They may be either symmetrical or asymmetrical, and their relative distribution and density depends on the type of neuron. The dendrites of some cells are covered with both types of synapse, whereas others have relatively few of one or the other type, and some have few of either type. Generally, the symmetrical synapses predominate on the larger dendritic trunks near

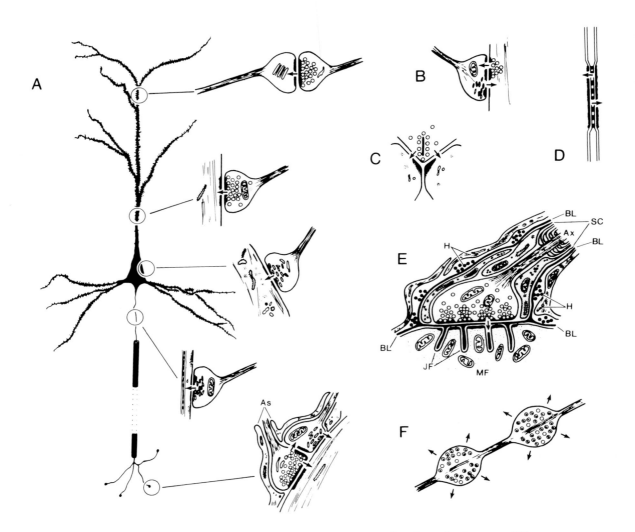

8–37 Types of synapse; **arrows** indicate direction of transmission. **A.** Types of synaptic contact received or made by pyramidal cell of cerebral cortex. From above, down: axospinous; axodendritic, axosomatic; initial segment synapse; axoaxonic, and serial synapse. **As,** astroglial covering. **B.** Reciprocal synapse of olfactory bulb. **C.** Ribbon synapse of retina. **D.** Electrical (gap junction) synapse. **E.** Motor end plate. **Ax,** myelinated axon; **BL,** basal lamina; **H,** fibroblast processes and collagen bundles forming sheath of Henle; **JF,** junctional folds; **MF,** muscle fiber; **SC,** Schwann cell processes; **T,** axon terminal. **F.** Adrenergic terminal in sympathetic nervous system.

the soma. Synapses on the perikaryon are known as *axosomatic synapses*. Again, their numbers and type vary from cell to cell; cells that receive few axosomatic synapses tend to have only symmetrical synapses on the soma; those that receive many tend to have both types. Where a synapse is found on the initial segment of the axon or adjacent axon hillock of a neuron, it may be referred to as an *initial-segment synapse*. Because of the critical role of the initial segment in impulse initiation, synapses located on or near it are in a unique position to influence the discharge of the cell. It is significant therefore that wherever such synapses have been observed, they have invariably been of the symmetrical type, and it is generally assumed that they exert an inhibitory effect on the postsynaptic cell. In some instances a terminal from one axon may form a synapse on a terminal of another: this arrangement is called an *axoaxonic synapse*. Axoaxonic synapses seem to be involved in the phenomenon of *presynaptic inhibition*, because their action tends to reduce the amount of transmitter released by the postsynaptic axon terminal. Occasionally axoaxonic synapses of this type are serially arranged so that one process is postsynaptic at one synapse and presynaptic (on another process) at a second synapse. Such arrangements are *serial synapses.*

The remaining classes of synapses are all rather unusual and have been demonstrated in only a few sites in the nervous system. In some cases dendrites have been found to contain clusters of synaptic vesicles and membrane specializations indistinguishable from those seen in axon terminals. Such processes are termed *presynaptic dendrites,* and because they usually contact other dendrites, the synapses they form are *dendrodendritic synapses.* Such dendrodendritic synapses have now been described in several sites such as the thalamus where they are of the symmetrical type and the presynaptic dendrite usually contains flattened vesicles. A special type of dendrodendritic synapse has been found in the olfactory bulb between the dendrites of the mitral cells and the processes of granule cells. In this case the mitral cell dendrites form asymmetrical synapses (associated with spherical synaptic vesicles) on the granule cell processes; usually within a few microns of such a contact, the same granule cell process forms a *reciprocal synapse* on the mitral cell dendrite. The granule cell processes usually contain flattenable synaptic vesicles and form symmetrical synapses (which are known to be inhibitory) on the mitral cells. *Somatodendritic* and *somatosomatic* synapses have also been described in certain amphibia and in the sympathetic ganglia of mammals. As the names suggest, the presynaptic element in both cases is the cell body of a neuron.

Another form of synapse is the so-called *ribbon synapse,* the best known examples of which are found in the retina. In these cases the axonal process of one type of cell makes synaptic contact with the juxtaposed processes of two other cell types (see Chap. 33). These "triad" synapses are characterized by the presence in the presynaptic element of an electron-dense synaptic ribbon. The synaptic ribbon is invariably aligned perpendicular to the presynaptic membrane and the synaptic vesicles are gathered about it instead of aggregated at the presynaptic membrane.

All the synapses described so far are chemical synapses because they act through the intermediary of a chemical synaptic transmitter. A final synaptic type (relatively infrequent in mammals but very common in other vertebrates and in invertebrates) is the so-called *electrical synapse.* In these synapses the pre- and postsynaptic elements are joined through low-resistance gap junctions so that the electrical activity set up in one cell readily spreads to the next cell without a significant delay. The gap junctions found between neuronal processes are identical to those found in other tissues in which electrical coupling occurs (*see* Chap. 3). In certain cases, an axon terminal may make both a conventional (chemical) and an electrical synapse with a postsynaptic element. The best-known example of such a mixed chemical and electrical synapse is in the ciliary ganglion of birds, but similar contacts have been found in the lateral vestibular nucleus and in the mesencephalic nucleus of the trigeminal nerve of mammals.

Neuroglia and Other Supporting Cells

Although neurons tend to dominate any microscopic section of nervous tissue, they form only a relatively small percentage of the total population of cells present in the section. In most regions they are far outnumbered by the generally smaller nonneuronal or supporting cells, which in the central nervous system are collectively referred to as *neuroglial cells.* Such cells may account for more than one-half the total weight of the brain, and they may outnumber the neurons by as much as 10:1 to 50:1.

The supporting cells are characterized by their generally small size, their ubiquity, and their large numbers. Because of their small size, only their nuclei are seen in routine preparations (Figs. 8–10, 8–22A, and 8–38). The nuclei vary in diameter from 3 to 10 μm, which is about the same size as the very smallest neurons. They are found between neuronal somata and within fiber tracts. Unlike neurons, probably all supporting cells retain the capacity to proliferate under appropriate circumstances.

The Supporting Cells of the Central Nervous System

Two main classes of supporting cell are recognized in the brain and spinal cord (Fig. 8–39). The first consists of *astrocytes* and *oligodendrocytes,* sometimes known collectively as the macroglia. The second class is a heterogeneous group of cells, including the *ependymal cells,* which form the epithelial linings of the choroid plexuses, of the ventricular system of the brain, and of the central canal of the spinal cord; a va-

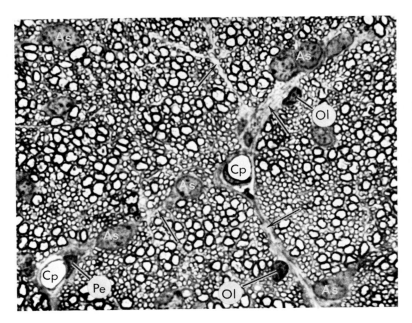

8–38 Cross section of monkey optic nerve showing myelinated axons, astrocytes **(As)**, and oligodendrocytes **(Ol)**. Septa **(arrows)** formed by astrocytic cytoplasm contain capillaries **(Cp)**, one of which is associated with a pericyte **(Pe)**. Toluidine-blue stained plastic section. × 1,600.

riety of vascular and perivascular cells; and cells commonly called *microglial cells*, once thought to be mesodermal rather than neurectodermal in origin but now regarded as immature, or resting, glioblasts.

Astrocytes. As the name implies, astrocytes are star-shaped when demonstrated by heavy metal preparations that impregnate the whole cell (Fig. 8–40A and B). A small, irregularly shaped cell soma gives rise to a number of pro-

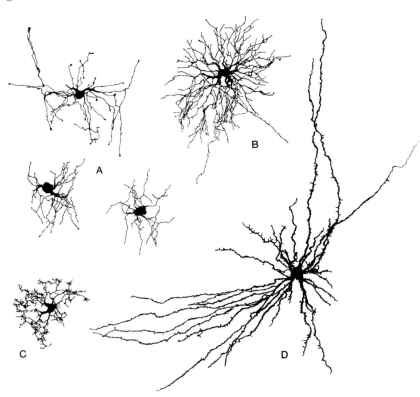

8–39 Camera lucida drawings at same magnification (× 1,000) showing oligodendrocytes **(A)**, protoplasmic astrocyte **(B)**, microglial cell **(C)** and fibrous astrocyte **(D)**. Golgi stain, cerebral cortex of monkey.

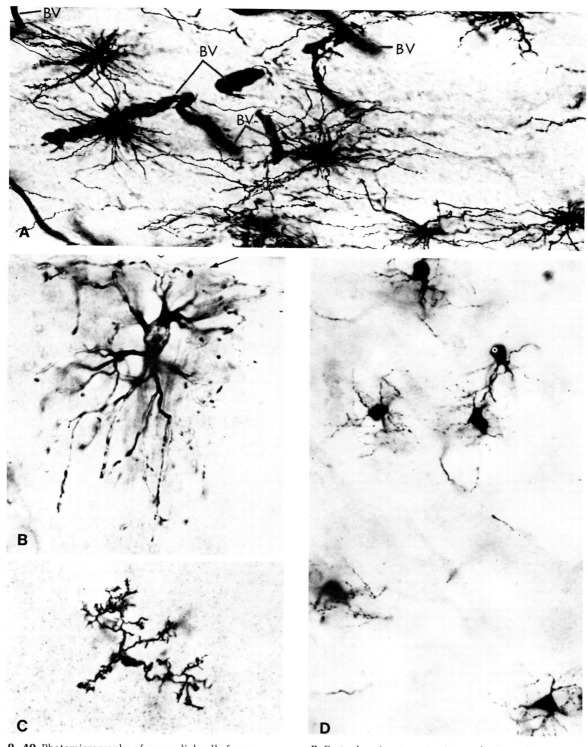

8–40 Photomicrographs of neuroglial cells from cerebral cortex of monkey, Golgi stain.
A. Fibrous astrocytes. **BV,** blood vessels. × 1,000.

B. Protoplasmic astrocyte. **Arrow,** brain surface.
× 1,900. **C.** Microglial cell. × 1,700.
D. Oligodendrocytes. × 1,900.

cesses of variable thickness, length, and branching pattern, which ramify between the perikarya and processes of nerve cells. Astrocytes near the surface of the brain or spinal cord usually have one or more processes extending to the pial surface where they expand to form "end feet;" others have similar end feet on the walls of blood vessels. Two types of astrocyte have traditionally been recognized: *fibrous astrocytes* and *protoplasmic astrocytes*. Fibrous astrocytes (Figs. 8–39, 8–40A, 8–42, and 8–43), found predominantly in white matter, have long, slender, generally unbranched processes containing many delicate fibrils when stained with the usual metallic methods. Protoplasmic astrocytes are found predominantly in gray matter and have shorter, stouter, much more highly branched processes that give to the cells a "fluffy" appearance (Figs. 8–40B, 8–41A, 8–42, and 8–43). These two types of astrocyte are, in fact, modulations in the form of a single cell type, and the appearance of the cells apparently depends on their location and possibly on their metabolic state.

Although the full extent of individual astrocytes can be demonstrated only by using special metallic stains, it is more common to see them in routine neurohistological preparations. In such preparations generally only the nuclei of the cells are seen, because the amount of perikaryal cytoplasm they contain is small and their cytoplasmic processes are thin. The nuclei are usually oval in shape, vesicular, and somewhat larger than the nuclei of oligodendrocytes (see below).

In electron micrographs, astrocytes are distinguished by their relatively organelle-free cytoplasm and their euchromatic nuclei (Figs. 8–44 and 8–45). Ordinarily the nucleus is oval and indented, and distinct nucleoli are not seen. Only a small amount of cytoplasm is usually seen around the nucleus in single sections; however, these sections give a very incomplete picture of the extent of the cytoplasm, for several irregularly shaped cytoplasmic processes emanate from the perikaryon and often extend for considerable distances. As they do so, they give rise to branches and protrusions that align themselves along blood vessels or along the pial surface and insinuate themselves between the somata and processes of nerve cells and other glial cells. Some of these processes are stout and lengthy, but others are thin and sheetlike.

The cytoplasm contains few free ribosomes and little rough-surfaced endoplasmic reticulum. A Golgi complex is always present, and lyso-

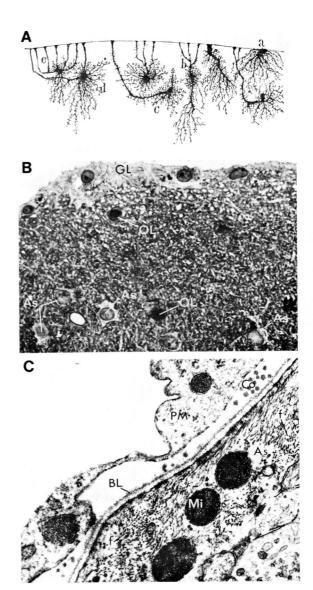

8–41 **A.** Protoplasmic astrocytes at surface of cerebral cortex in a Golgi preparation. **B.** Protoplasmic astrocytes forming the glia limitans **(GL)** at surface of cerebral cortex of a monkey. Other astrocytes **(AS)** and oligodendrocytes **(OL)** are more deeply situated. Toluidine-blue-stained plastic section. × 800. **C.** Electron micrograph showing cell process **(PM)** and collagen bundles **(Co)** of pia mater lying loosely on basal lamina **(BL)** of monkey cerebral cortex. Beneath the basal lamina lie astrocytic processes **(As)** containing mitochondria **(Mi)** and many microfilaments **(f)**. × 30,000. (Part A from Cajal, S. Ramón y. 1909. Histologie de Système Nerveux de l'Homme et des vertébrés, vol. 1. Republished 1952. Madrid: Consejo Superior de Investigaciones Cientificas.)

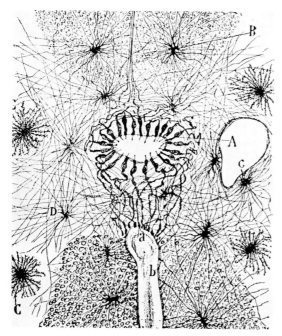

8–42 Astrocytes and ependymal cells in human spinal cord, Golgi stain. Ependymal cell foot processes reach surface at **a**. (From Cajal, S. Ramón y. 1909. Histologie de Système Nerveux de l'Homme et des Vertébrés, vol. 1. Republished 1952. Madrid: Consejo Superior de Investigaciones Cientificas.)

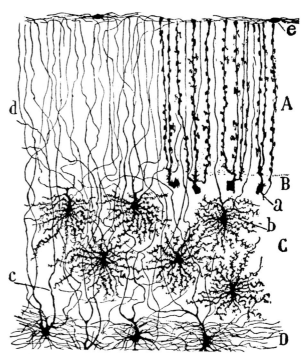

8–43 Astrocytes in human cerebellar cortex, Golgi stain. **a**, Bergmann glial cells; **b**, protoplasmic astrocytes; **c**, fibrous astrocytes. (From Cajal, S. Ramón y. 1911. Histologie de Système Nerveux de l'Homme et des Vertébrés, vol. 2. Republished 1952. Madrid: Consejo Superior de Investigaciones Cientificas.)

somes and glycogen granules are common. The most distinctive astrocytic organelles are the glial filaments, which are similar in appearance to the neurofilaments of nerve cells (Figs. 8–41C and 8–44). Variably sized bundles of these filaments are found in the perikaryal cytoplasm and in most of the processes of all astrocytes. Such bundles of filaments clearly form the basis of the fibrils that are seen with the light microscope.

Two special types of modified astrocyte are known. One is the *Müller cell* of the retina, which is an elongated columnar cell extending across the thickness of the neural retina (*see* Chap. 34). Müller cells have expanded foot processes that form the inner and outer limiting membranes of the retina. The second type is the *Bergmann glial cell* of the cerebellum (Fig. 8–43). The somata of Bergmann glial cells lie at the Purkinje cell layer, and each glial cell has several processes with short side branches that ascend and envelop the Purkinje cell dendrites.

The functions of astrocytes in the normal central nervous system are unknown, but some features about their distribution are suggestive.

Many of their processes are aligned at interfaces between the nervous system and other tissues. Such interfaces occur at the surface of the brain and spinal cord where neural tissue abuts the meninges and along the walls of blood vessels within the central nervous system (Figs. 8–41A to C, 8–46, and 8–47). The largest concentration of astrocytic processes is found beneath the pial surface where many astrocytic foot processes form the *glia limitans*. The outer surface of this zone of astrocytic processes is in contact with the *basal lamina*, which surrounds the brain and spinal cord and derives from the original basal lamina of the embryonic neuroepithelium (Fig. 8–41C). Similarly, as the larger blood vessels enter or exit from the central nervous system, they are invariably separated from the neural tissues proper by the basal lamina and by a *perivascular space* that is continuous with the subarachnoid space surrounding the brain and spinal cord (Fig. 8–46). Again, the basal lamina

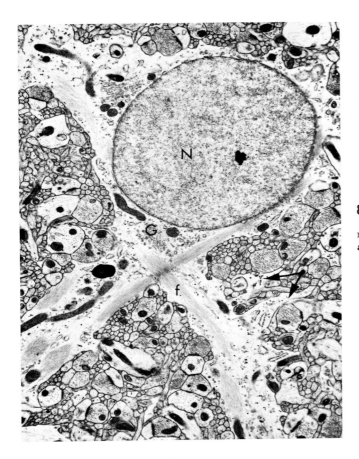

8–44 Electron micrograph of an astrocyte from cerebral cortex of a cat. **N,** nucleus; **f,** filaments; **G,** Golgi complex; **arrows,** cell processes. × 8,000.

is underlain by stacked astrocytic processes. As the vessels penetrate farther into the brain or spinal cord, they progressively lose their muscle coats and the perivascular space becomes obliterated (Fig. 8–47). Finally the capillaries, deep within the substance of the brain or cord, are invested by a continuous basal lamina, which remains ensheathed by astrocytic end feet.

The presence of astrocytic processes at these interfaces suggested to earlier workers that they might serve as diffusional barriers and, in particular, that they might represent the morphological basis of the well-known blood–brain barrier. However, we now know that the intercellular spaces within the brain and spinal cord freely communicate with the subarachnoid space through channels between the astrocytic foot processes; and even though there are occasional gap junctions between adjoining processes, they do not prevent passage of even large molecules between the cerebrospinal fluid and the neural parenchyma. The structural basis of the blood–brain barrier clearly consists of occluding tight junctions between the capillary endothelial cells.

Astrocytes and their processes also divide the brain and spinal cord into sectors of varying distinctiveness, in some places, such as the spinal cord and optic nerve (Fig. 8–38), actually forming septa. It has been suggested, therefore, that their major role is to provide a form of scaffolding, or structural support, on which the neurons and their processes are assembled. It is doubtful that this could be their sole, or even principal, purpose, although in some parts of the nervous system they may serve to isolate groups of neurons or, more often, groups of synapses from their neighbors. Interestingly, the initial segments of most axons and the "bare" segments at nodes of Ranvier are usually ensheathed in astrocytic processes; in many situations, groups of axon terminals ending on a particular neuron, or part of a neuron, are separated from other cells and their processes by an almost complete enve-

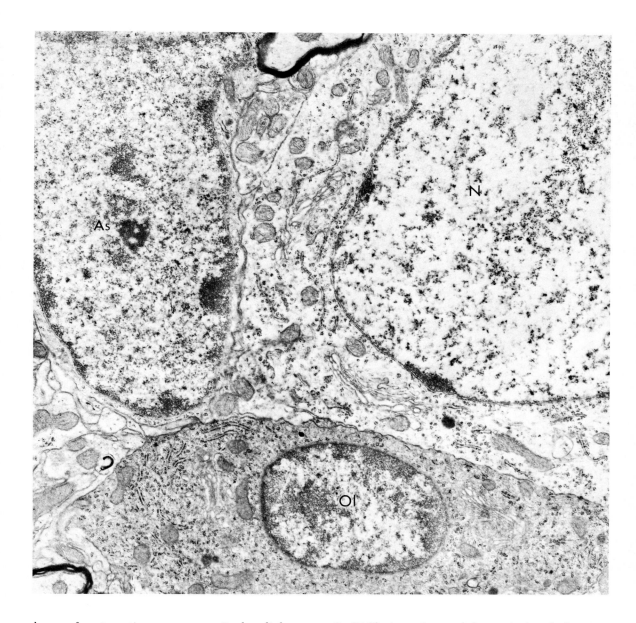

8–45 Electron micrograph from spinal cord of a rat showing distinguishing features of neuron **(N)**, astrocyte **(As)**, and oligodendrocyte **(Ol)**. Label is on nucleus in each case. × 15,000.

lope of astrocytic processes. Such glial-ensheathed synaptic aggregations are sometimes called *glomeruli* (Fig. 8–37).

Some astrocytes undergo a slow depolarization when neighboring nerve cells are repeatedly activated. This depolarization appears to be due to the uptake by astrocytes of excess potassium from the extracellular space, which accumulates during prolonged neuronal activity. The ability to serve as a "potassium sink" is extremely important, although we should point out that at least some invertebrate neurons can be stripped

of their glial ensheathment and yet continue to function for considerable periods of time.

Finally, under various pathological conditions astrocytes play a key role in removing neuronal debris and in sealing off damaged brain tissue (see p. 327).

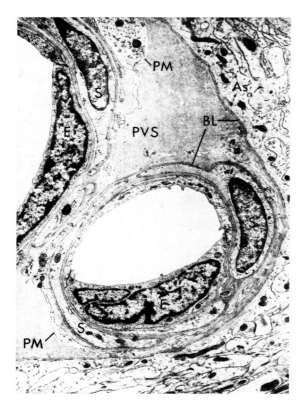

8–46 Electron micrograph of two blood vessels lying in a perivascular space **(PVS)** as they enter cerebral cortex of a cat. **E,** endothelial cells; **S,** smooth muscle cells; **BL,** basal lamina; **PM,** pia mater; **As,** astrocytic processes. × 7,500. (From Jones, E. G. 1970. J. Anat. [Lond.] 106:507.)

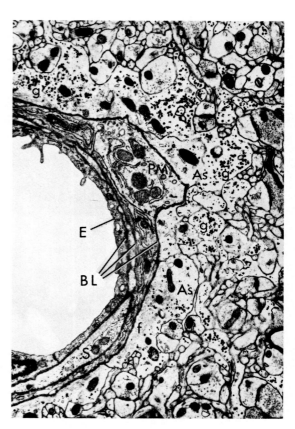

8–47 Electron micrograph showing a small blood vessel with a cell process of the pia mater **(PM)** caught between it and basal lamina of brain. **As,** astrocyte foot processes containing filaments **(f)** and glycogen **(g); BL,** basal lamina; **E,** endothelial cell. Cat cerebral cortex. × 17,500. (From Jones, E. G., and Powell, T. P. S. 1970. Philos. Trans. R. Soc. Lond. [Biol. Sci.] 257:1.)

Oligodendrocytes. Oligodendrocytes are small neuroglial cells with relatively few processes. In light-microscopic preparations (Fig. 8–38) their nuclei are smaller, more irregular, and more deeply staining than those of astrocytes. There are two main types of oligodendrocytes, *interfascicular oligodendrocytes* and *perineuronal satellite* cells (Figs. 8–39 and 8–40D). As the names suggest, interfascicular oligodendrocytes are found among the bundles of axons constituting the white matter of the brain and spinal cord. Perineuronal satellite cells, on the other hand, are found in close association with the perikarya of neurons in areas of gray matter. Although the interfascicular form tends to be more elongated than the perineuronal satellite form, the two types are essentially similar.

In electron micrographs, the oligodendrocyte is generally a much denser cell than the astrocyte

(Figs. 8–45 and 8–48). The nucleus is heterochromatic and the cytoplasm is filled with organelles, especially large numbers of free and attached ribosomes, the latter associated with numerous short cisternae of endoplasmic reticulum. The Golgi apparatus is also extensive, and many mitochondria are present. Perhaps the most striking cytoplasmic feature is the large number of microtubules that permeate the perikaryal cytoplasm and extend into the processes of the cell.

The close association of perineuronal satellite oligodendrocytes with neurons has suggested to some workers that these oligodendrocytes may be in some way involved in maintaining the metabolic state of the neurons with which they are

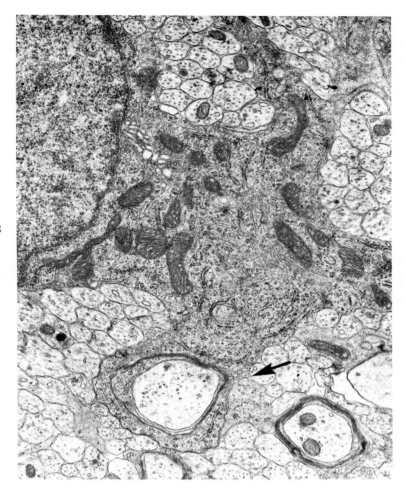

8–48 Electron micrograph of a myelin-forming oligodendrocyte in the developing optic nerve of a rat. **Arrow** indicates mesaxon. × 12,500. (From Vaughn, J. E. 1969. Z. Zellforsch. Mikrosk. Anat. 94:293; courtesy of J. E. Vaughn.)

associated. However, this has never been satisfactorily demonstrated. Only one function can be attributed with confidence to the oligodendrocytes. Both interfascicular and perineuronal oligodendrocytes are the *myelin-forming* cells of the central nervous system (Fig. 8–49).

In a myelinated axon, the sheath begins at the end of the initial segment, usually a few microns from the axon hillock, and ends near the region of termination of the axon (Figs. 8–50 and 8–51). With the light microscope the myelin sheath appears as an elongated tube that is interrupted at regular intervals along its length at the *nodes of Ranvier*. The segments of myelin between consecutive nodes of Ranvier are termed *internodal segments,* or *internodes.* The thickness of the myelin sheath and the length of the internodal segments are fairly constant for a given axon and have been found to be proportional to the diam-

eter (or more strictly, the circumference) of the contained axon.

In the central nervous system, each internodal segment of myelin is formed by a cytoplasmic process of an oligodendrocyte wrapping itself around the axon in a spiral fashion (Figs. 8–48 and 8–49). The process becomes extremely attenuated as it approaches the axon, and this portion of the process is known as the *external tongue* (Fig. 8–50). As the process spirals around the axon, the cytoplasmic faces of its plasma membrane fuse to form what appears in section as a dense line (about 25 to 30 Å thick), called the *major dense line.* A myelin internode is made up of repeated wrappings or lamellae of the oligodendrocytic process and therefore appears as a regularly arranged, repeating series of major dense lines. They are separated from one another by an electron-lucent zone approximately 90 Å

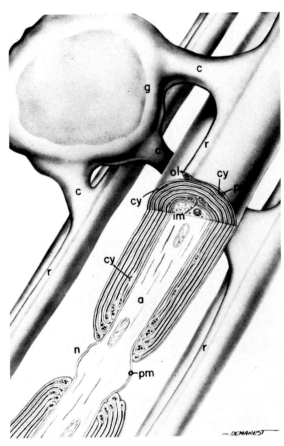

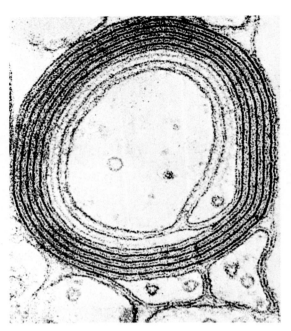

8–50 Electron micrograph of a small myelinated axon in the central nervous system showing inner and outer tongues of oligodendrocytic cytoplasm and major and minor dense lines of myelin sheath. × 161,000. (From Hirano, A., and Dembitzer. H. M. 1967. J. Cell Biol. 34:555; courtesy of A. Hirano.)

8–49 Schematic drawing of an oligodendrocyte forming internodes on three adjacent axons. **r,** outer tongue; **n,** node of Ranvier. (From Bunge, M. B., Bunge, R. P., and Ris, H. 1961. J. Biophys. Biochem. Cytol. 10:67; courtesy of M. B. Bunge and R. P. Bunge.)

wide—referred to as the *intraperiod line*—that contains a faint line somewhat thinner than the major dense line. The intraperiod line is formed by the fused outer faces of the plasma membranes of adjoining wrappings of the oligodendrocytic process.

The outermost major dense line of a myelin internodal segment is directly continuous with the external tongue of the oligodendrocytic process. The innermost major dense line splits apart as it approaches its end to form a similar tongue of cytoplasm known as the *internal tongue*. The intraperiod line disappears as the inner and outer tongues emerge. The internal tongue is the leading edge, as it were, of the oligodendrocytic process. The thickness of a myelin sheath is de-

termined by the number of wrappings of oligodendrocytic cytoplasm and in axons of increasing diameter, the number of major dense lines and intraperiod lines becomes progressively greater. In myelinated axons, one lamella is added for approximately every 0.2-μm increase in axonal diameter. The great concentration of plasma membranes in the myelin sheath accounts for the high concentration of lipids and lipoproteins that gives it a high affinity for fat stains (Fig. 8–51) and also accounts for its intense staining in electron-microscopic preparations.

Oligodendrocytes have several processes and, therefore, unlike Schwann cells in the peripheral nervous system (see pp. 329–330), can each form several internodal segments. In the optic nerve of the rat, a single oligodendrocyte may give rise to as many as 40 or 50 internodal segments. If the portions of an oligodendrocyte that form myelin internodes could be unwrapped, they would appear as extensive flattened sheets roughly trapezoidal in shape. The extent of the cell is there-

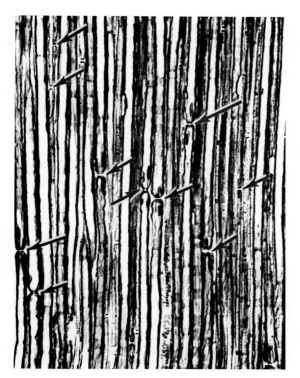

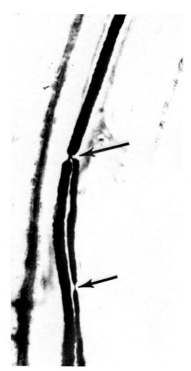

8–51 Osmium-tetroxide–stained longitudinal section of peripheral nerve of cat showing myelin sheaths and nodes of Ranvier **(arrows).** × 300.

8–52 Gold-chloride–stained, teased preparation of myelinated nerve fiber branching at a node **(upper arrow).** Thinner branch has shorter internodal distance (to **lower arrow**). Muscle nerve of a marsupial. × 500.

fore actually much greater than is shown in even the best specimens impregnated with metallic salts, for here the tenuous connections between the parent oligodendrocytic processes and the myelin internodal segments are not visualized. Even in electron micrographs, clear demonstrations of the continuity are limited to occasional fortuitous examples.

The "naked" portions of the axon at the nodes of Ranvier (Figs. 8–52 and 8–53) are highly specialized regions of high capacitance and low electrical resistance, responsible for the self-regenerative capacity of the conducted action potential. During the passage of an action potential, significant changes in membrane conductance occur almost exclusively at the nodes; thus, the wave of depolarization leaps from node to node, a form of conduction known as "saltatory." The structure of the axonal membrane is modified at the node by the addition of a dense membrane undercoat similar to that seen at the initial segment. The outer surface of the membrane is free of any oligodendrocytic covering and is usually

separated from astrocytic processes by the 200-Å wide extracellular cleft seen between all processes in the central nervous system. The remainder of the axon is unchanged at the node, although occasionally a typical axon terminal may bulge from its side, and when myelinated axons branch, the branching always occurs at a node (Fig. 8–52). In such cases, three or more internodal segments come together.

At the nodes of Ranvier the edges of the spirally wrapped myelin lamellae separate at each major dense line and form a series of tonguelike processes. These processes, of course, contain oligodendrocytic cytoplasm; microtubules and other organelles are usually seen in each tongue. The tongues of cytoplasm are best visualized in longitudinal sections where they collectively form the *paranodal region* of the myelinated fiber (Figs. 8–49 and 8–53). In the paranodal region, each tongue is in contact with the axolemma; thus the tongue arising from the most

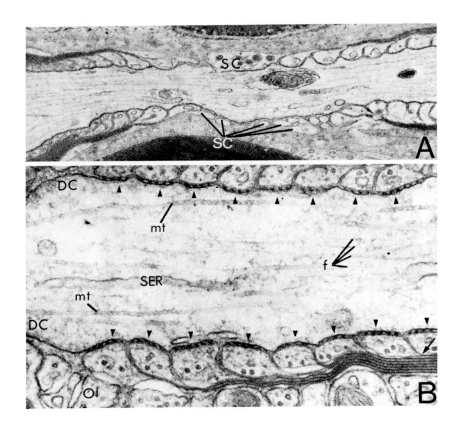

8–53 A. Electron micrograph of node of Ranvier in trigeminal nerve of rat. **SC,** Schwann cell processes. × 25,000. **B.** Electron micrograph of paranodal region of myelinated axon in inferior colliculus of cat. **Arrowheads** indicate dense bars joining tongues of oligodendrocytic cytoplasm to axon. **Arrow** indicates formation of major dense line. **DC,** dense undercoating of naked part of axonal membrane; **f,** neurofilaments; **mt,** microtubules; **Ol,** oligodendrocytic processes; **SER,** smooth endoplasmic reticulum. × 54,000.

superficial major dense line adjoins the naked part of the axon at the node, whereas the tongue arising from the innermost major dense line is the deepest and lies farthest from the node. Because of the spiral nature of the myelin wrapping, the tongues are continuous with one another; and if they could be displayed three-dimensionally they would appear as a helix spiraling around the paranodal segment of the axon.

The tongues of oligodendrocytic cytoplasm at the paranodal region are much more intimately associated with the axolemma than is the innermost myelin wrapping of the rest of the inter-node. At the paranodal region the gap between the tongues and the axolemma is reduced at intervals to a form of close junction in which the adjoining plasma membranes are separated by a gap no more than 20 to 30 Å wide. Within this gap, a series of regularly spaced, short, dense bands are seen extending from the axolemma to the oligodendrocytic tongues (Fig. 8–53B). These dense bands appear to form a continuous spiral around the paranodal region, with about 3 to 5 bands associated with each tongue. Despite the close proximity of the membranes of the oligodendrocyte tongues and the spiral bands, there seems to be fairly free diffusion of ions and even larger particles between the axon and the innermost lamella of the myelin sheath, for electron-dense markers such as lanthanum can readily penetrate between them.

When first formed, all nerve fibers are unmyelinated. In the human embryo, myelination begins at about the fourteenth week of intrauterine life and accelerates in the last trimester of pregnancy. However, a considerable amount of myelination occurs postnatally; and in some animals, such as the rat, which is born in a relatively immature state, the brain may be largely devoid of myelin at birth. In fiber pathways that normally myelinate after birth, the process of myelination is in general related to the functional maturation of the system to which the pathway belongs. For example, in the human infant the myelination of the major descending pathways that control voluntary movements starts at birth, and essentially all of the fibers have acquired a myelin sheath by the time of walking. Thereafter, no new internodal segments are added, but existing internodes increase in length as the brain and spinal cord grow and the nerve fibers elongate.

Other Neuroglial Cells and Pathology of Neuroglia

When the central nervous system is injured or diseased, glial cells proliferate, become phagocytic, and may form a scar. The extent to which astrocytes and oligodendrocytes are involved in these three processes is still much debated, and the role of blood-borne and other macrophages is also uncertain. For some time it was believed that a specific class of cells, the so-called microglia, was the major source of phagocytes in the central nervous system. In light-microscopic preparations, this cell is usually described as being the smallest of the glial elements, with a deeply staining, angular nucleus. When impregnated with heavy metal salts, it resembles a small oligodendrocyte, but with rather more spikelike projections from its slender processes (Fig. 8–40C). Microglia are said to be present in small numbers in the normal central nervous system. The neuropathologist del Rio Hortega believed that they were mesodermal rather than neurectodermal in origin, and that they invaded the brain and spinal cord with the capillary network during the period of vascularization. In areas of neural damage, or during inflammatory disease processes, the microglial cells have been thought to proliferate and become actively phagocytic. As they ingest more and more debris, such as degenerating myelin, they enlarge and become globular in shape and filled with large vacuoles, lipid droplets, and other inclusions; they are then termed *compound granular corpuscles*, or *Gitterzellen*.

At the electron-microscopic level, it has been extremely difficult to identify microglia. Many workers, finding that virtually all glial cells can be fairly readily classified as either astrocytes or oligodendrocytes, would prefer to regard the resting microglial cell of convential light microscopy as simply a variety of oligodendrocyte. If this is the case, unless the vasculature of the nervous system is damaged, all the phagocytes in an area of neuronal death will be derived from astrocytes and oligodendroyctes. If the integrity of the vascular system is damaged, extraneous cells may invade the damaged or diseased central nervous system. Many of these cells are blood-borne phagocytes, but some appear to be vascular pericytes associated with the walls of blood vessels. In experiments in which the brain was subjected to heavy-particle irradiation, it was found that the pericytes (Fig. 8–38), which are normally surrounded by the basal lamina of the capillaries, can break through the basal lamina, invade the brain, and become phagocytic. The pericytes are thus regarded by some as being the source of microglial cells. Another possible source is the meninges, for the presence of infective agents or other foreign material in the subarachnoid space may cause many of the cells of the pia and arachnoid to detach themselves and to invade the brain, particularly by way of the perivascular spaces.

Several recent studies have led to the suggestion that there may be a third class of glial cell normally resident in the central nervous system that, under the appropriate stimulus, may proliferate and become the major source of phagocytic cells in pathological states. These cells are more or less intermediate in fine structure between oligodendrocytes and astrocytes. The developing optic nerve may contain a considerable proportion of such cells, but their numbers decline as astrocytes and oligodendrocytes become more prominent. It has been claimed that they are a form of glial precursor cell derived from the neurectoderm, or the subventricular zone, which persists in small numbers into adulthood and retains the capacity to produce both oligodendrocytes and astrocytes. In regions of axonal degeneration, these precursor cells may become phagocytic and for this reason are regarded by some researchers as the source of the phagocytic microglia.

The Ependyma and the Choroid Plexus

The central canal system of the brain and spinal cord is lined by a layer of closely packed cuboidal or columnar epithelial cells known collectively as the *ependyma* (Fig. 8–42). These cells are the remnants of the embryonic neuroepithelium and retain their original position after the neuroblasts and glioblasts have migrated into the mantle layer. The ependymal cells have many microvilli at their luminal surfaces and commonly have one or more cilia, although the distribution of cilia is patchy and large areas of the lining of the central canal system may be devoid of them. The ependyma is only one cell thick, but its thickness varies because the constituent cells are of variable height in different regions. In parts of the third ventricle overlying the median eminence of the hypothalamus and over certain specializations of the ventricular walls (such as the subcommissural organ and the area postrema) the cells may be very attenuated and even absent. Elsewhere, they are tall and columnar. The ependymal cells are bound to their neighbors near their luminal surfaces by the usual junctional complexes, including close junctions and zonulae adhaerentes. There are, however, no occluding junctions (except in the modified ependymal lining of the choroid plexus): solutes, and even moderately large protein molecules seem to be able to reach the brain parenchyma by passing between the ependymal cells. In this way the cerebrospinal fluid of the ventricular system can communicate freely with the intercellular spaces of the central nervous system.

Ependymal cells usually have a pronounced apical accumulation of mitochondria, but in most other respects their fine structure resembles that of astrocytes. Rough endoplasmic reticulum is not prominent and the cells contain bundles of filaments 60 to 80 Å in diameter. Many ependymal cells have lengthy processes extending from their basal aspects. In the embryo, these processes often reach the surface of the developing brain and spinal cord; but in the mature nervous system, this arrangement is rare except in certain sites such as the anterior median fissure of the spinal cord, where the central canal is relatively close to the surface (Fig. 8–42).

In the four ventricles of the brain, the ependyma is modified to form the special secretory epithelium of the choroid plexuses (Figs. 8–54 and 8–55). The choroid plexuses are formed at regions where the roof plate of the developing neural tube becomes extremely attenuated so that the ependyma and the overlying pia mater come into direct contact with one another over an area known as a choroidal tela. The portion of the pia mater entering into the formation of the choroidal tela becomes richly vascularized,

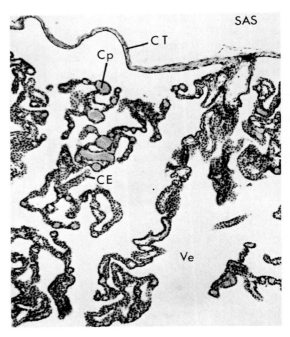

8–54 Choroidal tela (CT) and choroid plexus from fourth ventricle (Ve) of a cat. Cp, capillary; CE, choroidal epithelium; SAS, subarachnoid space. Hematoxylin and eosin stain. × 32.

and this highly vascular tissue becomes invaginated into the ventricle as a mass of villous-like processes collectively known as the choroid plexus. The line of invagination of the choroidal tela is the choroid fissure.

Electron micrographs of the choroid plexus reveal an essentially trilayered structure (Fig. 8–55): (1) At the ventricular surface there is a row of closely packed, columnar ependymal cells with many microvilli but no cilia. The sides and bases of the cells are thrown into numerous interdigitating cytoplasmic processes, and near their luminal surfaces the cells are joined by zonulae adhaerentes and true tight junctions (zonulae occludentes) that encircle the cells so as to occlude the intercellular cleft. (2) The basal surfaces of these modified ependymal cells rest on a basal lamina continuous with that covering the rest of the brain. (3) Deep to this is a thin connective tissue space containing free-lying pia-arachnoid cells, small irregular bundles of collagen fibers, and many small blood vessels. The endothelial cells lining the choroidal capillaries are highly fenestrated and the constituents of blood plasma, including proteins, can pass freely

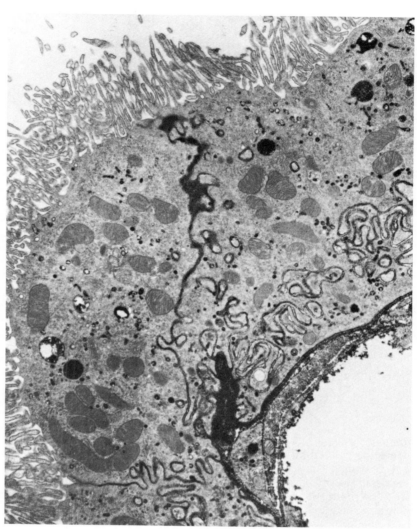

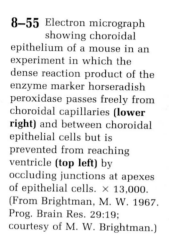

8–55 Electron micrograph showing choroidal epithelium of a mouse in an experiment in which the dense reaction product of the enzyme marker horseradish peroxidase passes freely from choroidal capillaries **(lower right)** and between choroidal epithelial cells but is prevented from reaching ventricle **(top left)** by occluding junctions at apexes of epithelial cells. × 13,000. (From Brightman, M. W. 1967. Prog. Brain Res. 29:19; courtesy of M. W. Brightman.)

into the connective tissue spaces. However, these materials are prevented from reaching the ventricles by the apical tight junctions surrounding the epithelial cells. Thus, despite the permeability of the choroidal capillaries to plasma proteins, the cerebrospinal fluid under normal conditions contains little or no protein.

The secretion of cerebrospinal fluid is an active process requiring energy and can be readily inhibited by carbonic anhydrase inhibitors and by ouabain, which blocks sodium transport. Moreover, it can continue despite an adverse pressure gradient, as in the case of an obstruction to its outflow (thus resulting in hydrocephalus).

Cerebrospinal fluid is produced in humans at the rate of approximately 0.5 liter/day. The fluid flows out into the subarachnoid space through the median and lateral apertures of the fourth ventricle and is absorbed primarily into the cranial venous sinuses through tufts of pia-arachnoid cells (arachnoid villi), which protrude through the walls of the sinuses into the lumen.

Supporting Cells in the Peripheral Nervous System

The supporting cells of the peripheral nervous system are the *Schwann cells,* associated with all peripheral nerve fibers and forming the capsular or satellite cells of the dorsal root and au-

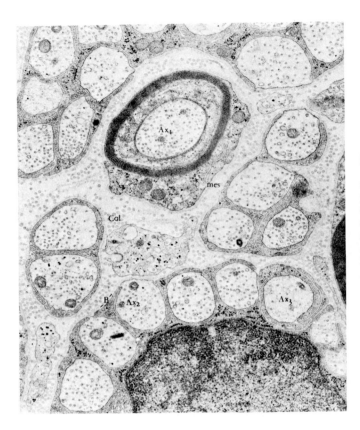

8–56 Electron micrograph of cross section of sciatic nerve of rat showing relationship of Schwann cells and their processes to myelinated and unmyelinated axons. **B,** basal lamina; **Col,** collagen; **mes,** mesaxon. × 21,000. (From Peters, A., Palay S. L., and Webster, H. deF. 1976. The Fine Structure of the Nervous System. Philadelphia: W. B. Saunders; courtesy of A. Peters.)

tonomic ganglia. They are derived from the neural crest. Like their counterparts in the central nervous system, all the peripheral supporting cells are small cells, and cytologically they are unexceptional. The outer surfaces of their plasma membranes are always associated with a basal lamina.

Schwann Cells in Peripheral Nerve Trunks. The Schwann cells of peripheral nerve trunks are sometimes known as neurilemmal or sheath cells because of the manner in which they enfold the constituent axons (Fig. 8–56). Every axon in the peripheral nervous system, from the dorsal and ventral roots to the most distal branches of the sensory or motor fibers, is surrounded over most of its length by a series of Schwann cells; in the case of axons with a diameter greater than about 1 μm each of these Schwann cells forms a single myelin internodal segment (Fig. 8–57). In two respects the association of Schwann cells with peripheral axons differs from that between the supporting cells of the central nervous system and central axons: (1) unmyelinated axons in the

central nervous system lack any form of ensheathment; and (2) whereas each Schwann cell forms only a single internodal segment, each oligodendrocyte may form 50 or more internodal segments and be associated with a comparable number of axons.

Peripheral nerves have several coverings, of which the Schwann cell constituent is most intimately related to the axons. Aside from the Schwann cells, there are three connective tissue coats (Figs. 8–58 and 8–59): an epineurium, perineurium, and endoneurium. An *epineurium* made up of dense fibrous connective tissue encloses the entire nerve as in a sleeve. This covering is sufficiently thick to be sutured in operations involving nerve repair. Within the epineurium the axons of the nerve are formed into longitudinally running bundles, or *fasciculi*, of variable size. These fasciculi are also enclosed in a sleeve of moderately dense fibrous connective tissue called the *perineurium*. This sheath is not completely limiting, however, since axons may leave one fasciculus to join another. Within the perineurium the axons and their as-

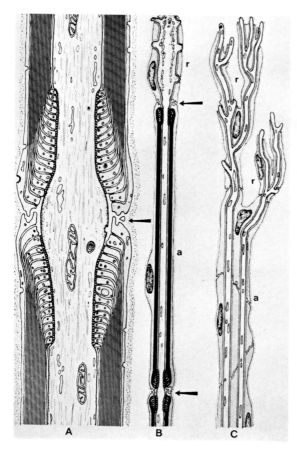

8–57 Schematic drawings of a node of Ranvier in
peripheral nervous system **(A)**, terminal
portion of a myelinated sensory nerve fiber **(B)**, and
terminal portions of two unmyelinated sensory nerve
fibers **(C)**, showing relationship of axon to investing
Schwann cells. (From Andres, K. H., and von Düring,
M. 1973. Handbook of Sensory Physiology, vol. 2.
New York: Springer-Verlag, New York, Inc.; courtesy
of K. H. Andres.)

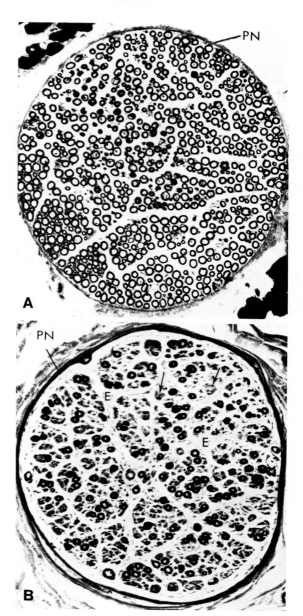

8–58 A. Cross section of part of a spinal ventral root
of a cat showing bimodal myelinated fiber
spectrum. **PN,** perineurium. Osmium tetroxide stain.
× 125. **B.** Cross section of a fascicle of a small
cutaneous sensory nerve showing unmyelinated
(arrows) as well as large and small myelinated fibers.
E, endoneurium. Osmium tetroxide stain. × 165.

sociated Schwann cells are surrounded by a
small amount of delicate, loose connective tissue
known as the *endoneurium*. Generally, a small
number of blood vessels, the *vasa nervorum*, are
also present; they penetrate the epineurial and
perineurial sheaths and break up into a loose
capillary plexus in the endoneurium.

Although Schwann cells are found along the
length of peripheral nerve fibers, any short segment of the fiber is associated with only a single
Schwann cell. To a greater or lesser degree, all
fibers are invaginated into the Schwann cells.

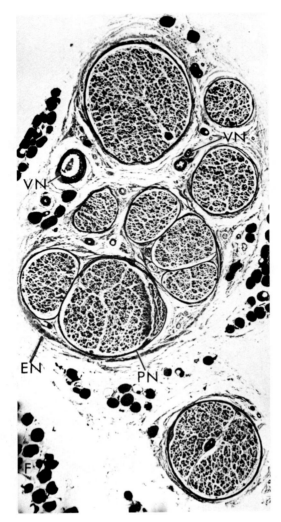

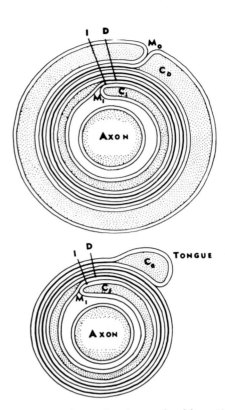

8–60 Schematic figure showing mode of formation of myelin in peripheral nervous system **(top)** and central nervous system **(bottom).** C_i, C_o, inner and outer cytoplasmic leaflets; **D,** major dense line; **I,** intraperiod line; M_i, M_o, inner and outer mesaxon. (From Peters, A. 1960. J. Biophys. Biochem. Cytol., 7:121; courtesy of A. Peters.)

8–59 Cross section of small peripheral nerve consisting of several fascicles surrounded by epineurium **(EN)** and perineurium **(PN). F,** fat cells; **VN,** vasa nervorum. Osmium tetroxide stain. × 50.

The line of the invagination, which usually forms a narrow cleft leading from the endoneurium to the enclosed axon, is known as the *mesaxon* (Fig. 8–56), by analogy with the mesenteries of the alimentary canal. *Schwann cells* associated with unmyelinated fibers may invest as many as 20 such fibers, and surrounding the whole cell and the associated fibers is the basal lamina. Where one Schwann cell comes to an end, it is overlapped by the next cell in the chain of Schwann cells (Fig. 8–57), and there is no gap comparable to the nodes of Ranvier of myeli-

nated fibers. In the case of myelinated fibers, each Schwann cell is associated with only a single fiber.

Although the general form of myelin in the peripheral nervous system is similar to that found in the central nervous system, its mode of formation is rather different. In the peripheral nervous system the axon to be myelinated first becomes invaginated into the Schwann cell. Then one of the lips of cytoplasm adjoining the mesaxon appears to insinuate itself between the adjoining lip and the axon; and by the continued elongation of the lips of the mesaxon, a spiral wrapping made up of many lamellae is formed (Fig. 8–60). By the alternate fusion of the inner leaflets of the plasma membranes (belonging to the same lamella) and of the outer leaflets of the plasma membranes (belonging to adjoining lamellae), the major dense and intraperiod lines are respectively established. The exact manner in which the spiral wrapping occurs is uncertain, but there is some evidence from observations in tissue culture that at least in the initial phase the whole Schwann cell may rotate around the axon.

The innermost major dense line expands to form an inner tongue of Schwann cell cytoplasm, and the cleft formed by the associated separation of the innermost intraperiod line is usually called the *inner mesaxon*. This cleft is originally continuous with the initial line of invagination of the fiber, which constitutes the *outer mesaxon*. At the outer mesaxon, the outermost major dense line splits and becomes continuous with what is usually a substantial amount of Schwann cell cytoplasm—far greater than the small outer tongue of oligodendrocytic cytoplasm seen in the central nervous system. If the myelin sheath is seen in a longitudinal section or in a cross section near the middle of an internode, the nucleus of the Schwann cell will also be present; and, as in the case of unmyelinated fibers, the cell is surrounded by a basal lamina.

Nodes of Ranvier are present in myelinated peripheral nerve fibers, as in the central nervous system (Fig. 8–53). The nodal portion of the axon has a dense membrane undercoat, and the Schwann cells of the two adjoining internodes form comparable tongues of cytoplasm in the paranodal regions. The spiral bands between the tongues and the outer leaflet of the axolemma are usually less distinct than in the central nervous system. However, the major difference between nodal regions in the central and peripheral nervous systems is that at peripheral nodes the nerve fiber is not completely bare. Although devoid of a myelin sheath, the nodal segment is covered by large overlapping processes of Schwann cell cytoplasm derived from the cells that give rise to the two adjoining internodes, and the whole region is surrounded by a basal lamina.

Myelin internodes in the peripheral nervous system often show a series of small clefts or splittings running obliquely for some distance across the thickness of the myelin sheath. They are called *Schmidt-Lanterman incisures*, or *clefts*, and they represent regions in which the major dense lines are separated over a short distance so that a small amount of Schwann cell cytoplasm is inserted into the myelin wrapping. Where the cleavage affects all lamellae, the cleft will form a helical wrapping around the sheath,

but sometimes only a few adjacent major dense lines are affected.

Supporting Cells in the Peripheral Ganglia. Schwann cells, often called *satellite cells*, are found in large numbers in both dorsal root ganglia and autonomic ganglia. In the dorsal root ganglia (Fig. 8–61A) and in the sensory ganglia of certain of the cranial nerves, they tend to surround the pseudounipolar neurons and are, therefore, sometimes called *capsular cells* (Fig. 8–61B). In autonomic ganglia, the investment of individual neurons is rarely so complete (Fig. 8–62), and most neurons are associated with a relatively small number of satellite cells.

The capsular cells are distinguished by their small size relative to the neurons and, in light micrographs, by their paucity of cytoplasm. In electron micrographs they usually appear to be embedded in depressions in the ganglion cell cytoplasm, and the neurons may invaginate finger-like extensions into the capsular cell. The cytoplasmic processes of adjacent capsular cells overlap to a variable extent, and the thickness of the capsular layer is usually proportional to the size of the ganglion cell. Because the cells are Schwann cells, it is not surprising that the entire "capsule" is invested by a basal lamina. No synapses are present in dorsal root ganglia, but in autonomic ganglia the capsule is deficient at several points to allow for the passage of the terminal portions of the preganglionic axons that form synapses on the cells. In some cases, capsular cells form myelin around the enclosed neurons. In mammals, this unusual situation is mainly confined to the ganglia of the vestibulocochlear nerve in which the somata of the bipolar cells commonly have a thin covering of loose myelin.

The capsular cells continue without interruption onto the initial segment of the axon, and portions of the same capsular cell may line both the perikaryon and the axon. In many animals, and particularly in humans, the initial stem processes of the dorsal root ganglion cells, before bifurcating into central and peripheral branches, are highly coiled, forming what is usually referred to as a *glomerular segment* (Fig. 8–62C). The enveloping cells follow the contours of this convoluted structure and normally give rise to one or more myelin internodes just before the point of branching. The branching occurs, as always, at a node.

The Schwann cells continue along the central processes of the sensory ganglion cells to the

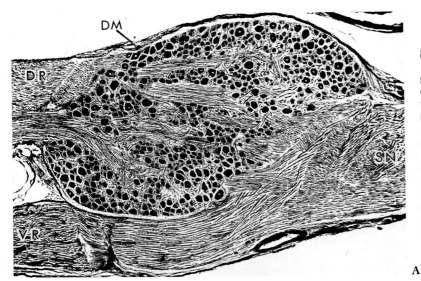

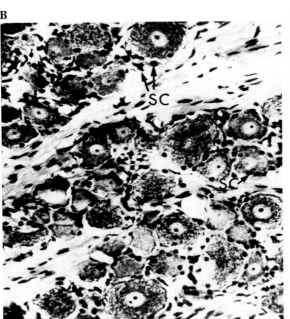

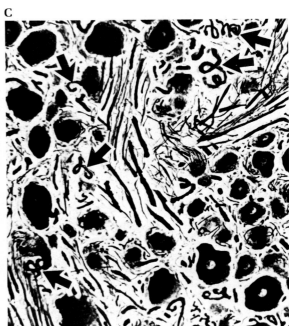

8-61 A. Bodian-stained preparation of dorsal root ganglion of a cat showing covering of dura mater **(DM)**, ventral root **(VR)**, dorsal root **(DR)**, and spinal nerve **(SN)**. × 90. **B.** Thionin-stained section showing dorsal root ganglion cells of varying size and enveloping Schwann (capsular) cells **(SC)**. × 480. **C.** Higher-powered view of a part of **A**, showing coiled initial axon segments of ganglion cells **(arrows)**. × 480.

spinal cord or brainstem. The point at which these cells disappear and the oligodendrocytes assume the responsibility for forming the myelin sheath of the central process has not been studied intensively. The changeover seems to occur not at a sharp boundary line but over a long region of transition.

Schwann Cells in Degeneration and Repair of Peripheral Nerves. Degeneration of a peripheral nerve after a transection or some injury at a more proximal level is always accompanied by reactive changes in the Schwann cells. The axons that are severed from their trophic center, the cell body, degenerate distal to a transection. This degenerative process is known as *Wallerian degeneration* after the neurologist A. V. Waller, who first described it in 1850. It includes the whole distal portion of an axon and its terminal ramifications. Although the earliest stages of de-

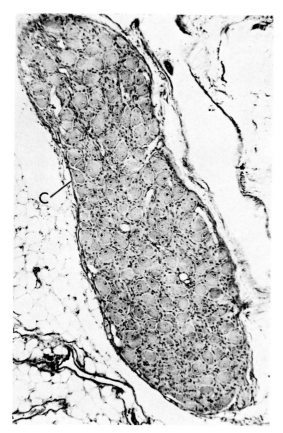

8–62 Longitudinal section of otic ganglion of a dog showing sympathetic neurons and intervening small nuclei of satellite Schwann cells. **C,** capsule. Hematoxylin and eosin stain. × 250.

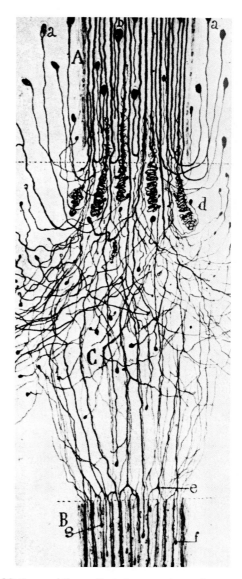

8–63 Some of the earliest degenerative and regenerative changes seen at the site of interruption of a nerve bundle. The proximal stump **(A)** in the upper part of the figure shows numerous retraction bulbs, convoluted spiral structures, and newly formed axon sprouts, some of which have grown toward the Schwann tubes of the distal stump **(B).** (From Cajal, S. Ramón y. 1928. Degeneration and Regeneration of the Nervous System. Republished 1958. New York: Hafner Pub. Co.)

generation may be seen close to the severed end, the changes affect the whole distal portion more or less simultaneously. The first changes are seen at the nodes of Ranvier, where the axon swells and the mitochondria are disrupted. Within a few hours the paranodal portions of the myelin sheath start to fragment and clefts resembling Schmidt-Lantermann incisures appear in large numbers in the internodes. This is followed by fragmentation of the whole myelin sheath, which appears in myelin-stained preparations as a chain of ovoid or vesicular masses. These masses become denser and further fragmented, and they and the fragments of degenerating axoplasm are phagocytosed by the Schwann cells and by macrophages that invade the degenerating portion of the nerve from the blood stream. These cells become filled with large heterogeneous dense bodies and vacuoles containing lipids derived from the further degradation of the myelin fragments.

The Schwann cells hypertrophy and markedly increase in number. The proliferation may continue for as long as 3 weeks and the number of cells may increase to more than 10 times the original population. Clearly, large portions of the plasma membrane of the Schwann cell are disrupted in the course of fragmentation of the myelin sheath, but few cells actually appear to die. The proliferating Schwann cells seem to free themselves from their surrounding basal laminae, which remain as a series of longitudinally oriented tubes. Along these tubes, the Schwann cells form a complexly interdigitated mass of cytoplasmic processes that, together with the tubes of basal lamina, appear to guide the regenerating axonal sprouts into the degenerated distal segment and toward their peripheral target (Fig. 8–63). The extracellular compartments formed by the interdigitating Schwann cell processes and the basal laminae are often referred to as *Schwann tubes*.

As regeneration of the axons proceeds, the Schwann cells become more orderly in their arrangement and gradually form linear arrays within the persisting tubes of basal laminae. The regenerated axons become invaginated within the Schwann cells and those larger than 1 μm become remyelinated. The new myelin internodes are generally shorter and thinner than those in the normal nerve. The shortness is perhaps to be expected, in view of the marked proliferation of Schwann cells, but it is uncertain what proportion of the newly produced Schwann cells survive to form internodes or to ensheath unmyelinated fibers.

The Peripheral Terminations of Nerve Fibers

In the peripheral nervous system, the processes of neurons either synapse with other nerve cells, as in the case of autonomic preganglionic neurons, or enter into a functional relationship with the cellular components of other tissues, as in the case of the dorsal root ganglion cells, the motoneurons of the spinal cord or the autonomic postganglionic neurons. The structure of autonomic ganglia is described below. Here we shall be concerned primarily with the peripheral terminations of dorsal root ganglion cells, of spinal motoneurons, and of autonomic postganglionic neurons.

The peripheral processes of dorsal root ganglion cells and of the cells in the sensory cranial ganglia terminate in association with specialized connective, epithelial or muscular tissues that in many cases facilitate the sensory transduction process leading to the discharge of action potentials in the nerve fiber and to their propagation toward the central nervous system. The pseudounipolar ganglion cells are, therefore, *receptor* neurons and their peripheral terminals are specialized sensory receptors. Motoneurons in the spinal cord and brainstem and the autonomic postganglionic neurons are *effector* neurons, and their axons terminate respectively on skeletal muscle cells and on smooth muscle or gland cells. In these cases, the peripheral terminal is an effector or "motor" ending, comparable in its general structure and function to a central synapse, although the effect on the target organ is, of course, to induce muscular contraction or glandular secretion.

The Structure and Function of Peripheral Sensory Receptors

The peripheral sensory receptors are concerned with the transduction of various forms of energy into neural activity, which, if of sufficient intensity, results in the discharge of nerve impulses whose frequency and pattern constitute the neural code that is interpreted centrally as a sensory experience. Before describing individual receptors three general points may be made. (1) For the most part, the type or *modality* of sensation mediated by a particular axon is specific for each axon, and its specificity resides within the axon itself. As a rule, each axon is concerned with only one sensory modality. (2) The sensory transduction process occurs within the axon itself rather than in the specialized end formations that may be associated with it. (3) Not all activity in sensory receptors is consciously perceived; much of it is concerned with various reflexes and other adjustments to changes in the external or internal environment, of which the subject is often wholly unconscious. The use of the term *sensory* is synonymous with *afferent* and does not necessarily imply conscious *sensation*.

Sensory receptors may be classified in several ways. Among the oldest is that of Sherrington, who spoke of (1) *exteroceptors*, specialized for the reception of stimuli on or beyond the surface of the body; (2) *interoceptors*, concerned with the reception of stimuli arising within the body itself; and (3) *proprioceptors*, which are a special group of interoceptors specialized for the reception of information about the position of the body, or its parts, in space; this group includes the receptors in the vestibular apparatus and those in muscles and joints. More recent physiological classifications tend to emphasize the nature of the stimulus that the receptors are equipped to deal with. Hence we may speak of *mechanoreceptors*, *thermoreceptors*, *nociceptors* (for pain), *chemoreceptors*, *photoreceptors* (in the retina), and so on.

A useful anatomical classification rests on the fact that in most parts of the body, the terminal portions of the peripheral processes of cranial or spinal ganglion cells fall into one of three groups: (1) *Free nerve endings*, which in this case, are the terminal branches of the processes that lose all their coverings (including their Schwann cell investment) and end without specialization among the epithelial, connective tissue, or other cells of the innervated region (Fig. 8–57). (2) *Expanded tip endings*, which are found more especially in the skin. Here the terminal branches end in a series of bulbous expansions that make contact with the bases of dome-like aggregations of specialized epithelial cells. (3) *Encapsulated endings*, in which the terminal axon ends inside a distinct connective tissue capsule in relation to either groups of connective tissue or muscle cells; such endings are apparently specialized for determining the direction or type of displacing force that acts on the contained sensory nerve terminal. We shall follow this classification but, for convenience, describe the sensory nerve terminals in relation to three main groups of tissues: skin and subcutaneous tissue, muscles and joints, and blood vessels and viscera.

Sensory Receptors in the Skin and Subcutaneous Tissues

As the peripheral branches of a cutaneous nerve penetrate the subcutaneous tissues and approach the skin, they form an intricate plexus of interconnected bundles just beneath the dermis (Fig. 8–64). Several branches of a single nerve, and branches of different nerves, usually contribute to this *subcutaneous plexus*. From the subcutaneous plexus, branches pass to deep receptors, and many fine bundles of axons ascend to form a second *dermal plexus* beneath the epidermal ridges. From this plexus, terminal branches pass into the dermal papillae and into the epidermis. Unless otherwise specified, what follows refers to both hairy and nonhairy (*glabrous*) skin, but it

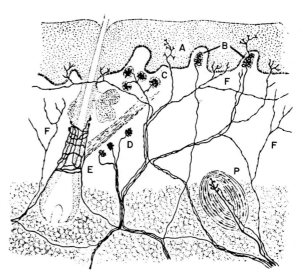

8–64 Schematic drawing showing innervation pattern of hairy skin. **A,** intraepithelial endings; **B,** Meissner corpuscles; **C,** Krause's end bulbs; **D,** Ruffini endings; **E,** endings associated with hairs; **F,** free endings; **P,** Pacinian corpuscle. (From LeGros Clark, W. E. 1965. The Tissues of the Body. Fairlawn, N. J.: Oxford University Press.)

should be noted that in addition to the sensory fibers, each plexus also contains sympathetic postganglionic fibers that supply the blood vessels, sweat glands, and arrector pili muscles of the skin.

Free Nerve Terminals. Free nerve terminals form the majority of the sensory receptors in the skin. All are derived from unmyelinated axons of small diameter (approximately 1 μm or less) and a single fiber often branches profusely over a wide area. On approaching the deepest layer of the epidermis, the basal lamina of the Schwann cells fuses with that beneath the epidermis, and the naked nerve fibers pass into the epidermis within deep invaginations in the epidermal cells. In this way they may penetrate the epidermis almost as far superficially as the stratum corneum. They display no obvious structural specialization, but evidence suggests that different fibers are functionally specialized to respond to painful stimuli, to warmth or cold, and to mechanical displacement of the skin. Such receptors are connected to unmyelinated (Fig. 8–57) or finely myelinated axons in the peripheral nerve trunks.

Sensory Nerve Endings in Relation to Hairs. Hairs are associated with such a rich innervation that they should probably be considered as one of the more elaborate forms of sensory receptor. At least 80% of the finely myelinated fibers in a cutaneous nerve terminate in relation to hairs. Different categories of hair may be identified, and each type is associated with sensory nerve fibers that signal different types of information to the central nervous system. In what follows, we shall be concerned only with the generalities of this system and shall not consider the details of the different types.

Every hair follicle receives several fine unmyelinated axons, most of which are ultimately derived from thinly myelinated parent axons 1 to 5 μm in diameter in the peripheral nerve trunk. Others appear to be branches of thicker myelinated fibers with diameters up to 12 μm.[3] A single parent fiber may branch many times and innervate several hundred follicles, so the *peripheral receptive field* from which the parent nerve fiber or its dorsal root ganglion cell can be activated may be very large. The various fibers innervating a single hair follicle form an encircling meshwork containing both longitudinally and circumferentially running branches that surround the greater part of the hair follicle as it traverses the dermis. Most of the terminal portions of the axons are enclosed in Schwann cells, but the ultimate portion is naked and embedded in the glassy membrane that forms the outermost covering of the follicle. The nerve endings are thus in a position to be activated when the hair is deflected.

Nerve Terminals with Expanded Tips. Two kinds of sensory receptor with expanded nerve terminals are found in glabrous and hairy skin. The most distinctive of these is the *Merkel's touch corpuscle* (Fig. 8–65). As a cutaneous nerve approaches one of these epithelial specializations, it gives rise to a number of unmyelinated branches that lose their Schwann cell covering and penetrate the basal lamina of the epidermis. Each terminal expands to form a flattened disc or plate that is closely applied to a modified epidermal cell (Merkel cell). These cells are attached to the neighboring cells by desmosomes, and they have many flattened cytoplasmic protrusions that enclose the terminal discs of the nerve fiber. Where it is in close contact with the nerve ending, the Merkel cell con-

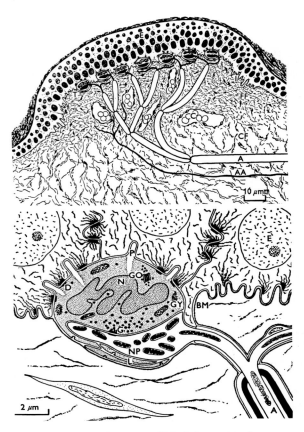

8–65 Schematic drawings of Merkel-type touch corpuscles from footpad of a cat. Merkel cell (indicated by shading in lower figure) contains granular vesicles **(G)** and is contacted by platelike axon terminal **(NP).** (From Iggo, A., and Muir, A. R. 1969. J. Physiol. [Lond.], 200:763; courtesy of A. Iggo.)

tains many large, dense-core vesicles approximately 1,000 Å in diameter. The nerve terminal itself does not contain vesicles. The myelinated nerves whose terminals end in Merkel's corpuscles are of large diameter (7 to 12 μm) and are usually excited by pressure applied directly to the touch corpuscles.

A simpler form of epithelial cell–nerve terminal complex, in which expanded terminals of an axon end in relation to normal basal epidermal cells, has been identified as a cold receptor. In these cases, the parent axons are myelinated and are about 1 to 6 μm in diameter; they are specifically activated by localized cooling of the epidermis over their terminals. No specialized receptors have yet been identified for the reception of warm stimuli.

---

[3]Fiber diameters indicated here refer to primates. Diameters of the largest fibers in some experimental animals (e.g., cats) may be up to 15–16 μm.

Encapsulated Nerve Terminals. Although numerically in the minority, encapsulated receptors have tended to dominate descriptions of the innervation of the skin and subcutaneous tissues because of their large size and distinctive appearance. Three main types are usually recognized: *Pacinian corpuscles, Ruffini endings,* and *Meissner's corpuscles.* Other types, less distinct and not recognized by all authorities, are *Krause's end bulbs* and *Golgi-Mazzoni corpuscles.* All these encapsulated endings are distinguished by the presence of a lamellated connective tissue sheath surrounding the nerve terminals. The form of the connective tissue ensheathment and of the nerve terminal is extremely variable but sufficiently characteristic for each type of receptor to be readily recognized. Each is innervated by a single myelinated axon, 6 to 12 μm in diameter, which is usually derived from a parent trunk that supplies many lamellated endings of the same type.

The Pacinian Corpuscle. This is one of the largest sensory receptors, often with a diameter of 1 mm. They are found in subcutaneous tissues below both hairy and glabrous skin and are especially numerous just beneath the dermis of the digits; they are also present in large numbers in the deep musculoskeletal tissues, especially in the periosteum, and in the mesenteries of the peritoneal cavity. The capsule is ellipsoidal and made up of 30 or more concentric rings of flattened fibroblast-like cells that are continuous with the endoneural sheath of the nerve terminating in the capsule (Fig. 8–66). The lamellae of the capsule are formed by the overlapping processes of several cells and each lamella is separated from its neighbor by a fluid-filled space. The nerve fiber enters one pole of the capsule and its last one or two myelin internodes are usually contained within the capsule. However, the greater part of the axon within the sheath is unmyelinated. This part is straight and terminates near the other pole of the corpuscle as a small spray of knoblike branches (Fig. 8–67). Like all other sensory nerve terminals, the axon endings display no unique structure at the electron-microscope level. The unmyelinated part of the axon is surrounded by multiple lamellae of flattened Schwann cells that are closely packed and form an *inner core* within the encircling fibrous connective tissue lamellae (the *outer core*). Pacinian corpuscles are exquisitely sensitive to mechanical displacement: the corpuscle can respond to vibratory stimuli up to about 700 per

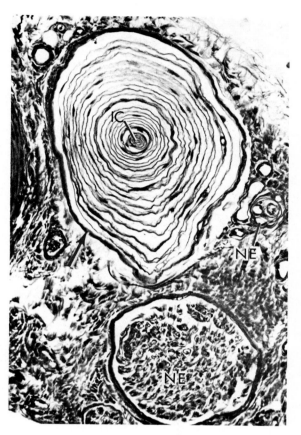

8–66 Pacinian corpuscle with numerous concentric lamellae and inner core **(IC)** containing the terminal part of the innervating axon that is usually derived from a nearby nerve bundle **(Ne)**. **Arrow** indicates capsule of Pacinian corpuscle. Hematoxylin and eosin stain. × 200.

second. The capsule is not essential for the responsiveness of the terminal (since all the outer core and much of the inner can be removed without affecting the response of the nerve terminal to directly applied mechanical stimuli). However, it seems to serve as a mechanical filter, and its elastic components ensure that the nerve responds in a rapidly adapting manner both when the stimulus is applied and when it is removed.

Meissner's Corpuscles. These receptors are found in the dermal papillae of glabrous skin (Fig. 8–68). They are particularly common near the tips of the fingers and toes. The corpuscle is smaller (approximately 150 μm long) and more cylindrical than the Pacinian corpuscle. The flat-

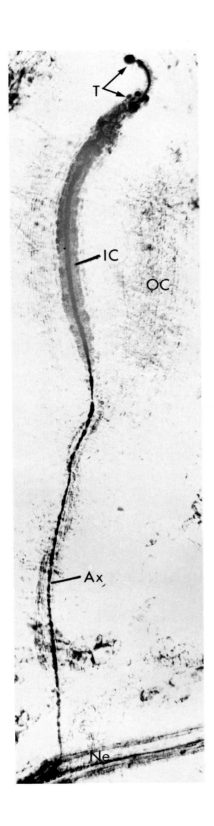

8–67 A myelinated nerve fiber **(Ax)** leaving a nerve bundle **(Ne)** to innervate a Pacinian corpuscle. The inner core of the corpuscle **(IC)** is clearly shown, as are the naked terminal expansions of the nerve fiber **(T)**. The outer capsular lamellae **(OC)** are lightly stained. Gold chloride stain. × 1,000.

tened cells form the greater part of its mass and are arranged in multiple-stacked lamellae within a thin, fibrous connective tissue outer coat. Most of the lamellar cells appear to be modified Schwann cells, and the unmyelinated terminal part of the axon threads its way among the lamellae to the superficial pole of the corpuscle. Commonly, more than one axon may enter a sin-

8–68 Schematic drawing of a Meissner corpuscle showing linkage by tonofibrils to overlying epidermis. **ax,** axons; **cp,** blood vessel; **pn,** perineurial sheath; **ra,** receptor part of axons; **SC,** Schwann cells. (From Andres, K. H., and von Düring, M. 1973. Handbook of Sensory Physiology, vol. 2. New York: Springer-Verlag, New York, Inc.; courtesy of K. H. Andres.)

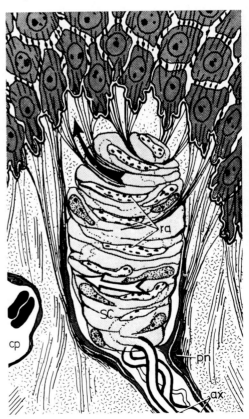

gle Meissner's corpuscle, but it is not clear whether they are branches of the same or of different parent axons. Meissner's corpuscles seem to be sensitive tactile receptors usually activated by moving the epidermal ridges of the glabrous skin over a surface. Although they too are rapidly adapting, they seem to respond best to low-frequency stimuli (approximately 30–40 per second).

Ruffini Endings. Although once considered artifacts of metallic impregnation, these endings are now regarded as one of the commonest forms of slowly adapting mechanoreceptor (Fig. 8–69). They are elongated fusiform structures, up to 1 to 2 mm in length, and are found in the dermis of both hairy and glabrous skin, in subcutaneous tissues, and in joint capsules. They are the least highly lamellated of the encapsulated receptors and consist of a thin connective tissue capsule enclosing a fluid-filled space. This space is traversed by bundles of collagen fibers that often pass through the capsule and are joined to other collagen fibers in the dermis and adjacent tissues. A single myelinated axon, 5 to 12 μm in diameter, enters the capsular space, loses its myelin sheath, and breaks up into a large number of unmyelinated branches that intertwine with the collagen bundles. The receptors are activated by displacement of the surrounding connective tissues and they usually respond with a regular, sustained discharge to a maintained mechanical stimulus.

Sensory Receptors in Muscles and Joints

Sensory Receptors in Muscle. Skeletal muscles contain some of the most highly organized encapsulated sensory receptors, together with many free nerve endings (Fig. 8–70). The encapsulated endings are the *muscle spindles* and the *Golgi tendon organs,* both of which are *proprioceptors.*

Muscle Spindles. *Muscle spindles* are found in all human striated muscles but are occasionally absent from some muscles, such as the tongue and the extraocular muscles, in other animals. Their numbers vary from muscle to muscle: in general, muscles that are capable of delicate movements and are subject to the highest degree of central nervous control contain the highest numbers of muscle spindles. For example, the intrinsic muscles of the hand, and the neck muscles at the base of the skull that are responsible for the delicate postural adjustments of the head on the spinal column contain a greater relative number of spindles than do such large muscles as the gluteus maximus and latissimus dorsi.

Each muscle spindle consists of an ovoid connective tissue capsule, about 1.5 mm long and 0.5 mm wide, enclosing a fluid-filled space (Figs. 8–71 and 8–72). This space is traversed from pole to pole by a bundle of special striated muscle fibers that are associated with specialized sensory and motor nerves. The capsule is composed of several circumferential lamellae of flattened fibroblasts (Fig. 8–72), joined to one another at intervals by desmosomes. At the poles of the spindle the lamellae are closely applied to the contained muscle fibers, but elsewhere they enclose a dilated *capsular space* containing tissue fluid, a little delicate endomysial connective tissue, and the neuromuscular apparatus of the spindle. The muscle fibers within the spindle are termed *intrafusal fibers* to distinguish them from the main contractile elements of the muscle, which are termed *extrafusal fibers.* The intrafusal fibers are much smaller, both in diameter and length, than extrafusal fibers, but their orientation is the same, so that the muscle spindles are said to be *in parallel* with the extrafusal fibers.

Each small bundle of intrafusal fibers contains

8–69 Camera lucida drawing of nerve terminal from a gold-chloride-impregnated Ruffini ending in knee-joint capsule of a cat. Capsule of ending and other connective tissue elements are not shown. (From Skoglund, S. 1956. Acta Physiol. Scand. 36 (Suppl.) 124:1)

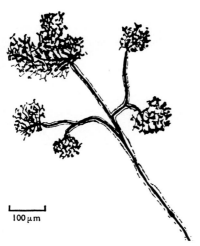

100 μm

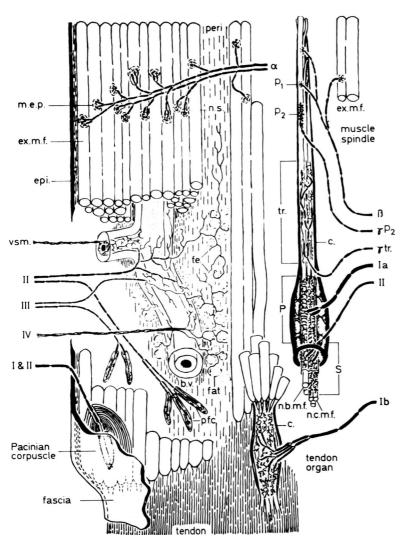

8–70 Schematic drawing showing pattern of innervation of skeletal muscle. Nerve fiber groupings indicated to left and right innervate structures shown. **bv,** blood vessel; **fe,** free endings; **pfc,** "Paciniform" corpuscles; **vsm,** vasomotor (sympathetic) endings. (From Barker, D. 1974. Handbook of Sensory Physiology, vol. 3, part 2. New York: Springer-Verlag, New York, Inc., Courtesy of D. Barker.)

from two to 20 or more intrafusal fibers. In most mammals they are of two main types: a longer, somewhat thicker form that extends well beyond the poles of the spindle capsule, its ends being inserted into endo- or perimysial connective tissue; and a shorter, thinner form whose ends do not extend much beyond the poles of the capsule. Every spindle contains one or two of the thicker type and many more of the smaller type. Both types are striated over much of their length and have dark-staining, peripherally placed nuclei. As they approach the widest part of the capsular space (the "equator" of the spindle) they usually lose their striations. In the larger form of intrafusal fiber, there is a large central aggrega-

tion of nuclei in the equatorial region; for this reason these fibers are known as *nuclear bag* fibers (Fig. 8–72). On each side of this central aggregation, the nuclei form a single row (the "myotube" region); beyond this, they are progressively replaced by myofibrils and peripheral nuclei. Some nuclear bag fibers may enter a second spindle capsule at some distance from the first and give rise to a nuclear bag in the second as well. This arrangement constitutes a *tandem spindle.*

The shorter and more numerous form of intrafusal fiber has only a single row of vesicular nuclei in its central nonstriated portion. It is thus known as a *nuclear chain fiber* (Fig. 8–72). Nu-

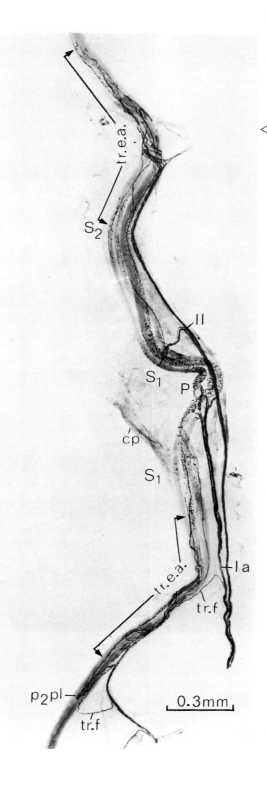

8–71 Silver-stained, teased, whole preparation of a muscle spindle from muscle of a cat. **cp,** capsule; **P** primary ending; **p₂pl,** plate ending; **S₁, S₂,** secondary endings; **tr.e.a., tr. f.,** trail endings and trail fiber. (From Barker, D., Stacey, M. J., and Adal, M. N. 1970. Philos. Trans. R. Soc. Lond. [Biol. Sci.] 258: 315; courtesy of D. Barker.)

clear chain fibers and some nuclear bag fibers have been found to be more rapidly contracting than other nuclear bag fibers and they usually have a less-regular pattern of myofilaments with much intervening sarcoplasm and well-developed M lines. The other nuclear bag fibers have a more orderly array of myofilaments, less intervening sarcoplasm, and no M lines. These nuclear bag fibers seem to contract in a tonic fashion, and their activation is not associated with a propagated action potential. They therefore resemble the "slow" muscles of lower vertebrates. The contraction of nuclear chain fibers is more twitchlike and is associated with propagated action potentials. Note that because of the lack of myofilaments in the equatorial regions, the cen-

8–72 A muscle spindle in cross section showing the appearance of the connective tissue capsule **(C),** the capsular space **(CS),** two large nuclear bag intrafusal fibers **(NB),** and several smaller nuclear chain fibers **(NC).** The spindle as a whole is in parallel with the extrafusal muscle fibers **(MF).** Van Gieson stain. × 350.

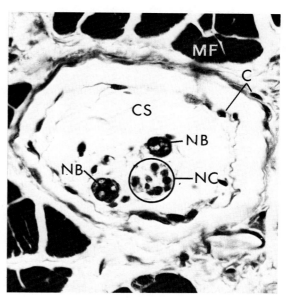

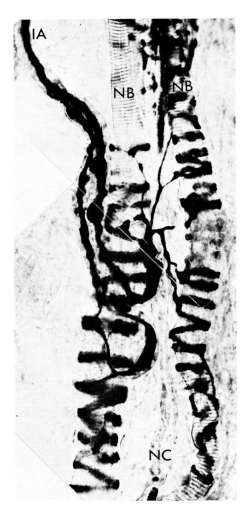

8–73 A group **IA** fiber terminating as spiral primary endings on two nuclear bag fibers **(NB)** in muscle spindle of a marsupial. Nuclear chain fibers **(NC)** do not appear to receive a primary ending in this methylene-blue-stained, teased preparation. × 400. (From Jones, E. G., 1967. J. Anat. [Lond.] 100:733.)

tral parts of the intrafusal fibers are essentially noncontractile.

The sensory nerves to a muscle spindle enter through the capsule and terminate near the equatorial region of the intrafusal muscle fibers (Figs. 8–71 and 8–73). Every spindle receives a single, large, myelinated afferent fiber about 12 to 20 μm in diameter. This fiber loses its myelin sheath close to the intrafusal bundle and gives rise to several branches that end in a series of ribbonlike spirals that partially or completely encircle the central portion of each nuclear bag and nu-

clear chain fiber (Fig. 8–73). Electron microscopy shows that the terminal spirals and rings may be deeply invaginated into folds in the sarcolemma of the intrafusal fibers without any intervening basal lamina. The whole terminal complex is known as the *primary sensory ending* of the spindle, and its parent fiber (which may supply primary endings to more than one spindle capsule) is usually called a *group Ia* afferent fiber.

Many spindles, although not all, also receive one or more smaller (group II) afferent fibers, about 6 to 8 μm in diameter. These fibers lose their myelin sheath as they branch within the spindle capsule and form terminal spirals, rings, and sprays similar to those of the primary ending but predominantly on the nuclear chain fibers. This complex constitutes the *secondary sensory ending* of the spindle. Both the primary and secondary endings of a spindle are activated by any stretching force acting on the muscle as a whole, which would tend to lengthen the intrafusal bundle. The primary ending responds most vigorously during the dynamic phase of the stretch; secondary endings are more responsive to maintained stretch. That is, the primary endings exhibit *dynamic sensitivity*, the secondary endings *static sensitivity*.

The spindles are also innervated by a number of small motor nerve fibers that end on the striated portions of the intrafusal fibers near both poles of the capsule (Fig. 8–71). The parent nerve fibers are small, myelinated axons 2 to 8 μm in diameter arising from a specific group of small motoneurons in the ventral horn of the spinal cord. These fibers innervate only intrafusal muscle fibers and are known as γ *motoneurons*, or *fusimotor neurons*; the axons that provide the motor innervation to the spindle are, thus, termed γ *efferents*, or *fusimotor fibers*. Less commonly, some of the large α motor fibers that supply the extrafusal musculature (see p. 346) also provide a branch to one or more intrafusal fibers in a neighboring spindle. Two types of motor nerve terminal are seen on the intrafusal fibers. Some are localized and closely resemble the motor end plates on extrafusal muscle fibers. Others are long, diffuse endings that ramify widely over the surface of the intrafusal fiber and make multiple *en passant* terminal contacts. The "plate" type of ending is found mainly on nuclear bag fibers, and the diffuse "trail" type, mainly on nuclear chain fibers; but both types can at times be found on the same fiber. Activity in the fusimotor fibers causes the intrafusal fibers to contract and thus effectively

organ lies (Fig. 8–74). The whole complex may be about 1 mm long, and since a variable number (3 to 25) of extrafusal muscle fibers are inserted into the collagenous tendon slips that make up the greater part of the tendon organ, these receptors are said to be *in series* with the extrafusal fibers. This arrangement permits the sensory nerve fibers to be activated during both contraction and stretching of the relevant muscle.

Each tendon organ receives a single, large, myelinated sensory nerve fiber having a diameter of 12 to 15 μm; afferent fibers of this type fall within the group Ib class of muscle afferents (see below). The terminal branches of the fiber lose their myelin sheaths after entering the capsule of the tendon organ and give rise to a number of longitudinally running unmyelinated branches that terminate in small sprays of naked terminals wrapped around, and insinuated between, the bundles of collagen fibers.

Sensory Receptors in Joints. The capsules and periarticular tissues of joints are richly endowed with proprioceptors, which, along with muscle receptors, are believed to contribute to the conscious awareness of movement and position (*kinesthesis*). The majority of receptors found in joints have already been described. There are many free nerve endings derived from both unmyelinated and finely myelinated parent fibers, some of which penetrate as far as the synovial membrane. The major type of encapsulated ending found in joint capsules is the Ruffini ending, but some Pacinian corpuscles are also present. In the ligaments associated with the joint capsule, Golgi tendon organs are common. The function of these different receptors in kinesthesis is not clear; recent evidence suggests that the stretch receptors of the muscles acting on a joint may signal small variations in joint angle. The Ruffini endings seem to discharge in response to movement in one direction, and some show a substantial response when the joint is held in a fixed position. The small Pacinian corpuscles seem to respond only to movements. The role of the free nerve terminals is uncertain, but many are thought to be nociceptive.

Sensory Nerve Endings in Blood Vessels and Viscera

The walls of the larger blood vessels, and all the thoracic and abdominal viscera, contain a fairly rich complement of mechanoreceptors. In many regions nociceptors are also present and individ-

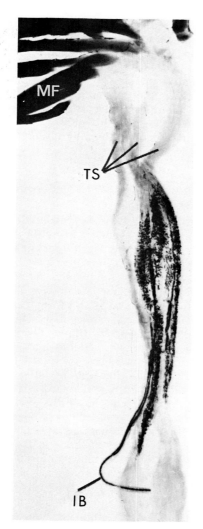

8–74 Gold-chloride-stained, teased preparation of a Golgi tendon organ from myotendinous junction of a marsupial. Group **IB** fiber branches widely among tendinous slips **(TS)** attached to several skeletal muscle fibers **(MF).** × 80.

stretch the nonstriated part of the fiber that carries the sensory endings. This leads to a state of increased sensitivity of the sensory endings so that they discharge more readily and at increased rates when the muscle in which they lie is stretched.

Golgi Tendon Organs. These receptors, found primarily at musculotendinous junctions, consist of a thin, fibroblastic capsule that is filled with a number of large, collagenous fiber bundles continuous with those of the tendon in which the

ual organs may have other special kinds of receptors that reflect their particular functions. Collectively, these receptors are termed *interoceptors*.

Most interoceptors are free, or relatively poorly organized, nerve endings that ramify beneath and between epithelial cells and in the submucosal, muscular, and serosal coats of hollow viscera. The parent nerves are usually of small diameter (unmyelinated or thinly myelinated) and are distributed with the autonomic nerves. In some sites, such as the mesenteries, encapsulated endings (and especially Pacinian corpuscles) are also seen.

The best-defined interoceptors are those associated with the aortic arch and with the carotid body and sinus. They monitor circulating blood gas levels and blood pressure and mediate a variety of cardiovascular and respiratory reflexes. The receptors that are sensitive to changes in oxygen and carbon dioxide tension and blood pH are called *chemoreceptors* and are found in the carotid body and in similar bodies on the arch of the aorta. Those sensitive to changes in blood pressure are called *baroreceptors* and are found in the walls of the carotid sinus and aortic arch. Each has a rather similar structure consisting of glomerular aggregations of large globular cells (which are thought to be the actual receptors) on which the highly branched afferent nerve fibers terminate. In the case of the chemoreceptors, the large cells are filled with dense-core vesicles 1,000 to 2,000 Å in diameter and contain rich stores of catecholamines. Many arteriovenous anastomoses are also present and apparently serve to regulate blood flow through the carotid and aortic bodies. Free nerve endings are also found in the subendocardial layers of the heart, particularly near the valves and in the atrial walls close to the point of entry of the great veins.

In the hollow viscera of the alimentary and genitourinary tracts the free nerve endings seem to be excited mainly by distension of the viscus or by peristaltic or other muscular activity. In certain regions, groups of free receptor terminals in the epithelium are thought to be specifically excited by changes in intraluminal pH, by changes in glucose concentration, or by the presence of certain amino acids and polypeptides.

In the respiratory tract, free nerve endings in and beneath the epithelium of the larynx, trachea, and bronchi are sensitive to irritant particles and gases, and when stimulated evoke a coughing reflex. In the lungs themselves, the pulmonary stretch receptors are mainly free nerve endings associated with the smooth muscle of the bronchi. Their afferent fibers are myelinated and are among the fastest conducting interoceptive afferents. Other free endings in the interstitial tissue around the alveoli are thought to be sensitive to changes in the interstitial fluid, particularly those brought about by vascular congestion and irritant vapors.

The Peripheral Terminations of Efferent Nerve Fibers

Motor Nerve Fibers to Skeletal Muscle. Striated muscles are innervated by the axons of motor nerve cells (motoneurons) situated in the ventral horn of the spinal cord or in the motor nuclei of certain of the cranial nerves. Two classes of myelinated fiber are involved: (1) large fibers with diameters of 12 to 20 μm, commonly termed α *motor fibers*, which innervate the extrafusal muscle fibers; (2) thinner fibers, 2 to 8 μm in diameter, termed γ *efferents*, or *fusimotor fibers*, which innervate the intrafusal fibers of the muscle spindles. Because the latter have already been described, the following account will be concerned solely with the α fibers.

The α motor axons, which are among the largest in the peripheral nervous system, seldom branch before entering the muscle they innervate. However, they branch profusely in the muscle so that a single parent axon may innervate anything from 1 or 2 muscle fibers to 500 or more. On the other hand, each muscle fiber is usually innervated by only one axon. A single motor axon and all the extrafusal fibers it supplies are referred to as a *motor unit*.

As the branches of an axon approach the muscle fibers they are to innervate, they lose their myelin sheaths; covered only by their Schwann cell investment, they form specialized terminal formations known as *motor end plates* (Figs. 8–37, 8–75A, 8–76, and 8–77). Typically a motor end plate is made up of the expanded terminal portion of an α motor axon and its sheath, a junctional cleft, and a specialized portion of the underlying extrafusal muscle fiber. On the surface of the muscle fiber, the axon forms a number of interconnected terminal bulbs of varying size within a fairly circumscribed round or oval zone (Fig. 8–77). In the light microscope this zone appears slightly elevated because the terminal bulbs are overlain by Schwann cells and by the

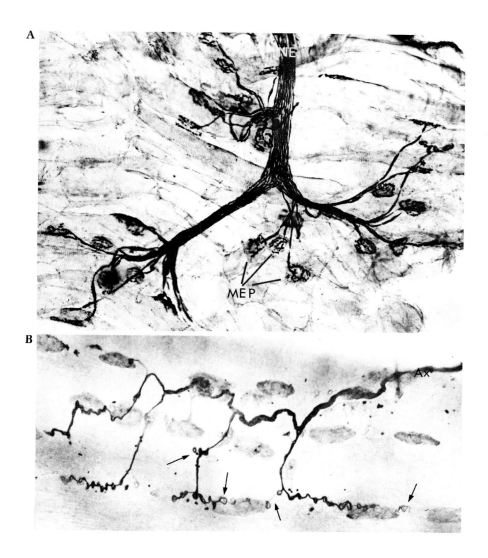

cells of the endoneurium, which become continuous with the endomysium. This connective tissue layer, external to the Schwann cells, is
termed the *sheath of Henle* (Fig. 8–37).

In electron micrographs the terminals resemble synaptic boutons, being filled with large
numbers of clear vesicles (approximately 400 Å
in diameter) and many mitochondria. Fingers of
Schwann cell cytoplasm cover the individual
terminal bulbs and may penetrate between them
and the muscle fiber (Fig. 8–76). The plasma
membranes of the axon terminal and the underlying muscle fiber are separated by an extracellular cleft approximately 500 Å in width, which
is filled with the basal lamina of the muscle fiber. The presynaptic membrane shows no dis-

8–75 A Gold-chloride-stained, teased preparation of
human intercostal muscle showing
intramuscular nerve **(NE)** branching to supply motor
end plates **(MEP)** on skeletal muscle fibers. × 70.
B. Silver-stained, teased preparation showing motor
axon **(Ax)** branching to supply diffuse multiterminal
endings in slow muscle of a tortoise. **Arrows** indicate
neurofibrillar rings. × 650.

tinctive specialization; but over the whole length
of its approximation to the sarcolemma, the latter
is thrown into a large number of folds that
deeply invaginate the underlying sarcoplasm.
Like the cleft, these infoldings are filled with
basal lamina (Figs. 8–37 and 8–76).

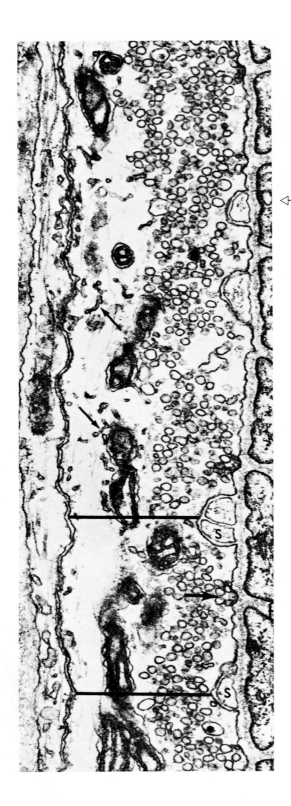

8–76 Electron micrograph of a frog neuromuscular junction. Terminal is separated by basal lamina from junctional folds of muscle fiber (to right). Schwann cell process covers it to far left and some Schwann cell processes **(S)** intervene between terminal and basal lamina. **Large arrow** indicates one of several aggregations of synaptic vesicles about a presynaptic density, site of active synaptic vesicle release. **Small arrows** indicate smooth endoplasmic reticulum. × 40,000 (From Heuser, J. E., and Reese, T. S. 1973. J. Cell Biol. 57:315; courtesy of T. S. Reese.)

The plasma membrane of the muscle fiber usually has a small amount of dense material attached to it along the crests between each infolding. This region thus resembles the postsynaptic specialization seen at central synapses and is thought to represent the "active site" of the neuromuscular junction. In the portion of the axon terminal immediately opposite each of the junctional folds, there is usually a ridge and a small accumulation of synaptic vesicles (Figs. 8–37, 8–76, and 8–78). During prolonged stimulation of a motor nerve, synaptic vesicles move toward these sites. The sarcoplasm beneath the nerve terminal is often called the *sole plate* and is usually devoid of myofilaments but rich in free ribosomes, rough endoplasmic reticulum, and mitochondria. There is also an accumulation of nuclei in this region that are somewhat larger

8–77 Gold-chloride-stained preparation of two motor end plates from a human intercostal muscle. Dark bulbs are terminal contacts. × 1,100.

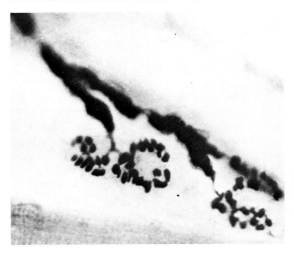

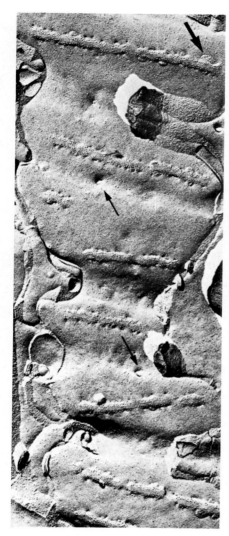

8–78 Freeze-fracture preparation showing surface of nerve terminal at a frog neuromuscular junction. Transverse ridges with membrane particles correspond to presynaptic regions indicated by large arrow in Fig. 8–76. Grooves between ridges correspond to regions occupied by Schwann cell processes. **Arrows** indicate presumed re-formation of synaptic vesicles by endocytosis. × 30,000. (From Heuser, J. E., Reese, T. S., and Landis, D. M. D. 1974. J. Neurocytol. 3:109; courtesy of T. S. Reese.)

and more vesicular than other muscle nuclei; they are the *sole plate nuclei*.

Motor end plates vary in structure, depending on the type of muscle in which they lie. In mammals, the motor end plates of *fast-twitch muscles* have many long and often branched sarcolemmal infoldings. In *slow-twitch muscles* the sarcolemmal infoldings are fewer and shallower; the axon terminals also contain fewer synaptic vesicles than do those ending on fast-twitch muscles. True *slow muscles*, which do not show propagated action potentials and which are capable of sustained, graded contractions, are uncommon in mammals. When present (for example, in the extraocular muscles) they are characterized by diffuse, multiterminal (or *en grappes*) motor endings; the terminal motor axon spreads diffusely over much of the surface of the muscle fiber and gives off terminal bulbs at intervals (Fig. 8–75B). Individual bulbs may be separated from one another by several hundred microns. Each of these bulbs contains synaptic vesicles and makes a contact in every way similar to a motor end plate, but there are no associated sarcolemmal infoldings.

The Peripheral Terminations of Autonomic Nerve Fibers

The axons of the neurons in sympathetic and parasympathetic ganglia are extremely fine (approximately 1 μm) and in most cases unmyelinated. The postganglionic fibers of the sympathetic division of the autonomic nervous system are distributed in peripheral nerves (which they join via the gray rami communicantes), or in plexuses associated with the larger blood vessels (Fig. 8–79A), or in the splanchnic nerves. In the autonomic plexuses of the abdominopelvic cavity, sympathetic preganglionic fibers are distributed with the postganglionic fibers, since not all preganglionic fibers synapse in the sympathetic chain. Parasympathetic preganglionic fibers derived from the vagus are also found in the visceral autonomic plexuses.

Although the sympathetic nervous system is in general a diffusely distributed system, the density and diffuseness of the innervation varies from organ to organ. For example, the postganglionic axons supplying the sphincter pupillae muscle branch little before entering the iris and give rise to a relatively sparse terminal plexus within it, whereas those innervating the gut branch profusely and give rise to a widespread plexus in the gut wall. The terminal ramifications of sympathetic postganglionic fibers in an organ are called the *sympathetic ground plexus*. This consists of a large number of fine, often interconnected, axons that ramify over the surfaces

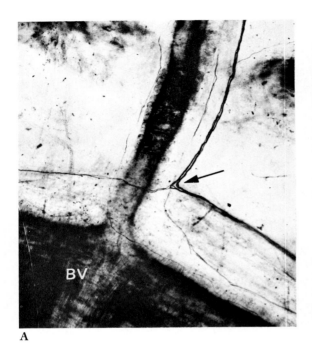

A

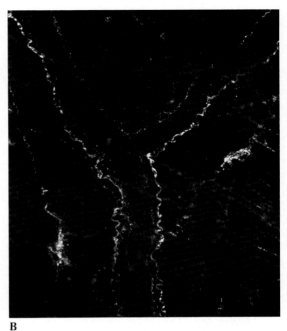

B

8–79 **A.** Silver-stained, teased preparation showing several unmyelinated axons accompanying a large blood vessel **(BV). Arrow** indicates point of bifurcation of certain fibers. × 500. **B.** Fluorescence photomicrograph showing a small branching blood vessel in the mucous membrane of the alimentary tract outlined by thin axons. The axons contain the peptide transmitter, substance P, and have been labeled immunocytochemically with a monoclonal antibody to this peptide. × 250. (Courtesy of A. C. Cuello and M. A. Matthews.)

of smooth muscle and gland cells. At regular intervals each terminal branch has a series of bulblike expansions that are regions of transmitter release (Fig. 8–37).

At the electron microscopic level, these bulblike expansions appear rather like synaptic boutons, because they contain large aggregations of synaptic vesicles and mitochondria. However, they are usually not in intimate contact with the underlying smooth muscle or gland cells, and the characteristic pre- or postsynaptic membrane densities seen at central synapses are rarely present. In some places such as the vas deferens and the sphincter pupillae, the terminal bulbs may approach to within 150 to 200 Å of the smooth muscle fibers and no Schwann cell processes in-

tervene: in these sites it is possible that all or most muscle cells are contacted by at least one terminal bulb. In other sites, such as the gut, most terminal varicosities lie at some distance (1,000 Å) from the target cells and are thought to exert their effects by releasing their transmitters into the general intercellular space. Because smooth muscle cells are electrotonically coupled by means of gap junctions, the excitation of one cell rapidly spreads from cell to cell throughout the tissue.

The terminals of most sympathetic postganglionic axons release *norepinephrine (noradrenaline)*, but some release *acetylcholine*. In the case of noradrenergic endings, most of the synaptic vesicles present are small (about 500 Å) and contain dense cores (Fig. 8–34). These dense cores are especially obvious if the tissue has been "loaded" with the transmitter or with an analog, such as 6-hydroxydopamine, or if it has been fixed in potassium permanganate. A few larger, dense-core vesicles (approximately 1,000 Å) are also found in adrenergic terminals. Both types probably contain norepinephrine and the final enzyme involved in its synthesis, *dopamine-β-hydroxylase*.

Cholinergic nerve terminals in the sympathetic system generally resemble the adrenergic terminals with the notable exception that the vesicles they contain are clear, comparable to those seen in motor nerve terminals in skeletal muscle. Although much less work has been done on the peripheral terminations of parasympathetic postganglionic fibers, they too appear to be of this type. Parasympathetic preganglionic fibers end in such sites as the sinoatrial and atrioventricular nodes and on the postganglionic neurons by means of terminals containing clear vesicles and with definite (asymmetric) pre- and postsynaptic membrane thickenings.

The walls of the alimentary tract possess extensive plexuses of nerve fibers that derive partly from pre- and postganglionic sympathetic and parasympathetic fibers and partly from neurons that are intrinsic to the gut wall (see Chap. 19). These plexuses are concerned with maintaining the rhythmic peristaltic activity of the alimentary canal, although the intrinsic neuronal system is itself capable of maintaining this activity when the sympathetic and parasympathetic nerves are destroyed.

The two major plexuses of the gut wall are the *myenteric* (or Auerbach's) *plexus,* which lies between the longitudinal and circumferential muscle coats, and the *submucosal* (or Meissner's) *plexus,* which lies in the submucosa. Each of these contains localized aggregations of moderately large, multipolar neurons resembling those of the sympathetic and parasympathetic ganglia. The adrenergic nerve terminals in these plexuses may be derived from sympathetic neurons situated in the sympathetic chain or in the ganglionated plexuses. They take the form of chains of bulbous terminals containing large numbers of small, dense-core vesicles. Such terminals form axodendritic and axosomatic synapses on the intrinsic neurons. Unlike adrenergic terminals elsewhere, definite membrane specializations are present. Other nerve terminals within the plexuses contain small, clear vesicles and also end axosomatically and axodendritically. These may be the terminals of both sympathetic and parasympathetic fibers. The intrinsic neurons themselves appear to have short axons that end as varicose, clear-vesicle-containing terminals among the smooth muscle cells adjacent to the plexus; they appear to utilize a variety of neurotransmitters.

A third smaller plexus of fine nerve fibers is found in the gut wall at the level of the muscularis mucosae. It contains relatively few nerve cells and seems to be composed predominantly of sensory fibers whose finer branches ramify beneath the epithelium, sending naked terminal processes between adjoining epithelial cells. The sensory nerve fibers supplying the mucous membrane have their cell bodies in the dorsal root ganglia, but they are distributed with the autonomic nerves and thus pass through the myenteric and submucosal plexuses en route to the mucosa.

The Fiber Spectra of Peripheral Nerves

In the foregoing accounts of sensory, motor, and autonomic nerves and their terminations, we have frequently pointed out that different types of nerve endings are customarily supplied by axons whose diameter and degree of myelination are fairly constant for a particular category of ending. Because the diameter of an axon is closely related to its conduction velocity, fibers in a particular diameter range will also fall within a fairly constant range of conduction velocities. The range of fiber diameters in a nerve is known as the *fiber spectrum* of that nerve (Fig. 8–58A and B), and because of the relationship between diameter and conduction velocity, such a fiber spectrum also effectively indicates the range of conduction velocities in the fibers of that nerve.

On the basis of their diameters, conduction velocities, and certain other properties that need not concern us here, peripheral nerve fibers have been grouped into several classes. A summary of the two main classifications in current use is given in Table 8–1. The alphabetic classification into groups A, B, and C was made in the 1930s by Erlanger and Gasser and is based on the conduction velocities of mixed peripheral nerve fibers as revealed by the peaks of the compound action potentials recorded after electrical stimulation of the various peripheral nerves. Group A contains fibers with the fastest conduction velocities, and within it two subgroups are now identified. These subgroups (in order of decreasing diameter) are the Aα and Aδ fibers. The B group is formed principally by autonomic preganglionic fibers, and the C group is composed of unmyelinated fibers (including both afferent fibers entering the spinal cord in the dorsal roots and autonomic postganglionic fibers).

A second widely used classification was originally introduced by Lloyd to describe the afferent fibers in muscle nerves. Four groups of fibers were recognized on the basis of their diameters: groups I, II, III, and IV. This is perhaps the more

Table 8–1 Classification of Peripheral Nerve Fibers

Fiber type	Aα		Aδ	C
	Group I	Group II	Group III	Group IV (unmyelinated)
Diameter (includes myelin sheath, where present)	5–20 μm 12–20 μm	5–12 μm	2–5 μm	0.1–1.5 μm
Conduction velocity	30–120 m/s 70–120 m/s	30–70 m/s	5–30 m/s	0.5–2 m/s
Receptor types	Primary endings in muscle spindles (Ia) Golgi tendon organs (Ib)	Secondary endings in muscle spindles Most other encapsulated endings Larger diameter mechanoreceptors and interoreceptors	Thermoceptors Nociceptors Smaller diameter mechanoreceptors and interoreceptors	
Other fiber types	α motor fibers, 12–20 μm	γ motor fibers, 2–8 μm	Autonomic preganglionic fibers 1.5–4 μm (B fibers)	Autonomic postganglionic fibers; olfactory nerve fibers, 0.1–1 μm

useful classification (since it also takes into account the peripheral terminations of sensory fibers). However, it is not usually applied to nonsensory nerves even though they can be made to fit into the scheme (Table 8–1).

Some Aspects of Neuronal Organization

Up to this point we have considered neurons more or less as isolated units. After their migration from the neuroepithelium or the neural crest, however, most neurons normally aggregate with other similar nerve cells to form characteristic neuronal populations. Here we shall consider some general principles of neuronal organization and indicate how the more common neural aggregates are constructed. The three most common types of neural aggregate are (1) the ganglia of the peripheral nervous system, including the sensory ganglia associated with the cranial and spinal nerves, and the ganglia of the autonomic nervous system; (2) various cellular groups in the central nervous system, usually re-

ferred to as *nuclei;* and (3) cortical formations, also found in the central nervous system.

Sensory Ganglia

The cells of all the spinal ganglia (Fig. 8–61A) and most of those in the sensory ganglia associated with the cranial nerves are derived from the neural crest. The cells of certain cranial nerve ganglia are derived from the associated placodal epithelia. The factors leading to the segregation of the neural crest cells that give rise to the sensory ganglia from those that give rise to other crest derivatives are not known. After migrating to their definitive location, they aggregate to form the presumptive ganglion. The key morphogenetic event—the coming together of cells of like kind—represents the first step in the formation of any neuronal population.

Subsequently, a high percentage of the neurons that were initially generated die, usually about the time that the cells in the population as a whole make their synaptic or peripheral sensory connections. This *histogenetic cell death* appears to be a general feature of the formation of most neuronal populations in both the peripheral and central nervous systems: in all populations that have been analyzed quantitatively, only about 30 to 60% of the cells survive to maturity. The factors responsible for the death of so many neurons are not known, but it is generally thought that the cells that die are unable to establish either the appropriate number or the appropriate type of synaptic or sensory connections.

At present the most complete accounts of the development of the sensory ganglia derive from the study of these structures in chick embryos. In these ganglia, two distinct neuronal populations appear: initially a large-celled ventrolateral group of neurons (thought to be proprioceptive) arises; and somewhat later in development a smaller-celled dorsomedially located population is generated. Although at a later stage the topographic segregation of the two populations is obscured, they are clearly different. For example, after the early removal of a developing limb, the larger cells degenerate extremely rapidly, whereas the small-celled population usually persists for a much longer period. Conversely, the developing small-celled population appears to be particularly sensitive to the action of the neurotrophic protein, nerve growth factor (NGF). The precursors of this population and the postganglionic sympathetic neurons are said to be the only cells that proliferate under the influence of NGF. A process of *functional specification* of the ganglion cells must then occur. This process determines not only the peripheral and central connections of the cells but also the sensory modality to which they will respond. The nature of this specification is poorly understood: we do not yet know whether it is an intrinsic property of the developing neurons or if it is imposed on them by the peripheral tissues they innervate. In the adult animal a number of different functional classes of ganglionic cell are present, corresponding to each of the various modalities of somatic sensibility, but except for variations in size (Fig. 8–61B) and in the relative amounts of Nissl material and other organelles that the cells contain, no distinct morphological differences exist within the population of ganglion cells. However, cells innervating closely adjacent peripheral receptive fields and projecting their central processes into the same dorsal root filament tend to lie together. This tendency for neurons that innervate a particular region to be closely related

to each other topographically is one of the fundemental prinicples of neuronal organization and is found at virtually all levels of the nervous system. Throughout the somatosensory system, the arrangement is commonly called the *somatotopic organization*, reflecting the systematic central nervous mapping of the body surface; but comparable patterns of organization are found in the other sensory systems where the organizing feature is either topographic (for example, the retinotopic organization of the visual system) or functional (for example, the tonotopic organization of the auditory system).

Interestingly, both the large and small neurons in the sensory ganglia undergo chromatolysis when their peripheral processes are interrupted but not when their central processes are cut. This may be related to the observation that substantially more of the materials synthesized in the perikaryon are transported into the peripheral than into the central processes. Because impulse transmission in these sensory neurons seems to proceed directly from the peripheral to the central process (either without invading the soma or by invading it only after some delay), and inasmuch as there are no synapses on the perikaryon, it appears that the principal role of the ganglion cell soma is trophic, in the sense that the soma serves primarily to maintain the integrity of the processes.

The Ganglia of the Autonomic Nervous System

The second major class of peripheral nerve cell aggregation comprises the ganglia associated with the sympathetic and parasympathetic divisions of the autonomic nervous system (Fig. 8–62). The structure of the para- and prevertebral sympathetic ganglia and the principal cranial and sacral parasympathetic ganglia is essentially the same. Certain of the ganglionic arrangements in the viscera (for example, the gut plexuses) are different and have already been briefly outlined.

Like the sensory ganglia, the ganglia of the autonomic nervous system are invested by a fairly dense fibrous connective tissue capsule that is continuous with the epineurium of the related pre- and postganglionic nerve trunks. Within the ganglia the nerve cells are surrounded by satellite cells, which, like the neurons, are of neural crest origin. However, these ganglia differ from the sensory ganglia in two important respects. First, the neurons are all *multipolar*, usually with several dendrites of varying length and with a single, usually unmyelinated, axon that passes out into the appropriate postganglionic trunk. Second, all the so-called principal ganglion cells (and these constitute most of the neurons in each ganglion) receive synapses from the preganglionic fibers. These synapses are all cholinergic in type. The great majority of them are distributed to the dendrites rather than to the cell soma. As a rule, each ganglion cell receives an input from several preganglionic fibers, and conversely each preganglionic fiber forms synapses with several neurons. There are exceptions to this pattern (for example, in the ciliary portion of the avian ciliary ganglion there is a one-to-one relationship between preganglionic fibers and postsynaptic cells), but such exceptions are rare in the mammalian autonomic nervous system.

The ganglion cells themselves are not uniform in type. In most ganglia there is a class of principal cells that are relatively large, with ovoid or spherical nuclei and an abundance of rough endoplasmic reticulum. Those cells that are adrenergic (as are most principal ganglion cells) contain large numbers of small, dense-core vesicles both in their somata and throughout their processes, but especially at the sites of presumed transmitter release from their axons. As we have seen, these dense-core vesicles contain the neurotransmitter norepinephrine (noradrenaline) and the last enzyme involved in its synthesis, dopamine-β-hydroxylase. The presence of these two substances provides the basis for two common methods for displaying postganglionic sympathetic fibers: namely, the Falck-Hillarp method in which the norepinephrine is condensed by formaldehyde vapor to form a highly fluorescent compound; and an immunohistochemical method, using a peroxidase or fluorescently labeled antibody to dopamine-β-hydroxylase (Fig. 8–35).

In many sympathetic ganglia a second, smaller cell type is found that is intensely fluorescent when treated with formaldelyde vapor. These so-called SIF (small, intensely fluorescent) cells appear to be a class of *dopaminergic* interneurons, but their functional role remains to be determined. At their most numerous they constitute only a small percentage of the total number of ganglion cells. Their nuclei are smaller, often ellipsoidal or convoluted, and more heterochromatic than those of the principal cells. They contain many large dense-core vesicles and are

presynaptic to the principal cells, but they may also release their contents directly into the blood stream (Fig. 8–16).

The Organization of Neuronal Aggregates in the Central Nervous System

Compared with the relatively simple organization of peripheral neural aggregates, the central nervous system presents a bewildering display of different neuronal patterns. No two regions of the central nervous system are identical in their organization, although from animal to animal within any species, and even between different species and different classes, homologous structures usually show a surprisingly consistent neural architecture. Only two of the more common patterns will be considered here. These are the so-called central *nuclei* and certain laminated or *cortical* structures. Each of these different types of neuronal aggregate can be readily recognized at a fairly gross level in preparations stained either by the Nissl method or by one of the common methods for myelinated fibers; the analyses of neural organization at this level are called *cytoarchitectonic* or *myeloarchitectonic* studies, respectively, and constitute an essential preliminary to any serious study of the central nervous system.

Central Cell Masses or "Nuclear Groups." Collections of neurons of similar type in the central nervous system are usually termed nuclei (a term that should not be confused with the nuclei of individual neurons) (Figs. 8–80 and 8–81). The neurons in such nuclei are usually generated over a restricted period of time in a well-defined region of the neuroepithelium. From this region the postmitotic, but still immature, neurons migrate to their definitive location where they aggregate with other neurons of the same type. The mechanisms responsible for this selective cell aggregation are generally thought to involve the presence on the surfaces of the cells of certain cell-type-specific macromolecules (probably glycoproteins) that serve to "recognize" other cells of similar type. This does not imply that all the cells in a given nucleus are absolutely identical in structure or function. In fact, in nearly every center that has been carefully studied in adult animals, two or more distinct cell types have been found. One type, which we may again refer to as the principal cell, usually gives rise to the efferent axons that connect the cell mass to other

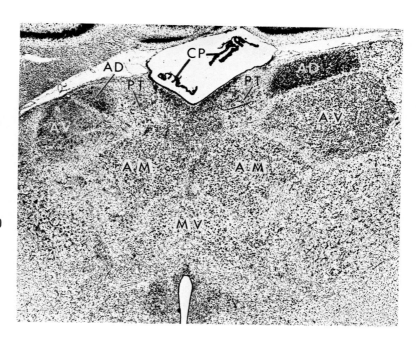

8–80 Frontal section of diencephalon of a rabbit brain from which cingulate region of cerebral cortex was removed several weeks previously. Anterodorsal **(AD)** and anteroventral **(AV)** nuclei of left thalamus have undergone profound retrograde degeneration characterized by cell death and gliosis. Other nuclei **(AM, PT, MV)** remain normal. **CP,** choroid plexus. Thionin stain. × 70.

parts of the central nervous system. These cells have relatively long axons and are usually the largest cells in the nucleus. Often, but not always, the afferent input to the nucleus ends on the dendrites or somata of the principal cells. There is usually a second population of cells, usually smaller than the principal cells. These cells are thought to serve as interneurons, being interposed either between the major source of af-

ferents to the cell mass and the principal cells or between axon collaterals of some principal cells and other, adjacent principal cells. In the first case, they are usually excitatory in nature; in the second, inhibitory. Such small cells are generally Golgi type II neurons with short, locally ramifying axons; but, evidently many of them may be axonless and act through "presynaptic dendrites."

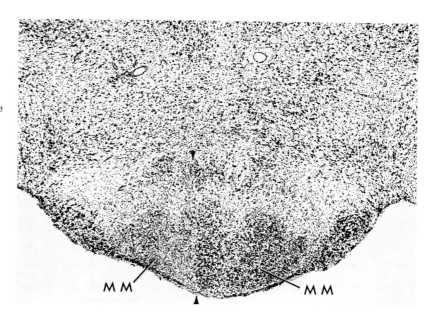

8–81 Mamillary body of same brain as in Fig. 8–80, retrograde transneuronal degeneration of cells in left mamillary nuclei **(MM)** that project their axons to degenerated area of thalamus. **Arrowheads** indicate midline. Thionin stain. × 140.

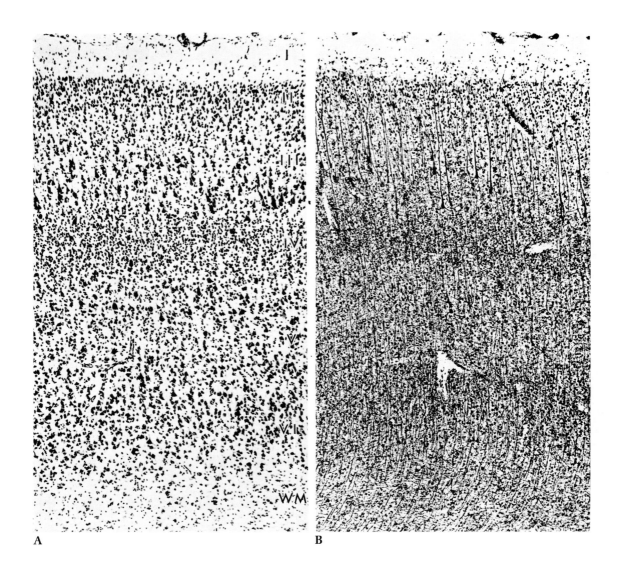

A

B

8–82 **A.** Nissl-stained preparation of paravisual cerebral cortex of a monkey showing cell layers. (I–VI) **WM,** white matter. × 70. **B.** Bodian-stained preparation of section adjacent to that shown in part A demonstrating cellular and fiber lamination. × 70.

"Cortical" and Other Laminated Structures.

Where nerve cells are found on the surface of the brain, the region is called a *cortex* (Fig. 8–82A and B). Here the neurons are arranged in a series of superimposed layers with cells of similar type tending to occupy the same layer. As in the case of the nuclear masses, each cortical area is, in some respects, morphologically distinct, so that

no general account can be given that is applicable to all.

In the simplest types of cortex (like that in certain parts of the olfactory system and in the hippocampal formation), the principal cells have their somata arranged in a single, compact lamina, while their principal dendrites are regularly oriented in a second overlying layer. The various extrinsic inputs to the cortex terminate on these dendrites and are so arranged that the afferents from different sources contact different segments of the dendritic tree (Fig. 8–83). Various inter-neurons, usually of an inhibitory kind, are found in a third, deeper layer and their axons usually terminate on the cell somata or the proximal

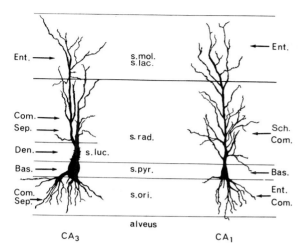

8–83 Drawings of two types of pyramidal cell found in the mammalian hippocampus to illustrate the principle that afferents from different sources are usually spatially segregated on the surface of complex neurons. **Ent, Com, Sep:** entorhinal, commissural, and septal afferents. (From Gottlieb, D. I., and Cowan, W. M. 1972. Z Zellforsch. Mikrosk. Anat. 129:413.)

parts of the dendrites of the principal cell type. This type of spatial segregation of afferent inputs is most clearly seen in simple cortical areas such as this, but it may well be the case in most neurons that receive synapses from two or more sources. The output from such a cortex is represented by the collected axons of the principal cells, which generally enter a zone of subcortical white matter.

Most cortical areas are considerably more complex than this. For example, in all but a few regions of the cerebral cortex (the so-called *neocortex*) there are five superimposed cellular layers and a relatively cell-free outer zone, or molecular layer, just beneath the surface (Fig. 8–82A). Within each cellular layer, there are often several different cell types, although for heuristic reasons it is convenient to regard them as belonging to only two major classes: *pyramidal cells*, so called because of the pyramidal form of the cell bodies, which lead superficially to a prominent ascending or apical dendrite; and nonpyramidal, or *stellate cells*, whose dendritic arborizations lack the rigid organization of the pyramidal cell (see Figs. 8–7, 8–8, and 8–11A and B). The pyramidal cell bodies are generally found in layers II, III, and V, and to a lesser extent in layer VI, and send their apical dendrites

into the supervening layers and their axons into the subcortical white matter. The nonpyramidal cells are found in all layers, but certain types are particularly concentrated in layer IV. Their axons are distributed within the cortex itself. Certain extrinsic inputs to the cortex (for example, those from the related thalamic nucleus) appear to terminate mainly on the nonpyramidal cells in layer IV, whereas others (such as the commissural fibers from the cortex of the opposite hemisphere) also end in layers I, II, and III. These and other inputs are then relayed to the pyramidal cells in the outer layers by nonpyramidal cells with vertical axons (Fig. 8–8). The axons of the pyramidal cells, in turn, project to other regions of the brain. Investigators have recently found that the pyramidal cells in different layers project to different parts of the nervous system: generally the cells in layers II and III were found to project to other parts of the cerebral cortex, those in layer VI to the thalamus, and those in layer V to the brainstem, basal ganglia, and spinal cord. A second important principle that has emerged from recent studies of the sensory areas of the cerebral cortex is that interrelated cells are arranged into vertical columns or slabs perpendicular to the cortical surface and passing through all layers. In each column all the cells appear to subserve one sensory submodality, or to be responsive to some special feature of a sensory stimulus. Thus, in the somatosensory cortex the cells in one column may all respond to movement of a particular joint, whereas those in another column may all respond to light tactile stimulation of the skin. Similarly, in the visual cortex, cells in one slab will respond preferentially to stimulation of the left eye, whereas those in the adjoining slab will respond to stimulation of the right eye. And within either "eye-dominance column," all the cells in a single, narrow, vertical column may respond only to visual stimuli with a particular spatial orientation. In the case of the motor cortex, the cells of a column are all connected to the same group of spinal motoneurons.

The cerebral cortex can be subdivided into a number of different areas, each having its own distinctive structure. These so-called cytoarchitectonic fields differ from each other in the number, density, and arrangement of the cells and fibers in their various layers, and the boundaries between adjoining fields are occasionally remarkably distinct (Fig. 8–84). Most of these cytoarchitectonically distinct fields also have dis-

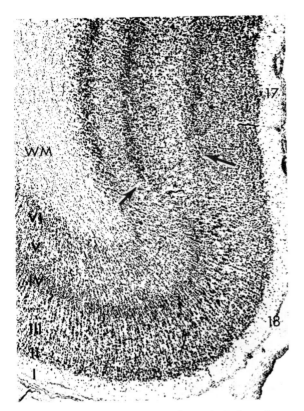

8–84 Junction of primary visual area **(17)** of monkey cerebral cortex with adjacent area **(18). Arrows** show region at which trilaminar layer **IV** of area 17 gives place to unilaminar layer **IV** of area 18. Latter area also has larger cells in layer **III,** and layers **V** and **VI** are less distinct. **WM,** white matter. Thionin stain. × 23.

tinctive patterns of afferent and efferent connections, and in a number of cases it has been possible to show that functionally they are equally distinct. How these striking differences are generated during the early development of the cortex is unknown. At present the only relevant evidence we have is that the cells in the different layers are generated at different times. The first-formed cortical cells are those that finally reside in the deepest lamina (layer VI); those in the progressively more superficial layers are generated at successively later times. In addition, because many of the cells appear to display their characteristic functional properties shortly after the cortex is developed, it seems likely that the formation of their connections is genetically determined. But the "wiring pattern" seems also to be modifiable by environmental manipulation (for example, by depriving the visual cortex of its normal functional input from one eye).

The Reaction of Neural Tissue to Injury

Because, among animal cells, neurons are distinguished by the number and variety of their processes, considerable attention has been paid to the trophic relationship between the nerve cell soma and its axonal and dendritic processes and to the long-term consequences of neuronal injury. More than a century ago the English physiologist Augustus Waller formulated what is perhaps still the only "law" in neuroanatomy when he pointed out that when an axon is interrupted, the distal segment invariably degenerates. However, it is not only in this part of the axon that degenerative changes occur. In many neurons comparably severe changes can be seen in the perikaryon; in several neuronal systems, an atrophy, or even degeneration, can be observed in the neurons that are related synaptically to the injured nerve cells.

Changes at the Site of the Lesion

After the uncomplicated interruption of an axon, there is a short period during which axoplasm leaks from the cut ends, since the axon appears to be in a state of some turgor owing to the continuous flow of axoplasm and axonal organelles. However, the leakage of axonal contents does not seem to be a serious matter, for within a short while there is a retraction of the axon and the axolemma appears to fuse over the severed ends and effectively seals them off. This is followed by a damming up of axonal material behind the fused membranes so that within 12 to 24 h there is a distinct swelling or dilatation of the axon. These swellings (which contain a variety of organelles, neurofilaments, vesicles of various kinds, mitochondria, and so forth, and stain deeply with most reduced silver methods) are termed *retraction bulbs.* The subsequent fate of the retraction bulbs depends on whether or not regeneration occurs in the cut axon. In most, if not all, parts of the central nervous systems of higher vertebrates (including reptiles, birds, and mammals) no significant regeneration occurs, and within a day or two the proximal end of the severed axon degenerates at least as far back as the axon's nearest collateral branch. In the peripheral nervous system (and to a lesser extent in the central nervous systems of fish and amphibians) numerous filopodia appear on the surface of the retraction bulb. Subsequently, large numbers of new axonal sprouts grow out from the bulb and make their way toward the distal segment of the nerve (Fig. 8–63).

At the site of the injury the supporting and certain other nonneural cells become activated and participate in the removal of the neuronal debris in the formation of a scar and possibly also in the process of regeneration. In the central nervous system the cells principally involved in this "mopping-up operation" are the local astrocytes and microglial which may be stimulated to proliferate and to become actively phagocytic. Oligodendrocytes and vascular pericytes also become reactive. And if there has been some damage to the neighboring capillaries, large numbers of blood-borne phagocytes (polymorphonuclear leukocytes and other macrophages) usually invade the tissue. After the necrotic tissue has been phagocytosed, the glial cells initiate a vigorous repair process. Astrocytic processes either expand to fill the vacated area to form a dense glial scar that bridges across the traumatized zone or, if this area is too large, they effectively seal it off as an encysted space. The oligodendrocytes, on the other hand, seem to be able to sequester large masses of cellular debris by forming myelin ensheathments around them. These glial responses, and especially the formation of a glial scar, most probably either prevent or seriously limit central neural regeneration.

In the peripheral nervous system, the Schwann cells show a similar prompt response by actively proliferating and phagocytosing the breakdown products of the neuronal degeneration. To what extent the reaction of the Schwann cells actually promotes regeneration is not known. To date, most attempts to demonstrate it experimentally have yielded equivocal results, but it is clear that they do form new sheaths for the regenerating axons.

The Reaction in the Distal Segment

In certain invertebrate nerves the surrounding sheath cells seem to be able to maintain the viability of the distal segment of a cut axon more or less indefinitely. But more often, and certainly in all vertebrates, the entire distal segment will, in time, undergo *Wallerian degeneration*. However, the earliest changes seem to appear not close to the injury, as might be expected, but at the axon terminals.

Terminal degeneration takes several forms.

The earliest changes, in the form of a swelling and possibly some loss of synaptic vesicles, can often be recognized within 12 to 24 h after axotomy. (The actual rate of appearance varies somewhat from system to system but, in general, appears to be a function of the distance of the nerve transection from the terminals: the closer to the terminals the axon is interrupted, the more rapidly the degenerative changes appear.) Subsequently, there may be a marked increase in the number of neurofilaments in the terminals, and a corresponding decrease in the number of synaptic vesicles (Fig. 8–85). The neurofilamentous hyperplasia (which is presumably a result of the polymerization of soluble filament precursor material in the axon) accounts for the increased argyrophilia of degenerating axon terminals; and because the filaments often appear as a tangled whorl around a central cluster of mitochondria and synaptic vesicles, in neurofibrillar preparations such degenerating terminals are often impregnated as ringlike structures. Later the whole terminal may become filled with filaments and, in silver preparations, appear as a swollen, degenerating end bulb.

A third reaction involves a progressive increase in the density of the axoplasmic matrix of the terminal and a concomitant loss of the remaining synaptic vesicles (Fig. 8–86). This "dark reaction" may occur as a primary response in certain nerve terminals or, in others, it may be secondary to the neurofilamentous change described above. The physicochemical nature of the axoplasmic change is unknown, but in time there is virtually a complete loss of synaptic vesicles and the mitochondria become increasingly dense and fragmented. A short while later the terminal appears to be "dissected" away from the postsynaptic membrane specialization and phagocytosed by the neighboring astrocytes; the engulfed fragments then resemble lysosomal dense bodies. Terminals undergoing this dense reaction are particularly susceptible to impregnation by certain silver methods, e.g., the Fink-Heimer modification of the Nauta technique, a feature that makes these methods extremely useful for determining the sites of termination of neural pathways.

With the exception of the neuromuscular junction, the degeneration of most peripheral nerve terminations has not been carefully studied. In the case of the neuromuscular junction, the degenerative changes are essentially comparable to those at central neuronal synapses. However, because of the more favorable circum-

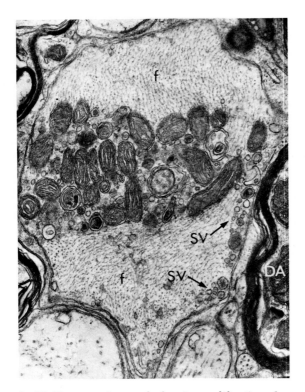

8–85 Electron micrograph showing proliferation of neurofilaments **(f)**, reduction in synaptic vesicles **(SV)**, and central clumping of mitochondria and lysosomes in an axon terminal following interruption of its parent axon. **DA,** degenerating axon. Inferior colliculus of cat. × 34,000. (From Jones, E. G., and Rockel, A. J. 1973. J. Comp. Neurol. 147:93.)

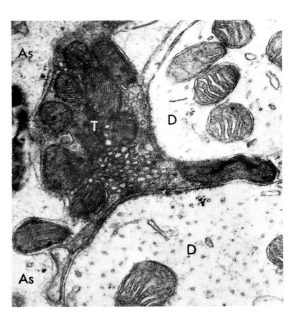

8–86 The electron-dense reaction in a degenerating axon terminal **(T)** that has been cut off from its cell soma. Note the dense clumping of the synaptic vesicles, the persistence of the postsynaptic membrane specializations on the dendrites **(D),** and the surrounding astrocytic processes **(As).** × 33,000. (From Jones, E. G., and Rockel, A. J. 1973. J. Comp. Neurol. 147:93.)

stances for experimental study, it has been easier to show that the cessation of transmission from nerve to muscle precedes the earliest morphological changes by several hours, and that the time required for transmission to fail varies directly with the length of the segment between the nerve section and the axon terminals.

Proximal to the terminals the axon—and in the case of myelinated fibers, the surrounding myelin sheath—seems to degenerate in a piecemeal fashion. Over most of its extent the axoplasm becomes progressively more electron-dense, the normally smooth contour of the axon becomes more and more irregular with fusiform swellings and constrictions every few microns along its length, and it finally breaks up into numerous short fragments. This accounts for the characteristic fragmented appearance of degen-

erating nerve tracts that has been used to such good effect in tracing pathways in the central nervous system (Fig. 8–93). Concurrently, the myelin lamellae (where present) are drawn away from the axolemma, and clefts appear between adjoining lamellae as the myelin sheath disintegrates. The fragmentation of the myelin sheath, and an alteration in its lipid composition, form the basis of yet another method for following neural pathways—the Marchi technique. The signal for the disintegration of the myelin sheath, when its enclosed axon degenerates, is unknown, but the fact that it occurs so consistently suggests that there is normally a close—perhaps even trophic—relationship between axons and the related myelin-forming cells.

Degenerative Changes in the Proximal Segment of the Axon

Depending on the reaction of the nerve cell soma, the axon proximal to the site of the transection may either degenerate completely or show only relatively minor changes in the region adjoining the traumatized zone. Should the parent cell die (see below), the axon will degenerate in a proximodistal sequence starting near the initial segment. Because the appearance of the degeneration is essentially the same as that seen in the distal segment, it is called *indirect Wallerian degeneration* (or, sometimes retrograde fiber degeneration, although this is misleading in that it suggests that the degenerative change proceeds backward from the lesion to the cell soma).

In cases in which the cell body survives the injury, the axon appears to degenerate only as far back as the nearest collateral branch. In the absence of regeneration of the main portion of the axon, this collateral may become hypertrophied and function as the principal conducting channel of the neuron. Regeneration, when it occurs, may begin either from near the origin of this collateral or, more often, from the retraction bulb, as described above. The actual process of axonal regeneration appears to be identical to the initial outgrowth of the axon with the interesting difference that usually several (up to 50) sprouts grow out from the cut end of the axon. The great majority of these sprouts subsequently degenerate; only one or two actually grow into the distal stump of the nerve.

The Reaction of the Nerve Cell Soma to Axotomy

Although it is commonly stated that the event termed *chromatolysis* is the characteristic response of nerve cells to interruption of their axons, a whole spectrum of reactions may in fact occur in the soma, from the death of the neuron at one end, to no discernible change at the other.

The reason for this variability is unknown: it is widely believed that the presence of axon collaterals proximal to the nerve section is responsible for preserving the integrity of the soma, and that chromatolysis is essentially a regenerative response.

Chromatolysis. This reaction is usually seen in motoneurons, in sensory ganglion cells, and in a number of large central neurons in the brainstem and spinal cord (Fig. 8–87). Characteristically it consists of a progressive breakdown of the Nissl material (from which the reaction gets its name), a tendency for the nucleus to become more and more eccentric (usually moving away from the axon hillock), and a variable amount of swelling of the perikaryon. In its fully developed state the cell appears globular, having lost its usual angular profile, with the nucleus pressing against the cell membrane and only a narrow rim of Nissl material around the perimeter of the cell or in a "cap" over the nucleus. The whole process takes about 2 weeks to develop, and if the axon regenerates the entire sequence of changes may be reversed over the next 4 to 6 weeks.

Cell Death. In many neural centers (such as the nuclei of the mammalian thalamus) and in the developing nervous sytem, axon section is followed within a few days by the death of the cell and its removal by glial action. The cytolog-

8–87 A normal motoneuron **(A)** and one showing advanced chromatolysis **(B)** after interruption of its axon. (From Bodian, D., and Mellors, R. C. 1945. J. Exp. Med. 81:469; courtesy of D. Bodian.)

A

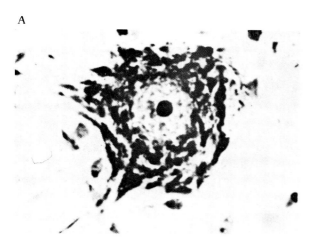

B

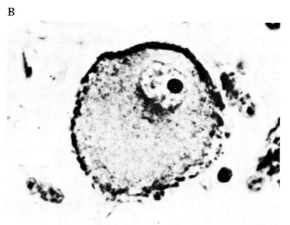

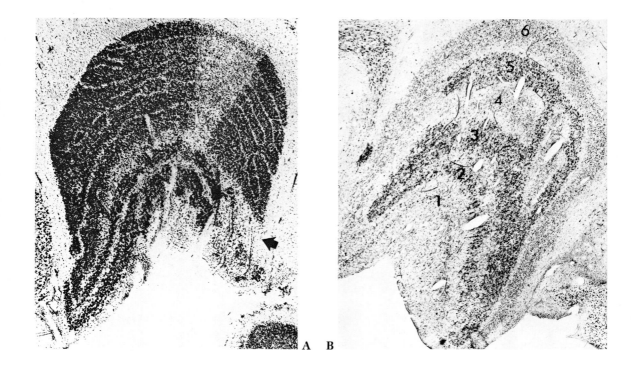

8–88 A. Retrograde cell degeneration involving a wedge-shaped area extending through all layers of the lateral geniculate nucleus of a monkey after destruction of a small portion of the visual cortex **(arrow).** Thionin stain. × 15. **B.** Anterograde transneuronal degeneration in monkey lateral geniculate nucleus which has resulted in severe cell shrinkage in the neurons of layers 1, 4, and 6, following removal of the contralateral eye some months earlier. Thionin stain. × 20. (Part A from Kaas, J. H., Guillery, R. W., and Allman, J. M. 1973. Brain Behav. Evol. 6:253; courtesy of J. H. Kaas.)

ical changes vary from case to case, but characteristically the nucleus becomes increasingly pyknotic, the Nissl material is lost, and the perikaryon shrinks dramatically. In the adult nervous system these changes are accompanied by a marked glial proliferation *(gliosis)*, which persists after the removal of the neuronal debris (Figs. 8–80 and 8–88A). On the other hand, in embryos the neuronal death not only occurs more rapidly but is seldom accompanied by an obvious glial reaction (Fig. 8–89).

Other Cellular Reactions. In some situations the neurons seem to persist more or less indefinitely after axon section, but in a shrunken, atro-

phied form. Whether this is because the cells have other axonal branches that escaped injury or because of some other reason remains to be determined. In still other cases, such as the large pyramidal neurons in the cerebral cortex, there may be no detectable reaction in the perikaryon even though the greater part of the axon has been amputated. In at least some instances the cell seems to be preserved by the hypertrophy of collateral branches given off close to the cell body.

Transneuronal (or Transsynaptic) Degeneration

In a few neuronal systems distinct degenerative (or atrophic) changes have been observed in the neurons that are synaptically related to those whose axons were interrupted. Depending on the direction of the transneuronal effects, they may be termed *anterograde* or *retrograde*. Such effects may extend beyond the first synapse so that secondary and even tertiary transneuronal effects are recognized.

Anterograde Transneuronal Degeneration. The classic site for this type of change is the dorsal lateral geniculate nucleus of the mammalian thalamus, which receives a substantial part of its

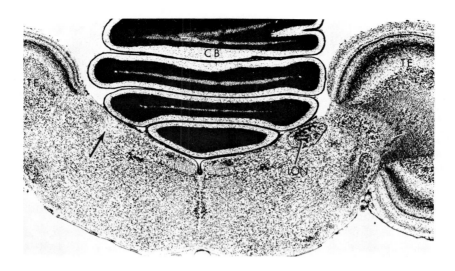

input from the ganglion cells of the retina (Fig. 8–88B). If an eye is removed, or if an optic nerve is cut, the related cells in the lateral geniculate nucleus undergo a progressive atrophy marked by the shrinkage of both the perikaryon and the nucleus, the loss of some Nissl material, and in adults, after many weeks or months, some degree of cell death. In younger animals the changes occur more rapidly, are more severe, and if sufficient time has elapsed, they may be associated with secondary changes in the neurons in the visual cortex to which the geniculate cells project. The most commonly described secondary transneuronal change in the cortex is a loss of dendritic spines, but a generalized thinning of the cortex with a loss of cells in certain layers has also been described.

Although the transneuronal changes in the visual system are the best-documented examples of this form of degeneration, it is now known to occur in many regions in both the central and peripheral nervous systems. Such degeneration is generally thought to be due either to the removal of some form of trophic substance passed from the pre- to the postsynaptic neuron or to the absence of appropriate functional activity in the postsynaptic cells.

Retrograde Transneuronal Degeneration. In some neural systems in which retrograde cell degeneration after axon section is particularly severe, such as the lateral geniculate and anterior nuclei of the mammalian thalamus, degenerative changes have also been observed in the cells that project to those nuclei (Fig. 8–81). Such retro-

8–89 Neurons whose axons are unable to form synaptic connections during development degenerate completely as shown by the absence of the nucleus of origin of the centrifugal fibers to the chick retina **(ION)** after early removal of the contralateral eye in the embryo. In the region usually occupied by the ION, there is a complete cell loss on the side opposite the eye removal **(arrow). CB,** cerebellum; **TE,** tectum. Thionin stain. × 28.

grade transneuronal changes are significantly more severe in young animals and become progressively more marked with increasing survival after the initial lesion. In the case of the anterior thalamic nuclei, it has been found in several species that if the primary lesion in the cerebral cortex occurs early enough, degenerative changes may be found not only in the mamillary nuclei (which project to the anterior thalamic nuclei) but also in one of the midbrain tegmental nuclei that sends its axons to the mamillary nuclei.

Why certain neural systems should show primary, or even secondary, retrograde transneuronal changes is not yet known; at present the only clue is that this type of degeneration is never seen unless there is appreciable cell death in the initial retrograde degeneration. This suggests that there may be a two-way interaction between neurons that are synaptically related: if a neuron is to reach full growth and survive, it must both form an adequate number of synapses on other neurons (or effector tissues such as muscle or gland cells) and receive an adequate number of synaptic inputs from other neurons. Whether these contacts are necessary simply to maintain an adequate level of activity or to provide an adequate exchange of trophic materials remains to be determined.

Methods Used in the Study of the Nervous System

Many techniques are used to study the nervous system. We shall consider only those more commonly used. Broadly, the methods fall into two classes: (1) those based on the study of *normal* neural tissue, and (2) *experimental* methods.

Methods for Normal Neural Tissue

In the study of normal neural tissue, five groups of techniques are in common use.

The Nissl Method. The staining of the Nissl material within neurons, by any one of a number of basic aniline dyes, has been used for almost a century to identify the somata of individual neurons and to analyze the distribution of populations of neurons. Several of the illustrations in this chapter (for example, Figs. 8–10, 8–84, and 8–89) are of Nissl-stained preparations; their use is essential for any cytoarchitectonic or cytological study of the nervous system.

8–90 Several weeks after interrupting a fiber bundle, all the axons degenerate and are removed by the phagocytic action of glial cells. In this section of the human spinal cord in a case of tabes dorsalis, the fibers in the gracile funiculi **(GF)** have completely disappeared. (Weigert method, to show myelinated fibers.) **AM,** arachnoid mater; **DR,** dorsal root; **VR,** ventral root. × 9.

Methods for Staining Nerve Fibers. A number of techniques more or less selectively stain the sheaths of myelinated axons. Most of them involve some prior treatment of the tissue in a mordant such as potassium dichromate, which serves to stabilize the lipids of the myelin sheaths, and subsequent staining of the pretreated myelin with a basic dye such as hematoxylin. Figure 8–90 shows a preparation stained in this way. Because of its high affinity for lipids, osmium tetroxide also provides an extremely intense stain for myelin (Fig. 8–51). Axons themselves and dendrites can be stained by various *reduced silver methods.* In a general sense these methods resemble certain photographic procedures in which silver salts are "developed" and the resulting metallic silver "fixed." In many of these methods, the tissue is pretreated in a silver nitrate solution at high pH followed by a reduction involving an acidified formalin solution. As a result, "nuclei" of metallic silver are deposited around certain cellular organelles (for example, the nuclear membrane, nucleoli, and so forth) but especially around clusters of neurofilaments. As we have pointed out, this appears to be the basis for the light-microscopic appearance of neurofibrils. These methods are sometimes called "neurofibrillar methods." Figures 8–24, 8–25, and 8–75B show preparations of this kind.

The Analytic Methods. Because of the difficulty of analyzing preparations in which all the neuronal perikarya or all the various processes are stained, two invaluable methods were developed in the latter part of the last century. They are the *supravital methylene blue method* of

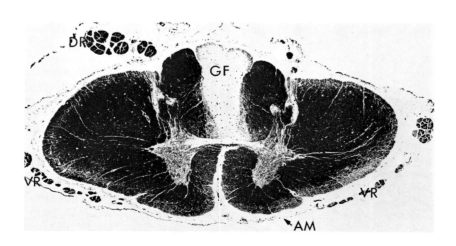

Ehrlich and the *Golgi method*. These methods have two major advantages: first, they stain only a small percentage of the neurons in any one area (commonly less than 1%); and, second, they usually stain the cells in their entirety. As Figs. 8–11 and 8–12 show, in a preparation of this kind, individual neurons stand out strikingly against a relatively clear, unstained background, and usually the full extent of the perikarya, the dendrites (including dendritic spines), and the unmyelinated segments of their axons are displayed. The reason for the selectivity of these methods is not known, nor is the mechanism of the actual staining procedures. In the case of the Golgi method (which has been the more intensively studied and is currently the more widely used of the two methods), the tissue is commonly pretreated with potassium dichromate and then impregnated in a silver nitrate solution. This results in the deposition of silver salts throughout most of the interior of the neuron, excluding the various membranous components. Despite a certain capriciousness, these methods are extremely valuable for studying dendritic organization and are among the few that are useful for analyzing local neuronal circuitry.

Intracellular Labeling of Physiologically Identified Neurons. This recent development in neurobiology represents an especially powerful addition to the older analytic methods, because it permits full visualization of neurons whose functional properties have previously been defined electrophysiologically. Briefly, the method involves using a micropipette to inject a cell with a fluorescent dye (such as Procion yellow), or an opaque substance (such as a cobalt salt), or a histochemically demonstrable enzyme (such as horseradish peroxidase). The label, usually injected into the perikaryon, diffuses or is actively transported into the dendrites and the initial portion of the axon (Fig. 8–95). In suitably prepared sections and with the appropriate optics (e.g., fluorescence microscopy is needed to visualize cells filled with Procion yellow), the entire geometry of the cell can be readily demonstrated. Alternatively, the marker molecule can be iontophoresed up the axon from its cut end and subsequently precipitated in the perikaryon and dendrites. This approach has proved especially effective for labeling motoneurons in invertebrates. A recent variant of the intracellular labeling procedure involves the use of tritium-labeled precursors of certain macromolecules (such as

[³H]amino acids or [³H]fucose), which are incorporated into proteins or glycoproteins and which are rapidly transported from the soma into the dendrites and axon of the labeled cell. After an appropriate interval to allow for the transport of the radioactive macromolecules, the distribution of the tritium label can be displayed autoradiographically.

Electron Microscopy. The introduction of the electron microscope to biology in the early 1950s added an entirely new dimension to neuroanatomical studies, not only because it offered increased resolution but, perhaps more importantly, because it displayed *all* the structures within a tissue. In this respect it differs from all the other methods commonly used. One of its earliest contributions was the demonstration that there is no extensive "ground substance" in the brain and spinal cord as was formerly believed; rather, the central nervous system resembles most other ectodermal derivatives, with only narrow (200 Å) clefts between adjoining cells and their processes. In addition, it made possible for the first time the critical study of such structures as synapses and their associated organelles, the substructure of myelin sheaths, the form of nodes of Ranvier, and the ultrastructural counterparts of such neuronal organelles as Nissl bodies, and neurofibrils. The preparation of neural tissue for electron microscopy generally involves fixation by perfusion with a buffered solution of aldehydes (formaldehyde and glutaraldehyde are commonly used), postfixation in osmium tetroxide, and embedding in an appropriate plastic. Because the sections used are generally of the order of 600 to 1,000 Å thick and the area available for study in any one section is usually only a few hundred square microns in extent, the amount of tissue that can be studied is rather limited. Within these limits, however, the method is the most critical available to the neuroanatomist. In recent years this approach has been significantly extended by the development of techniques for preparing large numbers of serial sections, by the application of the electron microscope to tissue previously stained by some other method (such as the Golgi technique or after intracellular labeling; see Fig. 8–95), and by the introduction of such special methods as freeze-etching, which permits the interior of membrane surfaces to be visualized (Fig. 8–31). The use of the high-voltage electron microscope has made it possible to study sections as thick as 1 or 2 μm; this has been particularly valuable in the analysis of Golgi-impregnated material.

Experimental Methods

Although the examination of normal material is an essential prerequisite for all neuroanatomical studies, it is seldom possible in such material to determine the connections between groups of neurons that are separated by more than just a few hundred microns. For this, one must resort to experimental material, which is basically of two kinds: the first is aimed at determining the *origin* of neuronal pathways, the second at mapping their sites of *termination*.

Retrograde Methods. For many years the method of choice for determining the origin of nervous pathways was based on the retrograde reaction seen in nerve cell somata after their axons were interrupted or their synaptic terminals destroyed (for example, see Figs. 8–80 and 8–88A). This method was particularly successful in elucidating the origin of the motor divisions of the cranial nerves, the location of spinal motoneurons supplying various muscle groups and certain of the connections of the cerebellum, and most strikingly, in establishing the pattern of projection of the various nuclei of the thalamus on the cerebral cortex and corpus striatum. Unfortunately, as we have pointed out above, not all neurons show a clear-cut reaction to axotomy, and in these cases the method not only is of little value but has often proved to be misleading. Another "retrograde" method is both more reliable and more generally applicable than the cell-degeneration approach. This method is based on the uptake of exogenous marker molecules (such as the enzyme horseradish peroxidase [Figs. 8–91 and 8–92], the reaction product of which can be readily demonstrated histochemically) by axons and especially by their terminals, and its transport back to the cell soma by the process of retrograde axonal transport. This method has proved to be invaluable for such difficult problems as the origin of the various efferent projections from the cerebral cortex, the projection of different populations of retinal ganglion cells, and the connections of various nuclear groups in the thalamus and brainstem.

Anterograde Methods. The alternative approach is aimed at determining the site and pattern of termination of the axons arising from a

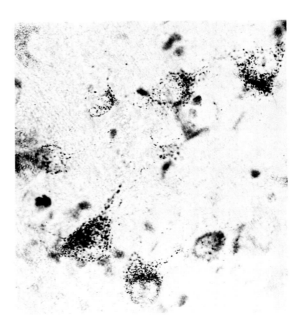

8–91 A group of neurons that have been labeled retrogradely with the enzyme marker horseradish peroxidase. Dark granules are reaction product in cell soma and dendrites. × 430. (From Jones, E. G., and Leavitt, R. Y. 1974. J. Comp. Neurol. 154:349.)

given population of neurons. Three fundamentally different strategies have been used. The first is based on the anterograde degenerative changes seen in the distal portion of axons after their interruption or the destruction of their parent nerve cell bodies by an experimental lesion. Because these changes have been described in the previous section, we need only add that the methods most widely used at present are variants of a silver technique introduced by Nauta and Gygax in 1951 and commonly called the *Nauta technique* (Figs. 8–93 and 8–94). This technique takes advantage of the increased argyrophilia of degenerating axons; and when the staining of the normal fibers is critically suppressed, the degenerating axons and axon terminals can be displayed against a relatively clear background. The most critical method for identifying degenerating axons and presynaptic processes is the use of the *electron microscope*. Indeed, this is the only method that enables one confidently to identify synaptic relationships; the presence of the various degenerative changes described on pages 359–360 (Figs. 8–85 and

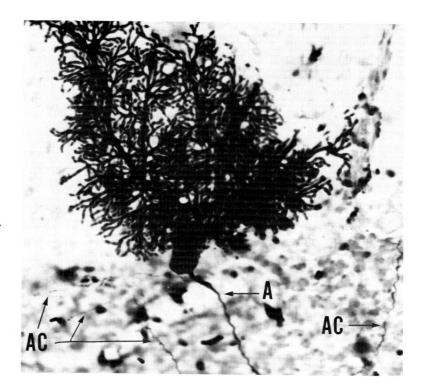

8–92 A Purkinje cell from the cerebellar cortex of a cat stained by the intracellular injection of horseradish peroxidase. **A,** axon; **AC,** axon collateral. × 25. (Courtesy of S. T. Kitai.)

8–86) in a presynaptic profile constitutes ineluctable evidence that the parent cell or its axons has been damaged.

An earlier method was introduced by Marchi in 1885 and was based on the increased affinity of disintegrating myelin sheaths for osmium tetroxide. However, because it was somewhat capricious and applicable only to myelinated pathways, the Marchi method is now only of historical interest. If enough time has elapsed between the causative lesion and the fixation of the brain, the anterograde degeneration of the pathways in question may have proceeded to the point where all the fibers have been removed by glial action. In this case their former location can

be identified, as it were negatively, by the absence of stainable fibers. Although this approach has little to commend it for experimental studies, it is still quite widely used in human neuropathology to follow the degeneration resulting from long-standing brain lesions (Fig. 8–90).

The second strategy is based on the axonal transport of materials synthesized in neuronal somata and distributed along the length of the axons to their terminals. Most commonly, various tritiated precursors, such as [^{3}H] fucose or [^{3}H] amino acids, are used. A concentrated solution of the labeled precursor is injected into the neuronal population whose connections are to be studied. The neurons in the immediate vicinity

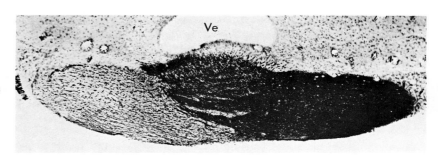

8–93 Degenerating axons become intensely argyrophilic, as seen in this photomicrograph of the optic chiasm of a guinea pig 6 days after removal of the left eye. **Ve,** ventricle, Nauta-Gygax method. × 80.

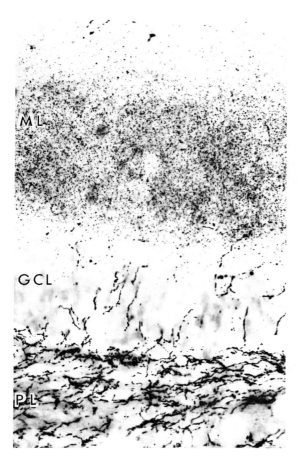

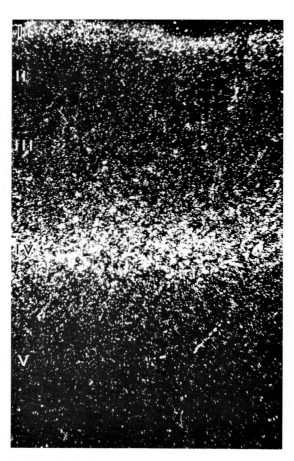

8–94 Silver-stained, degenerating axons ascending from the polymorph layer **(PL)** of the dentate gyrus through the granule cell layer **(GCL)** to end in a dense mass of terminal fragments in the deeper part of the molecular layer **(ML).** Fink and Heimer stain, marsupial brain after destruction of hippocampal commissure. × 200. (From Heath, C. J., and Jones, E. G. 1971. J Anat. [Lond.] 109:253.)

8–95 Dark-field photomicrograph from an autoradiograph demonstrating axoplasmically transported label in axon terminals in layers I and IV of the cerebral cortex following an injection of tritiated amino acids in the thalamus. × 165.

of the injection (but not axons passing through it) take up the precursor and incorporate it into certain macromolecules (such as proteins, glycoproteins, or glycolipids), which are then transported at various velocities down their axons. The labeled axons and axon terminals can then be identified in serial light-microscopic autoradiographs (or electron-microscopic autoradiographs) of the relevant areas (Fig. 8–95). Because this method is based on an established physiological property of nerve cells and does not involve the destruction of the tissue being studied, it has a number of advantages over the degeneration methods and, in addition, appears to be somewhat more sensitive.

The third strategy is aimed at identifying specific neural pathways that act by the release of certain identified neurotransmitters. These methods are based either on the inherent fluorescence of such biogenic amines as dopamine, norepinephrine, and serotonin when exposed to formalin vapor or, for example, in the case of cholinergic and noradrenergic fibers, on the binding of fluorescent-labeled antibodies to the enzymes choline acetyltransferase and dopamine-β-hydroxylase, which are the key enzymes in the biosynthesis of acetylcholine and norepinephrine, respectively (Fig. 8–35). A somewhat different method in this category is based on the finding that neurons that release certain transmitter substances (such as γ-amino butyric acid or glycine) have a high-affinity uptake system for the transmitter. When exposed to a radioactively labeled solution of the transmitter, the neurons, and especially their axon terminals, take up the label in high concentrations; its presence in the cell or axon terminals can subsequently be demonstrated autoradiographically. Since their introduction in the late 1960s, these methods have proved extremely useful, in both the central and peripheral nervous systems, and clearly presage the development of a new phase in neuroanatomical studies that should lead in time to a complete account of the "chemical architecture" of the brain and spinal cord.

References and Selected Bibliography

General

Brodal, A., 1981. Neurological Anatomy in Relation to Clinical Medicine, 3rd ed. New York: Oxford University Press.

Cajal, S. Ramón y. 1909–1911, Histologie du Système Nerveux de l'Homme et des Vertébrés, 2 vol. Republished 1952. Consejo Superior de Investigaciones Cientificas, Madrid.

Cooper, J. R., Bloom, F. E. and Roth, R. M. 1978. The Biochemical Basis of Neuropharmacology. Third ed. New York: Oxford University Press.

Fawcett, D. W. 1981. The Cell, 2nd ed. Philadelphia: W. B. Saunders.

Jones, E. G. 1982. The Structure of Nervous Tissue, four-part tape–slide course. New York: Audio Visual Mktg., Inc.

Kandel, E. R. (ed.). 1977. Handbook of Physiology. Section I. The Nervous System, vol. I, Pts. 1 and 2, Cellular Biology of Neurons. Bethesda, Md.: American Physiological Society.

Kandel, E. R., and Schwartz, J. H. 1981. Principles of Neural Science. New York: Elsevier North-Holland.

Kuffler, S. W., and Nicholls, J. G. 1976. From Neuron to Brain. Sunderland, Mass.: Sinauer Associates Inc.

Scientific American. The brain. Vol. 241 pt. 3 (1979).

Schmitt, F. O., and Worden, F. G. (eds.). 1974. The Neurosciences Third Study Program. Cambridge, Mass.: MIT Press.

Schmitt, F. O., and Worden, F. G. (eds.). The Neurosciences Fourth Study Program. Cambridge, Mass.: MIT Press.

Shepherd, G. M. 1979. The Synaptic Organization of the Brain, 2nd ed. New York: Oxford University Press.

Siegal, G. J., Albers, R. W., Agranoff, B. W., and Katzman, R. 1981. Basic Neurochemistry, 3rd ed. Boston: Little, Brown, and Co.

Development

Angevine, J. B., 1970. Critical cellular events in the shaping of neural centers. In F. O. Schmitt (ed.), The Neurosciences Second Study Program. New York: Rockefeller University Press, pp. 62–72.

Cowan, W. M., 1978. Aspects of neural development. Int. Rev. Physiol. 17:149.

Cowan, W. M., (ed.). 1981. Studies in developmental neurobiology. Essays in Honor of Viktor Hamburger. New York: Oxford University Press.

Dennis, M. J. 1981. Development of the neuromuscular junction: Inductive interactions between cells. Ann. Rev. Neurosci. 4:43.

Hamburger, V., Brunso-Bechtold, J. K., and Yip, J. 1981. Neuronal death in the spinal ganglia of the chick embryo and its reduction by nerve growth factor. J. Neurosci. 1:60.

Hamburger, V., and Levi-Montalcini, R. 1949. Proliferation, differentiation and degeneration in the spinal ganglia of the chick embryo under normal and experimental conditions. J. Exp. Zool. 111:457.

Jacobson, M. 1978. Developmental Neurobiology, 2nd ed. New York: Plenum Press.

Rakic, P. 1974. Neurons in Rhesus monkey visual cortex: Systematic relation between time of origin and eventual disposition. Science 183:425.

Rakic, P. 1977. Prenatal development of the visual system in Rhesus monkey. Phil. Trans. Roy. Soc. Ser. B. 278:245.

Sidman, R. L. 1974. Cell-cell recognition in the developing nervous system. In F. O. Schmitt and F. G. Worden (eds.), The Neurosciences Third Study Program. Cambridge, Mass.: The MIT Press, pp. 743–758.

Sidman, R. L., and Rakic, P. 1974. Neuronal migration, with special reference to the developing human brain: A review. Brain Res. 62:1.

Tuchman-DuPlessis, H., Auroux, M., and Haegel, P. 1974. Illustrated Human Embryology, vol. III. Nervous System and Endocrine Glands. New York: Springer-Verlag New York, Inc.

Neurons

Barr, M. L., Bertram, L. F., and Lindsay, H. A. 1950. The morphology of the nerve cell nucleus, according to sex. Anat. Rec. 107:283.

Bray, D., and Gilbert, D. 1981. Cytoskeletal elements in neurons. Ann. Rev. Neurosci. 4:505.

Chan-Palay, V., and Palay, S. L. 1972. High voltage electron microscopy of rapid Golgi preparations. Neurons and their processes in the cerebellar cortex of the monkey and rat. Z. Anat. Entwicklungsgesch. 137:125.

Jones, E. G. 1975. Varieties and distribution of non-pyramidal cells in the sensory-motor cortex of the squirrel monkey. J. Comp. Neurol. 160:205.

Jones, E. G., and Powell, T. P. S., 1969. Morphological variations in the dendritic spines of the neocortex. J. Cell. Sci. 5:509.

Palay, S. L., and Palade, G. E. 1955. The fine structure of neurons. J. Biophys. Biochem. Cytol. 1:69.

Palay, S. L., Sotelo, C., Peters, A., and Orkand, P. M. 1968. The axon hillock and the initial segment. J. Cell Biol. 38:193.

Peters, A., Palay, S. L. and Webster, H. DeF. 1976: The Fine Structure of the Nervous System, 2nd ed. Philadelphia: W. B. Saunders.

Pfenninger, K. H., 1978. Organization of neuronal membranes. Ann. Rev. Neurosci. 1:445.

Schwartz, J. H. 1979. Axonal transport: Components, mechanisms, and specificity. Ann. Rev. Neurosci. 2:467.

Synapses

Bodian, D. 1937. The structure of the vertebrate synapse. A study of the axon endings on Mauthner cells and neighboring centers in the goldfish. J. Comp. Neurol. 68:117.

Cold Spring Harbor Symposia on Quantitative Biology. 1976. The Synapse, Vol. 40. Cold Spring Harbor Laboratory, New York.

Gray, E. G. 1959. Axo-somatic and axo-dendritic synapses of the cerebral cortex: An electron microscope study. J. Anat. (Lond.) 93:420.

Heuser, J. E., and Reese, T. S. 1973. Evidence for recycling of synaptic vesicle membrane during transmitter release at the frog neuromuscular junction. J. Cell Biol. 57:315.

Heuser, J. E., Reese, T. S., and Landis, D. M. D. 1974: Functional changes in frog neuromuscular junctions studied with freeze-fracture. J. Neurocytol. 3:109.

Landis, D. M. D., and Reese, T. S. 1974. Differences in membrane structure between excitatory and inhibitory synapses in the cerebellar cortex. J. Comp. Neurol. 155:93.

Uchizono, K. 1965. Characteristics of excitatory and inhibitory synapses in the central nervous system of the cat. Nature, 207:642.

Supporting Cells

Brightman, M. W., and Palay, S. L. 1963. The fine structure of the ependyma in the brain of the rat. J. Cell Biol. 19:415.

Brightman, M. W., and Reese, T. S. 1969. Junctions between intimately opposed cell membranes in the vertebrate brain. J. Cell Biol. 40:648.

Bray, G. M., Rasminsky, M., and Aguayo, A. J. 1981. Interactions between axons and their sheath cells. Ann. Rev. Neurosci. 4:127.

Bunge, R. P. 1968. Glial cells and the central myelin sheath. Physiol. Rev. 48:197.

Jones, E. G. 1970. On the mode of entry of blood vessels into cerebral cortex. J. Anat. 106:507.

Penfield, W. 1932. Neuroglia: Normal and pathological. In W. Penfield (ed.), Cytology and Cellular Pathology of the Nervous System, vol. 2. New York: Hoeber, pp. 421–479.

Peters, A. 1966. The node of Ranvier in the central nervous system. Quart. J. Exp. Physiol. 51:229.

Peters, A., Palay, S. L. and Webster, H. DeF. 1976. The fine structure of the nervous system. The Neurons and Supporting Cells. Philadelphia: W. B. Saunders.

Vaughn, J. E. 1969. An electron microscopic analysis of gliogenesis in rat optic nerves. Z. Zellforsch. Mikr. Anat. 94:293.

Vaughn, J. E., Hinds, P. L., and Skoff, R. P. 1970. Electron microscopic studies of Wallerian degeneration in rat optic nerves. I. The multipotential Glia. J. Comp. Neurol. 140:175.

Uzman, B. G. 1964. The spiral configuration of myelin lamellae. J. Ultrastruct. Res. 11:208.

Webster, H. De F. 1975. Development of peripheral myelinated and unmyelinated nerve fibers. In P. J. Dyck, P. K. Thomas, and E. H. Lambert (eds.), Peripheral Neuropathy. Philadelphia: W. B. Saunders.

Peripheral Nervous System

Barker, D.: The morphology of muscle receptors. In C. C. Hunt (ed.), Handbook of Sensory Physiology, vol. III/2, chap. 2. New York: Springer-Verlag New York, Inc., pp. 1–190.

Gershon, M. D. 1981. The enteric nervous system. Ann. Rev. Neurosci. 4:227.

Hubbard, J. I. (ed.). 1974. The Peripheral Nervous System. New York: Plenum Press.

Iggo, A. (ed.). 1974. Somatosensory system. Handbook of Sensory Physiology, vol. 2. New York: Springer-Verlag New York, Inc.

Loewenstein, W. R. 1960. Biological Tranducers. Sci. Am. 203:98.

Central Nervous System

Eccles, J. C., Ito, M., and Szentágothai, J. 1966. The Cerebellum as a Neuronal Machine. Berlin: Springer-Verlag.

Hubel, D. H., and Wiesel, T. N. 1977. Functional architecture of macaque monkey visual cortex. Proc. Roy. Soc. Lond. Ser. B. 198:1.

Jones, E. G. 1981. Functional subdivision and synaptic organization of the mammalian thalamus. In R. Porter (ed.), Int. Rev. Physiol., vol. 25, Neurophysiology IV. Baltimore, Md.: University Park Press, pp. 173–245.

Palay, S. L., and Chan-Palay, V. 1974. Cerebellar Cortex: Cytology and Organization. New York: Springer-Verlag New York, Inc.

Schmitt, F. O., Worden, F. G., Adelman, G., and Dennis, S. G. (eds.). 1981. The Organization of the Cerebral Cortex. Cambridge, Mass.: The MIT Press.

Willis, W. D., and Coggeshall, R. E. 1978. Sensory Mechanisms of the Spinal Cord. New York: Plenum Press.

Degeneration and Regeneration

Bodian, D., and Mellors, R. C. 1945. The regenerative cycle of motoneurons with special reference to phosphatase activity. J. Exp. Med. 81:469.

Cajal, S. Ramón Y. 1928. Degeneration and Regeneration of the Nervous System, W. May, (trans.). 2 vols. Oxford, England: Oxford University Press.

Gray, E. G., and Guillery, R. W. 1966. Synaptic morphology in the normal and degenerating nervous system. Int. Rev. Cytol. 19:111.

Tsukuhara, N. 1981. Synaptic plasticity in the mammalian central nervous system. Ann. Rev. Neurosci. 4:351–380.

The Cardiovascular System

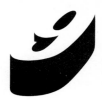

Nicolae Simionescu and Maya Simionescu

The normal activity of cells requires a continuous equilibrium between the inflow of nutrient material and outflow of cell products and wastes. Unicellular organisms exchange such materials continually with the external medium by means of simple diffusion and various transport systems through their cell membranes. In multicellular organisms, the need for a mechanism to transport these substances to different parts of the body is met by the circulation of a fraction of the internal medium. This function is carried out in a specialized circuit of continuous and closed branching tubes (vessels), the *circulatory system*. In vertebrates, humans included, the body fluid is partitioned by semipermeable boundaries into four compartments: blood plasma, lymph, interstitial fluid, and intracellular fluid. For a human being weighing 160 lb, the circulating fluid amounts to approximately 17 liters, and, in relatively steady state, it is distributed as follows: the blood plasma, is approximately 3 liters; the lymph, approximately 3 liters; and the interstitial fluid, approximately 11 liters. An almost equal amount of fluid, approximately 15 liters, is contained in cells. The blood plasma and the lymph circulate in a unidirectional flow in the blood circulatory system and the lymphatic circulatory system, respectively.

The *blood circulatory system* includes a muscular pump, the heart, and the blood vessels. (Together they are frequently called the *cardiovasular system*.)

The *heart* is a modified blood vessel, specialized as a double pump for propulsion. Its right side receives blood from the whole body and this blood circulates through the lungs; its left side collects blood from the lungs and distributes it to all other organs and tissues of the body. Vessels that carry blood to and from the lungs constitute the *pulmonary circulation*, whereas those that distribute and collect blood from the rest of the body form the *systemic circulation*. In both circulations, blood is pumped into and conducted through arteries, which by successive branching increase in number and decrease in caliber until they become *arterioles* that resolve into a network of *capillaries*. It is at the level of these fine vessels that the major exchanges between blood plasma and interstitial fluid take place. Blood returns via confluent *venules* and veins to the heart.

The *lymphatic circulatory system* carries lymph from tissue interstitia to the veins located at the base of the neck. This circulation drains the interstitial fluid and its movable cellular elements into the blindly ending *lymphatic capillaries*. The latter converge in various-sized *lymphatic vessels* (that may or may not be provided with organized collections of lymphocytes, the *lymph nodes*), which return lymph to the blood venous system (see Chap. 15).

By ensuring the distribution of cell metabolites throughout all the tissues and cells, the circulatory system, in association with the nervous system, contributes to communication among, and the integration of, all body constituents.

Structural Plan and Components

In the histogenesis of the blood circulatory system, one can postulate the influence of a genetic pattern as well as adaptive differentiations that modulate the basic organization of the system to meet various local functional requirements.

Physiological and biophysical conditions of the blood circulation are reflected in the tissue composition and structural organization of the cardiovascular system.

General Functional–Structural Correlations

The blood is confined to a closed circuit of vessels lined by a thin layer of simple squamous epithelial cells, the *endothelium*. The latter is differentiated to fulfill the role of physical partition and semipermeable porous membrane between the blood and the interstitial fluid.

Propulsion of the blood is carried out by the heart, whose muscular wall has become largely augmented and differentiated for intermittent contraction. During the systole, the heart ventricles eject the blood under considerable pressure into the large arteries, the aorta and pulmonary. Because of the *elastic tissue* in the walls of these vessels, some of the pressure is converted into increased wall tension; the tension is partially released during diastole, when the vessels passively contract. Hydrostatic pressure within the arterial system is thus maintained (at a lower level) during diastole, and the blood is conducted downstream.

The branches arising from the large arteries supply different parts of the body. The volume of the circulatory system is considerably larger than the blood volume, and the regional functional conditions vary. Therefore, to adjust the amount of blood to local metabolic requirements, a distributing system becomes necessary. This distribution is accomplished by circularly or helically arranged muscle cells amply supplied in all *muscular*, or *distributing*, *arteries*. These vascular smooth muscle cells can contract in response to nervous stimuli. As the vessels become smaller, the blood flow is progressively converted from an intermittent series of propulsions generated by the rhythmic contraction of the heart into a steady, continuous stream. This effect is primarily accomplished in elastic and muscular arteries.

Downstream, two mechanical conditions have to be met: (1) a relatively high hydrostatic pressure must be maintained in arteries to ensure sufficient quantities of blood to various organs and tissues; (2) the blood must be delivered into capillary beds under low pressure to protect the capillary wall, which is extremely thin to allow rapid and extensive exchanges through it. Both conditions are ensured in the smallest arterial ramifications, the arterioles, where relatively thick muscular layers have been differentiated. Smooth muscles of arterioles have the peculiarity of responding not only to nervous sympathetic impulses but also to metabolic stimuli that express the local needs of the tissues *(autoregulation)*. Owing to these factors, about half the resistance to blood flow resides in arterioles that are the major regulators of blood flow.

At the level of capillaries, the speed, magnitude, and nature of the blood–tissue exchanges require a thin, semipermeable partition, which is achieved by the reduction of the vascular wall to a single layer of flat cells, the endothelium. The exchanges occur also in the postcapillary (pericytic) venules, which have a comparable wall structure. In some tissues, the blood approaching the microvascular beds may bypass the exchange vessels (capillaries and pericytic venules) by using shunts, or *arteriovenous anastomoses*, that directly connect the arterioles with venules.

In the slightly larger venules at the beginning of the return circulation, the blood enters under a very low pressure and flows slowly. As a result, the veins exhibit larger lumina and thinner walls than the corresponding arteries. In their walls, connective tissue is more extensive than muscular tissue as structural material. The veins represent low-pressure vessels that are largely distensible and easily compressible. These properties pose particular problems for the venous circulation, problems that are partially solved by special devices called *valves*. Owing to their distensibility, the veins play an important role as a variable blood reservoir *(capacitance vessels)*. At normal hydrostatic pressure in human beings, the blood volume in the systemic veins is approximately four to five times greater than it is in the corresponding arteries.

Tissue Components

Three basic structural constituents may be recognized in the wall of the blood vessels: the *endothelium* (a specialized epithelial tissue), the *muscular tissue*, and the *connective tissue* with a large elastic component. Along the blood circulatory system, these tissues are unevenly distributed in the vascular wall.

The Endothelium. The sheet of thin squamous epithelial cells lining the heart is called *cardiac endothelium*, and that lining the blood vessels is called *vascular endothelium*. The heart and the great majority of blood vessels (arteries, arterioles, capillaries of somatic tissues, venules, and veins) are provided with *continuous endothelium*. In contrast, the endothelium in visceral capillaries displays a relatively large number of small transcellular openings called *fenestrae*; this endothelium is designated *fenestrated endothelium*. In organs where extensive exchanges of relatively large particles (liver) or cells take place between the vessel lumen and interstitia, large gaps may occur in the endothelium, which is then called *discontinuous*. As is the case with other epithelia, the endothelium rests on a *basal lamina* (basement membrane) that varies in thickness and continuity (Table 9–1). The endothelium and its basal lamina constitute the main *permeability barrier*, and the regional differences in their tightness and completeness impart a manifest porosity to the entire vascular wall. In some parts of the microvasculature, the endothelium is surrounded by satellite cells of still unknown function, the *pericytes*. In vessels where smooth muscle cells exist in the vicinity of the endothelium, *myoendothelial junctions* occur.

The Muscular Tissue. In the heart the muscular tissue consists of a special type of *striated muscle cells (cardiac muscle)* that constitute the myocardium; in the wall of blood vessels, *smooth muscle* cells appear. The latter are encountered either (1) as organized concentric layers helically arranged (well developed in muscular arteries and arterioles) or (2) as lon-

374

Table 9–1 Functional and Structural Characteristics of Series-Coupled Segments of the Blood Circulatory System

Functions	Morphological Equivalents	Pump — Heart	Conducting Vessels — Elastic arteries	Distributing Vessels — Muscular arteries
Physical partition; semipermeable barrier	Endothelium	Continuous	Continuous	Continuous
	Basal lamina	Thin, continuous	Thin, continuous; largely reticular	Thin, continuous; inconspicuous in small arteries
Contraction; phagocytosis	Pericytes	Absent	Absent	Absent
Support; diffusion regulator medium; local vasoactive mediators; defense system	Subendothelial layer	Thick connective tissue, smooth muscle— subendothelial layer. Subendocardial layer—loose connective tissue, conducting system, vessels, nerves	Thick connective tissue smooth muscle (longitudinal)	Thick connective tissue, smooth muscle (longitudinal) at branching sites; thin or absent in small arteries
Elastic tension	Internal elastic lamina	Absent	Less distinct in light microscopy; distinct in electron microscopy	Prominent, fenestrated
	Elastic lamellae	Dense, compact fibrous tissue (cardiac skeleton)	50 to 70 thick superposed lamellae	Present in large arteries; rare in small arteries
Active tension (contraction)	Muscle tissue heart striated vessels smooth	(Striated fibers; cardiac muscle)	Alternating with but fewer than elastic lamellae	30 to 40 concentric layers
Elastic tension	External elastic lamina	Absent	Not distinct as separate feature	Present in large arteries, thin or absent in small arteries
Support, vessels and nerves on the wall	Adventitial layer	Subepicardial layer—connective tissue vessels, nerves	Thin, connective tissue, smooth muscle (longitudinal) vessels, nerves	Thick, connective tissue, smooth muscle (longitudinal) vessels, nerves
Gliding surface	Serosa	Mesothelial cells of visceral pericardium		

Table 9–1 *(continued)*

Regulating and Resistance Vessels	Exchange Vessels		Returning and Capacitance Vessels		Tunics
Arterioles	Capillaries	Pericytic venules	Muscular venules	Veins	
Continuous	Continuous, fenestrated, or discontinuous	Continuous, (occasionally fenestrated)	Continuous	Continuous	Tunica intima heart = endocardium
Less conspicuous in arterioles >50μm; present in terminal arterioles	Continuous; discontinuous or absent in sinusoids	Thin, continuous	Thin, continuous	Inconspicuous	
Absent	Present	Frequent (almost complete layer)	Rare	Absent	
Thin, connective tissue	Connective tissue (pericapillary space), variable	Thin, connective tissue	Thin, connective tissue	Thin, connective tissue	
Thin, fenestrated in arterioles >50μm; absent in terminal arterioles	Absent	Absent	Absent	Inconspicuous or discontinuous in small veins; present in large veins	
Absent	Absent	Absent	Absent	Absent	Tunica media heart = myocardium
1 to 2 layers	Absent	Absent	1 to 2 thin layers	Few, weak layers	
Not distinct	Absent	Absent	Absent	Absent	
Thin, connective tissue, nerves	Thin, connective tissue	Thin, connective tissue	Thick, connective tissue, nerves	Very thick, connective tissue, smooth muscle (longitudinal) vessels, nerves	Tunica adventitia heart = epicardium

gitudinally disposed *bundles* of muscle cells, intercalated with other structures in the vascular wall.

The Connective Tissue. Because of its diverse composition (collagen and reticular fibers, fixed and wandering cells, and ground substance), the connective tissue fulfills a complex role (see Table 9–1). Topographically, it is spread throughout the vessel wall with two especially large accumulations: beneath the endothelium, the *subendothelial layer;* and outside the tunica media, the *adventitial layer.* In both locations, elements of the connective tissue are interspersed with bundles of smooth muscle; in adventitia the connective tissue also houses the blood vessels, lymphatics, and nerves of the myocardium or the large vessels. An additional concentration of connective tissue is encountered in endocardium as the *subendocardial layer* (Table 9–1). The adventitial layer of connective tissue is relatively much thinner in the microvasculature than in large vessels. All cellular and fibrillar components of the cardiovascular wall are embedded in a highly hydrated gel-like matrix of glucosaminoglycans, the ground substance of the local connective tissue. The heart is covered by a coat of *mesothelial cells* representing the visceral leaflet of the pericardium.

The Elastic Elements. Two types of elastic structures may be found: (1) *isolated elastic fibers* dispersed within the layers of the vascular wall, and (2) *elastic sheets,* organized either as separate units *(internal elastic lamina and external elastic lamina)* or as a system of concentric lamellae *(elastic lamellae)* developed in media of large arteries only (see Table 9–1). In the heart, a dense fibroelastic tissue forms the *cardiac skeleton.*

Basic Organization

Layered Structure (Tunics). The entire cardiovascular system follows a common plan of histological organization: the tissue components described above are arranged in concentric layers. As a result of particular local adaptations, some features of this basic plan are accentuated, reduced, or omitted; moreover, to meet some special local mechanical or metabolic requirements, certain additional structures may be introduced. Basically, however, the layered organization remains. For descriptive purposes, these concentric layers have been classified as three tunics, the boundaries of which are determined by convention. Considered from the lumen outward, the tunics are:

(1) *Tunica intima,* or simply the *intima,* containing, at most, the endothelium, the basal lamina (with pericytes), the subendothelial connective tissue, and the internal elastic lamina; in the heart the equivalent of the intima is the *endocardium.*

(2) *Tunica media,* or *media,* which is composed of muscular cells, elastic lamellae, and the external elastic lamina; in the heart the media is represented by the *myocardium.*

(3) *Tunica adventitia,* or adventitia, which contains the adventitial connective tissue with its various components; in the heart this outermost layer, together with the visceral pericardium, is called *epicardium.*

Segmental Differentiations: Cardiovascular Segments. Certain physiological conditions differentially prevail along the cardiovascular system. Accordingly, segmental specializations occur that are reflected in some relevant features characterizing each part of the system (Table 9–1). Several criteria (size, prominent structure, or function) have been used alternatively to define and classify these sequential segments, but each classification used is somewhat arbitrary and thus should not be taken rigidly. There are various transitional forms of vessels, one of which may be transformed with changing local conditions. The following classification will be used throughout this chapter:

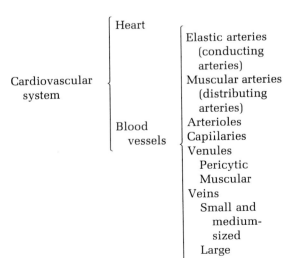

Large vessels and their branches larger than 100 μm are visible with the naked eye and accordingly are considered the *macrovasculature*. All blood vessels with diameters smaller than 100 μm may be seen only through the microscope. This is the case with the arterioles, capillaries, and their emerging venules, as well as with the arteriovenous anastomoses; together they are referred to as the *microvasculature*.

The Blood Vessels

Tissue Components of Vascular Wall

The layered structure of blood vessels undergoes segmental differentiations under the influence of the following two groups of functional factors. (1) *Mechanical factors*, primarily the blood pressure, act essentially on large vessels (conducting and distributing arteries and veins) and determine the amount and arrangement of their elastic and muscular tissue constituents. (2) *Metabolic factors*, reflecting the local needs of the tissues,

operate especially on the microvessels that are instrumental in blood–tissue exchanges (i.e., the capillaries and the postcapillary pericytic venules). At this level, the only structural elements represented are the endothelium and its basal lamina. Unlike large vessels that occur as rather isolated anatomical entities, the capillaries and the pericytic venules appear structurally and functionally as part of the tissue they supply (Fig. 9–1).

Endothelium

The vascular endothelium represents a special epithelium interposed as a partially selective diffusion barrier between two compartments of the internal medium, the plasma and the interstital fluid. Endothelium is highly differentiated to mediate and monitor the extensive bidirectional exchange of small molecules and to restrict some of the transport of macromolecules. Among the characteristic features associated with the extensive transport carried out by the vascular endo-

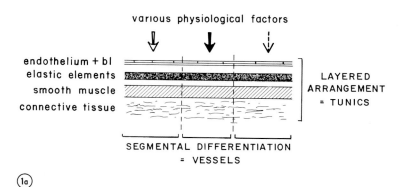

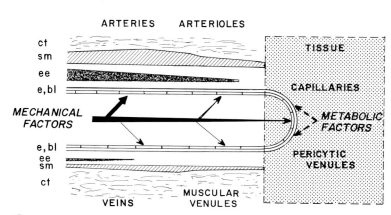

9–1 Diagrammatic representation of the functional factors associated with the layered organization and segmental differentiation of vessel wall. **a.** Under the influence of various physiological conditions, the basic tissue layers of the vascular wall have undergone characteristic segmental differentiations. **bl**-basal lamina. **b.** The mechanical factors act primarily on the large vessels, whereas the metabolic factors are essentially related to the structural characteristics of the intratissular vessels (capillaries and pericytic venules especially), which are involved in the blood–tissue exchanges.

thelium are its extreme attenuation (with a thickness of about 0.2–0.4 μm) and the very large population of *plasmalemmal vesicles* (about 5,000 to 10,000 per cell). The endothelial cells are linked to one another by *intercellular junctions* of two basic types: *occluding* (tight) *junctions* and *communicating* (gap) *junctions*.[1] As in other epithelia, the occluding junctions are presumably involved in the mechanical link between adjacent endothelial cells and in the control of permeability along the intercellular spaces. Communicating (gap) junctions allow direct two-way communication between cells. Each vascular segment has characteristically organized endothelial junctions that reflect various degrees of tightness and intercellular coupling along the vasculature (Table 9–2). The morphological evidence indicates that the endothelial junctions are generally more elaborate in arteries than in veins; the strongest junctional organization occurs in arterioles, whereas the loosest is found in venules, and endothelial junctions of capillaries are structurally similar to the occluding junctions of the arterioles.

The *endothelial cell* is an approximately uniform repeating unit, polygonal in shape, about 10 to 15 μm wide by 25 to 50 μm long. The cells and their elongate prominent nuclei are oriented in the long axis of the vessel and are presumably arranged in longitudinal vector fields generated by shearing effects of the blood flow. The most characteristic feature is the presence of numerous, uniform (60–70 nm in diameter) infoldings of cell membrane called *plasmalemmal vesicles* by Palade. They are often called pinocytotic vesicles, but the term is questionable inasmuch as the vesicles are not engaged in true pinocytosis; in general, the endocytosis appears to be a secondary activity in most of the endothelial cells. Plasmalemmal vesicles are open either on the blood front or on the tissue front, or they lie free in the cytoplasm of the endothelial cells; their fractional frequency in these three locations is almost even. As established for the capillary endothelium, the fractional volume occupied by vesicles may amount to about one-third of the to-

tal cell volume. Vesicles are active in the transendothelial transport of some water-soluble molecules. They either can function as isolated units shuttling from one cell front to another or can fuse and form patent transendothelial channels (see Fig. 9–25A). As suggested by the occurrence of transitional forms, the vesicles seem capable of forming *fenestrae* (Fig. 9–2). All these features—vesicles, channels, and fenestrae—represent different aspects of a common dynamic system. By their considerable aggregate inner volume, the vesicles may also serve as a sort of transient and dispersed reservoir for plasma. In some capillaries, the endothelial cell displays several openings appearing either as uniform fenestrae or nonuniform large gaps (see Fig. 9–25B and C, and section on Capillaries).

Besides the nucleus, the endothelial cells contain the common set of *organelles*: rough endoplasmic reticulum, attached and free ribosomes, Golgi complex, a few mitochondria, a few cisternae of smooth endoplasmic reticulum, centrosphere regions with two centrioles, lyosomes (more frequent in arteries), multivesicular bodies, and glycogen. Thin and thick *filaments* are occasionally concentrated either in the junctional zone or at the albuminal cell membrane; the thick filaments are sometimes in phase with similar extracellular fibrils. Intermediate-sized filaments (10 nm) are frequently encountered in the perinuclear region (Blose et al., 1977) and appear to be predominantly of the vimentin type (Franke et al., 1979). Indirect evidence (nuclear pinching and cellular shortening with intercellular gaps) suggests that in response to certain stimuli, the endothelial cells may contract. Peculiar rod-shaped granules, 0.1 μm thick by 3 μm long, consisting of several tubules (approximately 15 nm thick) embedded in a dense matrix, have been described by Weibel and Palade in arterial endothelia of human beings, rats, and amphibia and were later found in other vessels and other species. The significance of these organelles is unknown, but they are a reliable tag for identifying isolated endothelial cells.

Qualitative *cytochemical* investigations revealed the presence in the endothelial cell of a relatively large spectrum of enzymes involved in activities such as anaerobic glycolysis, oxidative phosphorylation, and desulfation. Some enzymes are preferentially detected in plasmalemmal vesicles, for example, ATPase, nucleoside phosphatase, and 5′-nucleotidase (this localization presumably reflects the vesicles' involve-

---

[1]In the special case of the endothelium, the term *gap junction* is particularly confusing, because junctions with a gap of 20 to 40 Å have been described as occurring instead of tight junctions in the capillary endothelium. Therefore, we use the term *communicating junction (macula communicans, maculae communicantes)*, which describes the macular geometry of the structure and relates to its main function so far established (M. Simionescu et al., 1975).

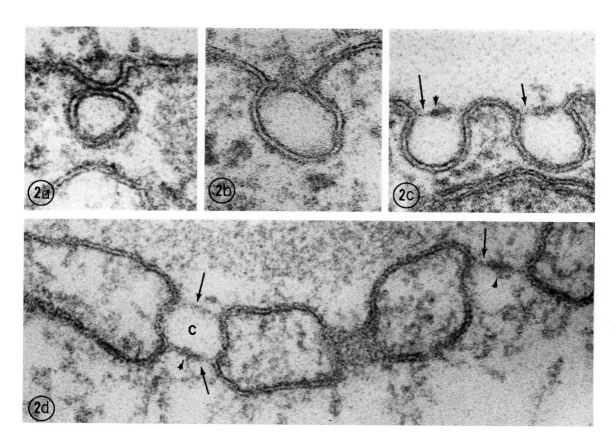

9–2 Blood capillary: endothelium (rat tongue).
Morphological modulations of plasmalemmal vesicles suggesting stages in the discharge process of vesicular contents. **a.** Fusion of vesicular membrane with the cell membrane forming a five-layered structure. **b.** Intermediary stage between (a) and (c) in the progressive elimination of membrane layers. **c.** Vesicles on the blood front of the endothelium: the openings are provided with diaphragms **(arrows),** which display a central knob **(arrowhead).** × 240,000. (From Palade, G. E., and Bruns, R. R. 1968. J. Cell Biol. 37:633.) **d.** Blood capillary (mouse intestinal mucosa): the attenuated part of the endothelium showing a channel **(c)** provided with two diaphragms **(arrows),** and a fenestra closed by a diaphragm **(arrow).** Note the presence of a central knob in each diaphragm **(arrowheads).** (From Clementi, F., and Palade, G. E. 1969. J. Cell Biol. 41:33.)

ment in the metabolism of some vasoactive substances). The catecholamine-sensitive adenyl cyclase found in both vesicles and junctions might be related to their participation in hormone transport.

The endothelium is a slowly renewing population of cells that rarely divide (for example, the estimated life span of aortic endothelial cells in rabbit is 100 to 180 days). Endothelial cells of veins have a greater mitotic potential than those of arteries. Regeneration of damaged (e.g., by injury) or missing endothelium (as in synthetic grafts) is assumed to occur from sources such as circulating blood cells, fibroblasts, smooth muscle cells, adjacent endothelium, or undifferentiated cells from the subendothelial layers.

At the tissue surface, a rather amorphous matrix 30 to 50 nm wide separates the endothelium from the fine microfibrillar *basal lamina.* This matrix is about 40 to 80 nm thick; and, as in other epithelia, it is probably produced by the endothelium itself. The basal lamina is made up chiefly of types IV and AB_2 collagen, and their inability to polymerize into striated fibrils may

result from their high carbohydrate content. In renal glomerular capillaries, the basal lamina is fairly thick and has special chemical characteristics. Owing to its high content of collagen, the basal lamina can be digested by collagenase. After treatment with collagenase, endothelial cells from various vessels (human umbilical vein, animal arteries, veins, and microvessels) can be isolated and grown in tissue culture for in vitro studies. Other constituents identified in the basal lamina are fibronectin, glycosaminoglycans, glycoproteins, and sialoglycoproteins. In glomerular basement membrane, anionic sites are particularly dense in the lamina rara externa and are contributed by heparin sulfate (Kanwar and Farquhar, 1979).

The endothelial cell may establish close apposition with the processes of neighboring *pericytes* (see Fig. 9–29). In vessels provided with an internal elastica, the endothelial cell may extend processes that penetrate the elastica and make close contact with the adjoining smooth muscle cells *(myoendothelial junction)* (Figs. 9–16 and 9–21).

The Blood–Endothelial Interface. As detected by immunocytochemistry and lectins coupled to peroxidase or ferritin, *the luminal endothelial cell surface* is provided with a cell coat (approximately 10–30 nm thick) made up of a fixed layer and a movable layer. The fixed layer consists largely of (1) sialic acid; (2) the oligosaccharide moieties of cell membrane glycoproteins and glycolipids (e.g., α-mannose, D-galactose, N-acetylglucosamine, and N-acetylgalactosamine), which might function as recognition sites for molecules to be transported by an active process across the endothelium; and (3) glycosaminoglycans (e.g., heparan sulfate). The movable layer is composed of adsorbed *plasma proteins*. One of them, α-2 macroglobulin, seems to protect endothelium against proteolysis; the existence of fibrinogen is still uncertain.

Both the circulating blood cells and the endothelial surface have a negative charge and thus repel each other. The *anionic sites* have been demonstrated mostly with catonized ferritin (for details, see Capillaries, p. 398). Because of its charge, metabolic activities, and molecular environment, the intact endothelium is *not attractive* for the blood cells and therefore is *nonthrombogenic*. Conversely, the subendothelial structures (basal lamina; collagen, especially type I and III; and microfibrils) are highly attractive for the blood cells; consequently they are thrombogenic. The intact vessel wall does not interact with normal platelets.

When subendothelial structures are exposed, as in *endothelial injury* (e.g., owing to hemodynamic stress; hyperlipoproteinemia, especially low-density lipoproteins; toxins; CO; antigen–

antibody complexes; excess epinephrine; viruses; or bacteria) or opening of endothelial junctions (e.g., by high concentrations of histamine or serotonin), platelets usually adhere to sites of vascular injury. Platelets release adenosine diphosphate (ADP), serotonin, and thromboxane A_2, which enhance platelet aggregation and thrombin deposition. A platelet plug is developed as part of the coagulation process. The plug can evolve into a thrombus that eventually can obstruct the vessel. In other conditions, the aggregated platelets can release a mitogenic factor that stimulates smooth muscle cell proliferation, a key step in the formation of the atherosclerotic plaque. Thrombin increases platelet aggregation; heparin prevents this effect and inhibits binding of low-density lipoproteins (LDL) to its receptors on the endothelial cell and smooth muscle cell of the vessel wall. Hence, disturbances in the structural and functional integrity of the blood–endothelial interface play a crucial role in the initiation and development of both atherosclerosis and thrombosis.

Metabolic Activities. Results obtained in most studies on cultures of endothelial cells indicate that these cells are capable of producing and secreting substances with a variety of actions.

1. Endothelial cells contribute in the metabolism of vasoactive substances.
   (a) by angiotensin-converting enzyme of kininase II, which converts angiotensin I (a decapeptide) into its more active derivative, angiotensin II (an octapeptide);
   (b) by enzymes (catechol-O-methyltransferase and monoamine oxidase) that inactivate norepinephrine, serotonin, and bradikynin; and
   (c) by synthesizing prostaglandins: among these, prostacyclin (PGI_2) is a very potent antagonist of thromboxane A_2 produced by platelets.
2. Endothelial cells participate in hemostasis:
   (a) by producing both *coagulant substances* (tissue factor, antihemophilic factor, and plasminogen inhibitor), and *anticoagulant substances* (plasminogen activator and prostacyclin). In normal conditions, the anticoagulant activity prevails. As detected with peroxidase-conjugated antibodies, small vessels show more plasminogen activator than do large vessels, and veins show more than do arteries.

3. Other products secreted by endothelium are:
   (a) blood group antigens A and B (apparently associated with the endothelial cell surface), and
   (b) collagen—types IV, and V—for its own basal lamina, fibronectin, elastin, and glycosaminoglycans.

Endothelial cells can take up and use long-chain saturated fatty acids; the arterial cells can incorporate more labeled ^{3}H-oleic acid than can the venous ones.

In situ studies have demonstrated that arterial endothelium take up LDL particles via receptor-mediated endocytosis which carries them to lysosomes, and also can transport such particles through transcytosis for delivery to the rest of the vessel wall.

Endothelium as barrier and transport system is discussed in the section on Functional–Structural Correlates in Capillary Permeability.

Vascular Smooth Muscle

This tissue occurs in all vessels, except capillaries and pericytic venules where its place is taken by pericytes (probably a variant of muscle cells). In contrast to other vertebrates, smooth muscle represents the only cellular element in the media of mammalian elastic arteries, and it is the prevailing component of muscular arteries and arterioles. Commonly, smooth muscle cells are frequent and arranged in helical layers in media, but they are less numerous and usually longitudinally oriented in intima and adventitia. Additional muscle cells can appear in the intima during aging and under certain pathological conditions. Each cell is surrounded by the basal lamina it secretes and by various amounts of collagen fibers, which may anchor the cell to neighboring elastic fibers (Figs. 9–3 and 9–4). Such attachments allow the contracting force to be transmitted to the network of elastic fibers. Vascular smooth muscle cells are frequently held together by *communicating (gap) junctions* (Figs. 9–3 to 9–5), generally more frequent in arterioles and small arteries than in large vessels. These junctions may be instrumental in the conduction of impulses and transmission of information among cells. For the organization of smooth muscle cells in general, see Chap. 7. The vascular smooth muscle cells are smaller (25–80 μm) than the smooth muscle cells in other locations. The large population of *sarcolemmal vesicles* increases the surface area by approximately 25%.

They are organized in characteristic longitudinal rows with vesicle-free areas in between (Fig. 9–6). The latter may correspond to regions of attachment of myofilaments and dense bodies. Salient components are the *lysosomes* that may accumulate cholesterol during the atheromatous process. Vascular smooth muscle cells behave phenotypically as fibroblasts during much of gestation; under various stimuli, they are capable of producing most components of vessel walls—elastic fibers, microfibrilar proteins, collagen (especially types I and III), glucosaminoglycans, and more muscle cells. Like that of skeletal muscle, the activity of vascular smooth muscle is initiated by nervous stimuli. Not all cells have an *innervation*; excitation may spread between adjacent cells through communicating (gap) junctions. The distance observed between the unmyelinated axon and sarcolemma is larger than in the motor end plate of striated muscle (approximately 50 nm). Perturbations of the vessel wall (e.g., hemodynamic stress, injury, ischemia, inflammation, excess LDL drugs, or hormones) may stimulate smooth muscle cells to migrate into the intima and proliferate, which leads, in turn, to an *intimal thickening*, a characteristic feature of the atheromatous plaque. A similar change occurs in aging, but the media itself is not altered.

In aging and in atherogenesis, large amounts of cholesteryl esters may accumulate in smooth muscle cells, forming inclusions of cholesteryl oleate. Intracellular lipid deposition can transform the smooth muscle cell into a "foam cell," a disfigured cholesterol-laden cell. Eventually, the excessive impairment of cellular metabolism can result in cell necrosis.

Vascular Connective Tissue

Eliminating muscle activity by treating aortic segments with potassium thiocyanate does not alter the static mechanical property of the media, which is provided mainly by connective tissue components. These components are present in the walls of the vessels in amounts and proportions that vary according to the local functional requirements and to the interrelationships with other tissues, especially the endothelium and smooth muscle.

Fibers. Elastic fibers ensure the resilient rebound of the stretched vascular wall. Collagen fibers impart the tensile strength that supports and

382

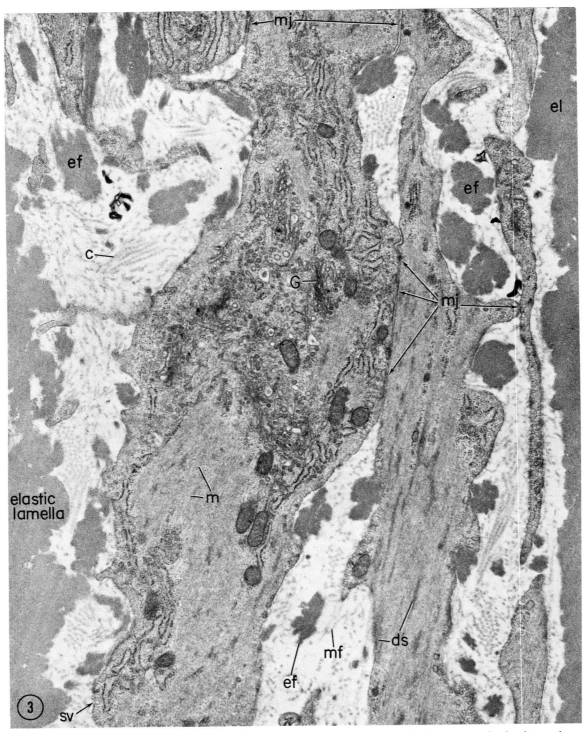

9–3 Smooth muscle cells of a tunica media of rat mesenteric artery; cells display frequent intercellular junctions **(mj)**. Elastic elements appear either as isolated elastic fibers **(ef)** or wide elastic lamellae **(el)**; microfibrils **(mf)** can also be detected. **c**, collagen; **sv**, sarcolemmal vesicles; **G**, Golgi complex; **ds**, dense segments of myofilaments **(m)**. × 18,000.

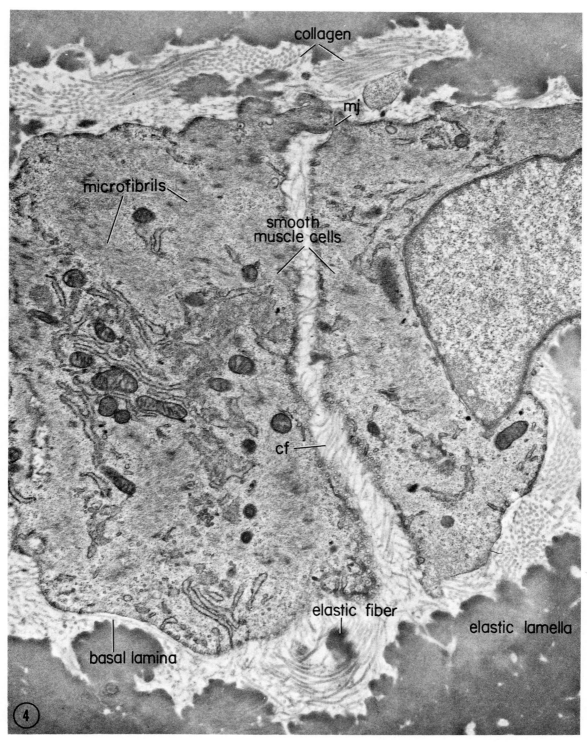

9–4 Structural connections between two neighboring smooth muscle cells (the media of rat aorta), represented in this preparation by a narrow junction **(mj)** and frequent bridges of collagen fibers **(cf).** × 18,000.

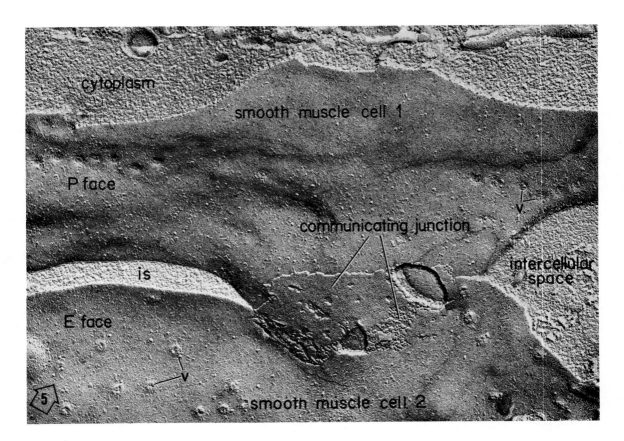

9–5 Freeze-cleaved preparation of aortic intima
    displaying a communicating (gap) junction
between two adjacent smooth muscle cells. The
junction appears as clusters of particles on the P face
and as complementary pits on the E face. **is,**
intercellular spaces; **v,** vesicle opening. × 75,000.

binds together coherent groups of other structural elements.

Elastic fibers are either *isolated* or, more frequently, in *sheets* several micrometers in diameter. The sheets appear either as a single feature (internal elastic lamina, external elastic lamina, or the scattered elastic bundles of the adventitia) or as lamellae organized in a regular alternating pattern with the muscle cells throughout the entire media. These lamellae are extensively fenestrated and partially connected in a three-dimensional network. Elastic fibers have two components: the amorphous-appearing *elastin,* which provides the elastometric properties of the fibers; and the *microfibrils,* the significance of which is less understood (Fig. 9–4). Elastic fibers

are oriented in different directions so that mechanical stresses are complexly balanced. The occurrence of elastic fibers along the vasculature is schematically tabulated in Table 9–1.

Collagen fibers are found throughout the vascular wall concentrated between muscle cells, in adventitia, and in some subendothelial spaces (Figs. 9–4, 9–10, and 9–25, respectively). In human aorta, collagen and elastin each represent 20% of the dry weight, whereas the vena cava contains about seven times more collagen (types I, III, and IV) than elastin. Preliminary information indicates that the collagen prevalent in arteries is collagen of type $\alpha 1$ [III], characterized by smaller quantities of galactose or glucosylgalactose linked to hydroxylysine. Disorders in elastic and collagen metabolism occur both in aging (increased cross-linking of collagen) and in major vascular disease such as atherosclerosis (abnormal pattern of elastin cross-linking) and arteriosclerosis (increased collagen synthesis caused by a high proline-hydroxylase activity).

In diabetes, the thickening of endothelial basal lamina is presumed to result from a slow-

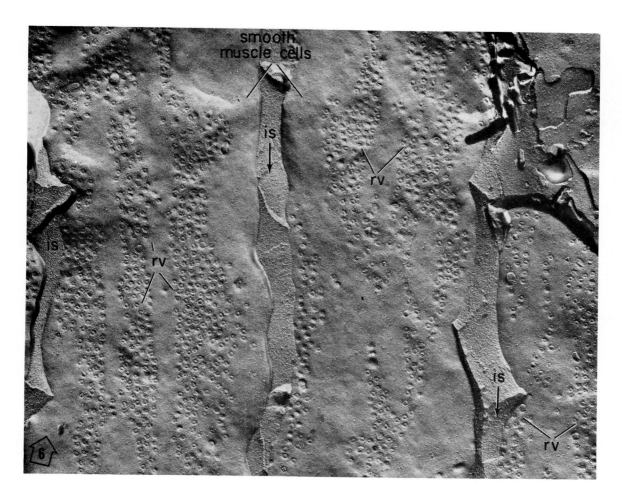

ing of collagen degradation due to a change in its glycosylation.

Ground Substance. Extracellular spaces of the vessel wall are occupied by a continuous but heterogeneous gel of proteoglycans. Some capillaries are surrounded by a relatively thin layer of ground substance; others can be considered embedded in the matrix gel, which may be responsible for the relative patency and apparent rigidity of capillaries under differential pressures in comparison with the distensibility of arteries and arterioles. The ground substance contains domains of different composition and hydration. The concentration of glucosaminoglycans is higher in arterial than in venous tissue. In the former, chondroitin sulfate prevails; and in the latter, dermatan sulfate. The ground substance contributes to the physical properties of the walls of the vessels and probably affects diffu-

9–6 Replica of freeze-cleaved sarcolemma of three adjacent smooth muscle cells of an arteriole. Vesicle openings are characteristically arranged in longitudinal parallel ribbons **(rv)** alternating with vesicle-free areas. Compare with Fig. 9–48. **is,** intercellular spaces. × 27,000.

sion differently from domain to domain and, hence, affects permeability across the wall.

In aging, there is an increased secretion of collagen types I and III (known for their high affinity for platelets) and an enhanced production of dermatan sulfate. The altered molecular conformation of elastin and glycoproteins may facilitate trapping of LDL, very low-density lipoproteins (VLDL), and calcium with subsequent calcification. On a larger scale, these perturbations also characterize the modified ground substance of the atherosclerotic plaque.

Connective Tissue Cells. Located in the partition between internal medium and surrounding tissues and organs, the connective tissue cells of the vascular wall constitute a pluripotential system. In locations where the adventitia is continuous with the connective elements of the surrounding tissue, the boundary between the two compartments is arbitrary. This complex population in the following important functions: (1) the production, storage, and secretion of local *vasoactive mediators*, such as histamine and serotonin, primarily by the mast cells (which are very frequently located along the microvasculature and seem to be particularly efficient on the pericytic venules); (2) *phagocytosis*, largely performed by the *macrophages* almost constantly patrolling along the vessels; (3) local *immunological reactions*, which may involve plasma

cells and eosinophils; (4) *secretion of connective tissue fibers*, carried out mostly by *fibroblasts*, which also represent a pluripotential pool for cell formation and local repair, for example, in endothelial regeneration. In human beings, the main cellular component of the arterial adventitia consists of the fibroblasts, which are absent in the media.

Nutrition of the Vascular Wall

Blood Vessels. The vascular wall is provided with its own nutrient vessels, called *vasa vasorum*. The extent of the intramural vascular bed is determined by (1) the tissue composition of the wall, (2) participation of the luminal blood in supplying the wall, and (3) the wall compression under the blood pressure. In large vessels with well-developed media, the intima receives its nutrient material by diffusion from the luminal blood, as does the microvasculature. On the adventitia (Fig. 9–7) and in some arteries, the outer layers of the media (in which tissue compression is lower than capillary blood pressure) are pro-

9–7 Low-power electron micrograph of the adventitia of a muscular artery (rat mesenteric artery) showing some connective tissue constituents, vasa vasorum, and nerves. × 5,000.

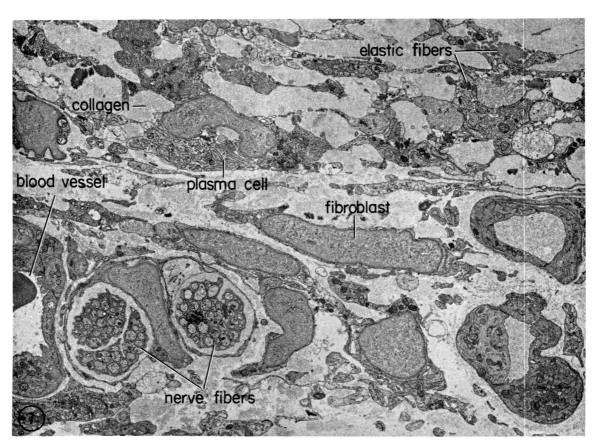

vided with vasa vasorum. The rest of the wall is nourished by diffusion. Vasa vasorum of veins are more abundant and penetrate much closer to the intima than do those of arteries.

Lymphatics. The lymphatic vessels are commonly encountered in the walls of large vessels where their distribution is similar to that of the intramural blood supply. Lymphatics are more frequent and go deeper into the media of veins than of arteries. The interstitial fluid circulates freely throughout fenestrated elastic lamellae. Favored by the prevailing blood pressure, both the interstitial fluids and the lymphatic flow go from within the wall outward.

Vascular Nerves. Except for capillaries (and probably pericytic venules), all blood vessels have a relatively rich supply of nerves. Bundles or single nerve fibers are found in the adventitia (Fig. 9–7) and may extend their terminal processes into the media; a few of them can be traced as far as the intima. *Unmyelinated axons,* which are vasomotor (arising from the sympathetic ganglia), form plexuses in adventitia; some of them end with fine knoblike terminations close to the muscle cells. A particularly rich innervation of the arterioles has been noticed. There is no accurate estimate of the ratio of nerve endings to muscle cells, and it is still questionable whether each muscle unit is innervated or whether the stimuli pass to neighboring muscle cells by other mechanisms. *Afferent myelinated fibers* (representing the dendrites of spinal or cranial ganglion cells) terminate in free sensory endings, found mostly in the adventitia. Small intraadventitial ganglia occur in the aorta, and

coronary, coeliac, and mesenteric arteries. Sensory features are particularly well developed in some arteries: they are especially sensitive to pressure changes *(baroreceptors)* or to modifications in the chemical composition of the blood *(chemoreceptors)* (see Special Sensory Tissues of Arteries).

Arteries

The dimensions of arteries and veins, unlike those of the microvascular components, are largely species-related and depend primarily on the total blood volume. In humans, despite the low number of arteries, their relatively large dimensions result in a blood volume of approximately 2% in the aorta and 9% in the rest of the systemic arteries, whereas the pulmonary arteries contain almost 8% of the whole blood volume.

According to their prevalent tissue component, the arteries can be classified as *elastic arteries* and *muscular arteries,* which continue the former.

Elastic Arteries. Large vessels conducting blood from the heart to the muscular (distribut-

9–8 Endothelial junction complex of the aorta as revealed by freeze-fracture preparations. The cleavage plane exposes an occluding junction with large communicating (gap) junctions fitted within its meshes. On the E face **(E)**, the grooves of the occluding junction **(arrows)** are marked by protruding, elongated particles, which tend to form continuous rows. **v,** openings of plasmalemmal vesicles. × 90,000. (From Simionescu, M., Simionescu, N., and Palade, G. E. 1976. J. Cell Biol. 68:705.)

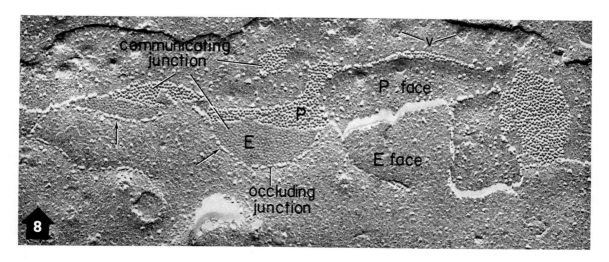

Table 9–2 Segmental Variations of the Endothelial Junctions Along the Vasculature
(Observations made on freeze-fracture preparations)

| Vascular segments | Occluding junctions | | Communicationg junctions (gap junctions) |
	Ridges/grooves predominantly with particles	Ridges/grooves predominantly without particles	
Arteries	2–4 continuous		Frequent, large, predominantly intercalated
Arterioles	2–6, continuous		Frequent, large, predominantly intercalated
Capillaries	2–5, continuous or staggered and quasi-continuous		Absent
Venules			
Pericytic		1–4, discontinuous	Absent
Muscular		1–5, discontinuous	Rare, small, isolated
Veins	2–5, continuous	1–4, discontinuous	Rare, small, predominantly isolated

Source: Adapted from Simionescu, M., Simionescu, N., and Palade, G. E., 1976. Thromb. Res. Suppl. II, 8:247.

ing) arteries have a high content of elastic fibers, hence, the name elastic arteries. To this category belong the aorta and the pulmonary, innominate (brachiocephalic), common carotid, subclavian (including its vertebral and internal thoracic branches), and common iliac arteries. In comparison with their large lumen, the wall is relatively thin, being less than one-tenth of the vessel diameter.

The *intima* is about 100 to 130 μm thick and represents approximately one-sixth of the wall thickness. The *endothelial* cells are rich in plasmalemmal vesicles and contain a variable amount of cytoplasmic filaments. The cells are extensively linked by a strongly organized combination of occluding (tight) junctions with closely intercalated communicating (gap) junctions (Figs. 9–8 and 9–12, and Table 9–2). The permeability characteristics of the arterial endothelium are not yet well defined, and conflicting observations have been reported, especially concerning a possible intercellular pathway for probe molecules as large as 5 to 6 nm (e.g., horseradish peroxidase). The vesicles appear to be active in the transendothelial transport of a large range of molecular species. Plasma macromolecules enter the intima in relatively large amounts. This process also involves the LDL, whose concentration in the intima (on a volumetric basis) is about 500 mg/100 cc, compared with their estimated value in plasma of about 500 mg/100 ml (Smith, 1974). (For the mechanisms of

LDL transport across endothelium, see below.) It has been reported that hypercholesterolemia (especially LDL) may injure the vascular endothelium; high-density lipoproteins (HDL) can inhibit this effect to a certain extent. The *basal lamina* is thin and of prominent reticular aspect. In humans, the endothelial layer constitutes about one-fourth of the total wall thickness. It contains loose connective tissue, elastic fibers oriented longitudinally, scattered fibroblasts, and a few elongated, mostly longitudinally running smooth muscle cells. The *elastica interna* is less distinct as a separate feature with light microscopy (Fig. 9–9); with electron microscopy, however, it appears as the first elastic lamella that merges with tunica media (Fig. 9–10).

The *media* is the thickest tunic: in humans it measures 500 μm and is essentially composed of 40 to 70 concentric elastic sheets, 5 to 15 μm apart. Each sheet is 2 to 3 μm thick and consists of broad interwoven fenestrated bands and a few connecting bundles located between sheets (Figs. 9–11 and 9–12). The latter are interspersed with the ground substance, in which elongated and branched smooth muscle cells lie bound to the adjoining elastic lamellae by microfibrils and collagen. (Types I, III, and IV are present in normal aortas.)

The *adventitia* is relatively thin and not highly organized. It contains bundles of collagen with longitudinal-helical courses, a few elastic fibers similarly arranged, fibroblasts, mast cells,

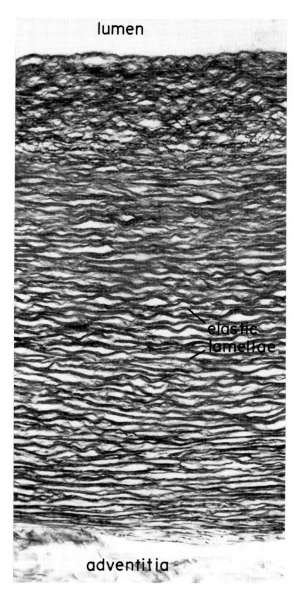

lumen

elastic
lamellae

adventitia

9-9 Photomicrograph of a cross section through the
wall of human aorta. Elastic tissue has been
darkly stained with resorcin–fuchsin. Note the high
frequency of concentric elastic lamellae. × 3,000.

sometimes accompanied by myelinated or non-myelinated *nerves*. The adventitia merges with the surrounding connective tissue. As elastic arteries branch into smaller vessels, their structure gradually changes to that of the muscular type.

Muscular Arteries. The general organization of the vessels that conduct blood to various regions and organs of the body resembles that of elastic arteries, but the proportions of cell types and fibers are distinctive. The most abundant component is the muscular tissue (Figs. 9–13 and 9–14), whose contraction and relaxation control the vascular lumen, thus regulating the blood flow. The great majority of arteries belong to this category. The popliteal artery, in spite of its distal location when compared to the femoral artery, has a predominantly elastic structure. In humans the muscular arteries vary greatly in diameter, from 1 cm to 0.3 mm. Without any clear-cut boundaries, they are often arbitrarily subdivided either into large, medium-sized, and small arteries, or into the last two categories only. In most cases, the wall thickness is one-fourth of the vessel diameter.

The *endothelium* of the intima is similar to that of elastic arteries. In small arteries, processes of the endothelial cells extend through the fenestrations of elastica interna and contact underlying smooth muscle cells (Figs. 9–15 and 9–16). Through the same openings, the ground substance of intima is in continuity with that of the media. Two types of junctions link the endothelial cells of muscular arteries: communicating (gap) junctions and occluding junctions that resemble those described in elastic arteries (Table 9–2). Junctions seem to undergo quickly reversible loosening or widening under various influences (diabetes, nicotine, epinephrine, angiotensin II, serotonin, and so forth). As a result, lipoproteins and other large molecules can be trapped by the vascular wall.

The *basal lamina* is thin and generally continuous in large arteries.

The *subendothelial layer* diminishes in thickness with the decreasing size of the vessel. It comprises collagen fibers and smooth muscle cells organized in longitudinal bundles in some specialized arteries (Fig. 9–15). At branching sites of some vessels (e.g., coronary, thyroid, renal, splenic, intracranial, and nasal mucosa), protruding "intimal cushions" have been described. The *elastica interna* is generally prominent and fenestrated.

and rare longitudinal smooth muscle cells (Fig. 9–11). The *elastica externa,* not always evident under light microscopic examination, appears at high magnification as a discontinuous lamella. The *vasa vasorum* and *lymphatics* are detected only as far as the outer half of the tunica media,

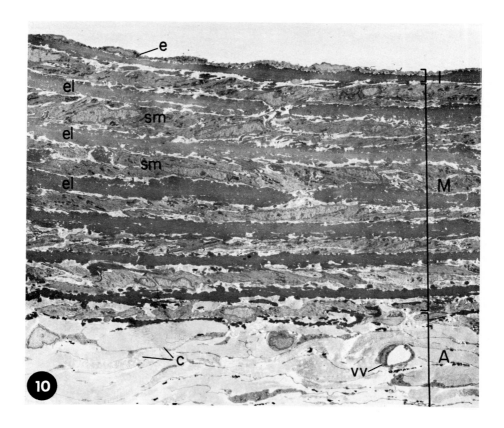

9–10 Low-power electron micrograph of a portion of the wall of rat aorta in cross section. The vessel wall is formed by interspersed layers of elastic lamellae **(el),** and smooth muscle cells **(sm).** e, endothelium; **A,** adventitia; **I,** intima; **M,** media; **vv,** vasa vasorum; **c,** collagen. × 1,000.

The *media* is mostly muscular; in humans it consists of 10 to 40 helical layers concentrically arranged. Their number can decrease to 3 to 4 in small arteries, and there are more layers in arteries of the legs than in arteries of the arms. *Muscular cells* are surrounded by basal laminae and collagen fibers and are interspersed with isolated *elastic fibers or lamellae,* fenestrated and helically oriented (Figs. 9–14 and 9–15). The smooth muscles are the only cellular component of media (see Vascular Smooth Muscle, above).

The *adventitia* is thick with an inner dense and an outer loose part; it contains bundles of collagen and elastic fibers longitudinal or helically arranged, sparse fibroblasts, adipose cells, and a few longitudinal smooth muscle fibers.

The *elastica externa* is thin and discontinuous, especially in small vessels. The adventitia is provided with *vasa vasorum, lymphatics,* and *nerves* that penetrate to the external layers of media.

Transitional Segments of Arteries. The gradual transition from elastic to muscular arteries is seen best in the so-called arteries of mixed type (e.g., axillary, carotid, and common iliac arteries). In some places an abrupt structural change occurs: arteries with such short transitional segments are called arteries of hybrid type (e.g., visceral branches of abdominal aorta). In their media, an internal muscular layer coexists over a certain distance with an external elastic layer.

Specialized Arteries. As a result of adaptations to local functional requirements, certain arteries display characteristic structural modifications: overall increase or decrease in the thickness of the vascular wall or particular development of either the muscular or elastic components.

An *overall augmentation* of the wall thickness occurs in the coronary arteries subjected to high pressure and in the arteries of the legs com-

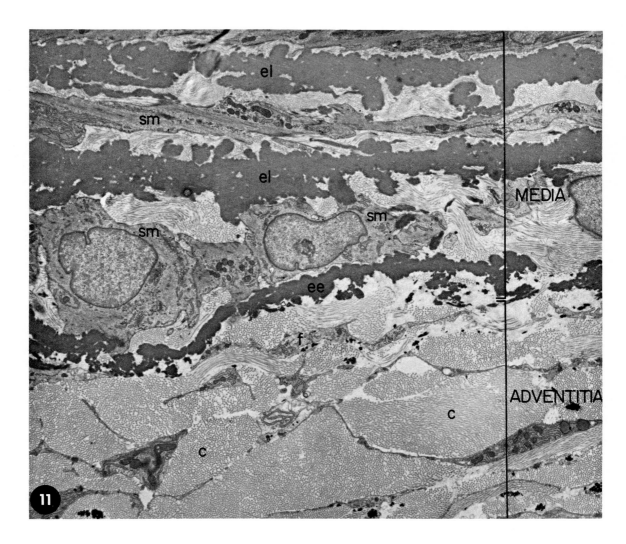

9–11 Electron micrograph of an area of the outer part of the aortic media. Note the interspersed layers of smooth muscle cells **(sm)**, which are the sole cellular component of this tunic, and the elastic lamellae **(el)**. The outermost lamella represents actually the external elastic lamina **(ee)**. **c,** collagen; **f,** fibroblast. × 6,000.

pared with their analogs in the arms. An overall reduction of the vessel wall thickness occurs in arteries protected by the skull from external mechanical forces (cerebral and dural arteries) and in regions of low blood pressure (arteries of the lung).

Well-developed bundles of *longitudinal muscle fibers* in both the intima and media are found in arteries subjected to repeated bending—carotid, axillary, common iliac, and popliteal arteries. Bundles of longitudinal muscle may be preferentially developed in the *intima* (occipital, palmar, uterine, and penile arteries after puberty), *media* (penile arteries, splenic, mesenteric superior, renal, and umbilical artery, the last exhibiting two layers, an inner longitudinal and an outer circular), or in the *adventitia* (lingual, splenic, and renal). *Cardiac muscle* extends into the wall of the roots of pulmonary artery and aorta.

Elastic components are relatively well developed in arteries within the skull and in renal and popliteal arteries; the elastica interna is lacking in the umbilical artery.

For a discussion of blood vessels, lymphatics, and nerves of arteries, see Nutrition of the Vascular Wall, above.

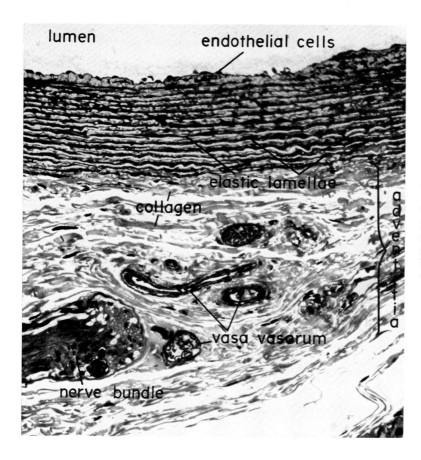

9–12 Cross section through carotid artery (monkey). The elastic lamellae are interspersed with layers of smooth muscle cells. The adventitia is relatively large and contains bundles of collagen, with vasa vasorum and nerves. × 120.

9–13 Longitudinal section through a muscular artery (rat external iliac artery). The vascular wall consists predominantly of layers of smooth muscle cells **(sm)** interspersed with discontinuous elastic lamellae **(el).** Note the conspicuous internal elastic lamina **(ie). A,** adventitia; **e,** endothelium; **rbc,** red blood cells; **I,** intima; **M,** media. × 600.

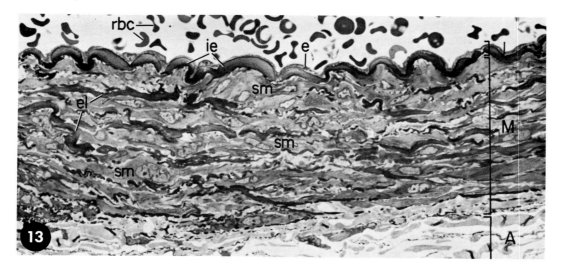

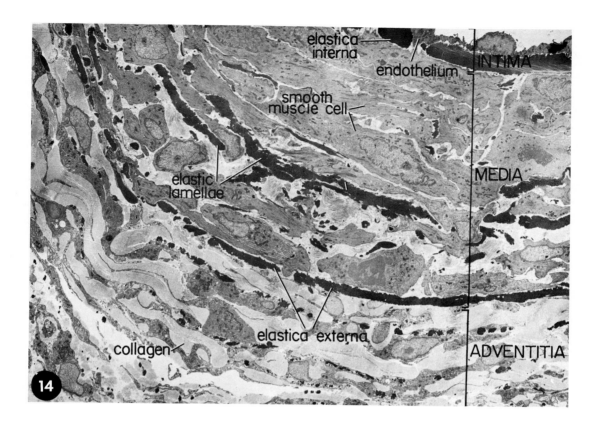

Special Sensory Tissues of Arteries. Along with sensory endings dispersed within the wall of arteries, there are in certain regions of the arterial tree highly specialized tissues that monitor the blood by sensors particularly receptive to changes in blood pressure (baroreceptors) or in blood chemical composition (chemoreceptors). In lower vertebrates, special vascular receptors are present in each of the branchial arch arteries; in human beings, such sensory organs are found in arteries that constitute persistent parts of the branchial arches.

As baroreceptor, the carotid sinus is an enlargement at the bifurcation of the common carotid and the origin of the internal carotid artery. At this level, the outer part of the thinned tunica media exhibits a rich network of large nerve endings. Most of these endings make contacts with the cells of adventitia. Pressure changes generate nerve impulses that are conducted by the glossopharyngeal nerve to the medulla. In addition to the carotid sinus, other similar but less easily recognizable areas have been described in the common carotid artery and great veins close to the heart. The pressor-receptor mechanisms re-

9–14 Low-power electron micrograph of a cross section through a muscular artery (rat mesenteric artery). Note the predominant muscular content of the media, the relatively rare and largely fenestrated elastic lamellae, and the wide adventitia, only a part of which is presented in this area. × 1,800.

spond to an increase in blood pressure by an inhibition of heart action and by general vasodilation.

Chemoreceptors are primarily represented by the *carotid bodies* located at the bifurcation of each common carotid, and by the *aortic bodies*. On the right side, the aortic body lies in the angle between common carotid and subclavian; on the left, it is found on the aorta, medial to the origin of the subclavian artery. These small organs consist of cords and clumps of epithelial-like cells richly supplied with nerve endings and intimately associated with numerous fenestrated or sinusoidal capillaries. Two types of parenchymal cells have been distinguished: the glomus cells, or *type I* which occur in clusters and contain many small cells, vacuoles and secretory-

394

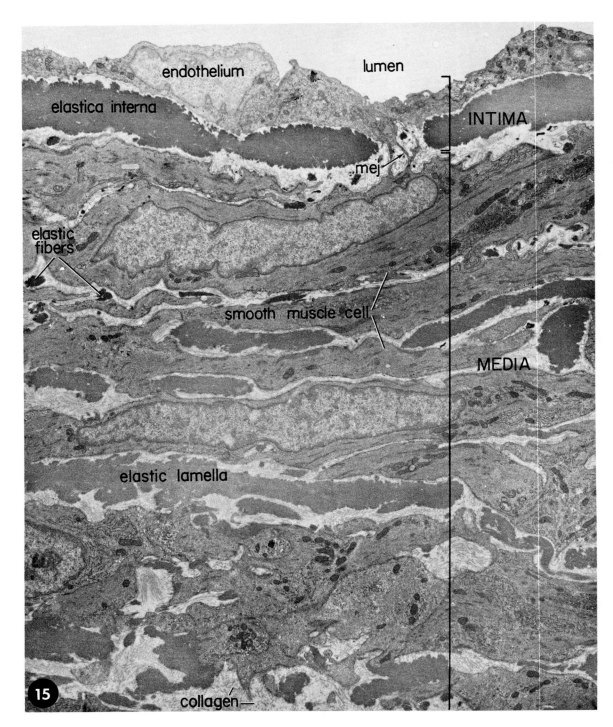

9–15 Muscular artery: detail of the inner part of the vascular wall. Through a fenestra of elastica interna, processes of the endothelial cell establish a myoendothelial junction **(mej)** with the adjacent smooth muscle cell belonging to the media. In the latter, the prevalent muscular tissue is interspersed with less frequent and discontinuous elastic lamellae. × 6,000.

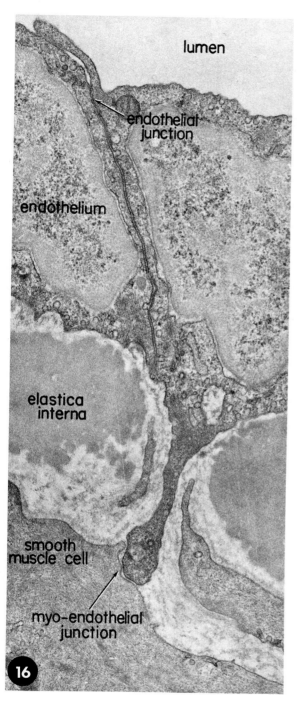

lumen

endothelial junction

endothelium

elastica interna

smooth muscle cell

myo-endothelial junction

16

9–16 Endothelial junction and myoendothelial junction in a muscular artery. The latter occurs through a fenestra of the elastica interna. × 25,000.

type granules (rich in catecholamines and 5-hydroxytryptamine); and *type II cells,* which are free of granules. The function of these two categories of cells is still unclear. Changes in blood pH, oxygen, and carbon dioxide tension generate nerve impulses that are conducted through the glossopharyngeal and vagus nerves to the central nervous system, which initiates adequate respiratory and cardiovascular responses.

Age-related Changes in Arteries. The structural pattern of arteries, as described above, is achieved gradually through a continuous process of differentiation that extends to the age of 20 to 25 in humans (for example, the aorta is a muscular vessel at birth). Starting with middle age, a relative increase commonly occurs in elastic fibers, collagen, and in glycosaminoglycans, with a concomitant reduction of smooth muscle and water content. These changes result in an overall stiffness, more pronounced in elastic than in muscular arteries, and minimal or absent in small muscular arteries and arterioles. Each artery has its own way and schedule of differentiation and aging. At old age, regressive physiological changes cannot be clearly distinguished from similar pathological changes that lead to arteriosclerosis or atherosclerosis. Modifications at the boundary between normal involution and pathological condition include an increase in thickness of the vascular wall; an increase in the number of cross-linkages between collagen fibers; a relative decrease in endoplasmic reticulum of smooth muscle cells; a patchy, irregular thickening of the intima (by migration and proliferation of smooth muscle and accumulation of their products); a deposition of calcium salts and lipids in the media of muscular arteries; and a splitting of the elastica interna (see also pages 381 and 384). The arteries most affected are the aorta, coronary, and brain vessels. It may thus be truly said that one is as old as one's arteries.

Microvasculature

The microvasculature connects arterial and venous vasculature. Small arteries branch into tiny ramifications, the *arterioles,* which resolve into a fine network of *capillaries,* from which the blood is drained by emerging *venules* (Figs. 9–17, 9–21, and 9–22). The blood can be also shunted from arterioles directly to venules via *arteriovenous anastomoses.* These sequential segments of the terminal vascular bed that con-

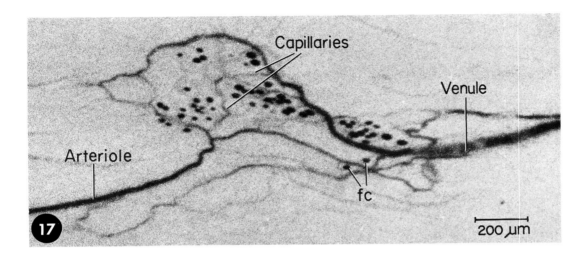

9–17 Photomicrograph of a microvascular unit in rat omentum. The arteriole branches into a network of capillaries that are collected by a venule. **fc,** fat cells. (From Simionescu, M., Simionescu, N., and Palade, G. E. 1975. J. Cell Biol. 67:863.)

stitute the microvasculature[2] may be seen only through the microscope.

In mammals, light-microscopic observations carried out in vivo under routine or special conditions (phase-contrast, interference, or fluorescence) show that the microvascular bed has a very complex architecture according to the nature and activity of the surrounding tissues to which the microvessels functionally belong. Usually the capillary bed is a network supplied by several arterioles and drained by multiple venules (mesentery). In some tissues (muscle), a terminal arteriole supplies groups, or "tufts," of capillaries. Besides the short arteriovenous anastomoses, some "preferential channels" that can shunt the true capillary network even earlier may also occur (e.g., as in muscle). The organization and the structure of the capillaries vary characteristically in the vascular beds of each organ (e.g., in the brain, heart, lung, liver, spleen, kidney, placenta, and so forth).

Various microvascular patterns are encountered: (1) commonly, arteriole–capillary–venule;

(2) a shunt, such as arteriole–arteriovenous anastomosis–venule (arteriovenous anastomoses can occur in a specific organ, the glomus); (3) a special pattern: capillaries–veins–capillaries (such vessels interposed between two capillary beds define a *venous portal system*, as in the liver and in the hypothalamo-hypophyseal complex); or (4) a variant of the latter in which the sequence is: arteriole (afferent)–capillaries–arteriole (efferent)–capillaries, termed an *arterial portal system*, or rete mirabile (renal glomeruli, pancreatic islands).

In humans, the microvasculature of the systemic circulation includes 10% of the blood volume: the corresponding figure for the pulmonary circulation is only 4%. The transition from macrovasculature to microvasculature is gradual and there is no general agreement about the limits between the two territories.

Arterioles

The arterioles are the smallest arteries. The media of arterioles is reduced to a single or double layer of muscle cells (Figs. 9–18 and 9–19). The vessels' diameter, commonly less than 300 μm, may decrease in the proximity of capillaries to 75 to 30 μm, especially when this terminal part has a muscular, sphincter-like structure (*precapillary sphincter area*) (Fig. 9–20). The wall thickness may be as much as one-half the inner diameter.

The *intima* includes endothelium, basal lamina, and a subendothelial layer. The endothelial

---

[2]According to other classifications, the microvascular system contains blood vessels below 500 μm diameter, the larger ones being assigned to the macrovascular system.

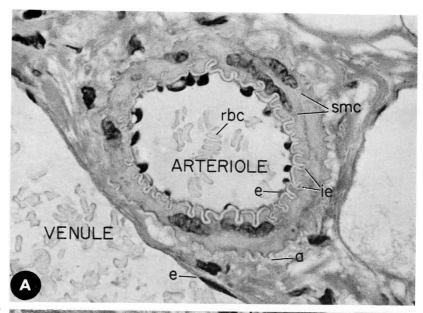

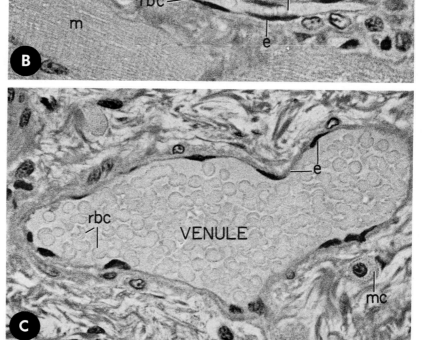

9–18 Photomicrographs of cross sections through an arteriole (actually the transition between small artery and arteriole) **(A)**, capillaries **(B, inset)**, and a venule **(C)**, and of a longitudinal section through a capillary **(B)**. **e,** endothelium; **ie,** internal elastic lamina; **m,** muscular fibers; **mc,** mast cell; **p,** pericyte; **rbc,** red blood cell. **A,** × 600; **B,** × 700; **B, inset,** × 750; **C,** × 500.

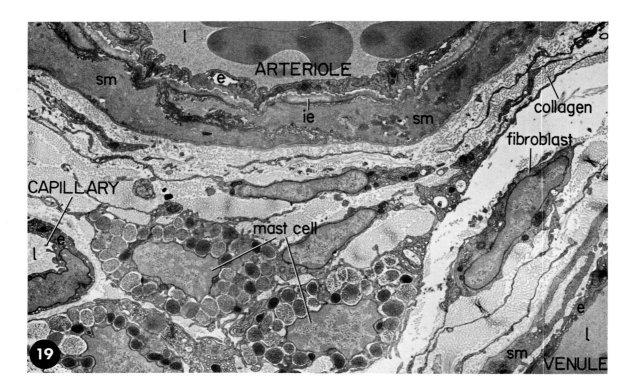

9–19 Low-power electron micrograph of a cross
section through rat messentery showing parts
of the vascular walls of an arteriole, a capillary, and a
venule. Note the frequency of mast cells closely
associated with the vessels. **e**, endothelium; **ie**,
internal elastica; **l**, vascular lumen; **sm**, smooth
muscle cells. × 33,000.

cells are linked by strongly organized junctions
basically similar to those found in arteries (Fig.
9–39a). Basal processes of the endothelial cells
penetrate through fenestrae of the elastic lamina
to form myoendothelial junctions with adjacent
smooth muscle cells (Fig. 9–21). The *basal lamina* is thin, and less distinct in arterioles larger
than 50 μm in diameter. The *subendothelial
layer* is usually thin, it is composed of loose connective tissue and a few collagen and elastic fibers. The *internal elastica* is thin and fenestrated
in arterioles larger than 50 μm; it disappears in
the small terminal arterioles (except in the kidney).

The *media* includes one or two layers of
smooth muscle cells helically arranged (Figs.
9–18 to 9–20). Most often there is a single layer;
rarely (and in large arterioles only), there are
two. They are surrounded by basal laminae and
collagen fibrils.

The terminal part of many arterioles (10–100
μm long), frequently called *metarteriole* or the
precapillary sphincter area, may have a cone-
shaped lumen progressively reduced down to 5
μm (Fig. 9–20). Its media contains a few smooth
muscle cells, some of them displaying myoendothelial junctions. The muscle contraction produces intermittent opening and closing of arteriolar–capillary communication, each phase of the
relaxation–contraction cycle lasting 2 to 8 sec.
This activity intermittently induces new intra-
capillary gradients of water and electrolytes.
Sympathetic stimulation increases arteriolar resistance more than venular resistance. *Intima
cushions* of the type described in arteries have
been found in some arterioles closely associated
with the precapillary sphincters.

The *adventitia* is thin and composed of loose
connective tissue with fibrilar elements and a
few macrophages, mast cells (Fig. 9–19), plasma
cells, fibroblasts, and unmyelinated nerve fibers.

Capillaries

The terminal ramifications of the arterioles are
called capillaries because Malpighi, who discovered them in 1661, called them "capilli" (hairs),
having been impressed by their thinness. The

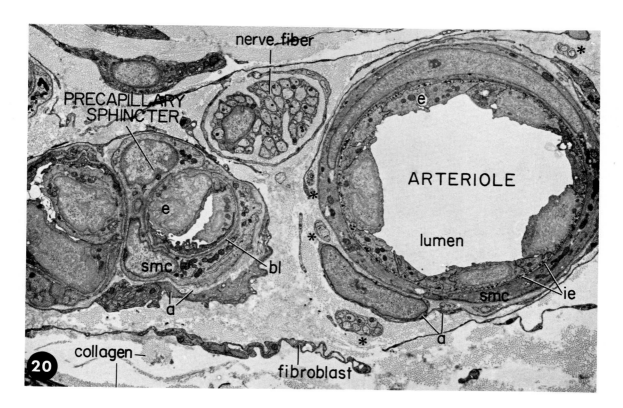

9–20 Low-power electron micrograph of cross-sectioned arteriole and precapillary sphincter (the adventitia of esophagus). Note the narrow lumen of the precapillary sphincter segment in contrast with its relatively thick layer of muscle cells **(smc)**, and the presence of the basal lamina **(bl)** instead of the internal elastica **(ie)** occurring in the arteriole proper. Frequent nerve fibers **(asterisks)** are located near the vessel. **a,** adventitia; **e,** endothelium. × 4,000.

term is restricted to vessels consisting only of endothelium, basal lamina, and a few pericytes. The inner diameter of blood capillaries ranges from 5 to 10 μm (Figs. 9–22 and 9–23) and their average length is 20 to 100 mm. Unlike the boundary between arterioles and capillaries, which is marked by the disappearance of the muscular tissue, the transition from capillary to venule is gradual and structurally less well defined. Capillary density in tissues reflects the magnitude of metabolic rates, especially the oxygen uptake. Oxygen is transported from plasma into cells by diffusion. An increase in the diffusion distance is associated with a decrease in the oxygen pressure. This is particularly important in some tissues, such as the myocardium, in which even small increases in the diffusion distance may lead to a considerable cellular hypoxia. Capillary density can be estimated by different methods, one of which is to count capillaries in tissue sections. The frequency of capillaries per square millimeter of tissue is significantly different among various tissues: 2,000 in myocardium, 600 to 1,200 in skeletal muscle, 1,000 in brain cortex, and only 50 in skin and connective tissue. These figures, however, may be affected by conditions of fixation (such as

shrinkage or swelling). *Capillary surface* area varies: it ranges from 0.9 to 2.4 m² per 100 cm³ of muscle tissue, and is approximately 4 m² per 100 g tissue in the lung. For humans, the total surface area has been estimated at 60 m² systemic capillaries and 40 m² in pulmonary capillaries. These values indicate that 1 ml of blood may be exposed to approximately 5,000 cm² of capillary surface for exchanging materials through the thin (less than 0.5 μm) capillary wall. The capillary bed contains, however, less than 8% of the blood.

The basic structure of blood capillaries is characterized by great simplification of tunics: *intima* is composed only of endothelium, basal lamina, and a few pericytes; *media* is virtually lacking; and *adventitia* consists of a thin peri-

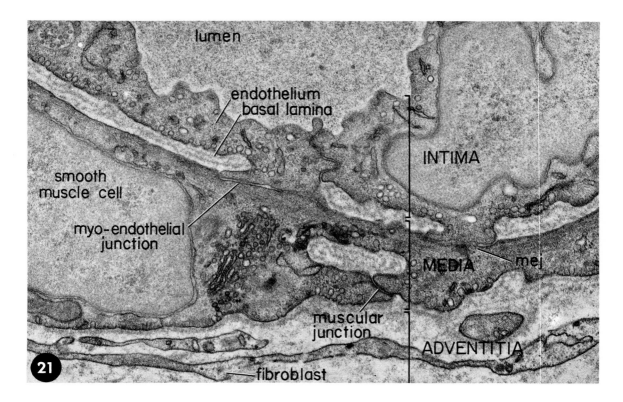

9–21 Detail of the wall of a terminal arteriole
showing the constituents of its tunics and the
presence of two myoendothelial junctions **(mej)**, and a
rather unusual junction between two processes of the
same muscle cell. × 25,000.

capillary layer of connective tissue continuous
with that of the surrounding tissue (Figs. 9–18B
and 9–24). The detailed structure of the layers
varies from one capillary bed to another, reflecting local differences in the nature and magnitude
of blood–tissue exchanges. Based mainly on
variations in the appearance and continuity of
the endothelium and its basal lamina, as revealed by electron microscopy, three principal
types of blood capillaries have been described:
continuous capillaries, fenestrated capillaries,
and *discontinuous capillaries (sinusoids)* (Fig.
9–25).

Continuous Capillaries. These capillaries are
characterized by a continuous endothelium similar to that found in the macrovasculature and a
continuous basal lamina. This most common
type of capillary is found in muscular tissue
(skeletal, cardiac, and smooth muscle), in connective tissue, in the central nervous system, and
in the exocrine pancreas, gonads, and so forth.
The endothelium is approximately 0.2 to 0.3 μm
thick and has a large population of plasmalemmal vesicles 60 to 70 nm in diameter (Figs.
9–25A and 9–26). A relatively thinner endothelium (approximately 0.1 μm) with fewer vesicles
characterizes the capillaries of the central nervous system, lung and haversian systems of the
bone. Plasmalemmal vesicles open on each front
of the cell or are enclosed in the cytoplasm (Figs.
9–24 and 9–25A). In fixed tissues, the great majority appear as isolated units, but some of them
can fuse and form patent transendothelial channels (Figs. 9–25A and 9–34). The intercellular
clefts are approximately 10 to 20 nm wide and
are interrupted by occluding (tight) junctions
(Figs. 9–24, 9–26, and 9–39). The appearance of
these junctions in thin sections varies from a
close apposition to a complete fusion and an
elimination of the outer leaflets of the neighboring cells. Open (2–4 nm) junctions are occasionally encountered.

We do not have enough information about the
molecular organization at the surface of the cell-

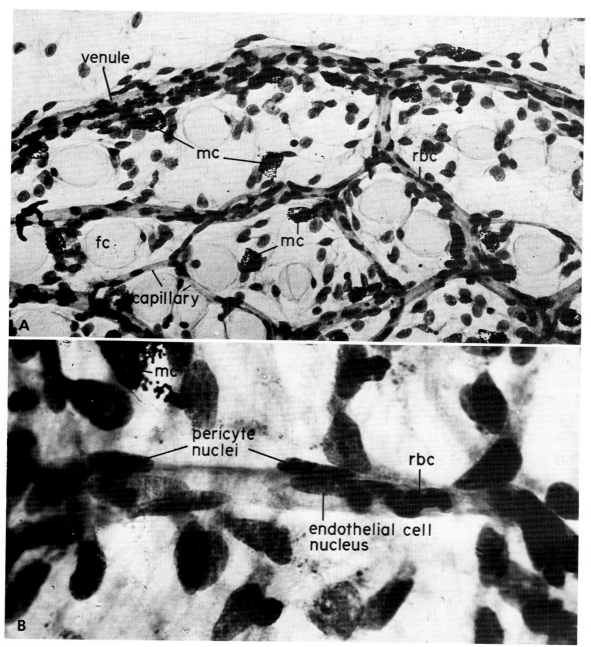

9–22 **A.** Mount of the whole omentum (rat). Area of the microvascular bed: the network of capillaries is collected in a postcapillary venule. Note the frequency of mast cells **(mc)** close to the microvessels. The pale nuclei in the avascular areas correspond to mesothelial cells of the peritoneum.

rbc, red blood cells, **fc,** fat cell. × 250. **B.** Same preparation as in part A. Blood capillary containing red blood cells **(rbc).** Note the position of an endothelial cell nucleus as compared with two adjoining pericyte nuclei. **mc,** mast cell. × 1,800.

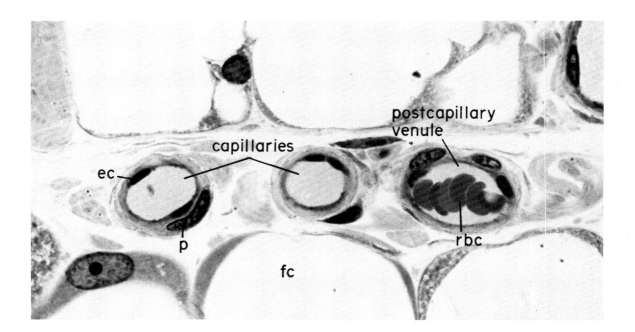

9–23 Cross section through omentum. Connective
tissue stroma surrounded by fat cells **(fc)** and
containing several microvascular profiles, as indicated
in the figure. **rbc,** red blood cells, **ec,** endothelial cell,
p, pericyte. × 700.

to-cell contact in this system. In freeze-cleaved
membrane, the occluding junctions display a different organization from that seen in other epithelia. Endothelial junctions of blood capillaries
consist of two to four strands of intramembranous particles; the strands are either continuous
and connected or staggered (Fig. 9–40B). It is difficult to ascertain whether they form complete
belts. Gap junctions seem to be absent at this
level.

Basal lamina is a continuous layer approximately 20 to 50 nm thick, which appears as a
lightly matted feltwork of poorly resolved fibrils
with a diameter of about 3 to 4 nm. This layer
splits to enclose the pericytes (or Rouget cells)
that come into close contact with the endothelial
cell (Figs. 9–24 and 9–27). The basal lamina is
inconspicuous in bone and lymphoid tissue (the
pericytes are also very scarce in these tissues).

The adventitia is arbitrarily limited to the
connective tissue components, which may remain in close association with the rest of the
capillary wall when experimental or pathological
interstitial edema occurs. Such elements include

fibroblasts, macrophages, mast cells, collagen
and elastic fibers, and ground substance (Figs.
9–24 and 9–25). The amount and nature of the
adventitial connective tissue may influence both
the vessel patency and the transcapillary fluid
exchanges.

Fenestrated Capillaries. The endothelium of
these vessels is attenuated (approximately
0.05–0.1 μm) and has several transcellular circular openings called the fenestrae, with diameters of approximately 60 to 80 nm. All around
their periphery, the cell membrane of the blood
front is continuous with the cell membrane of
the tissue front. Therefore, the fenestrae cut
across the endothelium without affecting the
continuity of the plasmalemma of individual
cells. Each fenestra is usually closed by a thin
single-layered diaphragm (approximately 4–6
nm) with a central knob about 10 to 15 nm in
diameter (Figs. 9–2 and 9–25). The chemical nature and porosity of these diaphragms are still
unknown. We assume, however, that there is no
hydrophobic barrier in these diaphragms. Their
frequency in some visceral capillaries is indicated in Table 9–3. In freeze-fracture preparations, the fenestrae can appear either randomly
distributed or in patches (Fig. 9–28).

The basal lamina is continuous. Fenestrated
capillaries are found in the mucosa of the gas-

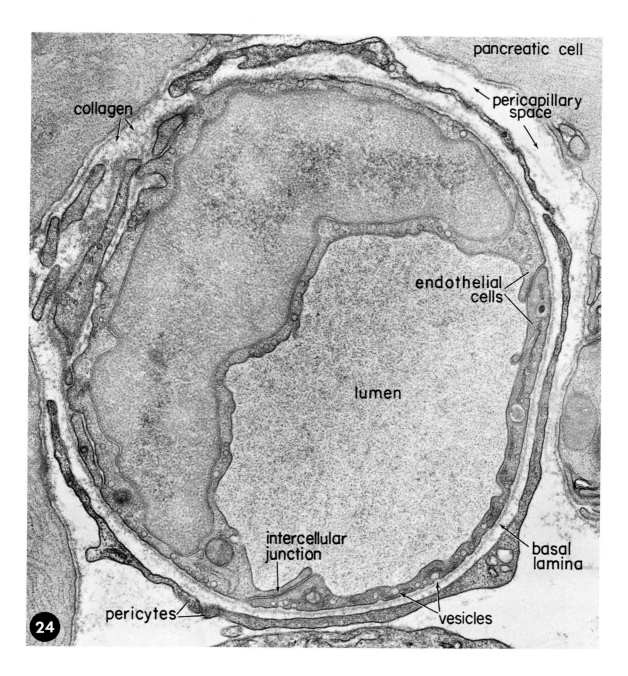

collagen

pancreatic cell

pericapillary space

endothelial cells

lumen

intercellular junction

basal lamina

pericytes

vesicles

24

trointestinal tract, endocrine glands, renal glomerular and peritubular capillaries, choroid
plexus, and ciliary body. In the glomerular capillaries, the fenestrae are usually not closed by
diaphragms, and the basal lamina is almost three
times thicker than that of other capillaries and
plays a crucial role in the permeability characteristics of the organ (see Chap. 24).

9–24 The most common feature of a blood capillary
characterized by continuous endothelium and
basal lamina (rat pancreas). In this case, the
endothelial lining is formed by two cells held together
by intercellular junctions of the occluding type.
× 40,000.

404

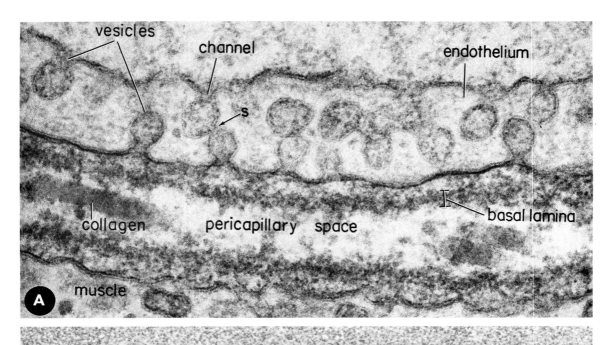

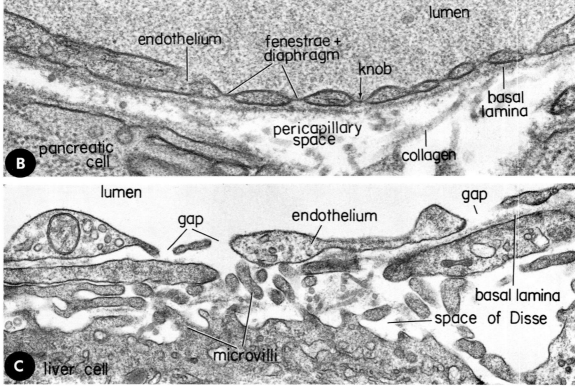

9–25 The three basic types of blood capillaries, differentiated by the continuity of the endothelial cell and the basal lamina. **A,** continuous capillary; **B,** fenestrated capillary; **C,** discontinuous capillary (sinusoid). Rat diaphragm, pancreas, and liver, respectively. **A,** × 120,000; **B,** × 70,000; **C,** × 30,000.

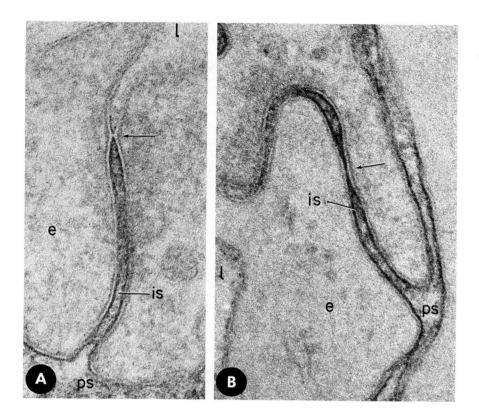

Discontinuous Vessels (Sinusoids or Vascular Sinuses). These vessels are thin-walled with irregular caliber and outline, molded on the neighboring epithelial cells.

The endothelium has large gaps (up to thousands of angstroms in diameter) and the basal lamina, in most species, is either discontinuous or entirely missing (Fig. 9–25C). Such capillaries are found in the liver.

Functional–Structural Correlates in Capillary Permeability

The partition between plasma and interstitial fluid is formed by several successive layers of various natures and functions as follows:

1. The *endothelial cell coat* is composed of the peripheral, exposed portions of cell membrane glycoproteins, glycolipids, and glycosaminoglycans. Among them is thought to be a certain amount of adsorbed plasma proteins (see p. 378). This coat is immersed within the outermost, immobile layer of plasma. This "unstirred" layer may facilitate the stabilization and access of plasma molecules to the en-

9–26 Endothelial junctions in blood capillaries (rat diaphragm). **A.** membrane fusion in which the outer leaflets are eliminated over a distance of about 8 nm **(arrow). B.** fusion of the two outer membrane leaflets of the opposed cells **(arrow). e,** endothelial cell; **is,** intercellular space; **l,** capillary lumen; **ps,** pericapillary space. **A, B,** × 175,000. (From Simionescu, M., Simionescu, N., and Palade, G. E. 1975. J. Cell Biol. 68:705.)

dothelial surface without disturbances from the blood flow.

2. The endothelium is the main barrier; a thin space filled with ground substance mediates its contact with the next layer.
3. The basal lamina and pericytes.
4. The adventitia (heterogeneous).

These layers form a functional and structural unit.

Comparing the blood circulation within the closed system of vessels with the invisible flow of water and dissolved substances across the vascular walls, we find that the latter is much greater. The filtration–absorption phenomenon represents a submicroscopic circulation through

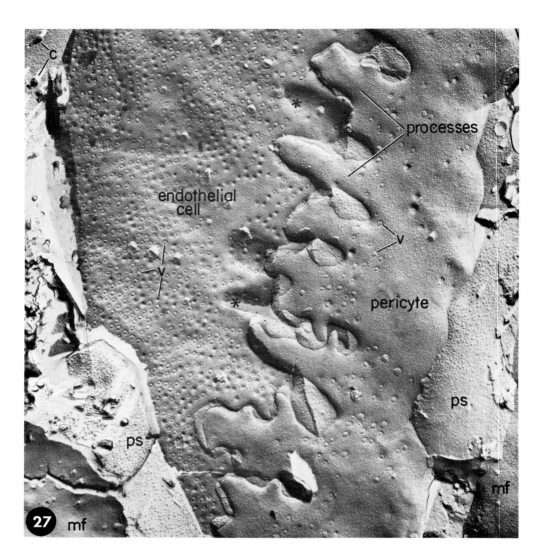

9–27 Freeze-fracture preparation of a blood capillary (rat diaphragm). The endothelial cell is partially covered by a pericyte, the processes of which were in some places removed by the fracture exposing complementary depressions **(asterisks)** left on the endothelium. Note the striking difference in the frequency of vesicular openings **(v)** between the endothelial cell and the pericytes. **mf,** muscle fiber; **c,** collagen; **ps,** pericapillary space. × 27,000. (From Simionescu, M., Simionescu, N., and Palade, G. E. 1974. J. Cell Biol. 60:128.)

the capillary wall: water and solutes get out of plasma at the arteriolar end of the capillary and enter back into it at the venular end. In addition to this, a more extensive fluid movement back and forth through the entire length of the capil-

lary wall is carried out by exchange diffusion, which is practically independent of the rate and direction, of the filtration–absorption flow.

The transcapillary exchanges are governed by the driving forces acting on each side of capillary wall and by the intrinsic activity of the endothelial cells. The driving forces are:

1. The hydrostatic pressure that drives water out of the capillary
2. The osmotic pressure of plasma proteins that draws water back into the capillary
3. Concentration gradients that enable molecules to diffuse by themselves toward lower concentration

The hydrostatic pressure is higher than osmotic pressure at the arteriolar end of the capil-

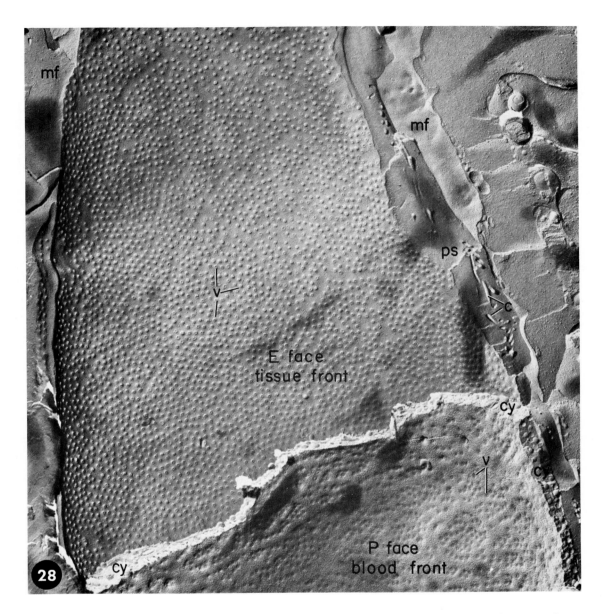

28

lary, but at its venular end, the osmotic pressure is predominant. As a result of these differences in the pressure, about 20 to 22 liters of plasma water and solutes filtrate daily through the capillary walls. The magnitude of the exchanges by filtration alone is, therefore, too small to cover the metabolic requirements of the tissues. Work with isotopes has established, however, that in 24 h the water and solute molecules moving in and out of capillaries actually amount to an equivalent of approximately 80,000 liters. Filtration carries small amounts of metabolites (for example, 20 g of glucose) into the tissues, amounts

9–28 Freeze-fracture preparation of a myocardium capillary. The cleavage plane exposes the P face of the blood front, breaks through the cytoplasm **(cy)** and continues on the E face of the tissue front of the same endothelial cell. Note the high frequency of vesicular openings **(v)**. × 21,000. (From Simionescu, M., Simionescu, N., and Palade, G. E. 1974. J. Cell Biol. 60:128.)

insufficient to keep the cells alive. Diffusion accomplishes an extensive and effective exchange between plasma and tissues; this mechanism supplies cells with metabolites much in excess for a large margin of safety. The exchange diffusion is possible owing to the high permeability of the endothelium: it is much higher than that of other cells and epithelia. Some aspects can be explained (permeability for lipid-soluble molecules); others require special adaptations to explain the high permeability for water and solutes and the high permeability for large water-soluble molecules. The latter could cross the endothelium only through some water-filled channels, or "pores."

Physiological experiments by Pappenheimer, Grotte, and their co-workers using molecules of graded size (dextrans) have indicated the presence of two types of pores:

Small pores: diameter, approximately 11 nm; frequency, 15 to 20 μm^2; aggregate area, 0.1%

Large pores: diameter approximately 50 to 70 nm; frequency, 1/15 to 20 μm^2

Unlike large pores, the small pores restrict diffusion with increasing molecular size. The electron microscope, however, has not revealed structures looking like true pores and displaying the exact dimensions and frequency postulated by the pore theory of capillary permeability. To identify the structural equivalents of these two categories of pores, probe molecules of known dimensions have been used.[3] The results obtained with such tracer experiments have shown that, in *fenestrated capillaries* (Figs. 6–29 and 6–30), large probe molecules (10–30 nm in diameter) pass primarily through a fraction of the fenestral population. Because molecules smaller than 10 nm in diameter penetrate through all fenestrae (Fig. 9–31), it is assumed that the size-limiting structures are part of the fenestral diaphragms. Molecules 2 to 30 nm diameter also cross these endothelia through vesicles and channels.

---

[3]Such molecules can be visualized with the electron microscope either directly as individual particles *(particulate tracers)* such as ferritin (approximately 11 nm), dextrans (approximately 5–20 nm), and glycogens (approximately 25–30 nm), or indirectly through a reaction product *(mass tracer)* obtainable after histochemical reaction of such molecular species as horseradish peroxidase (approximately 5 nm), cytochrome c (approximately 3.3 nm), or hemepeptide (approximately 2 nm). All these molecules have peroxidatic activities. The former group has been used as a probe for the larger pores and the latter, primarily for the small pores.

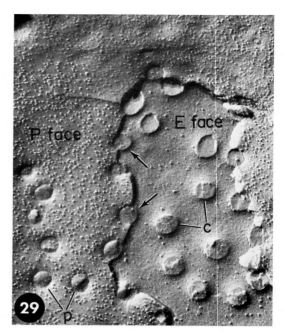

9–29 Freeze-fracture preparation of a fenestrated capillary (rat pancreas). The fenestrae appear as papillae **(p)** on the P face and as craters **(c)** on the E face of the cleaved membrane of the endothelial cell. Note the change in feature from crater to papilla for the fenestrae located along the fracture line through the endothelium **(arrows).** × 68,000. (From Simionescu, M., Simionescu, N., and Palade, G. E. 1974. J. Cell Biol. 60:128.)

In *continuous capillaries,* molecules larger than 10 nm cross the capillary wall only via plasmalemmal vesicles and transendothelial channels (Fig. 9–32), which have been recognized as the structural equivalent of the large pores provided that they open completely (full diameter) at loading or discharging. Investigators still disagree about the small pores, the main pathway followed by molecules smaller than 10 nm in diameter. According to some investigators, they are located in the intercellular junctions; according to others, plasmalemmal vesicles are involved in the passage of molecules of diameter larger than 2 nm. Work with small hemepeptides (MW, 1550–1,900; diameter, 1.7–2 nm) favors a route through chains of vesicles that form patent transendothelial channels (simple or in chains) connecting the two endothelial fronts (Fig. 9–34). The size-limiting structure may be either the strictures at the fusion points of vesicles (di-

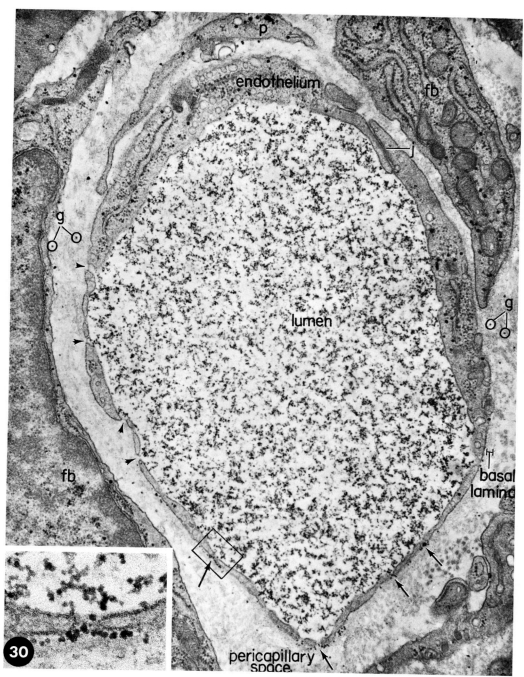

9–30 Fenestrated capillary (rat jejunal mucosa) 4 min after an intravenous injection of a tracer solution of shellfish glycogen. Tracer particles are in high concentration and even distribution in the lumen, and some of them have penetrated many endothelial fenestrae. Some fenestrae do not exhibit particles **(arrowheads);** at the level of others, the tracer is accumulated against the basal lamina **(arrows).** The intercellular junction **(j)** is free of tracer particles. **g,** individual particles in the pericapillary space. × 28,000; inset, × 160,000. (From Simionescu, N., Simionescu, M., and Palade, G. E. 1972. J. Cell Biol. 53:365.)

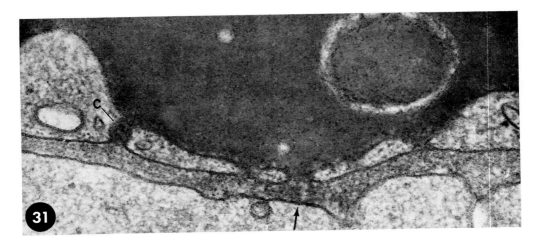

9–31 Blood capillary (mouse intestinal mucosa) 1
△   min, 15 sec after an intravenous peroxidase
injection. In the pericapillary spaces the reaction
product forms a gradient with its maximum opposite
the fenestra **(arrow)** of the endothelium. **c,** channel.
× 110,000. (From Clementi, F., and Palade, G. E.
1969. J. Cell Biol. 41:33.)

9–32 Continuous capillary (rat diaphragm), 10 min
       after an intravenous injection of a tracer
solution of shellfish glycogen. Tracer particles are
present in the lumen and in vesicles open on the
blood front or tissue front **(arrowheads),** or free in the
cytoplasm **(double arrow)** of the endothelial cell.
Some vesicles are closed by their diaphragms
(arrows). × 94,000. (From Simionescu, N.,
Simionescu, M., and Palade, G. E. 1976. Thromb. Res.
(Suppl II) 8:257.)   ▽

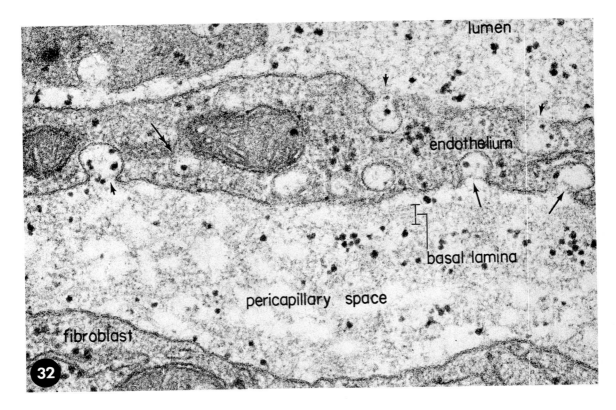

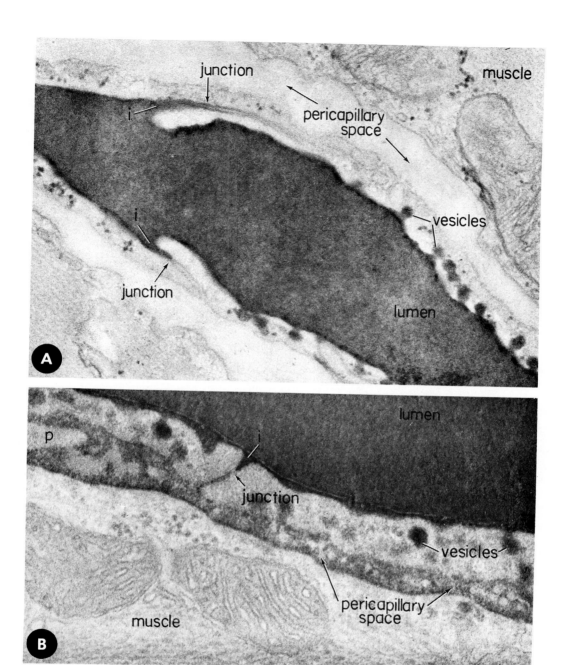

9–33 Blood capillaries of rat diaphragm after intravenous injection of a tracer solution of heme-octapeptide. **A.** 35 sec after tracer injection; the reaction product marks the infundibula leading to the endothelial junctions; the intercellular spaces beyond the junctions are free of reaction product, whereas many plasmalemmal vesicles are labeled **B.** 60 sec after tracer injection at the time when most vesicles are labeled (including those opened on the tissue front), the reaction product is present within the infundibulum **(i)** in the same concentration as in the capillary lumen, but shows a sharp stop at the level of tight junction. The intercellular space beyond this junction contains reaction product in concentration equal to that found in the adjacent pericapillary space. A, × 36,000; B, × 48,000. (From Simionescu, N., Simionescu, M., and Palade, G. E. 1975. J. Cell Biol. 64:586.)

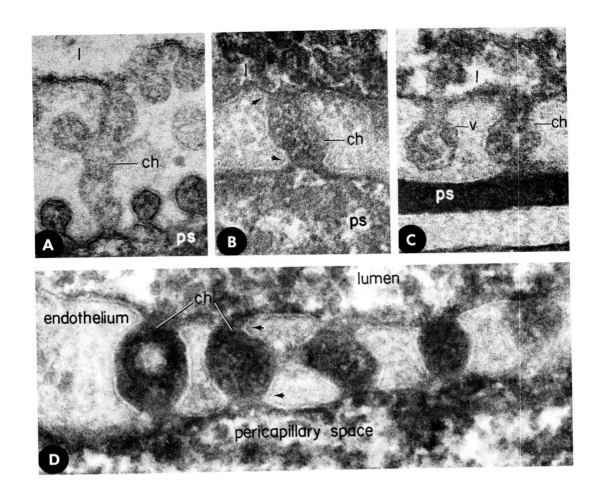

9–34 Transendothelial channels in muscle capillaries (rat diaphragm) from control animals **(A)** and after intravenous injection of heme-undecapeptide tracer solution **(B).** In **C** and **D**, blood capillaries of rat cremaster after local interstitial injection of an identical tracer solution. The channels are formed either by a single vesicle (part C), by two fused vesicles (B and probably some of the features in D), or by a chain of more vesicles (A). Note that the plasmalemma and the vesicle membranes are in continuity on both sides of the channels **(arrowheads).** A, × 150,000; B, C, D, × 200,000. (From Simionescu, N., Simionescu, M., and Palade, G. E. 1975. J. Cell Biol. 64:586.)

ameter, approximately 8–10 nm) or diaphragms at their openings (Fig. 9–25A). According to these experiments and within the limitations of the methods used, the endothelial junctions are not permeable to molecules larger than 2 nm (Fig. 9–33). However, other investigators claim that at least some endothelial junctions are permeated by such tracers.

Similar findings were also obtained by back-diffusion experiments in which the tracer was injected into interstitia from which it partially crossed the endothelium to enter the blood.

Transcytosis. When tracers pass across endothelial cells, the lysosomal apparatus is bypassed and remains unlabeled. This shortcut directly coupling endocytosis to exocytosis is called transcytosis (Simionescu, 1979) and can carry molecules across endothelia both in quanta via discrete vesicles (dissipative transcytosis) and through transient channels and fenestrae (convective transcytosis). The process is bidirectional. The two modes of transcytosis may be intercovertible, thus imparting to the transport process a broad adaptability to the metabolic needs and the local conditions of plasma–interstitial fluid exchanges.

Studies with isolated endothelial cells (e.g., rabbit myocardium) have revealed that the uptake of macromolecules is an intrinsic property of these cells, largely independent of the physical forces operating in vivo. Moreover, vesicular uptake discriminates in favor of anionic proteins (which is the case with most plasma proteins).

Investigations with cationic ferritin (CF) indicate the existence of a differentiated distribution of anionic sites on the luminal front of capillary endothelium: they occur in characteristic high amounts on fenestral diaphragms, whereas vesicle and channel diaphragms are practically devoid of anionic sites (Fig. 9–35). Enzymatic digestions performed in situ prior to CF injection revealed that the anionic sites of fenestral diaphragms are primarily contributed by heparin sulfate, because they are removed by heparinase but not by neuraminidase or other glycosaminoglycan-degrading enzymes (Fig. 9–35).

Work with peroxidase-coupled lectins has shown that plasmalemmal vesicles, transendothelial channels, and their diaphragms are particularly rich in β-D-galactose and β-N-acetylglucosamine. (Fig. 9–36).

This preferential distribution of some glycosaminoglycans and monosaccharide moieties demonstrates the existence of microdomains of glycoconjugates on the luminal front of capillary endothelium. They occur especially on features involved in transcytosis: *fenestral diaphragms are anionic* and contain mostly heparin sulfate, whereas *vesicle and channel diaphragms* are *neutral* and particularly rich in galactose and N-acetylglucosamine (Fig. 9–37). It appears that plasmalemmal vesicles and channels are devised to favor the transcytosis of anionic proteins while fenestrae are primarily associated with elevation of permeability to water and small solutes.

Recent physiological data and information on the cellular biology of capillary endothelium indicate that transport processes in various capillaries no longer can be analyzed with the simplicity of the initial formulation of the pore theory. The high permeability of capillary endothelium to water and solutes can be associated with the unusual development of a *modulating transport system* (vesicles, channels, fenestrae, and diaphragms) and with its capability to efficiently and extensively couple endocytosis with exocytosis *(transcytosis)*. As such, capillary endothelium appears to be provided with a *dynamic hydrophylic system* that, under characteristic segmental and local differentiations, im-

parts a great variety to capillary structure and function.

Various modes of transport differ in relative importance from one capillary bed to another. At one extreme are the so-called blood–tissue barriers (e.g., brain, eyes, thymus, and gonads): they are characterized by extensive tight junctions and few plasmalemmal vesicles, indicating that these elements participate to a lesser extent in exchanges. At the other extreme are the fenestrated or largely discontinuous capillaries, which are freely and extensively permeable to molecules or particles larger than 70 nm (liver) or to cells (spleen and bone marrow).[4]

Endocytosis. In physiological conditions, true endocytosis is a relatively secondary occurrence, largely overwhelmed by transcytosis. Three endocytic processes can take place in endothelium: *phagocytosis, pinocytosis* (in which uncoated vesicles deliver substances to lysosomes), and *adsorptive endocytosis* (e.g., receptor-mediated endocytosis of LDL particles).

The extent of endocytosis and transcytosis and the ratio between them vary among different endothelia. For example, phagocytosis is well developed in the endothelium of liver and in hematopoietic tissues; pinocytosis is prominent in the high endothelium of the postcapillary venules of lymph nodes; active transcytosis is the salient event in the endothelium of both somatic and visceral capillaries.

Venules

The transition from capillaries to venules occurs gradually. The immediate postcapillary venules, ranging in diameter from 10 to 50 μm and in length from 50 to 700 μm, are characterized by the presence of pericytes *(pericytic venules)*. They are drained by venules of increasing diameter from 50 to 200 μm, which contain in their media one or two thin layers of smooth muscle cells *(muscular venules)*.

Pericytic Venules. The *intima's* endothelium, 0.2 to 0.4 μm thick, is generally continuous, but occasionally a few clusters of fenestrae with diaphragms may be seen. The cells are joined by loosely organized intercellular junc-

---

[4]In the kidney the process of filtration and absorption occurs in two distinct sets of capillaries (glomerular and peritubular capillaries, respectively) connected by the efferent arteriole.

414

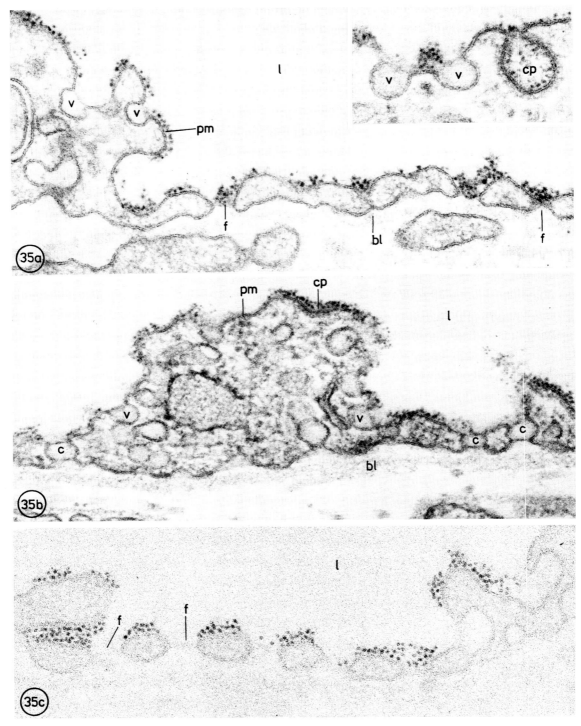

Figure 9–35

9–35 Differential distribution of anionic sites on the luminal front of fenestrated endothelium (pancreas capillaries), as detected by labeling with cationic ferritin (CF). Vessels were cleared out of blood before the administration of the ligand. **a.** Within 1 min after its perfusion in situ, CF bound to plasma membrane (**pm**) and with a characteristic high density on fenestral diaphragms (**f**); CF is absent from vesicle membrane and vesicle diaphragms (**v**). × 110,000. **Inset:** CF marks intensely a coated pit (**cp**) (on its way to be internalized as coated vesicle), in contradistinction to lack of CF on plasmalemmal vesicles and their diaphragms (**v**). **l**, lumen, **bl**, basal lamina. × 130,000. **b.** Same as part a: note three transendothelial channels (**c**), the membranes as well as the diaphragms of which lack CF labeling. **cp**, coated pit, **pm**, plasma membrane, **v**, vesicle. × 100,000. **c.** CF distribution on a capillary endothelium: before CF administration, vessels were perfused with heparinase (reported to be able to remove primarily heparan sulfates and heparins). Note the almost complete absence of CF from fenestral diaphragms (**f**), indicating that the anionic sites are primarily contributed by sulfated glycosaminoglycans, probably heparan sulfate. × 120,000.

tions characterized in freeze-fracture preparations by discontinuous low-profile ridges and grooves frequently devoid of particles. They represent the loosest endothelial junctions encountered along the entire vascular system. Communicating (gap) junctions are usually missing (Table 9–2).

In thin-sectioned specimens, about 30% of venular junctions are open to a gap up to 6 nm and are permeated by molecules up to 5 to 5.5 nm in diameter (e.g., hemepeptides, and horseradish peroxidase). The venules seem to be particularly labile and sensitive to histamine, serotonin, bradykinin, and some prostaglandins, all of which induce the opening and leakage of their junctions (Figs. 9–38 and 9–39). Recent work using a histamine–ferritin conjugate has revealed that venular endothelium contains characteristically high-affinity histamine receptors, predominantly of the H_2 type. They are frequently located on domains of cell membrane that correspond to conspicuous accumulations of filaments in the underlying cytoplasm (Heltianu, Simionescu, Simionescu, 1980).

The basal lamina is thin and penetrated by pericytes that make an almost continuous layer and also establish frequent contacts of unclear

9–36 Preferential distribution of wheat germ agglutinin-peroxidase conjugate (WGA-P) on the luminal domain of the fenestrated endothelium (pancreas capillary). WGA-P binds relatively uniformly to plasma membrane (**p**) while it decorates intensely plasmalemmal vesicles and their diaphragms (**v**). Fenestral diaphragms (**f**) usually contain negligible amounts of residues such as *N*-acetylglucosaminyl for which WGA has a reported specificity. **l**, lumen, **e**, endothelium, **bl**, basal lamina. × 92,000.

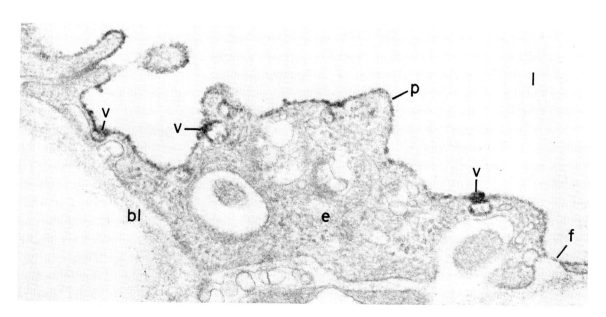

416

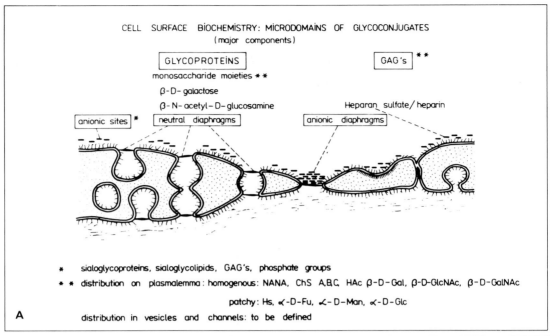

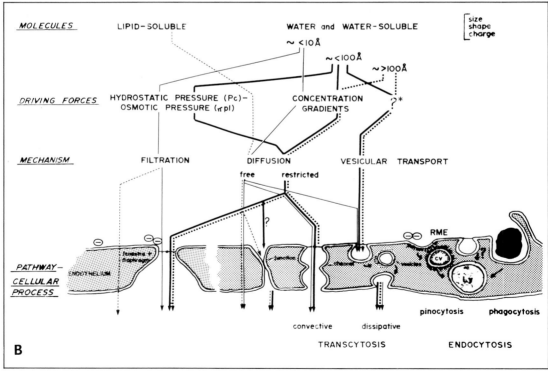

9–37 A. Diagrammatic representation of some microdomains of glycoconjugates so far detected on the luminal surface of fenestrated capillary endothelium (for details, see text). **B.** Simplified diagram of the driving forces and mechanism involved in the pathway taken by plasma molecules across the capillary endothelium including transcytosis, as well as the three modes of endocytosis: receptor-mediated endocytosis **(RME),** pinocytosis, and phagocytosis.

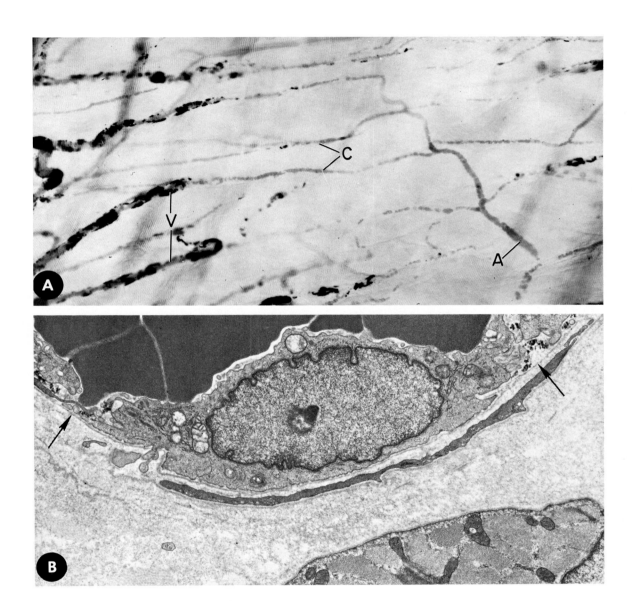

morphological nature with the endothelium. The subendothelial layer is poorly developed as a thin coat of loose connective tissue.

A true *media* is lacking. In larger venules, the pericytes contain more cytoplasmic filaments and even dense bodies that make them resemble smooth muscle cells, to which they are assumed to be related.

The *adventitia* is relatively thin with few connective tissue fibrillar elements and scattered fibroblasts, macrophages, plasma cells, and mast cells. In lymph nodes, the venules may contain a relatively large number of lymphocytes within their walls.

9–38 A. The phenomenon of vascular labeling. Rat cremaster muscle, cleared in glycerine, 1 h after a local injection of histamine and an I.V. injection of colloidal carbon black. **A,** arteriole; **C,** capillaries. Carbon deposits occur almost exclusively in the venules. × 180. (From Majno, G., Palade, G. E., and Schoefl, G. I. 1961. J. Biophys. Biochem. Cytol. 11:607.) **B.** Wall of a venule in a similar experiment as seen by electron microscopy. Note bulging endothelial cell with tight nuclear folds (suggestive of cellular contraction). **Left arrow:** gap between two endothelial cells. **Right arrow:** particles of carbon escaping along an intercellular junction. × 4,100. (Courtesy of Isabelle Joris and G. Majno.)

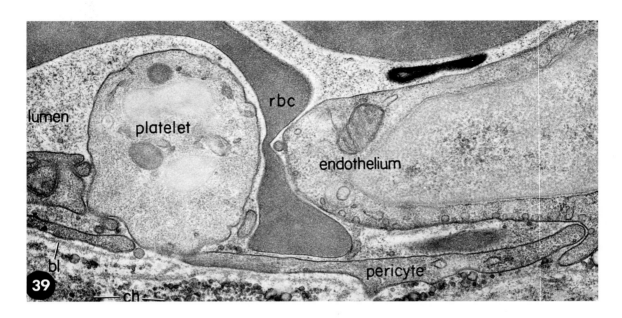

9–39 Cross section of a pericytic venule (rat omentum) 10 min after its exposure to air. Under these stressing conditions, large openings of some endothelial junctions occur. In this specimen, the open junction is occupied by a platelet and part of a red blood cell (**rbc**), both adhering to the subendothelial structures. **bl,** basal lamina; **ch,** chilomicrons. × 32,000.

The immediately postcapillary venules most probably play an important role in the blood–interstitial fluid exchanges. In contrast to capillaries, these venules are easily affected by extreme temperature, inflammation, and allergic reactions, to which they respond by opening the junctions for an augmented extravasation of water, solutes, and blood cells (Figs. 9–38 and 9–39).

Muscular Venules. These venules usually accompany arterioles, from which in sectioned specimens they are easily distinguished because of their thinner wall and irregular and collapsed lumen (Fig. 9–18C).

The *intima* has a continuous endothelium slightly thicker than in pericytic venules. Two types of intercellular junctions have been found in these venules (Fig. 9–40C): (1) the occluding-type junctions, identical to those observed in pericytic venules (Table 9–2); and (2) the communicating (gap) junctions, which may appear as

rare, small, and isolated patches. A thin basal lamina is perforated only in areas of myoendothelial junctions. The scarce subendothelial layer is composed of connective tissue elements (Fig. 9–41).

The *media* is marked by the presence of one or two layers of flat smooth muscle cells (forming an incomplete coat in venules of spleen and kidney). They are surrounded by basal laminae, little ground substance, a delicate network of collagen, and elastic fibers.

The *adventitia* is relatively thick (Fig. 9–41) and contains connective tissue elements among which thin flat fibroblasts, termed for this reason veil cells, are encountered. Unmyelinated nerve fibers occasionally occur.

9–40 The characteristic organization of the endothelial junctions in three segments of the microvasculature. **A.** arteriole: elaborate occluding junctions with intercalated large communicating (gap) junctions. **B.** capillary: only occluding junctions are present, as branching or staggered strands. **C.** muscular venule: discontinuous, low-profile ridges and grooves usually devoid of particles are seen on the P face and E face, respectively; also note a small, isolated communicating (gap) junction. **v,** vesicle openings. A, × 140,000; B, × 160,000; C, × 145,000. (From Simionescu, M., Simionescu, N., and Palade, G. E. 1975. J. Cell Biol. 68:863.)

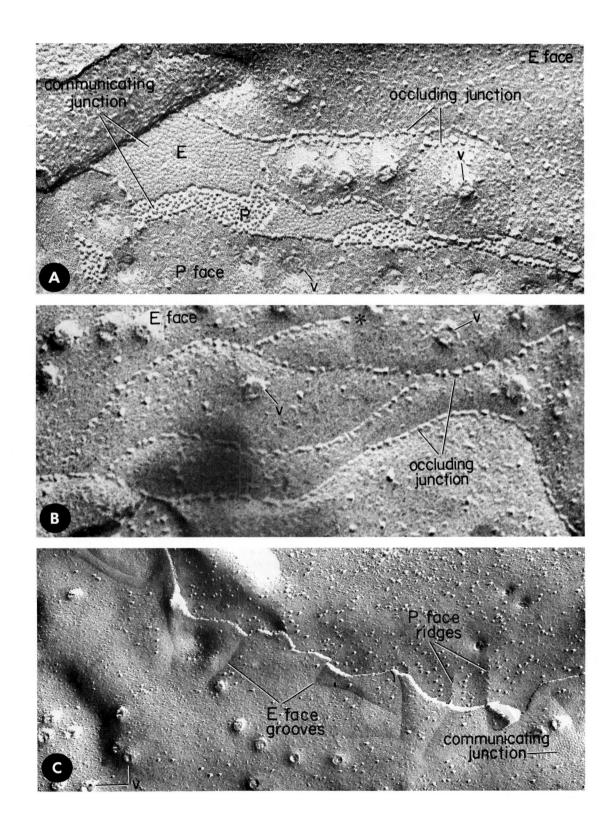

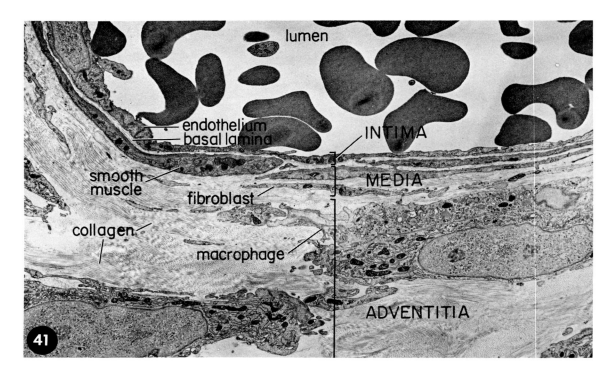

9–41 Cross section through a muscular venule showing the tissue composition of the three tunics. Note the relatively wide adventitia. × 4,600.

Arteriovenous Anastomoses

In certain regions, particularly those where the blood flow varies largely in time, many arterioles are directly connected to venules by short, coiled shunts, the *arteriovenous anastomoses*. These vessels have a thick wall, an average diameter of 12 to 15 μm, and may vary from 300 to 100 μm in length. Such shunts are frequent in the microvascular bed of the skin of the fingertips and toes, nail beds, lips, nose, intestinal tract, thyroid, and erectile tissue. Shunts also represent an essential part of the carotic, aortic, and coccygeal bodies. The last consists of a group of coiled anastomoses arranged in a mass 2.5 mm wide and embedded in connective tissue. In the skin, the arteriovenous anastomoses are frequently convoluted and surrounded by a condensation of connective tissue, forming a glomus that also contains a part of the arteriole. The endothelium lies directly on a specialized muscular media, whose cells are rather short and thick, forming a sphincter that in section resembles a stratified cuboidal epithelium (epitheloid cells). The ad-

ventitia of these anastomoses contains a large number of both myelinated and nonmyelinated nerve fibers.

Veins

From venules, the blood is collected in veins of increasing size, arbitrarily classified as small, medium, and large. Unlike arteries, a correspondence between the size and structure in veins cannot be systematically established. In human beings and other mammals, the veins are very distensible and compressible because of the predominant elastic component of their vascular wall. In the systemic circulation, about 65 to 70% of the blood is contained in the veins (not counting the blood in the reservoirs of the portal venous system, the liver, and spleen). In the pulmonary circulation, the figure is approximately 50 to 55%. The three basic tunics—media, intima, and adventitia—can be recognized in the wall of veins, although their boundaries are less distinct than in arteries. Roughly speaking, the veins of the upper (supercardiac) regions of the body are essentially draining veins that return blood to the heart by gravity; their walls contain mostly elastic and collagen fibers. The veins of the lower (infracardiac) regions of the body are predominantly propulsive veins that actively

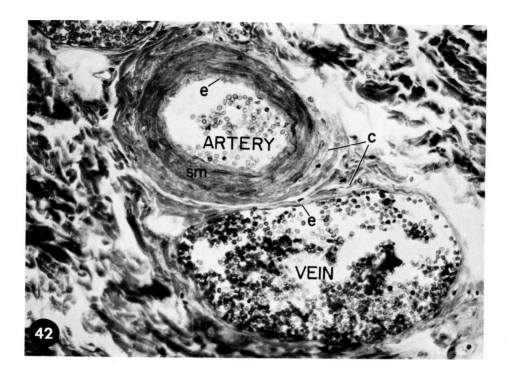

propel the blood to the heart by contracting their muscle fibers. The structure may be different in veins of the same caliber and even in separate regions of the same vein.

9–42 Cross section through small artery and vein.
Note the difference in wall thickness between the two vessels. **e**, endothelium; **sm**, smooth muscle layer; **c**, collagen fibers. × 130.

Small- and Medium-sized Veins. Small veins measure approximately 0.2 to 1 mm in diameter. The *intima* is formed by endothelium and a thin basal lamina. The *media* contains two to four layers of smooth muscle fibers interspersed between a thin network of elastic and collagen fibers (Fig. 9–42). The *adventitia* has delicate bundles of collagen and elastic fibers longitudinally oriented and few fibroblasts and macrophages.

Medium-sized veins have a diameter that may vary from 1 to 10 mm. The wall thickness represents only one-tenth of the vascular diameter. Except for the main trunks, all named veins of the viscera and distal part of the extremities belong to this category.

The *intima* is rather thin, the endothelium being made up of short polygonal cells; some of them extend processes to form myoendothelial junctions with neighboring muscle cells. The basal lamina is thin. The subendothelial layer contains delicate collagen and scattered elastic fibers. The poorly defined elastica interna is found in veins that conduct blood against the force of gravity (in the legs). The intima extends into the lumen pairs of semilunar folds (called valves), which are formed by a connective core covered on both surfaces by endothelium. The free margins of these valves are directed toward the heart. The space between the concave aspect of the valve and the vein wall in called the sinus of the valve. At this level the venous wall is thick. Usually located just distally to the entry of a tributary vein, the valves help to prevent gravitational backflow of blood.

The *media* is thinner than in arteries of similar caliber: two to four circular layers of smooth muscle are separated by bundles of longitudinal collagen fibers interspersed with a delicate network of elastic fibers and a few fibroblasts (Fig. 9–43). The circumferential distensibility of the veins is due in large measure to the circular-helical arrangement of muscle fibers. They are closely related to the elastic fibers, which make a network with longitudinal cracks, and with the collagen fibers, which form another network in a crimped pattern. The changes in length are facilitated by the longitudinal orientation of some

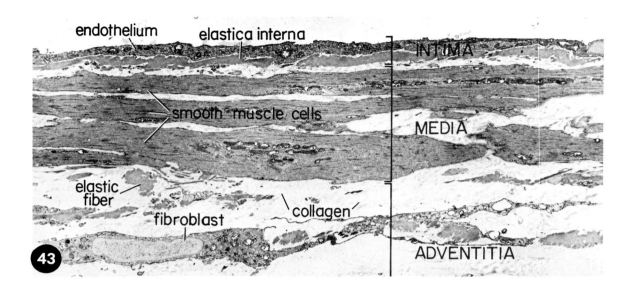

9–43 Longitudinal section through a medium-sized vein (rabbit) showing the tissue composition of the three vascular tunics. Only part of the adventitia is shown in this picture. × 4,000.

smooth muscle, elastic, and collagen fibers. The elastica externa is poorly defined.

The *adventitia* is thicker than the media and is composed of loose connective tissue with collagen and elastic fibers, and smooth muscle cells frequently oriented longitudinally. Vasa vasorum, lymphatics, and unmyelinated nerves are consistently present.

Large Veins. In human beings, these veins are larger than 9 to 10 mm (external jugular, innominate, azygos, pulmonary, external iliac, renal, adrenal, superior mesenteric, splenic, portal, and vena cava). Their wall is extremely thin: one-twentieth of the vascular diameter.

The *intima* has the same configuration as in the medium-sized veins. The endothelial cells are linked together by two types of intercellular junctions: occluding junctions and communicating (gap) junctions. The latter are smaller and less frequent than those found in arteries (Table 9–2). Little is known about the permeability characteristics of the venous endothelium. Widening of the intercellular clefts has been observed after administration of angiotensin, serotonin, epinephrine, and bradykinin. The basal lamina is thin in comparison with the rest of the intima (45–70 μm thick), which contains loose

connective tissue interposed with a network of collagen fibers, scattered elastic elements, and bundles of longitudinal muscle fibers. The elastica interna is largely fenestrated or fragmented.

The *media* is thin and in some areas of vena cava may be absent; otherwise the general organization is similar to that found in medium-sized veins, with few layers of muscle fibers. Rare processes of endothelial cells penetrate the elastica interna to establish myoendothelial junctions. Elastica externa is either poorly defined or missing (Fig. 9–44).

The *adventitia* represents the greatest part of the wall. It contains loose connective tissue with thick bundles of elastic and collagen fibers longitudinally oriented; smooth muscle fibers have a similar arrangement, and in humans they are numerous in vena cava inferior. Vasa vasorum and lymphatics are more developed than in arteries and can sometimes be traced as far as the intima. A rich nervous plexus is also encountered.

Specialized Veins. Functional adaptations have introduced augmentation or reduction of structural elements especially in the muscular composition of some veins.

Veins rich in smooth muscle: longitudinally oriented muscle bundles may be encountered in all three tunics: in the intima; internal jugular, veins of forearm, saphenous, popliteal, femoral, mesenteric, and uterine (of pregnancy); in the media: limbs and umbilical; or in the adventitia: veins of the abdominal cavity. In some regions of the vena cava, the extreme thinning of

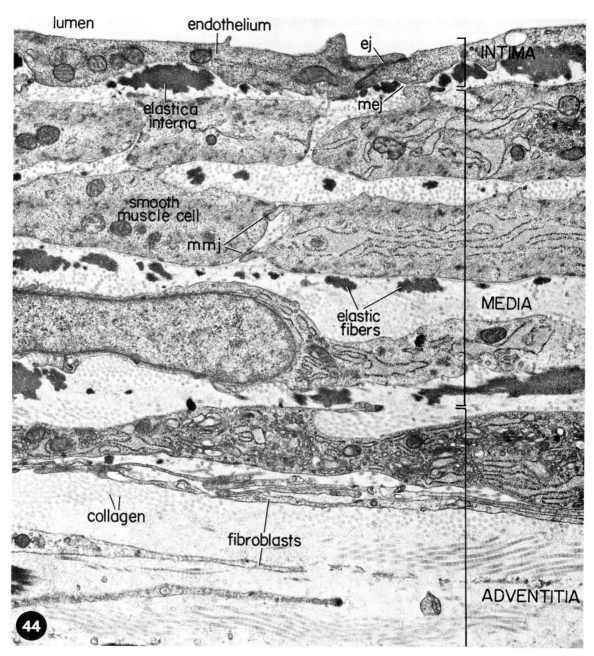

lumen
endothelium
ej
INTIMA
elastica interna
mej
smooth muscle cell
mmj
elastic fibers
MEDIA
collagen
fibroblasts
ADVENTITIA

44

the media brings the longitudinal muscle of the adventitia in contact with the intima. Cardiac muscle extends over a short distance in the adventitia of pulmonary veins and venae cavae.

Veins devoid of smooth muscle: Meningeal and dural sinuses, veins of retina, bones, splenic trabeculae, maternal placenta, and nail bed.

Blood vessels, lymphatics, and nerves of veins have been discussed previously (see page 386).

9–44 Cross section through the wall of a large vein (rat vena cava inferior). The elastica interna is discontinuous and largely fenestrated; a myoendothelial junction **(mej)** can be seen through one of such fenestrae. In this area, the media contains three layers of smooth muscle cells interspersed with rare isolated elastic fibers and bundles of collagen. The adventitia is only partially shown in this figure. **ej,** endothelial junction; **mmj,** muscle junction. × 15,000.

The Heart

The heart is basically a segment of the vascular system, highly specialized as a pump made of striated muscle. It is capable of spontaneous rhythmical contractions, which propel blood through the blood vessels.

The heart displays the three basic tunics of a blood vessel, but a distinctive name has been given to each. The inner layer, homologous to the intima, is called the *endocardium*. The middle layer, corresponding to the media, is termed the *myocardium*; it is particularly differentiated and represents the main mass of the organ. The outer coat, representing the adventitia, is called the *epicardium*; it also contains the visceral sheet of the serous pericardium. (See Table 9–1 and Fig. 9–45.) The endocardium lines separately the right and the left pairs of the heart chambers and is continuous with the intima of the corresponding great vessels entering and leaving the heart. The atrial myocardium inserts on the upper aspect and the ventricular myocardium on the lower aspect of the annuli fibrosi of the cardiac skeleton. No morphological continuity occurs between these two parts of the myocardium, the only connection being the atrioventricular node of the conducting system of the heart. The epicardium functions as a continuous coat that almost completely covers the heart and part of the roots of the large vessels.

Endocardium

The endothelium is of the continuous type like that encountered in large vessels and lies on a thin but continuous basal lamina. Beneath the basal lamina, the subendothelial layer of connective tissue is particularly dense in its inner part owing to a relatively large number of elastic and collagen fibers and smooth muscle cells. Nearer and contiguous with the myocardium, additional loose connective tissue with collagen fibers marks the subendocardial layer: it contains small blood vessels, nerves, and, in ventricles, branches of the conducting system; it is continuous with the interstitial tissue of the myocardium (Fig. 9–46).

Cardiac Valves. Cardiac orifices are provided with valves consisting of folds of endocardium reinforced with a central flat sheet of dense connective tissue continuous with that of the fibrous ring from which they emerge. There are three cusps in the *tricuspid valve*, which lies in the

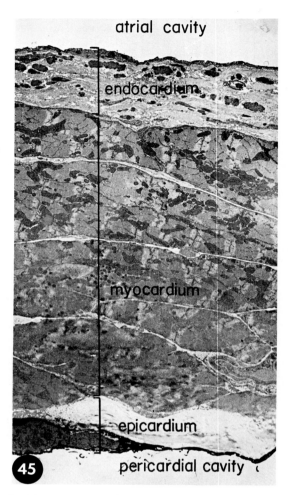

9–45 Cross section through the atrial wall of rat heart showing the three major tunics. Note the relative thickness of both endocardium and epicardium. × 5,000.

right atrioventricular orifice and two cusps in its left counterpart, the *mitral valve*. Near the base of these valves, sparse smooth muscle fibers, blood capillaries, and macrophages may exist. The free borders of the cusps are connected to the papillary muscles by several fibrous cords, the chordae tendinae. These cords restrain the valves from everting when the intraventricular pressure increases during systole. Valves at the orifices of the aorta and pulmonary artery have three semilunar cusps each. At the middle of the free border, each cusp exhibits a small ovoid thickening, the nodule. In the semilunar cusps, the aspect toward the artery is strengthened with collagen and elastic fibers that withstand the

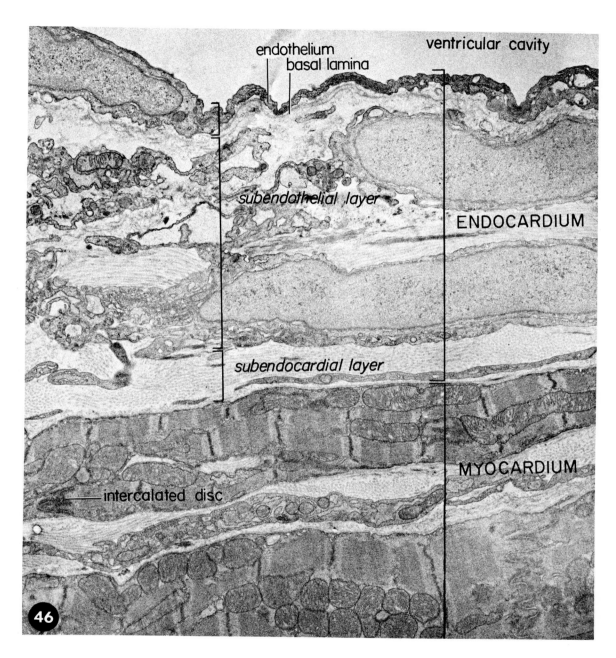

9–46 Cross section through the inner part of the ventricular wall (rat heart). In addition to the endothelium and its basal lamina, the endocardium consists of a relatively large subendothelial layer and the subendocardial layer of loose connective tissue and collagen that continues with the interstitial spaces of the myocardium. × 9,500.

backflow of blood when the valves close. The cardiac valves contain neither lymphatics nor nerves.

Myocardium

The middle tunic of the heart contains mainly three types of tissues: the myocardium proper, the impulse-conducting system of the heart, and the bulk of the cardiac skeleton. The entire wall

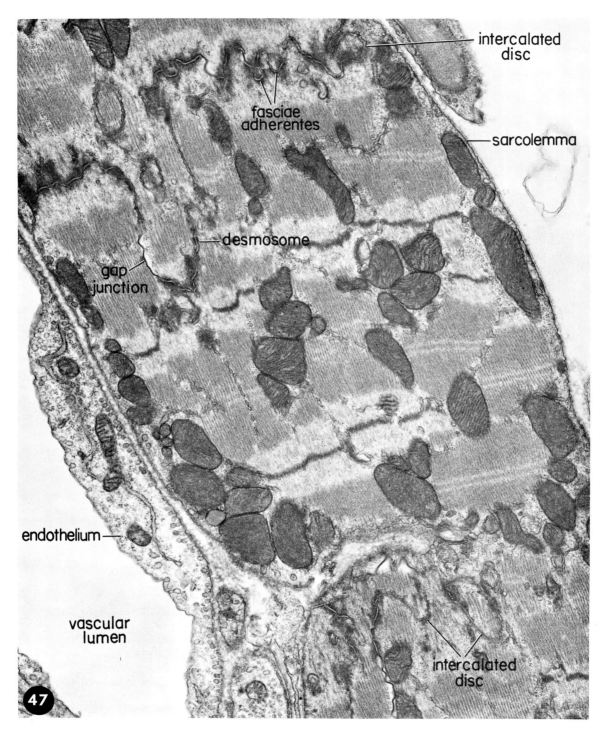

intercalated disc

fasciae adherentes

sarcolemma

desmosome

gap junction

endothelium

vascular lumen

intercalated disc

47

9–47 Longitudinal section of cardiac muscle (left ventricle) displaying on its full length a myocardial cell connected with neighboring myocytes by an intercalated disc at each end. Notice the three types of junctions in the latter. × 20,000.

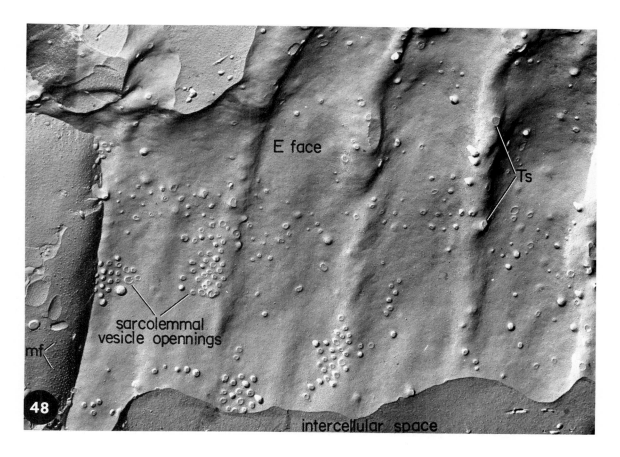

9-48 Replica of freeze-cleaved sarcolemma of a cardiac muscle cell. Vesicle openings are organized in irregular clusters or appear randomly distributed. **Ts,** entry into a T system; **mf,** myofibrils in cross fracture. Compare with Fig. 9–6. × 26,000.

is thinnest in atria and thickest in the left ventricle. Textbooks of anatomy should be consulted for the macroscopic and topographic description of these structures. The general histology and ultrastructure of the cardiac muscle and of the conducting system are described in Chap. 10. The myocardium is arranged in layers and bundles of complex pattern that are embedded in connective tissue together with a large number of capillaries (Figs. 9–47 and 9–50). In atria, the muscles form a latticework and locally appear as prominent ridges resembling a comb (pectinate muscles) intercalated with relatively large amounts of collagen and elastic fibers connecting the endocardium and epicardium. In ventricles, the muscle bundles circumscribe the chambers in a complex, predominantly helical fashion. Superficial muscle layers surround both ventricles, whereas the deep layers encircle each ventricle and form in between the interventricular septum. A similar arrangement occurs in atria. Elastic fibers are scarce in ventricular myocardium. Most of the muscle fibers are inserted on the cardiac

skeleton, mainly the fibrous rings (annuli fibrosi), which separate completely the muscle of atria from that of ventricles. Compared with the ventricular muscle cells, atrial cells are smaller, with a less elaborate T system (Fig. 9–48) and with more frequent communicating (gap) junctions (Fig. 9–47), containing numerous *granules* (Fig. 9–49) of unknown chemical composition. Some of these characteristics may contribute to a higher rate of conduction and greater intrinsic rhythmicity in atrial contractile cells than in those of ventricles. Physiological data suggest that ventricular myocardium has significant metabolic differences between its inner and outer layers. Connective tissue components surround the muscle cells as perimysium (continuous with the interfibrillar endomysium) that houses fre-

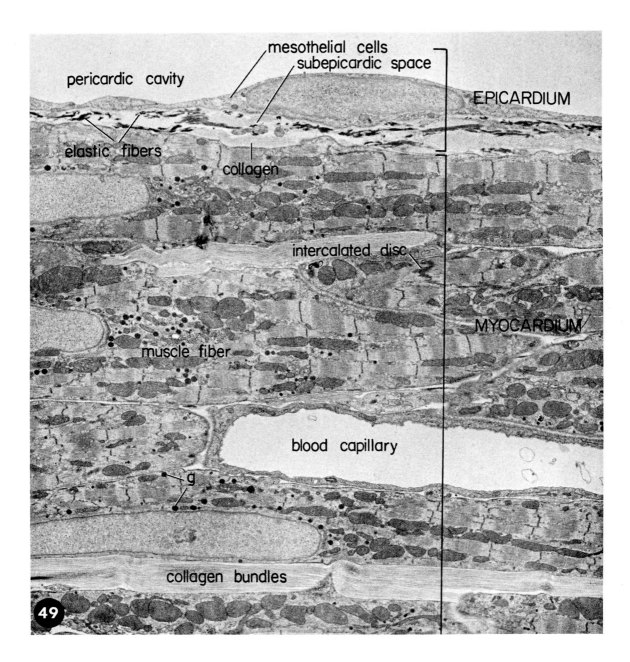

9–49 Longitudinal section of the right atrium of rat
    heart showing the general tissue organization
of epicardium and myocardium. The atrial muscle
cells contain characteristic granules (**g**); relatively
large bundles of collagen occur in some regions of the
atrial myocardium. × 6,000.

quent fibroblasts. The latter may become very
numerous during focal repairs of heart injuries.
The regenerative ability of cardiac muscle itself
is negligible.

Conducting System. Mammals, humans included, have a system of peculiar cardiac muscle
cells specialized for initiating and conducting

the rhythmical electrochemical impulses that generate the coordinated contraction and relaxation of the four chambers of the heart. This conducting tissue—called the *sinoatrial (SA) node*—is represented by a small mass (approximately 5 × 2 mm) that lies in the median wall of the right atrium close to the orifice of the superior vena cava. From this pacemaker, the impulses spread through common cardiac muscle (although the possibility of some specialized conducting cells in atria is not ruled out) at a rate of approximately 1 m/sec. The wave of excitation reaches another mass of conductive cells, the *atrioventricular (AV) node*, located on the right side of the interatrial septum. The slow conduction along the atrial fibers that contact the AV node induces a delay of 0.08 to 0.12 sec, during which time the atrial contraction is completed. Leaving the AV node, the impulses pass rapidly (approximately 4 to 5 m/sec) along an *atrioventricular bundle* (approximately 15 mm long by 2–3 mm wide) that passes into the interventricular septum and gives off a subendocardial branching trunk to each ventricle. Trunk ramifications, primarily described as *Purkinje fibers*, contact the ordinary muscle fibers. Three types of cells compose the conducting system of the heart: *nodal cells, bundle cells (Purkinje cells)*, and *transitional cells* that connect with the myocardial cells (see Chap. 10). Bundles of conducting tissue are characteristically isolated from the surrounding myocardium by a sheet of connective tissue. The activity of the pacemaker system is regulated by complex feedback mechanisms involving nerves, baroreceptors, chemoreceptors, hormones, and so forth.

Cardiac Skeleton. The fibrous base on which cardiac valves and muscle insert is inappropriately, but customarily, called the *cardiac skeleton*. Its main part consists of a mass of dense fibrous tissue organized in rings, the *annuli fibrosi*, which surround the atrioventricular canals and the origins of the aorta and pulmonary artery. Between the two groups of fibrous rings, additional masses of fibrous tissue constitute the *trigona fibrosa*. The upper part of the interventricular septum is formed by a fibrous partition, the *septum membranaceum*. Fibrous rings also contain elastic fibers and few adipocytes, whereas in the trigona fibrosa, islands of chondroid tissue may occur. During aging, these structures may become focally calcified.

Epicardium

Its outermost coat is formed by the mesothelial cells of the visceral pericardium; their smooth, wet surface minimizes friction during heart contraction. Beneath a thin basal lamina, the subepicardial layer (composed of areolar connective tissue, elastic and collagen fibers, adipocytes, vessels, and nerves) attaches the epicardium to the myocardium (Fig. 9–49).

Intrinsic Vessels of the Heart

The overall density of the blood microvascular bed is greater in myocardium than in skeletal muscle (see Capillaries, and Fig. 9–50). The amount of blood passing through the coronary arteries is about 225 ml/min, representing approximately 4 to 5% of all the blood pumped by the heart. Unlike other parts of the circulation, coronary flow is greater during diastole than during systole. Myocardium capillaries are morphologically similar to skeletal muscle capillaries, but they are more permeable than the latter. The structural substrate of such differences is not clear. Controversial data suggest that macromolecules cross the endothelium of myocardial capillaries either through the intercellular clefts or via plasmalemmal vesicles. The frequency of the latter is remarkably high (Table 9–3). It has also been indicated that in regions with high oxygen tension (such as subendocardial coat) capillaries are more permeable to probe molecules (such as horseradish peroxidase) than are the subepicardial capillaries.

Table 9–3 Frequency of Vesicle Openings and Fenestrae on Endothelial Surfaces[a]

Type of capillary	Vesicular openings/μm^2		Fenestrae/μm^2
	Blood front	Tissue front	
Muscular			
Diaphragm	60	100	
Myocardium	70	110	
Visceral	30	20	15
Pancreas	10	10	25
Jejunal mucosa			

[a]Adapted from M. Simionescu, N. Simionescu, and G. E. Palade, *J. Cell Biol.*, 60:128,1974.

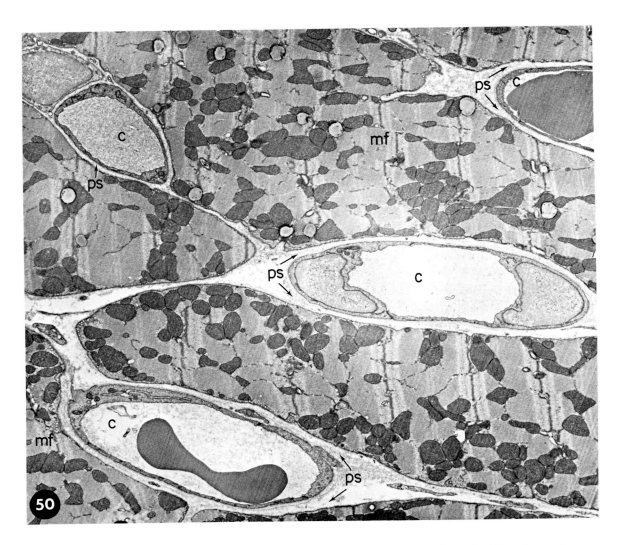

9–50 Longitudinal section through the cardiac
muscle (guinea pig heart ventriculum) showing
the general organization of muscle fibers **(mf)**, the high
frequency of blood capillaries **(c)**, and the relative
thinness of pericapillary spaces **(ps)**. × 6,000.

Lymphatics are richly represented in myocardium. Small lymphatic capillaries (approximately 8–10 μm in diameter) originate near muscle fibers and endocardium; they drain protein-
rich fluid into the larger lymphatics of the epicardial coat.

Intrinsic Nerves of the Heart

The heart receives numerous myelinated and unmyelinated nerve fibers of sympathetic and par-

asymphathetic (vagal) origin. They form plexuses
in each major layer of the heart wall and many
small ganglia occur in some of them (e.g., subepicardial and perinodal networks). Sensory
nerve fibers have their cell bodies either in the
vagal or spinal ganglia (first to fourth pair). Nerve
endings make myoneural junctions, presumably
cholinergic, with the atrial myocardium. Sensory
unencapsulated end organs (baroreceptors) associated with 4 to 9 μm thick nerve fibers have
been recently identified in the atrial endocardium. Despite many fine branches passing into
the interstitia of ventricular myocardium, no
neuromuscular junctions have been described in
ventricles. At this level, the nerve processes lie
within more than 20 nm of the sarcolemma,
which does not exhibit any local specialization.

The innervation, however, participates significantly in the complex mechanisms that regulate the heart's performance by making the adjustments necessary to meet the shifting circulatory needs of various organs and tissues of the body.

References and Selected Bibliography

Blood Vessels in General

Benninghoff, A. 1939. *In* W. von Möllendorf (ed.), Handbuch der Microskopischen Anatomie des Menschen, Vol. 6, Part 1, Blutgefässe und Herz. Berlin: Springer Verlag, p. 1.

Blose, S. H., Shelanski, H. L., and Chacko, S. 1977. Localization of bovine filament antibody on intermediate (100Å) filaments in guinea pig vascular endothelial cells and chick cardiac muscle cells. Proc. Natl. Acad. Sci. U.S.A. 74:662.

Copley, A. L., and Scheinthal, B. M. 1970. Nature of the endo-endothelial layer as demonstrated by ruthenium red, Exp. Cell Res. 59:491.

Cotran, R. S. 1965. Endothelial phagocytosis: An electron-microscopic study. Exp. Mol. Pathol. 4:217.

Franke, W. W., Schmid, E., Osborn, M., and Weber, K. 1979. Intermediate-sized filaments of human endothelial cells. J. Cell Biol. 81:570.

Jaffe, E., Nachman, R., Becker, C., and Minik, C. R. 1973. Culture of human endothelial cells derived from umbilical veins. J. Clin. Invest. 52:2745.

Kefalides, N. A. 1978. Current status of chemistry and structure of basement membranes. *In* Biology and Chemistry of Basement Membranes. N. Kefalides (ed.), New York: Academic Press, p. 215.

Kresse, H., Filipovic, I., Iserloh, A., and Buddecke, E. 1970. Comparative studies on the chemistry and the metabolism of arterial and venous tissue. Angiologica 7:321.

Majno, G. 1970. Two endothelial novelties: Endothelial contraction; collagenase digestion of the basement membrane. *In* F. Koller, K. M. Brinkhous, R. Biggs, N. F. Rodman, and S. Hinnom (eds.), Vascular Factors in Thrombosis. Stuttgart: F. K. Schattauer Verlag, p. 23.

Majno, G., and Joris, I. 1978. Endothelium 1977: A review. *In* A. B. Chandler et al. (eds.), The Thrombotic Process in Atherogenesis (Adv. Exp. Med. Biol. 104). New York: Plenum Press, p. 169.

Ross, R., and Bornstein, P. 1969. The elastic fiber. 1. The separation and partial characterization of its macromolecular components. J. Cell Biol. 40:366.

Ryan, V. S., Ryan, J. W., Whitaker, C., and Chiu, A. 1976. Localization of angiotesin converting enzyme (Kininase II). Immunocytochemistry and immunofluorescence. Tissue Cell 8:125.

Skutelsky, E., and Danon, D. 1976. Redistribution of surface anionic sites on the luminal front of blood vessel endothelium after interaction with polycationic ligand. J. Cell Biol. 71:232.

Somlyo, A. P., and Somlyo, A. V. 1968. Vascular smooth muscle. 1. Normal structure, physiology,

biochemistry and biophysics. Pharmacol. Rev. 20:197.

Zeldis, S. M., Nemerson, Y., Pitlick, F. A., and Lenz, T. L. 1972. Tissue factor (thromboplastin): Localization to plasma membranes by peroxidase-conjugated antibodies. Science (Wash., D.C.) 175:766.

Arteries and Arterioles

Biscoe, T. J. 1971. Carotid body. Structure and function. Physiol. Rev. 51:437.

Giacomelli, F., and Weiner, J. 1974. Regional variation in the permeability of rat thoracic aorta. Am. J. Pathol. 75:513.

Gozna, E. R., Marble, A. E., Shaw, A., and Holland, J. G. 1974. Age-related changes in the mechanics of the aorta and pulmonary artery of man. J. Appl. Physiol. 36:407.

Hüttner, T., Boutet, M., and Moore, R. H. 1973. Studies on protein passage through arterial endothelium. 1. Structural correlates of permeability in rat arterial endothelium. Lab. Invest. 28:672.

Rhodin, J. A. G. 1967. The ultrastructure of mammalian arterioles and precapillary sphincters. J. Ultrastruct. Res. 18:181.

Schwartz, S. M., and Benditt, E. P. 1972. Studies on aortic intima. 1. Structure and permeability of rat thoracic aortic intima. Am. J. Pathol. 66:241.

Schwartz, S. M. and Benditt, E. P. 1973. Cell replication in the aortic endothelium. A new method for study of the problem. Lab. Invest. 28:699.

Simionescu, M., Simionescu, N., and Palade, G. E. 1975. Segmental differentiations of cell junctions in the vascular endothelium. The microvasculature. J. Cell Biol. 67:863.

Simionescu, M., Simionescu, N., and Palade, G. E. 1976. Segmental differentiations of cell junctions in the vascular endothelium. Arteries and veins. J. Cell Biol., 68:705.

Simionescu, N., Demetrian, S., Abramescu, N., and Abagiu, N. 1962. Coussinets endartériels des artères segmentaires et sous-segmentaires de la rate chez l'homme. Arch. Anat. Pathol. 10:215.

Smith, E. B. 1974. The relationship between plasma and tissue lipids in human atherosclerosis. Adv. Lipid Res. 12:1.

Stein, Y., and Stein, O. 1979. Interaction between serum lipoproteins and cellular components of the arterial wall. *In* A. M. Scanu et al. (eds.), The Biochemistry of Atherosclerosis. New York: M. Dekker, Inc., p. 313.

Trelstad, R. L. 1974. Human aorta collagens: Evidence for three distinct species. Biochem. Biophys. Res. Commun. 57:717.

Vasile, E., Nistor, A., Nedelcu, S., Simionescu, M., and Simionescu, N. 1980. Dual pathway of low density lipoprotein transport through aortic endothelium, and vasa vasorum, in situ. Eur. J. Cell Biol. 22:181.

Weibel, E. R., and Palade, G. E. 1964. New cytoplasmic components in arterial endothelia. J. Cell Biol. 23:101.

Wight, T. N., and Ross, R. 1975. Proteoglycans in primate arteries. 1. Ultrastructural localization and distribution in the intima. J. Cell Biol. 67:660.

Wright, H. P. 1971. Areas of mitosis in aortic endothelium of guinea-pigs. J. Pathol. 105:65.

Capillaries

Bennett, H. S., Luft, J. H., and Hampton, J. C. 1959. Morphological classification of vertebrate blood capillaries. Am. J. Physiol. 196:381.

Brightman, M. W. 1977. Morphology of blood–brain interfaces. Eye Res. Suppl. 1.

Bruns, R. R., and Palade, G. E. 1968. Studies on blood capillaries. I. General organization of muscle capillaries. J. Cell Biol. 37:244.

Bruns, R. R., and Palade, G. E. 1968. Studies on blood capillaries. II. Transport of ferritin molecules across the wall of muscle capillaries. J. Cell Biol. 37:277.

Clementi, F., and Palade, G. E. 1969. Intestinal capillaries. Permeability to peroxidase and ferritin. J. Cell Biol. 41:33.

Crone, C., and Christensen, O. 1979. Transcapillary transport of small solutes and water. In A. C. Guyton and D. B. Young (eds.), Cardiovascular Physiology III. (Int. Rev. Physiol. 18). Baltimore: University Press, p. 149.

Farquhar, M. G. 1978. Structure and function in glomerular capillaries. Role of the basement membrane in glomerular filtration. In N. Kefalides (ed.), Biology and Chemistry of Basement Membrane. New York: Academic Press, p. 43.

Fawcett, D. W. 1963. Comparative Observations on the Fine Structure of Blood Capillaries in Peripheral Vessels, Int. Acad. Pathol. Monogr. 4. Baltimore: Williams and Wilkins.

Grotte, G. 1956. Passage of dextran molecules across the blood–lymph barrier. Acta. Chir. Scand. (Suppl.) 211:1.

Johansson, B. R. 1978. Permeability of muscle capillaries to interstitially microinjected horseradish peroxidase. Microvasc. Res. 16:340.

Johansson, B. R. 1979. Size and distribution of endothelial plasmalemmal vesicles in consecutive segments of the microvasculature in cat skeletal muscle. Microvasc. Res. 17:107.

Kanwar, Y. S., and Farquhar, M. G. 1979. Anionic sites in the glomerular basement membrane. In vivo and in vitro localization to the laminae rara by cationic probes. J. Cell Biol. 81:137.

Kanwar, Y. S., Linker, A., and Farquhar, M. G. 1980. Increased permeability of the glomerular basement membrane to ferritin after removal of glycosaminoglycans (heparan sulfate) by enzyme digestion. J. Cell Biol. 86:688.

Karnovsky, M. J. 1967. The ultrastructural basis of capillary permeability studied with peroxidase as a tracer. J. Cell Biol. 35:213.

Karnovsky, M. J. 1970 Morphology of capillaries with special reference to muscle capillaries. In C. Crone and N. A. Lassen (eds.), Capillary Permeability; Alfred Bezon Symposium, II. New York: Academic Press, Inc., p. 341.

Landis, E. M., and Pappenheimer, J. R. 1963. Exchange of substances through the capillary walls. In W. F. Hamilton and P. Dow (eds.), Handbook of Physiology, Vol. II, Sec. 2. Washington, D.C.: American Physiological Society, p. 961.

London, M. F., Michel, C. C., and White, I. F. 1979. The labeling of vesicles in frog endothelial cells with ferritin. J. Physiol. (Lond.) 296:97.

Luft, J. H. 1966. Fine structure of capillary and endocapillary layer as revealed by ruthenium red. Fed. Proc. 25:1773.

Majno, G. 1965. Ultrastructure of the vascular membrane. In W. F. Hamilton and P. Dow (eds.), Handbook of Physiology, Vol. III, Sec. 2. Washington, D.C.: American Physiological Society, p. 2293.

Maul, G. G. 1971. Structure and formation of pores in fenestrated capillaries. J. Ultrastruct. Res. 36:768.

Paaske, W. P., and Sejrsen, P. 1977. Transcapillary exchange of ^{14}C-inulin by free diffusion in channels of fused vesicles. Acta Physiol. Scand. 100:437.

Raviola, E., and Karnovsky, M. J. 1972. Evidence for a blood–thymus barrier using electron opaque tracers. J. Exp. Med. 136:466.

Reese, T. S., and Karnovsky, M. J. 1967. Fine structural localization of a blood–brain barrier for exogenous peroxidase. J. Cell Biol. 34:207.

Palade, G. E. 1953. Fine structure of blood capillaries, J. Appl. Physiol. 24:1424.

Palade, G. E. 1960. Transport in quanta across the endothelium of blood capillaries. Anat. Rec. 136:254.

Palade, G. E. 1961. Blood capillaries of the heart and other organs. Circulation 24:368.

Palade, G. E., and Bruns, R. R. 1968. Structural modulations of plasmalemmal vesicles. J. Cell Biol. 37:633.

Palade, G. E., Simionescu, M., and Simionescu, N. 1979. Structural aspects of the permeability of the microvascular endothelium. Acta Physiol. Scand. (Suppl.) 463:11.

Renkee, H. G., Cotran, R. S., and Venkatachalam, M. A. 1975. Role of molecular charge in glomerular permeability. Tracer studies with cationized ferritins. J. Cell Biol. 67:638.

Renkin, E. M. 1977. Multiple pathways of capillary permeability. Circ. Res. 41:735.

Simionescu, M. 1979. Transendothelial movement of large molecules in the microvasculature. In Pulmonary Edema. Washington, D.C.: American Physiological Society, p. 39.

Simionescu, M., Simionescu, N., and Palade, G. E. 1974. Morphometric data on the endothelium of blood capillaries. J. Cell Biol. 60:128.

Simionescu, N. 1979. The microvascular endothelium: Segmental differentiations; transcytosis; selective distribution of anionic sites. In G. Weissman et al. (eds.), Advances in Inflammation Research, Vol. 1. New York: Raven Press, p. 61.

Simionescu, N. 1981. Transcytosis and traffic of membranes in the endothelial cell. In Cell Biology 1980–1981. Heidelberg: Springer Verlag (in press).

Simionescu, N., and Simionescu, M. 1980. The hydrophilic pathways of capillary endothelium, a dynamic system. *In* A. Benzon Symposium 15 on Water Transport Across Epithelia. Copenhagen: Munksgaard.

Simionescu, N., Simionescu, M, and Palade, G. E. 1972. Permeability of intestinal capillaries. Pathway followed by dextrans and glycogens. J. Cell Biol. 53:365.

Simionescu, N., Simionescu, M., and Palade, G. E. 1973. Permeability of muscle capillaries to exogenous myoglobin. J. Cell Biol. 57:424.

Simionescu, N., Simionescu, M., and Palade, G. E. 1975. Permeability of muscle capillaries to small heme-peptides. Evidence for the existence of patent transendothelial channels. J. Cell Biol. 64:586.

Simionescu, N., Simionescu, M., and Palade, G. E. 1978. Structural basis of permeability in sequential segments of the microvasculature. Microvasc. Res. 15:1.

Wagner, R. C., Kreiner, P., Barrnett, R. J., and Bitensky, M. W. 1972. Biochemical characterization and cytochemical localization of a catecholamine-sensitive adenylate cyclase in isolated capillary endothelium. Proc. Natl. Acad. Sci. U.S.A. 69:3175.

Wissig, S. L., and Williams, M. C. 1978. Permeability of muscle capillaries to microperoxidase. J. Cell Biol. 76:341.

Venules and Veins

Azuma, T., and Hasegawa, M. 1973. Distensibility of the vein from the architectural point of view. Biorrheology, 10:409.

Buccianti, L. 1966. Microscopie optique de la paroi veineuse. *In* Symp. Int. Morphologie Histochim. Paroi Vasculaire (Fribourg), 1963, pt. II. Basel: S. Karger, p. 211.

Cho, Y., and De Bruyn, P. P. 1979. The endothelial structure of the postcapillary venules of the lymph node and the passage of lymphocytes across the venule wall. J. Ultrastruct. Res. 69:13.

Heltianu, C., Simionescu, M., and Simionescu, N. 1980. Identification of histamine receptors by using a histamine-ferritin conjugate: Characteristic high affinity binding sites in venular endothelium. J. Cell Biol. 87:156a.

Hulström, D., and Svensjö, E. 1977. Simultaneous fluorescence and electron microscopic detection of bradykinin induced macromolecular leakage. Bibl. Anat. 15:466.

Majno, G., Palade, G. E., and Schoefl, G. I. 1961. Studies on inflammation. II. The site of action of histamine and serotonin along the vascular tree: A to-

pographical study. J. Biophys. Biochem. Cytol. 11:607.

Majno, G., Shea, S. M., and Leventhal, M. 1969. Endothelial contraction induced by histamine-type mediators. An electron microscopic study. J. Cell Biol. 42:647.

Rhodin, J. A. G. 1968. Ultrastructure of mammalian venous capillaries, venules, and small collecting venules. J. Ultrastruct. Res. 25:452.

Simionescu, N., Simionescu, M., and Palade, G. E. 1978. Open junctions in the endothelium of the postcapillary venules of the diaphragm. J. Cell Biol. 79:27.

Svensjö, E., and Arfors, K. E. 1975. Bradykinin-induced macromolecular permeability: Repeated application and potentiation by PGE_1, PGE_2, and PGE_{21}. Microvasc. Res. 10:235.

van Deurs, B. 1978. Endocytosis in high-endothelial venules. Evidence for transport of exogenous material to lysosomes by uncoated "endothelial" vesicles. Microvasc. Res. 16:280.

Heart

Abraham, A. 1969. Microscopic Innervation of the Heart and Blood Vessels in Vertebrates Including Man. New York; Pergamon Press.

Ellison, J. P., and Hibbs, G. R. 1976. An ultrastructural study of mammalian cardiac ganglia. J. Mol. Cell. Cardiol. 8:89.

McNutt, N. S., and Fawcett, D. W. 1974. Myocardial ultrastructure. *In* G. A. Langer and A. J. Brady (eds.), The Mammalian Myocardium New York: John Wiley & Sons, Inc., p. 1.

Mochet, M., Moranec, L. Guillemot, H. and Hatt, R. Y. 1975. The ultrastructure of rat conductive tissue: An electron microscopic study of the atrioventicular node and the bundle of his. J. Mol. Cell Cardiol. 7:869.

Rakusan, K. 1971. Quantitative morphology of capillaries of the heart. Number of capillaries in animal and human hearts under normal and pathological conditions. Meth. Achievm. Pathol. 5:272.

Viragh, S., and Challice, C. E. 1973. The impulse generation and conduction system of the heart. *In* A. J. Dalton and C. E. Challice (eds.), Ultrastructure in Biological Systems, Vol. 6, Ultrastructure of the Mammalian Heart. New York: Academic Press, p. 43.

Weihe, E., and Kalmbach, P. 1978. Ultrastructure of capillaries in the conductive system of the heart in various mammals. Cell Tissue Res. 192:77.

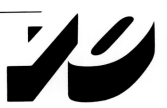

The Heart

Eva Griepp

The heart is a highly specialized part of the vascular system whose function is to pump blood to the lungs for oxygenation and to the whole of the body to meet its metabolic needs. The complex demands made on the heart are reflected in the differences between cardiac and skeletal muscle, the modifications of cardiac muscle in different parts of the heart, the characteristics of the specialized condition tissues, the organization of the heart's blood supply, and its innervation.

General Organization and Function

Like the other components of the vascular system, the heart consists of an intima, the *endocardium;* a media, the *myocardium;* and an adventitia, the *epicardium,* which are in continuity with the appropriate layers of the great veins and arteries. During embryological development, the heart evolves from fusion of a pair of vessels to form a single tube that folds upon itself and subsequently is divided into four chambers. In the normal adult heart (Fig. 10–1), venous blood enters the *right atrium* from the *superior* and *inferior vena cavae,* then flows through the *tricuspid valve* into the *right ventricle.* With ventricular contraction, or *systole,* blood is ejected from the *right ventricle* via the *pulmonary valve* and *pulmonary artery* into the lungs, where gas exchange occurs. Oxygenated blood returns via the *pulmonary veins* to the *left atrium* and goes through the bicuspid *mitral valve* into the *left ventricle.* During systole it is propelled from the left ventricle through the *aor-*

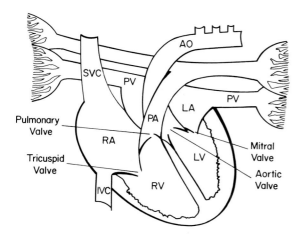

10–1 Diagrammatic representation of the normal heart. Desaturated blood returns via the superior vena cava **(SVC)** and inferior vena cava **(IVC)** to the right atrium **(RA).** From the right ventricle **(RV)** it is pumped to the lungs via the pulmonary artery **(PA)**. Oxygenated blood returns from the lungs through the pulmonary veins **(PV)** to the left atrium **(LA)**. From the left ventricle **(LV)** it is pumped via the aorta **(AO)** to the body.

tic valve into the *aorta* and is then distributed throughout the systemic circulation. The pressures in both atria under normal circumstances are quite low throughout the cardiac cycle, because atrial contraction occurs during ventricular *diastole*, when the ventricle is relaxed. Consequently, the walls of the atria are much thinner than those of the ventricles, and the muscle of atrial myocardium differs from that of ventricular myocardium. Similarly, because the resistance of the pulmonary circuit to ejection is much lower than systemic resistance, right ventricular pressure is usually lower than left ventricular pressure, and the right ventricular has a thinner wall than the left.

Endocardium

The interiors of the cardiac chambers and the surfaces of the valves are covered by a thin endothelium with a continuous basement membrane. The bulk of the endocardium, however, is in the subendothelial layer, composed of varying amounts of elastic elements, collagen fibers, and connective tissue containing smooth muscle cells. Between the endocardium and myocardium lies loose connective tissue, the subendocardial layer, which is continuous with the ex-

tracellular matrix of myocardial cells and, eventually, with the connective tissue underlying the epicardium.

Epicardium

The subepicardial region on the outer aspect of the myocardium is continuous with the connective tissue of the myocardium and contains fat cells and nerves in addition to elastic and collagen fibers. It is covered by a thin mesothelium whose free surface is moist and slippery, allowing the heart to move within the pericardium with minimal friction.

Cardiac Valves

The valves of the heart, which separate the atria from the ventricles and the ventricles from the great arteries, are composed of rings of dense fibrous tissue, from which projections of fibrous tissue covered by endothelium, called the valve leaflets, arise. Both the aortic and pulmonic valves have three cusps, as does the tricuspid valve; the mitral valve has only two cusps. The free edges of the atrioventricular valve leaflets are prevented from eversion by fibrous attachments, the *chordae tendineae*, which attach to the papillary muscles of the ventricles. The valve rings are connected to one another by more fibrous tissue; together with the fibrous upper part of the ventricular septum, the *septum membranaceum*, they constitute the so-called *cardiac skeleton*.

Myocardium

General Features of Cardiac Muscle–Comparison with Skeletal Muscle

The myocardium is composed chiefly of a type of striated muscle unique to the heart and therefore called *cardiac muscle* (Fig. 10–2). Like skeletal muscle, its intracellular functional unit is a *sarcomere*, an orderly arrangement of thick filaments composed of myosin, thin filaments containing actin, and the regulatory proteins troponin and tropomysin. Each sarcomere, as in skeletal muscle, is demarcated by two Z lines, in which the thin filaments are thought to be anchored and where the protein α-actinin has been found. Z lines of adjacent sarcomeres are linked by 10-nm intermediate filaments composed of desmin. Contraction of cardiac muscle is thought

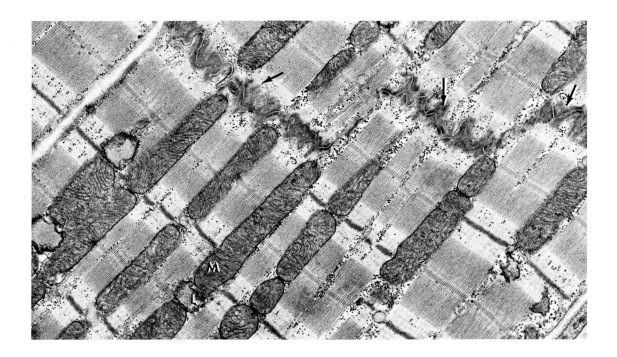

10–2 Electron micrograph of a longitudinal section from the ventricular papillary muscle of the cat. The transverse banding pattern is similar to that of skeletal muscle. Paired mitochondria are absent from the I bands, but large mitochondria **(M)** form almost continuous longitudinal rows, and lipid droplets **(L)** are closely associated with them. A transverse cell junction is arranged in the typical stepwise pattern that constitutes the intercalated disc. Parts of three transverse portions **(arrows)** of the intercalated disc are included in the section, together with the longitudinal portions that connect them. × 15,000. (From D. W. Fawcett and N. S. McNutt, 1969.)

to occur by a sliding filament mechanism like that of skeletal muscle.

Unlike skeletal muscle, however, cardiac muscle is not a syncytium, but is composed of individual branching cells containing many parallel myofilament bundles, each with a single, usually centrally placed nucleus. The cells of heart muscle are joined together by a characteristic structure called the *intercalated disc* which contains intercellular junctions that permit both mechanical and ionic coupling between cells, allowing the individual cardiac muscle cells to function together as an integrated whole. This coordinated function is of obvious importance in assuring that the cells within each cardiac chamber contract synchronously under normal conditions and enables them to act in concert in response to stress. In contrast to skeletal muscle, all fibers within heart muscle are already activated in the baseline state, and the demand for additional output must be met by changes in the function of the heart as a whole rather than by recruitment of additional muscle fibers. In an acute situation, the heart can increase its mechanical advantage by dilating (augmenting stroke volume), the heart rate can be increased (positive chronotropic effect), and the contractility of the muscle can be improved by means of adrenergic hormones or drugs such as digitalis (positive inotropic effect). If an increased work load must be met chronically, cardiac cells can hypertrophy, increasing the number of sarcomeres, but the cells cannot divide.

Cardiac muscle contains many more mitochondria than does skeletal muscle (35% of cell volume vs. 2%), reflecting the extreme dependence of cardiac muscle on aerobic metabolism. The mitochondria are evenly distributed, dividing cardiac muscle cells into apparent myofibrils, and have projections that are thought to maximize the mitochondrial membrane area while minimizing the distance over which diffusion to a bundle of myofilaments must occur. The sarcoplasm of cardiac muscle is also characterized by numerous lipid droplets and glycogen particles, correlating with the known use by cardiac muscle (as well as some skeletal muscles) of fatty acids, glucose, and lactose as sources of energy. Reserves of these nutrients are present to ensure the uninterrupted function of the heart should the exogenous supply of substrates for oxidation be lost. If isolated cardiac muscle cells are examined after having been stimulated to contract in a medium free of nutrients, first the lipid and then the glycogen in the tissue are seen to be depleted.

As in skeletal muscle, excitation–contraction coupling in cardiac muscle is regulated by the availability of calcium ions, but unlike the situation in skeletal muscle, magnesium ions cannot be substituted for extracellular calcium in cardiac muscle. It is thought that the network of smooth membranes known as the *sarcoplasmic reticulum* is the site of uptake and storage of the calcium needed for contraction. In cardiac muscle the sarcoplasmic reticulum is less abundant and less evenly distributed than in skeletal muscle, probably reflecting a more limited capacity for calcium storage and therefore explaining the greater dependence of cardiac muscle on extracellular calcium. As in skeletal muscle, the plasmalemma of the muscle cell, or *sarcolemma,* invaginates into the interior of the cell in a network of tubules known as *T tubules,* which in cardiac muscle are lined with a protein–polysaccharide glycocalyx. In cardiac muscle, the T-tubular network is simpler and wider than that in skeletal muscle, perhaps allowing for more rapid equilibration across the membranes. The sites of contact of T tubules with the sarcoplasmic reticulum are characterized by flattened *subsarcolemmal cisternae*; these so-called "couplings" are fewer and smaller than comparable structures in skeletal muscle, usually forming *dyads* rather than triads. The abundance and even distribution of the mitochondria in cardiac muscle has led to the hypothesis that mitochondria may also participate in storage and release of calcium in cardiac muscle.

The intercalated disc (Fig. 10–3) is the means by which individual cardiac cells are electrically and mechanically linked, allowing the heart to function in an integrated fashion. The intercalated disc is found in regions of the membrane where two cardiac cells are joined end to end and occurs in place of a Z line. In longitudinal sections of cardiac muscle the discs are seen as transverse structures running between cells in a steplike fashion. Within the intercalated disc are intercellular junctions, specialized regions of membrane that provide electrical coupling and mechanical adhesion.

The gap junction (discussed at some length in Chap. 3) provides a low-resistance pathway across the membranes of adjoining cells, allowing the unrestricted passage of ions required for the synchronous beating of heart cells. Gap junctions are usually found in the longitudinal rather than the transverse protions of a typical intercalated disc.

The second junction within the intercalated disc, called the *fascia adherens,* resembles the zonula adherens of epithelium and is thought to carry out a similar function: anchoring the actin cytoskeletal elements within each cell (in this case the myofilaments) to the plasma membrane, while providing a bond between plasma membranes of adjacent cells. Each of these extensive desmosome-like junctions in cardiac muscle consists of a submembranous network of 7-nm actin filaments and a space between membranes of 15 to 20 nm. The fasciae adherentes occur primarily in the transverse portion of the intercalated disc.

In addition, typical desmosomes with 10-nm tonofilaments are occasionally seen in both the longitudinal and transverse portions of the intercalated disc. These desmosomes probably serve to anchor the plasma membranes to nonactin cytoskeletal structures within the cardiac muscle cells as well as to provide adhesion between plasma membranes of adjacent cells.

Differences Between Atrial and Ventricular Muscle

Because the functional characteristics of atrial and ventricular myocardium differ, it is not surprising that structural and biochemical differences between atrial and ventricular muscle have been detected.

Atrial muscle cells are generally smaller in diameter than their ventricular counterparts (in the cat averaging 5 to 6 μm in diameter compared with 10 to 12 μm in ventricular myocardium); this difference is consistent with the need for ventricular muscle to eject against a much higher resistance than atrial muscle. Another striking difference in most mammals studied is the virtual absence in atrial muscle cells of a T-tubular network. It has been speculated that the smaller diameter of the atrial cells may allow rapid equi-

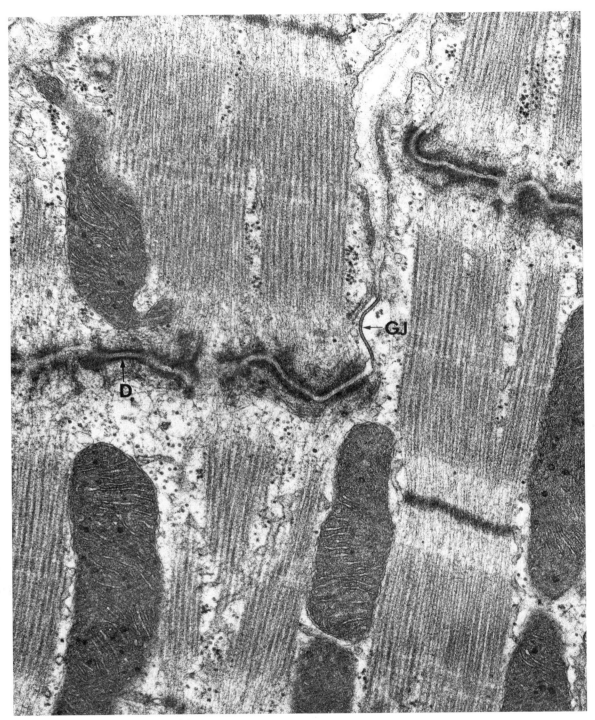

10–3 Thin-section electron micrograph of an intercalated disc from cat ventricle. A gap junction **(GJ)** can be seen in the longitudinal portion of the disc. In the transverse portions, the thin filaments of the sarcomere can be seen inserting into the filamentous web underlying the extensive fascia adhaerens junction. An occasional spot desmosome **(D)** is also visible. (From McNutt, N. S., and Fawcett, D. W. 1974. In Langer, G. A., and Brady, A. J. (eds.), The Mammalian Myocardium. New York: Wiley, p.1.)

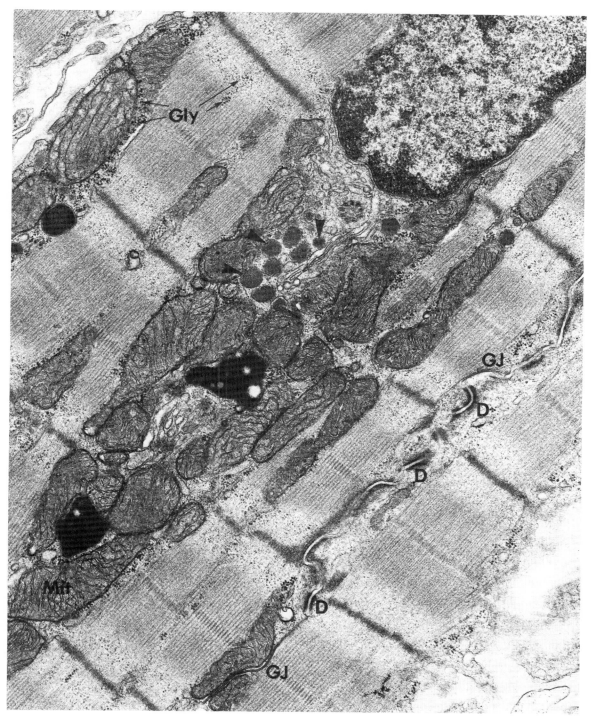

10–4 Thin-section electron micrograph of cat atrium, showing the characteristic atrial granules **(arrowheads)** in the perinuclear Golgi region of the cell. Desmosomes **(D)** and gap junctions **(GJ)** in the longitudinal portion of the intercalated disc are also beautifully shown. As is characteristic of cardiac muscle, glycogen particles **(Gly)** are abundant, and many mitochondria **(Mit)** are present. The heavily stained areas are lipofuchsin granules. (From McNutt, N. S., and Fawcett, D. W. 1969. J. Cell Biol. 42 (1):1.)

libration of calcium between the cell and the extracellular space with each contraction, obviating the need for calcium storage in T tubules. The absence of the extra capacitance contributed by the membranes of the T-tubular system in atrial tissue may be an important factor in allowing impulse conduction to proceed at a faster rate than in ventricular muscle, as has been shown electrophysiologically (the opposite would be expected on the basis of the smaller size of the atrial cells). Another factor contributing to the faster conduction between atrial cells than ventricular cells is the somewhat increased number of gap junctions within the intercalated discs between atrial myocytes.

Atrial cells also differ from ventricular cells in having distinctive electron-dense granules in their cytoplasm that are associated with the Golgi complex (Fig. 10–4). The composition and function of these vesicles is not known: it has been suggested that they may be storage sites for catecholamines.

Specialized Conduction Tissue

Although the heart is innervated by branches from both the sympathetic and parasympathetic nervous systems, the stimulus for initiating the cardiac impulse comes from within the heart itself and is propagated via specialized cells of the conduction system to the working muscle cells of the myocardium. There are several cell types within the conduction system whose physiological, biochemical, and morphological character-

10–5 Diagram of the course of the conduction system, correlated with the intracellular recordings of action potentials from different cell types within the heart and their contribution to the surface electrocardiogram. Note the variation in both the timing and the configuration of the action potentials from various cell types within the heart. The P wave originates from the SA node and from atrial contraction, the P-R interval is determined by conduction through the AV node, and the QRS complex is the result of activation of ventricular cells. Note that only in the recordings from the SA and AV nodes is there a change in the resting potential during phase 4, and that the upward slope during phase 4 is steeper in the SA than in the AV node. It is this gradual depolarization that confers pacemaker activity on the cells from these regions. The His-Purkinje system that connects the AV node with ventricular cells is shown but not labeled: His-Purkinje cells do not have pacemaker activity. (Adapted from an original painting by Frank H. Netter from the Ciba Collection of Medical Illustrations, copyright by CIBA Pharmaceutical Company, Division of CIBA-GEIGY Corporation.)

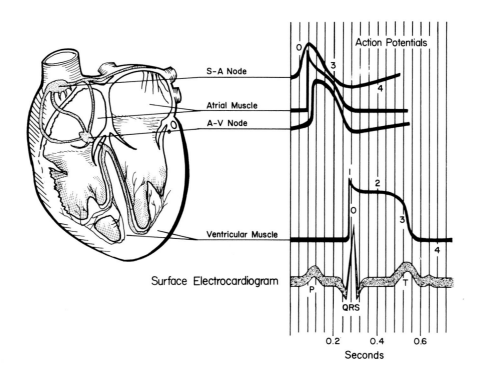

istics differ not only from those of the cardiac muscle cells surrounding them, but also from one another. It is worth distinguishing these different cell types within the heart in order to make sense of the complex and otherwise confusing effects of autonomic hormones and cardioactive drugs on various portions of the heart.

The heartbeat is normally initiated by the cells of the *sinus* or *sinoatrial (SA) node*. This group of cells is located near the entrance of the superior vena cava into the heart, in close proximity to a single large arterial branch, usually from the right coronary artery, which provides its blood supply. The pacemaker activity of the cells of the SA node is explained by the characteristics of electrophysiological recordings from them (Fig. 10–5). These cells differ from adjacent atrial cells (and from ventricular cells) in showing a gradual depolarization during phase 4 of the action potential, which allows them spontaneously to reach the threshold at which a new action potential is automatically triggered. The cells of the SA node are smaller than atrial muscle cells and contain fewer and more poorly organized myofilaments (Fig. 10–6). The endomysium of the SA node contains more elastic tissue than adjacent atrial tissue. There are no intercalated discs within the SA node, although intercellular junctions are present. Nerve endings, mainly parasympathetic, are frequent, but no

specialized myoneural junctions have been described.

From the SA node, the impulse travels through the atrium via several pathways that have not been identified anatomically to the *atrioventricular* or *AV node*, which is located between the tricuspid valve and the coronary sinus. The cells of the AV node are very similar to those of the SA node: they are smaller than atrial muscle cells, have few organized myofilaments, and are separated by connective tissue. There are rare junctions not organized into intercalated discs, and nerve endings are frequent (Fig. 10–7). Intracellular recordings from the AV node, like those from the SA node, show a gradual depolarization in phase 4 of the action potential (Fig. 10–5), but the rate of depolarization is slower than that in the sinus node. Thus, the AV

10–6 Electron micrograph of a longitudinal section through a typical SA nodal cell of a rabbit heart. Note that the myofilament bundles show poorly organized sarcomeres, with interrupted Z lines **(Z)**. Numerous thin actin-like filaments **(a)** and occasional thick myosin-like filaments **(m)** are found seemingly at random within the cytoplasm. × 20,700. (From Tranum-Jensen, J. 1976. In Wellens, H. J. J., Lie, K. I., and Janse, M. J., The Conduction System of the Heart. Philadelphia: Lea and Febiger.)

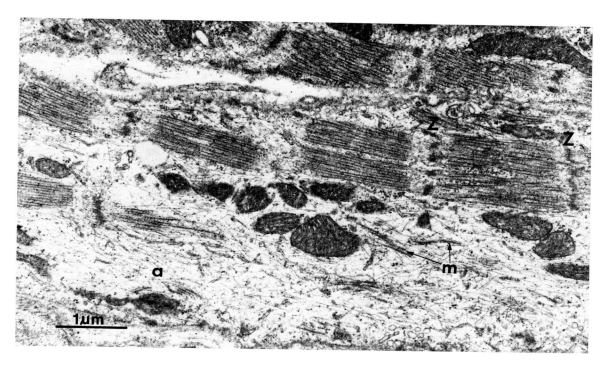

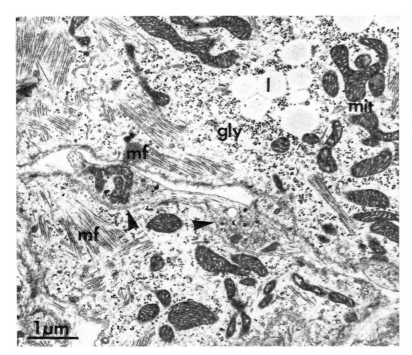

10–7 Thin section electron micrograph of AV nodal tissue from rabbit heart. The **arrowheads** indicate two varicosities of an axon making close contact with a myocardial cell without evidence of any subsynaptic specialization. Note the poorly organized microfilament bundles **(mf)** and the abundant mitochondria **(mit)**, glycogen granules **(gly)** and lipid droplets **(l)** × 14,700. (From Tranum-Jensen, J. 1976. In Wellen, H. J. J., Lie, K. I., and Janse, M. J. (eds.), The Conduction System of the Heart. Philadelphia: Lea and Febiger.)

node is normally triggered by the impulse emanating from the SA node rather than by its intrinsic pacemaker mechanism. However, if the sinus node is damaged (e.g., by interruption of its blood supply) the AV node, which is supplied by branches from both the right and left coronary arteries, can take over as the heart's pacemaker. The AV node normally slows conduction of the impulse as it travels from the atria to the ventricles, providing a delay between activation and contraction of the upper and lower chambers of the heart.

The impulse travels from the AV node to the *AV bundle* or *bundle of His.* This bundle divides into one *right* and two *left bundle branches,* which conduct the impulse via *Purkinje fibers* and *transitional cells* to the working myocardium of the ventricles. The cells of the proximal AV bundle are smaller than ventricular cells, but as one proceeds distally, the cells of the conduction system gradually take on the appearance typical of *Purkinje cells.* Purkinje cells are bigger than ventricular muscle cells and contain a larger amount of glycogen. They have few organized myofilaments, which usually occupy only their periphery, and an abundance of intermediate filaments. Within Purkinje fibers, as in other parts of the conduction system, there are no T

tubules. Intercalated discs are present but are characterized by broad, irregular Z bands (Fig. 10–8). Impulse conduction along the Purkinje fibers is extremely rapid, consistent with the large size of the cells, their abundant glycogen, the presence of frequent gap junctions, absence of T tubules, and insulation from the surrounding myocardium by a sheath of connective tissue. Distally, the Purkinje cells evolve into "transitional cells," which are smaller than Purkinje cells, lack intercalated discs (although a few gap junctions are present), and have a very slow speed of conduction.

The progress of the impulse through the various parts of the conduction system is mirrored in the surface electrocardiogram: activation of the atria is reflected by the P wave, a delay is seen as the impulse travels through the AV node (the P-R interval), and then the ventricles are activated in an orderly sequence beginning with the septum (q wave), as is predicted by the distribution of the conducting fibers.

The Coronary Circulation

Because the heart depends on aerobic metabolism, an adequate blood supply is essential for cardiac muscle. As in skeletal muscle, there is

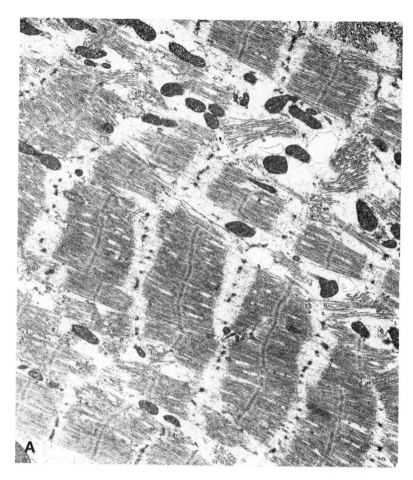

10–8 **A.** Thin section electron micrograph of a Purkinje cell from rabbit heart. Note the disorganization of the myofilaments, the patchy, irregular, and occasionally broadened Z-lines, and the abundance of glycogen. × 14,000. (From Thornell, L. E. 1973. J. Ultrastruct. Res. 44.) **B.** Higher power thin section of a Purkinje cell from avian heart. The presence of intermediate filaments, the disorganization of the sparse myofilaments, and the abundance of glycogen are evident. × 19,000. (From Bogusch, G. 1974. Cell Tiss. Res. 150.)

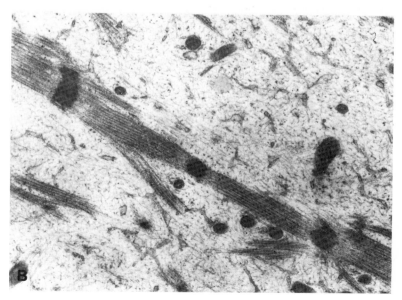

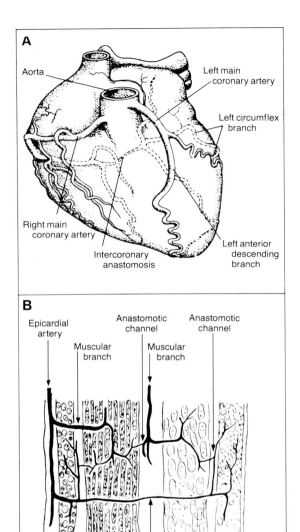

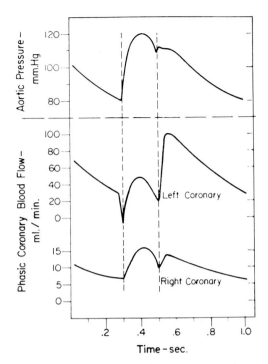

10–10 Graph of the flow in the coronary arteries during the phases of the cardiac cycle. Ventricular systole occurs between 0.3 and 0.5 sec, (indicated by the vertical **broken lines**) and is reflected in the rapid rise and peaking of aortic pressure. Left coronary blood flow is seen to be greatest in early diastole. (From Berne, A. M., and Levy, M. N. 1977. Cardiovascular Physiology, 3rd ed. St. Louis: Mosby.)

10–9 Diagram of the most common configuration of the major coronary arteries in man **(A)** and the distribution within the myocardial wall of the branches of these arteries **(B)**, which enter from the epicardial surface. Note particularly the presence of many interconnecting anastomatic channels. (From Katz, A. M. 1977. Physiology of the Heart. New York: Raven Press.)

one capillary per muscle fiber; these capillaries are supplied by the coronary arteries. The ramifications of the coronary system vary, but usually there is a dominant left coronary artery that splits into several main branches, and a smaller right coronary artery (Fig. 10–9). In view of the critical importance of maintaining the blood supply to the heart, it is reassuring to note that between the branches of the coronary arteries there are multiple collateral vessels, as large as 300 μm in diameter even under normal circumstances; in the event of coronary occlusion or narrowing, these collateral vessels usually increase in size and number, providing alternative routes for blood flow to areas distal to an obstruction. As is true for the rest of the systemic circulation, blood flow to the heart is subject to complex *autoregu-*

lation at the level of the small muscular arterioles, which dilate to allow for increased flow during hypoxia.

Because the ventricular myocardium is compressed during systole, most coronary flow occurs during diastole, when ventricular muscle is relaxed (Fig. 10–10). Normally, flow is evenly distributed throughout the thickness of the myocardium. Under certain circumstances, however, coronary flow may be compromised, especially to the subendocardial regions (which experience higher pressures because of geometric factors). Situations predisposing to inadequate coronary blood flow include tachycardia, which shortens diastole; hypotension, which lowers perfusion pressure; and high left ventricular end-diastolic pressure, which increases resistance to flow.

Innervation of the Heart

The heart has direct sympathetic and parasympathetic innervation, and there is a constant interplay between these usually opposite influences on heart rate and force of contraction. The sympathetic nerves arise from the superior and inferior cervical and the first thoracic ganglia; the parasympathetic innervation comes from the medulla via the vagus nerve. There is particu-

larly rich sympathetic and parasympathetic innervation of the SA and AV nodes (Fig. 10–11), but working myocardial cells of both the atria and ventricles are also supplied by autonomic fibers. As has been emphasized earlier, however, the role of the nervous system is regulatory rather than essential for the initiation and maintenance of cardiac function. Much of the autonomic effect can be achieved indirectly via humoral pathways, as can be demonstrated by the response of the transplanted heart to exercise: denervation affects the immediacy and the rate of cardiovascular response, but not its final magnitude.

10–11 Thin-section electron micrograph of a bundle of axons between cells of the SA node in rabbit heart illustrating its rich sympathetic (adrenergic) and parasympathetic (cholinergic) innervation. Adrenergic varicosities (**A**) can be identified by the presence of both large (**lcv**) and small dense-core vesicles (**scv**). Adrenergic varicosities are in close proximity to cholinergic nerve endings (**C**), in which large dense-core vesicles and small empty vesicles (**sev**) are seen. × 18,300 (From Tranum-Jensen, J., 1976, In Wellens, H. J. J., Lie, K. I., and Janse, M. J. (eds.), The Conduction System of the Heart. Philadelphia: Lea and Febiger, p. 55.)

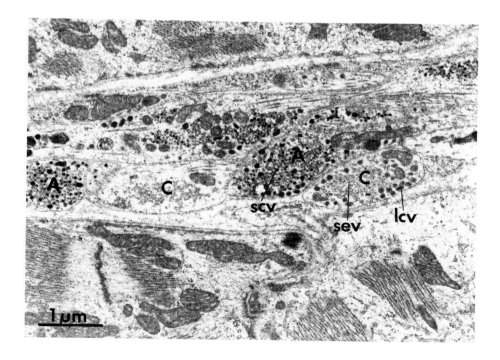

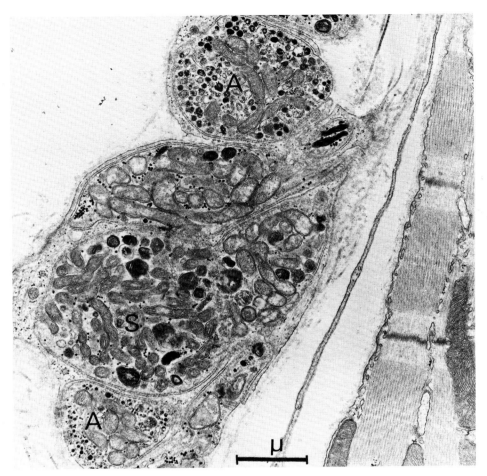

10–12 Thin section electron micrograph of a presumptive chemoreceptor sensory nerve ending from guinea pig atrium. Note the abundant small mitochondria, glycogen granules, large granular vesicles, and the dark lamellar bodies (which are characteristic and are assumed to be lysosomal). On either side are adrenergic nerve endings **(A)** whose small dense vesicles are easily visualized as a result of administration of the false transmitter 5-hydroxydopamine. × 19,000. (From Chiba, T. 1973. *In* Ultrastructure of the Mammalian Heart. New York: Academic Press, Inc.)

There are also afferent nerve fibers from the heart (Fig. 10–12) to the central nervous system, which allow the perception of ischemic cardiac pain, or *angina pectoris*.

References and Selected Bibliography

General

Challice, C. E., and S. Viragh (eds.). 1973. Ultrastructure of the Mammalian Heart. New York: Academic Press, Inc.

McNutt, N. S., and Fawcett, D. W. 1974. Myocardial ultrastructure. *In* Lander and Brady (eds.), The Mammalian Myocardium. New York: John Wiley & Sons, Inc., pp. 1–49.

Simpson, F. O., Rayns, D. G., and Ledingham, J. M. 1974. Fine Structure of Mammalian Myocardial Cells. Adv. Cardiol. 12:15.

Sommer, J. R., and Johnson, E. A. 1979. Ultrastructure of cardiac muscle. *In* Berne (ed.), Handbook of Physiology—The Cardiovascular System I. Pages 113–186.

Conduction System

Tranum-Jensen, J. 1976. The fine structure of the atrial and atrioventricular (AV) junctional specialized tissues of the rabbit heart. *In* Wellens, Lie, and Janse (eds.), The Conduction System of the Heart. Leiden: Steufert-Kroese, pp. 55–81.

Viragh, S., and Challice, C. E. 1973. The impulse generation and conduction system of the heart. *In* Challice and Viragh (eds.), Ultrastructure of the Mammalian Heart. New York: Academic Press, Inc.

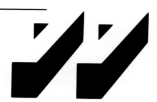

The Blood

Leon Weiss

The blood is a fluid tissue, which constitutes about 7% of body weight and 5 liters in volume in human beings, containing blood cells, which lie free in a protein rich liquid intercellular substance, the *blood plasma*. The blood is enclosed in blood vessels and flows through the body, propelled by the contraction of the heart, the recoil of the great vessels, the movement of muscles, the excursion of the lungs, and the force of gravity. Components of the blood regularly cross the walls of blood vessels and enter the perivascular tissues. Fluid, representing a protein-poor filtrate of the plasma, diffuses in massive volume through the walls of fine blood vessels and enters the perivascular tissue carrying nutrients, hormones, and other regulatory compounds to virtually every cell of the body. Most of this fluid diffuses back into the blood vessels carrying wastes and other metabolites. Some of the fluid flows into lymphatic vessels and thereby forms *lymph* (Chap. 15). Although red blood cells remain within blood vessels, white blood cells regularly leave them by passing through their walls into the perivascular tissues.

Freshly drawn blood is a red fluid of specific gravity 1.052 to 1.064. On standing, it rapidly clots into a jelly-like mass. However, if clotting is prevented, the blood cells settle, leaving the plasma supernatant. There are three layers in settled or centrifuged blood (Fig. 11–1). The lowermost layer, about 45% of the blood volume, is red and consists of erythrocytes, or red blood cells. A thin gray-white layer, the buffy coat, lies

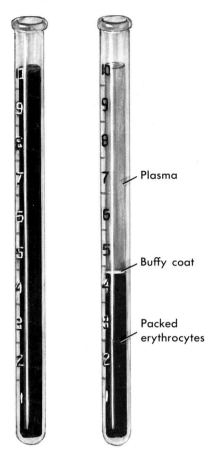

Plasma

Buffy coat

Packed
erythrocytes

11–1 Blood before and after sedimentation. The
volume of packed erythrocytes is almost 45%
of the total blood volume. The leukocytes and
platelets form a buffy coat, accounting for about 1% of
the blood volume. The remainder of the blood is the
supernatant plasma.

above the erythrocytes and accounts for about 1%
of the blood volume. The buffy coat is formed of
platelets and leukocytes, or white blood cells, of
which there are five types in human beings and
many vertebrates: lymphocytes, monocytes, polymorphonuclear neutrophils, polymorphonuclear
eosinophils, and polymorphonuclear basophils.
The uppermost layer of centrifuged blood is the
plasma.

The volume of packed red blood cells is
called the packed cell volume (PCV) or hemocrit
(H). There are approximately 10×10^6 red blood
cells per mm³ of human blood. They far outnumber leukocytes, whose concentration is normally
approximately 5×10^3 per mm³. The mean num-

bers of the different leukocyte types per milliliter
of blood are: neutrophils, 4,400; eosinophils,
200; basophils, 5; lymphocytes, 2,500; and
monocytes, 300. The normal level of platelets is
200,000 to 400,000/mm³.

The Structure of Blood Cells

Living Blood Cells

Living blood cells may be studied microscopically outside the body in hanging drops or in tissue culture and, in whole animals, in such favorable places as the web of the toe, the tongue, or
the mesentery, and in specially designed chambers inserted into accessible sites such as the ear
or skin (Figs. 11–2 and 11–3). Living cells may
be studied unstained by phase-contrast microscopy (Fig. 11–6) or interference microscopy, or
they may be stained supravitally (Fig. 11–4). Our
discussion, although applicable to many mammals, is concerned primarily with human blood.

Unstained Blood Cells. Living red cells are
orange-yellow, remarkably deformable, and without intrinsic motion. Their biconcavity is striking. They tend to stack into columns, similar to
stacks of coins, called *rouleaux*. Erythrocytes in
hypertonic media lose water by osmotic pressure
and shrink. The plasma membrane is thrown
into folds, and the cells assume a burrlike or *cre-
nated* appearance. In hypotonic solutions, on the
other hand, water enters erythrocytes. Their hemoglobin is leached out and they become enlarged colorless structures, termed *ghosts*.

Living leukocytes are motile. As they move on
a flat surface, they typically show an active anterior end that produces pseudopodia, a central
portion containing the nucleus and the bulk of
the cell, and a trailing cytoplasmic tail called the
uropod. A lymphocyte in motion looks like a
hand mirror, its round nucleus rimmed by cytoplasm and the uropod trailing like a handle (see
Fig. 11–13). Polymorphonuclear cells contain
distinctive cytoplasmic granules, the larger ones
in unstained cells seen as refractile structures.
They show nicely in phase-contrast, interference,
or dark-field microscopy.

Supravitally Stained Blood Cells. Certain organelles may be stained while living and observed in the surviving cells (Fig. 11–5, here and
color insert). Mitochondria are selectively revealed by their ability to maintain Janus green B

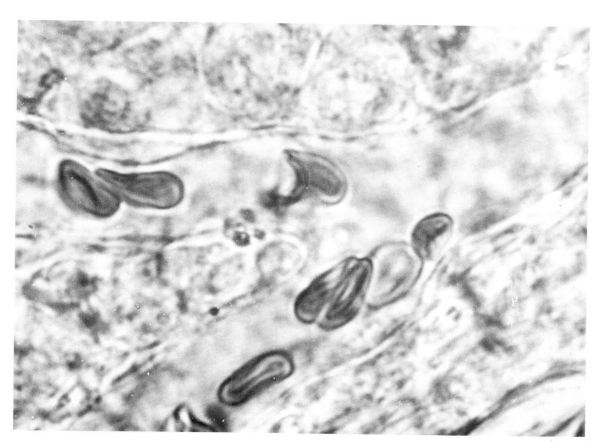

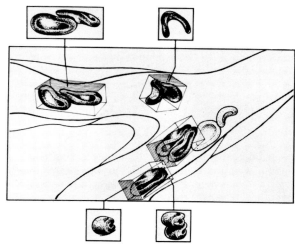

11–2 Deformation of erythrocytes in venule with an explanatory diagram illustrating Brånemark's interpretation of the mode in which each red cell has been stretched, bent, and twisted. Intravital photomicrograph of a human microvessel in connective tissue. × 2,750. (From Brånemark, P.-I. 1971. Intravascular Anatomy of Blood Cells in Man. Basel, Switzerland: S. Karger AG.)

in its oxidized or colored state. The granules of each of the polymorphonuclear leukocytes take up the dye neutral red, a pH indicator. One can thereby use color to differentiate the granules of neutrophils, eosinophils, and basophils. Neutral red also stains lysosomes and phagolysosomes. A rosette of neutral-red stained granules characteristically surrounds the centrosome in monocytes and probably represents lysosomal staining. Supravital staining is now seldom used, but

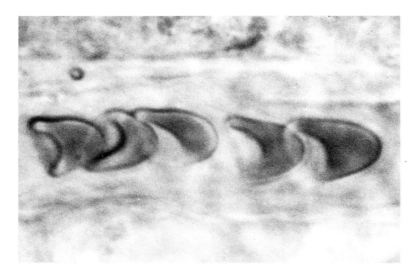

11–3 Deformation of human erythrocytes flowing in single file in a small venule. Intravital photomicrograph of a human microvessel. × 3,000. (From Brånemark, P-I. 1971. Intravascular Anatomy of Blood Cells in Man. Basel, Switzerland: S. Karger AG.)

it remains a valuable procedure for staining freshly produced erythrocytes, called *reticulocytes* (discussed in Chap. 12).

The Structure of Blood Cells in Romanovsky-Stained Smears

Smears of blood stained with Romanovsky-type stains are invaluable in research and clinical practice (Fig. 11–4, here and color insert). A blood smear is made by spreading a drop of blood to a thickness of one cell on a slide or a coverslip. The dried smear is fixed by methanol and stained with the Romanovsky dye mixture. Blood cells lie flat and are richly and subtly stained because of the many dyes and dye combinations in this type of stain. In addition to the ionized dyes eosin$^-$, methylene blue$^+$, and the azures$^+$ (oxidation products of methylene blue), Romanovsky mixtures contain neutral dyes (nondissociated eosinates of methylene blue and the azures). Commonly used Romanovsky stains are Wright, Giemsa, and May-Grünwald stains.

Human erythrocytes in such preparations are round or slightly oval, their diameter ranging from 6.5 to 8.0 μm. They bind eosin deeply around their thick periphery but the color gradually becomes very faint in their thin central zone (Fig. 11–5, here and color insert).

Polymorphonuclear neutrophils, approximately 12 to 15 μm in diameter, contain a heterochromatic nucleus segmented into three to five lobes joined by thin strands. Nucleoli are absent. The cytoplasm is stained pink and contains a moderate number of *azurophilic* granules that can just be resolved.

Eosinophils, 12 to 15 μm in diameter, often contain a trilobed heterochromatic nucleus with two large lobes joined by a strand from which a third small lobe hangs. The cytoplasm is dominated by striking eosinophilic granules. These granules are large, spherical, closely packed, uniform in size, and stained a deep bright red or orange.

Basophils measure 12 to 15 μm in diameter. Their nuclei contain two or three heterochromatic lobes, often less segmented than those of neutrophils or eosinophils. Cytoplasmic granules are most prominent, strongly stained violet, and often overlie the nucleus.[1] Well-preserved granules are nearly spherical and rather uniform in size, but their appearance varies because they are difficult to preserve.

Lymphocytes vary in size. Small lymphocytes, 5 to 8 μm in diameter, have a round or slightly indented heterochromatic nucleus without visible nucleoli, surrounded by a thin rim of clear blue cytoplasm containing a few small granules (Figs. 11–5 and 11–6). Large lymphocytes, up to 15 μm in diameter, have proportion-

---

[1]These granules, because of their content of sulfate groups, avidly bind basic dye and induce a spectral shift in the dye. They are therefore *metachromatic* (see Chap. 2). Strictly speaking, it is inappropriate to characterize a structure as metachromatic in a Romanovsky-type stain because such a stain is mixture of dyes, some of which are violet. To establish the presence of metachromasia, one should use a single dye such as toluidine blue.

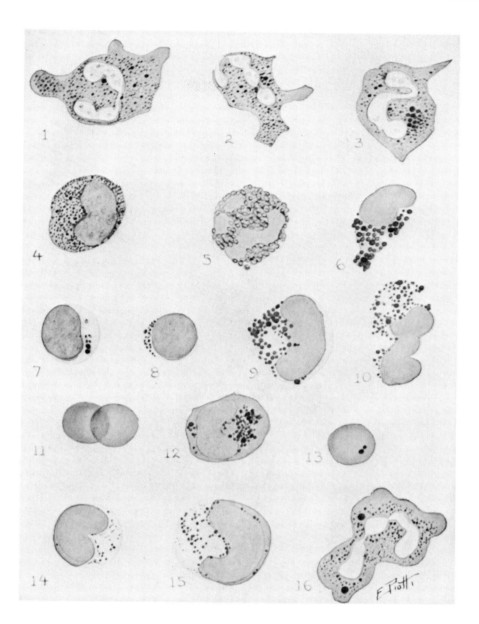

ally more cytoplasm. Their nucleus may be flattened or indented and it is less completely heterochromatic than in smaller cells. Nucleoli may be visible.

Monocytes, whose diameter is 12 to 18 μm, are among the largest of the white blood cells. The nucleus is often horseshoe-shaped but may appear only slightly indented. In contrast to the coarse chromatin of lymphocytes, the chromatin forms a delicate network. Nucleoli are typically not visible. Cytoplasm is abundant, gray or blue

11–4 Human blood cells stained supravitally. See special section for four-color illustration and lengthy caption.

in color, and "dusty" owing to many very fine, barely resolvable particles. A prominent centrosome lies in the nuclear indentation or *hof.*

Platelets are ovoid bodies, 2 to 4 μm in diameter, that tend to aggregate. They contain a central blue granular zone, the *granulomere,* and a lighter clear periphery, the *hylomere.*

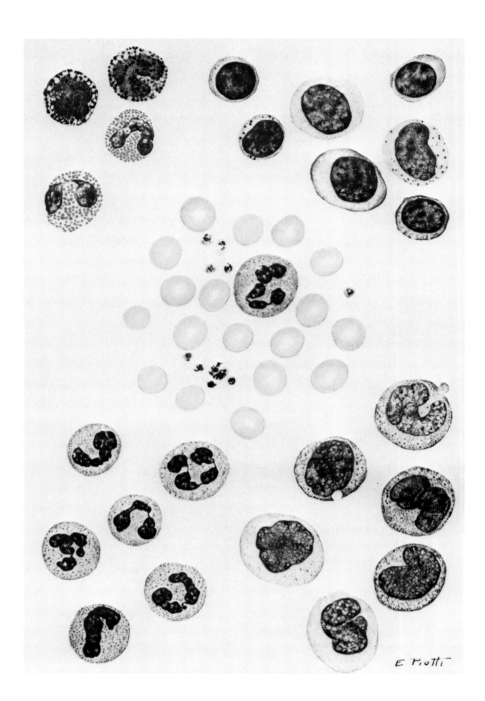

11–5 Cells from a smear preparation of normal human blood. See special section for four-color figure and lengthy caption.

A few dead or dying leukocytes are always present in blood smears. They are more fragile than viable cells and, partly because of the mechanical stress in preparing the smear, they may be spread out, torn, and appear reticulated or spongy. They are called, simply *smudge cells*.

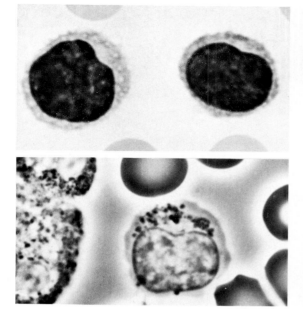

11–6 Lymphocytes of human blood. **Top.** Blood film
has been fixed and stained with Wright's
stain. Two small lymphocytes are present. **Bottom.**
Small blood lymphocyte is seen in a phase-contrast
photomicrograph. × 2,400. (From the work of G. A.
Ackerman.)

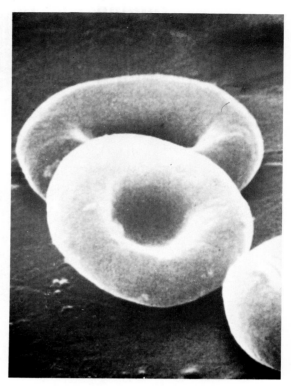

11–7 Human erythrocytes; scanning electron
micrograph × 10,000. (From Morel, F. M. M.,
Baker, R. F., and Wayland, H., 1971. J. Cell Biol.
48:91.)

Electron Microscopy of Blood Cells

In thin sections examined by transmission electron microscopy, erythrocytes contain a uniformly granular density representing hemoglobin. Some ferritin may be present. Ribosomes,
mitochondria, endoplasmic reticulum (ER), Golgi
complexes, and lysosomes are absent in mature
cells. Clear vesicles may be present. Spectrin, a
protein distinctive to erythrocytes, occurs as a
network of filaments beneath the plasma membrane. It may be masked in normal hemoglobin-
containing cells, but visible in hemolyzed cells.
The plasma membrane is trilaminar in section
(see Fig. 1–24) but contains many descrete structures shown in freeze-fracture etch preparations
(Fig. 1–26). In scanning electron microscopy
the biconcave shape of erythrocytes is striking
(Fig. 11–7).

Neutrophils (Fig. 11–8) possess two types of
granules that are membrane-bounded and together number about 200. *Primary, type A* granules, corresponding to the azurophilic granules
of light microscopy, account for about 20% of the
granules. They are relatively large (approximately 0.4 μm), dense, and homogeneous when
well fixed. Often some extraction occurs during
the processing, however, leaving less-dense irregular structures. Approximately 80% of the
granules are *definitive, secondary,* or *type B.*
They are smaller, less than 0.3 μm, less dense
than primary granules, and may contain a crystalloid (Fig. 11–8). Type B granules are often invisible by light microscopy so that only the relatively few azurophilic granules can be seen.[2]

---

[2]The term neutrophil designates the human cell. In rabbits
and certain other species, the secondary granules are eosinophilic, large, and spherical. In birds the granules are eosinophilic and rod-shaped. To distinguish these cells from true eosinophils, they are termed *pseudoeosinophils.* The generic
term for this cell type regardless of species and staining reaction is *heterophil.* By electron microscopy, heterophils of rabbits (pseudoeosinophils) and human beings (neutrophils) are
remarkably alike. But these terminological distinctions are
being lost in usage. The term heterophil is being used to refer
to those granulocytes, in birds, for example, that are the counterparts of the neutrophil.

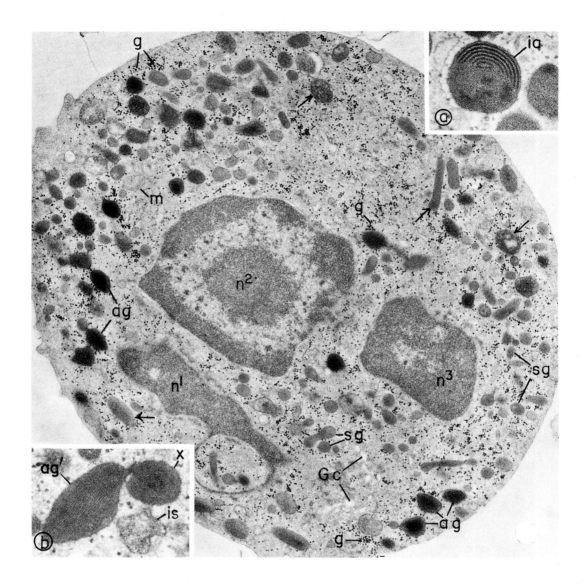

11–8 Mature human polymorphonuclear neutrophil (PMN). Several lobes of the nucleus are present (n^1 to n^3), and numerous granules, as well as glycogen **(g)**, are scattered throughout the cytoplasm. A few mitochondria **(m)** and a small Golgi complex **(Gc)** are also visible. Some of the granules present are large and dense **(ag)**, whereas others are small and less dense **(sg)**. However, many granules are intermediate in size and density. Elongated forms, including football and dumbbell shapes, are also present **(arrows)**. The insets depict internal structure within the large, dense (azurophilic) granules. **Inset a** shows a spherical granule **(ia)** containing concentric half-rings. **Inset b** illustrates the crystalline lattice with periodicity of approximately 100 Å, which is commonly seen in football or ellipsoid forms **(ag')**. A cross section **(X)** of the ellipsoid form and an immature specific granule **(is)** are also present in this field taken from a PMN myelocyte. The sequence of development of these cells together with additional electron micrographs (Fig. 12–15) is presented in Chaps. 12 and 13. **a,** × 45,000; **b,** × 45,000. (From Bainton, D. F., Ullyot, J. L., and Farquhar, M. G. 1971. J. Exp. Med. 134:907.)

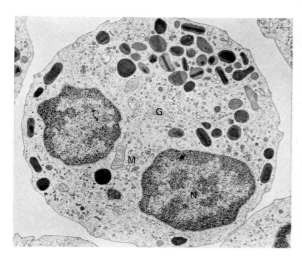

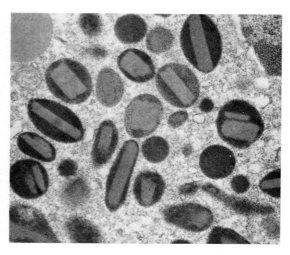

11–9 Eosinophil obtained from the peripheral blood of a normal human subject. Fixed with glutaraldehyde and osmium tetroxide. Note that the granules have an electron-dense "core" and a less electron-dense "matrix." **N,** bilobed nucleus; **G,** Golgi body; **M,** mitochondria. × 7,742. (From Zucker-Franklin, D. 1974. Adv. Intern. Med. 19:1.)

11–10 Eosinophil granules treated with phosphotungstic acid during dehydration. Note that the electron density of the core and matrix is reversed. × 27,160. (From Zucker-Franklin, D. 1974. Adv. Intern. Med. 19:1.)

Eosinophils have large (0.16 to 1.0 μm), spherical, membrane-bounded granules that contain an angular, dense, and lamellated crystalloid (Figs. 11–9 and 11–10). They also contain a few smaller dense nonspecific granules.

The specific granules of basophils are membrane-bounded structures about 0.5 μm in diameter (Fig. 11–11, A and B) that contain granular material, myelin figures, lucent zones, and crystalloids. A few nonspecific granules may also be present. Specific granules are similar but not identical to the granules of mast cells, (Chap. 4).

Lymphocytes (Figs. 11–12 and 11–13) contain a number of lysosomal granules and small-to-moderately sized Golgi complexes. They may contain polyribosomes and some profiles of smooth ER, but, unless undergoing "blast" transformation or proliferation (discussed under Lymphocytes, below), they possess little rough ER. Lymphocytes, as other cells, have distinctive molecules on their cell surface. They are not evident in conventional transmission electron micrographs, but may be visualized by special stains (see following section on Cytochemistry).

Monocytes contain moderate numbers of lysosomes, prominent Golgi complexes, and rough ER. The centrosome is large and may be surrounded by microtubules.

Platelets (Fig. 11–14) have a plasma membrane with a heavy glycocalyx. The plasma membrane dips into the cytoplasm to become continuous with a system of canaliculi (the open canalicular system). Electron-microscopic markers such as thorium dioxide placed in the plasma have ready access to the canaliculi. Microfilaments of the actin–myosin system lie directly beneath the plasma membrane and among microtubules. A bundle of microtubules runs as a hoop around the periphery of the platelet and probably accounts for its lenticular shape. Platelets contain a variety of membrane-bounded granules. *Dense-core granules* 0.5 to 1.5 μm in diameter, similar to a class of synaptic vesicles, contain serotonin, ADP, ATP, and calcium. *Alpha granules,* somewhat larger and more numerous, contain various substances related to blood clotting: platelet factor 4, which neutralizes heparin; factors that increase vascular permeability and are chemotactic for neutrophils, platelet fibrinogen, actin and myosin, and ADP, ATP, and ATPase. The alpha granules are lysosomal in character, moreover, because they contain many of the acid hydrolytic enzymes characteristic of lysosomes. A few staightforward lysosomes, *lambda granules,* are present as well. There are a few mitochondria. Small profiles of smooth membrane that represent the dense tubular system are present. They concentrate calcium and

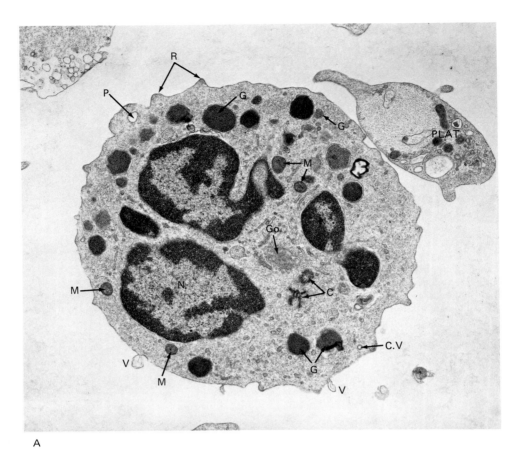

A

11–11 A. Electron micrograph of a normal human basophil leukocyte. This cell was taken from a person who suffered from allergic rhinitis on exposure to grass pollen, but not on exposure to ragweed pollen. When an aliquot of washed blood cells was incubated in vitro with a ragweed extract, there was no release of histamine and the basophils looked normal as shown here. The cell surface is smooth, showing only small ridges **(R)**, pockets **(P)**, and vesicular protrusions **(V)**. One platelet is adherent to the cell surface **(PLAT)**. The cytoplasm contains many typical basophilic granules **(G)**, which vary in size and shape. Also shown are the polymorphous nucleus **(N)**, four mitochondria **(M)**, the Golgi apparatus **(Go)**, the two centrioles **(C)** and a coated vesicle **(C.V)**. × 15,000. **B.** Electron micrograph of a degranulated human basophil leukocyte. This cell was taken from the same donor as that shown in part A. In

synthesize prostaglandins. Particles of glycogen are also present.

Cytochemistry of Blood Cells

Much may be inferred of the chemical composition of blood cells from their appearance in Romanovsky-type preparations, such as the strongly anionic nature of eosinophilic granules and the strongly cationic nature of basophilic granules. The use of selective or specific cytochemical reagents can extend this information at both the light- and electron-microscopic levels (Chap. 2). There are many chemical moieties common to many blood cells, such as ribonucleoprotein and actin. The most significant use of cytochemistry, however, has been to reveal compounds distinctive to a cell type, or to certain phases in the cycle of that cell type, or to certain subtypes; thus cytochemistry provides the basis for identifying a cell type and for understanding its function and life history.

Erythrocytes are positive for hemoglobin, gradually synthesized during their development.

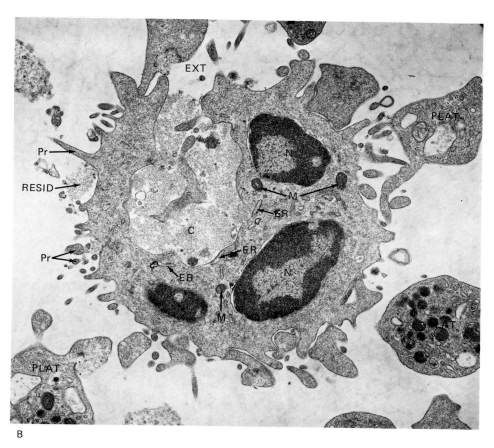

B

the same experiment, an aliquot of washed blood cells was incubated in vitro with a grass extract. Secretion of more than 95% of the histamine in the cells resulted and the basophils appeared degranulated as shown here. The cell surface is irregular, showing numerous projections of variable appearance (**Pr**). Other leukocytes and platelets (**PLAT**) are adherent to the surface of the basophil. No basophilic granules can be seen in the cytoplasm, but a large membrane-bounded cavity (**C**) is evident, which contains residual granular material and communicates widely with the exterior (**Ext**). Further residual granular material can be seen at the cell surface (**Resid**). Also shown are the polymorphous nucleus (**N**), three mitochondria (**M**), and cisternae of smooth endoplasmic reticulum (**ER**). × 15,000. (From Hastie, R., Levy, D., and Weiss, L. 1977. J. Lab. Invest. 36:173.)

Spectrin can be localized by immunocytochemistry. The azurophilic granules of neutrophils are lysosomal in nature because they contain lysosome-associated enzymes. The specific granules contain a cytochemically demonstrable peroxidase. The granules of neutrophils contain many other enzymes and metabolically active compounds (page 462), most of which can be demonstrated cytochemically. The pronounced eosinophilia of the eosinophilic granule is largely due to a major basic protein (MBP) present in the crystalloid. This protein accounts for more than 50% of granule protein, has a molecular weight of 11,000, and is quite rich in the amino acid arginine, which bears a strongly cationic, terminal guanidonium group (pK > 11). The capacity of the granules to bind eosin or other anionic dyes seems to be due to MBP. The granules contain lipid, reactive both with Sudan black B and with methods for phospholipid. Myeloperoxidase is present and can serve as a marker. Other granule enzymes are arylsulfatase, phospholipases, acid phosphatase, β-glucuronidase, ribonuclease, and cathepsin. The intense metachromatic basophilia

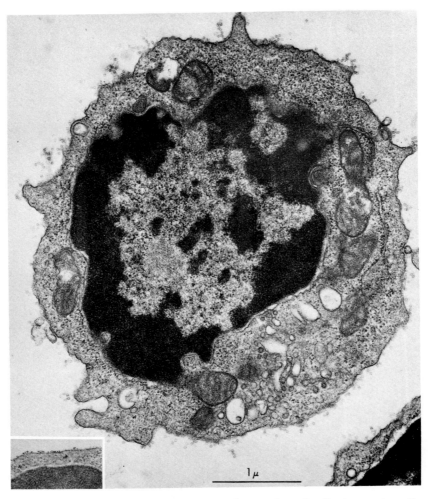

1μ

11–12 Electron micrograph of mouse B lymphocyte.
The antibody receptors on the surface of this cell have been revealed by an antibody to the mouse antibody receptors prepared in a rabbit (rabbit antimouse immunoglobulin, RAMG). The RAMG has been linked to a large hemocyanin molecule, and this molecule, which looks like a little box under the electron microscope, serves as a label indicating the presence of the mouse antibody receptors. Note that the label is distributed rather uniformly over the surface of the B lymphocyte. This preparation was labeled at a temperature of 4° C. At this temperature the antibody receptors, which are mobile, are fixed in their uniform distribution on the cell surface. At higher temperatures, after being linked with RAMG, the antibody receptors would move to one pole of the cell and concentrate there—a phenomenon known as *capping.* In the **inset,** at the same magnification, is a portion of another mouse B lymphocyte treated in the same way, except that ferritin, an iron-bearing compound is conjugated to the RAMG. The disposition of ferritin, visualized as dense particles, indicates the distribution of antibody receptors on the surface of the mouse B lymphocyte. (From Karnovsky, M. 1972. J. Exp. Med. 136:907.)

of the specific granules of basophils is due to heparin, a strongly anionic, sulfated mucopolysaccharide. These granules are periodic acid–Schiff-positive (Chap. 2). The staining reactions of basophilic granules are quite similar to those of mast cell granules. Monocytes contain lysosomes and therefore show reactions for acid phosphatase and other lysosome-related enzymes. Platelets and the granulocytes can be stained for glycogen, and the dense-core granules of platelets for serotonin.

It has proved of great value to characterize molecules on the surface of blood cells because many critical cellular interactions are initiated

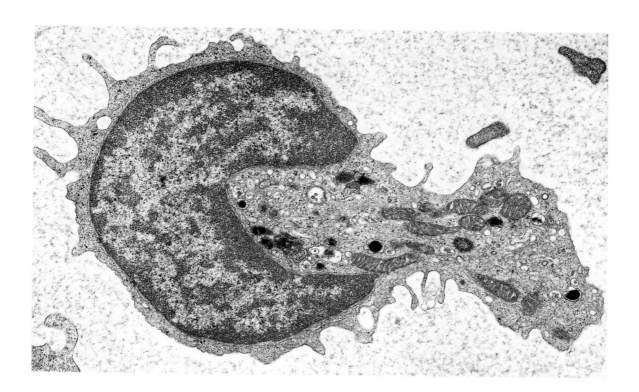

by structures there. Some of these molecules may be present in a number of cell types, as, for example, those on the surface of monocytes and some lymphocytes that bind the Fc component of antibody. Others are quite specific to a given cell type. Thus, erythrocytes have a molecule on their surface that binds transferrin, the serum protein that transports iron. This transferrin receptor permits iron to be taken up by red cells and translocated into the cell where it is used in hemoglobin synthesis. As would be expected, immature erythroid cells synthesizing hemoglobin have more of this receptor than those in which hemoglobin synthesis is complete.

On the basis of molecules on the cell surface that can be stained by immunocytochemical methods (see Chap. 2), lymphocytes may be divided into three classes: B cells, T cells, and null cells. This division, which underlies our understanding of the immune system, is discussed in the section on Lymphocytes, below.

Cytochemical data, especially from enzyme histochemistry and immunocytochemistry, are increasingly important in understanding the blood cells and hematopoietic tissues, and they will be further discussed, in this and following chapters.

11–13 Human lymphocyte. A motile lymphocyte contains a moderate number of membrane-bounded granules. Note the microvilli on the cell surface. It is likely that the lymphocyte is moving to the left, advancing with its nuclear pole. The cell assumes a hand-mirror configuration. The tail of cytoplasm has been termed a *uropod*. × 9,200. (From the work of G. A. Ackerman.)

Functions of Blood Cells

Erythrocytes

Erythrocytes transport oxygen from pulmonary alveoli to the tissues and carbon dioxide from the tissues to pulmonary alveoli. In alveoli, oxygenated blood has an oxygen tension of approximately 96 mm of Hg, whereas in systemic venous blood coming from the tissues, the oxygen tension is approximately 40 mm of Hg. Venous blood also carries carbon dioxide at a pressure of almost 50 mm of Hg, far greater than that in alveoli. As a result, oxygen diffuses through the alveolar wall into erythrocytes where it is loosely bound by the heme of hemoglobin. At the same time, carbon dioxide leaves the plasma and hemoglobin where it travels as bicarbonate and carbaminohemoglobin and diffuses into the al-

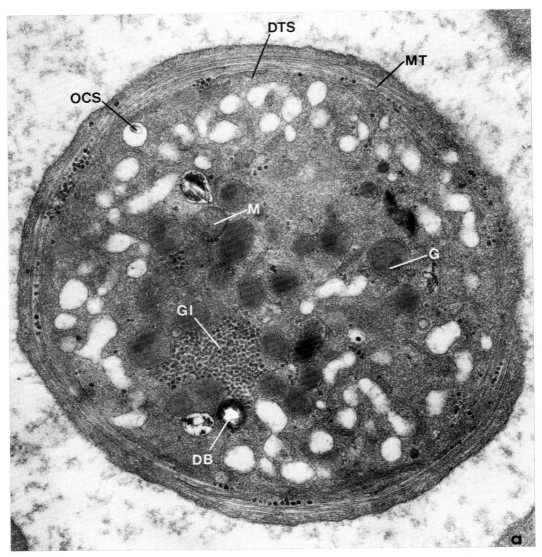

11–14 Human platelet blood. **a.** Cross section through the equatorial region of a discoid platelet. The microtubules **(MT)** form a peripheral ring. Several dense bodies **(DB)**, granules **(G)**, glycogen **(Gl)**, and mitochondria **(M)** are present. The open canalicular system **(OCS)** lies as a system of connecting tubules. In this section their surface connection is not evident, but see part a. Elements of the dense tubular system **(DTS)** are also present. × 41,000. **b.** Longitudinal section through a discoid platelet. The open canalicular system **(OCS)** lies in the center, its connection to the outside evident on the lower surface **(arrow).** The microtubules **(MT)** are present in cross section at the poles of the platelet. Elements of the dense tubular system **(DTS)** are also present. × 41,000. (From the work of James G. White.)

veoli. When blood reaches capillaries, oxygen dissociates from the hemoglobin and diffuses through the plasma and capillary wall and out into the surrounding tissues, while carbon dioxide diffuses from the tissues into the plasma and into erythrocytes.

Hemoglobin, a globular chromoprotein of 68,000 daltons, is a tetramer, each unit consisting of a heme group associated with a polypeptide chain, the globin. The heme group is a protoporphyrin composed of four pyrrole rings coordinated through their N atom with iron.

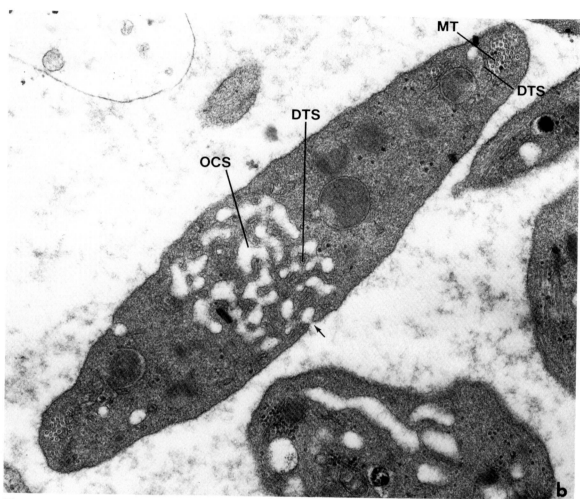

Figure 11–14b

Heme occurs not only in hemoglobin, but in myoglobin and such enzymes as catalase, peroxidase, and the cytochromes as well. Normal adult human globin consists of two alpha chains (each 241 amino acids long) and two nonalpha chains. The major adult hemoglobin, hemoglobin A (HbA) contains 2 beta chains (246 amino acids long). Each of these four chains has eight helical segments; the four chains, arranged in two pairs, are coiled in a distinctive quaternary structure into a globular molecule with the hemes lying in pockets in the center. Here the iron of heme associates with oxygen. The iron must be maintained in a ferrous form in order to transport oxygen. The oxidized form, *methemoglobin,* is inactive. Erythrocytes contain an enzyme, *methemoglobin reductase,* that maintains hemoglo-

bin in its reduced state. Hemoglobin constitutes about 33% of the weight of the cell and is in so concentrated a solution that it approaches the crystalline state. It may, in some pathological conditions, become so viscous as to reduce the plasticity of red cells and prevent efficient blood flow. The biconcave shape of erythrocytes, maintained by the subplasmalemmal framework of spectrin, efficiently makes the interior of the cell quite accessible to oxygen and carbon dioxide. In flow, the central biconcavity is commonly drawn out and the erythrocyte circulates in the shape of a cone, apex forward (Fig. 11–2). The spectrin framework also stabilizes the red cell membrane against the shearing forces encountered in flow. In spectrin-deficient animals, erythrocytes lose their biconcave shape and are short-lived. Ma-

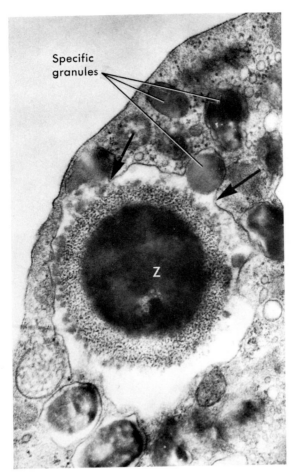

Specific granules

11–15 Phagocytic polymorphonuclear heterophil of the rabbit. This cell, harvested from the peritoneal cavity, has ingested zymosan particles **(Z)**. The specific granules of the heterophil discharge their content of hydrolytic enzymes into the phagocytic vacuole. The granule moves toward the phagocytic vacuole; its membrane fuses with the membrane of the vacuole **(arrows)**; and the contents of the granule enter the phagocytic vacuole. × 30,000. (Courtesy of D. Zucker-Franklin.)

ture erythrocytes, lacking nucleus, ribosomes, and mitochondria, have lost their capacities for protein synthesis and aerobic metabolism. They depend on glycolysis for energy, most of which is used to maintain hemoglobin in the reduced state and to maintain the internal ion concentration through active transport of ions across their semipermeable plasma membrane. Mature erythrocytes have lost the capacity to synthesize new cell membrane. They have even lost the capacity to control fully the chemical composition of their

plasma membrane. For example, the cholesterol concentration in the red cell membrane is determined by the cholesterol concentration in the plasma and not by the metabolism of the red cell. This is important because membrane plasticity, which is necessary for red cell survival, is affected by the cholesterol content of the membrane.

Neutrophils

Antimicrobial Actions. Neutrophils phagocytize and often kill bacteria and other infectious organisms that enter the body. Neutrophils are necessary to life: an individual without them or with impaired neutrophils dies of infection. A neutrophil moves toward bacteria because they release an attractant that diffuses into the surrounding tissue and interacts with the leukocyte membrane (chemotropism). There are also host factors, such as *complement* released in an inflammatory response, that attract neutrophils. The phagocytic system of neutrophils, eosinophils, and basophils has been called the *microphage system* to distinguish it from the *macrophage system* (Chap. 4). Phagocytosis is facilitated by a surface against which the microorganisms can be pinioned: bacteria suspended in a fluid-filled body cavity may escape. Phagocytosis may be enhanced by certain antibodies called *opsonins*, which neutrophils can bind to their surface.

Phagocytosis by neutrophils and other granulocytes is associated with the fusion of granules and phagosomes (Fig. 11–15, and Chap. 4). In neutrophils the specific granules usually fuse first with the phagosome, often within 30 sec of its formation. Later the azurophilic granules may combine with the phagosome. Phagocytosis requires energy and causes increased oxygen consumption.

Because they are lysosomal in character, azurophilic granules contain acid hydrolytic enzymes. They also contain *lysozyme*, an enzyme complex that hydrolyzes glycosides in the cell wall of bacteria, and a myeloperoxidase that complexes with H_2O_2 producing activated oxygen, which is bacteriocidal. Specific granules also contain lysozyme, as well as *lactoferrin*, a protein that binds ferric iron. Lactoferrin is bacteriostatic as bacteria require iron, which is unavailable when bound to lactoferrin. Lactoferrin also inhibits the production of neutrophils. This property is the basis of a feedback loop in neutrophil production: as more neutrophils are produced, more lactoferrin is produced, and thereby more inhibition is exerted on neutrophil production. Specific granules also contain cationic compounds rich in arginine and lysine, which are bacteriocidal. These granules, moreover, can generate iodides, chlorides, fatty acids, and lecithins, all of which inhibit or kill microorganisms.

Because many of the functions of neutrophils and other leukocytes are revealed in the phenomenom of inflammation, we shall next consider certain phases of inflammation. If chemical irritants or bacteria or other foreign substances penetrate the body, a series of reactions is initiated that constitutes inflammation. Inflammation is largely a phenomenon of vascular and connective tissues. The ground substance is depolymerized and becomes much less viscous. Capillaries and venules supplying the affected area become dilated, increasing its blood supply and hence its temperature. The permeability of the vascular wall is increased and plasma pours into the surrounding connective tissues, causing swelling and increased pressure on nerve endings. Cells in the locale respond. Mast cells degranulate, further intensifying inflammation. The macrophages may become hypertrophied or "activated." Circulating polymorphonuclear leukocytes, monocytes, and lymphocytes escape from capillary and postcapillary vessels and move into the site. Bacteria are phagocytized. Lymphocytes, as discussed below, may release factors called *lymphokines* with far-reaching effects on other cells and on the inflammatory process. Monocytes are transformed into macrophages and they and other cells may release kines similar to lymphokines (termed *monokines* and *cytokines*). Neutrophils, eosinophils, basophils, and macrophages may degranulate and release a large variety of substances with microcidal inflammatory and diverse further effects, as discussed under each of these cell types. Immune reactions may supervene, augmenting the population and activities of macrophages, lymphocytes, plasma cells, mast cells, eosinophils, and related cell types.

Systems of factors that are derived largely from blood plasma and consist of polypeptides and proteins, many of which are enzymes, are complexly interrelated in inflammation, blood coagulation, and immunity. The *complement system* consists of at least 10 plasma components that, when activated, react sequentially with multifold consequences. Components of complement, in conjunction with certain antibodies,

cause cell lysis. Other components induce the release of histamine from mast cells and basophils (see below), are chemotactic for neutrophils, enhance phagocytosis, induce smooth muscle contraction, and can initiate the coagulation of blood. The *kinins*, another plasma system, include compounds such as the *kallikreins* that are chemotactic for neutrophils and that induce activation of the *Hageman factor*. This factor is a plasma globulin that can convert prekallikreins to their active form and it is also both able to initiate blood coagulation and to induce lysis of the blood clot *(fibrinolysis)*. One product of the kinin system is the nonapepetide *bradykinin*, which is as potent as histamine in inducing increased capillary permeability and the contraction of vascular and other smooth muscle. This system is also tied to the coagulation of blood. Other humoral substances, *prostaglandins*, have inflammatory effects, such as inducing pain, fever, and muscular contraction. The efficiency of acetylsalicylic acid (aspirin) depends on its antagonism to prostaglandins.

The ancients recognized these characteristics of inflammation: *tumor, rubor, dolor,* and *calor.* They constitute the cardinal clinical features of the acute inflammation. Leukocytes, largely neutrophils, are the preponderant cells in the immediate or acute phase of inflammation. They die after a short time. Dead and dying leukocytes mixed with serum and tissue fluids, yellow in color and creamy in consistency, are called *pus.* The activity of leukocytes underlies the swelling, redness, pain, and heat of a boil. As the acute phase of inflammation subsides and the process becomes subacute and chronic, the production and accumulation of neutrophils diminishes and macrophages come into the affected zone in larger numbers. They clear away cellular remnants and persisting irritants by phagocytosis and by releasing lytic enzymes. Most macrophages in inflammation come from circulating monocytes that leave blood vessels, move to the site of inflammation, and, as they do, are transformed into macrophages. Macrophages may in some instances accumulate and undergo further transformation into epithelioid cells and multinucleate giant cells. Indeed, the *granulomatous diseases,* which include tuberculosis and brucellosis, are characterized by nodular accumulations of macrophages and related cells.

Inflammation represents a major mechanism for controlling infectious disease, tumors, and other derangements. Inflammation is regulated by many feedback loops (for example, that of lactoferrin), but the process can escape control, become exaggerated, and can damage or kill the host. Further information related to inflammation is presented in the subsequent sections on basophils, eosinophils, and lymphocytes, and in the chapters on the connective tissues, bone marrow, thymus, lymph nodes, and spleen.

Basophils

Basophils are phagocytic motile granulocytes. Because their granules contain hydrolytic enzymes and form heterolysosomes, they undoubtedly share phagocytic-related antimicrobial features with neutrophils. Basophilic granules and those of mast cells are similar morphologically and physiologically.

Basophil granules contain heparin and histamine. Heparin is a sulfated mucopolysaccharide responsible for the metachromasia of the granules. It is an anticoagulant of blood and disperses lipid. Histamine, formed by the decarboxylation of the amino acid histidine; serotonin, which occurs in rodent basophil granules; and slow reacting substance (SRS) are vasodilating agents that induce increased vascular permeability. Unlike histamine, whose effects are prompt and transient, SRS acts in a more sustained fashion after a latent period. Slow reacting substance is lipid, possibly related to the prostaglandins. Thus the granules of basophils (and of mast cells) contain powerful mediators that affect blood vessels and intensify inflammation.

Basophils may degranulate in response to a variety of stimuli and can be important in general inflammation. However, a specific antibody-induced type of degranulation does occur. Certain antigens induce plasma cells to produce a distinctive class of antibody, immunoglobulin E (IgE), which quickly becomes fixed to the cell surface of basophils and mast cells. Loaded with IgE, basophils and mast cells remain apparently undisturbed. However, when the antigen that stimulated the production of IgE reenters the body, it combines with the IgE bound to the cell surfaces. The cells now undergo acute degranulation, releasing histamine and other mediators (Fig. 11–11, A and B). The reaction may be localized to certain shock organs such as the skin (the so-called *Prausnitz-Küstner reagenic response*) and the lungs (as in bronchial asthma); or it may be widespread and severe, as in the anaphylactic response after a bee sting or an injection of penicillin in allergic individuals.

These reactions that depend on degranulation of basophils and mast cells occur quickly and are classified as *immediate hypersensitivity.*

Basophils are also part of the initial response in a class of immunological reactions that take some time to develop, the so-called *delayed hypersensitivities* (see the section below on Cellular Immunity). Examples of delayed hypersensitivities that involve an initial basophil response are those associated with worm and viral infections, the allergic reaction in the skin after contact with certain chemicals (*cutaneous basophil hypersensitivity*), and that in tick infestations. In these reactions, basophils appear to induce inflammation, prepare the way for further immunological response, and, in the case of parasites, induce expulsion. In many cases where basophils occur, eosinophils are also present because basophils may release at least six factors chemotactic for eosinophils. These factors include eosinophilic chemotactic factor of anaphylaxis (ECF-A), tetrapeptides, and histamine. Basophils release additional substances that, on interaction with tissue factors, become chemotactic for eosinophils. Eosinophils are killer cells in certain parasitic infections. These infections induce a mast cell or basophil response that then calls in the eosinophils.

Basophils share many cytochemical and pharmacological characteristics with mast cells. However, they have a polymorphous nucleus unlike the round nucleus of mast cells. The ultrastructure of the granules of these two cell types, moreover, is similar but not the same. Some species have one cell type and not the other. Mice, for example, have mast cells and not basophils; turtles, basophils and not mast cells. Mast cells and basophils appear to have evolved as separate systems to meet similar needs and in many animals, as in human beings, supplement one another.

Eosinophils

Eosinophils, like neutrophils, are motile phagocytic granulocytes, but they lack the phagocytic capacity of neutrophils.

Eosinophils have a distinctive function: they kill the larvae of parasites that invade tissues, as in schistosomiasis, trichinosis, and ascariasis. In each of these diseases the level of circulating eosinophils may be driven to 90% of that of leukocytes. In experimental schistosomiasis in immune animals, a response involving mast cells and basophils occurs within about 5 min of the invasion of the parasite, and within about 15 min large numbers of eosinophils are on the scene. Within 2 h, eosinophils surround the larvae, virtually encapsulating them; degranulate on them, releasing MBP and other antilarval substances; and destroy them. If the eosinophil response is aborted, as can be done by administering an antieosinophilic antiserum, the parasitic invasion goes unchecked. The ability of the eosinophils to kill requires a specific antiparasitic antibody of the IgG type. In nonimmune animals (lacking an antiparasite antibody) the parasite may cause severe disease before immunity develops. Components of the host's complement systems can augment the eosinophils' antiparasite role. The parasitic larvae directly attract complement to their surface and thereby become chemotactic for eosinophils.

Basophils (and mast cells) summon eosinophils not only in parasitic infections where the eosinophil is a killer cell but in nonparasitic inflammation where the role of the eosinophil is less clear. Eosinophils do possess certain antiinflammatory capacities and can degrade inflammatory mediators released by basophils. For example, eosinophils can inactivate histamine because they contain the enzyme *histaminase.* However, the antibasophil role of the eosinophil must remain in doubt because in vitro assays show that the capacity of basophils to excite inflammation far exceeds the capacity of eosinophils to dampen it.

Lymphocytes are also important in eosinophil functions. Some of the lymphokines produced by lymphocytes in immune responses are chemotactic for eosinophils. Thus in inflammatory reactions where immune mechanisms are also activated, as in parasitic infections, both basophils (and mast cells) and lymphocytes elaborate factors chemotactic for eosinophils, bringing them to the site of reaction. Further, the increased production of eosinophils that occurs in the course of parasitic infection requires that a thymic-produced lymphocyte (T cell) serve as a helper cell (Chap. 15).

Lymphocytes

Lymphocytes are the central cell types of the immune system. The three types of lymphocytes (T cells, B cells, and null cells) look alike both with the Romanovsky stains and by conventional transmission electron microscopy, but they can be distinguished by cytochemical markers. B cells are the precursors of plasma cells, the cells that produce humoral or circulating antibody. These cells can be recognized microscopically by cytochemical demonstration of antibody molecules that cover their surface. T cells, comprising several subtypes, have both a primary role in cellular immunity and a role in the regulation of hematopoiesis, including control of the differentiation of B cells into plasma cells. T cells can be identified by distinctive marker molecules on their surface and in their interior. Null cells are lymphocytes that lack T- or B-cell markers. As expected, they represent a variegated group of cells including lymphocyte killer cells and hematopoietic stem cells. In order to understand the biology of lymphocytes and of the tissues—bone marrow–thymus, spleen, lymph nodes—of which they are an intrinsic part, a knowledge of immunity is necessary.

Immunity. The idea of immunity is rooted in infectious disease. If an individual survives an infection, he may thereafter be resistant or immune to disease caused by the infecting organism. Implicit in this phenomenon are both specificity (for the individual is resistant to the microorganism he has survived and not to others) and memory (because the immunity is long-lasting, or remembered). The immune system is a means of recognizing genetic relatedness. Thus, an individual will mount an immune response against foreign tissue but not against his own or genetically identical tissue. The immune system recognizes even slight differences between what is native to an individual and what is foreign, what is "self" and what is "nonself," and reacts against nonself. An intriguing speculation is that some forms of cancer represent a mutation that the host's immune system recognizes as nonself and therefore reacts against. The development of cancer may thus represent a failure of the immune system. Indeed, when an individual's immune system is suppressed by x rays or other means, the incidence of cancer is greatly increased. However, the immune system may in some cases lose the ability to distinguish between self and nonself and attack the host's own tissues. The process results in *autoimmune disease.* There are many such diseases of which certain thyroid, kidney, and connective tissue diseases and hemolytic anemias are examples.

The two major types of immunity are humoral immunity and cellular immunity.

HUMORAL IMMUNITY. Humoral immunity tends to be elicited by invading microorganisms that live outside of host cells and by toxins released by such microorganisms. The basis of humoral immunity is the secretion of antibody by plasma cells and by B lymphocytes undergoing transformation into plasma cells. The antibody diffuses through the blood plasma, lymph, and other fluids of the body. The large-scale secretion of antibody is triggered by antigen, and the presence of antibody throughout the fluids of the body constitutes a protective presence that eliminates or limits antigen. Antigens are particulate or colloidal substances, typically foreign to the host, which may be immunogenic (that is, capable of inducing an immune response). The surface of an invading microorganism, for example, bears many descrete antigens or *antigenic determinants*. Antibodies are proteins, for the most part gamma globulins. They are classified as immunoglobulins (Ig) and are of several types. Immunoglobulin M is a large pentameric molecule (molecular weight approximately 1,000,000) and is typically, in human beings and many animals, the first produced in an immune response. It is too large to cross the placenta and other vascular barriers. As an immune response proceeds, IgM production wanes and it is succeeded by IgG, a smaller (molecular weight approximately 160,000), more efficient, higher-affinity antibody capable of crossing the placenta (Fig. 11–16). Immunoglobulin G accounts for most of the antibodies in plasma. In secondary responses (that is, in responses occurring after reintroduction of antigen) IgG is the immunoglobulin produced. Immunoglobulin A is a secretory immunoglobulin produced in the mucosa of the respiratory tract, the gut, the genitourinary tract, mammary glands, and other places where a mucous membrane separates the body from the environment. It is produced by plasma cells beneath the epithelium and then passes through the epithelium, which secretes it into the lumen of the viscus. As it passes through the epithelium, two molecules of IgA are "dimerized" by a protein *secretory piece*, synthesized, and added by the epithelial cells of the mucosa. This dimerization may make the antibody more resistant to breakdown. Immunoglobin E is the class of immunoglobulin called *homocytotrophic*; that is, it becomes affixed to the surface of mast cells and basophils. Immunoglobin D, together with monomeric IgM, serves as receptor antibody on the surface of B lymphocytes. Its further roles have

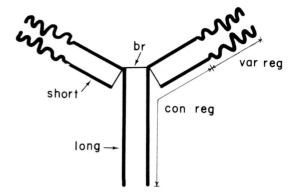

11–16 Schema of an antibody molecule of the immunoglobulin G (IgG) class. Paired long chains **(long)** diverge at the disulfide bridge **(br),** which joins them. At the site of divergence each long chain is joined to a short chain **(short)** by a disulfide bridge. Each long chain and each short chain has a variable region **(var reg)** and a constant region **(con reg)** that lie in register. The constant region, like the handle of a key, is the same—has the same amino acid sequence—for each class of immunoglobulin. The variable region, like the part of the key inserted into the lock, is different—has a different amino acid sequence—for different antigens. The variable region of the long and short chains lying in register is that part of the antibody molecule that engages the antigen, and has been referred to as the **fab** fragment of the molecule. Because this antibody molecule possesses two fab fragments, it is divalent, that is, capable of combining with two molecules of antigen. The constant region consists of paired portions of the long chains (below the bridge) and paired portions of long chain and short chain (beyond the bridge). The constant portion of the antibody molecule, referred to as the **fc** fragment, can combine with such substrates as complement or the cell surface of macrophages, and thereby confers certain distinctive biological properties upon its antibody class.

not been well defined. Humoral immunity may be transferred from an immune to a nonimmune animal by transferring either serum (which contains antibody) or antibody-producing cells.

Plasma cells are, in essence, unicellular glands that secrete antibody. They contain the organelles associated with the synthesis and secretion of protein, namely, nucleoli, rough ER, Golgi complexes, and the secretory vesicles. They are free cells, concentrated in lymphatic tissues (lymph nodes and spleen) but found in connective tissues throughout the body. They are ovoid, measuring 10 to 20 μm in diameter.

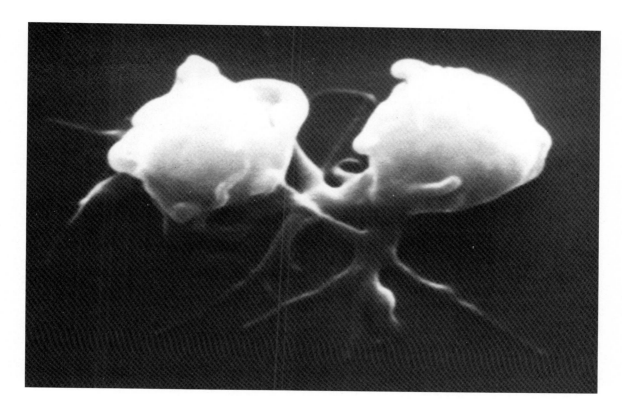

Plasma cells vary in appearance depending on phases in their life cycle (Fig. 12–17). Their distinguishing feature is the presence of antibody, which can be stained by immunocytochemical techniques, in cisternae of ER and perinuclear membranes. The Golgi apparatus of plasma cells is large. It "packages" the antibody and synthesizes and affixes a carbohydrate moiety to it. After the antibody is packaged in membrane, it travels to the cell surface in secretory vesicles and is released. The nucleus tends to lie eccentrically in the cell, displaced by the large cytocentrum. Its heterochromatin is often arranged in a pattern resembling the spokes of a wheel.

The precursors of plasma cells are B lymphocytes or, simply, B cells, which circulate in the blood (accounting for as few as 5–10% of the lymphocytes there) and also lie in characteristic loci in spleen, lymph nodes, and other lymphatic tissues. B cells can be recognized by immunocytochemical methods, which reveal molecules of immunoglobulin (types IgM and IgD) covering their surface. The antibodies lie in the plasma membrane of these B cells and readily move about in the plane of the membrane, with their antigen-combining sites directed outward and

11–17 Scanning electron micrograph of transformed platelets, displaying pseudopodia. × 30,000. (From the work of James G. White.)

free to react. These antibody molecules act as receptors for antigen. Each of the molecules of antibodies on the surface of a B cell, whether IgM or IgD, has the same antigen specificity. This specificity is very restricted, and in practice the antibody on a given B cell is capable of binding to only a single antigen. It is this narrowly focused capacity to combine with specific antigen that confers specificity on B cells and on the humoral immune system.

B lymphocytes function as follows: An antigen enters the body and, via lymph or blood, reaches sites of B-cell concentration (Chaps. 13 and 14). In these sites the antigen will "find" or "select" those B cells whose surface antibodies fit determinants on the surface of the antigen. The antigen will then link to immunoglobulin molecules on the cell surface. These antigen–antibody surface complexes now move to one pole of the B cell, at the uropod (Figs. 11–12 and 11–13) and are then taken up by endocytosis. Thus the production of plasma cells is initiated. It is a phenomenom associated with two concomitant processes. One process is the differentiation of B cells into plasma cells with concomitant high-level secretion of antibody. Curiously, those cells intermediate between B cells and the definitive small plasma cells, the *transitional cells*, produce the greatest amount of antibody. They have the appearance of large, activated lymphocytes or young plasma cells. The other process is proliferation of B cells, resulting in a B-cell clone. Indeed, it is a portion of this B-cell clone that differentiates into the plasma cells. However, a portion remains as B cells, thereby increasing the population of B cells with a given antigenic specificity. This larger pool of B lymphocytes provides the immunological memory of humoral immunity and is the basis of the heightened, brisker, and more sustained antibody response when the antigen is reintroduced, *the secondary response*. B lymphocytes may be long-lived cells, surviving months and even years. Plasma cells, on the other hand, live only about 2 weeks. Humoral immunity is an efficient process because clusters of antibody-producing cells in strategic locations produce prodigious amounts of antibodies, which, diffused through the fluids of the body, provide protection against the antigen that stimulated their production.

Some antigens, particularly those having polymeric or repeating structure, can directly induce B cells to convert into plasma cells. Most antigens cannot do this without the help of T lymphocytes. The sequence is this: a T cell recognizes and combines with antigen by means of receptors on its surface; the T cell then moves to an appropriate B cell, perhaps with the help of a macrophage (see below), and presents the antigen to the immunoglobulin receptors of the B cell.[3] Alternatively, the T cell may release lymphokines, which affect B cells. T cells may also inhibit antibody formation. Those T cells that help to convert B cells into plasma cells are a subclass, *T helper cells* (T_H). T cells that suppress the conversion are another subclass, *T suppressor cells* (T_S).

Macrophages are important in antibody formation. They have multiple roles in immunity but they do not have the narrow antigenic specificity of lymphocytes. As a rule, only antigens that are processed by macrophages are immunogenic. When sheep erythrocytes are injected into mice and elicit an immune response, they must be broken up into colloidal or small-sized particles. Macrophages do this. In addition, macrophages may hold antigen on their surface for long periods and present it to lymphocytes.

There is now recognized a class of cells, *antigen-presenting cells*, that includes stromal cells in lymphatic tissues, the *follicular dendritic cells* and the *interdigitating cells*, and the *Langerhans cells* of the epidermis. Their roles, and that of macrophages—which have long been accorded the function of antigen presentation—are being sorted out. These cells hold Ag on their surface, probably by cell surface receptors that bind the fc portion of the Ab molecule (fc receptors) and present the Ag to the immunocompetent lymphocytes. Without antigen-presenting cells, it is believed that many antigens would fail to reach the immunocompetent lymphocytes and that immunity would therefore fail to develop.

Macrophages destroy excess antigen. Antigen in very high (or very low) concentration causes the immune system to be unresponsive—a type of immune paralysis or *tolerance*. By phagocytizing a portion of antigen and destroying it or isolating it from immunocompetent cells, macrophages may bring the level of antigen to immunogenic levels.

Humoral antibody forms complexes with the antigen that stimulated its production and these Ag-Ab complexes will initiate a variety of responses (such as phagocytosis, lysis, activation of the complement and kinin systems, and inflammation) that tend to limit and eliminate antigen. The protective functions of the immune system are thereby accomplished.

MONOCLONAL ANTIBODIES. The immunoglobulin molecules that serve as receptors on B lymphocytes are capable, as are all antibodies, of combining quite selectively with complementary molecular conformations or *antigenic determinants* on the surface of antigens. Such complex antigens as foreign erythrocytes, viruses, bacteria, and even proteins, present many antigenic determinants on their surface. Any given B lymphocyte characteristically responds to only one antigenic determinant by producing immunoglobin molecules whose antigen-combining groups are identical (of the same *idiotype*). Therefore, as many B lymphocytes may participate in an antibody response as there are antigenic determinants on the surface of the antigen. Further, more than one B

---

[3]To become activated, a T cell must have two cell-surface receptors satisfied, as discussed below under Cellular Immunity. One of these receptors is a receptor for "self," which the macrophage as an accessory cell may satisfy.

lymphocyte may be activated by a single antigenic determinant, the idiotype produced by one lymphocyte fitting the antigenic determinant to greater or lesser degree than that produced by another—that is, with greater or lesser *affinity*. Because each lymphocyte and its clone (the lymphocytes and plasma cells derived from it by proliferation and differentiation) produce antibody molecules (of the same idiotype), this immune response is *monoclonal*. But, since an antigen bears many antigenic determinants, many different monoclonal lymphocytes are elicited in an immune response. The response is therefore *polyclonal*. If one isolates a single lymphocyte in an antibody response, it is difficult to obtain any useful amount of monoclonal antibody because the lymphocyte does not produce much antibody and does not live very long. Until recently, therefore, it has been possible to obtain monoclonal antibody in significant quantities only in unusual situations. The disease *multiple myeloma* is one such situation: A B lymphocyte differentiates into a malignant plasma cell, the *myeloma cell*, and proliferates intensely. This single malignant clone expands to completely fill the bone marrow, crowding out—with lethal consequences—all of the other hematopoietic cells and in the process producing large amounts of monoclonal antibody. Although myeloma antibody is not stimulated by a known antigen and it is abnormal, much fundamental knowledge of antibody has been learned from it.

Recently it has become possible, by an extraordinarily clever and remarkably simple means, to produce in large amount monoclonal antibody to known antigenic determinants. A single B lymphocyte obtained by micropipetting minced spleen from an animal undergoing an antibody response is fused with a myeloma cell taken from a standard laboratory strain of myeloma cells which has lost its capacity to produce antibody but which maintains its capacity for unlimited proliferation. The result of this fusion is a hybrid cell that partakes of the myeloma's capacity for unlimited proliferation—*immortality*—and of the lymphocyte's capacity for monoclonal antibody production. The hybrid cell produces much more antibody than that of the starting B lymphocyte, perhaps because the myeloma cell confers not only immortality but a heightened capacity for protein synthesis on the hybrid. Cell fusion technology can regularly be done by exposing cells to propylene glycol. The clones or *hybridomas* thus produced are the source of wholesale quantities of monoclonal antibodies.

They may be maintained in tissue culture or transplanted to the peritoneal cavity of a mouse where they form an ascites tumor producing prodigious amounts of monoclonal antibody.

Because each of the different lymphocyte idiotypes contributing to an immune response may be hybridized to a myeloma cell, one may obtain that array of monoclonal antibodies that reflects the array of antigenic determinants in the antigen. Antigens can thereby be "fingerprinted." For example, otherwise identical strains of poliomyelitis virus in an outbreak of polio may be differentiated and epidemiological studies carried out. Cell types, and subtypes, as varieties of lymphocytes or macrophages and their developmental and functional state, may be distinguished by distinctive varieties and patterns of cell surface antigens. Monoclonal antibodies prepared against antigenic determinants in such significant biological entities as the plasma membrane may be isolated and conjugated to a horseradish peroxidase or other cytochemical markers (see Chap. 2 on cytochemical methods) and an arsenal of powerful cytochemical reagents thereby created. This topic is presented more fully in the discussion in Chap. 14 of major histocompatability complex (MHC)–determined cell surface antigens on the plasma membranes of the epithelial cells of the thymus.

Monoclonal antibodies are becoming valuable in the clinic. If monoclonal antibodies are prepared against antigenic determinants that are distinctive to a tumor, the presence of that tumor and its metastases can be demonstrated by administering to the patient monoclonal antibodies tagged with radioactive isotopes. The distribution of the isotope, and inferentially of the tumor, can then be determined by scanning the whole body by using newer imaging techniques, as computer assisted axial tomography (CAT scanning) and nuclear magnetic resonance (NMR) imaging. Therapeutic use of monoclonal antibodies against tumors (immunotherapy) may be possible by conjugating a tumoricidal agent to the antibodies, which would deliver the agent specifically and in high concentration to the tumor.

CELLULAR IMMUNITY. In contrast to humoral immunity, which by the dispersion of antibody molecules has systemic scope, *cellular immunity* depends on immunologically competent cells working over short range in restricted sites where antigen is lodged. Cellular immunity is elicited by microorganisms (certain bacteria, protozoa, fungi, and viruses) that do not lie free in the host but lie intracellularly within macrophages and other cells, by diffusible products elaborated by these microorganisms, by grafts of tissue, by tumors, and by certain compounds applied to skin and other surfaces (contact hypersensitivity). In each of these varieties of cellular immunity the manifestations of the response to antigen by an immune or sensitized individual are not immediate, as they are in humoral immunity (see discussion of Arthus reaction, below), but delayed several hours. For this reason the term *delayed hypersensitivity* has been applied to cellular immunity, particularly to that variety elicited by products of the microorganisms causing cellular immunity.

Cellular immunity depends on T cells. T cells account for about 80–90% of the lymphocytes circulating in the blood and in thoracic duct lymph. They have surface receptors that are as specific for antigen as the immunoglobulin receptors of B cells. The molecular nature of the T-cell receptor for antigen is not known. However, there are functional immune response (ir) genes in T lymphocytes[4] and it is suspected that a low-molecular-weight compound with antigen-specific receptors may be coded by these genes, produced in the cell, and may move to the cell surface to serve as the antigen receptors of the T cell. T cells bear another receptor coded by the same gene complex. This receptor expresses "self." For a T cell to be activated, each of these receptors must be satisfied. In addition to presenting the Ag to the T cell, satisfying the T cell's Ag receptors, macrophages present their own surface molecules to satisfy the T cell's "self" receptors. Other distinctive substances can be demonstrated on the surface of T cells. Although the function of these substances is not known, they serve as markers. Antibodies—nowadays often monoclonal antibodies—to these substances may be prepared and, when suitably labeled, are the basis of immunocytochemical tests to detect T cells (Figs. 15–19 and 16–22). Because they may be recognized by antibody-conjugated reagents, these surface molecules are often termed *cell surface antigens*.

The cell surface antigens on T cells vary in kind and in concentration with the development of the T cell in bone marrow, thymus, and spleen (Chap. 12). Among the antigens that mark the surface of mouse T cells are varieties of the H-2 antigens. Certain H-2 Ag also occur on the surface of many other cells and seem to be responsible for exciting the host's cellular immune response to a graft, leading to rejection of the graft. The TL or thymic leukemia antigen is a cluster of several antigens on the surface of T cells during their thymic phase of development. These antigens are not present on T cells of every strain of mouse but do appear when leukemia develops. Mouse leukemia is virally induced, so that this surface antigen may well represent the product of a viral genome integrated into a mouse chromosome. *GIX* is another such antigen. It represents a glycoprotein component of the envelope of a mouse leukemia virus and is present in the thymic phase of T-cell differentiation but not in fully differentiated T cells. One of the first discovered of the T-cell surface markers in the mouse is the Θ antigen (also termed Thy-1). It is in both immature and mature T cells, but in somewhat lesser amount in the mature cell. This antigen is also present on certain brain cells, fibroblasts, and epithelia. The Ly-1 and Ly-2,3 antigens and surface markers are found on mature T cells in mice, human beings, and other species and are valuable because they correlate with T-cell function: the Ly-1 marks T_H cells and the Ly-2,3, marks both T_s cells and T cells that kill target cells bearing a specific antigen (T_C).[5] The markers so far discussed lie on the cell surface. Other markers of T cells may be internal, such as the nuclear enzyme *terminal deoxynucleotydl transferase (Tdt)*, an enzyme distinctive to thymic T cells. This enzyme adds nucleotides to segments of DNA and may play a role in inducing T-cell mutation and immunological diversity. Another internal enzyme that marks the adult T cells of many species is an *α-naphthyl-acid esterase* located in lysosomes. Some efforts have been made to differentiate T cells from other lymphocytes morphologically, i.e., by the presence of a smooth microvillus-free surface or by nuclear shape; but these "easy methods" have proved unreliable and we are left with having to use specialized immunocytochemical and enzyme cytochemical techniques to demonstrate the markers described above.

Cellular immunity depends on the specific interaction of antigen and T cell, often at the site

---

[4]These genes are part of an extensive gene complex, a "supergene," known as the *major histocompatability complex (MHC)* a name derived from transplantation immunology (page 524). In the mouse the MHC is known as the H-2 complex and is in chromosome 17. In human beings it is termed the HL complex and lies in chromosome 6.

[5]B cells possess an Ly-4 surface antigen.

of antigen, as in the bed or vasculature of a skin graft undergoing rejection. The antigen, somewhat denatured or altered, is held on the surface of antigen presenting cells and thus presented to T cells. Again, as in B-cell stimulation, the antigen must "select" the appropriate T cell. The stimulated T cell then undergoes clonal expansion and a portion of that clone probably engages in the cellular immune response, i.e. the production of lymphokines. The remaining cells of the clone constitute a bank of memory cells. Clonal selection, memory, and specificity are inherent in the phenomenon of cellular immunity, parallel to the B-cell response in humoral immunity. The fate of the activated lymphokine-producing T cells is unknown. They may die or become part of the memory pool.

Lymphokines have been identified on the basis of biological activity. Almost one hundred types have been postulated! Most probably, when they are chemically characterized, single lymphokines will be found to have multiple activities and, therefore, the total number of lymphokines will be considerably reduced. As the biology of lymphokines is further studied it is becoming evident that monocytes and macrophages can produce similar factors (hence, the term *monokine*), as can other cell types (hence, the term *cytokine*). Quite possibly, these small nonimmunoglobulin molecules represent a general way by which cells may affect one another. Lymphocytes, of course, are distinctive because their lymphokine production can be specifically activated by antigen.

The actions of lymphokines may be appreciated in an example of cellular immunity, the rejection of a homograft of skin.[6] After such skin is grafted, T lymphocytes (which, as discussed in Chap. 12, circulate and recirculate through the tissues) enter the bed of the graft, flowing through its blood vessels. Those T cells bearing surface receptors specific for the foreign antigen encounter and interact with that antigen held on the surface of macrophages. The antigen is often associated with blood vessels of the graft, the first foreign place the host T cell reaches at the graft site. The lymphocytes become activated and

produce and release lymphokines. One of the best characterized of the lymphokines is *macrophage migration inhibition factor* (MIF). Macrophages normally wander in and out of tissues. However, if they are exposed to MIF, they cease wandering and accumulate—in this example, in the bed of the graft. *Macrophage activation factor* (MAF), another lymphokine (perhaps overlaping MIF in activity) would activate these macrophages (see Chap. 4), making them "irate." *Lymphotoxin* (LT) damages or destroys cells other than lymphocytes. *Lymphocyte blastogenic factor* (BF) induces "blast formation" and division in lymphocytes. Other lymphokines released by the antigen-stimulated T cells are chemotactic for basophils and eosinophils and bring these granulocytes to the scene. Some lymphokines affect vascular permeability; others are generally cytotoxic. The net effect of this complex process is the rejection of the graft.

A classic type of cellular immunity serving as an example of delayed hypersensitivity occurs in tuberculosis as the *tuberculin reaction*. A purified protein derivitive (PPD) of tubercle bacilli is injected into the skin of a tuberculous animal. This animal is sensitive to many antigens in the bacilli, including PPD. The site of injection is first apparently unreactive, and then in 4 to 8 h redness and induration (hardness) appear. The reaction builds to a peak in 24 to 48 h, thus "delayed hypersensitivity," and then subsides. It may consist only of redness and some swelling, but if severe it can be painful and ulcerated. The basis of the reaction is that circulating T lymphocytes sensitive to the PPD, i.e., having surface receptors for the PPD, enter the site where tubercle bacilli lie; there they react through intermediary macrophages with the bacilli's PPD and liberate lymphokines. These lymphokines immobilize local and passing macrophages, call in lymphocytes and other cells, and induce the inflammation and cell damage characteristic of the tuberculin reaction. Despite the fact that sensitized lymphocytes initiate the process, the major cell types present and effecting the reaction are monocytes and macrophages. Thus this process, like that of the skin graft presented above, depends on sensitized lymphycytes moving to the site and acting locally.

In contrast, an example of humoral antibody-mediated immunity is the *Arthus reaction*. In this case, an antigen is injected into the skin of an individual who is immunized against that antigen and carries circulating antibody to it.

---

[6]A homograft is within the same species but between different strains, such as the different strains of inbred mice (AKR to C57B). An *isograft* is a graft from donor to recipient of the same strain (e.g., AKR to AKR). Because individuals of the same strain (and same sex) are the same genetically, isografts are not rejected. Humans, being outbred, may have isografts only between identical twins.

Within minutes after injection, the skin is inflamed: red, painful, hot, and hard. This reaction is initiated by injected antigen combining with circulating antibody at the site. The antigen–antibody complex combines with complement and other serum factors and causes local injury, inducing inflammation and an accumulation of large numbers of neutrophils.

In summary, lymphocytes are central in the immune response. B lymphocytes are precursors to plasma cells. They synthesize antibody and underlie humoral antibody production. T lymphocytes are the basis of cellular immunity, a complex of immune reactions directed toward intracellular bacteria, viruses, protozoal parasites and fungi, tumors, tissue grafts, and certain soluble, diffusible compounds. In addition, T cells may regulate humoral antibody production. T_H lymphocytes, a subset of T cells, permit B lymphocytes to mount a humoral response; T_s lymphocytes, another subset, suppress B-cell maturation and forestall a humoral response. Because of their specificity for antigen and their capacity for establishing immunological memory (immunity), lymphocytes are called "immunologically competent cells."

THE DEVELOPMENT OF IMMUNOLOGICAL COMPETENCE. At birth most mammals are immunologically quiet, both because their immunological capacities are not fully developed and because the placental barrier has shielded them from foreign material. The newborn, moreover, is protected against many infectious diseases by maternal antibodies that cross the placental barrier and circulate in its body. Such transplacental antibody constitutes a *passive immunization*. The immunological competence of a fetus increases as the time of parturition approaches, and within a few days of birth the newborn's own immunological mechanisms become active because of exposure to antigens. That the fetus does possess increasing immunological capacity can be shown experimentally by its production of antibody after direct injection of antigen.

Lymphocyte Control of Hematopoiesis. T lymphocytes appear to play a significant role in the production of blood cells (hematopoiesis). Intact animals will generate high levels of eosinophils when infected with nematode parasites whose larvae encyst in host muscle, but athymic animals lacking T cells are unable to bring their eosinophils over basal levels. When supplied with T cells, however, animals deficient in T cells can generate high levels of eosinophils. Under certain conditions, moreover, heightened neutrophilopoiesis also seems to depend on the thymus. With regard to erythrocytes, colonies derived from cell precursors in tissue culture increase in number and size when cocultured with T cells. Certain anemias, such as the Diamond-Blackfan syndrome, may be due to T_s cells inhibiting erythropoiesis. The best known and best understood example of T-cell control of hematopoiesis concerns the differentiation of B cells into plasma cells after stimulation by antigen. T_H and T_s cells regulate this process, as described above. Thus T lymphocytes may exert a general control over hematopoiesis, of which the differentiation of B lymphocytes into plasma cells is but an example.

Monocytes

Monocytes are the precursors of macrophages. Their functions are discussed in Chap. 4.

Platelets

Platelets are essential in preventing and staunching hemorrhage. They seal off small breaks in blood vessels, they participate in blood coagulation, and they maintain the competence of endothelium. If a blood vessel is cut and its endothelial continuity broken, certain plasma proteins—notably *Von Willebrand's factor*—are absorbed upon the exposed subendothelial collagen and other extracellular connective tissues. Within seconds circulating platelets establish contact with this subendothelial tissue and adhere to it. The platelets spread out over the damaged zone and their surface becomes altered, so that newly arrived platelets adhere to them and a hemostatic *platelet plug* is formed. As circulating platelets join the plug, they change from the discoid or lenticular form to a flattened or spherical shape with spicule-like pseudopodia (Fig. 11–17). These pseudopodia undoubtedly facilitate plug formation. This *primary aggregation* of platelets is induced by a number of factors: ADP (adenosine diphosphate) released from adherent platelets, epinephrine, and the plasma protein *thrombin*. Aggregation, moreover, is dependent upon *plasma fibrinogen* and *calcium*. As the process unfolds, the adherent platelets undergo a *release reaction*, a type of secretion wherein the platelets discharge first their dense granules and then their alpha and lambda granules. Non-granular platelet substances are also released. The release reaction causes even a larger build-up of aggregated platelets, or *secondary aggregation*.

Directly after vascular injury, during platelet aggregation, *blood clotting* or *coagulation* is initiated by plasma factors and factors released from the damaged vessel. Blood coagulation is the consequence of the sequential interactions, or *cascade*, of perhaps thirteen plasma proteins. The last step in this cascade is the conversion of the monomer plasma protein *fibrinogen* to the linear polymer *fibrin* through the action of the plasma enzyme *thrombin*. Fibrin forms an interlacing network of slender fibers, running among the platelets and trapping erythrocytes and other blood cells. The result is a jelly-like bulky clot that, with the platelet plug, serves to block bleeding. Although the blood clot may be initiated without platelets, the adherent platelets are essential to the production of a useful clot. They display great procoagulant activity by which they accelerate and magnify the process of blood coagulation. The platelet surface, exposing phospholipids such as platelet factor-3 and other substances, serves to collect coagulation proteins and facilitate their cascade. Moreover, many platelet factors secreted in the release reaction promote coagulation.

A blood clot may not only block bleeding, it may also obstruct the flow of blood by bulging into the vascular lumen. Such bulging is considerably reduced by the contraction of the clot, *clot retraction*. This platelet function is accomplished by the contractile proteins actin and myosin and adenosine triphosphate (ATP) and ATPase contained in platelets. With its injury covered by the clot, the vessel heals and its endothelium is regenerated. The clot is no longer needed. A plasma protein *plasminogen* is converted to the hydrolytic enzyme *plasmin* by *plasminogen activators* secreted by endothelial cells, and plasmin dissolves the clot.

Related to their role in hemostasis, platelets maintain the competence of endothelium. When the level of circulating platelets is reduced below about 60,000/ml^3, *(thrombocytopenia)*, fine blood vessels lose their competence and blood seeps out of them *(thrombocytopenic purpura)*. Restore platelets to normal levels and vascular competence is restored.

[See Chap. 12 for References and Selected Bibliography.]

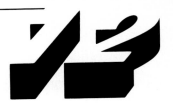

The Life Cycle of Blood Cells

Leon Weiss

Origin and Development of Blood Cells

Blood cells, like keratinocytes in skin and epithelium in gut, have a short life span. But they are constantly renewed in specialized centers, *hematopoietic tissues*, and their numbers are thereby kept constant. The system, moreover, is responsive. In infection, for example, hematopoiesis may be intensified and large numbers of leukocytes produced. Blood cells are normally released to the circulation only when sufficiently mature. They circulate within blood vessels but may temporarily stop circulating and become marginated cells. Erythrocytes and platelets remain within the vasculature. However, leukocytes will leave blood vessels and enter the perivascular tissue where they function, undergo cellular transformation, or are destroyed. Or, apparently unchanged, they may reenter the circulation, often via lymphatic vessels.

Sites of Production of Blood Cells

The major discrete hematopoietic tissues are bone marrow, spleen, lymph nodes, and thymus. There are other large concentrations of hematopoietic tissue, notably in the walls of the gastrointestinal tract. Prenatally hematopoiesis also occurs in yolk sac and liver and other sites. Except for the thymus, which has entodermal, mesenchymal and, perhaps, ectodermal components, the major hematopoietic organs in mammals are of mesenchymal origin. They contain a stroma made up of reticular cells and fibers, are supplied by vessels and nerves, and are enclosed by a capsule and trabeculae. The stroma holds free cells, including the blood cells and their precursors, macrophages, plasma cells, and mast cells.

Prenatal Hematopoiesis

Hematopoiesis in the human embryo begins in the second week of life, extraembryonically, in the wall of the yolk sac. Small nests of hematopoietic cells, largely erythroblastic (that is, producing erythrocytes), lie in mesenchyme surrounded by developing blood vessels. These foci constitute *blood islands*. The vessels enlarge and form a network within the wall of the yolk sac, connect to the systemic intraembryonic vessels through the vitelline vasculature, and become part of the circulation. By the sixth week of embryonic life erythropoietic foci appear in the liver, which becomes the major hematopoietic center. Hepatic granulocytopoiesis is minor, but there is moderate production of platelets and macrophages. Bone marrow appears in the clavicle in the second month and, with increased formation of bone, becomes extensive. It becomes the dominant hematopoietic organ in the latter half of gestation, when hematopoiesis in the liver wanes, and throughout postnatal life. All of the blood cells except T lymphocytes are produced in the marrow, and even T cells originate in marrow as stem cells and migrate to the thymus where they differentiate. From the second month of gestation the thymus engages in restricted hematopoiesis, the production of T cells.

A minor level of hematopoiesis, largely erythropoietic, becomes established in the spleen in the third fetal month and fades in the fifth. The spleen and lymph nodes receive and stock T cells from the thymus as early as the second fetal month, but only in the first postnatal weeks do the stocks become large. Although the liver is inactive hematopoietically after birth, it does retain its potential for hematopoiesis. In cases of bone marrow failure, hematopoiesis may be resumed there (and in the spleen), a phenomenon called *extramedullary hematopoiesis*.

Hematopoietic Stem Cells

A hematopoietic stem cell is capable of both sustained proliferation (producing a clone) and differentiation into mature blood cells. If only a portion of the clone differentiates into blood cells a population of stem cells is maintained. A stem cell may be multipotential, able to differentiate into any of the blood cells, or it may be of more limited potential, such as the stem cell capable of differentiating only into monocytes and neutrophils.

The existence of a pluripotential hematopoietic stem cell, which had been in doubt, has been demonstrated largely by the work of Till and McCulloch and their associates. The demonstration, although secure, is rather indirect because the stem cell has no distinguishing characteristic or marker, like, for example, the hemoglobin of red blood cells or the immunoglobulin receptor on B cells. It depends upon injecting cells that bear distinctive chromosomal markers (revealed in a metaphase karyotype) into lethally irradiated hosts, in the following type of experimental model.

After lethal irradiation (more than 900 rads) a mouse dies with all of its blood cells profoundly depleted (pancytopenia). Death may be averted if the mouse is given a suspension of living bone marrow cells from another mouse of the same inbred strain. The recipient mouse survives and in early stages of its recovery shows in both bone marrow and spleen, against a background of irradiation-induced devastation, grossly visible nodules that represent colonies of proliferating hematopoietic cells (Fig. 12–1). These colonies will grow and differentiate, and within weeks bone marrow and spleen are restored. The cellular composition of the hematopoietic colonies varies. Many of them contain only one or two types of blood cell but a significant number contain each of the blood cell types (Fig. 12–2). There is evidence that each of these colonies, including those with multiple blood cell types, is a clone (i.e., derived from a single hematopoietic cell precursor).

The evidence for such clones is obtained by irradiating the donor marrow cells severely, but not lethally, to induce chromosomal damage. This damage occurs in a widespread unpredictable way and results in cells each with uniquely or highly distinctively abnormal chromosomes (Fig. 12–3). Becker, Wu, Till, and McCulloch found that when such irradiated donor cells containing uniquely damaged chromosomes form splenic or bone marrow colonies in lethally irradiated recipients, different hematopoietic cell types within a given colony bear the same distinctive karyotype. This finding reveals that different blood cell types, such as erythrocytes, granulocytes, and monocytes, can originate trom

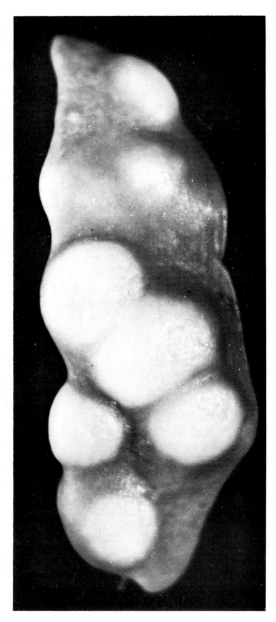

12-1 Splenic nodules. This spleen was removed
from an animal given lethal irradiation and
then a "rescuing" injection of bone marrow cells. The
stem cells, which constitute a portion of the marrow,
circulated to the irradiated spleen where they
remained, proliferated, and formed these macroscopic
colonies. Later these colonies will coalesce and the
normal structure of the spleen will be restored. (From
the work of J. Till and E. McCulloch.)

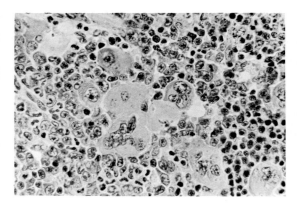

12-2 Splenic nodule. A number of splenic nodules
have a diverse hematopoietic population
including virtually all hematopoietic cell types. This
light-microscopic field is from such a nodule. (From
the work of W. T. Wu, J. Becker, J. Till, and E.
McCulloch.)

12-3 "Unique" mouse karyotype. The clonal nature
of the splenic colonies exemplified in Fig.
12-1 is revealed by distinctive or unique karyotypes
in the donor marrow cells. These karyotypes are
induced by lightly irradiating the donor cells (see
text). **Arrow** points to the distinctively damaged
chromosomes that serve as a marker. (From the work
of W. T. Wu, J. Till, and E. McCulloch.)

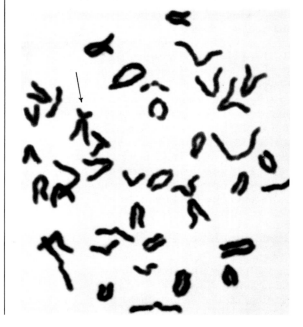

the same stem cell. Further evidence supporting the clonal nature of splenic colonies includes a linear relationship between the number of nucleated donor cells and the number of splenic and bone marrow colonies, and the resemblance of the irradiation–survival curve of colony-forming cells to that of single cells in tissue culture or tumor transplants.

The greatest concentration of multipotential stem cells in the adult, as determined by spleen colony assay, is in the bone marrow. The total number in the marrow of the mouse may be 40,000 stem cells. In contrast, the spleen may have only 2,000. The vastly greater capacity of the marrow relative to the spleen to restore an irradiated recipient is explicable by its 20-fold superiority in stem cell content. But even its relatively high content of stem cells does not represent, for the marrow, a high concentration; in the mouse it is 1 per 10,000 nucleated cells. Stem cells circulate, and there are approximately 10 in each milliliter of blood, which represents 1 per million nucleated blood cells, one-hundredth the concentration in the marrow. Stem cells circulate in the fetus and are present in fetal liver and bone marrow. When hepatic hematopoiesis declines, the number of circulating stem cells becomes unusually high, suggesting their large-scale emigration from liver to marrow.

Although no direct evidence of the structure of the multipotential hematopoietic stem cell exists, indirect evidence strongly indicates that structurally it is a lymphocyte, although many investigators eschew that term and prefer to call it a *candidate stem cell* (Figs. 12–4 and 12–21). The indirect evidence of its appearance is garnered from experiments carried out by Van Bekkum and his colleagues, using the Till and McCulloch spleen colony assay to measure the number of stem cells in a bone marrow suspension. The relative number of multipotential stem cells is greatly increased if dividing hematopoietic cells are destroyed by treating the suspension with vincristine, a drug whose action is like that of x rays.[1] The number of multipotential stem cells is further increased by subjecting the marrow suspension to density-gradient centrifu-

gation and obtaining a number of fractions, one of which can be determined to be rich in stem cells by spleen colony assay. By these methods, the stem cell concentration in a marrow suspension may be increased by a factor of 40 or more. In proportion to the increase in stem cells is the presence of a cell type, the candidate stem cell, which is lymphocytic in appearance (as seen in Fig. 12–4). Because the existence of multipotential stem cells was first clearly demonstrated on the basis of colonies in the splenic assays of Till and McCulloch, this cell has been termed the colony forming unit–spleen (CFU-S). It circulates in the blood as one of the *null cells*, one of the lymphocyte types that is neither T cell nor B cell.

The above discussion has been confined to the multipotential stem cell (CFU-S). There are stem cells derived from CFU-S capable of differentiating only into red cells or into white cell types. These more restricted stem cells, revealed by specialized tissue culture techniques, are discussed below under Culture of Erythrocyte Stem Cells and under Culture of Granulocyte and Monocyte Stem Cells.

The Life Cycle of Erythrocytes

The earliest erythroid cell recognizable in Romanovsky-stained smears of bone marrow is a fully endowed cell having nucleus, ribosomes, mitochondria, Golgi apparatus, and so forth. It serves as a stem cell for erythropoiesis, the production of erythrocytes. The nucleated precursor cells of erythrocytes are called *erythroblasts*.

In Romanovsky preparations, hemoglobin binds the anionic dye eosin because its globin is strongly cationic; RNA binds the cationic dye methylene blue[+] and the azures[+] because its phosphate groups are strongly anionic.[2] Accordingly, in early-stage erythroblasts with many ribosomes and little hemoglobin, the cytoplasm is stained deeply with basic dyes (blue in Romanovsky stains). In late stages of development, on the other hand, with few ribosomes and abundant hemoglobin, the cytoplasm is deeply stained with acid dyes (red in Romanovsky stains). Therefore, early erythroblasts are called

---

[1]Multipotential stem cells divide infrequently. They are, in fact, held in reserve and are not even in the cell cycle, being in G_0 (Chap. 1). It is left to the more differentiated stem cells to proliferate and differentiate, carrying on the normal business of the bone marrow, and these dividing cells are highly sensitive to x rays or to *radiomimetic* drugs.

[2]Positively charged dyes are termed *basic dyes* and negatively charged dyes are termed *acid* by histologists. Tissue components that bind basic dyes are called basophilic and those that bind acid dyes, acidophilic. See Chap. 2.

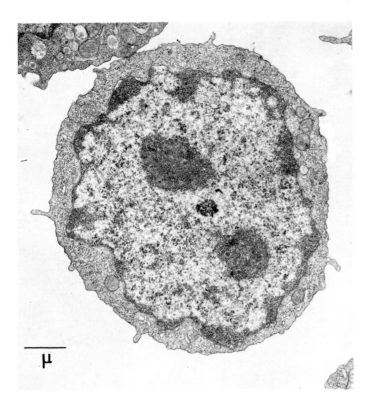

12–4 Candidate stem cell. There are no obvious morphological signs indicating cellular differentiation. The cytoplasm is rich in free ribosomes. × 15,130. (From the work of Van Bekkum et al. 1971. Blood 38:547.)

μ

basophilic erythroblasts,[3] and late erythroblasts having almost the true color of mature red cells are called *orthochromatic erythroblasts.* (The term *normoblast* is commonly applied to orthochromatic erythroblasts.) In intermediate stages, the hue of the cytoplasm represents a combination of the colors of the acid and basic dyes, and the cells are therefore termed *polychromatophilic erythroblasts* (Figs. 12–5 [here and color insert] to 12–7). Cell diameter decreases as erythroblasts differentiate, the basophilic erythroblast being about 15 μm in diameter, the orthochromatic erythroblasts or normoblasts, only 8 to 10 μm. The erythroblast pool is maintained by proliferation of basophilic and polychromatophilic erythroblasts. Normoblasts are postmitotic, that is, they do not divide.

By electron microscopy the cytoplasm of erythroblasts contains polyribosomes, small Golgi complexes, mitochondria, a few lysosomes, hemoglobin, ferritin, scanty endoplasmic reticulum

(ER), some microtubules, actin, and spectrin. Basophilic and early polychromatophilic erythroblasts contain abundant polyribosomes. By the orthochromatic stage, the polyribosomes are considerably reduced in both concentration and ribosomal number. The density of the cytoplasm, owing to the hemoglobin, increases throughout maturation. *Ferritin,* a protein able to store as many as 2,500 iron atoms, may be scattered as single molecules or in the aggregated form, *hemosiderin.* Hemosiderin may be collected into membrane-bound granules, *siderosomes.* Iron is transported by a plasma iron-binding globulin, *transferrin,* to transferrin receptors on the surface of erythroid cells. Here the iron flips to the inside of the cell for storage (as ferritin or hemosiderin) or for use in hemoglobin synthesis (Chap. 11). In basophilic erythroblasts a bit of rough ER is present, but even this rapidly diminishes. One or more Golgi complexes occur, and these too become quite small and disappear by the orthochromatic phase. Mitochondria diminish in number and size in polychromatophilic cells. A few remain in orthochromatic erythroblasts (normoblasts) and they are absent in mature erythrocytes (see Fig. 12–21).

---

[3]Some authors recognize a *proerythroblast* as less differentiated than the basophilic erythroblast. It is a similar cell but somewhat larger.

Cells from bone marrow.

Cells from spleen.

Cells found in circulating blood.

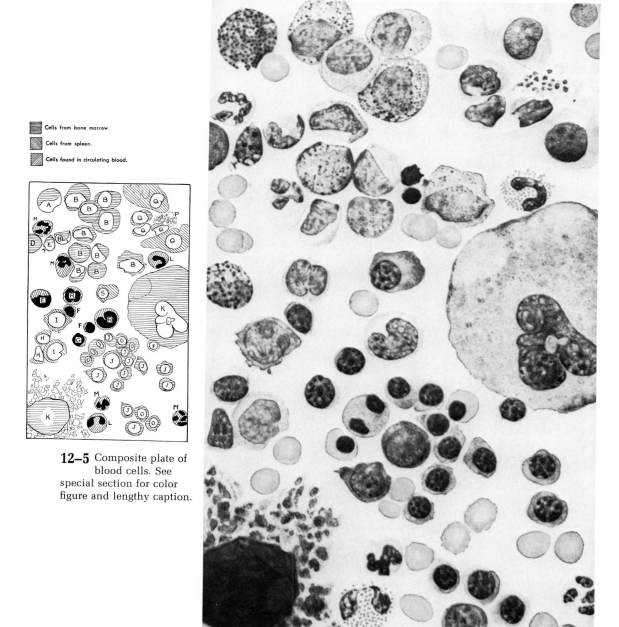

12–5 Composite plate of blood cells. See special section for color figure and lengthy caption.

With maturation, the nucleus becomes smaller, markedly heterochromatic, and nearly spherical and loses nucleoli. Just before nuclear loss, the nucleus with a thin rim of cytoplasm occupies one pole of the cell, and at the other pole is the bulk of the cytoplasm. The poles break apart and the fragment containing the nucleus is rather rapidly phagocytized. The freed anucleate pole is an erythrocyte (see following section on Reticulocytes). The thin layer of cytoplasm surrounding the discarded nucleus carries on its plasma membrane certain cell surface receptors that may

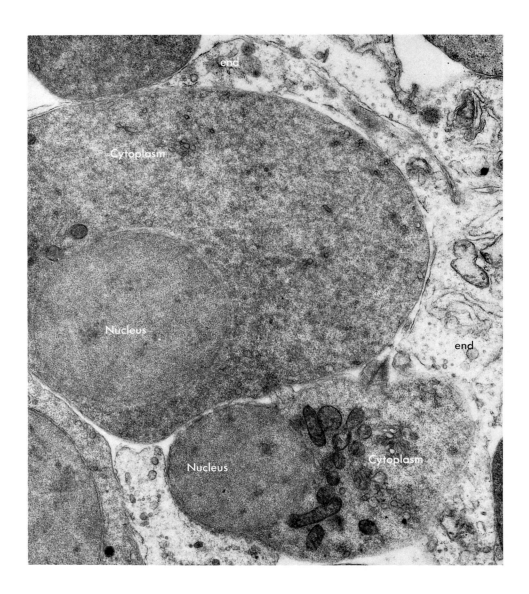

12–6 Polychromatophilic erythroblasts, bone marrow of the rat. Two polychromatophilic erythroblasts press against different points of the endothelium (end) of vascular sinuses of the marrow. The erythroblasts are markedly polarized. The cytoplasm, at one pole, contains ribosomes and mitochondria as well as hemoglobin. The nuclear pole is surrounded by a thin rim of hemoglobinized cytoplasm. The nuclear pole will be detached and phagocytized, and the cytoplasmic pole will become a reticulocyte. × 40,000. (From Weiss, L. 1965. J. Morphol. 117:467.)

be useful in erythroblast maturation but not in discarded erythrocytes. Nuclear loss regularly occurs near the orthochromatic stage. The nucleus may be lost at earlier stages, particularly in intensified erythropoiesis, resulting in polychromatophilic or even basophilic erythrocytes.

Reticulocytes

Freshly produced erythrocytes normally contain some ribosomes, yet fewer than 1% have enough to be polychromatophilic or basophilic in Ro-

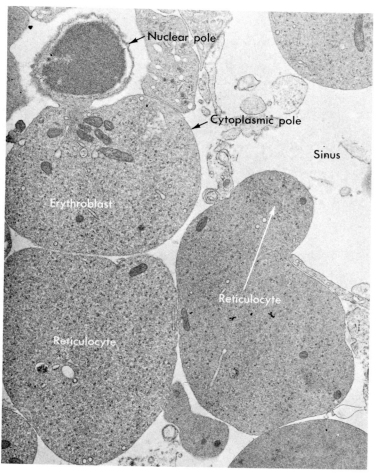

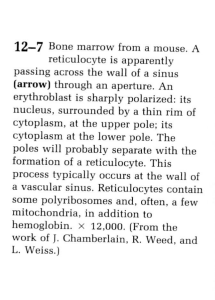

12–7 Bone marrow from a mouse. A reticulocyte is apparently passing across the wall of a sinus **(arrow)** through an aperture. An erythroblast is sharply polarized: its nucleus, surrounded by a thin rim of cytoplasm, at the upper pole; its cytoplasm at the lower pole. The poles will probably separate with the formation of a reticulocyte. This process typically occurs at the wall of a vascular sinus. Reticulocytes contain some polyribosomes and, often, a few mitochondria, in addition to hemoglobin. × 12,000. (From the work of J. Chamberlain, R. Weed, and L. Weiss.)

manovsky stains. A more sensitive method for revealing ribosomes in erythrocytes is supravital staining (Chap. 11). A drop of freshly drawn blood is mixed with a drop of brilliant cresyl blue or other suitable dye and then made into a smear. Ribonucleoprotein (RNP) appears as a striking blue web or reticulum. (In leukocytes RNP is not revealed because the supravital dye cannot penetrate the plasma membrane of living leukocytes.) These smears may be further stained with a Romanovsky stain and the blue web will lie within a pink erythrocyte. Such supravitally stained cells, called *reticulocytes*, constitute about 2% of circulating erythrocytes in normal human blood, 1% in canine, 0.1% in feline, and are absent in equine blood. The enhanced sensitivity of supravital staining over conventional Romanovsky staining in demonstrating RNP in

erythrocytes is due to the distribution of ribosomes. In Romanovsky staining the ribosomes remain so finely dispersed as to be below the limit of resolution of the light microscope. In supravital staining they are clumped into visible masses (the reticulum).

Reticulocyte maturation is characterized by decreasing cell size and loss of mitochondria and ribosomes. The reticulum in young reticulocytes is an abundant skein-like structure. In old reticulocytes it is scanty and punctate. In mature erythrocytes it is, of course, absent.

Kinetics

Human erythroid cells may be divided into four categories as shown in the following chart from Donahue et al. (1958).

Erythroid cells	Number of cells per kg of body weight
Erythroblasts (of marrow)	5.59×10^9
Marrow reticulocytes	5.73×10^9
Circulating reticulocytes	3.22×10^9
Circulating mature erythrocytes	309.0×10^9

Most of this population circulates. As a ready reserve, the marrow has a population of reticulocytes somewhat greater than the number in the blood.

The turnover rate of circulating erythrocytes can be calculated, since their number is constant and their life span (see below) is about 120 days. In a 70-kg man, the turnover rate being 0.83 to 1.0% daily, 17.9 to 21.6×10^{10} erythrocytes are produced each day and the same number destroyed. The mean life span of marrow reticulocytes is 36 to 44 h, and that of the circulating reticulocytes 25 h. The time required for erythroblasts to double by mitotic division is 36 to 44 h. Thus the total marrow turnover time is about 72 to 88 h from late-stage erythroblasts to mature erythrocytes. The differentiation of a basophilic erythroblast involves 16 to 32 cell divisions taking a total of approximately 96 h. Therefore, the time to produce a mature erythrocyte from a basophilic erythroblast is approximately 1 week.

Regulation

Cellular and humoral factors are associated with erythroid maturation. In the bone marrow macrophages, lymphocytes, and adventitial cells of the vascular sinuses are associated with erythroblasts. The macrophages are of greatest importance in erythropoiesis. Certain tissues favor certain types of hematopoiesis. For example, bone marrow preferentially supports granulocytopoiesis over erythropoiesis, and the reverse is true of spleen. The concept of distinctive *hematopoietic inductive microenvironments* has been advanced by Trentin and his colleagues with the thought that the stromal cells of a given hematopoietic tissue may decisively determine the nature of the microenvironment.

Humoral factors drive erythropoiesis. The best known, *erythropoietin*, is a glycoprotein of molecular weight 70,000, largely produced in the kidney. Erythropoietin stimulates the last three to five divisions in erythroid maturation. Other factors, as yet poorly characterized, regulate the early stages.

Life Span

Erythrocytes do not show clear morphological change as they age. However, they become more mechanically fragile, and the activity of certain enzymes, such as glucose-6-phosphate dehydrogenase, declines. The changes that trigger the destruction of an erythrocyte are not known, but about 120 days after a human red cell is released into the blood stream it is withdrawn from the circulation and destroyed.

Erythrocyte life span may be determined by several methods, the most common being radioactive chromium (^{51}Cr) tagging. A few microliters of red cells are removed from an individual, mixed with a solution of $Na_2^{51}CrO_7$, and then returned to the circulation. The ^{51}Cr adheres tenaciously to hemoglobin without doing appreciable damage, and the life span of erythrocytes is estimated by the level of persistent circulating radioactivity.

Destruction

At the end of their life span erythrocytes are withdrawn from the circulation, notably in the spleen, and are then phagocytized by macrophages. The hemoglobin is quickly degraded. Iron enters a labile pool from which it may be taken by transferrin to the marrow, where it is reused. The portion of hemoglobin that does not contain iron is transformed into the bile pigment bilirubin.

Culture of Erythrocyte Stem Cells

On the basis of tissue cultures of hematopoietic tissue grown in clots, two major types of erythrocyte stem cells have been described: erythroid burst forming units (BFU-E) and erythroid colony forming units (CFU-E). The presence of BFU-Es is recognized and quantitated by counting bursts or colonies of erythroid cells. The BFU-E itself has not been identified, but only its clonal descendants clustered in the bursts. The BFU-E is a descendant of the multipotential stem cell, CFU-S, and is considered the earliest of the cell types committed to erythropoiesis. It may be found in the circulation, in bone marrow, and in spleen. It either does not respond or responds

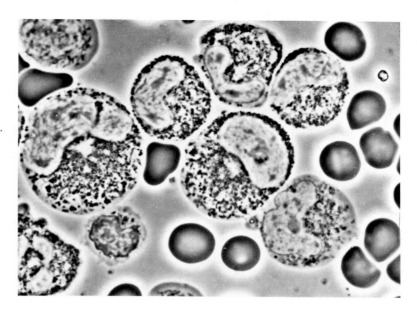

12–8 Human bone marrow cells. This field contains myelocytes together with erythrocytes. × 1,300. (From the work of G. A. Ackerman.)

poorly to erythropoietin. The CFU-E, a later stage than the BFU-E, proliferates to form smaller, relatively tight clusters of erythroid cells. CFU-Es are present in marrow and spleen but do not circulate. They are responsive to erythropoietin. Like the BFU-E, the CFU-E has not been identified. Its existence is inferred only by the colony it forms. Because CFU-E and BFU-E have not been identified microscopically it is difficult to indicate where they would fit into the morphological sequence of development discussed above. They undoubtedly come early, probably between the CFU-S and the basophilic erythroblast (see Fig. 12–21).

The Life Cycle of Polymorphonuclear Leukocytes

Differentiation

When granulocytes are formed from their precursors, called *myeloblasts*, the cytoplasm progressively acquires granules and the nucleus becomes flattened, indented, and then lobulated (Figs. 12–5 [here and color insert], 12–8 to 12–15, and 12–21). The myeloblast, the first recognizable precursor, in Giemsa stains, is approximately 10 to 15 μm in diameter and contains a large euchromatic nucleus, three to five nucleoli, and a basophilic cytoplasm without evident granules. The first clear evidence of differentia-

tion is a coarsening of chromatin (heterochromatin), flattening of the nucleus, and the appearance of a few granules in the cytoplasm. Gradually, cytoplasmic basophilia decreases and more granules accumulate. Neutrophils produce two types of granules: a large primary or azurophilic granule and a small definitive or secondary granule barely resolvable by light microscopy (see discussion of electron microscopy below). Basophilic and eosinophilic granules usually can be recognized soon after they appear. As the nucleus becomes heterochromatic, it begins to flatten on one aspect and then becomes more and more deeply indented until two to five lobes are produced (Figs. 12–10 and 12–21). The neutrophil precursor with slight nuclear flattening or indentation and only primary granules is called a *promyelocyte*. The later stage with a flattened or indented nucleus and both primary and secondary granules is a *myelocyte*. When nuclear indentation becomes significantly advanced to result in a **U**, **V**, or **T** shape, the cells are called *metamyelocytes* or *juvenile cells*. Further indentation results in nuclear lobes, the early stages of which have been termed *band forms*. Finally, when nuclear lobulation is completed, mature granulocytes exist. Myeloblasts, promyelocytes, and myelocytes are mitotic forms, whereas metamyelocytes, band forms, and mature granulocytes are postmitotic cells. A few metamyelocytes may normally be present in circulating

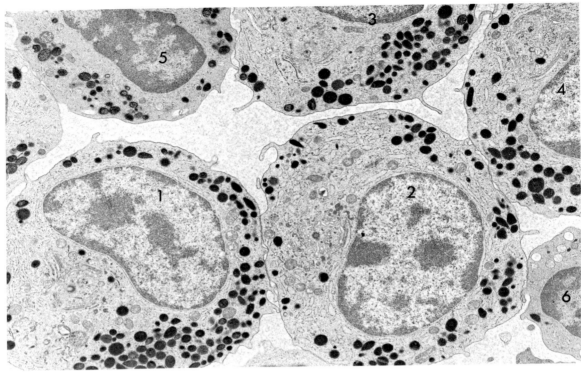

12–9 Human bone marrow cells. Myelocytes are
△ present in this electron micrograph. Cells 1 to
4 are early myelocytes; 5 and 6, late. × 9,200. (From
the work of G. A. Ackerman.)

MARROW
(development, 14 days)

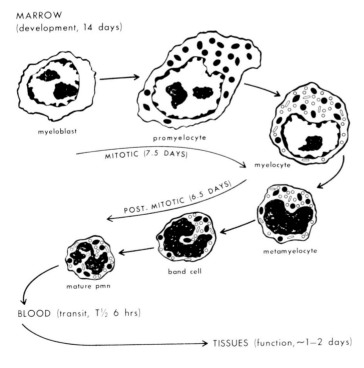

myeloblast

promyelocyte

MITOTIC (7.5 DAYS)

myelocyte

POST-MITOTIC (6.5 DAYS)

metamyelocyte

band cell

mature pmn

BLOOD (transit, T½ 6 hrs)

TISSUES (function, ~1–2 days)

12–10 Diagrammatic representation of the
polymorphonuclear neutrophil
(PMN) life cycle and stages of PMN
maturation. The myeloblast has a large oval
nucleus, large nucleoli, and cytoplasm
lacking granules. It is followed by two
granule-producing stages: the promyelocyte
and the myelocyte. During each of these
stages a distinct type of granule is produced:
azurophils **(solid black),** formed only during
the promyelocyte stage, and specific
granules **(white)** produced during the
myelocyte stage. The metamyelocyte and
band forms are nonproliferating, nongranule-
producing stages that develop into the
mature PMN. The latter is characterized by a
multilobulated nucleus and cytoplasm
containing primarily glycogen and granules.
The times indicated for the various
compartments were determined by isotope-
labeling techniques. (From Bainton, D. F.,
Ullyot, J. L., and Farquhar, M. G. 1971. J.
Exp. Med. 134:907.)

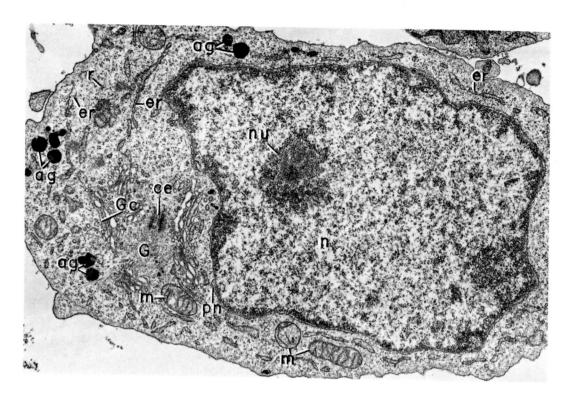

blood. Nuclei of eosinophils show two major lobes and often have a small central median lobe. Nuclear polymorphism of basophils is not pronounced.[4] In mature granulocytes the nucleus is markedly heterochromatic. Nucleoli are evident through the myelocyte stage but not in postmitotic cells. Some mitochondria are present in myeloblasts but become reduced in number and size until in the mature cell there are only a few. Metamyelocytes show ameboid movement, but such movement is absent in earlier forms, a change that favors the release of only mature cells to the circulation. Knowledge of granule production has been provided by the electron-microscopic studies of Bainton and colleagues and of G. A. Ackerman (Figs. 12–8 to 12–15).

The promyelocyte in humans is larger (approximately 15 μm) than the myeloblast from

12–11 Human polymorphonuclear neutrophil; promyelocyte (early), reacted for peroxidase. The nucleus **(n)** with its prominent nucleolus **(nu)** occupies the bulk of this very immature cell. The surrounding cytoplasm contains a few azurophilic granules **(ag)**, a large Golgi complex **(G)**, several mitochondria **(m)**, scanty rough endoplasmic reticulum **(er)**, many free polysomes **(r)**, and a centriole **(ce)**. All the azurophilic granules appear dense, since they are strongly reactive for peroxidase. The granule-producing apparatus (the perinuclear cisterna **[pn]**, rough endoplasmic reticulum **[er]**, and some of the Golgi cisternae **[Gc]**) is also reactive, although less so than the granules. × 21,000. (Legend and figure from Bainton, D. F., Ullyot, J. L., and Farquhar, M. G. 1971. J. Exp. Med. 134:907.)

---

[4]It had been thought that nuclear lobulation increased with age so that older cells had more nuclear lobes. This is not the case. Mature neutrophils are released from the marrow to the circulation with three to five nuclear lobes and live their entire life with their initial number. Some diseases such as pernicious anemia are characterized by hypersegmented nuclei containing six or more lobes. There is, on the other hand, a harmless congenital anomaly, the *Pelger-Huet* anomaly, with reduced nuclear lobulation.

which it derives and contains peroxidase-positive granules that correspond to the azurophilic granules of light microscopy. A large Golgi complex, mitochondria, and moderate amounts of rough ER are present. The granules are of two principal shapes. Most are round, approximately 500 nm in diameter: they contain flocculent material initially and dense homogeneous material when mature. Less common are football-shaped forms, approximately 300 × 900 nm, which fre-

486

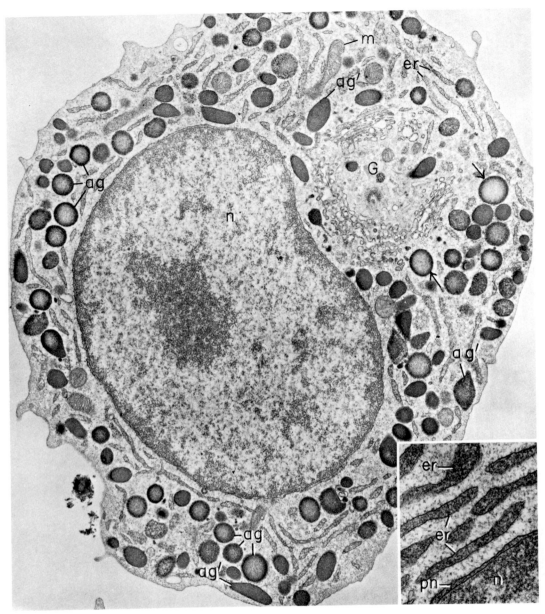

12–12 Human polymorphonuclear neutrophil; promyelocyte, reacted for peroxidase. This cell is the largest (approximately 15 μm) of the neutrophilic series. It has a sizable, slightly indented nucleus (n), a prominent Golgi region (G), and cytoplasm packed with peroxidase-positive azurophilic granules (ag). Note the two general shapes of azurophilic granules, spherical (ag) or ellipsoid (ag′). The majority are spherical, with a homogeneous matrix, but a few ellipsoid forms containing crystalloids are also present. Many of the spherical forms (arrows) have a dense periphery and a lighter core, owing presumably to incomplete penetration of substrate into the centers of granules. Peroxidase reaction product is visible in less concentrated form within all compartments of the granule-producing apparatus (endoplasmic reticulum [er], perinuclear cisterna [pn], and Golgi cisternae). No reaction product is seen in the cytoplasmic matrix, mitochondria (m), or nucleus (n). The **inset** depicts a portion of another promyelocyte at higher magnification, showing to better advantage flocculent deposits of peroxidase reaction product in the rough ER (er) including the perinuclear cisterna (pn). × 15,000; inset, × 34,000. (From Bainton, D. F., Ullyot, J. L., and Farquhar, M. G. 1971. J. Exp. Med. 134:907.)

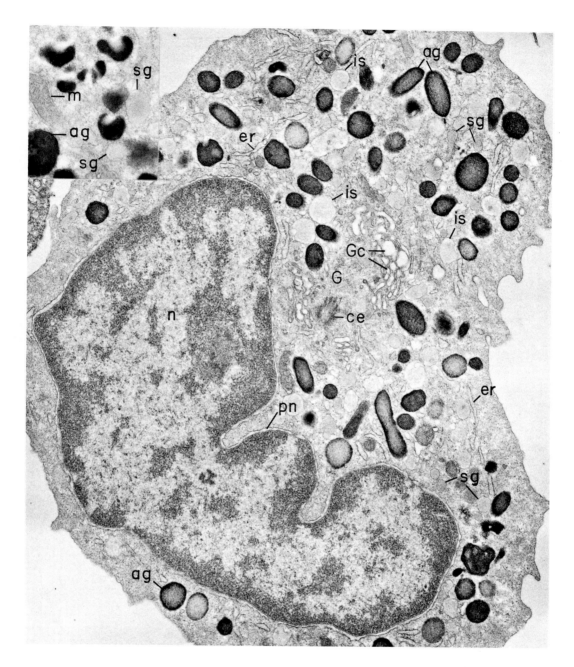

12–13 Human polymorphonuclear neutrophilic myelocyte, peroxidase reaction. At this stage the cell is smaller (approximately 10 μm) than the promyelocyte (see Fig. 12–12), the nucleus is more indented, and the cytoplasm contains two different types of granules: (1) large, peroxidase-positive azurophils **(ag)** and (2) the generally smaller specific granules **(sg),** which do not stain for peroxidase. A number of immature specifics **(is)**, which are larger, less compact, and more irregular in contour than mature granules, are seen in the Golgi region **(G).** The **inset,** a portion of a myelocyte, depicts a cluster of peroxidase-positive granules, most of which are smaller and more pleomorphic than the surrounding specifics **(sg)** and azurophils **(ag).** These granules are presumed to represent azurophil variants, since they appear during the promyelocyte stage. × 20,000; inset × 41,000. (From Bainton, D. F., Ullyot, J. L., and Farquhar, M. G. 1971. J. Exp. Med. 134:907.)

quently contain crystalline inclusions. The Golgi cisternae, the perinuclear space, and the rough ER—all of which are part of the secretory apparatus—often contain peroxidase-positive material, a precursor of the azurophilic granules.

The myelocyte is smaller than the promyelocyte. The Golgi complex is prominent and the granules now are of two types: newly produced peroxidase-negative granules and the peroxidase-positive azurophilic granules formed in the pro-

myelocyte stage. The new granules are specific. They are spheres approximately 200 nm in diameter, or rods 130 × 1,000 nm, with homogeneous, low-density content. These granules are produced at the convex surface of the Golgi complex, in distinction to the azurophilic granules, which are produced at the concave surface.

The metamyelocyte, band form, and mature neutrophil no longer appear to produce granules. The Golgi complex is small, and a mixed population of 200 to 300 granules is present. The ratio of specific to primary granules is 3 or 4 to 1. Relatively few primary granules are present in mature neutrophils because they are produced only in the promyelocyte stage. In the myelocyte stage, where the specific granules are produced in large number, there is active cell proliferation. The primary granules are thereby distributed to many daughter cells, and their number in any given cell is consequently reduced.

The primary or azurophilic granules are lysosomal; they contain myeloperoxidase as indicated above, acid phosphatase, β-galactosidase, 5′-nucleotidase, and other enzymes characteristic of lysosomes. The secondary or definitive

12–14 Higher-power view of the Golgi region of polymorphonuclear neutrophilic myelocyte similar to the cell shown in Fig. 12–13. As in the preceding figure, peroxidase reaction is seen in azurophils **(ag)** but not in specific granules **(sg)**. The stacked, smooth-surfaced Golgi cisternae **(Gc)** are oriented around the centriole **(ce)**. Note that the outer cisternae have a content of intermediate density **(arrows)** that is similar to the content of the specific granules. The images are compatible with the view that specific granules arise from the convex face of the Golgi complex. × 33,000. (From Bainton, D. F., Ullyot, J. L., and Farquhar, M. G. 1971. J. Exp. Med. 134:907.)

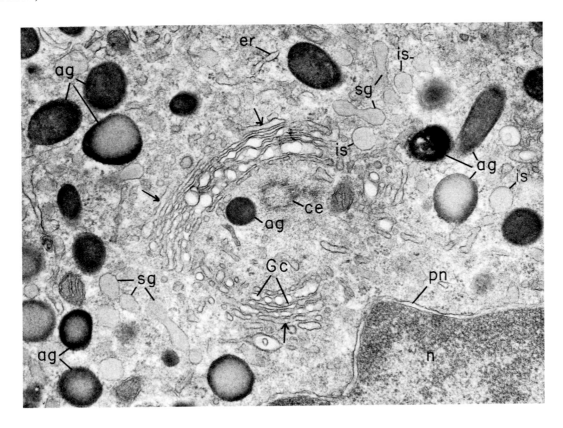

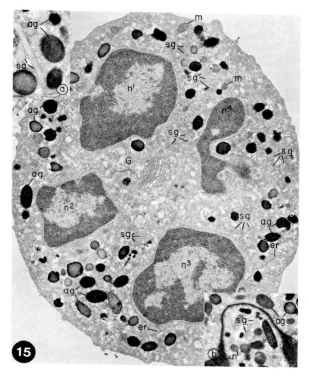

12–15 Human polymorphonuclear neutrophil
◁   (PMN), reacted for peroxidase. The cytoplasm
is filled with granules; the smaller peroxidase-negative
specifics **(sg)** are more numerous, azurophils **(ag)**
having been reduced in number by cell divisions after
the promyelocyte stage. Some small, irregularly
shaped azurophilic granule variants are also present
(arrow). The nucleus is condensed and lobulated **(n¹
to n⁴)**, the Golgi region **(G)** is small and lacks forming
granules, the ER **(er)** scanty, and mitochondria **(m)**
few. Note that the cytoplasm of this cell has a rather
ragged, moth-eaten appearance because the glycogen,
which is normally present, has been extracted. The
insets depict portions of the cytoplasm of mature
PMN reacted for peroxidase. Inset **(a)** demonstrates
that the peroxidase-positive azurophils **(ag)** can be
easily distinguished from the unreactive specifics **(sg)**.
Note that one of the specifics is quite elongated
(approximately 1,000 μm). Inset **(b)** illustrates the
narrow connection between two lobes **(n₁ and n₂)** of
the PMN nucleus. Inset, specimen preparation as in
Fig. 12–13. × 21,000; inset (a), × 36,000; inset (b),
× 14,000. (From Bainton, D. F., Ullyot, J. L., and
Farquhar, M. G. 1971. J. Exp. Med. 134:907.)

12–16 Physical and functional changes in
▽   polymorphonuclear neutrophils during
maturation. (From M. Lichtman and R. Weed, Blood
39:301, 1972.)

granules contain a variety of bactericidal compounds (Chap. 11).

The specific granules of eosinophils contain
flocculent material soon after they are produced
at the Golgi complex. As they mature, the dense
cystalloid element appears. Eosinophilic granules contain a myeloperoxidase somewhat different from that of the neutrophil, acid phosphatase, alkaline phosphatase, and a major basic
protein (MBP) (Chap. 11). Both eosinophils and
basophils contain a few primary granules in addition to their specific granules.

As neutrophils mature they undergo important physical and functional changes. Their negative surface charge density decreases and they
become less resistant to deformation, showing an
increased capacity for spreading and pseudopod
formation. They become more adhesive, motile,
and phagocytic (Fig. 12–16).

Kinetics and Distribution

Although the bulk of the erythroid complex is in
the circulation, granulocytic forms (which under
normal circumstances may be considered neutrophils) in the bone marrow far outnumber those
in the circulation, as shown in the table below

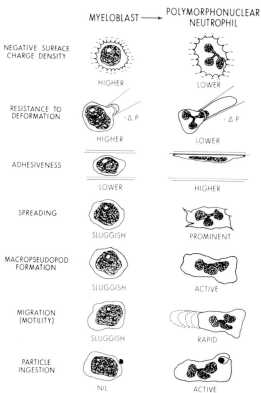

from the work of Donahue et al. (1958). A ready reserve of adult granulocytes and metamyelocytes, about 5×10^9 cells per kg body weight, is in human marrow. This represents more than 16 times the number of circulating cells. Counting all marrow granulocytes, the ratio of cells in marrow to those in blood is 38:1.

Granulocyte (neutrophils)	Number per kg of body weight
Circulating	0.3×10^9
Total marrow granulocytes	11.4×10^9
Segmented forms	1.6×10^9
Band forms	3.6×10^9
Myelocytes	2.6×10^9
Metamyelocytes	2.7×10^9
Adult granulocytes	2.5×10^9

Studies of the distribution and kinetics of granulocytes have been carried out with radioactive tags (e.g., diisopropyl fluorophosphate, which couples irreversibly with esterase). Two populations of granulocytes lie within blood vessels. The first circulates, the second constitutes a marginated pool. The latter consists of cells within blood vessels lying out of flow or marginated against the walls. Granulocytes, once released from the bone marrow, remain within blood vessels only hours (about 8–12 h in human beings). It is likely, moreover, that few granulocytes that leave the vasculature return. Most of them die in the perivascular tissues. There are then two major sources of ready reserve granulocytes, those in the marrow and those in marginated pools. The model shown below modified from the work of Mauer and colleagues indicates the relationship of the several granulocyte compartments.

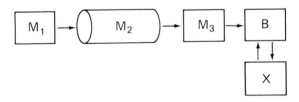

M_1 = pool of mitotically active cells in the marrow, including myeloblasts and myelocytes

M_2 = maturation phase, from which cells are not normally released until mature

M_3 = storage pool of mature granulocytes in marrow

B = granulocytic pool in blood

X = marginating cells in equilibrium with B

The Life Cycle of Monocytes

Monocytes are circulating blood cells whose life cycle includes promonocyte, monocyte, macrophage, epithelioid cell, and multinucleate giant cell. The life cycle of monocytes is discussed in Chap. 4.

Culture of Granulocyte and Monocyte Stem Cells

By means of tissue cultures of bone marrow grown in a gelated medium containing methyl cellulose it has been possible to identify a stem cell for eosinophils, *colony forming unit–eosinophil (CFU-Eo)*, another for megakaryocytes *(CFU-Meg)*, and still another that gives rise to both neutrophils and macrophages *(CFU-GM)* as well as separate stem cells for neutrophils, *colony forming unit–granulocytes (CFU-G)*, and for macrophages *(CFU-M)*. As is the case for their erythroid counterparts, *BFU-E* and *CFU-E*, these leukocytic CFU are stem cells derived from the multipotential stem cell, CFU-S. These derived stem cells remain stem cells in that they retain the capacities for both cell division and differentiation, but their capacity for differentiation is quite restricted, i.e., CFU-Eo can differentiate only into eosinophils.

A number of factors have been identified that stimulate colony growth. They are designated colony stimulating factors (CSF) and are low-molecular-weight protein or polypeptide moieties with an associated carbohydrate. Macrophages, lymphocytes, and perhaps other cells produce these CSFs. Substances that inhibit granulocytopoiesis have been discovered. They include prostaglandins produced by macrophages and lactoferrin (Chap. 11) produced by neutrophils themselves and thereby providing a negative feedback loop.

The Life Cycle of Lymphocytes

Stem cells destined to become T cells originate in bone marrow. They then leave the marrow and circulate to the periphery of the cortex of the thymus. There they undergo proliferation and differentiation toward T lymphocytes, moving deeper into the thymic cortex toward the center or the medulla of the gland. Many thymic lymphocytes die during development (Chap. 14). Moreover, the receptors on T cells change in

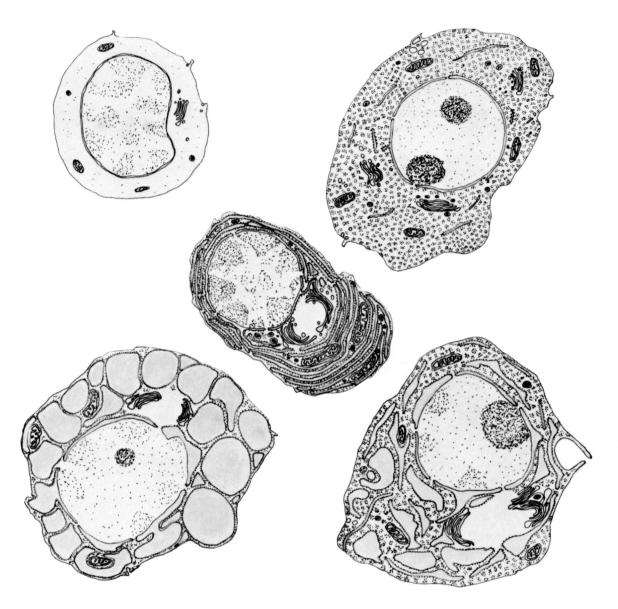

12–17 In this schematic view several stages of the life cycle of plasma cells are shown. At the upper left is a plasma cell precursor, the B lymphocyte. Antibody is present on the cell surface. The upper right-hand cell is a "blast" form. It has polyribosomes, segments of RER, nucleoli, nuclear pores, and other cellular elements indicative of protein synthesis. Antibody may be present in the perinuclear space and in the lumen of the RER. Antibody is no longer present on the cell surface. The lower cells, right and left, are clearly plasmacytic, of intermediate or transitional character. They have dilated perinuclear spaces and dilated ER, both containing antibody. Indeed, the continuity of the outer nuclear membrane and the ER is shown. The cell in the center is the classic small plasma cell, displaying polarized nucleus and cytoplasm, distribution of heterochromatin in chunks along the inner nuclear membrane, prominent cytocentrum including Golgi and centrioles, and deeply basophilic or pyroninophilic (= RNA) cytoplasm. This cell is a near-terminal form, past the peak of antibody production. The intermediate cells turn out most of the antibody. (From Weiss, L. 1972. The Cells and Tissues of the Immune System. Englewood Cliffs, N.J.: Prentice-Hall, Inc.)

character and concentration on maturation (Chap. 11). When released from the thymus, T cells travel to the spleen where the last phase of their maturation takes place. This may well depend on an encounter with antigen. From the spleen fully mature T cells are released. They are long-lived, small lymphocytes capable of years of life in humans and months in rodents. They are migratory cells, part of the recirculating pool of lymphocytes that circulate and recirculate through blood, lymph, and characteristic compartments in the spleen, lymph nodes, and other antibody-producing lymphatic tissues (Chaps. 15 and 16).

In birds, stem cells for B cells travel from the bone marrow to the *bursa of Fabricius*, a cloacal lymphoepithelial organ in which much of B-cell differentiation takes place. In mammals, B cells seem to be produced largely in bone marrow and complete their development in the spleen. B cells have a life span of 6 or more weeks in the rat and probably at least several months in humans. Like T cells, they circulate and recirculate through blood, lymph, spleen, lymph nodes, and other antibody-producing lymphatic tissues as part of the recirculating pool of lymphocytes (Chaps. 15 and 16). B cells themselves are stem cells that, when appropriately stimulated, differentiate into plasma cells (Figs. 12–7 and 12–21 and Chap. 11).

The migration pathways of the recirculating pool of lymphocytes facilitate the meeting of B and T cells with antigen, setting in motion immune responses (Chap. 11).

The Life Cycle of Platelets

Platelets originate as portions of the cytoplasm of giant cells, megakaryocytes, which may measure more than 50 μm in diameter. In humans, megakaryocytes are restricted largely to the bone marrow. In rodents they may also be found in the spleen. The megakaryocyte nucleus is a large, lobulated structure. It is polyploid, having doublings of ploidy up to 64n (see Chap. 1 for discussion of ploidy).

Megakaryocytes originate from stem cells. The first morphologically identifiable precursor of megakaryocytes is a cell 25 to 40 μm in diameter with a large oval or spherical nucleus and a cytoplasm containing ribosomes and other organelles, but without hint of platelet formation. This cell, called a *megakaryocytoblast*, undergoes DNA replication to its final level of ploidy before the nucleus becomes polymorphic. It has become

possible to recognize smaller (and earlier) megakaryocyte precursors by the use of cytochemical stains for acetylcholinesterase. In a population of megakaryocytoblasts ploidy varies from 2n to 64n. Two-thirds of the cells are in the 16n class, one-sixth in the 8n and 32n classes, and a few in 64n. In achieving polyploidy a cell will undergo successive incomplete mitosis without nuclear division (endomitosis). The result is a large nucleus (and cytoplasm), sized in proportion to the level of polyploidy. A concomitant of this nuclear division is the elaboration of abundant cytoplasmic membranes. These membranes outline platelet zones as the *demarcation system of membranes*. They are continuous, as invaginations, with the megakaryocyte plasma membrane. When platelets separate from the megakaryocyte, the demarcation membranes fuse and become the surface membranes of the platelets and the surface-connected canalicular system within platelets. Penington found that with increased ploidy there is increased membrane, fewer platelet organelles, and decreased platelet size.

The abundant cytoplasm of mature megakaryocytes is divisible into three zones: (1) The perinuclear zone contains Golgi, ER, polyribosomes, and some granules—in short, the organelles required for large-scale protein, granule, and membrane synthesis. (2) The intermediate zone consists of putative platelets demarcated to varying degrees of completeness by demarcation membranes. (3) The outermost zone resembles

12–18 Megakaryocyte from the bone marrow of a kitten, showing pseudopodia or platelet ribbons extending into a blood vessel **(V)** and giving rise to blood platelets **(bp)**. (From Wright, J. H. 1910. J. Morphol. 21:263.)

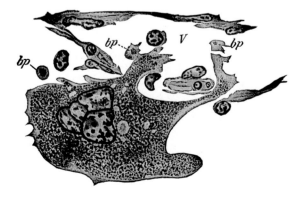

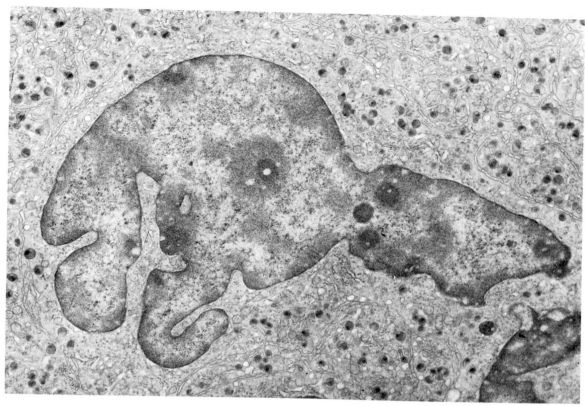

12–19 Electron micrograph of a megakaryocyte in human bone marrow. The nucleus is large and polymorphous. The cytoplasm contains granules of varying density and small mitochondria. The arresting cytoplasmic characteristic is the extensive system of demarcation membrane, which loculates platelet zones in the peripheral cytoplasm. (See Fig. 12–20.) Later the platelets will separate from the megakaryocyte and become free circulating structures. × 9,300. (From the work of I. Berman.)

12–20 Electron micrograph of megakaryocyte in rat bone marrow. A portion of the nucleus and central cytoplasm is at the upper margin. Most of the peripheral cytoplasm is clearly demarcated into platelet zones. × 10,500.

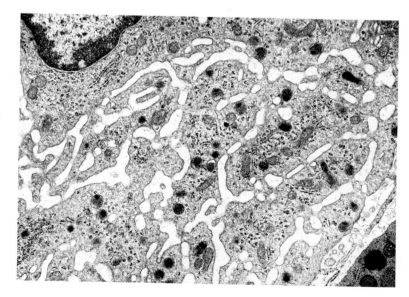

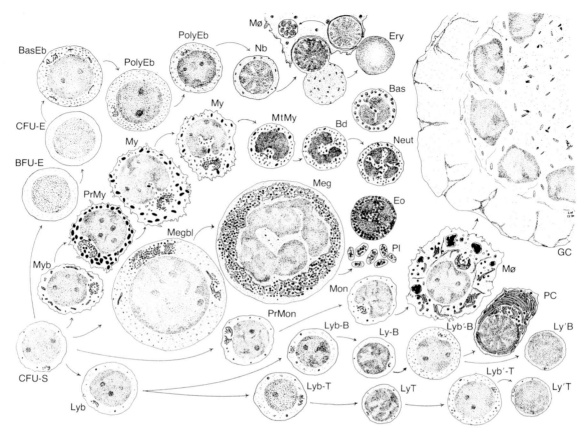

12–21 This schema shows stages in the differentiation of each of the blood cell lines as seen by electron microscopy. The multipotential stem cell (*colony forming unit–spleen*, **CFU-S**) is in the lower left corner and the various blood cell types radiate from it.

Along the topmost arc are the developing red cells. The first stages in erythrocyte differentiation are *erythroid burst forming units* (**BFU-E**) and *erythroid colony forming units* (**CFU-E**). These forms have not been seen as such; they are recognized by the colonies that derive from them in tissue culture. Their structure in this schema is, therefore, inferred. The *basophilic erythroblast* (**BasEb**) is rich in ribosomes and therefore would be deeply basophilic in Romanovsky preparations. Hemoglobin becomes evident in *polychromatophilic erythroblasts* (**PolyEb**), the early forms being relatively rich in ribosomes and poor in hemoglobin, and the later forms rich in hemoglobin and poor in ribosomes. Hemoglobin is almost fully developed and ribosomes quite depleted in *orthochromatic erythroblasts* or *normoblasts* (**Nb**). At this stage, moreover, the cells are postmitotic. Nuclear and cytoplasmic poles separate. The nuclear pole, surrounded by a rim of cytoplasm, is phagocytized by a macrophage (**Mφ**). The anucleate erythrocytes, still containing ribosomes and some

mitochondria, called *reticulocytes* after supravital staining, differentiate into a mature erythrocyte (**Ery**). Both reticulocytes and mature erythrocytes circulate.

The differentiation of neutrophilic leukocytes from the CFU-S is shown in the next arc. The first stage is the myleoblast (**Myb**). Then, in the *promyelocyte* (**PrMy**) primary granules appear, the nucleus begins to indent, and the cell grows larger. In the *myelocyte* stage (**My**) primary granule formation stops and secondary granule formation starts. The nucleus is increasingly indented, heterochromatic, and segmented. The metamyelocyte (**MtMy**) is smaller and postmitotic. The granule composition is definitive and the nucleus is increasingly heterochromatic and segmented. In the band form (**Bd**) and the mature neutrophil (**Neut**), nuclear segmentation is completed. An eosinophil (**Eo**) is shown below the neutrophil and a basophil (**Bas**) above.

Megakaryocyte development, presented in the third arc, depends on the development of polyploidy by endomitosis in a large mononuclear cell, a *megakaryocytoblast* (**Megbl**). Then, in its postendomitotic phase, the megakaryocyte (**Meg**) develops, undergoing cytoplasmic maturation and nuclear polymorphism. Platelets (**Pl**) are produced from the cytoplasm of megakaryocytes.

Monocytes (**Mon**), presented in the fourth

ectoplasm; it is finely granular and contains packets of microfilaments but is largely free of organelles (Figs. 12–5 [here and color insert], and 12–18 to 12–21). Megakaryocytes lie against the outside of vascular sinuses in bone marrow, delivering platelets through mural apertures directly into the vascular lumen (Figs. 12–18 and 13–4). They may deliver individual platelets or ribbons of platelets (as tickets unwinding from a spool) that subsequently separate into individual platelets in the vascular bed. Platelets are released as cytoplasmic fragments in which microtubules are present only in short segments and granules seem randomly located. Later, perhaps in the spleen, the microtubules link to form the definitive peripheral ring, the platelets assume their mature lenticular shape, and their granules lie centrally. Circulating platelets in human beings have a life span up to about 10 days. Platelets are most likely used randomly, that is, without reference to age.

There is good evidence that a humoral substance (or substances), *thrombopoietin*, stimu-

lates the maturation of megakaryocytes and the rate of platelet production. Platelet-stimulating activity is increased in the serum of individuals who have low blood platelet levels *(thrombocytopenia)*. The assay for thrombopoietin depends on the uptake of radioactive selenium (as selenomethionine-75) or sulfur (as $Na_2{}^{35}SO_4$) by megakaryocytes and the determination of the rate at which radioactive platelets appear in blood.

References and Selected Bibliography

General

Abramson, S., Miller, R. G., and Phillips, R. A. 1977. Identification of pluripotent and restricted stem cells of the myeloid and lymphoid systems. J. Exp. Med. 145:1567.

Bloom, W., and Bartelmez, G. W. 1940. Hematopoiesis in young human embryos. Am. J. Anat. 67:21.

De Bruyn, P. P. H. 1944 and 1946. Locomotion of blood cells in tissue culture. Anat. Rec. 89:43; 95:177.

Goldstein, G. 1978. Polypeptides regulating lymphocyte differentiation. *In* Differentiation of Normal and Neoplastic Hematopoietic Cells, Clarkson, B., Marks, P. A., Till, J. E. (eds.). Cold Spring Harbor Laboratory, New York: Vol A, p. 455.

Isaacs, R. 1930. The physiological histology of bone marrow. Folia Haematol. (Leipzig) 40:395.

Jaffe, R. H. 1938. The reticuloendothelial system. *In* H. Downey (ed.), Handbook of Hematology, vol. 2. New York: Paul B. Hoeber, Inc.

Jordon, H. E. 1933. The evolution of blood-forming tissues. Q. Rev. Biol. 8:58.

Kindred, J. E. 1942. A quantitative study of the hematopoietic organs of young adult albino rats. Am. J. Anat. 71:207.

Metcalf, D., and Moore, M. A. S. 1971. Haemopoietic Cells. North-Holland Research Monographs, Front. Biol. 24. Amsterdam: North-Holland Publishing Co.

Metchnikoff, E. 1893. Lectures on the Comparative Pathology of Inflammation. Starling, F. A. and E. H. (trans.). London: Kegan Paul, Trench, Trubner and Co.

Miklem, H. S., Ford, C. E., Evans, E. P., and Gar, J. 1966. Interrelationships of myeloid and lymphoid cells: Studies with chromosome-marked cells transfused into lethally irradiated mice. Proc. R. Soc. Lond. (Biol.) 165:78.

Strominger, J. L., Ferguson, W., Fuks, A., Kaufman, J., Orr, H., Parham, P., Robb, R., Terhorst, C., Giphart, M., and Mann, D. 1978. Isolation and structure of HLA antigens. *In* Differentiation of Normal and Neoplastic Hematopoietic Cells, Clarkson, B., Marks, P. A., Till, J. E. (eds.). Cold Spring Harbor Laboratory, New York: Vol A, p. 467.

Trentin, J. J. 1970. Influence of hemopoietic organ stroma (hematopoietic inductive microenvironments) on stem cell differentiation. *In* Regulation of Hematopoiesis, vol. I, Red Cell Production, Gordon, A. S. (ed.). New York: Appleton-Century-Crofts, p. 161.

progression, are derived from the multipotential hematopoietic stem cells **(CFU-S)** through the promonocyte **(PrMon)**, the difference between monocytes and promonocytes being quite subtle. Monocytes may differentiate further into macrophages **(Mφ)** and later, by fusion, into multinucleate giant cells **(GC)**. There is a stem cell *CFU-GM*, derived from the multipotential stem cell CFU-S, capable of differentiating either into the monocyte line or into the neutrophil line. It is not shown in this schema, but is discussed on p. 490.

Lymphocyte differentiation, presented in the lowermost progression, appears to depend on a lymphoid cell, a *lymphoblast* **(Lyb)**, derived from the multipotential stem cell. The lymphoblast differentiates into a *T lymphoblast* **(Lyb-T)**, which produces *T lymphocytes* **(Ly-T)** and *B lymphocytes* **(Ly-B)**. When appropriately stimulated, as by antigen, T and B lymphocytes become larger and develop nucleoli, polyribosomes, and other organelles associated with protein synthesis and mitosis. These altered T and B lymphocytes are said to have undergone *"blast" formation* **(Lyb'-T and Lyb'-B)**. They can go on to produce *plasma cells* **(PC)** and more **(Ly'-B)**-memory cells, in the case of B lymphocytes, and more **(Ly'-T)**-memory cells, in the case of T lymphocytes. The differentiation of CFUS into the lymphocyte lines is not evident (except in the case of plasma cells) in electron micrographs or in Romanovsky-stained material. Recognition of T and B cells depends on the visualization of distinctive cell-surface receptors by fluorescence microscopy or other means.

Basophilic Leukocytes

Dvorak, A. M. 1978. Biology and morphology of basophilic leukocytes. *In* Immediate Hypersensitivity, Modern Concepts and Development, Immunology Series, vol. 7, Bach, M. K. (ed.). New York: Marcel Dekker, Inc., p. 369.

Dvorak, A. M., Galli, S. J., Morgan, E., Galli, A. S., Hammond, M. E., and Dvorak, H. F. 1981. Anaphylactic degranulation of guinea pig basophilic leukocytes. I. Fusion of granule membranes and cytoplasmic vesicles: Formation and resolution of degranulation sacs. Lab. Invest. 44:174.

Terry, R. W., Bainton, D. F., and Farquhar, M. G. 1969. Formation and structure of specific granules in basophilic leukocytes of the guinea pig. Lab. Invest. 21:65.

Eosinophilic Leukocytes

Archer, G. T. 1963. Motion picture studies on degranulation of horse eosinophils during phagocytosis. J. Exp. Med. 118:276.

Beeson, P. B., and Bass, D. A. 1977. The eosinophil. Philadelphia: W. B. Saunders, Inc.

Erythrocytes

Brookoff, D., and Weiss, L. 1982. Adipocyte development and the loss of erythropoietic capacity in the bone marrow of mice after sustained hypertransfusion. Blood 60: December.

Harrison, P. R. 1976. Analysis of erythropoiesis at the molecular level. Review article. Nature (London) 262:353.

Howell, W. H. 1890. The life history of the formed elements of the blood: Especially the red corpuscles. J. Morphol. 4:57.

Johnson, G. R., and Metcalf, D. 1977c. Pure and mixed erythroid colony formation *in vitro*: Stimulation by spleen conditioned medium with no detectable erythropoietin. Proc. Natl. Acad. Sci. U.S.A. 74:3,879.

Rifkind, R. A., and Marks, P. A. 1975. The regulation of erythropoiesis. Blood Cells 1:417.

Lymphocytes

(See References and Selected Bibliography, Chapter 14 and Chapter 15)

Megakaryocytes and Platelets

Evatt, B. L., Levine, R. F., and Williams, N. T. 1981. Megakaryocyte Biology and Precursors: *in vitro* Cloning and Cellular Properties. New York: Elsevier-North Holland.

Metcalf, D., MacDonald, H. R., Odartchenki, N., and Sordat, B. 1975. Growth of mouse megakaryocyte colonies *in vitro*. Proc. Natl. Acad. Sci. U.S.A. 72:1744.

Paulus, J. M., Bury, J., and Grosent, J. C. 1979. Control of platelet territory development in megakaryocytes.

Penington, D. G. 1979. The cellular biology of megakaryocytes. Blood Cells 5:5.

Shattil, S. J., and Bennet, J. S. 1981. Platelets and their membranes in hemostasis: Physiology and pathophysiology. Ann. Intern. Med. 94:108.

Weissman, G., and Rite, G. A. 1972. Molecular basis of gouty inflammation: Interaction of monosodium urate crystals with lysosomes and liposomes. Nature (New Biol.) 240:167.

White, J. G., and Clawson, C. C. 1980. Overview article: Biostructure of blood platelets. Ultrastruct. Pathol. 1:533.

Williams, N., McDonald, T. P., and Trabellino, E. M. 1979. Maturation and regulation of megakaryocytopoiesis. Blood Cells 5:43.

Wright, J. H. 1910. The histogenesis of blood platelets. J. Morphol. 21:263.

Monocytes and Macrophages

(See References and Selected Bibliography, Chap. 4)

Neutrophilic Leukocytes

Bainton, D. F. Ullyot, J. L., and Farquhar, M. G. 1971. The development of neutrophilic polymorphonuclear leukocytes in human bone marrow. Origin and content of azurophil and specific granules. J. Exp. Med. 134:907.

Cohn, Z. A., and Morse, S. I. 1960. Functional and metabolic properties of polymorphonuclear leukocytes. I. Observations on the requirements and consequences of particle ingestion. J. Exp. Med. 111:667.

Craddock, C. G., Jr., Perry, S., Ventzke, L. E., and Lawrence, J. S. 1960. Evaluation of marrow granulocytic reserves in normal and disease states. Blood 15:840.

Hirsch, J. G., and Cohn, Z. A. 1960. Degranulation of polymorphonuclear leukocytes following phagocytosis of microorganisms. J. Exp. Med. 118:1005.

Johnson, G. R., and Metcalf, D. 1978. Characterization of mouse fetal liver granulocyte-macrophage colony-forming cells (GM-CFC) using velocity sedimentation. Exp. Hematol (Copenhagen). 6:246.

Johnson, G. R., and Metcalf, D. 1978. Sources and nature of granulocyte-macrophage colony stimulating factor in fetal mice. Exp. Hematol. (Copenhagen) 6:327.

Lisiewicz, J. 1980. Human Neutrophils. Bowe, Md.: The Charles Press Publishers.

Murphy, P. 1976. The Neutrophil. New York: Plenum.

Ramsey, W. A. 1972. Locomotion of human polymorphonuclear leukocytes. Exp. Cell Res. 72:489.

Spitznagel, J. K., Dalldorf, F. G., and Leffell, M. S. 1974. Characterization of azurophil and specific granules purified from human polymorphonuclear leukocytes. Lab. Invest. 30:774.

Weissman, G., and Rite, G. A. 1972. Molecular basis of gouty inflammation: Interaction of monosodium urate crystals with lysosomes and liposomes. Nature (New Biol.) 240:167.

Stem Cells

Abramson, S., Miller, R. G., and Phillips, R. A. 1977. Identification of pluripotent and restricted stem cells of the myeloid and lymphoid systems. J. Exp. Med. 145:1567.

van Bekkum, D. W., van Noord, M. J., Maat, B., and Dicke, K. A. 1971. Attempts at identification of hematopoietic stem cell in mouse. Blood 38:547.

Dexter, T. M., Allen, T. D., Lajtha, L. G., Krizsa, F., Testa, N. G., and Moore, M. A. S. 1978. In vitro analysis of self-renewal and commitment of hematopoietic stem cells. In Differentiation of normal and Neoplastic Hematopoietic Cells, Clarkson, B., Marks, P. A., Till, J. E., (eds.). Cold Spring Harbor Laboratory, New York: Vol A, p. 63.

Dicke, K. A., van Noord, M. J., and van Bekkum, D. W. 1973. Attempts at morphological identification of the hematopoietic stem cell in rodents and primates. Exp. Hemat. 1:36.

Donahue, D. M., Gabrio, B. W., and Finch, C. A. 1958. Quantitative measurements of hematopoietic cells of the marrow. J. Clin. Invest. 37:1,564.

Fowler, J. H., Wu, A. M., Till, J. E., McCulloch, E. A., and Siminovitch, L. 1967. The cellular composition of hematopoietic spleen colonies J. Cell Physiol. 69:65.

Johnson, G. R., and Moore, M. A. S. 1975. Role of stem cell migration in initiation of mouse foetal liver haemopoiesis. Nature (London) 258:726.

Moore, M. A. S., and Johnson, G. R. 1976. Stem cells during embryonic development and growth. In Cairnie, A. B., Lala, P. K., and Osmond, D. G. (eds.). Stem Cells of Renewing Cell Populations. New York: Academic Press, Inc., p. 323.

Moore, M. A. S., and Metcalf, D. 1970. Ontogeny of the haemopoietic system: Yolk sac origin of in vivo and in vitro colony forming cells in the developing mouse embryo. Br. J. Haematol. 18:279.

Siminovitch, L., McCulloch, E. A., and Till, J. E. 1963. The distribution of colony-forming cells among spleen colonies. J. Cell Comp. Physiol. 62:327.

Wu, A. M., Till, J. E., Siminovitch, L., and McCulloch, E. A. 1967. A cytological study of the capacity for differentiation of normal hematopoietic colony-forming cells. J. Cell Physiol. 69:177.

Wu, A. M., Till, J. E., Siminovitch, L., and McCulloch, E. A. 1968. Cytological evidence for a relationship between normal hematopoietic colony-forming cells and cells of the lymphoid system. J. Exp. Med. 127:455.

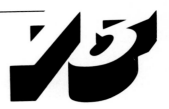

Bone Marrow

Leon Weiss

The bone marrow is a richly cellular connective tissue within the bones of the body, specialized to produce blood cells and deliver them to the circulation. It is the major hematopoietic tissue in human beings from the fifth month of fetal life through adulthood and accounts for about 5% of adult body weight. It attracts and holds hematopoietic stem cells in far greater number than any other tissue and provides diverse hematopoietic microenvironments for their maintenance and differentiation into each of the blood cell types. The differentiation of each of the blood cell types is initiated in the bone marrow. Erythrocytes, granulocytes, platelets, and monocytes develop almost completely in the marrow, with perhaps some terminal development occurring in the spleen before they are released to the general circulation. B lymphocytes undergo much of their development in marrow but mature in the spleen before entering the circulation. T lymphocyte development is initiated in marrow, occurs largely in the thymus, and is completed in the spleen.

Structure of Bone Marrow

Gross Characteristics

Bone marrow can be red, because of the presence of erythrocytes and their precursors, indicative of active hematopoiesis, or yellow, owing to fat and indicative of reduced hematopoiesis. Red and yellow marrow may be interconvertible, as demands for hematopoiesis change.

All marrow in newborn humans is red. Fat appears in long bones from the fifth to seventh years, and by the eighteenth year almost all limb marrow is yellow. Patches of red marrow persist only around the joints. Hematopoietic marrow in adults is virtually restricted to the skull, clavicles, vertebrae, ribs, sternebrae, and pelvis. Blood vessels and nerves reach marrow by piercing its bony shell. Particularly at the end of long bones, the internal surface of bone may be ridged with shelves and spicules of bone, the *trabeculae*, which protrude into the marrow cavity (Fig. 13–1).

Vascular Arrangements

There may be multiple small arterial twigs penetrating bone, or a major vessel, the *nutrient artery*, that enters marrow about midshaft in long bone and sends branches, *central longitudinal arteries*, that run in the central longitudinal axis of the marrow to the diaphyses. Slender branches of these arteries run radially through marrow toward the encasing bone and connect with venous vessels throughout the marrow cavity. Small arterial vessels actually enter the bone where they may become part of osteones or curve back toward the marrow and open into venous vessels.

The *venous* or *vascular sinuses* of marrow, the first vessels in the venous system, are thin-walled vessels 50 to 75 μm in diameter that anastomose richly. In long bones they run radially and empty into the central longitudinal vein, which runs in company with the corresponding artery (Figs. 13–2 to 13–4).

The circulation in marrow, in contrast to the spleen, is "closed" in that arteries connect directly to veins. Such direct connections have been demonstrated by vital microscopy and scanning electron microscopy (Fig. 13–5) and by the absence of blood from hematopoietic perivascular tissue.

The prominent system of venous sinuses and veins together with the system of arterial vessels constitutes the *vascular compartment* of the marrow. The remainder of the marrow lies between these vessels as irregular and anastomosing cords, the *hematopoietic cords*, and constitutes the *hematopoietic compartments* (Figs. 13–2 to 13–6). Hematopoiesis is most active in the periphery of the marrow near bone. Some fat always occurs in the center of the marrow in the hematopoietic compartment around the great vessels. In yellow marrow, the hematopoietic compartment is predominantly fatty.

Marrow lacks lymphatic vessels. The nerves in marrow are associated with the vasculature and appear to be vasomotor. The internal surface of the bone enclosing the marrow is lined with endosteum, composed of osteoblasts, osteoclasts and other bone lining cells (Chap. 6).

13–1 Bone marrow from central femur of human fetus, 200 mm crown rump length (22 weeks gestational age). The marrow tissue occurs in the spaces within bone. In the adult the bone will be removed from much of the center of the shaft of the femur, remaining only to form a cortical shell. The marrow will therefore become a solid cylindrical plug of tissue. The marrow contains large, thin-walled vascular sinuses (S) containing blood. Outside the sinuses lie the hematopoietic compartments. Some of them (H) are filled with hematopoietic cells. Note the large megakaryocyte (M) characteristically set on the outside wall of the sinus (see text). In some sites, the hematopoietic compartments have not yet filled with hematopoietic cells but contain fibrous connective tissue (H'). × 1,000. (From L-T. Chen and L. Weiss.)

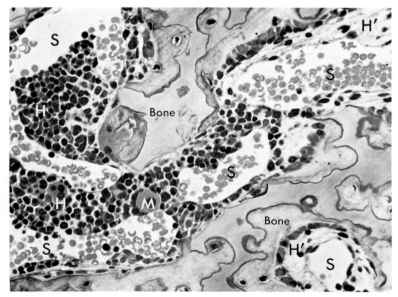

500

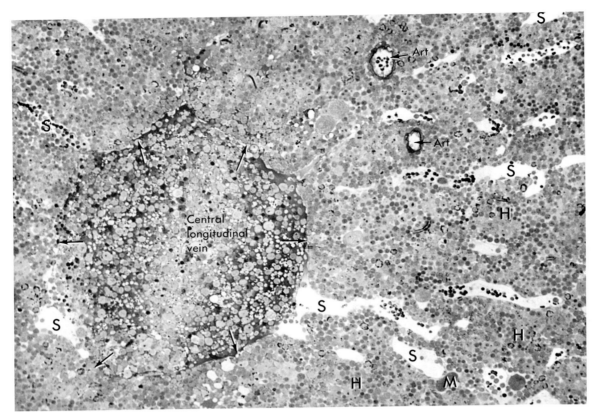

13-2 Rat bone marrow. This is a cross section of the marrow showing the relationships of major structural elements. The central longitudinal vein and branches of the nutrient artery **(Art)** are cut in cross section. The lumen of the vein is filled with cells: its wall is indicated by **arrows.** The sinuses **(S)** constitute a thin-walled radial system of venous vessels running into the vein. They are cut in longitudinal section. They are separated by hematopoietic compartments **(H)** containing the developing blood cells packed together. Megakaryocytes **(M)** lie characteristically against the outside wall of a sinus. × 750. (From Weiss, L. 1965. J. Morphol. 117:481.)

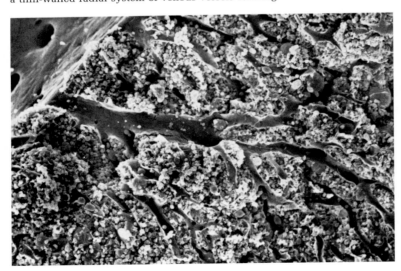

13-3 Rat bone marrow. This is a scanning electron micrograph of the cut surface showing a system of vascular sinuses originating at the periphery of the marrow (right side of field) and draining into a large vein (left upper corner). The large vein has several apertures in its wall, representing the entry of tributary venous sinuses. Hematopoietic tissue lies between the vascular sinuses. × 800. (From Weiss, L. 1976. Anat. Rec. 186:161.)

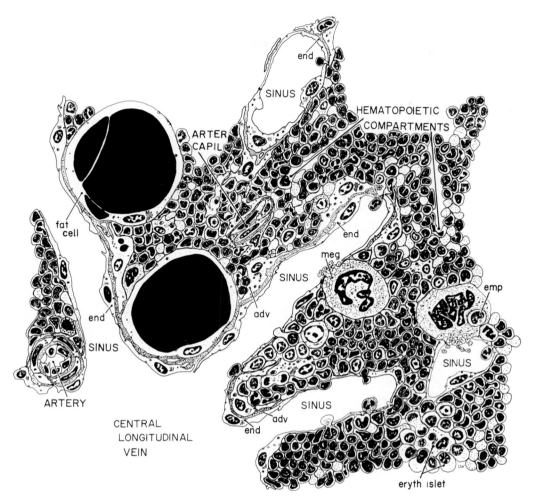

13–4 Bone marrow, schematic view of cross section near central longitudinal vein. Several sinuses drain into the central longitudinal vein. The sinuses are cut along their long axis, the vein, in cross section. A portion of the nutrient artery is present, as is an arterial capillary. Hematopoietic cells lie between the sinuses, constituting the hematopoietic compartment. Where hematopoiesis is relatively quiet, the wall of the sinus and of the central longitudinal vein is trilaminar consisting of endothelium **(end),** a basement membrane, and adventitial cell **(adv).** The adventitial cell may become voluminous, encroaching upon the hematopoietic space and thereby displacing hematopoietic cells. The increased volume of the adventitial cell may be due to a gelatinous change wherein its cytoplasm becomes rarefied, presumably because of hydration. If this change is widespread, the marrow may become grossly white and gelatinous. A second and more common basis for the large bulk of adventitial cells is fatty change, where they become fat cells. Contrariwise, when hematopoiesis is active the hematopoietic compartment is large and packed with myelocytes, erythroblasts, and megakaryocytes. The sinus wall becomes thin, reduced to an endothelial layer alone as the adventitial cells are displaced or lifted from the wall by infiltrating hematopoietic cells. Apertures appear in the endothelium, moreover, as maturing hematopoietic cells cross the sinus wall and enter the sinus lumen. Megakaryocytes **(meg)** characteristically lie against the outside of the sinus wall, discharging platelets into the lumen through an aperture. Occasionally the cytoplasm of megakaryocytes is entered by other cell types, which remain visible and later leave the megakaryocyte. The phenomenon is known as emperipolesis **(emp).** Erythroblasts tend to be present in clusters near the sinus wall. Erythroblastic islets (see text) may be present. Granulocytes usually develop near the center of the hematopoietic space. Lymphocytes occur throughout the marrow. Macrophages are common, and mast cells, plasma cells, and other connective tissue cells are also present.

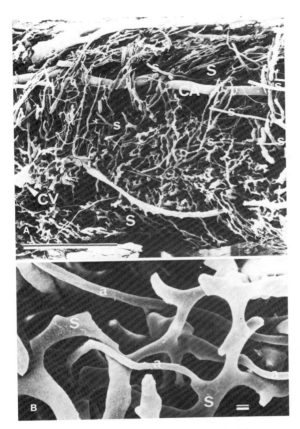

13–5 A. A scanning electron micrograph of the vascular cast of longitudinally cut rat's femur. Numerous fine terminal arterioles are seen arising from side branches **(s)** of the central artery **(CA). CV,** cut edge of the central vein; **S,** marrow sinusoid. Bar = 1 mm. **B.** A closer view of the vascular cast of the rat's bone marrow. Two terminal arterioles **(a)** are seen connecting with the sinusoids **(S).** Bar = 10 μm. (From the work of Osamu Ohtani.)

Vascular Sinuses

Blood cells are produced in the hematopoietic compartments and reach the circulation by crossing the wall of vascular sinuses. The sinus wall is therefore the barrier between hematopoietic tissue and the blood. In its fullest development the wall has three layers: endothelium, basement membrane, and adventitia (Figs. 13–4, and 13–6 to 13–9).

The endothelium is a thin, simple layer of flat cells connected to one another by circumferential zonulae adherens, probably associated with gap junctions. Endothelial cells contain many small vesicles, microfilaments, microtubules,

some ribosomes, small Golgi complexes, lysosomes, and heterolysosomes. The basement membrane is variably seen both because it may be absent physiologically, and because, when present, it is difficult to preserve by most electron-microscopic methods. Adventitial cells normally cover most of the outside surface of the endothelium. In the femoral marrow of the rat, more than 60% is covered. Adventitial cells vary in appearance but contain most of the organelles present in endothelium. These cells lie on the outside surface of the vascular sinuses as the most peripheral of the vascular layers and branch out into the surrounding hematopoietic cords. By their branching they form a meshwork, which supports the hematopoietic cells of the cords. The adventitial cells are therefore related to the reticular meshworks in the splenic cords and in lymph nodes, except that reticular fibers in marrow are much slighter and may be absent. Hence, the adventitial cells are a type of reticular cell and are termed *adventitial reticular cells.*

The reticular meshwork of the hematopoietic cords holds the developing blood cells. Reticular cells may play a further role in sorting hematopoietic cells into characteristic locations. They may well contribute to the hematopoietic microenvironments of marrow and thereby influence hematopoietic differentiation.

Adventitial reticular cells may become swollen, voluminous, and "empty" in appearance, probably because of marked water uptake. If this change occurs on a large scale, the marrow may become grossly white and gelatinous. Adventitial reticular cells, moreover, may become fatty; when this occurs extensively, the marrow becomes yellow (Figs. 13–4 and 13–9). These gelatinous or fatty cells protrude deeply into the perivascular hematopoietic cord and decrease the space available for hematopoiesis. Gelatinous or fatty marrows, therefore, are reduced in hematopoietic activity. As indicated above, the marrow is normally yellow in certain locations, as in the appendicular skeleton; but after exposure to certain toxins, normally hematopoietic red marrow may become fatty, resulting in reduced marrow hematopoietic capacity and anemia (*aplastic anemia*). In contrast, when hematopoietic volume must increase, as it does in response to severe blood loss and in certain diseases (such as leukemia or infection), it displaces normally fatty marrow. The fatty adventitial cells lose their fat, thereby decreasing in volume and providing additional space for hematopoiesis. Gelat-

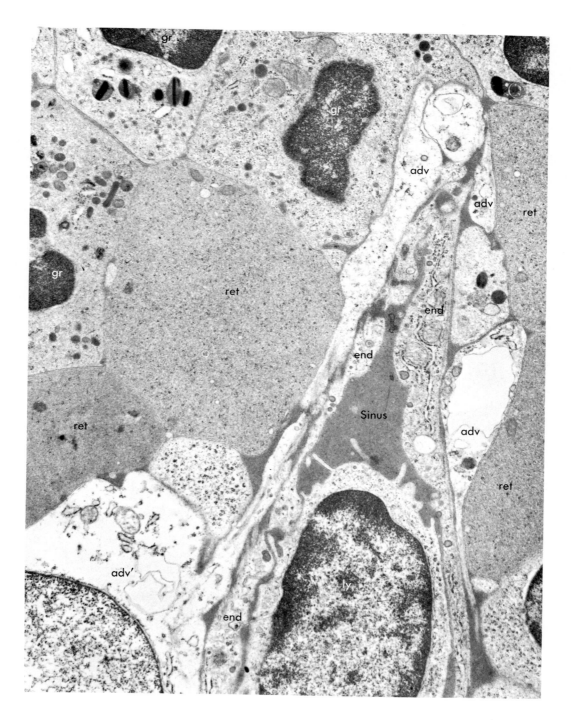

13–6 Rat bone marrow. A sinus is present, closely surrounded by hematopoietic cells. The lumen of the sinus contains a lymphocyte **(ly).** Its wall consists of endothelial **(end)** and adventitial **(adv)** layers. At the lower left corner of the field, the cytoplasm of an adventitial cell **(adv′)** is voluminous and extends into the surrounding hematopoietic space. Reticulocytes **(ret)** and granulocytes **(gr)** surround the sinus. × 15,200. (From Weiss, L. 1970. Blood 36:189.)

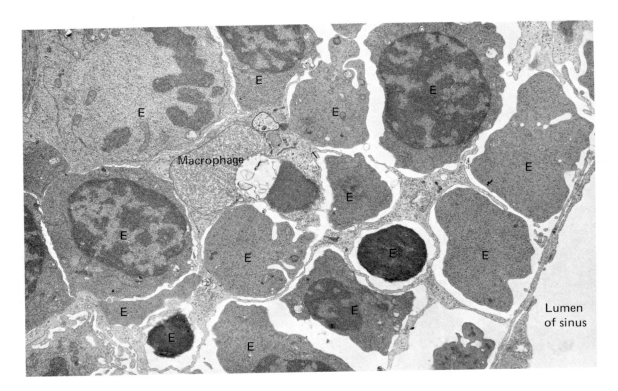

13–7   Rat bone marrow, erythroblastic islet. A macrophage lies amid a cluster of red cells **(E)**. It sends out a system of slender branching cell processes that enclose the surrounding red cells and reach to the wall of a vascular sinus on the upper right. (This tissue was perfused and the cells, as a result, are separated from one another, thereby revealing the extensive branching of the macrophage clearly.) × 7,300. (From Weiss, L. 1976. Anat. Rec. 186:161.)

inous and fatty transformations of adventitial reticular cells constitute mechanisms to change the volume of hematopoietic space in an organ which, because its "capsule" is bone, does not readily change and which, therefore must have a rather constant total volume.[1]

Fat cells do more than control hematopoietic space. They are active in the metabolism of steroid hormones, aromatizing testosterone to estrogens, as shown by Frisch. It also appears from Dexter's studies of bone marrow in tissue culture that fat cells induce granulocyte differentiation.

---

[1]In certain pathological states where hematopoiesis is abnormally intense for long periods, the bone in trabeculae and the cortex may thin considerably, even breaking as a result of minor trauma (pathological fracture).

The Hematopoietic Compartment

The hematopoietic tissue in marrow lies between vascular sinuses and consists of hematopoietic cells, mast cells, and related cell types of connective tissue held in a reticular meshwork formed by branches of reticular cells. The relative numbers of nucleated marrow hematopoietic cells are given in Table 13–1.

There is a pattern to the arrangement of hematopoietic cells in the hematopoietic compartments. Megakaryocytes lie close against the adventitial surface of vascular sinuses (Figs. 13–1, 13–2, and 13–4). They lie over apertures in the vascular wall and discharge platelets directly into the lumen. By lying over such an aperture, the megakaryocyte efficiently delivers platelets into the vascular lumen and, by its large size, both resists being swept into the circulation and prevents vascular leakage.

Erythrocytes are produced near sinuses. As they mature to the point where nuclear polarization is marked (Fig. 12–7) the cytoplasmic pole is typically directed toward a vascular sinus. Nuclear and cytoplasmic poles separate, and the cytoplasmic portion, now a freshly produced reticulocyte, remains near the wall. It becomes part of the reticulocyte reserve of the mar-

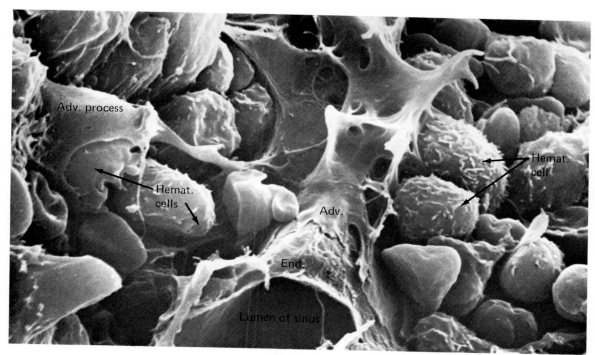

13–8 Rat bone marrow, scanning electron micrograph. A vascular sinus opens at the lower margin. The outside surface of its endothelium **(End)** is clothed by a reticular cell in adventitial position **(Adv)** in the vascular wall. The adventitial cell branches into the surrounding hematopoietic tissue. On the left a branch **(Adv process)** partially envelops a hematopoietic cell **(Hemat cell)**. On the right, two hematopoietic cells bearing microvilli press against the outside surface of the vessel. Cells appear to develop microvilli preparatory to passing across the vascular wall into the lumen. × 4,000. (From Weiss, L. 1976. Anat. Rec. 186:161.)

13–9 Rat bone marrow, scanning electron micrograph. A sinus lies at the right, with the luminal surface of its endothelium **(End surface)** and the torn edge of its endothelium **(End edge)** on view. The adventitial reticular cells have become fatty **(Fat cell)** and extend into the hematopoietic space, occupying space that would otherwise be available for hematopoiesis. × 4,050. (From Weiss, L. 1976. Anat. Rec. 186:161.)

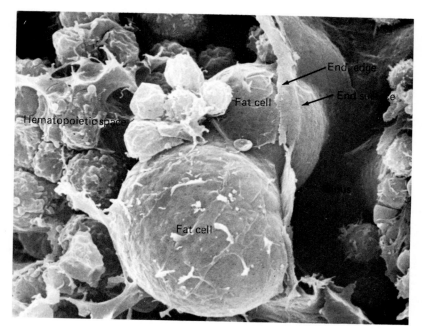

Table 13–1 Relative Number of Nucleated Cells in Normal Bone Marrow

	Range	Average
Myeloblasts	0.3–5.0	2.0
Promyelocytes	1.0–8.0	5.0
Myelocytes		
Neutrophilic	5.0–19.0	12.0
Eosinophilic	0.5–3.0	1.5
Basophilic	0.0–0.5	0.3
Metamyelocytes ("juvenile" forms)	13.0–32.0	22.0
Polymorphonuclear neutrophils	7.0–30.0	20.0
Polymorphonuclear eosinophils	0.5–4.0	2.0
Polymorphonuclear basophils	0.0–0.7	0.2
Lymphocytes	3.0–17.0	10.0
Plasma cells	0.0–2.0	0.4
Monocytes	0.5–5.0	2.0
Reticular cells	0.1–2.0	0.2
Megakaryocytes	0.03–3.0	0.4
Pronormoblasts	1.0–8.0	4.0
Erythroblasts (basophilic, polychromatophilic, and acidophilic)	7.0–32.0	18.0

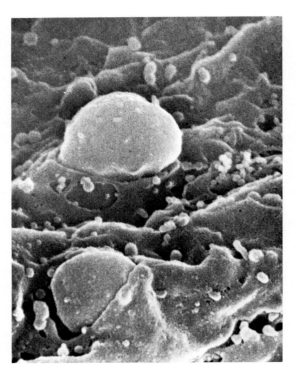

13–10 Rat bone marrow, scanning electron micrograph. This is a view of a vascular sinus on its luminal surface. Two cells are passing through the endothelium, probably entering the lumen of the sinus and the circulation. The upper cell is constricted as it squeezes through the endothelium. The lower one has a cowl of endothelium around it as it appears to emerge. × 3,000. (From Weiss, L., and Chen, L.-T. 1975. Blood cells, 1:617.)

row; after a variable time, an aperture in the wall is formed, and the reticulocyte squeezes through into the lumen of the sinus. Alternatively, a reticulocyte can be released to the circulation as it is being produced. The nuclear pole is phagocytized (Chap. 12). Macrophages are regularly associated with developing erythroblasts, phagocytizing nuclear poles, secreting factors that regulate erythropoiesis, and, perhaps, facilitating the delivery of reticulocytes to the circulation. Macrophages may lie among erythroblasts in no apparent arrangement, but often a macrophage lies in the center of an *erythroblastic islet*, its cytoplasm extending out and enclosing surrounding erythroblasts (Fig. 13–7). There may be one or more circlets or tiers of erythroblasts in an islet. The outer tiers consist of more mature cells than do the inner ones. Other cell types are associated with erythropoiesis, particularly when it is heightened as, for example, in response to severe blood loss. Then characteristic branched dense stromal cells and lymphocytes may be seen in company with macrophages and erythroblasts.

Granulocytes are typically produced in nests or as dispersed sheets of cells, somewhat away from the vascular sinus. On maturation, at the metamyelocyte stage, they become motile and join the reserve of marrow granulocytes, ready to move toward the vascular sinus and exit across

the wall of the sinus into the circulation (Figs. 13–10 and 13–11). As granulocyte precursors mature, they are regularly associated with other cell types. This is seen clearly during heightened granulocytopoiesis as, for example, in the intensified eosinophilopoiesis that occurs after infection with the nematode worm *Ascaris suum*. Then branched stromal cells, macrophages, and lymphocytes similar to those attending heightened erythropoiesis are present in proximity to the eosinophils (Fig. 13–12).

Delivery of Blood Cells to the Circulation

Maturing blood cells move from the hematopoietic compartment into the circulation through apertures in the walls of vascular sinuses. As

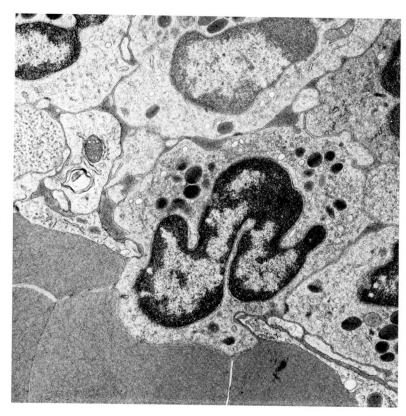

13–11 Mouse bone marrow. An eosinophil is crossing the wall of a vascular sinus, passing from the hematopoietic compartment above into the blood, below. × 9,500. (From N. Sakai and L. Weiss.)

blood cells mature they move to the adventitial surface of the vascular sinus. Adventitial cells move away from the wall, and the basement membrane depolymerizes, leaving the endothelium as the only barrier to the lumen of the sinus. The maturing blood cells press against the basal surface of the endothelium and apertures appear in the endothelial cells near (but not at) endothelial cell junctions. The blood cells then squeeze through into the lumen of the sinus. Apertures normally develop only in relationship to cell passage; they are either occupied by a cell in transit or absent. The integrity of the endothelial barrier between blood and hematopoietic compartments is thereby maintained (Figs. 13–4, 13–10, and 13–11).

Hematopoietic Microenvironment

Several lines of evidence suggest that hematopoietic organs provide a distinctive microenvironment that can influence the differentiation of blood cells. When an animal whose hematopoietic tissues have been destroyed by irradia-

tion is given a suspension of multipotential hematopoietic stem cells (CFU-S), the stem cells "home" to the hematopoietic tissues and, by proliferating and differentiating there, restore hematopoietic activity. The CFU-Ss going to the spleen differentiate mostly into erythroblasts, whereas those going to bone marrow differentiate into granulocytes and macrophages and, to a lesser extent, erythroblasts. Within the spleen and bone marrow, moreover, there are separate zones that favor erythroid, lymphocytic, or granulocytic differentiation. A pair of mouse congenital anemias further supports the concept of the hematopoietic microenvironment. The Wv/Wv strain of mouse has a mild anemia due to a deficiency in CFU-Ss; when stem cells are provided the anemia is cured. However, in the clinically similar anemia of the Sl/Sl^d mouse there are normal numbers of CFU-Ss, as shown by spleen colony assay, and the anemia cannot be cured by administering hematopoietic cells. The deficiency in this animal is considered to be due to a defect in the stroma, vasculature, or associated cells—in short, to the microenvironment.

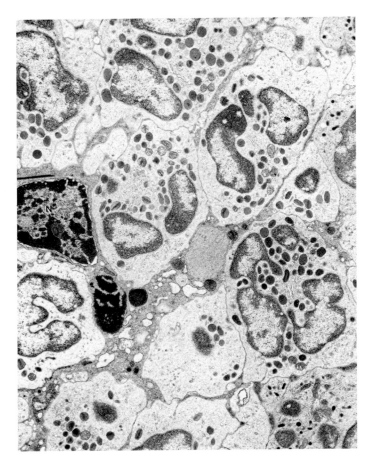

13–12 Mouse bone marrow stimulated to heightened eosinophilopoiesis. Many eosinophils in various stages of differentiation lie in the field. A large, branched stromal cell extends among them, its nucleus **(N)**. A similar stromal cell may be found among developing blood cells during heightened hematopoiesis affecting any blood cell type. (From Weiss, L., and Sakai, N. 1981. Microenvironments in hematopoietic and lymphoid differentiation, London: Pitman.)

Pathology

Hematopoietic activity of bone marrow may increase (hyperplasia) or decrease (hypoplasia or aplasia). Such change may affect every blood cell type or selected types. Increased hematopoietic activity may be due to an increase of essentially normal cells (such as in increased production of red cells after hemorrhage) or to abnormal cells (such as in the leukemias). In the leukemias, abnormal leukocytes are produced and may crowd the normal cells out. Leukemias occur in the different white blood cell types, as monocytic leukemia, lymphocytic leukemia, and so forth. A related malignancy of bone marrow is *multiple myeloma*. Here the marrow is crowded with myeloma cells that represent abnormal plasma cells. The myeloma cells in any given case constitute a clone that produces an abnormal incomplete antibody molecule. Knowledge of the amino acid sequence of such molecules has been valuable for elucidating normal antibody structure.

In *polycythemia vera* there is hypertrophy of the erythroblastic mass but the number of leukocytes and megakaryocytes may also be increased. Erythropoiesis may be so intense in certain anemias (as in the thalassemias) that the internal surface of the bone is eroded and trabeculae become reduced in size and number as the marrow cavity expands. Despite this considerable increase in erythropoiesis, the number of erythrocytes in the circulation is usually quite low because the erythrocytes in these conditions are markedly defective cells with considerably shortened life spans. There are many animal models of hematological disease. A congenital hemolytic anemia in the deer mouse appears similar to a congenital hemolytic anemia in children. Hemolytic anemias due to spectrin deficiencies have been shown in mice and in human beings.

In contrast, the bone marrow may become hypoplastic. Marrow may be reduced to a fatty state by starvation. Many chemicals are toxic to marrow. Lead and benzene may produce an aplastic anemia. Certain toxins may be used therapeutically, such as the nitrogen mustards, which suppress or destroy abnormal bone marrow like that in leukemia. Aplastic anemia may be genetically determined, and some animal models, such as the Wv/Wv and Sl/Sl^d strains discussed above, are providing insight into the mechanisms. In a rare human condition, the Diamond-Blackfan syndrome of congenital aplastic anemia, T$_s$ lymphocytes may suppress erythropoiesis. Malignant tumors may metastasize to bone marrow and create aplastic marrows by suppressing or displacing normal hematopoietic tissue. In some instances, vascular sinuses may become widely dilated with blood, encroaching on hematopoietic tissue and, paradoxically, conferring a brilliant red color on a hematopoietically inactive tissue. Hormones and humoral substances in addition to those (such as erythropoietin) specifically directed toward hematopoietic tissues influence hematopoiesis. Estrogens inhibit erythropoiesis and testosterone stimulates it. Unchecked production of calcitonin may result in bony overgrowth and a decrease in the volume of the marrow cavity, leading to a reduced output of blood cells.

References and Selected Bibliography

General

Bloom, W., and Bartelmez, G. W., 1940. Hematopoiesis in young human embryos. Am. J. Anat. 67:21.

Bråanemark, P. I. 1959. Vital microscopy of bone marrow in rabbit. Scand. J. Clin. Lab. Invest. (Suppl. 38) 11:1.

Donahue, D. M., Gabrio, B. W., and Finch, C. A. 1958. Quantitative measurement of hematopoietic cells of the marrow. J. Clin. Invest. 37:1564.

Gilmour, J. R. 1941. Normal hematopoiesis in intrauterine and neonatal life. J. Pathol. Bact. 52:25.

Weiss, L. 1965. The structure of bone marrow. Functional interrelationships of vascular and hematopoietic compartments in experimental hemolytic anemia. J. Morphol. 117:481.

Weiss, L. 1972. The Cells and Tissues of the Immune System. Englewood Cliffs, N.J.: Prentice-Hall.

Weiss, L., and Chen, L. T. 1975. The organization of hematopoietic cords and vascular sinuses in bone marrow. Blood Cells 1:617.

Wickramasinghe, S. N. 1975. Human Bone Marrow. Oxford: Blackwell Scientific Publications, Ltd.

Hematopoiesis

Allen, T. D., and Dexter, T. M. 1976. Cellular interrelationships during in vitro granulopoiesis. Differentiation. 6:191.

Huggins, C., and Blocksom, B. H. 1936. Changes in outlying bone marrow accompanying a local increase of temperature with physiological limits. J. Exp. Med. 64:253.

Iscove, N. N. 1977. The role of erythropoietin in regulation of population size and cell cycling of early and late erythroid precursors in mouse bone marrow. Cell Tissue Kinet. 10:323.

Lichtman, M. A. 1979. Cellular deformability during maturation of the myeloblast. Possible role in marrow egress. N. Engl. J. Med. 283:943.

Sakai, N., Johnstone, C., and Weiss, L. 1981. Bone marrow cells associated with heightened eosinophilopoiesis: An electron microscope study of murine bone marrow stimulated by Ascaris suum. Am. J. Anat. 161:11.

Trentin, J. J. 1970. Influence of hemopoietic organ stroma (hematopoietic inductive microenvironments) on stem cell differentiation. In Regulation of Hematopoiesis, vol. I: Red Cell Production, Gordon, A. S. (ed.). New York: Appleton-Crofts, p. 161.

Stroma

LaPushin, R. W., and Trentin, J. J., 1977. Identification of distinctive stromal elements in erythroid and neutrophil granuloid spleen colonies: Light and electron microscopic study. Exp. Hemat. 5:505.

McCuskey, R. S., and Meinke, H. A., 1973. Studies of the hematopoietic microenvironment. III. Differences in the splenic microvascular system and stroma between Sl/Sl^d and W/W^v mice. Am. J. Anat. 137:187.

Tavassoli, M. 1976. Marrow adipose cells-histochemical identification of labile and stable components. Arch. Pathol. Lab. Med. 100:16.

Weiss, L. 1976. The hematopoietic microenvironment of the bone marrow:An Ultrastructural study of the stroma in rats. Anat. Rec. 186:161.

Vasculature

Campbell, F. 1972. Ultrastructural studies of transmural migration of blood cells in the bone marrow of rats, mice and guinea pigs. Am. J. Anat. 135:521.

Doan, C. A. 1922. The capillaries of the bone marrow of the adult pigeon. Bull. Johns Hopkins Hosp. 33:222.

Fleidner, T. M. 1956. Research on the architecture of the vascular bed of the bone marrow of rats. Z. Zellforsch. Mikrosk. Anat. 45:328.

Lichtman, M. A., Chamberlain, J. K., and Santillo, P. A. 1978. Factors thought to contribute to the regulation of the egress of cells from marrow. In The Year in Hematology, Gordon, A. S., Silber, R. and Lobue, J. (eds.). New York: Plenum, p. 243.

Zamboni, L., and Pease, D. C. 1961. The vascular bed of red bone marrow. J. Ultrastruct. Res. 5:65.

Pathology

Hoshi, H., and Weiss, L. 1978. Rabbit bone marrow after administration of saponin. Lab. Invest. 38:67.

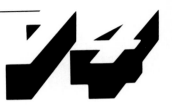

The Thymus

Leon Weiss

The human thymus is a lymphoepithelial organ derived both from the epithelium of the third branchial pouch and from lymphoid stem cells that enter from the blood. It is pyramidal, rests on the pericardium in the superior mediastinum, and achieves its greatest absolute weight, approximately 40 g, at puberty. It is bilaterally symmetrical, consisting of halves that meet in the midline except at the apex, where it extends into the neck and diverges around the trachea.

The thymus produces the T lymphocytes of the body from stem cells that migrate to it via the circulation from the bone marrow. The stem cells enter the thymus, proliferate, and mature there, presumably under the influence of the epithelial cells. The thymus also appears to monitor T-cell production, destroying those T cells capable of attacking self, that is, the body's own tissues, in contrast to foreign substances, such as bacteria or grafts or genetically different tissues. T cells are released by the thymus to complete their maturation in the spleen or lymph nodes. They then circulate and recirculate through the body, accumulating in spleen, lymph nodes, and other lymphatic tissues. Because the thymus does not itself directly participate to a significant degree in immune reactions, but rather releases cells to other tissues that do, it is, like bone marrow, classified as a *central immune organ*.

The thymus develops early compared with other lymphatic organs. It is well developed before birth, and before puberty it is round and fleshy. After puberty the thymus begins a remarkable *involution* or atrophy, its parenchyma

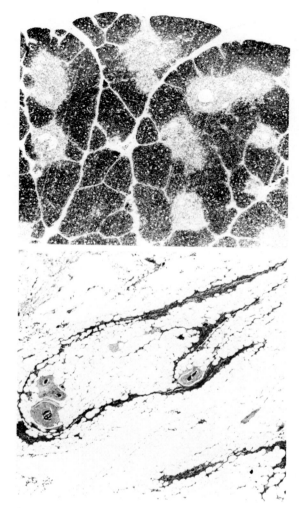

14–1 Human thymus before and after involution.
The tissue in the **upper** micrograph is from an infant 3 mos. old; the **lower**, from a 72-year-old person. Note the lobular pattern in the upper micrograph. The medulla is a branching structure. The cortex surrounds the lobular projections of the medulla. A thin fibrous capsule is present. Involutional changes are evident in the lower micrograph. The cortex is markedly diminished, and the organ is fatty. The blood vessels display thickened sclerotic walls (see Fig. 14–12). × 25. (From the work of Robert Rouse.)

being gradually replaced by fatty and fibrous tissue (Fig. 14–1). This *age involution* may be greatly accelerated by certain types of stress; it is then called *accidental involution*. (See section on Involution, page 521.)

Structure of the Thymus

The thymus is divided into lobes and lobules by septae that extend into the organ from the surrounding connective tissue capsule. The lobules, 0.5 to 2.0 mm in length, are roughly rectangular in outline. Each lobule is divided into a peripheral zone relatively rich in lymphocytes, called the *cortex*, and a central zone relatively rich in epithelial cells, called the *medulla* (Figs. 14–1 and 14–2).

Major Cell Types

Epithelial Cells. Epithelial cells assume several forms in the thymus. A major epithelial conformation is a meshwork or *cytoreticulum* made of richly branched cells attached to one another by desmosomes. In contrast to the reticulum of mesenchymal organs such as the spleen, this meshwork is made of epithelial cells alone, without reticular fibers, and the cells are called *epithelial-reticular cells*. The interstices of this cytoreticulum are tightly packed with lymphocytes, and the plasma membrane of each lymphocyte is closely surrounded by the plasma membrane of an epithelial cell (Fig. 14–3). Epithelial-reticular cells have tonofilaments and desmosomes indicative of their epithelial character, and membrane-bounded cytoplasmic inclusions suggesting a secretory capacity. Indeed epithelial cells produce *thymosin* and other humoral factors that control thymic function (see below). Although epithelial-reticular cells are best seen in the cortex, which contains 95% of the lymphocytes of the thymus, they are also present (less fully branched) in the medulla. Epithelial cell sacs that completely enclose clusters of 50 or more lymphocytes are reported in the cortex of the thymus. They are saclike structures that have been found after disruption of the thymus and are quite difficult to visualize in sectioned material. It is possible, however, that the sacs are artifacts caused by disruption.

Another major group of epithelial cells forms *thymic corpuscles*, or *Hassall's corpuscles*, structures unique to the medulla (Figs. 14–2, and 14–5 to 14–7). When well developed, these corpuscles consist of epithelial cells rather tightly wound upon one another in a concentric pattern. The central cells are prone to become swollen, calcified, and necrotic. They may undergo lysis, leaving a cystic structure. The corpuscle may become markedly keratinized, resembling the epi-

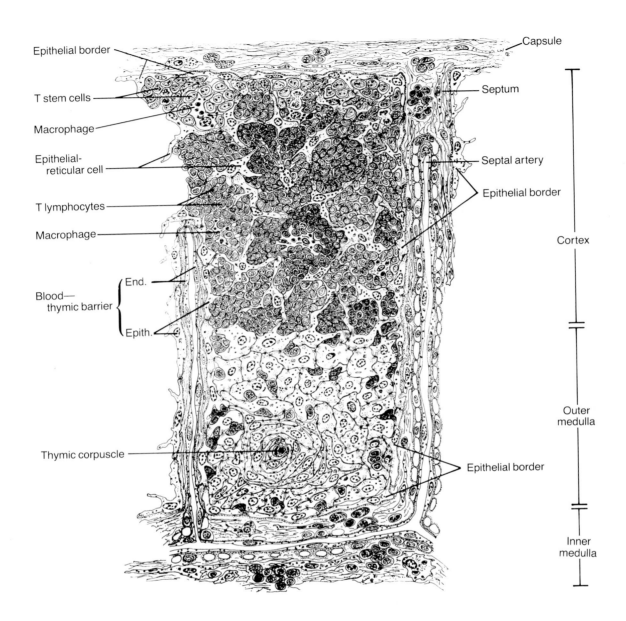

Epithelial border

T stem cells

Macrophage

Epithelial-
reticular cell

T lymphocytes

Macrophage

Blood—
thymic barrier { End.

Epith.

Thymic corpuscle

Capsule

Septum

Septal artery

Epithelial border

Cortex

Outer
medulla

Inner
medulla

Epithelial border

14–2 Schema of portion of thymus lobule. The cortex is heavily infiltrated with lymphocytes. As a result, the epithelial cells become stellate and remain attached to one another by desmosomes. The medulla is closer to a pure epithelium, although it, too, is commonly infiltrated by lymphocytes. A large thymic corpuscle, consisting of concentrically arranged epithelial cells, is shown. The capsule and trabeculae are rich in connective tissue fibers (mainly collagen) and contain blood vessels and variable numbers of plasma cells, granulocytes, and lymphocytes. A border of somewhat flattened epithelial cells surrounds the cortex and outer medulla.

dermis. Lymphocytes, eosinophils, and macrophages—usually degenerated—may lie within a thymic corpuscle. The peripheral epithelial cells within a corpuscle blend into the cytoreticulum. A thymic corpuscle may actually be present as a single cell, swollen, calcified, and degenerated, or it may be a huge multiform structure several hundred microns in one direction. Thymic corpuscles are well developed in human beings, dogs, and guinea pigs, and poorly developed in mice and rats. The number of thymic corpuscles in human beings reaches its maximum at about

they surround blood vessels and make up a major component of the blood–thymic barrier (Figs. 14–8 to 14–12 and see below). They also lie along the perimeter of the gland, forming a slender epithelial border that encloses both the cortex and the medulla and thereby "seals off" the thymus from many outside influences (Fig. 14–2 and see below).

Lymphocytes. Before its involution, the thymus contains vast numbers of developing T lymphocytes. More than 95% of them lie in the cortex, dominating its appearance. Approximately 10% of thymic lymphocytes are large. These cells are concentrated in the outer cortex beneath

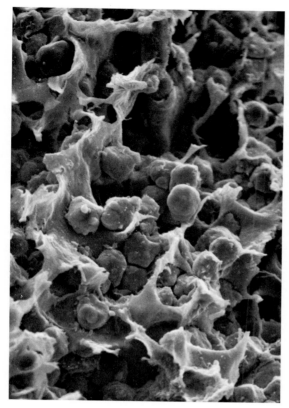

14–3 Rat thymus cortex, scanning electron micrograph. Many cortical lymphocytes have been washed away, revealing the broad branchings of the epithelial-reticular cells. Note that some of the lymphocytes remain, lying on the epithelial-reticular cells. × 5,700. (From the work of L.-T. Chen, B. W. Wetzel, and L. Weiss.)

14–4 Human thymus, infant. In this field a large epithelial cell **(Epith. cell)** lies among lymphocytes **(Ly)**. The surface of the epithelial cell reacts positively **(arrows)** in a cytochemical reaction labeling the Dr region of the major histocompatibility complex (the HLA complex in humans). The reaction depends on a monoclonal antibody reactive against the cell-surface antigens determined by the Dr region of the HLA complex. This antibody is linked to a horseradish peroxidase marker as discussed in Chap. 2. The HLA antigens on the surface of thymus cells are probably important in the cellular interactions underlying T-cell maturation and homing. See text for discussion. (From the work of Robert Rouse)

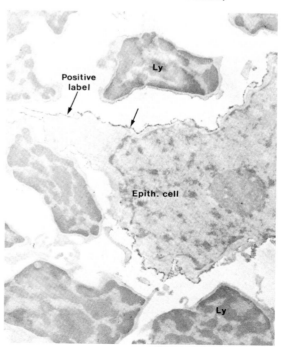

the time of puberty; from then on, they decrease in number, especially the smaller ones. With age, however, the remaining corpuscles become larger, and, as the thymus involutes, more prominent. The functions of thymic corpuscles are not known.

Epithelial cells in the thymus may occur as a simple cuboidal epithelium or a columnar ciliated mucus-producing epithelium lining the walls of cysts. Cysts are occasionally present in adult human thymus and may represent remnants of diverticuli of the fourth branchial pouches.

Epithelial cells in the thymus may also assume a barrier function. Somewhat flattened, and linked to one another by junctional complexes,

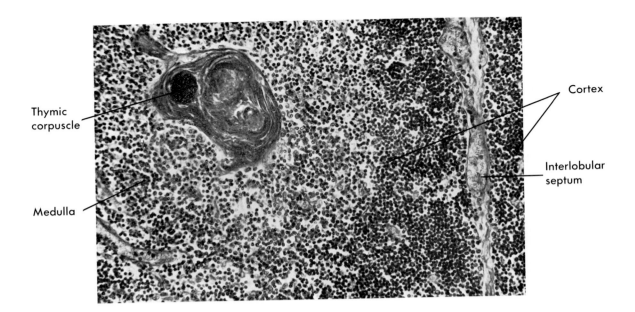

Thymic corpuscle

Medulla

Cortex

Interlobular septum

14–5 Thymus of a 20-year-old person. Lymphocytes are concentrated in the cortex. They are present in the medulla as well but are scattered loosely among epithelial-reticular cells. A large, multicentric thymic corpuscle is present in the medulla. The interlobular septum is slender and contains lymphatic vessels, blood vessels, and nerves. × 200. (Preparation from B. Castleman.)

the capsule and they actively proliferate. They represent stem cells recently arrived from bone marrow. The deeper part, and the bulk of the cortex, contains small thymic lymphocytes, about 85% of all thymic lymphocytes. They are maturing cells derived from the large subcapsular lymphocytes. As they mature they move deeper into the cortex, so that lymphocytes at the cortical–medullary junction and in the medulla are the most mature. Approximately 5% of thymic lymphocytes lie among the epithelial cells of the medulla. As thymic lymphocytes mature, they acquire distinctive markers on the cell surface and within the cytoplasm that are revealed by special staining. By standard light and electron-microscopic stains, developing T cells look like other lymphocytes. Small thymic lymphocytes, however, are somewhat smaller than small lymphocytes found elsewhere in the body. Degenerating lymphocytes are numerous but inconspicuous throughout the thymus. They may lie free or may be phagocytized by macrophages.

The kinetics of T-lymphocyte development can be followed by autoradiography after a single injection or pulse of tritiated thymidine. Lymphocytes in the outer cortex are labeled within 15 to 30 min. A shift of labeled cells then occurs, for in 12 to 24 h lymphocytes in the deep cortex and medulla become maximally labeled and the labeling of subcapsular lymphocytes is quite decreased. The total generation time of most thymic lymphocytes is about 9 h. The G_1 period is thought to be quite short. Thus the maturation of T lymphocytes, including their proliferation, differentiation, and migration from the subcapsular regions into the medulla, may occur within 24 h. Mature T lymphocytes leave the thymus by way of blood vessels and lymphatics.

Other Cells. Macrophages are invariably present within the thymus, lying among lymphocytes and epithelial cells of cortex and medulla. In addition to their evident phagocytic capacity, macrophages may secrete factors that stimulate T-cell mitosis or differentiation.

Antigen-presenting cells, similar to those present in white pulp of spleen and cortex of lymph nodes and related to the Langerhans cells of epidermis, are present in the thymic medulla. They bear Ia antigens on their surface and can contain Birbeck granules (see Langerhan Cells, Chap. 17, and discussion of antigen-presenting cells, p. 535). The *myoid cell* is present in the thymus of many species. It is more abundant in human fetuses than in adults. It contains myofilaments and in some species may appear as a well-developed muscle cell. Sarcomeres are not

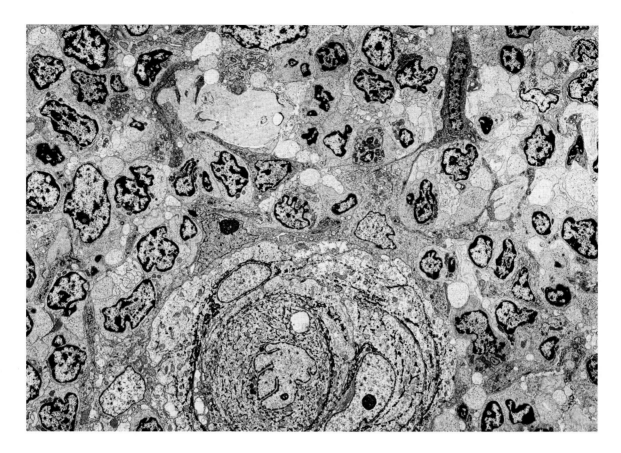

well developed in human beings. Eosinophils and other granulocytes are present in the young thymus; erythroblasts have also been reported. Mast cells may be present in large number in aged thymuses, where they are largely confined to the inner medulla, septae, and capsule. In NZB mice, mast cells may be massively produced within the cortex, presumably from thymic lymphocytes (see below). Plasma cells may occur in the thymus, again largely restricted to surrounding connective tissues but within the parenchyma of the gland as well. Lymphatic nodules may occur pathologically in the thymus. They are restricted to the capsule, septae, and inner medula.

Organization of Parenchyma and Vasculature

The line between the cortex and the medulla of the thymus often appears abrupt. The cortex contains most of the lymphocytes and the medulla contains all of the thymic corpuscles, but both the cortex and the medulla are lymphoepithelial

structures and should be regarded as a continuum. In fact, a simple layer of epithelial cells and their basal lamina runs as a boundary line around both cortex and medulla, thus enclosing both. The connective tissues of the capsule and septae lie outside the lymphoepithelial cortex and medulla, peripheral to the epithelial boundary line (Fig. 14–2). Thymic arteries (branches of the subclavian artery) enter the thymus from the surrounding connective tissues, pass down the septae, and enter the medulla. The vessels that enter the gland and ramify carry in with them a sheath of connective tissue that is continuous with the capsule and septae. As these vessels penetrate the lymphoepithelial cortex and outer medulla (see below), they bring with them a

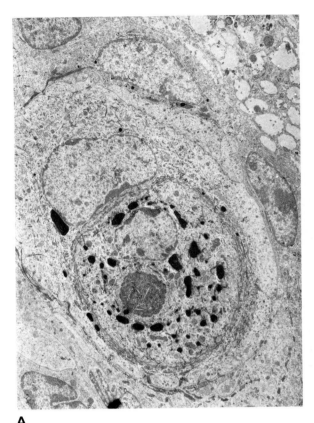

A

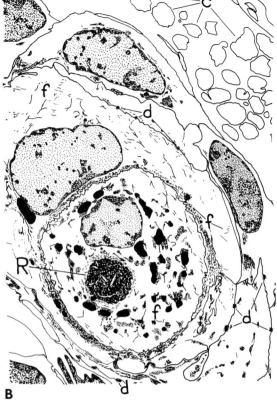

B

14–7 Thymus of a guinea pig. **A.** Electron micrograph of a thymic corpuscle. There is a small compressed central cell (labeled R in the accompanying tracing). Note the concentric pattern of the cells. The inner cells have droplets, probably keratohyaline droplets. Cytoplasmic filaments and desmosomes contribute to this corpuscle. A portion of an epithelial cell in the cytoreticulum in the right upper corner contains intracytoplasmic vacuoles. (From Kohnen, P., and Weiss, L. 1964. Anat. Rec. 148:29 [Fig. 1]). **B.** Tracing of the corpuscle shown in part A. Desmosomes are indicated by **d**, cytoplasmic filaments by **f**, and intracytoplasmic vacuoles by **c**. **R** is degenerated nucleus. × 5,000.

layer of epithelial cells that lies on a basal lamina continuous with the epithelial boundary layer described above (Figs. 14–2 and 14–8 to 14–9). Thus the vessels are surrounded by an epithelial sheath. The connective tissue sheath becomes attenuated as it extends along the smaller ramifications, and is quite slight around the fine cortical vessels. The vascular lumen in the lym-

phoepithelial zones is thereby separated from thymic lymphocytes by a number of layers that are, in order: endothelium (and in arteries and veins, a muscular coat), endothelial basal lamina, perivascular connective tissue, epithelial basal lamina, and epithelium. (See Figs. 14–2, 14–8, and 14–9.) These layers constitute the blood–thymus barrier.

The endothelium of thymic blood vessels and its basal lamina are continuous. There are no high endothelial venules of the sort present in lymph nodes. The connective tissue sheath can be quite thick and cellular around the larger vessels, which enter the gland in the central medulla. In fact, Pereira and Clermont recognize an *inner medulla* that is vascular and made of mesenchymal tissues in distinction to an *outer medulla*, which is lymphoepithelial and enclosed within an epithelial boundary layer. It is within the connective tissue of the inner medulla—and in its extensions throughout the gland as it runs along blood vessels—that many of the plasma cells, granulocytes, mast cells,

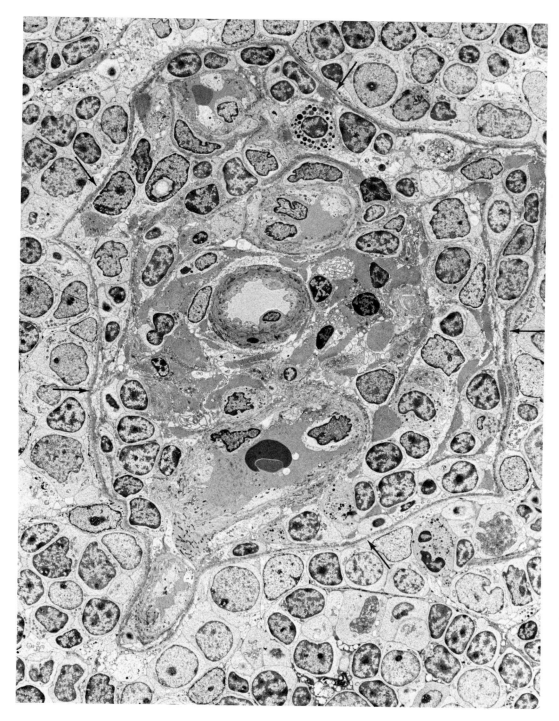

14–8 Human thymus, near the border of the cortex and the medulla. An arteriole with several branches as surrounded by a perivascular connective tissue space limited by epithelial–reticular cells **(arrows)**. × 1,850. (From Bearman, R. M., Bensch, K. G., and Levine, G. D. 1975. Anat. Rec. 183:485.) See Fig. 14–6.

518

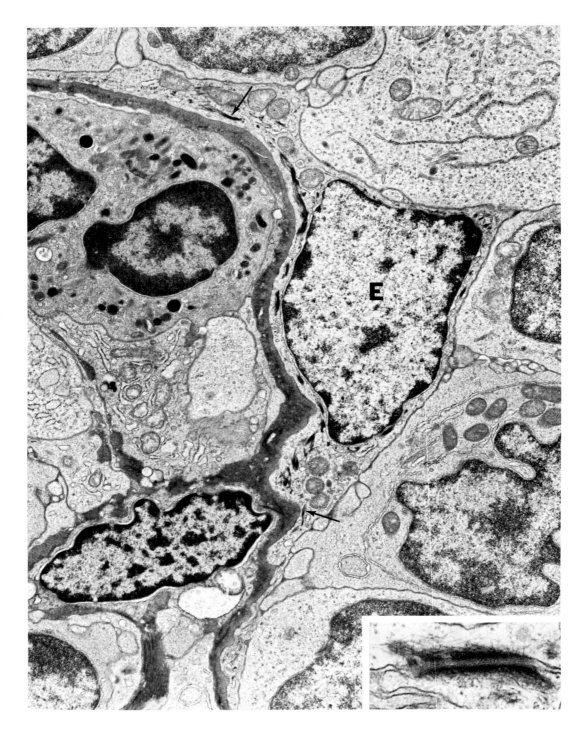

14–9 Human thymus: a higher magnification of the border of the perivascular space and the thymic parenchyma. An epithelial-reticular cell **(E)** delineates the space, which is to the left of the cell. The epithelial-reticular cell contains prominent tonofilaments **(arrows)**. × 16,500. **Inset.** Desmosome between two epithelial-reticular cells. × 50,000 (From Bearman, R.M., Bensch, K.G., and Levine, G. D. 1975. Anat. Rec. 183:485.)

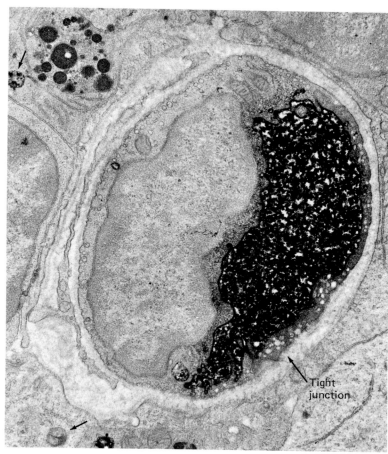

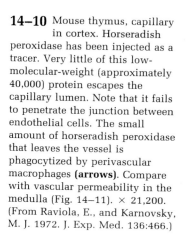

14–10 Mouse thymus, capillary in cortex. Horseradish peroxidase has been injected as a tracer. Very little of this low-molecular-weight (approximately 40,000) protein escapes the capillary lumen. Note that it fails to penetrate the junction between endothelial cells. The small amount of horseradish peroxidase that leaves the vessel is phagocytized by perivascular macrophages (**arrows**). Compare with vascular permeability in the medulla (Fig. 14–11). × 21,200. (From Raviola, E., and Karnovsky, M. J. 1972. J. Exp. Med. 136:466.)

Tight junction

macrophages, and other connective-tissue cell types are concentrated. The inner medulla is laced with reticular fibers and contains a mesenchymal reticulum in contrast to the cytoreticulum of the lymphoepithelial portion of the thymus. Levine and Bearman recognize epithelial and mesenchymal components of the thymus. They define an *intraparenchymal compartment* (IPC) composed of lymphoepithelial cortex and medulla and an *extraparenchymal compartment* (EPC) composed of blood vessels and surrounding connective tissue. The epithelial boundary layer with its basal lamina described above excludes the EPC. It is, in fact, the border of the IPC and is continuous with the subcapsular epithelial border around the perimeter of the gland.

A *blood–thymus barrier* exists that is impervious to such particulate and protein tracers as lanthanum, ferritin, and horseradish peroxidase. The epithelial cell layer surrounding the vascu-

lature is evidently a major element in this barrier. Raviola and Karnovsky have described the barrier as tight in most of the cortex but leaky in the juxtamedullary cortex (Figs. 14–10 and 14–11). Pereira and Clermont, however, have found the barrier to be tight throughout the thymus, except in the inner medulla.

The major blood vessels branch from the medulla and the corticomedullary junction. Slender arterial vessels run high in the cortex, breaking into capillaries beneath the capsule. Venules run back toward the corticomedullary junction and drain into veins there or in the inner medulla. The stem cells of T lymphocytes probably come into the gland through blood vessels and leave the vasculature beneath the capsule, selectively crossing the blood–thymus barrier and entering the intraparenchymal compartment high in the cortex. There they begin to proliferate and differentiate into T cells, which move deeper into the gland toward the corticomedullary junction.

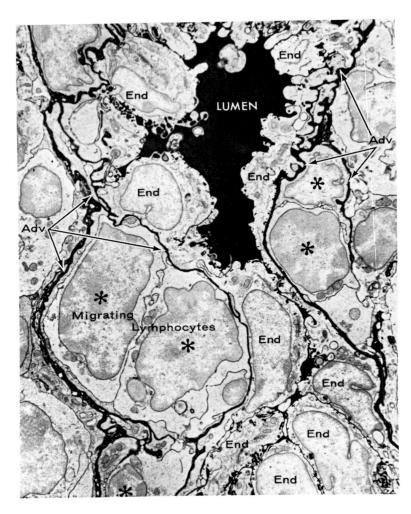

14–11 Mouse thymus, venule in medulla. Horseradish peroxidase has been injected as a tracer. In less than 5 min there has been an impressive leakage, staining the epithelial basal lamina and the adventitia **(Adv)** with the same intensity as the plasma in the lumen of the vessel. Note the irregular endothelium **(End)** bearing many pinocytotic vesicles containing the peroxidase tracer. The thick connective tissue adventitial layer **(Adv)** is traversed by migrating lymphocytes **(asterisks)** which are probably moving toward the lumen and into the circulation. Compare with Fig. 14–10. × 7,100. (From Raviola, E., and Karnovsky, M. J. 1972. J. Exp. Med. 136:466.)

Lymphatic Vessels. Efferent lymphatic vessels lie in the inner medulla of the thymus, run through septae and drain into mediastinal lymph nodes. They, as do veins, carry T lymphocytes from the thymus. There appear to be no afferent lymphatic vessels.

Nerve Supply. The capsule of the thymus is moderately rich in small myelinated and unmyelinated nerves from the vagus, cardiac plexus, first thoracic ganglion, and ansa hypoglossi. Vasomotor nerves enter the organ alongside its blood vessels.

Development

The human thymus develops bilaterally from the third branchial pouches. There may be small contributions from the fourth. The thymic rudiment in embryos of 10-mm crown–rump length (CRL) is a slender, tubular prolongation of branchial epithelium which extends caudad and mediad. The epithelium is of endodermal origin, but it is likely that an ectodermal contribution occurs. There may also be a contribution from the neural crest. The rudiment reaches into the mediastinum just caudal to the thyroid and parathyroid rudiments. The tip of the thymic prolongation proliferates, becoming bulbous. The intermediate portion, constituting the connection to the pharynx, vanishes and leaves the proliferating terminal bulb free in the mediastinum at 35-mm CRL. The epithelial rudiment becomes surrounded by a layer of mesenchyme. Soon afterwards, lymphocyte stem cells penetrate the mesenchyme, enter the epithelium, and lymphocytes and epithelial cells proliferate. The lobular pattern of the thymus becomes evident at

40-mm CRL. Thymic corpuscles appear at 60 to 70 mm.

The development of the thymus outstrips that of the remaining lymphatic organs. Whereas the thymus is rather fully developed prenatally, the spleen and lymph nodes are not.

The thymus may fail to develop normally. Defective thymic development in human beings is found in the Di George syndrome and Swiss-type agammaglobulinemia. A valuable animal model in which the thymus fails to develop normally is the nude (nu/nu) mutant mouse.

Involution

Involution, the process of atrophy and depletion, is related to age. After puberty the thymus gradually decreases in weight and suffers a considerable loss of cortical lymphocytes and of epithelial cells, both of which are replaced by fat.

Table 14–1 Age and Thymus Weight

Age, years	Weight, g
Newborn	13.26
1–5	22.98
6–10	26.10
11–15	37.52
16–20	25.58
21–25	24.73
26–35	19.87
36–45	16.27
46–55	12.85
56–65	16.08
66–75	6.00

There is a decrease in the number of the thymic corpuscles but an increase in their size. The septae show a proportionate increase in width as the lobules atrophy (Table 14–1 and Figs. 14–1 and 14–12).

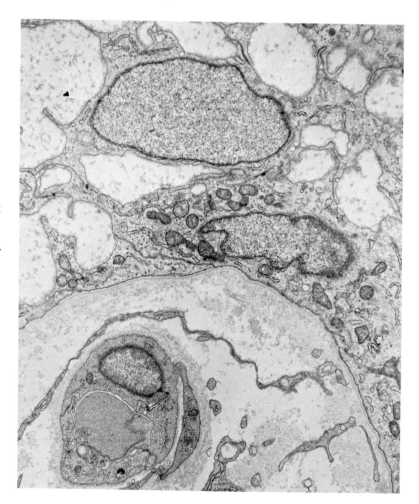

14–12 Human thymic cortex involution. A capillary at the bottom of the field lies in a perivascular space and is surrounded by an atrophic cortex. Lymphocytes have dropped out and the epithelial-reticular cells that remain form a fluid-filled meshwork. × 1,700. (From the work of G. D. Levine.)

Normal age-associated involution of the thymus should not be unduly emphasized, however, since the organ remains substantive and functional even in late adulthood. On the other hand, involution induced by stress may be severe and sudden. Such stress or accidental involution is caused by cortisone and related steroid hormones. The circulating levels of these hormones are increased in stress, and they have a lytic effect on immature T lymphocytes in the thymus. Stress involution is characterized by extensive cortical lymphocyte death and phagocytosis. The thymus in infants who die suddenly may be large and has been considered a cause of death, a condition called *status thymolymphaticus*. However, the thymus in this condition is a normal organ and is undiminished by stress involution.

Comparative Anatomy

Thymic tissue is present in every vertebrate. In lower forms it remains associated with the branchial arches, failing to move caudad. In mammals thymuses are remarkably alike, although differences in the development of thymic corpuscles, myoid cells, cysts, and other such structures may be found.

Functions of the Thymus

T-Lymphocyte Production

The thymus receives stem cells from the bone marrow (and from fetal liver before the marrow develops) and provides the microenvironment for them to develop into immunologically competent T cells. These T cells are released to undergo final maturation in the spleen and then begin a long life circulating and recirculating through blood and lymph, slowly passing through T-cell zones in peripheral lymphatic tissues. A large component of spleen and lymph nodes consists of T cells, and after neonatal thymectomy, these organs fail to develop fully (Fig. 14–13). The level of small lymphocytes circulating in the blood may be reduced by 60% or more; that in thoracic duct lymph may be reduced to an even lower level. The differentiation and migrations of T cells and their functions are discussed under Lymphocytes in Chaps. 11, 12, 15, and 16.

Thymectomy (or congenital athymia) results in severe immunological defects due primarily to a deficiency of T cells, if the operation is performed in the neonatal period before the thymus is able to carry out large-scale seeding of peripheral lymphatic organs with T cells (Fig. 14–13). Cellular immunity is impaired. Thus, after thymectomy in the newborn, homografts (a graft from a genetically different animal but one within the same species, as mouse to mouse) may persist indefinitely instead of being rejected within a week or two. Interference also occurs with antibody production against antigens that depend on cooperation of T cells with B cells. These deficiencies can be fully corrected with thymic grafts.

Thymectomy in adults causes no such clear-cut changes because the extrathymic lymphatic tissues and circulation are already stocked with T cells. The weight of spleen and lymph nodes is significantly reduced after thymectomy in adult rats, but 6 to 8 weeks are required for the change to develop. However, if adult rats are thymectomized and then irradiated to deplete stores of T cells in their lymphatic tissues, a condition emerges similar to that of the neonate after thymectomy.

Humoral Factors

The thymus secretes a number of immunological regulatory factors whose presence was first deduced from experiments involving neonatal thymectomy. As discussed above, a newborn mouse thymectomized at birth becomes deficient in both lymphocytes and immunological capacity. If a thymus wrapped in a cell-tight filter is inserted into the peritoneal cavity of such a mouse, the animal will have partial restoration of lymphocytes and suffer no immunological deficiencies. Factors appear to diffuse through the wrapping and largely substitute for the thymus. Further support for thymic humoral factors comes from experiments in which immunological competence is restored in thymectomized immunologically deficient female mice when they become pregnant, even though the placenta does not permit cells to move from fetus to mother. The best characterized of thymic humoral factors is *thymosin*, which may be separated into low-molecular-weight glycoprotein fractions (3,100 and 5,250 daltons). Thymosin restores T-cell deficiencies in thymectomized mice, thereby substituting for a thymus. Thymosin has been demonstrated in thymic epithelial cells by immunocytochemistry and is presumably se-

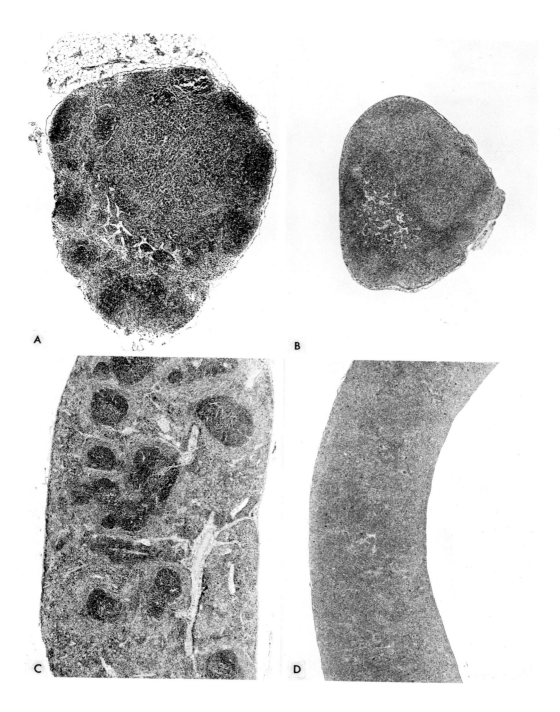

14–13 This plate illustrates the dependence of the lymph nodes and spleen on the thymus. The tissues are taken from C57BL mice. **A.** Lymph node of 8-week-old mouse sham-operated at birth. ×32. **B.** Lymph node of 8-week-old mouse thymectomized at birth. ×32. **C.** Spleen of 7-week-old mouse sham-operated at birth. ×32. **D.** Spleen of 7-week-old mouse thymectomized at birth. ×32. Thymectomy is followed by a decrease in size of the lymph nodes and spleen, due primarily to depletion of small lymphocytes (T cells). (From the work of J. F. A. P. Miller.)

creted by them. *Thymopoietin* (5500d) induces T cell maturation. *Thymic humoral factor* enhances the graft vs. host reaction. The *serum thymic factor* (847d) induces the development of markers in T cells. Secretion of a factor mitogenic for developing T cells has been ascribed to the thymic macrophages, a function related to the production of granulocyte colony stimulating factors (CSF-G) by macrophages (see Chap. 12).

Major Histocompatibility Complex Antigens

Epithelial-reticular cells, lymphocytes, and, indeed, virtually every cell in the body express an array of MHC antigens on their surface distinctive to cell type and development. These antigens are gene products whose background is as follows: There is a "supergene" known as the *major histocompatibility gene complex (MHC)*. It is on chromosome 17 in mice and chromosome 6 in human beings. The MHC complex is called the H-2 system in mice and the HLA (histocompatibility linked antigens) system in human beings. This supergene is subdivided into four major subdivisions: K, I, S, and D; each of them is subdivided so that, for example, subregions of the I region are Ia and Ib. The MHC contains genes that direct the production (through the usual processes of transcription, translation, and protein synthesis) of gene products, which may move to a position on the cell surface or be released to the extracellular environment. Through such gene products the MHC controls a number of immunological functions; and it is possible to correlate the activity of a given MHC subregion with a given immunological function. For example, the genes of the I region control a variety of phenomena associated with cellular recognition as well as with recognition of antigenic foreignness. Mouse T cells that help B cells (T_H or helper T cells) bear surface determinants coded in the Ia region and cytotoxic T cells (T_S or suppressor T cells) have cell-surface determinants coded in the K or D region. Similar arrangements occur in human beings and in other species tested. Rouse et al. and others have found that in the thymus the epithelial-reticular cells, which are intimately associated with developing T cells, have MHC gene products on their surfaces. The gene products of different regions of the MHC complex, moreover, are expressed in different patterns on the thymic cytoreticulum formed by the epithelial-reticular cells. The gene products of the Ia region are present throughout the thymic cortex, whereas those of the rest of the I region and of the K and D regions are expressed only variably. Thus, developing T lymphocytes are exposed, during their intimate association with epithelial-reticular cells, to a highly specific gene product expressing self. This exposure may well be a factor in determining which T cells are induced to divide and be released (those that recognize and react against foreign materials or nonself) and which are destroyed or not permitted to proliferate (those that would react against self and induce autoimmune disease). Monoclonal antibodies may be prepared against MHC antigens and, when coupled to horseradish peroxidase or another marker, may be used as the basis of a cytochemical test for demonstrating MHC antigens in tissue section (Fig. 14–14).

Mast Cell and Eosinophil Differentiation

Mast cells may be present within the thymus; in certain strains of mice, such as the NZB, they are present in massive numbers. In tissue culture of thymus, Ginsburg and Sachs showed large-scale differentiation of mast cells from thymic lymphocytes. The Ishizakas demonstrated that IgE receptors appeared on the surface of these cells at about the time cytoplasmic granules began to appear in their cytoplasm. Moreover, the thymic cells undergoing transformation into mast cells, were not T cells. Therefore, the thymus contains stem cells for mast cell differentiation.

The thymus is necessary for heightened eosinophilopoiesis. Nude mice and thymectomized animals have normal basal levels of eosinophils but are unable to produce increased numbers after such stimuli as infection with helminths.

Bursa of Fabricius

The bursa of Fabricius is a cloacal lymphoepithelial organ in birds that receives stem cells from bone marrow and induces them to differentiate into B cells. It is analogous to that other gut-derived lymphoepithelial organ, the thymus, which receives stem cells from the bone marrow and induces their differentiation into T cells. The letters T and B are taken from Thymus and Bursa.

The bursa originates as an epithelial diverticulum of the cloaca and becomes infiltrated by immigrated lymphocytes. In the bursa, the epithelial diverticulum retains connection with the cloaca and forms follicles around which the lymphocytes are organized. The bursa involutes markedly on sexual maturation. In fact, its development may be entirely suppressed by applying male sex hormones to the shell of embryonated eggs. In mammals, the bursal equivalent appears to be bone marrow.

References and Selected Bibliography

General

Bearman, R. M., Levine, G. D., and Bensch, K. G. 1978. The ultrastructure of the normal human thymus. Anat. Rec. 190:755.

Chapman, W. L., Jr., and Allen, J. R. 1971. The fine structure of the thymus of the fetal and neonatal monkey (Macaca mulatta). Z. Zellforsch. Mikrosk. Anat. 114:220.

Clark, S. L., Jr. 1973. The intrathymic environment. In A. J. S. Davies and R. L. Carter (eds.), Contemporary Topics in Immunobiology, Vol. 2, Thymus Dependency. New York: Plenum Press, p. 77.

Defendi, V., and Metcalf, D. (eds.). 1964. The Thymus. Philadelphia: Wistar Institute Press.

Hwang, W. S., Ho, T. Y., Luk, S. C., and Simon, G. T. 1974. Ultrastructure of the rat thymus. A transmission, scanning electron microscope, and morphometric study. Lab. Invest. 31:473.

Janossy, G., Thomas, J. A., Bollum, F. J., et al. 1980. The human thymic microenvironment: An immunohistological study. J. Immunol. 125:202.

Kendall, M. D. (ed.). 1981. The Thymus Gland. Academic Press. London.

Kindred, J. E. 1940. A quantitative study of the hematopoietic organs of young albino rats. Am. J. Anat. 67:99.

Kohnen, P., and Weiss, L. 1964. An electron microscopic study of thymic corpuscles in the guinea pig and the mouse. Anat. Rec. 148:29.

Parrott, D. M. V., De Sousa, M. A. B., and East, J. 1966. Thymus-dependent areas in the lymphoid areas of neonatally thymectomized mice. J. Exp. Med. 123:191.

Pereira. G., and Clermont, Y. 1971. Distribution of cell web-containing epithelial reticular cells in the rat thymus. Anat. Rec. 169:613.

Porter, R., and Whelan, J. 1981. Microenvironments in hematopoietic and lymphoid differentiation. Ciba Foundation Symposium 84. London: Pitman.

van Haelst, U. J. G. 1967. Light and electron microscopic study of the normal and pathological thymus of the rat. I. The normal thymus. Z. Zellforsch. Mikrosk. Anat. 77:534.

van Haelst, U. J. G. 1969. Light and electron microscopic study of the normal and pathological thymus of the rat. III. A mesenchymal histiocytic type of cell. Z. Zellforsch. Mikrosk. Anat. 99:198.

Cellular Migration

Harris, J. E., and Ford, C. E. 1964. Cellular traffic of the thymus: Experiments with chromosome markers. I. Evidence that the thymus plays an instructional part. Nature (Lond.) 201:884.

Harris, J. E., Ford, C. E., Barnes, D. W. H., and Evans, E. P. 1964. Cellular traffic of the thymus: Experiments with chromosome markers. II. Evidence from parabiosis for an afferent stream of cells. Nature (Lond.) 201:886.

Linna, J., and Stillstrom, J. 1966. Migration of cells from the thymus to the spleen in young guinea pigs. Acta Pathol. Microbiol. Scand. 68:465.

Sainte-Marie, G., and Peng, F. S. 1971. Emigration of thymocytes from the thymus. A review and study of the problem. Rev. Can. Biol. 30:51.

Toro, I., and Olah, I. 1967. Penetration of thymocytes into the blood circulation. J. Ultrastruct. Res. 17:439.

Weissman, I. L. 1967. Thymus cell migration. J. Exp. Med. 126:291.

Development and Regeneration

Downey, H. 1948. Cytology of rabbit thymus and regeneration of its thymocytes after irradiation, with some notes on the human thymus. Blood 3:1315.

Haar, J. L. 1974. Light and electron microscopy of the human fetal thymus. Anat. Rec. 179:463.

Hirokawa, K. 1969. Electron microscopic observation of the human thymus of the fetus and the newborn. Acta Pathol. Jpn. 19:1.

Mandel, T. 1970. Differentiation of epithelial cells in the mouse thymus. Z. Zellforsch. Mikrosk. Anat. 106:498.

Moore, M. A. S., and Owen, J. J. T. 1967. Experimental studies on the development of the thymus. J. Exp. Med. 126:715.

Immunological Role

Aranson, B. G., and Wennersten, C. 1962. Role of the thymus in immune reaction in rats. II. Suppressive effect of thymectomy at birth on reactions of delayed (cellular) hypersensitivity and the circulating small lymphocyte. J. Exp. Med. 116:177.

Jankovic, B., Waksman, B. H., and Aranson, B. G. 1962. Role of the thymus in immune reactions in rats. I. The immunologic response to bovine serum albumin (antibody formation, arthus reactivity and delayed hypersensitivity) in rats thymectomized or splenectomized at various times after birth. J. Exp. Med. 116:159.

Metcalf, D. 1966. The thymus: Its role in immune responses, leukaemia development and carcinogenesis. In Recent Results in Cancer Research, Vol. 5. Berlin: Springer-Verlag OHG.

Miller, J. F. A. P. 1962. Effect of neonatal thymectomy on the immunological responsiveness of the mouse. Proc. R. Soc. Lond. (Biol.) 156:415.

Waksman, B. H., Aranson, B. G., and Jankovic, B. D. 1962. Role of the thymus in immune reactions in rats. III. Changes in the lymphoid organs of thymec-tomized rats. J. Exp. Med. 116:187.

Mast Cells

Ginsburg, H., and Sachs, L. 1963. Formation of pure suspensions of mast cells in tissue culture by differentiation of lymphoid cells from the mouse thymus. J. Natl. Cancer Inst. 31:1.

Ishizaka, T., Okadaira, H., Mauser, L. E., and Ishizaka, K. 1976. Development of rat mast cells in vitro. I. Differentiation of mast cells from thymus cells. J. Immunol. 116:747.

MHC Antigens

Rouse, R. V., van Ewijk, W., Jones, P. P., and Weissman, I. L. 1979. Expression of MHC antigens by mouse thymic dendritic cells. J. Immunol. 122:2508.

van Ewijk, W., Rouse, R. V., and Weissan, I. L. 1980. Distribution of H-2 microenvironments in the mouse thymus. J. Histochem. Cytochem. 28:1089.

Pathology

Levine, G. D., Rosai, J., Bearman, R. M., and Polliack, A. 1975. The fine structure of thymoma, with emphasis on its differential diagnosis. A study of 10 cases. Am. J. Pathol. 81:49.

Rosai, J., and Levine, G. D. 1975. Tumors of the Thymus, 2nd Ser., Atlas of Tumor Pathology. Washington, D. C.: Armed Forces Institute of Pathology.

Wolstenholme, G. E. W., and Porter, R. (eds.). 1966. The Thymus: Experimental and Clinical Studies, a Ciba Foundation Symposium. Boston: Little, Brown and Company.

T Cells

Bevan, M. J., and Fink, P. J. 1978. The influence of thymus H-2 antigens on the specificity of maturing killer and helper cells. Immunol. Rev. 42:3.

Scollay, R., Jacobs, S., Jerabek, L., Butcher, E., and Weissman, I. 1980. T cell maturation: Thymocyte and thymus migrant subpopulations defined with monoclonal antibodies to MHC region antigens. J. Immunol. 124:2845.

Takatsu, K., and Ishizaka, K. 1976. Reagenic antibody formation in the mouse: VIII. Depression of the on-going IgE antibody formation by suppressor T-cells. J. Immunol. 117:1211.

Thymic Humoral Factors

Bach, J.-F., and Papiernik, M. 1981. Cellular and molecular signals in T-cell differentiation. In Ciba Foundation Symposium 84. Microenvironments in haemopoietic and lymphoid differentiation. Porter, R., and Whelan, I. (eds.). Pitman, p. 215.

Levey, R. H., Trainin, N., and Law, L. W. 1963. Evidence for function of thymic tissue in diffusion chambers implanted in neonatally thymectomized mice. J. Natl. Cancer Inst. 31:199.

Osoba, D., and Miller, J. F. A. P. 1964. The lymphoid tissues and immune responses to neonatally thymectomized mice bearing thymic tissues in millipore diffusion chambers. J. Exp. Med. 119:177.

Vasculature

Bearman, R. M., Bensch, K. G., and Levine, G. D. 1975. The normal human thymic vasculature: An ultrastructural study. Anat. Rec. 183:485.

Raviola, E., and Karnovsky, M. J. 1972. Evidence for a blood–thymus barrier using electron-opaque tracers. J. Exp. Med. 136:466.

Bursa of Fabricius

Jolly, J. 1915. La bourse de Fabricius et les organes lympho-épithéliaux. Arch. Anat. Microbiol. 16:363.

Moore, M. A. S., and Owen, J. J. T. 1966. Experimental studies on the development of the bursa of Fabricius. Dev. Biol. 14:40.

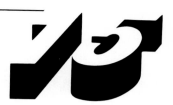

Lymphatic Vessels and Lymph Nodes

Leon Weiss

Lymphatic Vessels

Lymphatic vessels originate in connective tissue spaces as anastomosing capillaries. The capillaries flow into larger *collecting vessels;* the largest and most proximal empty into veins in the base of the neck as the left and right thoracic ducts. Like blood vessels, lymphatic vessels are an arborized system of endothelial-lined tubes that carry cellular elements suspended in a fluid intercellular substance. Unlike blood vessels, they do not form a circular system but carry their contents, called *lymph,* in only one direction, toward the base of the neck. Lymphatic vessels recover fluids that escape into the connective tissue spaces from blood capillaries and venules and return them to the blood. In mammals, dense encapsulated collections of lymphocytes called *lymph nodes* lie across lymphatic vessels, and lymph percolates through them. Lymph nodes filter lymph and serve as stations for traffic of T and B cells and their immunological activities.

Distribution

Lymphatic capillaries are most numerous beneath body surfaces: the skin; the mucous membranes of the gastrointestinal, respiratory, and genitourinary tracts; and subserous tissues. Lymphatic capillaries may be arranged in superficial and deep plexuses (Figs. 15–1 to 15–3), each of which is deeper than blood capillaries. Parts of the body are not supplied with lymphatics. The central nervous system, globus oculi, and the

528

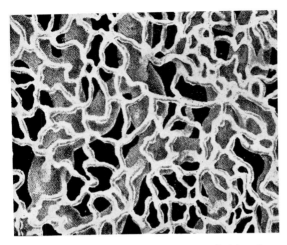

15–1 Lymphatic vessels of a dog. Superficial and deep vessels in the wall of the stomach as viewed from the surface. × 30. (From Teichmann.)

15–2 Lymphatic network in the human appendix as viewed from the surface. Note the enlargement of vessels over the lymphoid nodules and in the valves in the larger vessels. × 40. (From Teichmann.)

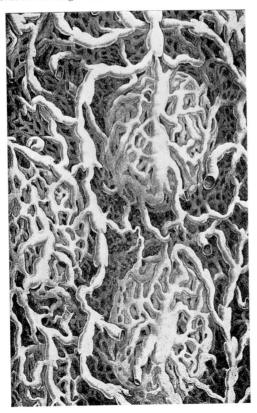

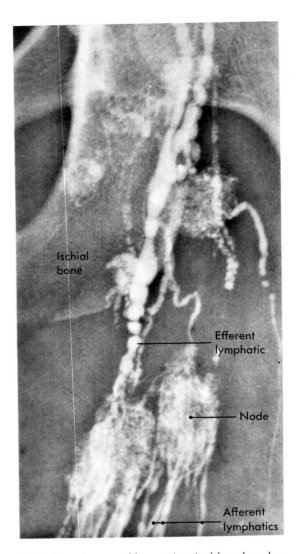

Ischial bone

Efferent lymphatic

Node

Afferent lymphatics

15–3 Lymphogram of human inguinal lymph nodes and lymphatics. A radiopaque dye injected into the lymphatic vessels in the thigh is carried by afferent lymphatic vessels into the draining lymph nodes of the inguinal region. The dye flows through the nodes and enters its efferent lymphatic vessels. The dye will continue centrally through the lymphatic system and eventually flow into the veins at the base of the neck. This lymphogram is an x-ray of the inguinal region several minutes after the injection of dye. Against the background of the soft tissues of the thigh and the pelvic bones, the lymphatic vessels and nodes are seen. Note the large number of slender afferent lymphatics. The nodes are oval, the dark zones within them representing lymphocytes and other cells around which the dye flows. The efferent lymphatics have a wide caliber. The beaded appearance of the largest vessel is due to the presence of valves.

bone marrow contain none. Striated (noncardiac) muscles contain lymphatic vessels only in the perimysium. Within the liver, lymphatic capillaries reach into the perilobular spaces and do not extend into the liver lobule. Loci in the liver, spleen, and bone marrow that are supplied by venous sinusoids lack lymphatics. The sinusoids appear to subserve functions of lymphatic vessels.

Structure

Lymphatic capillaries may reach 100 μm in diameter. Their walls are made of flattened endothelium (Figs. 15–4 to 15–6). Endothelial cells are attached to one another along their perimeter by zonulae adhaerens, and contiguous cells may overlap in flap-like fashion. The endothelium forms a complete layer but in some cases, such as in the lacteals of the intestinal villi, small apertures are present. The basement membrane is poorly developed. Fine *anchoring filaments* run from perivascular bundles of collagen and attach

15–4 Skin of guinea pig. A lymphatic capillary is present in the dermis. A small blood-filled venule is nearby. (From D. Chou and L. Weiss, in Weiss, L. 1972. Cells and Tissues of the Immune System. Englewood Cliffs, N.J.: Prentice-Hall, Inc.)

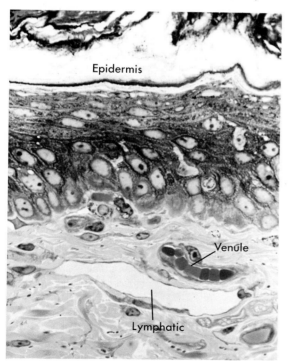

Epidermis

Venule

Lymphatic

to the outer surface of the endothelium. In inflammation, the pressure on perilymphatic tissues increases, but the anchoring filaments pull on the lymphatic vessel wall like a guy rope on a tent and help keep the vessel open (see Fig. 15–5). *Collecting vessels* are structurally similar to veins but without definite layers. Like the pattern seen in blood vessels, three coats or tunics are present: *intima*, *media*, and *adventitia* (Fig. 15–7). Even in the largest and best-developed lymphatic vessel, the left *thoracic duct*, it is difficult to delineate these layers. This thoracic duct, 4 to 6 μm in diameter, has an internal elastic membrane and is supplied by blood vessels and nerves that penetrate its adventitia and media, as do vasa vasorum and nerves of blood vessels.

Collecting vessels contain valves (Figs. 15–3 and 15–7), paired cusps each originating from opposite endothelial surfaces and extending into the lumen. The base of a single valve cusp takes up approximately 180° of circumference, so that the entire circumference of the vessel wall provides attachment for a valve. Occasional tricuspid valves are found. Cusps are formed as folds of endothelium. A few connective tissue fibers and even muscle fibers extend between the folded endothelial surfaces of the cusps from the subendothelial tissue. The cusps project in the direction of lymph flow and prevent back-flow. A valve in each of the great lymphatic channels at its junction with the systemic veins prevents the gurgitation of blood into the lymphatic system. Valves are responsible for the beaded appearance of lymphatic vessels; the vessel is constricted at the attachment of the base of the valve and dilated beyond.

Lymphatic vessels anastomose with one another and tend to travel in company with blood vessels (usually veins), which may be girdled by lymphatics. Lymph is carried to lymph nodes by afferent lymphatic vessels and from them by efferent vessels (Figs. 15–3). It is likely that no lymph reaches venous blood without flowing through at least one node.

Function

Lymphatic vessels return to the blood material that has escaped blood vessels. The walls of blood capillaries and venules are semipermeable membranes that permit the diffusion of small-molecular-weight materials through them and retain larger molecules (such as proteins and fatty complexes) and the cellular elements of the

530

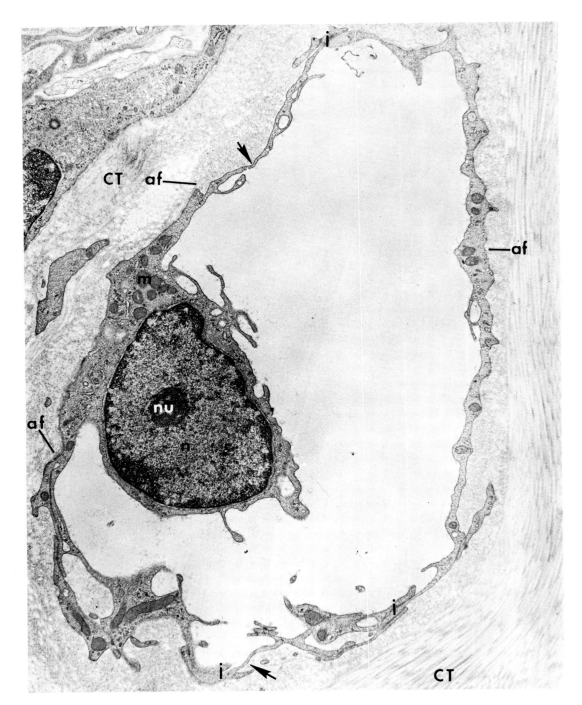

15–5 Cross section of lymphatic capillary. A close association of the surrounding interstitial elements **(CT)** with the capillary wall is maintained by numerous anchoring filaments **(af),** which appear as a network of small filaments in this low-power micrograph. The extreme attenuations **(arrows)** achieved by the endothelium are illustrated in various regions of the capillary wall. The nucleus **(n)** with its nucleolus **(nu)** protrudes into the lumen, and several intercellular junctions **(i)** are observed. Mitochondria **(m)** occur in the perinuclear regions and also throughout the thin cytoplasmic rim of the endothelial wall. × 11,000. (From the work of L. Leak and J. Burke.)

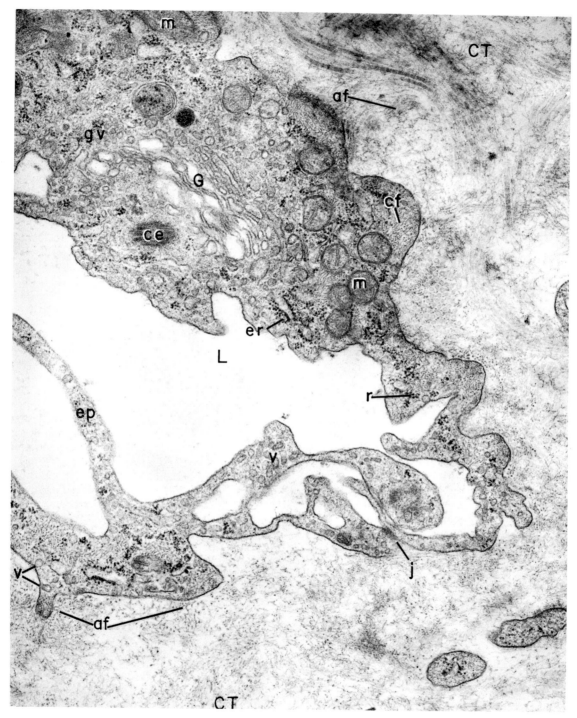

15–6 Lymphatic capillary. In this electron micrograph, the wall of the lymphatic capillary lies in its connective tissue bed. The lymphatic endothelium contains mitochondria **(m)**, a Golgi complex **(G)**, Golgi vesicles **(gv)**, ribosomes **(r)**, rough ER **(er)**, a centriole **(ce)**, luminal endothelial processes **(ep)**, and pinocytotic vesicles **(v)**. Anchoring filaments **(af)** are present. **L**, lumen; **CT**, connective tissue; **j**, junction complex of endothelial cells. (From the work of L. Leak and J. Burke.)

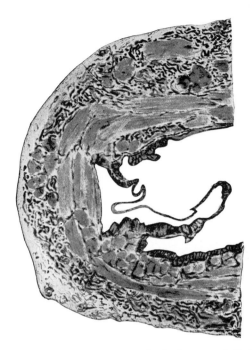

15–7 Lumbar lymphatic trunk of a human adult. A valve is present. Weigert's resorcinfuchsin and picroindigo carmine stain. (From the work of Kajava.)

blood. Small but cumulatively significant amounts of plasma protein do escape from blood vessels, however, with large volumes of fluid. The bathing of perivascular connective tissues by this transudate constitutes an essential physiological process. This is the means by which hormones, antibodies, enzymes and other macromolecules, low-molecular-weight molecules, and fluids reach the cells and intercellular matrix of the body. At least a part of this protein-containing fluid is absorbed into lymphatic capillaries and carried back to the blood. The importance of conserving plasma protein is shown by the following case report from Crandall, et al. (1943).

A 30-year-old woman was shot in the left side of the neck, 1 hour before admission to the hospital. The left jugular vein was ligated 2 days after admission. During the operation straw-colored fluid steadily welled up in the wound so that the skin was not closed. After the operation the dressings were rapidly saturated with this fluid and, for the next 6 weeks, a ceaseless leakage of what was unquestionably thoracic duct lymph continued. The patient at once took the regular hospital diet; after she had eaten, the leaking fluid became milky. But she lost weight at the rate of 5 lb. a week

and her plasma protein fell to 3.5 gm per 100 ml in just a month. A diet high in protein brought this to 4.6 gm per 100 ml in 13 days, but weight loss continued. Accordingly, in a second operation the thoracic duct was ligated and the wound closed. For 2 weeks after this ligation, the patient had cramps after eating but she gained 16 lb. in a month and was discharged free of complaints. The concentration of protein in the lymph ranged from 3.19 to 5.28 per 100 ml.

As suggested by the above report, lymphatic vessels absorb fat, especially neutral fat, from the intestine. The patient ingested olive oil stained with Sudan IV. Approximately 90 min after she swallowed the labeled olive oil, the dye appeared in thoracic duct lymph. In the resting state, probably 95% of the volume of thoracic duct lymph comes from the liver and intestine. Most of the protein in thoracic duct lymph originates in the liver.

There is a small but significant loss of cells from the blood (including red blood cells). Most of these cells function and are lost in the perivascular tissue. Some are picked up by lymphatics and returned to the blood. In addition, there is regular traffic of fluid and cells, especially macrophages, from serosal cavities (such as the peritoneal, and pericardial) via lymph into blood.

The permeability of lymphatic vessels increases greatly under certain mild conditions that occur normally or that represent at most, only a slight departure from the normal. Pressure sufficient to obstruct the flow of lymph causes permeability to increase before visible dilation of the lymphatic occurs. Stroking the skin with a blunt wire or scratching the skin without breaking the epidermis causes an immediate great increase in lymphatic permeability. Warming the ears of mice to 43°C increases permeability. Histamine also heightens lymphatic permeability. Particles and fluids cross the lymphatic endothelium by transcytosis, as is also characteristic of the endothelium of blood vessels (see Chap. 9). Cells cross through interendothelial-cell junctions.

Larger lymphatic vessels are supplied by vasomotor nerves and respond to such powerful constrictor agents as epinephrine or pituitrin. Lymphatic capillaries probably do not respond. They are, however, highly elastic, distensible by one-third without rupture. The flow of lymph is promoted by remitting compression of lymphatic vessels by surrounding structures (particularly muscles and pulsating blood vessels), respiratory movements, propulsive actions of the lymphatic walls (by smooth muscle), and the force of gravity (in the lymphatics above the thoracic duct). The direction of flow is controlled by valves. The rate of flow varies considerably. Trypan blue injected into the hind foot of a dog reaches thoracic duct lymph in seconds. The volume of lymph entering the blood stream from the thoracic duct in resting human subjects averages 1.38 ml per kg per h (range: 3.9–0.38). Flow is increased by ingesting food or water or by abdominal massage.

Lymph Nodes

Lymph nodes are ovoid encapsulated filters of lymph ranging from a few millimeters to more than a centimeter in their largest dimension (Figs. 15–8 to 15–10). They are best developed in mammals where they lie across collecting lymphatic vessels, and lymph flows through them as it moves toward the junctions of lymphatic vessels and veins. Sites rich in nodes are at the base of the extremities, the neck, retroperitoneum, and mediastinum. In birds, lymph nodes consist of loosely organized lymphatic tissue lying alongside lymphatic vessels. Birds have relatively few such nodes, however, and collections of lymphocytes lie scattered through

the pancreas, liver, kidney and other organs. Fish, amphibia, and reptiles lack lymph nodes.

Structure

A lymph node consists of a *capsule* that encloses lymphocytes and other free cells, which are arranged on a reticulum and supplied by blood and lymphatic vessels and nerves.

The capsule is composed of dense collagenous tissue and some muscle. Its outer surface is convex but contains an indentation, the *hilus,* through which lymphatic vessels leave the node and blood vessels enter. Afferent lymphatic vessels pierce the convex surface of the capsule and empty into the node. Trabeculae project from the inner surface of the capsule into the node.

The reticulum is a delicate meshwork composed, as in the spleen, of reticular fibers and reticular cells. The reticular cells are large branched cells that evidently secrete reticular fibers. The fibers lie on the surface of the reticular cells and form a branching meshwork, the *fibrous reticulum,* which can be selectively stained with silver (argyrophilia) and by the periodic acid Schiff (PAS) reaction.

Lymphocytes are the most numerous of the cells within the reticulum. In the periphery of a node they are closely packed, forming a layer

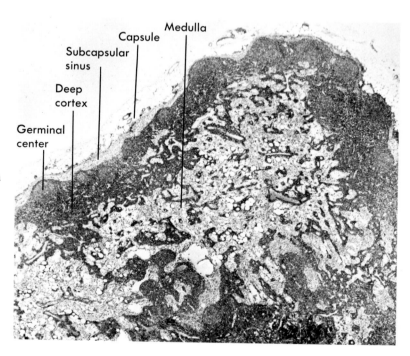

15–8 Human lymph node. Giemsa stain. × 30.

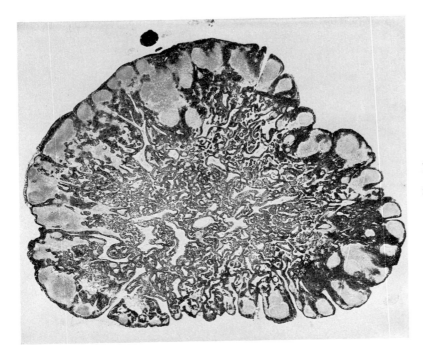

15–9 Lymph node injected with India ink. The sinus system is well outlined. × 10.

15–10 A. Popliteal lymph node of dog; scanning electron micrograph of cut surface of cortex. The capsule is prominent, and trabeculae extend from it into the node. Both the subcapsular sinus and the radial sinuses, which run along the trabeculae, are crisscrossed by the processes of reticular cells and reticular fibers. A germinal center, consisting of compactly organized cells, lies within a lymphatic nodule. × 111. **B.** A higher magnification showing details of capsule, subcapsular sinus, mantle zone of secondary lymphatic nodule and germinal center. × 370. (From Irino, S., Ono, T., Hiraki, K., and Murakami, T. 1974. Blood and Vessel 5:595 [in Japanese].)

A

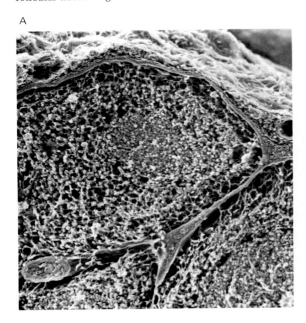

B

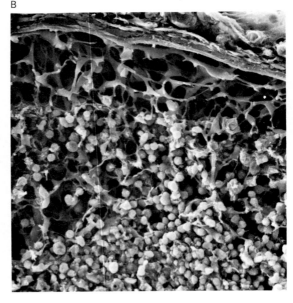

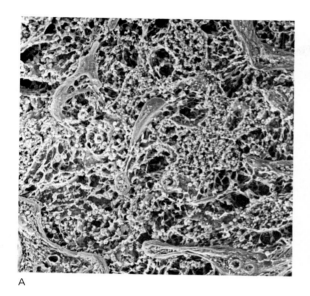

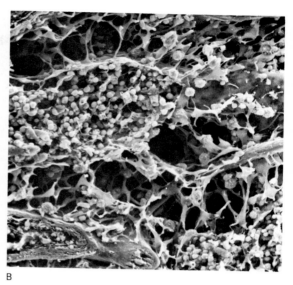

A

B

called the cortex. The medulla lies central to the cortex and extends to the hilus. Lymphocytes in the medulla lie in branching cords, the *medullary cords* (Fig. 15–11). Within the cortex at its periphery, groups of lymphocytes form spherical or ovoid lymphatic nodules (sometimes termed *follicles*). Lymphatic nodules that consist of uniform, tightly packed small lymphocytes are called *primary nodules*. Other nodules contain a central zone of larger lymphocytes and macrophages, relatively lightly stained because the larger cells have more voluminous pale-staining cytoplasm and a euchromatic nucleus that stains less densely than the heterochromatic nucleus of small lymphocytes. This central zone is the *germinal center*, and nodules having a germinal center are called *secondary nodules*. The zone of small lymphocytes surrounding the germinal center of the secondary nodule constitutes the *mantle zone*, sometimes termed the *crescent*.

Macrophages are always plentiful throughout lymph nodes and can quickly increase in number as needs arise. Macrophages tend to be most common in the medulla and may occur in large number in germinal centers after antibody formation declines. Macrophages are, of course, phagocytic, but they carry out other functions of secretion, antigen modification, etc., as discussed in Chap. 4.

A system of peripatetic cells has been recognized whose main function appears to be to capture and hold antigen on their surface and to present it to lymphocytes, thereby ensuring an

15–11 A. Popliteal lymph node of dog; scanning electron micrograph of cut surface of medulla. Trabeculae lie in the parenchyma, surrounded by lymphatic sinuses whose lumen is crisscrossed by a reticular meshwork. Medullary cords are also present. × 110. **B.** A higher magnification showing a cell-packed medullary cord surrounded by a lymphatic sinus. × 358. (From Irino, S., Ono, T., Hiraki, K., and Murakami, T. 1974. Blood vessel 5:595 [in Japanese].)

immune response. They may also cluster lymphocytes about them. These cells are neither fibroblastic nor phagocytic and are rather large and branched, with ruffled cytoplasmic surfaces. Certain cells in this system may possess a singular cytoplasmic marker known as the *Birbeck granule*.

Antigen presenting cells (APC), which originate in bone marrow, have been seen in many sites in the body and undoubtedly will be found in additional places. In the epidermis a cell long known as the *Langerhans cell* (Chap. 17) has been shown to capture antigen penetrating the skin. The Langerhans cell then moves out of the skin to the regional lymph nodes, carrying the antigen to the lymphocytes there. Langerhans cells, particularly those high in the epidermis, contain Birbeck granules (Chap. 17). An immune response distinctive to the skin, *contact hypersensitivity*, depends upon Langerhans cells. APC lie within the cortex of lymph nodes and the white pulp of the spleen in both B-cell and T-cell zones (see below and Chap. 16). APC in T-cell zones have been referred to as *interdigitating cells*, those in B cell zones as *follicular dendritic cells*. Interdigitating cells have also been observed in the thymus (Chap. 13). Interdigitating cells have Ia antigen of the major histocompatibility complex on their surface, an antigen associated with the capacity to cluster T cells. This capacity appears to facilitate immune responses and to contribute to the development of T cell zones and the phenomena of T-cell homing and sorting.

In addition to the APC of the tissues, there seems to be a cell in this system which travels in blood and lymph. By the usual cytological techniques it is likely identified as a monocyte, but Balfour has identified a rich array of veil-like cytoplasmic surface processes and has termed it the *veil cell*. This cell occasionally shows Birbeck granules. The M cell of the gut epithelium (Chap. 19) may be a candidate for this system of cells.

The presence of lymphatic nodules in the superficial cortex of lymph nodes establishes three cortical zones: (1) the *nodular cortex*; (2) the *internodular cortex*, which lies between nodules; and (3) a *deep* or *tertiary cortex*, which lies below the first two zones and above the medulla. The internodular and teritary cortexes may be taken together as the *diffuse cortex*. B lymphocytes are concentrated in primary nodules and T lymphocytes in the diffuse cortex (see Fig. 15–19). Germinal centers are sites of B-cell differentiation and high-level antibody formation. They are concerned with the development of B memory cells. They also contain T cells and macrophages. Plasma cell formation is initiated there, but few plasma cells are present in germinal centers because as B cells differentiate into plasma cells, they leave germinal centers and move toward the medulla. Medullary cords contain plasma cells, macrophages and lymphocytes, and some granulocytes. They are branching partitions of tissue that extend from the underside of the cortex and converge toward the hilus.

The interactions of the various zones of lymph nodes are discussed below under Immunological Functions.

Vascular Supply

Lymphatic Vessels. Afferent lymphatic vessels, carrying lymph from the connective tissue spaces or from a more peripheral lymph node, pierce the capsule and empty into a large *subcapsular sinus*, which lies directly beneath the capsule and is coextensive with it. *Cortical* or *radial sinuses* run radially from the subcapsular sinus through the cortex, often along trabeculae. They become *medullary sinuses* as they pass between the medullary cords and converge toward the hilus. There they drain into efferent lymphatic channels.

Lymphatic sinuses are lined by reticular cells, which provide a rather irregular surface that often contains apertures. The lining reticular cells extend cytoplasmic processes that crisscross the lumen (Figs. 15–10 and 15–11), retarding the lymph flow and causing turbulence.

Blood Vessels. Blood vessels enter a node at the hilus. (A few enter at the convex surface of the capsule.) Arterioles reach the cortex through trabeculae and break up into the capillaries, which empty into venules. These venules enter veins that run from cortex to medulla and then leave the node via the hilus. Postcapillary venules lie in the diffuse cortex. They have a cuboidal endothelium and therefore have been called high endothelial venules (HEV). The walls of the HEVs are often infiltrated with small lymphocytes (Figs. 15–12 to 15–18). Gowans and colleagues, using radioactively labeled lymphocytes and autoradiography, showed that these lymphocytes pass from the blood into the parenchyma of the node. They pass between endothelial cells, deeply indenting their lateral plasma membranes. High endothelial venules represent a major pathway by which small lymphocytes, both T and B cells, enter a node. Unmyelinated nerves enter the node at the hilus and run with blood vessels.

Other Lymphatic Tissue

In addition to such discretely organized tissue as lymph nodes and spleen, lymphatic tissue is associated with other tissues throughout the body. The wall of the alimentary tract is infiltrated with lymphatic tissue, evocative of the fact that developmentally this was the site where hematopoiesis first evolved. Lymphatic tissue, such as Peyer's patches, in the small intestine and the tonsils is well demarcated, whereas elsewhere it may diffusely infiltrate lamina propria and other layers. In addition to standard sites, lymphocytes, being migratory cells, may enter virtually any place in the body and with appropriate stimulation set up lymphatic loci.

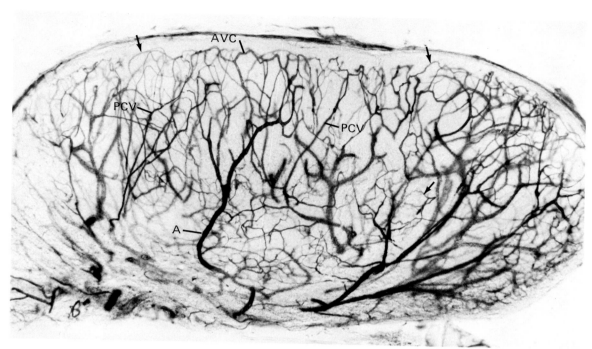

15–12 Lymph node of rat. This axillary lymph node has been perfused arterially by alcian blue and then sectioned and cleared to reveal the vasculature. Arteries **(A)** exhibit dense staining. Arteriovenous communications **(AVC)**, cortical and medullary capillaries **(arrows)**, and the high endothelial post capillary venules **(PCV)** are shown in the preparation. × 47. (From Anderson, A. D., and Anderson, N. D. 1975. Am. J. Pathol. 80:387.)

15–13 Schema of lymph node.
Afferent lymphatic vessels, some showing valves, pierce the capsule, and efferent lymphatics leave the node at the hilus. The nodular cortex consists of spherical lymphatic nodules, some of which contain germinal centers. The diffuse cortex lies between the nodules and deep to them. Within the center of the node lie the linear medullary cords, converging on the hilus. A subcapsular sinus, into which the afferent lymphatic vessels empty, lies beneath the full expanse of capsule. Radial sinuses run from the subcapsular sinus toward the hilus. They run along trabeculae, and, in the medulla, between medullary cords. Arteries enter the node at the hilus and branch richly, penetrating the node. Postcapillary venules tend to lie in the diffuse cortex. Veins leave the node at the hilus.

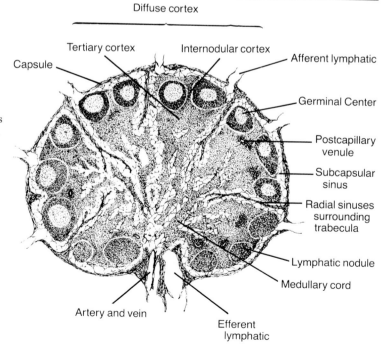

Diffuse cortex

Tertiary cortex — Internodular cortex — Afferent lymphatic — Capsule — Germinal Center — Postcapillary venule — Subcapsular sinus — Radial sinuses surrounding trabecula — Lymphatic nodule — Medullary cord — Artery and vein — Efferent lymphatic

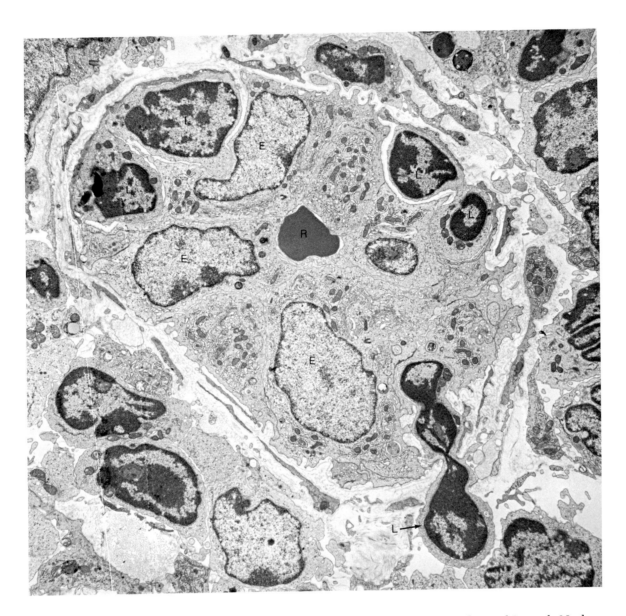

15–14 Postcapillary venules, mouse lymph node.
The vessel has a high endothelium containing lightly euchromatic nuclei **(E)**. The lumen is small and contains an erythrocyte **(R)**. The wall of the venule is infiltrated by a number of lymphocytes whose nuclei are heterochromatic and thus dense **(L)**. Note that one lymphocyte, its protoplasm beaded as a result of being squeezed by the endothelium, appears emerging from the venule and entering the perivascular lymphatic cortex **(L→)**. × 1,200. (From the work of G. D. Levine.)

Development and Decline of Lymph Nodes

Lymph nodes appear in the human embryo during the third month along the course of lymphatic vessels. Lymphatic vessels at sites of lymph node development become plexiform (*lymphatic sacs*) and lymphocytes aggregate around these sacs. Lymph nodes are not fully developed until several weeks postpartum, when cortex and medulla differentiate and germinal centers appear.

Lymph nodes and spleen begin to atrophy at the same time as thymus (Chap. 14), but the

15–15 **A.** Postcapillary venule, rat lymph node; scanning electron micrograph. Many lymphocytes lie on the endothelium, presumably about to penetrate between endothelial cells and through the wall of the venule into the surrounding cortex. Preparatory to crossing the wall, the lymphocytes appear to develop microvilli. × 563. **B.** At higher magnification, a lymphocyte is seen lying on the endothelium. The lymphocyte's microvilli appear to probe the endothelial surface. ×1,760. (From the work of A. O. Anderson and N. D. Anderson.)

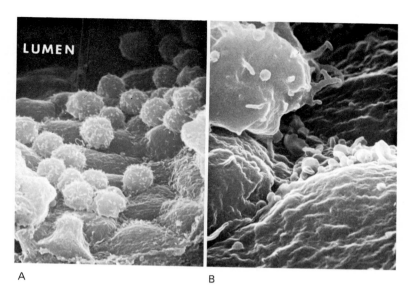

A   B

changes are quite gradual and subtle. In humans most nodes go on for 60 years or more with only slight atrophy, and they retain the capacity to enlarge throughout life.

Functions of Lymph Nodes

Filtration and Phagocytosis. Lymph nodes constitute extensive filtration beds. The reticular meshwork, crisscrossing the sinuses and the parenchyma, acts as a mechanical filter. Flow in the lymphatic sinuses of lymph nodes is quite slow

15–16 Postcapillary venule in a mesenteric lymph node 15 min after the initiation of a transfusion. Labeled cells have penetrated the endothelium of the vessel but have not yet migrated into the node. **L,** lumen of the vessel. Exposure, 28 days. Methyl green–pyronin stain. × 1,200. (From Gowans, J. L., and Knight, E. J. 1964. Proc. R. Soc. Lond. [Biol.] 159:257.)

15–17 Autoradiograph of thoracic duct cells that had been incubated in vitro with tritiated adenosine for 1 h at 37°C. Exposure, 14 days. Leishman stain. × 2,250. (From Gowans, J. L., and Knight, E. J. 1964. Proc. R. Soc. Lond. [Biol.] 159:257.)

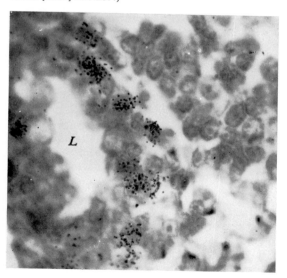

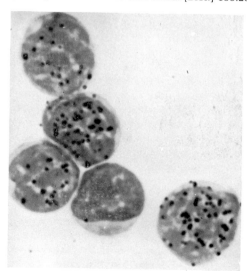

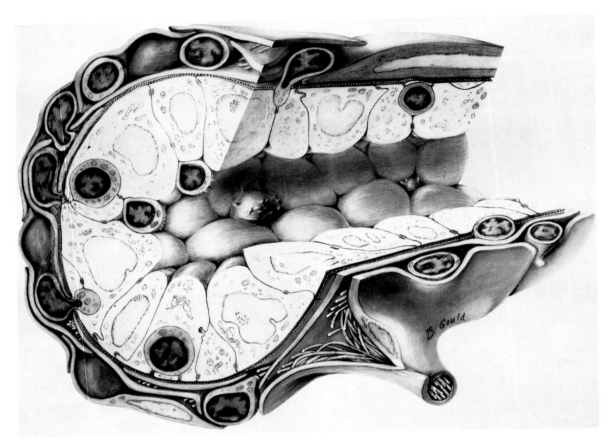

15–18　Postcapillary lymph node, artist's reconstruction. The high endothelium and the infiltration of the wall by lymphocytes are shown. (From the work of A. O. Anderson and N. D. Anderson.)

with many eddies, which favors phagocytosis. Fluid readily escapes the sinuses, moreover, and percolates through the parenchyma. Macrophages lie in the sinuses and in the parenchyma, and they can rapidly multiply and become activated. As they phagocytize, macrophages increase in volume; their bulk further impedes flow and thus enhances phagocytosis. Lymph nodes produce antibody (see below) and other substances that help to immobilize and agglutinate or lyse bacteria, facilitating filtration and phagocytosis. Drinker et al. (1934) perfused 5 ml of a serum-broth culture containing 600 million colonies per ml of hemolytic streptococci through a lymph node and collected perfusate at the efferent lymphatic vessels. When the perfusate was cultured, it was found to contain 4.5 million colonies/ml. The filtration efficiency was,

therefore, 99%. The efficiency of filtration makes lymph nodes vulnerable. If they fail to destroy the infectious agents or malignant cells that they concentrate, nodes become new foci and facilitate the spread of disease throughout the body.

Recirculation of Lymphocytes. Small T and B lymphocytes are part of the recirculating lymphocyte pool, traveling repeatedly through blood and lymphatic vessels and through lymph node, spleen, and other lymphatic tissue. Recirculating cells may enter a node through its arterial vessels, pass through capillaries, and reach postcapillary venules. They then pass through the walls of these venules into the parenchyma of the node. If they are T cells, they move to the diffuse cortex. B cells move to lymphatic nodules (Fig. 15–19). The lymphocytes remain in their characteristic sites for several hours and, if they do not engage in antibody production, they migrate to the medulla and leave the node through efferent lymphatics. Recirculating lymphocytes may also enter a node through afferent lymphatics, especially if the node is central and receives

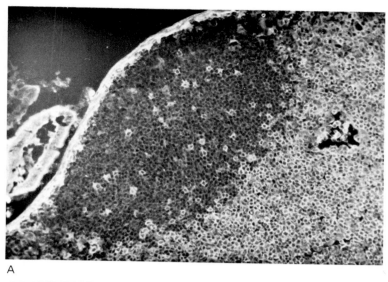

A

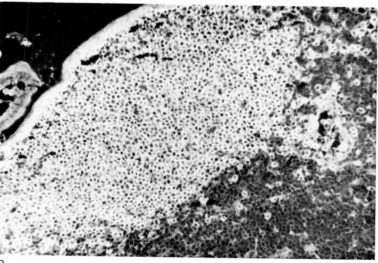

B

15–19 Lymph node, mouse. Distribution of T and B lymphocytes as revealed by fluorescence immunocytochemistry. The T and B cells are specially stained in these frozen sections by antibodies to the surface of T and B cells, respectively. The antibody is conjugated to a fluorescent marker, visible by fluorescence microscopy. In **A,** the lymphatic nodules in the cortex are largely unstained, whereas the deep or tertiary cortex is deeply stained, indicating that it is the site of concentration of T lymphocytes. Note that the postcapillary venule is stained. In **B,** the cells of the lymphatic nodules are deeply stained, indicating that B lymphocytes are concentrated there. Note that the postcapillary venule is also stained, as are some cells in the tertiary cortex. This staining pattern reflects B-cell traffic from the postcapillary venule toward the lymphatic nodule. (See Fig. 16–22 for distribution of T and B lymphocytes in the spleen.) (From Weissman, I. L. 1975. Transpl. Rev. 24:159.)

lymphocytes from more peripheral nodes. Transit time through a node in rodents is 4 to 6 h for T cells and somewhat longer for B cells. The recirculating lymphocytes enter veins through the thoracic ducts. They circulate in the blood stream until they eventually reach a lymph node (or other lymphatic tissue) and repeat the cycle. When T and B cells become engaged in antibody formation in a node, the pattern of recirculation is altered, as discussed below.

Immunological Functions. Lymph nodes produce antibody and engage in cellular immunity to regional antigen. Thus, antigen introduced into a footpad elicits an antibody response in a popliteal lymph node. This responsiveness of the lymph node to regional antigen complements that of the spleen, which responds to systemic (blood-borne) antigen. That lymphatic tissue produces antibody was shown by McMaster and Hudack in 1935, who injected antigen into the ears of rats and recovered antibody from the draining lymph nodes before it could be detected elsewhere. Two antigens were injected, one in each ear, and the antibody to each of the antigens was detected first in the isolateral node.

When antigen is first administered, a primary immune response follows that varies with the character of antigen, dose, and route of administration. With particulate antigens, such as bacteria or parts of bacteria, phagocytosis by macrophages is one of the earliest responses in a lymph node. The antigen is engulfed in the sinuses and in the medullary regions most conspicuously. However, antigen becomes concentrated rather rapidly around the primary nodules at the interface to T- and B-cell zones and then within the nodules. Soon the antigen disappears from other sites but remains in and around the lymphatic nodules, affixed to local macrophages and to antigen-presenting cells. Antigen thus held would seem able to interact with recirculating T and B cells as they move and sort themselves in the cortex of the node. This antigen processing enhances *clonal selection*, whereby the antigen *selects* T and B cells whose surface receptors "fit" with it. Selected T cells in the diffuse cortex and selected B cells in nodules proliferate to form *clones* by undergoing "blast transformation." These events occur within 24 h in a primary reaction.

Within several days, in a mounting reaction, antigen becomes more concentrated in the mantle zone and in germinal centers, held primarily by antigen-presenting cells. T cells undergoing blast transformation and proliferation in the diffuse cortex move into lymphatic nodules. There they interact both with B cells that have the appropriate receptors and with macrophages. These cell types proliferate and form a *germinal center*. As this happens, the small lymphocytes that have made up the primary nodule are forced to the periphery of the nodule and become the *mantle* or *crescent*. The resulting mantle and germinal center constitute a secondary nodule. By the fifth day of an active response, most of the activity may be in germinal centers. There, *effector B cells* undergoing transformation into plasma cells (the so-called *transitional cells*) produce considerable antibody and move toward the medullary cords as they complete their differentiation to plasma cells. Lymphocytes with immunological "memory" are produced (see below). Activated lymphocytes, both T and B, also release lymphokines, which have many actions. Lymphokines summon, detain, and activate macrophages and other cell types. They cause an increased vascular permeability, perhaps through intermediary mast cells and basophils, which leads to accumulation of perivascular fluid. The node is now tense and swollen. Over the next week or more the activity diminishes. Germinal centers remain for several weeks but show both an increasing proportion of macrophages that mop up and a decreasing proportion of activated lymphocytes. Plasma cells continue to accumulate in the medullary cords and live about 2 weeks, but their antibody output is low compared with that of transitional cells. In the process of antibody formation by effector B cells, there is increased production in the node of *memory B cells* (those which were not transformed to plasma cells) and of *memory T cells*. These cells join the recirculating pool of lymphocytes, augmenting the lymphocytes in the pool that had been initially responsive to the stimulating antigen.

On reexposure to antigen, a secondary reaction ensues. This time the lymph node reaction is more rapid, intense, and sustained, and the dominant feature is germinal center formation. As in the primary reaction, but after a longer period of time, the secondary reaction subsides: transitional cells synthesizing antibody in the germinal center die or are dispersed, macrophages increase in number and clean up, and the titer of antibody begins to fall. Macrophages within germinal centers contain a distinctive type of phagolysosome, called the *tingible* body, which includes nuclear material of phagocytized cells. When large numbers of macrophages containing tingible bodies are present in a germinal center they give an appearance that has been compared to a starry sky.

References and Selected Bibliography

General

Crabb E. D., and Kelsall, M. A. 1940. Organization of the mucosa and lymphatic structures in the rabbit appendix. J. Morphol. 67:351.

Fujita, T. 1978. Microarchitecture of reticular tissues. Reevaluation of the RES by scanning electron microscopy. Recent Adv. RES Res. 18:1.

Fujita, T., Miyoshi, M., and Murakami, T. 1972. Scanning electron microscope observation of the dog mesenteric lymph node. Z. Zellforsch. 133:147.

Porter, R., and Whelan J. (eds.). 191. Microenvironments in haemopoietic and lymphoid differentiation. CIBA Foundation Symposium 84.

Yoffey, J., and Courtice, F. 1956. Lymphatics, Lymph, and Lymphoid Tissue. Cambridge, Mass.: Harvard University Press.

Immune Response

Coons, A. H., Leduc, E. H., and Connolly, J. M. 1955. Studies on antibody production. I. A method for the histochemical demonstration of specific antibody and its application to a study of the hyperimmune rabbit. J. Exp. Med. 102:49.

Gastkemper, N. A., Wubbena, A. S., and Nieuwenhuis, P. 1979. Germinal centres and the B cell system: A search for the germinal centre precursor cell in the rat. In Adv. Biol. Med. 114:43. New York: Plenum Press.

Hanaoka, M. Nomoto, K., and Waksman, B. H., 1970. Appendix and IgM-antibody formation. I. Immune response and tolerance to bovine-Ig-globulin in irradiated, appendix-shielded rabbit. J. Immunol. 104:616.

Humphrey, J. H. 1976. The still unsolved germinal centre mystery. In Adv. Exp. Biol. Med. 66:711. New York: Plenum Press.

Klaus, G. G. B., Humphrey, J. H., Kinkl, A., and Dongworth, D. W., 1980. The follicular dendritic cell: Its role in antigen presentation in the generation of immunological memory. In Moller, G. (ed.), Imm. Rev. 53:3–28. Copenhagen: Munksgaard.

McMaster, P. D., and Hudack, S. 1935. The formation of agglutinins within lymph nodes. J. Exp. Med. 61:783.

Milstein, C. 1980. Monoclonal antibodies. Sci. Amer. 243:66.

Nieuwenhuis, P., and Lennert, K., 1980. Histophysiology of normal lymphoid tissue and immune reactions. In Van den Tweel et al. (eds.), Malignant Lymphoproliferative Diseases. The Hague: Martinus Nijhoff Publ., p. 3–12.

Ortega, L., and Mellors, R. 1957. Cellular sites of formation of gamma globulin. J. Exp. Med. 106:627.

Walesman, B. M., Ozer, M., and Blythman, M. 1973. Appendix and IgM antibody formation V. The functional anatomy of the rabbit appendix. Lab. Invest. 28:614.

Weissman, I. L. 1975. Development and distribution of immunoglobulin-bearing cells in mice. Transplant. Rev. 24:159.

Lymphocytes

Cho, Y., and De Bruyn, P. P. H. 1981. Transcellular migration of lymphocytes through the walls of the smooth surfaced squamous endothelial venules in the lymph node: Evidence for the direct entry of lymphocytes into the blood circulation of the lymph node. J. Ultrastruct. Res. 74:259.

De Sousa, M., Freitas, A., Huber, B., Cantor, H., and Boyse, E. A. 1979. Migratory patterns of the Ly subsets of T lymphocytes in the mouse. In Adv. Exp. Biol. Med. 114:51. New York: Plenum Press.

Gowans, J. L., and Knight, E. J. 1964. The route of recirculation of lymphocytes in the rat. Proc. R. Soc. Lond. (Biol) 159:257.

Gowans, J. L., McGregor, D., and Cowen, D. 1962. Initiation of immune responses by small lymphocytes. Nature (Lond). 196:651.

Nieuwenhuis, P. and Ford, W. L. 1976. Comparative migration of B- and T-lymphocytes in the rat spleen and lymph nodes. Cell. Immunol. 23:254.

Parrott, D. M. V., De Sousa, A. B., and East, J. 1966. Thymic dependent areas in the lymphoid organs of neonatally thymectomized mice. J. Exp. Med. 123:191.

Lymph Nodes

Clark, S. 1962. The reticulum of lymph nodes in mice studies with the electron microscope. Am. J. Anat. 110:217.

Drinker, C. K., Field, M. E., and Ward, H. K. 1934. The filtering capacity of lymph nodes. J. Exp. Med. 59:393.

Drinker, C. K., Wislocki, G. B., and Field, M. E. 1933. The structure of the sinuses in the lymph nodes. Anat. Rec. 56:261.

Han, S. 1961. The ultrastructure of the mesenteric lymph node of the rat. Am. J. Anat. 109:183.

Lymphatic Vessels

Crandall, L. A., Barker, S. B., and Graham, D. G. 1943. A study of the lymph flow from a patient with thoracic duct fistula. Gastroenterology 1:1040.

Forkert, P. G., Thliveris, J. A., and Bertalanffy, F. D. 1977. Structure of sinuses in the human lymph node. Cell Tissue Res. 183:115.

Leak, L. V., and Burke, J. F. 1968. Ultrastructural studies on the lymphatic anchoring filaments. J. Cell Biol. 36:129.

Vasculature

Anderson, A. O., and Anderson, N. D. 1975. Studies on the structure and permeability of the microvasculature in normal rat lymph nodes. Am. J. Pathol. 80:387.

Marchesi, V. T., and Gowans, J. L. 1964. The migration of lymphocytes through the endothelium of venules in lymph nodes: An electron microscope study. Proc. R. Soc. Lond. (Biol.) 159:283.

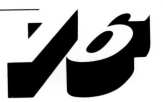

The Spleen

Leon Weiss

The spleen, weighing approximately 150 g in adult human beings, contains a specialized vasculature that modifies the circulating blood. There is no element of the blood, cellular or plasmal, that the spleen does not affect. It provides the proper hematopoietic microenvironment for the final differentiation of reticulocytes, platelets, T and B cells, and monocytes. It monitors the red blood cells of the circulation and destroys or modifies imperfect ones. It removes damaged or aged blood cells of all types. It sequesters monocytes from the blood, facilitates their transformation into macrophages, and holds them; they then impart enormous phagocytic capacity and other macrophage functions to the spleen. It receives T and B cells of the recirculating pool from the blood and sorts them into compartments, enabling them to interact with macrophages and antigen and to participate in immune responses. It stores as many as a third of the platelets of the body in a ready reserve. In certain species, it can also function as a reservoir for erythrocytes and granulocytes, delivering them rapidly to the blood when needed. The adult spleen is not essential to life, although its loss makes one more vulnerable to overwhelming infection. In some pathological conditions it may, in fact, eliminate or sequester circulating blood cells with such avidity that it must be removed to save life.

Structure of the Spleen

Capsule and Trabeculae

The human spleen is enclosed by a capsule of dense white connective tissue, a few millimeters in thickness. From the internal capsular surface a rich branching network of trabeculae subdivides the organ into communicating compartments several millimeters in each dimension (Fig. 16–1). The capsule contains relatively little muscle and is therefore incapable of the profound contraction that the muscular capsule of the spleen in dogs and cats exhibits. The capsule is indented medially at the hilus, where it is penetrated by blood vessels, lymphatic vessels, and nerves. Arterial vessels branch into the trabeculae and from there into the pulp or parenchyma of the organ. Veins and lymphatics also travel in the trabeculae, entering from the pulp and running out.

Splenic Pulp

The tissue enclosed within the capsule and trabeculae is the splenic pulp (Figs. 16–2 to 16–4). Much of it is red, owing to the presence of erythrocytes, and it is called *red pulp*. There are two types of spleen, those that contain vascular sinuses and those that do not. In sinusal spleens, of which the human spleen is an example, red pulp is made up of four vascular structures: slender nonanastomosing arterial vessels; large, branching thin-walled venous vessels called *venous sinuses* (or sinusoids); and thin plates or partitions of cellular tissue lying between the sinuses, called *splenic cords*. The venous sinuses flow into *pulp veins*. In nonsinusal spleens, like that of the cat, venous sinuses are absent. Blood flows through arterial vessels, *pulp spaces*, and veins.

Grossly visible zones of tightly packed lymphocytes also occur in the pulp and constitute the *white pulp* of the spleen. White pulp assumes two formations. One is cylindrical and surrounds major arterial branches of the splenic pulp as *periarterial lymphatic sheaths*. The other form is nodular and comprises the *lymphatic nodules*, which lie within the periarterial lymphatic sheaths (Fig. 16–4). Immune responses in the spleen are initiated in the white pulp. The splenic pulp at the junction of white pulp and red pulp is called the *marginal zone*. It is the site of high blood traffic where the distinctive blood cell processing of the spleen is begun.

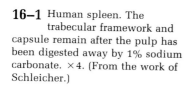

16–1 Human spleen. The trabecular framework and capsule remain after the pulp has been digested away by 1% sodium carbonate. ×4. (From the work of Schleicher.)

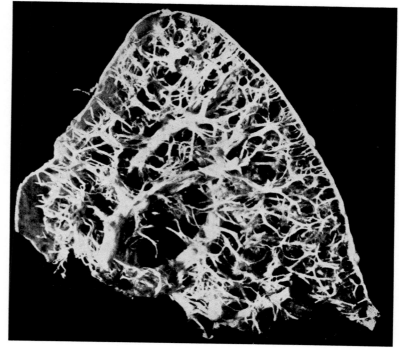

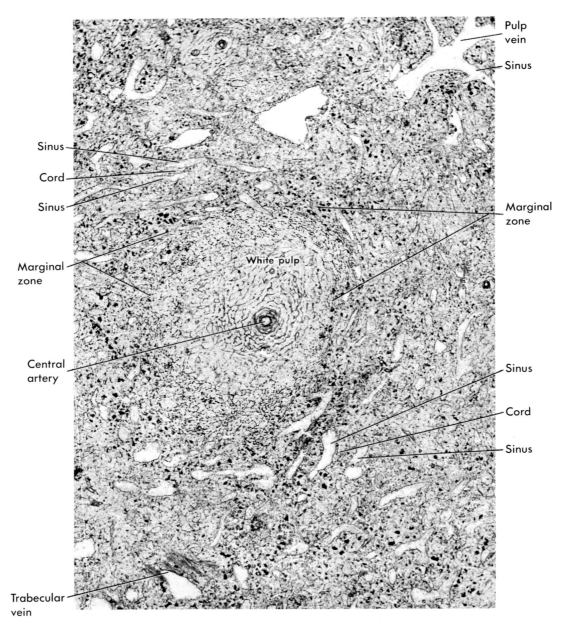

Pulp
vein

Sinus

Sinus

Cord

Sinus

Marginal
zone

Marginal
zone

White pulp

Central
artery

Sinus

Cord

Sinus

Trabecular
vein

16–2 Spleen of a rat. The extracellular reticulum is stained by the PAS reaction. The white pulp contains a darkly outlined central artery. Note the circumferential pattern of the reticulum of white pulp. A marginal zone surrounds the white pulp and contains a relatively dense meshwork of reticulum and many darkly stained cells. Beyond the white pulp and marginal zone lies the red pulp, accounting for most of the splenic volume. The clear spaces represent splenic sinuses, for the most part, but also pulp veins and trabecular veins. The splenic cords constitute the relatively solid tissue lying between the sinuses. × 225. (From Weiss, L. 1959. J. Anat. 93:465.)

16–3 Spleen of a hedgehog. In this low-power field, the white pulp, red pulp, blood outflow tract, and splenic mesentery are shown. The white pulp, occupying a relatively small volume, surrounds a central artery. The red pulp occupies most of the field. It is made up almost entirely of relatively clear spaces, the splenic sinuses, which form an anastomosing system of venous vessels. The splenic cords, darkly stained tissue lying between the sinuses, consist of a reticular meshwork that contains blood cells and macrophages and receives arterial terminations. Blood is carried out of the spleen through trabecular veins, which drain into the splenic vein. Splenic veins leave the spleen at the hilus and enter the splenic mesentery. At the **arrow,** splenic sinuses empty into a pulp vein that drains into a trabecular vein. The marginal zone lies between white pulp and red pulp. The mesentery contains a branch of the splenic artery that will enter the spleen at the hilus. × 150. (From Janout, V., and Weiss, L. 1972. Anat. Rec. 172:197.)

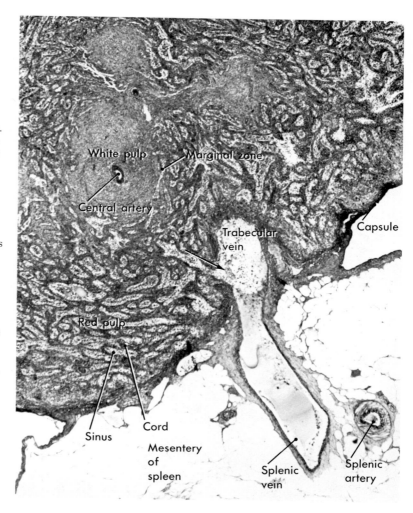

Blood Flow

Blood enters the spleen by way of splenic arteries that pass through the hilus. A splenic artery branches into trabeculae as *trabecular arteries,* which turn out of the trabeculae and enter the pulp. In the pulp, they are surrounded by *periarterial lymphatic sheaths.* As an artery travels through the periarterial lymphatic sheath as the *central artery,* it sends out many branches; some supply the lymphatic nodules within the sheath. In the human spleen, most branches travel to the periphery of the sheath and terminate in the marginal zone. The central artery itself runs out into the red pulp and terminates in cords. In the red pulp and in the marginal zone, blood flows through cords and enters splenic sinuses, which are tributaries of veins of the pulp. These veins enter trabeculae as trabecular veins. At the hilus, the trabecular veins are continuous with splenic veins, which drain the organ. The circulation of the spleen has been difficult to analyze and it will be discussed more fully below, after the structure of the pulp is described.

Lymphatic vessels lie in white pulp, girdling the central artery (Figs. 16–4 and 16–5). Lymphatics run into trabeculae and out of the spleen to drain into lymph nodes in the splenic mesentery.

White Pulp

The white pulp of the spleen is a lymphatic tissue analogous to the cortex of lymph nodes. It consists of lymphocytes, macrophages, and other free cells lying in a specialized reticular mesh-

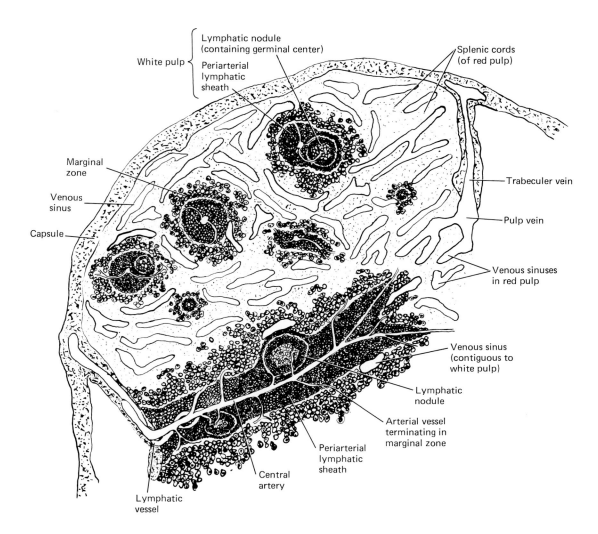

White pulp
- Lymphatic nodule (containing germinal center)
- Periarterial lymphatic sheath

Splenic cords (of red pulp)

Marginal zone

Venous sinus

Capsule

Trabeculer vein

Pulp vein

Venous sinuses in red pulp

Venous sinus (contiguous to white pulp)

Lymphatic nodule

Arterial vessel terminating in marginal zone

Periarterial lymphatic sheath

Central artery

Lymphatic vessel

16–4 Schematic view of the organization of the human spleen. The white pulp has two components: periarterial lymphatic sheaths and lymphatic nodules. The latter may be made up of a germinal center and a surrounding mantle zone. The white pulp is surrounded by the marginal zone. The remainder of the tissue depicted is the red pulp, which consists primarily of splenic sinuses separated by splenic cords. The pattern of blood flow is as follows. A trabecular artery enters the white pulp and becomes the central artery. The central artery passes through white pulp and gives rise to many branches. A few end within white pulp; some supply the germinal center and mantle zone of the secondary nodule. Most terminate at the periphery of the white pulp, emptying in or near the marginal zone. A number of arterial vessels emerge from the white pulp, pass into the marginal zone, reach the red pulp, and curve back to empty into the marginal zone. Some arterial branches, in addition to the main stem of the central artery, run into the red pulp. Almost all terminate in the cords. Here, too, variation exists. Some arterial vessels terminate in a cord close against a sinus wall, whereas others terminate in the midst of a cord, away from any sinus. Arterial vessels may terminate as capillaries or as somewhat larger vessels. Some arterial vessels may bear sheaths shortly before termination. The sinuses drain into pulp veins, which, in turn, drain into trabecular veins. A sinus may abut the white pulp and receive lymphocytes or other free cells that migrate from white pulp across its wall and into its lumen. Efferent lymphatic vessels lie about the proximal portion of the central artery and run out of the spleen through the trabeculae. (From Weiss, L., and Tavossoli, M. 1970. Semin. Hematol. 7:372.)

16–5 Spleen of a hedgehog. Lymphatic vessels are shown in this field. They lie within the periarterial lymphatic sheath **(PALS)** of white pulp in relation to the central artery, two branches of which are shown. The PALS consists of a reticular meshwork obscured by many lymphocytes crowded together. Outside the PALS is the marginal zone **(MZ)**. ×950. (From Janout, V., and Weiss, L. 1972. Anat. Rec. 172:197.)

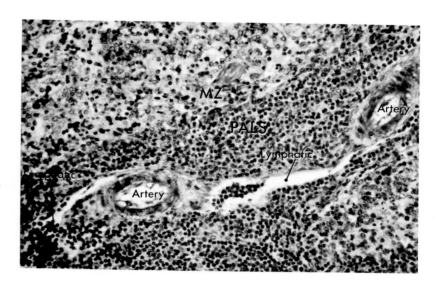

work. The periarterial lymphatic sheaths are cylinders that axially surround the central artery. Their reticular meshwork tends to be arranged in circumferential layers around the central artery, with a more prominent circumferential reticulum at their periphery (Figs. 16–6, 16–9, and 16–10). Lymphocytes are the most numerous of the free cells packed in these sheaths. They are predominantly T cells of the recirculating pool.

Periarterial lymphatic sheaths persist around arterial vessels, tapering down as the vessels branch and become finer. The sheaths are quite attenuated when the arterial vessels they surround become small arterioles. Lymphatic nodules are spherical or ovoid, resembling nodules of the cortex of lymph nodes. They lie within the periarterial lymphatic sheath, often at arterial branchings. B cells are concentrated in nodules.

16–6 A sketch of the meshwork of white pulp. Lymphocytes and other free cells are not included. The reticular cells are indicated as nucleated outlines. The reticular fibers, such as are stained in Fig. 16–2, are stippled. Virtually the entire field is taken by a cross section of the periarterial lymphatic sheath (PALS), in the center of which is the cross section of the central artery. Near the central artery the reticular meshwork may not be markedly specialized, while at the periphery it is circumferential (see Figs. 16–2 and 16–9). To the left of the central artery, the reticular meshwork supports a small lymphatic nodule supplied by several arterioles. A large branch of the central artery curves down and to the right, reaching the red pulp where it bifurcates **(1)**. (See Fig. 16–11.) Another large branch travels toward 12 o'clock and ends in the marginal zone as a sheathed capillary **(2)**. Another vessel arches toward 2 o'clock and opens into the marginal zone **(3)**. (From Weiss, L. 1972. Cells and Tissues of the Immune System. Englewood Cliffs, N.J.: Prentice-Hall, Inc.)

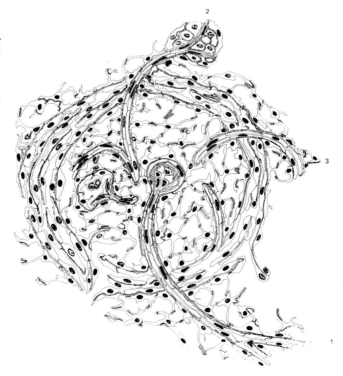

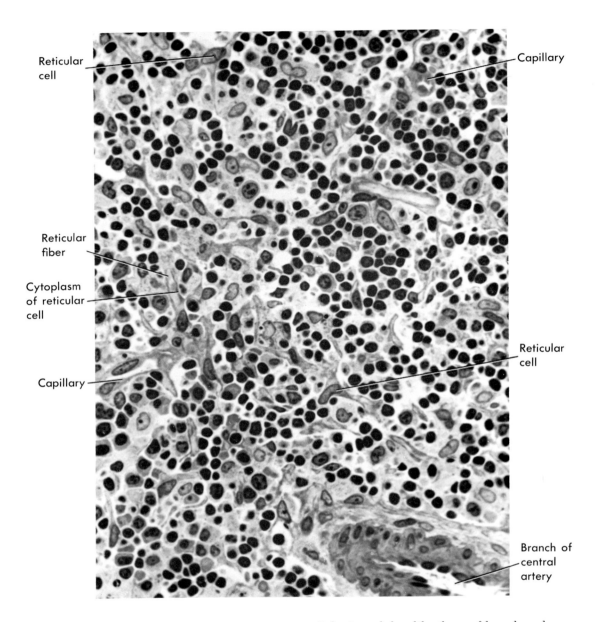

Reticular cell

Capillary

Reticular fiber

Cytoplasm of reticular cell

Reticular cell

Capillary

Branch of central artery

16–7 Spleen of a rabbit, periarterial lymphatic sheath of white pulp. A large branch of the central artery lies in the right lower corner. The larger part of the field consists of a reticular meshwork within which lies the small, densely stained round lymphocytes and related free cells. The meshwork is made of branching reticular cells and reticular fibers. The reticular cells ensheath the more lightly stained reticular fibers. Small blood vessels are present in places in this field. Their adventitial layers are continuous with the reticular meshwork, as are the adventitial layers of the branch of the central artery in the right lower corner. × 600. (From Weiss, L. 1964. Bull. Johns Hopkins Hosp. 115:99.)

Splenic nodules, like those of lymph nodes, may become secondary nodules by developing germinal centers. Antigen-presenting cells (page 535) are present in the white pulp. Lymphatic nodules cause periarterial lymphatic sheaths to bulge unevenly and thus force the central artery to assume an eccentric position.

Vascular Supply of White Pulp

The central artery is a medium-sized muscular artery that gives off branches as it runs through the periarterial lymphatic sheath (Figs. 16–3,

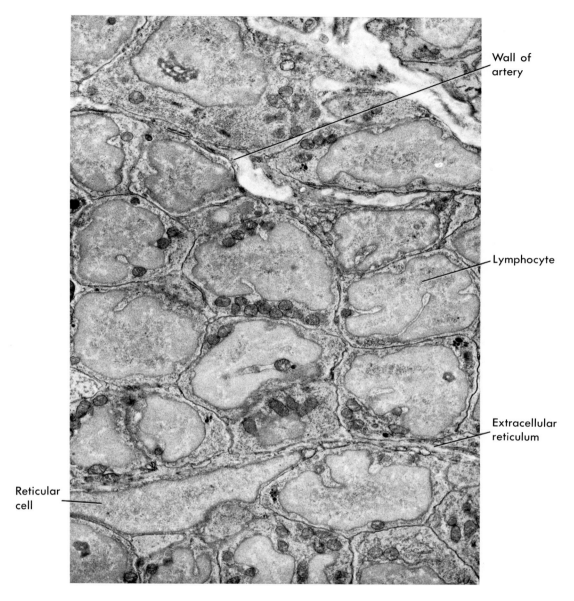

Wall of
artery

Lymphocyte

Extracellular
reticulum

Reticular
cell

16–4, 16–6, and 16–7 to 16–9). The branches tend to run radially toward the periphery of the white pulp. Many go beyond the white pulp and empty into the marginal zone. Some travel farther, reach red pulp, and terminate there. Lymphatic nodules are supplied by a deep and superficial set of branches from the central artery. Snook has described a distinctive arrangement in human spleen wherein lymphatic nodules are supplied by recurrent arteries curving back from red pulp. Efferent lymphatic vessels originate deep in white pulp. They converge on the central artery and its branches and wind around them,

16–8 Spleen of a rat, periarterial lymphatic sheath of white pulp. This electron micrograph illustrates the relationships of an arterial vessel, lymphocytes, and the reticular meshwork. The adventitia of a large branch of the central artery is in the upper part of the field. Small lymphocytes are present, tightly packed together. Note that their scanty cytoplasm is rich in ribonucleoprotein and in mitochondria but lacks endoplasmic reticulum. These cells are preponderantly T lymphocytes (see Fig. 16–22). A reticular cell in the lower part of the field is associated with a small segment of extracellular reticulum. × 15,000. (From Weiss, L. 1964. Bull. Johns Hopkins Hosp. 115:99.)

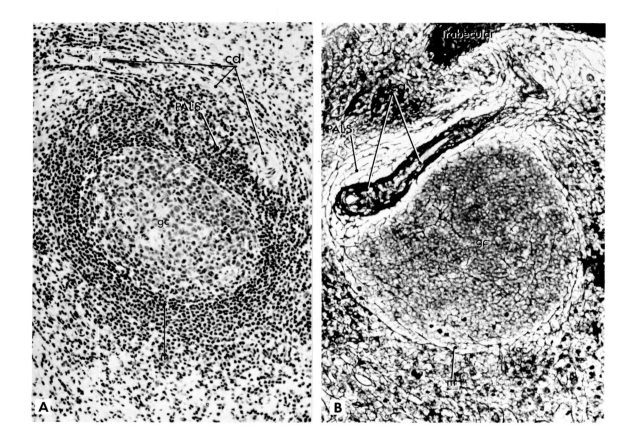

16–9 Human spleen, white pulp. **A.** Where the cells are stained with Giemsa stain, a central artery **(ca)** surrounded by the small lymphocyte-rich periarterial lymphatic sheath **(PALS)** curves into the field from the left. At the left leader it is cut in longitudinal section; at the right leader, in cross section. Hanging from the lower border of the PALS is a large lymphatic nodule, consisting of a large germinal center surrounded by a dense mantle **(m)** of small lymphocytes. **B.** In a reticulum preparation, in which the extracellular reticulum is blackened by silver, a similar field is shown. A central artery **(ca)** curves in from the right. It probably comes from the nearby trabecula. The central artery is surrounded by a PALS. Note the circumferential pattern of the reticulum of the PALS around the central artery. Again, a large lymphatic nodule hangs from the PALS. The periphery of the nodule, constituting the mantle **(m)** of small lymphocytes, actually represents the PALS, which has been carried out by the presence of the large germinal center **(gc)**. × 450. (From the preparation of K. Richardson.)

moving toward the trabeculae with their contents flowing into trabecular lymphatics. These lymphatic vessels are tributaries of larger collecting vessels that leave the spleen and empty into lymph nodes in the splenic mesentery and near the celiac plexus.

Marginal Zone

The marginal zone, lying between white pulp and red pulp, is bound centrally (on its white pulp aspect) by the outermost circumferential lamella of the white pulp. On its periphery or red pulp aspect it blends into the cords of red pulp. The reticular meshwork of the marginal zone is quite fine in human spleen. Many arterial vessels open into the marginal zone. They may terminate in a funnel-shaped orifice and often bifurcate just before ending. Venous sinuses regularly come near or into the marginal zone. The marginal zone is a site of heavy blood traffic and filtration, and much of the splenic processing of blood begins there.

Red Pulp

Red pulp in human spleen is a reticular mesh-work supplied by arteries and drained by venous sinuses (Figs. 16–3, 16–4, and 16–10 to 16–19). The venous sinuses form an anastomosing system in the meshwork. As a result, the reticular meshwork takes the form of a branching system of cords lying between the sinuses. After it distributes branches to the white pulp and marginal zone, the attenuated main stem of the central artery runs on into the cords of red pulp and branches into straight nonanastomosing slender vessels, about 25 μm in outside diameter, called *penicilli*. Arterial vessels open into the reticular meshwork of the cords. They do not open into the venous sinuses.

Shortly before they terminate, arterial capillaries may be modified by running through a sheath of macrophages supported in a reticular meshwork. (Figs. 16–20 and 16–21). The most commonly used term for these sheaths has been *ellipsoid* because the sheaths may have that shape, but they are often spherical, cylindrical, or irregular. Blue and Weiss have suggested the term *periarterial macrophage sheath* because it is anatomically and functionally descriptive and it is consistent with the useful term *periarterial lymphatic sheath*, which describes an analogous structure. Sheaths may be spongy because cells are loosened by plasma infiltration, or they may be tightly compressed. Erythrocytes, granulocytes, and other blood cells may be present in the sheath. The periarterial macrophage sheaths may represent a major population of macrophages in the spleen. Well-developed sheaths possess extraordinary phagocytic capacity and are major sites of clearance of blood-borne particles in the red pulp. They may, moreover, play a role in controlling blood flow in the spleen. Sheaths vary in development depending on the species. In the dog and cat they are very prominent. In rabbits they are absent. Periarterial macrophage sheaths in the human spleen are relatively small, and not every arterial capillary bears one. In spleens that lack periarterial macrophage sheaths, clearance functions are handled by macrophages in the marginal zone and red pulp. In some species, such as the horse, sheaths contain antigen-presenting cells.

Splenic cords, as indicated, are part of the vascular pathway, receiving blood from arterial vessels and conveying it to venous sinuses. The vascular pathway through the cords may be long,

where arterial vessels terminate some distance from the vascular sinus, or it may be short, where arterial vessels terminate close to the wall of vascular sinuses. Functions other than blood flow may occur in splenic cords. Erythropoiesis and, to a lesser degree, granulocytopoiesis may occur there. This hematopoiesis is not unusual in rodents but happens only pathologically in human spleen. Destruction of blood cells, in particular, old or damaged erythrocytes, also occurs in splenic cords and may be evident by the presence of erythrophagocytic macrophages.

16–10 Spleen of a rat. The periphery of white pulp (the periarterial lymphatic sheath, PALS) is present. On the left are the closely packed cells of the PALS. A large macrophage may be seen. Its location at the periphery of white pulp is characteristic. The PALS has a well-defined rim of concentric strands of reticulum, running from top to bottom of this field (between **arrows**). This rim is well shown in silver preparations in which the extracellular reticulum is stained (see Fig. 16–9). The marginal zone is on the right. × 19,000. (From Weiss, L. 1964. Bull. Johns Hopkins Hosp. 115:99.)

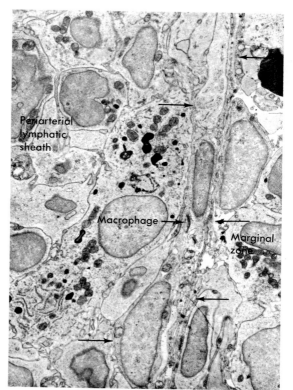

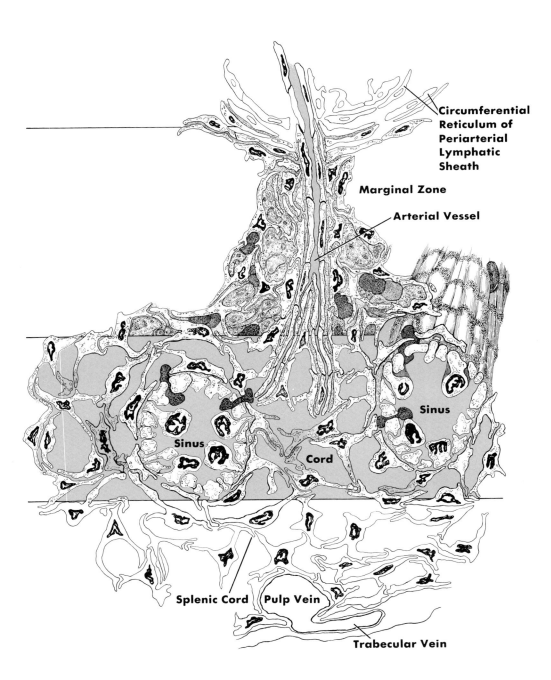

Circumferential Reticulum of Periarterial Lymphatic Sheath

Marginal Zone

Arterial Vessel

Sinus

Sinus

Cord

Splenic Cord   **Pulp Vein**

Trabecular Vein

16–11 Spleen. Schematic view of artery leaving the periarterial lymphatic sheath white pulp and entering red pulp. It enters a splenic cord and bifurcates between two sinuses. (From Weiss, L. 1972. The Cells and Tissues of the Immune System. Englewood Cliffs, N.J.: Prentice-Hall, Inc.)

Splenic Sinuses

Splenic sinuses (Figs. 16–2 to 16–4 and 16–11 to 16–19) are long, anastomosing vascular channels, 35 to 40 μm in diameter, with a unique endothelium and basement membrane. The endothelial cells are elongate with tapered ends and lie parallel to the long axis of the sinus. In cross section through sinuses, therefore, the endothe-

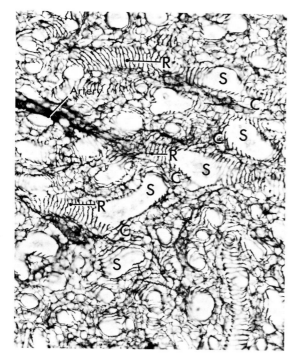

16–12 Red pulp of human spleen, reticulum stain.
△   Sinuses are present as clear spaces **(S).** Their
basement membrane is exposed as consisting
primarily of "ring fibers" **(R),** deeply stained. This
membrane is continuous with the reticular fibers of
the cords **(C).** An artery entering from the left appears
to open into the cord. × 600. (From the preparation of
K. Richardson.)

lial cells are cut in cross section. They lie side
by side and are separated by a slitlike space.
Tight junctional complexes occur regularly along
their lateral surfaces. Endothelial cells contain
bundles of microfilaments that run longitudinally in the basal cytoplasm. Intermediate (100
Å) filaments are distributed basally and throughout the cytoplasm. The luminal surface of endothelium is rich in micropinocytotic vesicles.
Blood cells flowing through the red pulp cross
the wall of splenic sinuses between endothelial
cells.

The endothelium lies on a basement membrane, which may be deeply stained in the periodic acid Schiff reaction or impregnated by silver. The basement membrane is perforated by
large, regularly arranged uniform polygonal apertures or fenestrae so that what little material
remains of the basement membrane is reduced to
slender strands that separate and outline the ap-

16–13 Rabbit spleen, red pulp. Sections of two
▽   sinuses with intervening cords are present in
this light micrograph. The basement membrane,
stained deeply with the PAS reaction, is interrupted
(see Figs. 16–11, 16–12, and 16–19) in this section
because of its fenestrated character. The cords are
crowded with macrophages. Reticular cells and PAS-
stained reticular fibers are present in the cords. An
arterial vessel that opens into a cord is also present.
PAS-hematoxylin stain. × 1,200. (From Weiss, L.
1959. J. Anat. 93:465.)

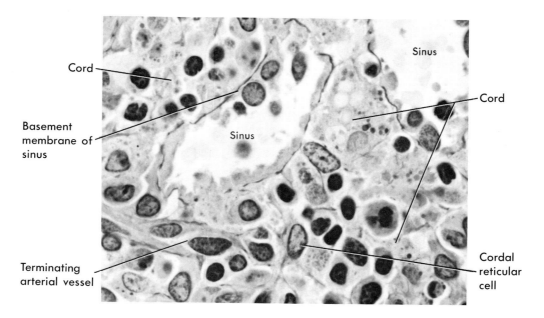

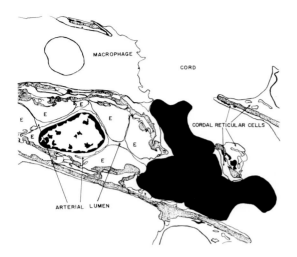

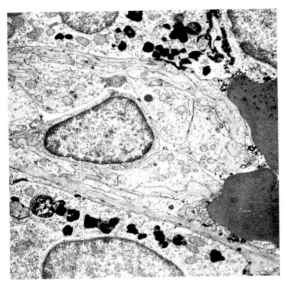

16–14 Spleen of a rabbit, red pulp. An arterial vessel ends in a cord. This vessel is typical of many terminating arterial vessels in red pulp. It is a small arteriole. Its endothelium (**E** in tracing) is high. Its lumen and the surrounding red pulp contain Thorotrast, which was injected intravenously several minutes before splenectomy. About two layers of extracellular reticulum (**stippled** in tracing) are present in the vessel wall. The inner one underlies the endothelium and constitutes a basement membrane. Portions of two macrophages lie above and below the vessel. The vessel opens to the right, and several erythrocytes lie just outside the orifice. × 18,000. (From Weiss, L. 1963. Am. J. Anat. 113:51.)

ertures (Figs. 16–11, 16–12, and 16–19). In a surface view, the basement membrane looks like a net. In human basement membrane, the transverse component is heavy and the longitudinal links relatively slight. The arrangement can be likened to a barrel in which the wooden staves correspond to the endothelium and the hoops to the basement membrane. With the electron microscope, the basement membrane is seen to consist of an extracellular granular material that may contain a few collagenous fibers. Its composition thus resembles that of reticular fibers and, indeed, reticular fibers of the cords surrounding splenic sinuses are continuous with the basement membrane of the sinuses (Figs. 16–11, 16–15, and 16–19). Reticular cells lie over the outside surface of the basement membrane of vascular sinuses, occupying an adventitial position. These reticular cells extend branches into the surrounding cords and are thereby part of the cordal reticular meshwork. They are associated with, and probably produce, reticular fibers.

The interendothelial slits of vascular sinuses constitute a major component in the vascular pathway through the red pulp. Blood passes out of arterial endings through the cords and through these interendothelial slits. From here it goes into the lumen of the vascular sinuses and then into splenic veins. In spleens without vascular sinuses, such as the cat's, blood flows from arterial terminations through the reticular meshwork of pulp spaces, a tissue comparable to splenic cords, and then is taken up by pulp veins.

Splenic Veins

Sinuses are tributaries of pulp veins. The transition of sinus into vein can be quite abrupt, the latter having a flat endothelium and a basement membrane without apertures. Blood cells do not cross the wall of pulp veins. These veins flow into trabecular veins that drain into the splenic veins, which leave the organ destined for the portal vein. Splenic vein blood may be rich in macrophages, which are undoubtedly filtered from the circulation by the liver and, should they pass the liver, by the lungs.

Embryology

The spleen originates in the dorsal mesogastrium at about 5-mm crown–rump length (CRL) in human embryos. At 40-mm CRL the spleen consists of an encapsulated cellular meshwork. By 55-

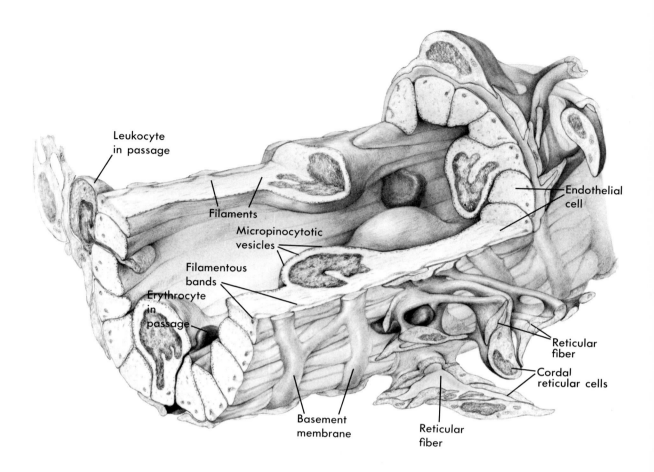

Leukocyte in passage

Filaments

Micropinocytotic vesicles

Filamentous bands

Erythrocyte in passage

Basement membrane

Reticular fiber

Endothelial cell

Reticular fiber

Cordal reticular cells

16–15 A schematic drawing of a human splenic sinus in red pulp. The endothelial cells are tapered rods that lie side by side with their long axis parallel to the long axis of the vessel. Virtually all arterial vessels end in the surrounding cords without direct connection to the sinuses. Accordingly, blood entering the vascular sinus must enter from the surrounding cord, squeezing through the slitlike spaces between sinus endothelial cells. Note that several blood cells in passage across the sinus wall are shown. The endothelial cells show several distinctive cytological features. These features include a row of pinocytotic vesicles just beneath the plasma membrane on the luminal and lateral surfaces, and two sets of cytoplasmic filaments. One set of filaments, rather loosely organized, runs longitudinally through the cytoplasm. The other set is tightly organized into dense bands in the basal cytoplasm. These bands arch between strands of the basement membrane. They appear to insert into the plasma membrane where it overlies the basement membrane and then continue through the plasma membrane into the substance of the basement membrane. These filaments are probably part of the cytoskeletal system, which stiffens the basal cytoplasm and maintains the shape of endothelial cells and the slitlike interendothelial space. They, or the other set of filaments, may be contractile. They play an important role in the spleen's capacity to recognize damaged blood cells and destroy or modify them (see text).

The basement membrane is fenestrated, having heavy strandlike transverse "ring" components and lighter longitudinal strands joining the rings. The large fenestrae or apertures in the basement membrane leave ample unimpeded space for blood cells to pass through the sinus wall. The cordal surface of the basement membrane is covered by cordal reticular cells, which branch into the surrounding cord. (From Chen, L. T., and Weiss, L. 1972. Am. J. Anat. 134:425.)

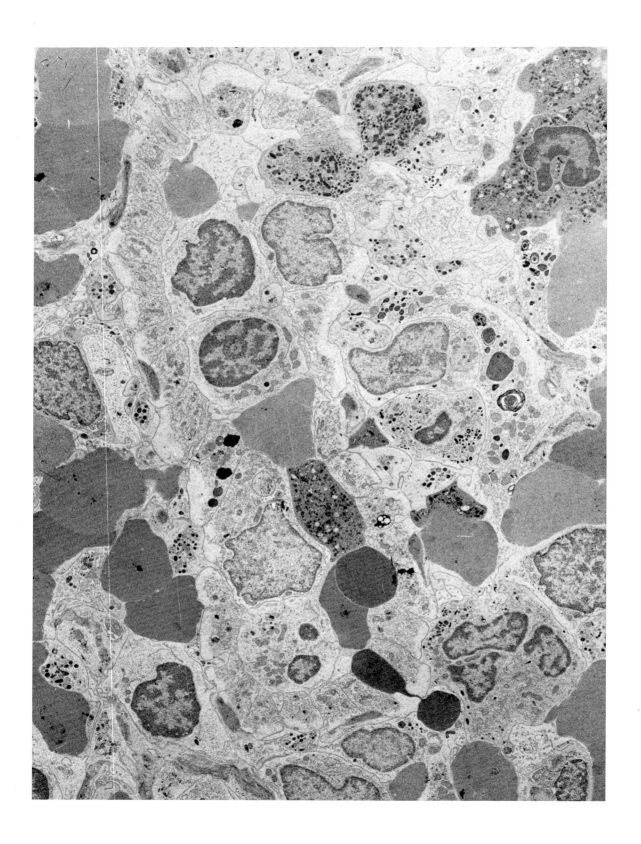

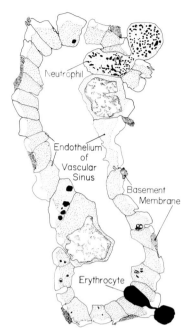

16–16 Human spleen, red pulp. A venous sinus occupies most of this field, but does not stand out because it is collapsed. Its wall is being crossed by an erythrocyte and neutrophil. Use above reduced tracing as key. Courtesy of Robert M. Powell

mm CRL, vascular sinuses are present and the meshwork is much looser, containing many free blood cells and macrophages. A rich vascular supply quickly develops. By 100-mm CRL, reticular cells tend to lay out the plan of the spleen and assume a circumferential pattern around arteries, defining the periarterial lymphatic sheaths and marginal zones. Soon thereafter, lymphocytes move into the periarterial sheaths, which are rather clearly developed after the first half of gestation. In the first trimester, the human fetal spleen is erythropoietic and myelopoietic. These activities fade after the fifth prenatal month, preempted successively by the liver and marrow.

Functions of the Spleen

The Circulation of Blood Through the Spleen

In most tissues of the body, blood flows through tubular blood vessels, and one can intuitively correlate the anatomy of the vascular bed with the physiology of actual blood flow. However, in some vascular beds, as in the cavernous tissue of the secondary sex organs and especially in the red pulp of the spleen, the anatomy is highly distinctive and correlations of structure and function are difficult to make. In order to understand the circulation of the spleen it is necessary to distinguish the structure of the vascular bed, determined by anatomical methods, from the nature of blood flow, determined by physiological methods.

Students of the spleen have wrestled with a major question about the anatomy of the vascular bed of red pulp: is the circulation open or closed? That is, do the arterial vessels connect directly to venous vessels, with endothelial continuity (closed circulation)? Or do the arterial vessels terminate and empty into the cords or pulp spaces, with the blood flowing through these spaces and then through the walls of venous vessels (open circulation)? Alternatively, is the circulation through the red pulp partly open and partly closed?

The overwhelming evidence is that the vascular pathway through the red pulp of the spleen, whether of the sinusal or nonsinusal type, is anatomically open. The key evidence is as follows: Arterial terminations can be seen by light microscopy and electron microscopy to open into the cords or pulp spaces, and blood is found there. Blood cells, moreover, may be regularly observed crossing the wall of vascular sinuses through interendothelial slits. No one has convincingly demonstrated endothelial continuity in sectioned material between arterial capillaries and venous sinuses or pulp veins.

Nonetheless, a number of investigators have concluded that the circulation through the red pulp of the spleen is closed, or that some arterial vessels do empty into sinuses. Let us consider the evidence for these conclusions. Knisely, whose work in the 1930s had great impact, studied the circulation in living spleen by exteriorizing the organ, maintaining its circulation intact, transilluminating it, and cooling it through a hollow quartz rod. He concluded that the circulation was closed. Several groups confirmed his work; others did not. But study of the living spleen is not primarily a study of the anatomical arrangements because this approach lacks the resolution to define endothelium and other cell structures critically. It is, rather, a study of blood flow. For example, Knisely studied circulation through the kitten spleen. This spleen contains no vascular sinuses. Arterial terminations are

560

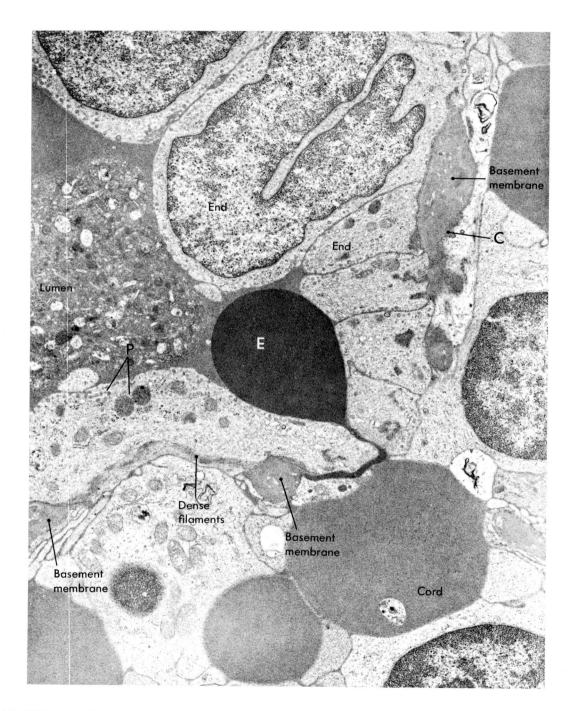

16–17 Human spleen, red pulp. An erythrocyte **(E)** passes from a cord and through the sinus wall between endothelial cells **(End)** into the lumen of the sinus. The erythrocyte is drawn into a thin strand as it passes through the mural slit. The endothelial cells contain many pinocytotic vesicles **(P)** at the luminal surface and dense filaments in the basal cytoplasm, which arches across the fenestrae of the basement membrane. Small portions of cordal reticular cells applied to the abluminal surface of the basement membrane are present. The cord is filled with erythrocytes and other free cells. × 10,000. (From Chen, L. T., and Weiss, L. 1972. Am. J. Anat. 134:425.)

16–18 Rat spleen, red pulp, showing the surface of the endothelium facing the lumen of a vascular sinus. The vessel runs from left to right, bifurcating on the right. The endothelial cells lie side by side, their long axis running from left to right. The cells bulge into the lumen in their nuclear zone. There appears to be no interendothelial space. At the curved **arrow** a red cell appears to be passing through the wall of the vascular sinus by squeezing between endothelial cells. Compare with Fig. 16–17 and see discussion in text. × 1,000. (From Weiss, L. 1974. Blood. 43:665.)

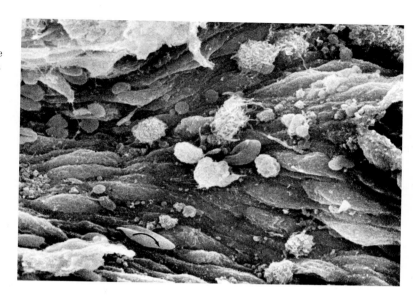

16–19 Human spleen. Reconstuction of extracellular reticulum of red pulp. Four sinuses are present in this field, outlined by the "ring fibers" of the basement membrane. The reticular fibers in the cords form a meshwork. In the human spleen the reticular fibers of the cords, as seen well between the upper two sinuses, form a collar or circlet around the sinus. The reader is referred to Koboth's work for additional valuable reconstructions of red pulp. (From Koboth, E. 1939. Beitr. Pathol. Anat. 103:11.)

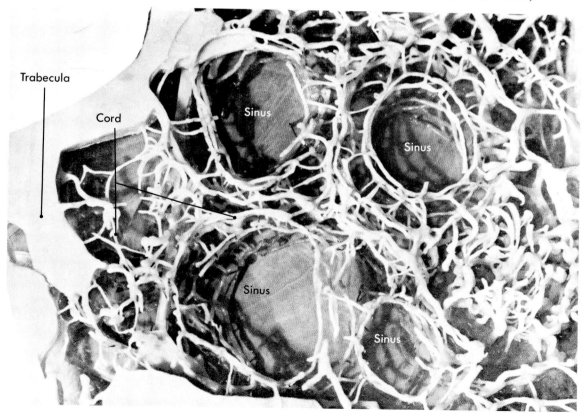

Trabecula

Cord

Sinus

Sinus

Sinus

Sinus

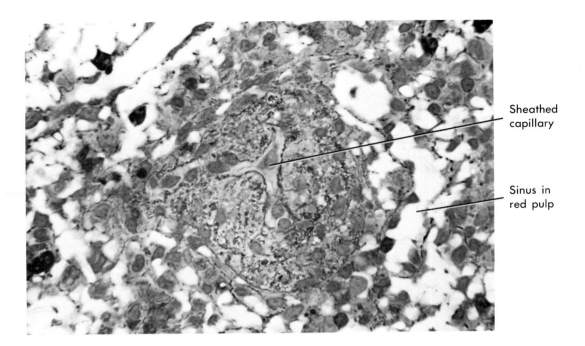

Sheathed
capillary

Sinus in
red pulp

16–20 Spleen of a dog, red pulp. In this light micrograph, an arterial vessel, which is actually a capillary, bifurcates within the sheath. Its endothelium is high, effacing the lumen. The sheath consists of phagocytes with strands of extracellular reticulum running between them. The sheath is about 75 μm in diameter. The surrounding red pulp contains sinuses. The darkly stained free cells in the red pulp are granulocytes. One, in the left upper corner of the field, is crossing the wall of a sinus. Erythrocytes, which abound in red pulp, are unstained in this preparation. PAS-hematoxylin stain. × 650. (From Weiss, L. 1962. Am. J. Anat. 111:131.)

widely separated from veins; and the walls of the veins, as seen by electron microscopy, contain apertures that open to the pulp spaces. It is hardly possible that such a spleen has an anatomically closed vascular bed, yet Knisely described the circulation as closed. In a sophisticated and fastidious study the McCuskeys correlated their observations on the living circulation, made using cool intense xenon light and recorded by motion picture, with fixed and sectioned spleen studies by electron microscopy. They found that blood flows out of arterial capillary terminations into the reticular meshwork of red pulp. However, in this reticular meshwork the blood is channeled by the cytoplasmic processes of reticular cells, which may form tubular structures. These channels convey the blood to

the walls of venous vessels. Thus, by correlating their two sets of observations, the McCuskeys concluded that the circulation through the red pulp of the spleen is anatomically open.

Snook, who provided evidence for an open circulation in many spleens, found that in some species, notably the guinea pig, arterial capillaries appeared to connect directly with venous vessels. However, his conclusion was based on silvered preparations, which stain extracellular material—specifically, basement membrane and reticular fibers. Endothelium and other cellular structures are not revealed, and it may not be possible to differentiate an arterial terminal that

16–21 Portion of a periarterial macrophage sheath. The arterial capillary at the center of the sheath (upper left corner) has a triangular shape because of oblique sectioning. Endothelial cells **(E_a)** impinge on the red cell in the lumen. A sinus **(S)** filled with red cells delimits the periphery of the sheath. Macrophages **(M)** containing ingested material are packed tightly into the sheath reticulum. Note the lucent centers in many residual bodies **(arrowheads).** Basement membrane outlines the arterial capillary and forms a broken line beneath the row of transversely sectioned sinus endothelial cells **(E_s)** at the bottom of the field. Reticular fibers of the same dense material run through the sheath and surround reticular cells **(RC).** × 3,400. (From Blue, J., and Weiss, L. The American Journal of Anatomy, 1981.)

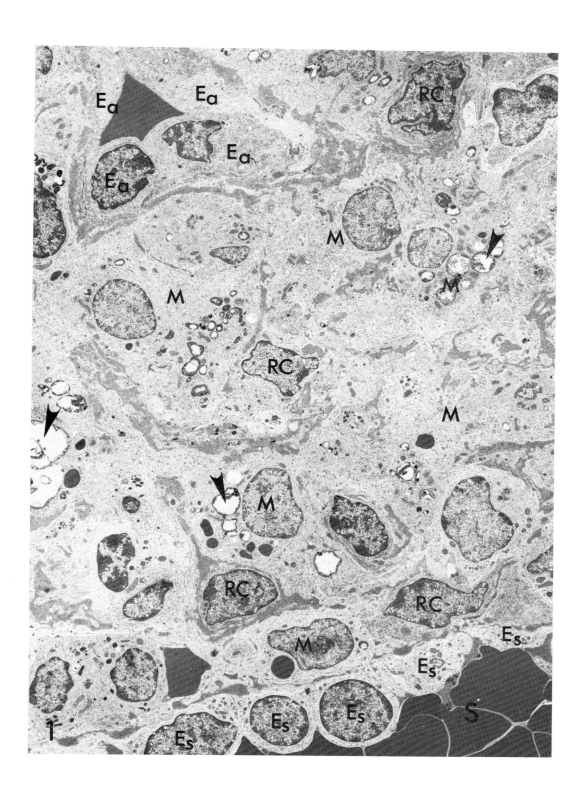

lies near a venous vessel from one that has actual endothelial continuity with a vein.

A number of scanning electron-microscopic studies have been done on casts of the spleen's vasculature. The casts have been made by injecting liquid plastic into splenic blood vessels, allowing it to harden, and then digesting away the tissue. Some investigators have concluded that the vasculature is open; others, that the vasculature is closed. With this technique, however, it is difficult to differentiate streams of plastic that had been enclosed by blood vessels from those that had not. Again, as in silver impregnation techniques for reticulum, this method does not seem suitable for determining whether the vascular bed of the spleen is anatomically open or closed.

In an ingenious approach to the question, Chen administered microspheres 3 to 4 μm in diameter intravenously to rabbits and found a portion of the spheres in the lumen of splenic sinuses. He concluded that there were some direct connections of arterial vessels to sinuses because, on the basis of earlier electron-microscopic observations of blood cell passage in the spleen, he believed that the interendothelial slits of vascular sinuses could not open wide enough to let through microspheres this large. However, intraendothelial slits 5 to 6 μm wide have been reported by Thomas in dog spleen perfused under physiological conditions. It appears, moreover, from Toghill and Prichard's work that spherocytes (spherical red blood cells larger than 3–4 μm in diameter) can cross the interendothelial slits of vascular sinuses with pressure generated by norepinephrine. Thus, the inference that interendothelial slits cannot open wide enough to allow microspheres 3 to 4 μm to pass through lacks sufficient experimental support.

Because there is an anatomically open vascular bed in the red pulp of the spleen, it must not be assumed that blood flow is delayed, irregular, or inefficient. A number of studies using red cells labeled with chromium-51 indicate that 98 to 99% of the blood entering human spleen flows through it in about 30 sec. In the spleen of dogs and cats, however, a component of the circulating blood passes through more slowly, indicating that these spleens have a reservoir function for erythrocytes. Groom and colleagues have carried out a kinetic analysis of red cell washout from perfused isolated spleens and have identified three functional compartments of blood flow in cat spleen. The first compartment offers fast flow. It receives 90% of total splenic blood flow and has a transit time of 30 sec, comparable to that of skeletal muscle. With respect to this fast compartment, the spleen may be said to have a circulation that is anatomically open and physiologically closed. It is likely that efficient blood flow is accomplished through the reticular meshwork of the red pulp by the formation of tubular conduits made of the sheetlike processes of reticular cells. A second compartment demonstrated by Song and Groom has an intermediate flow. It receives 9% of blood flow and has a transit time of 8 min. This compartment accounts for the blood-storage capacity of cat spleen and largely disappears when the spleen is induced to contract and expel the stored blood cells. The last compartment is slow, handling approximately 1% of blood flow with a transit time of 1 h. This compartment contains reticulocytes and perhaps some granulocytes that are held in the spleen for a short time to finish their maturation before they are released to the general circulation.

In conclusion, the circulation of the spleen is anatomically open where blood passes from arterial endings through the reticular meshwork and then into venous sinuses or veins. There does appear to be some variation in blood pathway, since the distance between arterial endings and venous walls may vary and the contents of the meshwork through which blood passes may include variable amounts of macrophages, hematopoietic cells, stored blood cells, plasma, etc. These anatomical arrangements in red pulp offer several types of flow. The principal flow is rapid, as rapid as that through other organs. But there is also (in some, but not in human spleens) a significant storage compartment, as well as a compartment that allows developing blood cells to finish their maturation. The reader is referred to the papers of Blue and Weiss for a full discussion of the splenic circulation.

Blood Processing

Plasma is separated from blood cells in the splenic circulation so that the cells are highly concentrated in red pulp, as shown both by direct puncture of the spleen and by microscopic study of the living circulation. The mechanism of separation depends on contraction of the splenic vein after sympathetic nerve stimulation, forcing plasma out of veins and vascular sinuses. The plasma crosses the spleen, is taken up by the deep lymphatics, and is carried out of the spleen to the thoracic duct. Barcroft and Poole abolished the spleen's capacity to remove plasma by cutting its vasomotor nerves. Concentration of blood cells in the spleen enhances its storage function. In animals with a muscular capsule, such as dogs and cats, a reserve mass of blood cells may be rapidly reintroduced into the circulation when adrenergic stimulation causes massive capsular contraction.

The spleen monitors circulating erythrocytes. It permits viable cells to pass through rapidly but detains and destroys or modifies damaged or aged erythrocytes. These functions are carried out in red pulp. The cords of sinusal spleens and the pulp spaces of nonsinusal spleens that consist of a reticular meshwork loaded with macrophages pose hazards to erythrocytes. Erythrocytes discharged into this meshwork from arterial terminations must travel through it in order to exit via the vascular sinuses and veins. The interstices of the meshwork are rather fine; when filled with bulky macrophages, they are even finer, and erythrocytes must be quite pliant to squeeze through. As an erythrocyte ages, it becomes more fragile and less apt to survive this cordal pathway. Indeed, the oxygen tension and the cholesterol and glucose concentrations of the cords make erythrocytes more rigid by affecting their hemoglobin, plasma membrane, and energy-producing capacity. This red cell conditioning may push a marginally viable erythrocyte toward phagocytosis. The unshielded presence of macrophages in the cordal pathway, moreover, not only places passing erythrocytes in direct range of these phagocytes but gives the extracellular fluids a high concentration of hydrolytic enzymes, which are secreted by the macrophages and bathe the cells in passage. An aged erythrocyte will lose sialic acid on its surface, exposing galactose residues. The spleen may recognize these galactose moieties, cause such erythrocytes to pool in the reticular meshwork, and phagocytize them. Passing through the interendothelial slit of vascular sinuses also constitutes a test for erythrocyte viability. Erythrocytes must be pliant to slip through the interendothelial slits. Rigid erythrocytes, like those in congenital spherocytic anemia, become "hung up" in the interendothelial slits and pool in the reticular meshwork, outside the vascular sinuses. Pliant erythrocytes that contain rigid inclusions, such as parasitic malarial organisms, may have the rigid inclusion "pitted out" at the sinus wall. The pliant portion of

the erythrocyte passes through the interendothelial slit while the rigid portion is held back. The pliant portion then snaps off; it enters the lumen of the sinus and thence the circulation as a smaller erythrocyte that tends to be spherical. The rigid part remains behind and is typically phagocytized by macrophages lying against the outside surface of the walls of vascular sinuses.

Monocytes of the blood passing through the spleen are selectively removed from the circulation and sequestered in the white pulp, the marginal zone, and the red pulp, where they may rapidly undergo conversion into macrophages. Large numbers of macrophages derived in this manner are always present in the spleen and are responsible for its great phagocytic capacity. In malaria and in other processes involving the reaction and enlargement of the spleen, the spleen appears to release humoral substances that induce the bone marrow to produce and release more monocytes. These cells come to the spleen and considerably augment its population of macrophages.

B and T cells of the recirculating lymphocyte pool enter the spleen and follow distinctive pathways, as determined experimentally in rodents. They are first distributed through red pulp and the marginal zone. Many go right on out of the spleen by way of veins, but a significant fraction migrates through the reticular meshwork into white pulp. T cells enter the periarterial lymphatic sheaths and move around there for approximately 4 to 6 h, whereas B cells enter lymphatic nodules and stay there for a somewhat longer time. T and B cells may engage in antibody production as discussed in the next section, but if they do not, they leave the spleen via efferent lymphatics or veins to continue migrating as part of the recirculating lymphocytic pool.

Granulocytes may also be stored in the spleen. Moreover, in the rat, eosinophils, which differentiate primarily in bone marrow, are released to the spleen for final maturation before they enter the general circulation. Approximately one-third of the platelets of the body are normally stored in the spleen in ready reserve, even in spleens like the human that lack a reservoir function for erythrocytes. Under certain pathological conditions, platelets may be trapped in the spleen with such avidity that there are too few in the circulation, and bleeding results. Similarly, the spleen may remove slightly damaged but functionally competent erythrocytes with such zeal that an anemic crisis is precipitated. These con-

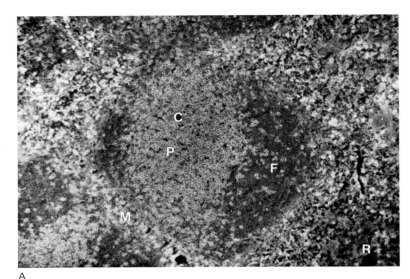

A

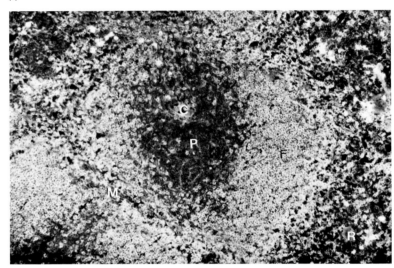

B

16–22 Spleen, mouse. Distribution of T and B lymphocytes as revealed by fluorescence immunocytochemistry. T and B cells are specifically stained in these frozen sections by a technique dependent on antibodies to the surface of T and B cells, respectively. The antibody is conjugated to a fluorescent marker, visible by fluorescence microscopy. In **A,** the central artery **(C)** is surrounded by the periarterial lymphatic sheath **(P),** which is stained by the anti-T-cell reagent, whereas the lymphatic nodule in the field **(F)** is largely unstained. The marginal zone **(M)** is stained. **R,** red pulp. Thus T lymphocytes are concentrated in the periarterial lymphatic sheath and marginal zone. In **B,** B lymphocytes are stained. Here the lymphatic nodule **(F)** and the marginal zone **(M)** are stained. Thus B lymphocytes are concentrated in lymphatic nodules and are largely absent from the periarterial lymphatic sheath. Both T and B cells are present in the marginal zone. See text and see Fig. 15–19 for distribution of T and B lymphocytes in lymph nodes (From Weissman, I. L. 1975. Transpl. Rev. 24:159.)

ditions, typically associated with a large spleen and designated *hypersplenism,* may be cured by splenectomy.

The capacity of the spleen to clear materials from the blood may be estimated by tagging test substances with radioactive isotopes and injecting them intravascularly. With this method it is possible to determine both the rate at which the isotope accumulates in the spleen (as inferred in human beings by counting radioactivity over the left upper quadrant of the abdomen) and the rate at which radioactivity disappears from the blood. Although lungs, liver, bone marrow, and other reticuloendothelial tissues also clear blood of particulate material, it is likely that the spleen's clearance capacity per gram of tissue is greatest.

Antibody Production

The spleen efficiently traps lymphocytes, monocytes, and antigen from the blood and permits them to interact and produce antibody. Antigen is first trapped and then phagocytized by macrophages in the marginal zone and red pulp. It subsequently moves into white pulp and surrounds lymphatic nodules, thereby lying at the junction of T- and B-cell zones (Fig. 16–22). Within the white pulp, antigen may be retained on the surface of antigen-presenting cells and macrophages.

In a primary immune response, antibody-producing cells appear first within the periarterial lymphatic sheaths as part of clusters of 20 to 100 or more cells. The cells migrate to the periphery of the sheaths and, at the same time, proliferate and secrete antibody. Then, traveling by routes that are not fully understood, they appear in red pulp as mature plasma cells and accumulate there. In secondary immune responses and in many primary responses that persist, germinal centers form and, as in lymph nodes, augment the antibody response and increase the number of memory cells.

References and Selected Bibliography

General

Barcroft, J., and Poole, L. T. 1927. The blood in the spleen pulp. J. Physiol. Lond. 64:23.

Blue, J., and Weiss, L. 1981a. Periarterial macrophages sheaths (ellipsoids) in cat spleen-an electron microscope study. Am. J. Anat. 161:115.

Crosby, E. H. 1959. Normal functions of the spleen relative to red blood cells: A review. Blood 14:399.

Fujita, T. 1974. A scanning electron microscope study of the human spleen. Arch. Histol. Jpn. 37:187.

Irino, S., Murkami, T., Fujita, T., Nagatani, T., and Kaneshige, T. 1978. Microdissection of tannin-osmium impregnated specimens in the scanning electron microscope: Demonstration of arterial terminals in human spleen. In O. Johari and R. P. Becker (eds.), Scanning Electron Microscopy/1978, pt. II. Chicago: SEM, Inc., p. 111.

Pereira, G. P. 1978. Evidence for a blood splenic white pulp barrier using a biologically inert electron-opaque tracer. In Johari and R. P. Becker (eds.), Electron Microscopy/1978, pt. II. Chicago: SEM, Inc. p. 649.

Pictet, R., Orci, L., Forssmann, W. B., and Girardier. 1969. An electron microscope study of the perfusion-fixed spleen. I. The splenic circulation and the RES concept. Z. Zellforsch. Mikrosk. Anat. 96:372.

Snook, T. 1950. A comprehensive study of the vascular arrangements in mammalian spleens. Am. J. Anat. 87:31.

Weiss, L. 1974. A scanning electron microscopic study of the spleen. Blood 43:665.

Circulation

Bjorkman, S. E. 1947. The splenic circulation with special reference to the function of the spleen sinus wall. Acta Med. Scan. 128 (Suppl. 191): 7.

Chen, L. T. 1978. Microcirculation of the spleen: An open or closed circulation? Science (Wash, D.C.) 201:157.

Groom, A. C., and Song, S. H. 1962. Effects of norepinephrine on washout of red cells from the spleen. Am. J. Physiol. 221:255.

Groom, A. C., Song, S. H., Lim, O., and Campling, B. 1971. Physical characteristics of red cells collected from the spleen. Can. J. Physiol. Pharmacol. 49:1092.

Irino, S., Murkami, T., and Fujita, T. 1977. Open circulation in the human spleen. Dissection scanning electron microscopy of conductive-stained tissue and observation of resin vascular casts. Arch. Histol. Jpn. 40:297.

Knisely, M. H. 1936. Spleen studies. I. Microscopic observations of the circulatory system of living unstimulated mammalian spleen. Anat. Rec. 65:23.

MacKenzie, D. W., Whipple, A. O., and Wintersteiner, M. P. 1941. Studies on the microscopic anatomy and physiology of living transilluminated mammalian spleens. Am. J. Anat. 68:397.

MacNeal, W. J. 1929. The circulation of blood through the spleen pulp. Arch. Pathol. Lab. Med. 7:215.

Mall, F. P. 1902. The circulation through the pulp of the dog's spleen. Am. J. Anat. 2:316.

McCuskey, R. S., and McCuskey, P. A. 1977. In vivo microscopy of the spleen. Bibl. Anat. 16:121.

Erythrocytes

Crosby, W. H. 1977. Splenic remodeling of red cell surfaces. Blood 50:643.

Lux, S. E., and John, K. M. 1977. Isolation and partial characterization of a high molecular weight red cell membrane protein complex normally removed by the spleen. Blood 50:625.

Song, S. H., and Groom, A. C. 1971b. The distribution of red cells in the spleen. Can. J. Physiol. Pharmacol. 49:734.

Song, S. H., and Groom, A. C. 1972. Sequestration and possible maturation of reticulocytes in the normal spleen. Can. J. Physiol. Pharmacol. 50:400.

Weiss, L., and Tavassoli, M. 1970. Anatomical hazards to the passage of erythrocytes through the spleen. Semin. Hematol. 7:372.

Immune Responses

Mitchell, J., and Abbot, A. 1971. Antigens in immunity. XVI. A light and electron microscope study of antigen localization in the rat spleen. Immunology 21:207.

Nossal, G. J. V., Austin, C. M., Pye, J., and Mitchell, J. 1966. Antigens in immunity. XII. Antigen trapping in the spleen. Int. Arch. Allergy 29:368.

Innervation

Heusermann, U., and Stutte, H. J. 1977. Electron microscopic studies of the innervation of the human spleen. Cell Tissue Res. 184:225.

Kudoh, G., Hoshi, K. and Murkami, T. 1979. Fluorescence microscopic and enzyme histochemical studies of the innervation of the human spleen. Arch. Histol. Jpn. 42:169.

Lymphocytes

Ford, W. L., and Smith, M. E. 1978. Lymphocyte recirculation between the spleen and blood. *In* Role of the Spleen in the Immunology of Parasitic Diseases. Tropical Diseases Research Series No. 1. Basel, Switzerland: Schwabe and Co. A.G., p. 29.

Mitchell, J. 1973. Lymphocyte circulation in the spleen. Marginal zone bridging channels and their possible role in cell traffic. Immunology 24:93.

Marginal Zone

Blue, J., and Weiss, L. 1981c. Species variations in the structure and function of the marginal zone: An electron microscope study of the cat spleen. Am. J. Anat. 161:169.

Sasou, S., Satodate, R., and Katsura, S. 1976. The marginal sinus in the perifollicular region of the rat spleen. Cell Tissue Res. 172:195.

Pathology

Bowdler, A. J. 1975. The spleen and haemolytic disorders. Clin. Haematol. 4:231.

Weiss, L. 1979. The spleen. *In* Role of the Spleen in the Immunology of Parasitic Diseases. Tropical Diseases Research Series No. I. Basel, Switzerland: Schwabe and Co. A.G., p. 7.

Red Pulp

Blue, J., and Weiss, L. 1981b. Vascular pathways in non-sinusal red pulp: An electron microscope study of cat spleen. Am. J. Anat. 161:135.

Chen, L. T., and Weiss, L. 1972. Electron microscopy of the red pulp of human spleen. Am. J. Anat. 134:425.

Chen, L. T., and Weiss, L. 1973. The role of the sinus wall in the passage of erythrocytes through the spleen. Blood 41:529.

Song, S. H., and Groom, A. C. 1971a. Storage of blood cells in the spleen of the cat. Am. J. Physiol. 220:779.

White Pulp

Galindo, B., and Imaeda, T. 1962. Electron microscope study of the white pulp of the mouse spleen. Anat. Rec. 143:399.

Satodate, R., Ogasawara, S., Sasou, S., and Katsura, S. 1971. Characteristic structure of the splenic white pulp of rats. J. Reticuloendothel Soc. 10:428.

Snook, T. 1946. Deep lymphatics of the spleen. Anat. Rec. 94:43.

Veerman, A. J. O., and van Ewijk, W. 1975. White pulp in the spleen of rats and mice. A light and electron microscopic study of lymphoid and non-lymphoid cell types in T- and B-areas. Cell Tissue Res. 156:417.

Weiss, L. 1974. The white pulp of the spleen. The relationships of arterial vessels, reticulum and free cells in the periarterial lymphatic sheath. Bull. Johns Hopkins Hosp. 115:99.

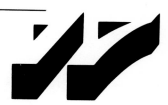

The Skin

Kurt S. Stenn

The skin serves as a protective and sensing buffer between the organism and the environment. Its importance is demonstrated by the problems of the patient who has lost his skin, as after a severe burn. He or she lacks sensation over the burned areas and is unable to detect pain, cold, and heat because cutaneous nerves are destroyed. When the outer impenetrable cutaneous layers are destroyed, microorganisms, insects, and chemicals penetrate through the burn into deeper tissues causing infections and toxic complications. Severe dehydration and electrolyte imbalance result from the loss of proteins and ionic fluids through the burned skin because the outer protective layer is gone. The burn patient's temperature may fluctuate widely because without the cutaneous vascular and sweat systems he or she is unable to conserve or dissipate heat adequately.

The outer skin, the *epidermis*, is a tightly bound, stratified squamous epithelium covered by *keratin*, a physically tough, insoluble protein product of epidermal cell differentiation. Keratin is particularly thick over some regions of the body subject to high friction forces, e.g., palmar–plantar surfaces. The epidermis overlies a dense collagenous tissue, the *dermis*, which is also highly resistant to physical injury. The dermis is richly endowed with sensory nerves and its blood vessels are exquisitely sensitive to temperature. The dermal appendages—hair and sebaceous and sweat glands—contain and dissipate heat and protect the body from physical injury. Finally, the compact epidermal–dermal complex lies on a soft insulating cushion of fibrofatty tissue, the subcutis (hypodermis or subcutaneous tissue), which also buffers trauma and temperature fluctuations.

Epidermis

Keratinocyte

The epidermis (Fig. 17–1) consists of four distinct cell types: keratinocyte, melanocyte, Langerhans cell, and Merkel cell. Because the epidermis is a stratified squamous epithelium, the predominant cell is an epithelial cell that differentiates to produce keratin and is therefore called the epidermal keratinocyte. There are

17–1 Epidermis from abdominal skin. Notice the loosely packed, basket-weave keratin layer **(ker)**, the thin granular layer in this region, the progressive flattening of the epidermal cells **(Epi)**, and the melanocytes **(M)** in the basal layer. Dermal papillae **(DP)** project into the epidermis.

three distinct phases to the life of a keratinocyte: (1) growth and proliferation, (2) maturation and outward displacement, and (3) dyshesion (or desquamation).

Keratinocyte growth begins in the basal layer of the epidermis where there is a population of proliferating cells. Most, if not all, normal keratinocyte cell divisions occur within this cell layer. The rate at which basal cells divide has been difficult to establish. Nevertheless, we know that at any given time about one or two mitoses are found per 1,000 basal cells and that it takes about 27 days for the epidermis to renew itself. Basal cells are columnar-cuboidal and have round euchromatic nuclei. They contain mitochondria and ribosomes as well as filaments ranging in width from 5 to 9 nm. They are firmly attached to the basal lamina by hemidesmosomes and to surrounding cells by desmosomes.

After division, a cell may remain in the basal layer or move outward. To maintain epidermal thickness, on the average, one of the daughter cells must move outward. The mechanism and

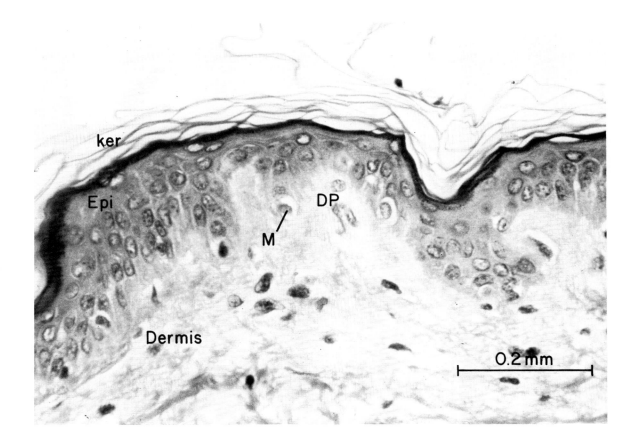

selection for vertical displacement is not known, and it has not been clearly demonstrated if vertical movement occurs independently of cell division. We do know that epidermal cells contain actin and may be actively motile and that basal cells may show active and rapid horizontal locomotion after wounding. It takes a keratinocyte about 12 to 14 days to pass from the basal layer to the surface. During this passage the cells flatten and align into columns (Fig. 17–2). This ordered arrangement becomes apparent in the outer spinous layer and is well defined in the horny layer. The most precisely ordered stacking of keratinocytes is best seen in the epidermis of rodent ear skin where the mitotic rate is normally rather low. In tissues where the mitotic rate is high, such as the palmar–plantar epidermis, there is less evidence of column formation among keratinocytes. Thus, it has been suggested that slow maturation of epidermal cells enables them to become arranged in stacks. Other studies suggest that the peripheral regions of the columns are significant in two respects: first, basal cell mitoses occur more frequently there; and, second, the upward movement of basal cells appears to originate at this site. In human skin the keratinocyte stacking pattern is less well defined than in rodents.

The keratinocyte differentiates into a nondividing, highly specialized cell. The successive changes from progenitor cell to final cell product can be viewed in one microscopic field. Early histologists recognized two epidermal regions: the nucleated or viable epidermis, which they called the stratum Malpighii, and the nonnu-

cleated or nonviable epidermis, the *stratum corneum*. Today the stratum Malpighii is divided into the *stratum germinativum* (basal layer), *stratum spinosum* (spinous layer, sometimes called the Malpighian layer), and *stratum granulosum* (granular layer) (Fig. 17–3).

In palmar–plantar skin an additional layer is occasionally seen between the stratum granulosum and the stratum corneum. This layer, the *stratum lucidum*, appears by light microscopy as a thin acellular lightly staining band probably because of unique keratin packing in this region.

As cells leave the basal layer, they flatten, covering more surface area, and develop many intercellular junctions. These junctions connect keratinocytes and form the coherent epidermal covering. The name of this layer, stratum spinosum, derives from the large number of desmosomes (Fig. 17–4), which appear as spines by light microscopy in these cells. In the spinous layer the filaments within keratinocytes, *keratin filaments* or *tonofilaments*, are plentiful and dense enough to form bundles or fibrils. There appears to be an important correlation between desmosomes and tonofilaments both in number (as the cell acquires more desmosomes it also fills with tonofilaments) and in strength of intercellular adhesion. In embryonic epidermis, desmosomes appear at the points of contact between cells. Then tonofilaments appear and extend from the desmosome into the cytoplasm. As keratinocytes mature, their cytoplasm fills with keratin filaments packed in an ill-defined matrix. Although it is not clear how the filaments add to the physical strength of the epidermis, a struc-

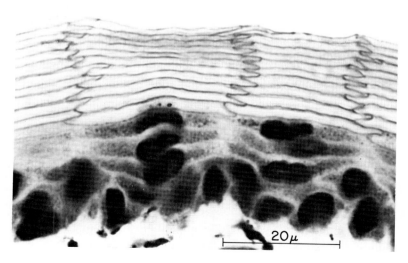

17–2 Frozen section of mouse ear epidermis showing the columnar patterning of cells in the upper epidermis. (From Mackenzie, I. C., 1975. Anat. Rec. 181:705.)

17–3 Schematic diagram showing the layering of the epidermis. The basal cells sit on the basal lamina and are mitotically active. As the cells move up, they acquire more cytoplasm and flatten. In the granular layer keratohyalin granules and membrane-coating granules **(MCG)** are found. The latter eventually appear extracellularly. In the keratin layer the cells lose cytoplasmic organelles, fill with keratin filaments, and acquire a cornified envelope. (From Montagna, W., and Parakkal, P. F. 1974. The Structure and Function of Skin. New York: Academic Press.)

tural function has been suggested by electron-microscopic studies where some tonofilaments are seen to course from one end of the cell to the other: they are believed to pass from a given desmosome, around the nucleus, and insert into desmosomes of the cell membrane beyond. In some disease states (e.g., Hailey-Hailey disease) where tonofilament–desmosomal association is disturbed, tonofilaments form aggregated masses instead of fibrillar arrays, and intercellular attachments break down.

X-ray diffraction studies reveal that the epidermis contains highly ordered molecules. The diffraction pattern, typical of keratins, represents a filamentous structure with regions of segmented, triple-chained, coiled-coil α helix. By convention, material with this physical property is referred to as keratin, and those tissues with an outer anuclear layer of keratin-filled cells are referred to as *keratinized* (other synonymous terms appearing in the literature include *horny* and *cornified*). Keratin can be extracted from the lower epidermis to a limited extent by denaturing agents (urea, sodium dodecyl sulfate) that do not break disulfide bonds. Recently, epidermal keratin has been isolated and reassembled into

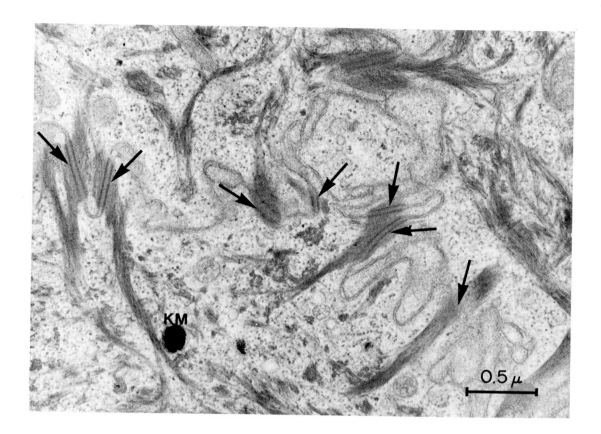

filaments 7 to 8 nm wide that are morphologically identical to those found in keratinocytes (Fig. 17–5). These filaments are made of six similar nonglycosylated polypeptide chains of 47,000 to 58,000 daltons, which are coded by distinct mRNAs. After the keratin species were chemically separated, it was found that certain recombinations are more effective in producing filaments in vitro than others. In all effective recombinations the stoichiometry involves two moles of one type of keratin chain and one mole of another. Although whole epidermis yields all six keratin chains, the concentration of individual keratins seems to vary with the stratum of the epidermis and the region of skin examined. The significance of the different keratins is not yet known.

Beginning in the upper spinous layer, epidermal cells accummulate irregular nonmembrane-bound electron-dense granules. In the granular layer these granules can become 1 to 5 μm in diameter. Two types of granules are apparent in mouse epidermis by electron microscopy. The smaller type shows uniform density and is called

17–4 Tonofilament–desmosomal structures between keratinocytes of the stratum spinosum. Note the complex interdigitations of the borders of adjacent cells and abundant desmosomes **(arrows)** shown in various planes of section. A single transferred melanin granule **(KM)** is present near the lower left corner. (Courtesy of G. Moellmann, Yale University.)

the *dense homogeneous deposit (DHD)*. Its chemistry is poorly defined but it seems to be rich in sulfyhydryl groups. The second type is larger, more irregular and granular. It is called the *keratohyalin granule (KG)*. The KG contains a mixture of substances: histidine-rich protein, RNA, polysaccharide, and lipids. In the granular layer an intimate reaction occurs between tonofilaments and keratohyalin granules. By electron microscopy, the filaments are seen to pass into the granules, where they lose their definition (Fig. 17–6).

These granules may provide the matrix that embeds keratin filaments in the horny layer. In support of this hypothesis is the finding that in

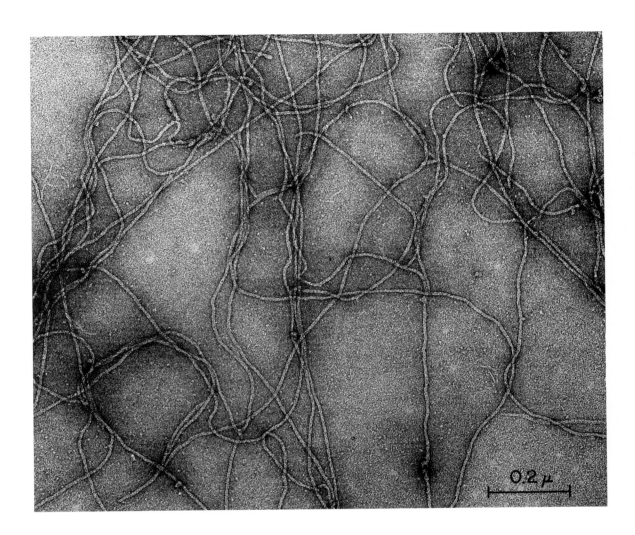

17–5 Keratin filaments reconstituted in vitro from an equimolar mixture of two isolated keratin polypeptides. (From Steinert, P. M., Idler, W. W., and Zimmerman, S. B. 1976. J. Mol. Biol. 108:547; courtesy of P. M. Steinert.)

vitro tonofilaments clump when mixed with a purified keratohyalin protein called filaggrin.

Within the uppermost granular layer, keratinocytes undergo a sudden and dramatic transition as virtually all of the cytoplasmic organelles, including nuclei, vanish (Fig. 17–1). The residual cellular shells are filled with tightly packed 7- to 8-nm electron-lucent filaments, each surrounded by an electron-dense matrix 3 to 4 nm wide. The KGs and the tonofilament bundles disappear as distinct structures. In contrast to the filament-forming keratin of the lower epidermis, that of the uppermost granular layer requires disulfide-reducing agents in order to be solubilized, indicating that more mature keratin is stabilized by disulfide bonds. Keratinocytes of this stratum have an altered inner cell membrane, which is called the *cornified envelope* or *horny cell membrane* (Figs. 17–7 and 17–8). In contrast to keratin fibrils and matrix of the stratum corneum cells, the cornified envelope is not solubilized by dissociating and reducing agents. In fact, in the presence of these agents, the envelope is the only element of the epidermis that remains. It forms a proteinaceous skeleton of the stratum corneum. Only when the envelope is hydrolyzed by proteolytic enzymes is it solubilized. In the resultant hydrolystate, a significant portion of the lysyl residues are not found as simple amino acids but as the cross-linking dipeptide ε-(γ glutamyl) lysine. Recently, a protein substrate of epidermal

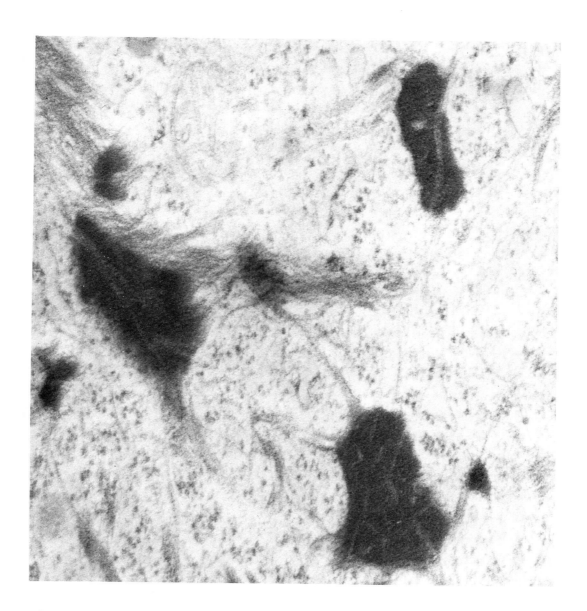

transglutaminase has been isolated from epidermis, which has a molecular weight of 92,000 and is immunologically and chemically distinct from the keratin proteins. Antibody to this protein, called involucrin, binds to the cornified envelope.

Keratinocytes of the upper spinous or granular layers contain unique round-to-oval granules, 100 to 500 nm in diameter, in their peripheral cytoplasm. These granules, bounded by a membrane and containing alternating dark and light lamellae each about 2 to 3.5 nm thick, are called *lamellar granules (Odland bodies, membrane-coating granules, keratinosomes).* In the granu-

17–6 Electron micrograph of keratinohyalin granules from human epidermis. Note keratin filaments passing into the granules. (Courtesy of R. M. Lavker and A. G. Matoltsy. 1971. J. Ultrastruct. Res. 35:575.)

lar layer these Golgi-produced structures are found in the cell periphery and become attached to the inner surface of the keratinocyte plasma membrane. Eventually the contents of the granules are secreted from the cell and deposited between keratinocytes (Fig. 17–8). The role of these organelles has not been entirely resolved. The most accepted hypothesis is that they form the primary intercellular barrier to water. The epi-

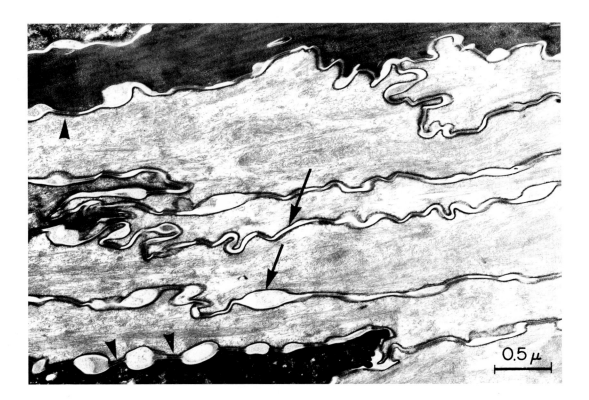

17–7 Interdigitating squamae in the stratum corneum (human epidermis). In the central scales of this picture the electron-dense matrix, visible in the upper and lower scales, has been lost during preparation of the tissue for electron microscopy, permitting the identification of the keratin filaments as positive rather than negative images. Note the dense cornified envelopes **(arrows)** and the altered desmosomes **(arrowheads)** in this layer. (Courtesy of G. Moellmann, Yale University.)

dermis is permeable to water in both its deeper and most superficial portions, but it is impermeable from either direction at the level of the granular layer. It is notable that there are no zonulae occludens in the epidermis and the lamellar granules are discharged at the level of the granular layer where the functional barrier to water is found.

The final step in epidermal maturation is desquamation. Cohesion, the critical characteristic of the epidermis in its protective role, and all the cellular features described above contribute to the impermeable, impenetrable, tightly coherent sheet. However, because epidermis grows continuously, its shedding is very important to the health of the organism. How epidermal dyshesion occurs is not known, but it is definitely inherent in the epidermal maturation process, for areas of normal skin experimentally covered and protected from physical trauma (e.g., under a plaster cast) do not thicken but desquamate. The patient with ichthyosis (fish skin) suffers because his thickly keratinized skin sheds epidermal cells inadequately. In one form of ichthyosis, the patient's cells lack steroid sulfatase. Because sulfated lipids are found in epidermal cells, one recently postulated mechanism of dyshesion is by the intercellular liberation of lipolytic enzymes at the level of the outer epidermis.

Melanocytes

Melanocytes arise in the neural crest and migrate to the dermis by the tenth week of embryonic development. They are found in the basal layer of the epidermis by the twelfth to fourteenth week. The density of melanocytes varies between body regions (e.g., about 2,000 melanocytes per mm^2 in forehead and scrotal skin, and about 1,000 per mm^2 in forearm and thigh skin) but is relatively constant between individuals and races. Charac-

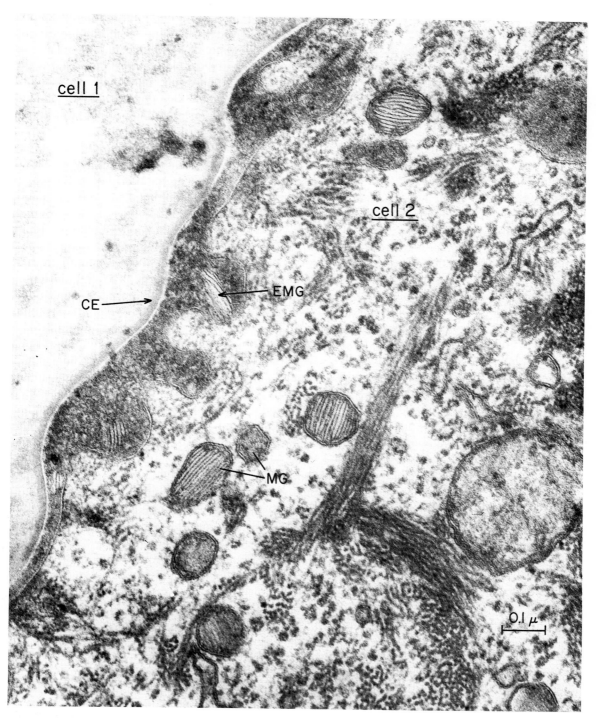

17–8 Junction between two keratinocytes of the upper granular layer. Note the membrane-coating granules within the cytoplasm of the cell to the right **(MG)**, the membrane-coating granules between the cells **(EMG)**, and the cornified envelope of the adjacent cell **(CE)**. (Courtesy of George Palade, Yale University.)

teristically, the melanocyte, a cell with a small round nucleus and numerous dendritic processes, sits on the basement membrane apart from other melanocytes and slightly below the basal keratinocytes (Fig. 17–1). Although it does not have desmosomal attachments to surrounding keratinocytes, the melanocyte adheres to the dermis by a junction similar to the keratinocyte–dermal junction. This melanocyte junction consists of hemidesmosome-like thickenings, a lamina lucida, a continuous basal lamina, and occasional subbasal laminar fibrous elements. The intracytoplasmic filaments of the melanocyte are 10 nm in diameter, are less numerous than tonofilaments in keratinocytes, and are not anchored in desmosomes.

The only known function of melanocytes is to produce melanin and to distribute it to keratinocytes and hair. Melanin is a pigment that protects skin from the ionizing effects of electromagnetic radiation. It is transferred from dendritic processes to basal keratinocytes. The melanin accumulates above the keratinocyte nucleus at the pole opposite the basement membrane. From this position, it is best able to protect the dividing nucleus of the basal cell from incoming radiation. An orderly functional association between one melanocyte and a group of keratinocytes, *the epidermal-melanin unit,* has been recognized (Fig. 17–9). Thus, although the ratio of melanocytes to keratinocytes varies with the body regions, only one melanocyte serves as the source of pigment for a given population of epidermal cells.

The melanins in human skin are eumelanin and pheomelanin. Although derived from a common intermediate, dopa-quinone (a product of the action of the aerobic oxidase, tyrosinase, first on tyrosine and then on dopa [3,4 dihydroxyphenylalanine]), eumelanins and pheomelanins differ in color. Eumelanins are brown-black pigments made of poorly characterized hydroxyindole polymers; pheomelanins, are red and yellow sulfur-containing polymers of cysteinyl dopa. People with blond or red hair and freckles carry the genetic trait to produce pheomelanin. The melanins absorb electromagnetic radiation over a broad spectrum ranging from 200 to 2,400 nm without a characteristic absorption maximum. The ability of melanin to form free radicals is thought to be significant to its radioprotective role.

Melanin formation and deposition occur within melanosomes, membrane-bounded granules that are found in the cytoplasm of melano-

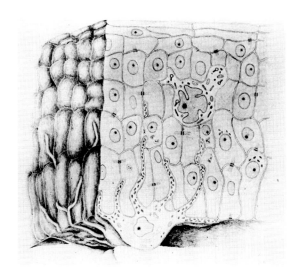

17–9 Sketch of epidermal-melanin unit showing the relationship between a basal melanocyte, higher-level Langerhans cell, and keratinocytes in mammalian epidermis. Notice the dendritic structure of the melanocyte and the accumulation of melanosomes in the distal dendritic processes. (From Jimbow, K., Quevedo, W. C., Fitzpatrick, T. B., and Szabo, G. 1976. J. Invest. Derm. 67:72; courtesy of W. C. Quevedo.)

cytes and that carry the enzyme tyrosinase. Tyrosinase is synthesized in ribosomes and transferred via the endoplasmic reticulum to the Golgi area. There the enzyme is packaged into vesicles that fuse with premelanosomes. Premelanosomes at first lack both ordered structure and melanin, but they mature through four defined stages into the melanin-packed melanosome or melanin granule (Fig. 17–10). Melanosomes are transported distally into dendritic processes of the melanocyte and are finally transferred to the keratinocytes of the epidermal-melanin unit. It has been shown in cell cultures that during the transfer of melanosomes to keratinocytes the entire tip of the melanocytic process is phagocytized by the keratinocyte, including its plasma membrane and cytoplasm.

The intensity of skin color is determined by the number and aggregation pattern of melanosomes present in keratinocytes. These properties, in turn, depend on the rate of melanin synthesis by melanocytes, the size of melanosomes, and the rate of melanosome transfer to keratinocytes. Thus, in heavily pigmented Negroes the melanosomes are larger than in Caucasians, are fully pigmented, and are dispersed in keratinocytes as

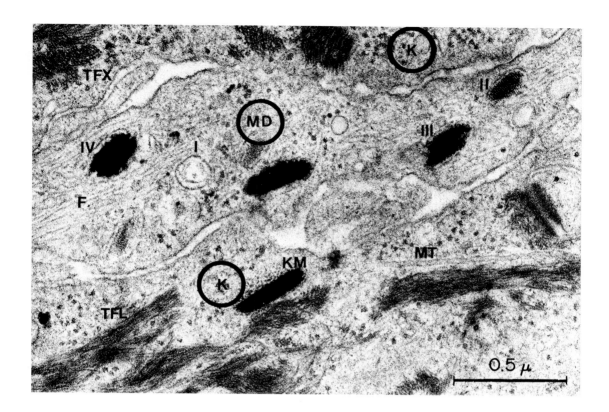

17–10 Melanosome dentrite **(MD)** between two keratinocytes **(K)**. This electron micrograph demonstrates the stages of melanosome maturation from the spherical relatively unlaminated, unpigmented form **(I),** to the laminated ellipsoidal, lightly pigmented form **(II and III,),** to the densely pigmented mature form **(IV). F,** 10-nm filaments in a melanocytic process; **TFL,** tonofilaments in longitudinal orientation; **TFX,** tonofilaments in cross section; **MT** microtubule. (Courtesy of G. Moellman, Yale University.)

separate units. In a lightly pigmented Caucasian on the other hand, melanosomes are few, small, and aggregated in groups around the keratinocyte nucleus.

Cutaneous pigmentation probably is controlled by hereditary, hormonal, and environmental factors. Genetic mechanisms appear to influence the size of the epidermal-melanin unit and of the melanosome, the pattern of melanosome aggregation, and the production of melanin. Hormones also influence human pigmentation; for example, MSH causes hyperpigmentation by stimulating the formation of highly dendritic melanocytes and the transfer of melanosomes to keratinocytes; in pregnancy, estrogen and progesterone stimulate increased pigmentation of facial, abdominal, and genital skin as well as the areola and nipple of the breast. Environmental factors such as trauma, ultraviolet light, or infection may also stimulate melanin production.

Langerhans Cell

In 1868 Paul Langerhans, then a medical student in Berlin, exposed sections of skin to a new gold chloride stain and discovered a distinct popula-tion of dendritic cells. A few of these cells are present in all epidermal layers. They are detectable with stains for ATPase and, like melanocytes, appear as "clear" cells by light microscopy. Recently, the Langerhans cell has been found to bear surface antigens common to most B and some T lymphocytes, monocytes, and macrophages (Fig. 17–11) and to carry receptors for immunoglobulin (Fc) and complement (C3). In part because of these properties, it is believed that the Langerhans cell belongs to the system of interdigitating cells that serves to fix and process cutaneous antigen (Chap. 15).

The density of Langerhans cells varies with

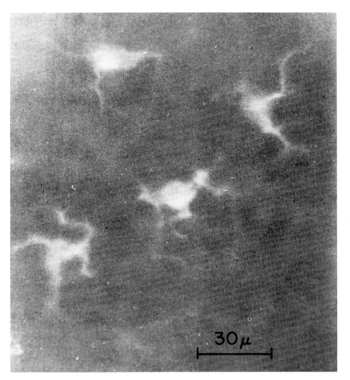

17–11 Langerhans cells within epidermis. In this preparation, epidermis was separated from the dermis and the preparation stained with fluorescent-labeled antibodies to Ia antigen. The only epidermal cells to stain are the Langerhans cells, which here show their dendritic structure. (Courtesy of J. Nordlund, Yale University.)
◁

17–12 Langerhans cell **(LC)** adjacent to a keratinocyte **(K).** Notice the cleft nucleus **(N),** and the numerous images of cross-sectioned Langerhans cell discs (Birbeck granules) **(arrows).** Many of the granules are still associated with their respective germinative vesicles **(arrowheads).** (Courtesy of G. Moellmann, Yale University.) ▽

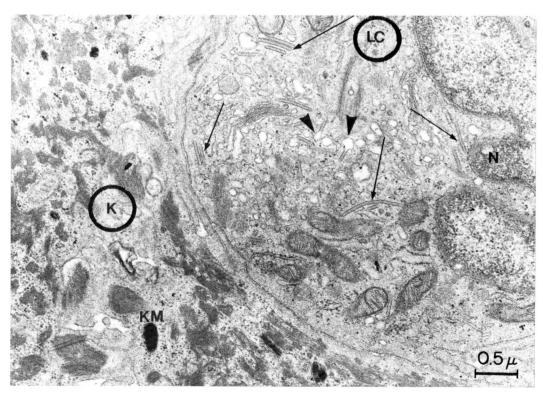

body region from 400 to 1,000 cells/mm². This regional variation is believed to reflect differences in epidermal thickness, since thicker skin contains more Langerhans cells. These cells have also been found in hair follicles, sebaceous glands, and apocrine glands. They are present in the mucosa of the mouth, tongue, tonsil, and esophagus. Unlike keratinocytes, a few Langerhans cells are normally found in the dermis and occasionally in regional lymph nodes and the thymus.

Compared to keratinocytes by electron microscopy (Fig. 17–12), the Langerhans cell has relatively clear cytoplasm without tonofilaments, desmosomes, or melanosomes. It has an irregularly indented nucleus and characteristic racket-shaped granules, *the Birbeck granules.* Birbeck granules are widely accepted as the sine qua non for identifying Langerhans cells. The biosyn-

thesis and function of this granule is completely unknown.

Merkel Cell

In mammalian epidermis adjacent to some hair follicles are thickened epidermal regions, the *hair discs.* Scattered among the basal keratinocytes in these areas are unique cells called *Merkel cells* (Fig. 17–13). Because they are associated with nerve terminations, they are thought to

17–13 Merkel cell. Adjacent to lower epidermal keratinocytes, the Merkel cell shows an irregularly folded nucleus and characteristic cytoplasmic granules. Characteristically these granules rest at one cytoplasmic pole of the cell. **Inset** shows higher magnification of the granules. (Courtesy of Sid Klaus, Yale University.)

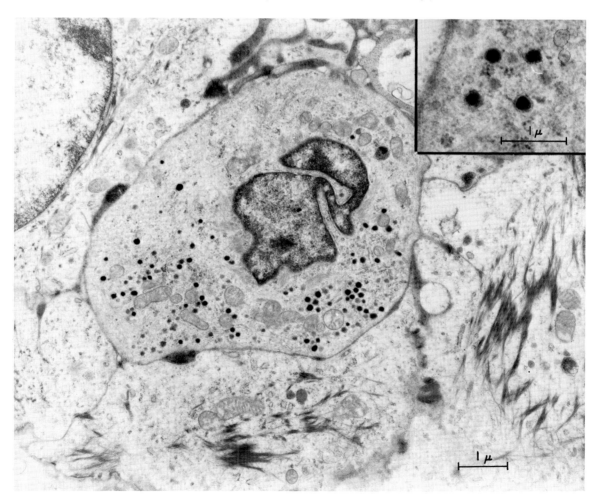

play a role in sensation. Merkel cells have lobated, irregular nuclei and their cytoplasm is less electron-dense than in adjacent keratinocytes. They contain numerous dense-core osmiophilic granules that are assumed to be formed in a prominent Golgi complex and are morphologically identical to the chromaffin granules found in the adrenal medulla. Although no secretory product has been associated with the Merkel cell granule, because of its granule it is considered an APUD (amine precursor uptake and decarboxylation) cell (Chap. 29). It is notable that Merkel cell granules are most concentrated at the basal side of the cell where neurites approach from the dermis. In contrast to melanocytes, Merkel cells are attached to adjacent keratinocytes by numerous desmosomes; in contrast to keratinocytes, their cytoplasmic tonofilaments are packed only into loose bundles. The role of this cell in skin is unknown.

Dermal–Epidermal Junction

The epidermis is attached to the dermis by a complex arrangement of epidermal and dermal components referred to collectively as the *dermal–epidermal (DE) junction*. The epidermis folds down as broad waves into the underlying dermis. The epidermal evaginations are called *rete ridges* and they surround small finger-like projections of dermis called *dermal papillae* (Fig. 17–14). Silver and PAS stains show a basement membrane at the apparent junction of epidermis and dermis (Fig. 17–15). The PAS-reaction suggests the presence of richly glycosylated proteins.

Electron microscopy reveals a more complex junction (Fig. 17–16). At this level of resolution, it is clear that the lower basal cell surface is remarkable for its irregular protrusions into the dermis and that the region of dermal attachment can be divided into three components: (1) the basal cell plasma membrane and its specialized attachment, the *hemidesmosome*; (2) the basal lamina (*lamina lucida* and *lamina densa*); and (3) the connective tissue fibers below the basal lamina, which include *anchoring fibrils, microfibril bundles,* and *collagen fibers*. Of these three components, it is primarily the connective tissue below the basal lamina that makes up the basement membrane seen by light microscopy with the PAS stain.

The basal plasma membrane of the basal cell is about 7 to 9 nm thick. At certain points it is

modified into an attachment site, the hemidesmosome. Along the cytoplasmic surface of the hemidesmosome there is an electron-opaque thickening of the inner leaflet of the plasma membrane called the *attachment plaque*, 20 to 40 nm thick, toward which tonofilaments converge. Tonofilament insertion, however, appears to occur in an electron-dense zone separated from the attachment plaque by a lucent zone. By high-resolution electron microscopy, the external leaflet of the plasma membrane is seen as a fine line on the outer surface of the attachment plaque.

The lamina lucida in most areas appears electron-lucent and amorphous. Adjacent to hemidesmosomes, however, the lamina lucida contains: (1) a centrally lying electron-dense line that parallels the plasma membrane, and (2) fine perpendicular filaments that course from the inner leaflet of the plasma membrane to the basal lamina. The latter have been called *anchoring filaments*. Recently, a glycoprotein unique to the lamina lucida has been characterized. It is a 900,000-dalton highly glycosylated multimeric protein that has been named *laminin*. Collagen has not been found in this layer. When proteolytic enzymes are used to separate the epidermis from the dermis experimentally, the lamina lucida is digested. In addition, in several diseases of the skin (e.g., bullous pemphigoid) the lamina lucida is destroyed, resulting in the separation of the epidermis from the dermis and the formation of blisters.

The basal lamina is a continuous electron-dense layer that may have an amorphous or a fibrillar character. Recent studies indicate that the basal lamina contains type IV (basement membrane) collagen and may contain various glycosaminoglycans.

Beneath the basal lamina are three types of fibers: anchoring fibrils, microfibril bundles, and collagen fibers (Fig. 17–16). *Anchoring fibrils,* which are found predominantly in the areas beneath hemidesmosomes, arise in the substance of the basal lamina and extend into the dermis. These fibrils demonstrate a characteristic periodicity not unlike that of the segment long spacings (SLS) of collagen. *The dermal microfibril bundles* usually arise at the tips of the basal cell protrusions into the dermis. These bundles course perpendicularly or obliquely from the DE junction deep into the dermis. With high-resolution electron microscopy, the individual fibers of these bundles show a regular beaded periodicity and a hollow tubular profile on cross section. Such features are reminiscent of the microfibril seen in elastic tissue and thus have led to the hypothesis that these bundles are extensions of dermal elastic tissue. Collagen in this area consists of randomly oriented single fibers that are not packed into dense bundles.

Three functions are ascribed to the DE junction: to bind the epidermis to the dermis, to support the epidermis, and to prevent the transfer of material and cells across the junction. The mooring role served by the components of the DE junction is demonstrated by the problems of the patient with epidermolysis bullosa dystrophica, who is born with defective epidermal–dermal attachments. This defect has been ascribed to an abnormal production of collagenase in this region or to a deficiency of anchoring fibrils. After the slightest cutaneous trauma such a patient develops blisters because of the separation of the skin below the basal lamina. Repair of these wounds leads to disfiguring scars. Experimentally, if the lamina lucida is removed with pro-teolytic enzymes, the remaining living epidermal basal cells show cytoplasmic blebbing at the disrupted surface. Such blebbing is reversible if the basal lamina is restored. This observation has been interpreted to indicate that the basal lamina also stabilizes the plasma membrane.

Although there is no evidence that the basal lamina serves as a barrier to water, electrolytes, or low-molecular-weight compounds, this layer seems to restrict the diffusion of larger molecules. Nevertheless, white blood cells do pass from the dermis into the epidermis, apparently by traversing a gap that the invading cell itself produces in the layers of the junction.

17–14 Rete ridge structure of epidermis. This section, taken predominantly tangential to the surface, shows clearly that the rete ridge **(RR)** is not a finger-like projection of epidermis into the dermis as it appears in the usual cross section of skin. Cross sections of dermal papillae **(DP)** with included capillary loops **(cap)** are easily seen. **ED**, eccrine duct; **ker**, keratin layer.

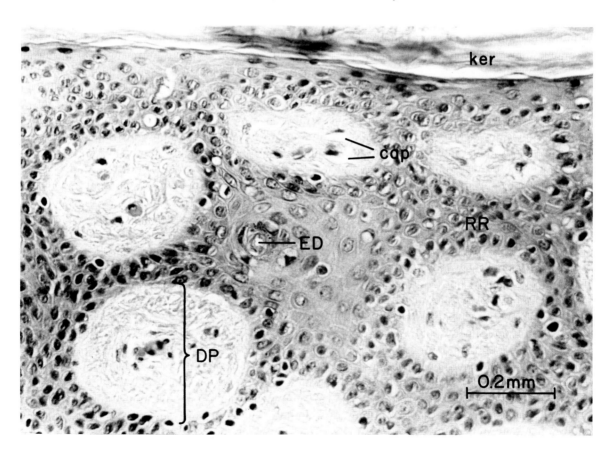

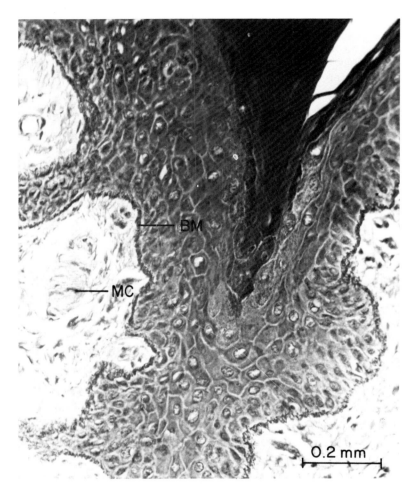

17-15 Dermal–epidermal junction by light microscopy. This silver preparation of plantar skin stains the basement membrane **(BM)** intensely. PAS stain highlights the basement membrane similarly. A Meissner corpuscle **(MC)** appears in a dermal papilla. Bodian stain.

Whereas the lamina lucida and lamina densa are probably synthesized by epidermal cells, the subbasal laminar fibers are believed to be synthesized by dermal elements.

Dermis

Dermal Structure

The important supporting layer of the skin is the dermis. It is made predominantly of connective tissue—collagen, elastic tissue, and ground substance—and, to a lesser extent, of cells and cellular structures. The cell that produces the connective tissue is the fibroblast. Collagen is laid down as bundles of varying size from fine to coarse, in a pattern that appears random. Varying in character and thickness with each body region, the dermis is composed of two layers: a superficial layer, the *papillary dermis,* which is made of loosely packed, fine fibrous tissue, and the *reticular dermis* which is made of densely packed, thick fibrous bundles. It is the reticular dermis that gives skin its leather-like character. The papillary dermis contains predominantly type III collagen and lesser amounts of type I. Conversely, the reticular dermis contains mostly type I collagen and lesser amounts of type III (Fig. 17–17).

The dermis also contains an elastic fiber network (Fig. 17–18). Fine elastic fibers are found in the papillary dermis, extending directly toward the epidermis and then splaying out under it. These fibers also may serve to bind the epidermis to the dermis. Coarse elastic fibers entwine the thick collagen bundles of the reticular dermis. The unique mechanical properties of the dermis probably depend on the extensible elastic

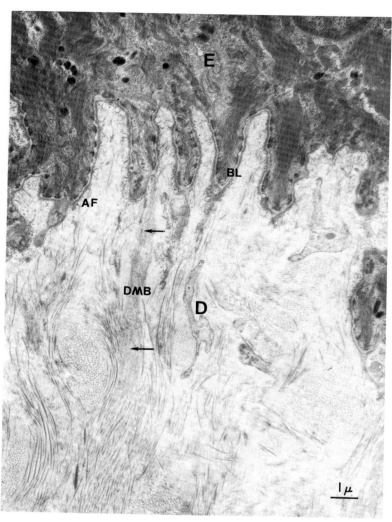

17–16 Dermal **(D)**–epidermal **(E)** junction by electron microscopy. Keratin or tonofilaments insert into hemidesmosomes of the undulating lower basal cell surface. This surface rests on the electron-lucent lamina lucida, which in turn is adjacent to the lamina densa or basal lamina **(BL).** Anchoring filaments **(AF)** and dermal microfibrillar bundles **(DMB** and **arrows)** extend from the basal lamina into the dermis. Collagen fibers are seen in the underlying dermis (From Briggaman, R. A., and Wheeler, C. E. 1975. J. Invest. Derm. 65:71; courtesy of R. A. Briggaman.)

fibers interwoven in the mesh of rather rigid collagen elements. Although elastic fibers are deformed by small forces, they recover their original dimensions even after considerable stretch. The orientation of dermal collagen and elastic fibers varies from area to area. The pattern of their orientation gives rise to certain lines of extensibility, *Langer's lines* (named after the German physician who first described them). The direction of these tension lines are demonstrable by removing a round piece of skin and observing the resultant elliptical hole.

The ground substance of the dermis is an amorphous matrix that embeds collagen and elastic fibers as well as the skin appendages. It is made up of (1) proteoglycans and other plasma constituents, (2) metabolic products of dermal cells, and (3) water and ions. Although there is no free fluid in the ground substance, the glycosaminoglycans of the proteoglycans are markedly hydrophilic and form a gel. Metabolites necessary for cutaneous survival and the migrant cells must pass through this gel. The three principal glycosaminoglycans of skin are hyaluronic acid, chondrotin sulfates, and dermatan sulfates. Because hyaluronic acid makes up to 70% of the dermal glycosaminoglycans, it is not surprising that hyaluronidase drastically alters the state of the ground substance. In contrast to hyaluronic acid, which is a huge molecule (several million daltons) that is loosely packed between collagen bundles, the chondroitin sulfates are smaller

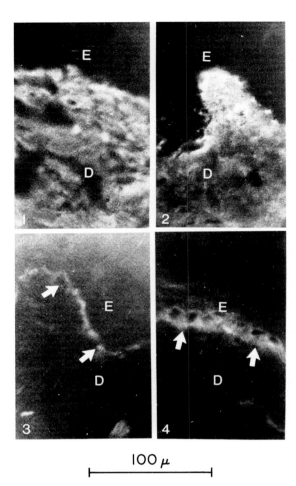

100 μ

17–17 Collagen types found in human skin. For this photograph, fresh human skin was stained with fluorescent-labeled antibodies to collagen types I **(1)**, III **(2)**, IV **(3)**, and V **(4)**. In most frames the epidermis **(E)** is difficult to distinguish from the dermis **(D)**. Notice that types I and III collagen are present in the upper dermis, type IV collagen is present at the dermal epidermal junction **(arrows)**, and type V collagen is present around the basal epidermal cells. (Courtesy of J. Madri, Yale University.)

(20,000 daltons) and firmly associated with collagen fibers.

Besides connective tissue, the dermis contains a scant cellular population, usually in perivascular distribution, consisting of fibroblasts, mast cells, macrophages, and a few lymphocytes. Also in the dermis are organized structures: the epidermal appendages (adnexa), vessels, lymphatics, and nerves.

In addition to its structural role, the dermis provides an important functional support for epidermal growth and maturation. It has been shown that isolated epidermis cannot be maintained in tissue culture for any length of time without some dermal elements. Embryologists have long recognized that developing epithelial systems depend on the underlying mesenchyme for inductive effects; for example, McLoughlin found in transplantation experiments that the epidermis of the chick embryo will grow as simple squamous epithelium on heart myoblasts, as simple nonkeratinizing squamous epithelium on proventriculus, and as keratinizing stratified squamous epithelium on limb-bud mesenchyme. A series of experiments by Billingham and Silvers suggested that even in the adult the dermis influences epidermal differentiation. When these workers transplanted hamster dermis from foot to chest, the chest epidermis that covered the foot dermis matured with characteristics of foot epidermis; conversely, when chest dermis was transplanted to the foot, the regenerating epidermis was chestlike. Studies such as these suggest that the dermis serves an important role in the normal dynamics of skin growth and differentiation.

Vascular Supply

Although varying in different body regions, the dermis is richly supplied with blood. As the blood supply far exceeds the metabolic demand of skin, the primary function of the rich dermal vascular network is thermal regulation.

Vessels of the skin arise from primary or secondary segmental branches of the aorta. From these arteries, perforating branches pass through muscle and fibrofatty tissue either as branching musculocutaneous vessels or as vessels going directly to the skin. Although the feeding vessels form two networks, one at the level of the dermal–subcutaneous junction and a second within the papillary dermis below the epidermis, the vessels anastomose extensively. Indeed, perfusion studies show vessels at all dermal levels (Fig. 17–19).

Arising from the superficial plexus, one small capillary loop enters each dermal papilla. This capillary serves all the nutritional needs of the epidermis, and electron-microscopically it is a typical capillary (Fig. 17–20). At the terminal arteriole, the extrapapillary portion of the capillary's ascending limb has characteristics of an ar-

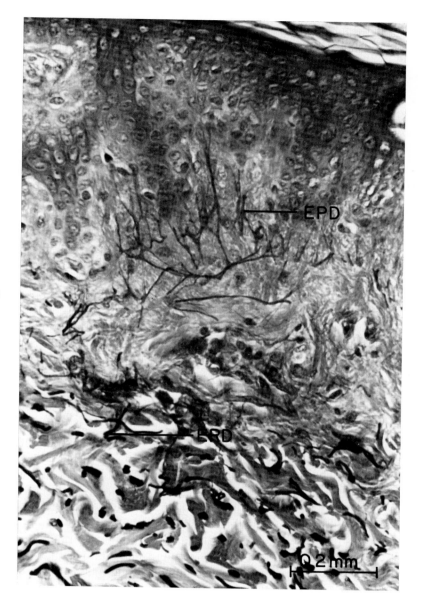

17–18 Elastic fiber structure of dermis. Notice the very fine arborizing elastic fibers of the papillary dermis **(EPD)** and the coarser, more fragmented fibers of the reticular dermis **(ERD)**.

terial capillary: the basement membrane material in its wall is homogeneous. When the loop enters the dermal papilla, although the outside diameter narrows, the basement membrane material in the wall retains its homogeneous arteriolar appearance. At the apex of the capillary loop, the basement membrane thins and, as it turns down, its diameter widens. As the capillary leaves the dermal papilla, the character of the basement membrane material changes abruptly: it loses its homogeneous appearance and develops multilayered features characteristic of venous vessels.

These structural differences are important because (1) the physiological properties of the arteriolar and venous portions of the capillary loop are quite different (e.g., it is known that white blood cell diapedesis occurs at the postcapillary loop and that the inflammatory mediators histamine, serotonin, and bradykinin act on this segment to increase permeability), and (2) in some cutaneous disease the venous portion of the dermal capillary loop increases (e.g., psoriasis).

Because the major role of the cutaneous vascular supply is to regulate heat, sensitive and

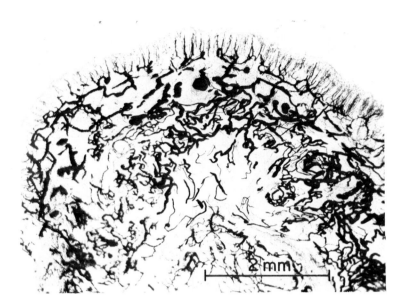

17–19 Dermal vascular supply. For this preparation skin was perfused with dye, then fixed and sectioned. Notice the rich vascular supply at all dermal levels. Very fine capillaries can be seen extending into the dermal papillae. The epidermis is poorly visualized. (From Winkelmann, R. K. 1961. Adv. Biol. Skin 2:3.)

powerful controls of blood flow must be present. Although the usual path of blood flow is from arteriole to capillary to venule, control is provided in the skin by means of multiple shunts that directly unite the arterial and venous vessels. Such shunts occur at two levels. First, direct arteriovenous (AV) shunts are found in small arteries of the deep dermis and, second, in the more superficial dermis, blood flowing from arterioles to capillary beds may pass directly through AV shunts when precapillary sphincters have closed. The latter function is assisted by the glomus body, described in Chap. 9. Such anastomoses are particularly rich in the upper reticular dermis of the fingertips, toes, nail bed, nose, and lips.

Lymphatics of the dermis follow the same vascular pattern as the blood vessels, although their density is greater in the upper reticular dermis. Lymphatics are not found in the epidermis or papillary dermis. They are distinguished in the dermis by their distended lumen, thin walls, and prominent valves.

Innervation

Skin is the largest sensory organ of the body and is richly innervated at all its levels. Sensory stimuli are conducted from the skin at various velocities by nerve fibers of different diameters and myelination. The sensory nerves arise as branches of the trigeminal and spinal nerves.

Each of these branches serves an area of skin, a *dermatome*, that varies in size, shape, and definition among body regions; however, in general, dermatomes form a horizontal, dorsal-ventral pattern. Sensory impulses pass to the dorsal root ganglion by spinal cord nerves or to the Gasserian ganglion by the trigeminal nerve. From there they pass to the thalamic centers and then to the sensory cortex.

Myelinated nerves associated with vessels enter the subcutis between fat lobules. As they progress upward they branch freely, intertwine with adjacent nerves, and form two networks. One network, the subcutaneous plexus, forms at the dermal–subcutis junction and the second, the dermal plexus, forms just below the epidermis. These networks contain sensory as well as sympathetic postganglionic fibers, which supply the blood vessels and skin appendages. Just as the density of dermal nerve fibers varies, the sensitivity of skin from region to region also varies (e.g., nerve density is high within the papillary dermis of the glans penis and finger, and low over the back). In the deep dermis nerve bundles are heavily myelinated and large in diameter, whereas in the superficial dermis they are minimally myelinated or nonmyelinated and thin. Thin nerve fibers occasionally extend into the epidermis to the level of the granular layer or approach the lower-lying Merkel cells.

The character of cutaneous nerve endings and the nature of sensory conduction are discussed in detail in Chap. 8.

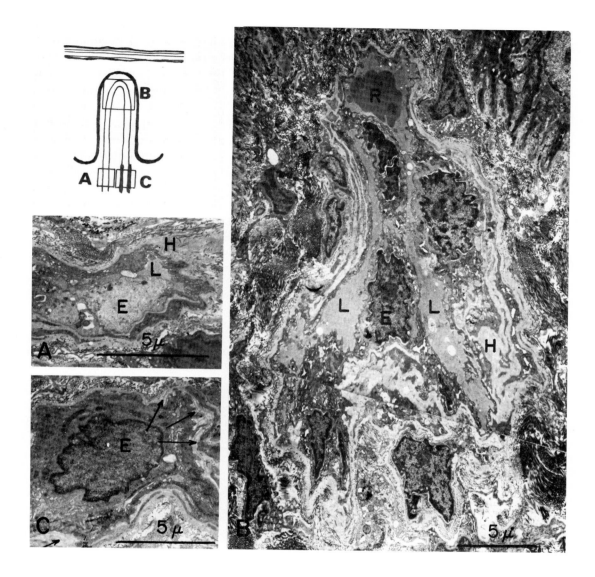

Development of Skin

The skin develops as a simple structure in the embryo, becomes more complex by birth, matures further at puberty, and atrophies in old age. The epidermal epithelial cell arises from ectoderm; the Langerhans cell, the dermis, and subcutis from mesoderm; and the melanocyte from neural crest. The primitive epidermis and the underlying dermis (mesenchyme) give rise to the skin appendages—the pilosebaceous apparatus, the eccrine gland, and the nail.

Until about the fourth week, the human embryo and fetus are covered by an epidermis made up of a single layer of flattened cells loosely arranged on a basal lamina and connected by infre-

17–20 Ultrastructure of a dermal capillary loop. The diagram at the upper left shows the levels at which sections were taken. Notice the homogeneous (H) basement membrane in **A** and **B** and the layered basement membrane in **C (arrows). L,** capillary lumen; **E,** endothelial cell; **H,** homogeneous basement membrane. (From Braverman, I., and Yen, A. 1977. J. Invest. Derm. 68:44; courtesy of I. Braverman.)

quent desmosomes. The dermis is a loose mesenchymal tissue rich in proteoglycans and glycogen. After the fifth week the epidermis becomes two-layered, with an inner or *basal layer* (stratum germinativum) and a nonkeratinized transient outer layer, the *periderm.* Although in early stages the periderm grows and keeps pace with the increasing fetal surface, its mitotic activity ceases, in the second trimester. The periderm cells are initially flat (Fig. 17–21) but soon become rounded and covered by a larger number of microvilli (Fig. 17–22). In early development, half the epidermal thickness is due to this simple columnar periderm layer, but with time the cells bleb and flatten. Meanwhile, the basal layer produces several layers of cells (*stratum intermedium*) between it and the periderm. By 160 days of gestation the cells of the stratum intermedium also begin to flatten, move upward, and keratinize. In this process the periderm cells are shed, leaving the epidermal surface much as it is found in the newborn.

Because the periderm remains associated with the developing epidermis until the latter matures, it may serve as the first embryonic cover until a keratinizing surface can be formed. The bleblike projections that seem to detach from the cells and the microvilli found on the outer cell surfaces suggest that the periderm may play a role in secretion, uptake, or conditioning of amniotic fluid. Supporting these hypotheses are in vivo and in vitro studies that show that early fetal skin transports isotopically labeled water better than older fetal skin and that these differences correlate with the morphological maturation of the

periderm. Moreover, the ionic character of amniotic fluid changes when the periderm is shed and the body skin keratinizes.

At approximately 5 to 6 months, as the periderm layer sheds, the epidermis consists almost entirely of stratified squamous epithelial cells, which are now present in the distinct layers seen in the adult: stratum germinativum, stratum spinosum, stratum granulosum, and stratum corneum.

In the third fetal month, anlagen for the skin appendages appear in a caudad–ventral sequence as downgrowths from the primitive epidermis. Each of the appendages—pilosebaceous apparatus (i.e., hair follicle, apocrine gland, and sebaceous gland), eccrine sweat gland, and nail—arises as an accumulation of basal cells that project or fold into the dermis. The growth, differentiation, and maturation of the appendages depends on an intimate and continuous interaction with the dermal mesenchyme. The cell cord forming a pilosebaceous apparatus grows at an oblique angle relative to the skin surface so that the erupted hair shaft generally projects caudad. At its deepest point, the epithelial portion of the hair follicle embraces a mesenchymal plug, the dermal papilla of the hair bulb. Cellular bulges appear at the posterior face of the pilosebaceous downgrowth (Fig. 17–23). The lowest

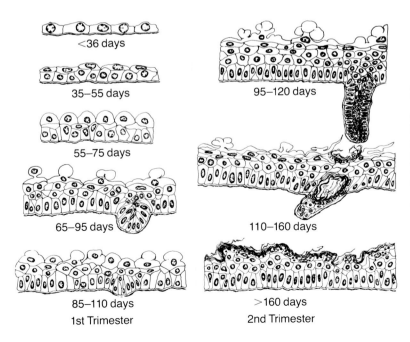

<36 days

35–55 days

55–75 days

65–95 days

85–110 days
1st Trimester

95–120 days

110–160 days

>160 days
2nd Trimester

17–21 Schematic diagram of periderm development and epidermal differentiation. Notice the progressing stratification of the epidermis, the intricate structure of the outer periderm layer, the loss of periderm by about 160 days, and the development of a skin appendage from the primitive epidermis. (From Holbrook, K. A., and Odland, G. F. 1975. J. Invest. Derm. 65:16.)

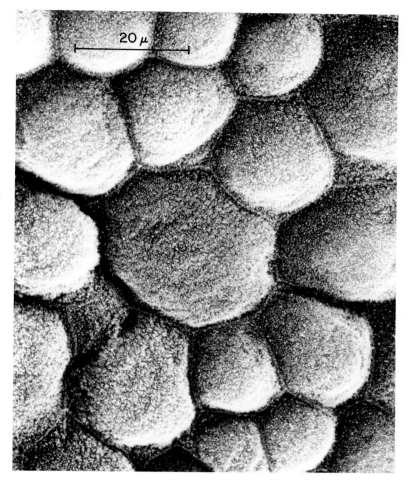

17–22 Scanning electron micrograph of skin surface from a 60-day-old human fetus. Notice the conspicuous cell boundaries, the elevated small and flattened broad cells, and the microvillous surface character of the cells. (From Holbrook, K. A., and Odland, G. F. 1975. J. Invest. Derm. 65:16.)

bulge serves as the attachment for the muscle of the hair follicle, the arrector pili; the middle bud, as the anlage for the sebaceous gland; and the highest, as the anlage for the apocrine gland.

Within the second month of fetal life nonkeratinizing cells are present in the epidermis. The melanocyte and Langerhans cells are distinguished from keratinocytes by their dendritic cytoplasmic processes, wider intercellular distances, lack of desmosomes, and distinctive cytological features. Melanocytes do not appear to be functionally mature until the second trimester. At approximately the fourth month, the Merkel cell appears in the epidermis of the fingertips, glabrous (hairless) skin, and nail beds.

By the end of the second trimester, the skin has matured into a structure that remains essentially unchanged to birth. There is some variation in the rate of development of skin, depending on location. For example, by the end of the first trimester the stratum intermedium is fully developed on the face but not elsewhere; in addition, although hair follicle anlagen are found in eyebrow, upper lip, and chin skin at 2 months, they are found elsewhere only later.

The structure of skin shows little change from birth through childhood, but in adolescence, under the influence of estrogenic and androgenic hormones, there are dramatic changes in the maturation of skin appendages. Apocrine glands of axillary and inguinal skin grow to their full extent and begin to liberate their secretions, ambosexual hairs appear, and sebaceous glands grow and secrete over the facial and neck regions. With advancing age, the size and secretions of the appendages decreases, and the epidermis, dermis, and subcutis thin.

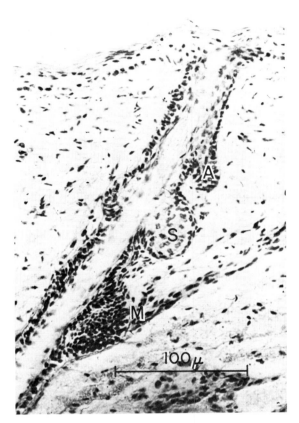

17–23 Developing pilosebaceous apparatus in a 17-week-old human fetus. The primitive pilosebaceous apparatus grows down from the fetal epidermis at an angle to the surface. From the side of the hair follicle that forms an obtuse angle with the surface emerge three structures: apocrine gland in the uppermost site **(A),** the muscle of the hair follicle in the lowermost site **(M),** and between these two the sebaceous gland **(S).** This picture shows the earliest formative stage of these three structures. (From Serri, F. 1962. J. Invest. Derm. 39:199.)

Regional Variation of Skin

The surface character, thickness, pliability, and color of skin, and the density and nature of appendages vary from region to region of the body, apparently serving the unique function of each area (Fig. 17–24). The skin is thicker on the dorsal and extensor surfaces than the ventral or flexor surfaces; in general, it is thicker in men than women. The epidermis varies in thickness over most of the body from 0.07 to 1.12 mm but attains a thickness of 0.8 to 1.4 mm over the palms and soles. The thickness of the dermis varies from 1 to 2 mm over most areas but may be less than 0.5 mm on the eyelids and greater than 5 mm over the back. The character, length, and density of hair also vary. Compare the coarse hairs of the beard, eyebrow, pubic, and axillary regions to the fine hairs of the forehead and nose. Sebaceous glands are particularly prominent in facial, upper back, and upper chest skin but scant over the trunk and extremities. Apocrine glands are prominent in the axilla, mammary line, and groin, sparse on the head and neck, and absent elsewhere. The thickness and constituents of the layers making up the subcutis also vary with body regions. For example, under the nail bed the dermis attaches directly to the aponeurosis of the bony digit, and over the muscle of the forearm the dermis attaches to a very thin subcutis made of loose connective tissue, the *tela subcutanea*. In contrast, over the buttocks and abdomen the subcutis is thick and fatty *(panniculus adiposus)*. Over the neck the subcutis contains small striated muscle fibers (the platysma). In other areas of the body (nipple, areola, scrotum, penis, and perianal regions), oriented smooth muscle fibers are found in the dermis and subcutis. Therefore, as there are impressive gross differences in regional skin, there are also distinctive histological differences in each of the cutaneous layers in each region.

Skin Appendages

Pilosebaceous Apparatus

Arising as a distinct skin structure in the embryo, the pilosebaceous apparatus is made up of a hair follicle, its attached smooth muscle, a sebaceous gland, and, in specific regions, an aprocrine gland (Fig. 17–25).

Hair Follicle. In more primitive mammals hair serves to conserve body temperature, protect against physical trauma, and sense the environment. Although still serving those functions for contemporary humans, hair is more important for personal adornment than protection.

The male and female human have at birth an equal number of hair follicles, approximately two million, 100,000 of which are on the scalp. The apparent difference in hair density between the sexes is due to the type of hair and its distribution—not to the number of hair follicles. Three hair types are recognized. Before birth the fetus is covered with a very fine unpigmented *lanugo hair*, which falls out shortly after birth. Before puberty the child is covered by two hair

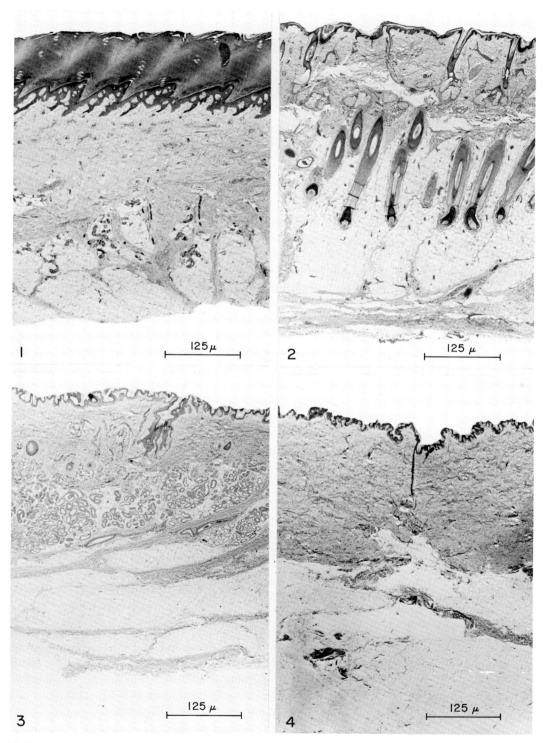

17–24 Comparative histology of regional skin. Differences in structure of the epidermis, dermis, and subcutis are readily apparent in the skin of plantar surface **(1)**, scalp **(2)**, axilla **(3)**, and abdomen **(4)** from a 20-year-old man.

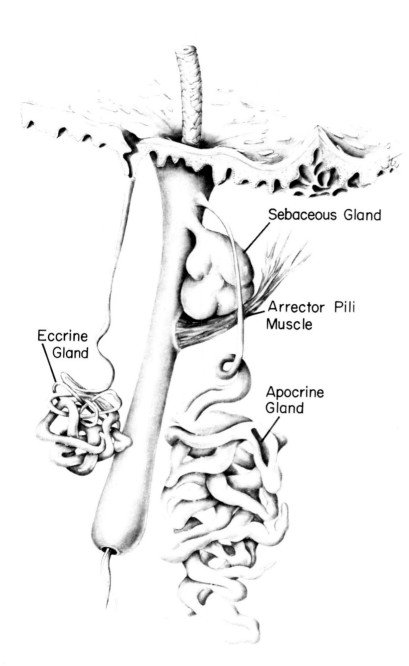

Sebaceous Gland

Arrector Pili
Muscle

Eccrine
Gland

Apocrine
Gland

17–25 Diagram of the cutaneous appendages: eccrine gland and pilosebaceous apparatus. Notice that both these structures communicate with the epidermis separately and that the apocrine gland, sebaceous gland, and arrector pili muscle attach to one side of the hair follicle. Compare this sketch to the embryonic follicle of Fig. 17–23. (From Montagna, W., and Parakkal, P. F. 1974. The Structure and Function of Skin. New York: Academic Press.)

types (Fig. 17–26): (1) a very fine, nonpigmented hair identical to the lanugo hair, now called *vellus hair*, which covers most of the body, and (2) a *terminal hair*, which is coarse, usually pigmented, and found on the scalp, eyelid (eyelash), and eyebrow areas. Vellus hair follicles are thin and extend only as deep as the middermis. The vellus hair shaft is correspondingly thin, colorless, and soft. The terminal hair follicle is wide and extends deeply through the dermis into the subcutis. The terminal hair shaft is pigmented and coarse, and it often contains an additional central structure, *a medulla*. After puberty, there is a maturation or conversion of vellus to terminal hair follicles in the axillary and anogenital regions in both sexes and over the face, extremities, and trunk in the male. The character and density of hair growth depends largely on ge-

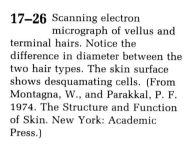 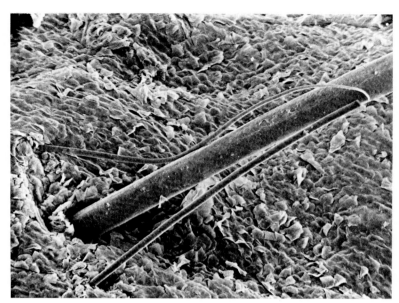

17–26 Scanning electron micrograph of vellus and terminal hairs. Notice the difference in diameter between the two hair types. The skin surface shows desquamating cells. (From Montagna, W., and Parakkal, P. F. 1974. The Structure and Function of Skin. New York: Academic Press.)

netic background. Although the hair shafts produced by follicles over the postpubertal trunk are considered terminal hairs, they differ somewhat from scalp hair in length, thickness, and tendency to curl; these hairs have been called *ambosexual hair.*

Hair length varies from region to region because there are differences in growth period and growth rate of hair follicles. All hair growth is cyclical, and in humans it is asynchronous so that in any specific area growing hair follicles will be adjacent to resting hair follicles. Three phases of the hair growth cycle are recognized: *anagen,* the growth phase; *catagen,* the regressing phase; and *telogen,* the resting phase (Fig. 17–27). In the human scalp the anagen phase varies from 2 to 6 years, catagen from 2 to 3 weeks, and telogen from 3 to 4 months. After telogen, the old hair shaft sheds and a new hair shaft appears. The growth cycle of the hair is reflected in dramatic morphological changes in the hair follicle.

As indicated above, the hair follicle arises as a downgrowth of the primitive epidermis, projecting at an angle with the epidermis so that the hair shaft usually points away from the head. In the obtuse angle of the follicle (relative to the epidermis) there are three noncycling structures: an apocrine gland (in axillary and anogenital areas), a sebaceous gland, and an arrector pili muscle (when this muscle contracts, the hair

17–27 Growth cycle of the hair follicle. Three stages of the hair growth cycle are recognized: the phase of active hair growth, anagen; the phase of hair follicle regression, catagen; and the phase of hair follicle rest, telogen. The follicle consists of three segments, two permanent (infundibulum and isthmus) and one cycling (the deep or inferior segment). (Adapted from Montagna, W., and Parakkel, P. F. 1974. The Structure and Function of Skin. New York: Academic Press.)

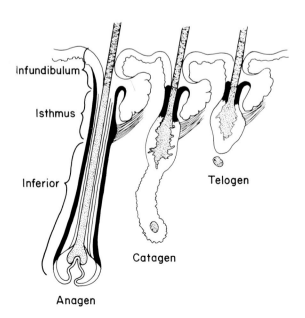

Infundibulum

Isthmus

Inferior

Anagen

Catagen

Telogen

shaft is brought upright). The portion of the hair follicle into which these structures insert is permanent, but the hair follicle below the arrector pili insertion undergoes changes as the follicle passes through its growth cycle. This cycling *inferior portion* of the hair follicle is distinguished from the noncycling middle portion, *the isthmus* (extending from the lower arrector pili muscle to the lower sebaceous duct), and the outer portion, *the infundibulum* (extending from the lower sebaceous duct to the surface opening of the follicle). In anagen, the deep portion of a terminal hair follicle extends into the subcutis. At its base the anagen follicle has a bulb-shaped expansion, the *follicular bulb,* which encloses a finger-like projection of connective tissue and blood vessels, *the dermal papilla of the hair follicle.* The densely packed epithelial cells of the bulb multiply rapidly, move outward in columns, and form characteristic layers. The innermost of these layers keratinize and form the hair shaft. During catagen, the cells of the deep follicle atrophy and the deep portion of the follicle shrinks. In telogen, the follicle ends at the insertion of the arrector pili muscle and very few cells of the deep follicle remain; in this phase there is neither active cell growth nor keratinization. Although the hair shaft remains within the telogen follicle, it does not grow. As anagen begins anew, the deep portion of the follicle grows, reassumes a mesenchymal papilla, and projects into the subcutis. In this process a new hair shaft forms, which grows out from under the old shaft and causes the latter to shed.

The histology of the hair follicle (Fig. 17–28) is best appreciated in terms of its embryology. As a finger of primitive epidermis projects into the dermis, it draws with it a keratinizing stratified squamous epithelium, a prominent basement membrane (the *glassy membrane*), and a surrounding loose connective tissue (the *adventitial dermis,* which is morphologically identical to the papillary dermis). Compared to the mature epidermis, the follicle wall is more complex. It is made up of three vertically oriented concentric cellular cylinders: the hair shaft, the internal follicular sheath, and the external follicular sheath. These cylinders grow from the rapidly dividing cell population of the hair follicle bulb and keratinize in the following order: hair shaft, internal sheath, and external sheath. For the cells of the internal and external sheaths the keratinization process seems very similar to that of the epidermis; but the cells of the hair shaft cortex keratin-

ize, like the nail, without forming cytoplasmic (keratohyalin) granules. It is notable that the cells forming the medulla of the hair shaft assemble cytoplasmic granules into their keratin. Keratinization of hair shaft cells begins in the upper bulb. A single layer of cells on the outer hair shaft forms a barklike cuticle that points toward the hair bulb. The polarity of this cuticle is easily appreciated by rubbing one's finger along a hair shaft. The internal follicular sheath, arising from cells of the bulb lateral to those forming the hair shaft, consists of three cell layers: a cuticle, which points toward the hair tip; a layer of cells (often two cells thick) with prominent cytoplasmic granules (trichohyalin granules) called *Huxley's layer*; and a layer of cells that keratinizes in the upper bulb, called *Henle's layer*. Some workers have suggested that the internal follicular sheath serves to shape the hair shaft. Interdigitation of the cuticle layers of the hair shaft and of the internal follicular sheath helps hold the hair shaft in the dermis. The outermost cell layer of the follicle is the external follicular sheath, which increases in thickness from the base to the follicle top. The cells making up this layer contain abundant cytoplasmic glycogen in the lower follicle and thus appear to have clear cytoplasm. In the upper follicle these cells appear more like epidermal cells.

Apocrine Sweat Gland. The apocrine gland arises first as a solid epithelial bulge along one side of most pilosebaceous apparatuses in the 5- to 6-month-old embryo. After this time the apocrine anlagen region atrophies except for specific areas: the axilla, mammary line, external auditory meatus, eyelids, and anogenital areas. By birth the gland in these areas is well defined but not mature. During adolescence the apocrine gland assumes adult histological features as the associated hair follicles also mature.

The apocrine gland is tubular, like the eccrine gland, and consists of a secretory coil (Fig. 17–29) in the deep dermis and a duct that transports the secretory product to the lumen of the pilosebaceous apparatus. Because the apocrine gland stores its secretions, the secretory coil varies in width depending on the secretory activity of the gland. Correspondingly, the epithelium of the coil is either cuboidal in the contracted gland or simple squamous in the distended gland. In either case, the glandular epithelial cells are single-layered and rest on a bed of large, loosely packed myoepithelial cells, outside of which is

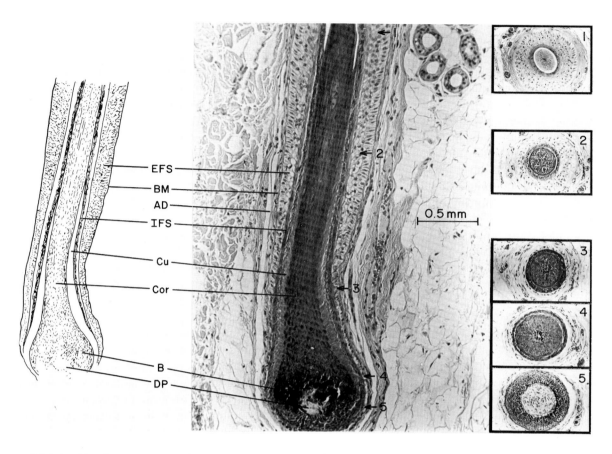

EFS
BM
AD
IFS
Cu
Cor
B
DP

0.5 mm

1
2
3
4
5

2
3
4
5

17–28 Anatomy of inferior segment of the hair follicle. A sketch of the longitudinal section of a deep hair follicle is shown on the left. Cross sections appear on the right, and the level of the section is indicated by short arrows with corresponding numbers. **EFS,** external follicular sheath; **BM,** basement membrane; **AD,** adventitial dermis; **IFS,** internal follicular sheath with its outer early keratinizing Henle layer and its inner richly granulated Huxley layer; **Cu,** cuticle layer, **Cor,** hair shaft cortex; **B,** bulb of the hair follicle; **DP,** dermal papilla of the hair follicle.

a thick hyaline basement membrane. By electron microscopy the cytoplasm of the secretory cells is filled with fine granules. Cytoplasmic elevations or apical caps of these cells project into the lumen and are covered with small microvilli (Fig. 17–30). These cytoplasmic elevations give the "apocrine" or "pinching-off" character to these cells. The upper part of the secretory segment narrows and emerges into a duct that runs a straight course parallel to the hair follicle and empties into the upper hair follicle above the sebaceous duct. This duct, morphologically most like the eccrine duct, occasionally consists of three concentric layers of epithelial cells. The innermost of these layers is made of cells with a keratinizing cytoplasmic border that appears as a cuticle by light microscopy. Unlike the eccrine duct, the apocrine duct has not been shown to modify apocrine secretions.

Apocrine secretion is a viscous, milky-to-clear substance that can be white, red, yellow, or black. This secretion contains protein, carbohydrate, ammonia, lipids, and ferric iron as well as chromogens, such as indoxyl, and fatty acids such as caprylic acid. This gland secretes slowly and afterwards undergoes a refractory period. Although the primary stimulus to secretion is believed to be adrenergic, apocrine glands secrete after both adrenergic and cholinergic stimuli.

The function of the apocrine gland has not been established. It is believed that the secretions are odorless when released but acquire the characteristic axillary-body smell after bacterial

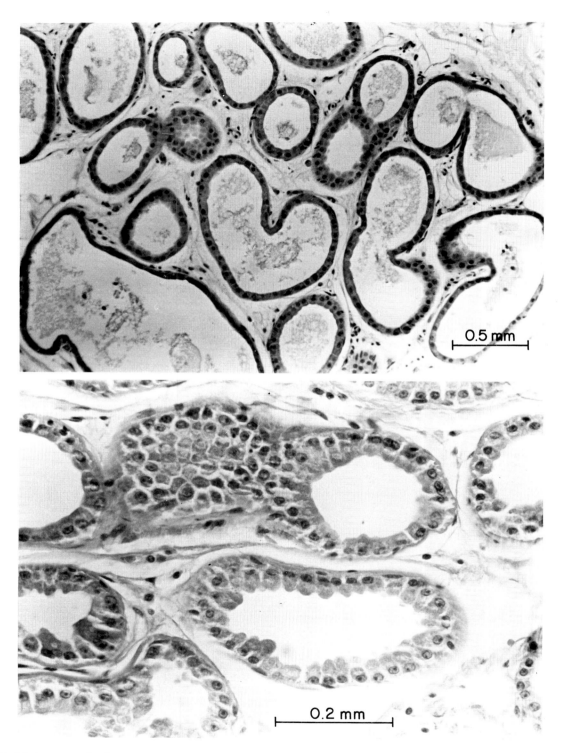

17–29 Apocrine gland, secretory portion. Top picture shows a dilated apocrine coil filled with secretions. Lower picture shows a relatively empty gland with prominent typical cytoplasmic budding (apical cap) into the gland lumen.

17–30 Electron micrograph of the secretory portion of the apocrine gland. Notice the villi over the apical cap, which projects into the gland lumen; the myoepithelial cells **(M)**; and the collagenous capsule **(C)**. (Courtesy of Ken Hashimoto, Wayne State University.)

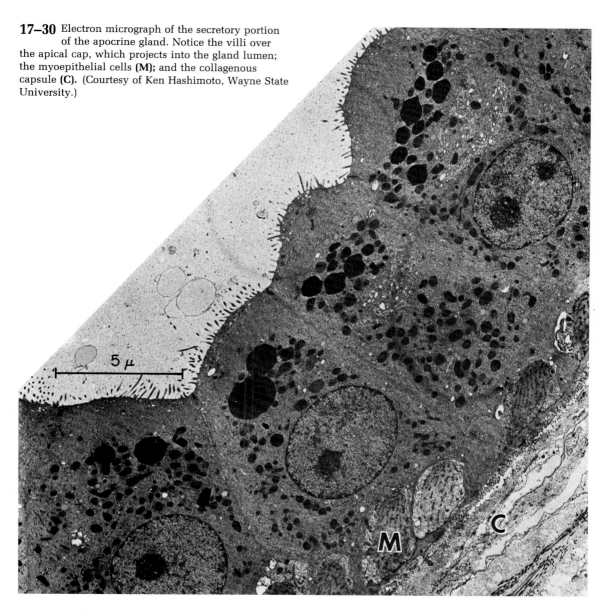

decomposition. The role this secretion plays in human intercourse, perhaps as a pheromone, has been postulated but not substantiated experimentally.

Sebaceous Glands. The sebaceous gland arises from the pilosebaceous apparatus just below the apocrine gland anlage and, although it is present in any body region where pilosebaceous structures are found, it varies in size in different body regions. Sebaceous glands are small within the pilosebaceous structures of the trunk and extremities, but they are prominent over the sebor-

rheic areas: face, neck, upper chest, and upper back. Indeed, in the latter areas the largest component of the pilosebaceous apparatus is the sebaceous gland and duct; for this reason, such a pilosebaceous apparatus is referred to as a *sebaceous follicle*.

The sebaceous gland (Figs. 17–25 and 17–31) consists of a lobular secretory portion and a ductal portion that empties into the upper hair follicle. The secretory portion is bordered by a single row of basaloid cells that rests on a basement membrane. The basal cells serve as the source of cells for the secretory function of this holocrine

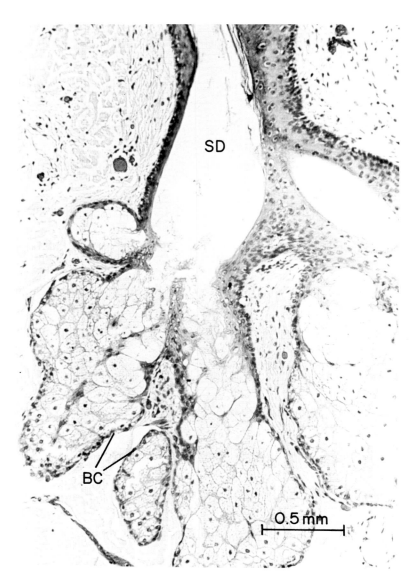

17–31 Sebaceous gland. This picture of a lower portion of a sebaceous gland shows sebum-filled cells maturing from the outerlying basal cells **(BC).** The mature sebaceous cells disintegrate, releasing sebum into the sebaceous duct **(SD).**

gland. Like the basal cells of the epidermis, these cells are attached to one another by desmosomes. Apparently, one daughter cell of a given cell division differentiates; in so doing it acquires a prominent Golgi apparatus, ribosomes, glycogen, and lipid (or sebum) vesicles. The pressure of cell division seems to push the maturing cells into the duct. As the cells mature they accumulate sebum vesicles until the cytoplasm is filled; at this point the cell breaks down and releases its contents into the duct.

Although the sebaceous gland secretion, sebum, is a whole cell product (holocrine secretion), it is almost entirely lipid. About 60% of

sebum (by weight) consists of glycerides and free fatty acids, but wax esters and squalene are also present. It is notable that although epidermis produces significant quantities of cholesterol, cholesterol esters, and phospholipids, sebaceous secretions contain relatively little of these lipids.

It is currently believed that sebum is secreted continuously without any obvious diurnal control of its release. The development and growth of sebaceous glands, particularly during puberty, are stimulated by androgens and inhibited by estrogens.

The role sebum plays in the health and physiology of skin is not known. It is not clear if se-

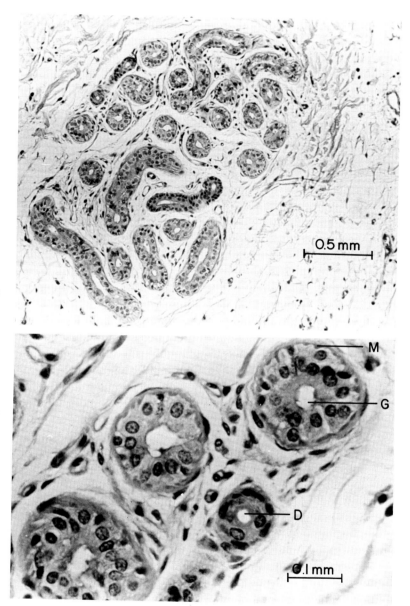

17–32 Eccrine gland. The top picture shows a cross section of an eccrine coil in the subcutis. The lower picture shows a higher power cross section of secretory **(G)** and ductal **(D)** portions of an eccrine gland with surrounding myoepithelial layer **(M)**.

bum serves as a permeability barrier, an emollient, or as a significant bacteriostatic or fungistatic agent. Because the scent gland of many mammals is sebaceous, it has been suggested that sebum acts as a pheromone.

Eccrine Sweat Gland

In humans the major source of evaporative heat loss is through eccrine sweat, and it is this mechanism that has enabled survival where ambient temperatures exceed the body temperature. In the adult, eccrine structures are found over most of the body. They are present in very high density on the palms and soles but absent on the glans penis, clitoris, and labia minora.

Eccrine structures arise independently of the pilosebaceous apparatus as a direct downgrowth of the primitive epidermis. Like the apocrine gland, the eccrine gland is a tubular structure and consists of ductal and secretory segments. The secretory portion is present in the deep der-

602

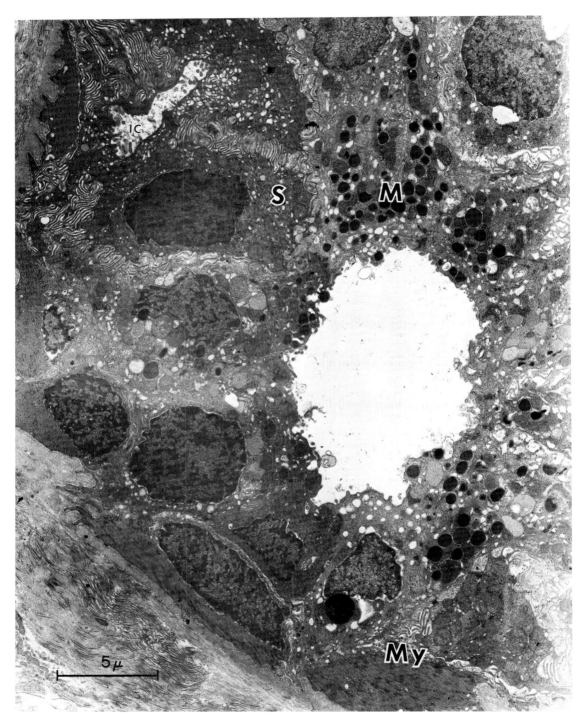

17–33 Electron micrograph of the secretory portion of an eccrine gland. Two types of glandular cells surround the gland lumen: serous cell **(S)** and mucous cell **(M).** Peripheral to the glandular epithelium are myoepithelial cells **(My).** Notice that intercellular canaliculi **(IC)** lined by villous processes are also present. (Courtesy of Ken Hashimoto, Wayne State University.)

mis or subcutis and consists of a coil lined by one layer of truncated pyramidal cells (Figs. 17–32 and 17–33). Two distinct eccrine secretory cells are recognized: a *clear serous cell*, which sits at the periphery of the tubule and has a large nucleus and pale cytoplasm, and a *dark mucous cell*, which is shaped like an inverted pyramid with its base toward the lumen and has a small nucleus and basophilic cytoplasm. The shape and arrangement of these two cells give the secretory portion a pseudostratified appearance. The clear cells contain in their cytoplasm many mitochondria, abundant glycogen, and an intricate system of intercellular canaliculi that extend between adjacent cells. The dark cells have cytoplasm rich in secretory granules, endoplasmic reticulum, Golgi apparatus, and acid mucoid substances. The plasma membranes at the luminal border of both cells form short microvilli. The secretory portion of the eccrine gland extends into the ductal portion that is morphologically similary to the apocrine duct. The lining of the lumen consists of two compact concentric layers of cuboidal cells; cytoplasm of its inner row of cells appears hyalinized because it contains densely packed cytoplasmic tonofilaments. The ductal cells are separated from the basement membrane by an incomplete layer of myoepithelial cells.

Eccrine sweat is made of a clear, hypotonic solution; its major solutes are sodium, potassium, chloride, lactate, and urea. Protein makes up less than 1% of sweat by weight. Although the greatest volume of sweat is made by the secretory coil, sweat is modified during its passage through the duct in that the ductal epithelium reabsorbs sodium and chloride. Sweat is believed to be a cell product and not a plasma filtrate, like urine. Therefore, unlike the kidney, the eccrine sweat gland does not function to regulate body fluid or to eliminate body wastes; indeed, under the proper stimulus, sweat gland secretion may lead to total body dehydration.

Functionally, eccrine glands can be separated into those found in palmer–plantar skin and those found elsewhere. The palmar–plantar skin glands increase their secretion as a result of mental and emotional stimuli and little, if at all, because of heat stress. In contrast, eccrine glands of the remaining body skin respond predominately to heat stress. In both cases stimulation appears to involve a cholinergic mechanism. Unlike apocrine gland secretion, eccrine secretion will persist as long as the stimulus lasts; in fact, under

severe heat stress an adult man may secrete 1 to 2 liters of sweat an hour.

Nail

The nail, a transparent keratinous sheet over the digit tip, serves in humans as a protective covering and as a support for the grasping function of the finger (imagine picking up a coin from a table top without the help of nails).

Looking at the dorsal surface of the thumb (or Fig. 17–34), one can see that the nail is made of a transparent, slightly curved covering, *the nail plate*. The nail plate rests on and is adherent to the *nail bed*. The nail bed epithelium looks like epidermis histologically but lacks a granular layer. The underlying dermis is densely collagenized and continuous with the aponeurosis surrrounding the distal digit bone. The epidermis underlying the tip (distal edge) of the nail is the *hyponychium*. The skin uplifted around the lateral edges of the nail is the *lateral nail fold* or *paronychium*.

The nail plate grows from the base or proximal nail bed, which develops in the 3-month-old-fetus as a lateral and proximal invagination of the epidermis. This specialized infolded epidermis that gives rise to the nail plate is called the *nail matrix* (Fig. 17–34). The nail matrix, then, is a **V**-shaped infolding of specialized epidermis without which a nail plate does not form. Microscopically, the epidermis of the matrix, like that of the nail bed, lacks a granular layer. The only part of the nail matrix that is apparent grossly is the *lunula*, a half moon-shaped whitish area at the nail base that varies in size from digit to digit. As an invagination of an epithelial sheet, the matrix epithelium has a ventral and dorsal portion. The ventral matrix is larger than the dorsal. The most distal portion of the ventral nail matrix corresponds to the outer edge of the lunula. The distal portion of the dorsal nail matrix reassumes a granular layer and grows out over the outer nail plate as the *proximal nail fold*. At the outer edge of the proximal nail fold is its keratinous product, the *eponychium*, or cuticle, which the manicurist assiduously pushes back.

Nail keratinization seems to involve the same elements as epidermal and hair keratinization. The keratinocyte fills with 7- 8-nm-wide filaments and an interfilamentous matrix. The cells flatten, their outer walls thicken, and they become firmly attached to one another. Nail plate

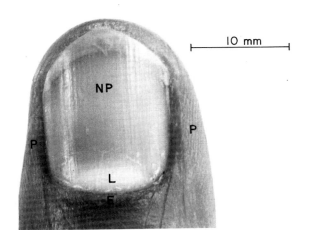

17–34 Nail. The top picture shows a thumb nail with the lateral nail fold **(P)**, eponychium and proximal nail fold, the lunula **(L)**, and nail plate **(NP)** labeled. The middle picture shows the saggital section of a toe with the nail plate **(NP)**, nail bed **(NB)**, eponychium and proximal nail fold **(E)**, dorsal **(DNM)** and ventral nail matrix **(VNM)** and hyponychium **(H)** labeled. Notice the proximity between the nail matrix and the distal digit bone and joint. The lower picture is a higher-power magnification of a nail matrix with the nail plate **(NP)**, nail bed **(NB)**, and dorsal **(DNM)** and ventral **(VNM)** nail matrix. Note the absence of a granular layer in the epithelium of the matrix.

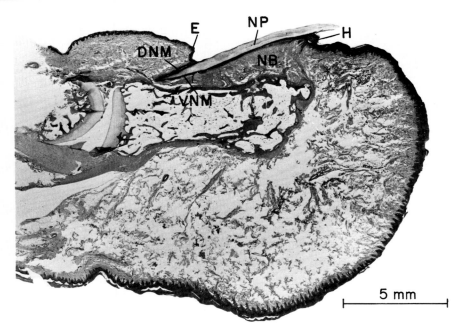

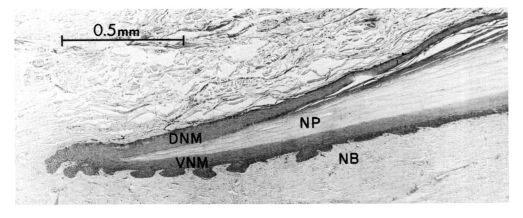

keratinocytes, like hair cortex keratinocytes, form hard keratin in the absence of a granular layer. Because this keratin does not desquamate, like hair shaft keratin, a nail must be worn down or trimmed in order to remain functional.

Unlike hair, the nail plate grows continuously without a resting phase. Nail growth is due to the addition of new cells at the matrix, resulting in a slow movement of the nail plate outward. Although the nail bed forms a tight adhesion to the plate, the nail bed contributes neither to the structure of the nail plate nor to its outward movement. The rate of nail growth is influenced by many factors. It is greatest in childhood and decreases slowly with aging. It is increased by trauma such as nail biting and playing a keyboard instrument. It is decreased by illness, immobilization, and inadequate nutrition. Fingernails grow faster than toenails; the nail of the middle finger grows fastest and those of the thumb and little finger, slowest.

References and Selected Bibliography

General Reference to Biology of the Skin

Montagna, W., and Parakkal, P. F. 1974. The Structure and Function of Skin, 3rd ed. New York: Academic Press.

Embryology of Skin

Holbrook, K. A. 1979. Human epidermal embryogenesis. Int. J. Dermatol. 18:329.

Holbrook, K. A., and Odland, G. F. 1975. The fine structure of developing human epidermis: Light, scanning and transmission electron microscopy of the periderm. J. Invest. Dermatol. 65:16.

Parmley, T. H., and Seeds, A. E. 1970. Fetal skin permeability to isotopic water (THO) in early pregnancy. Am. J. Obstet. Gynecol. 108:128.

Epidermis and Keratinization

Bernstein, I. A., and Seji, M. 1980. Biochemistry of Normal and Abnormal Epidermal Differentiation. Current Problems in Dermatology, Vol. 10. Basel: S. Karger.

Dale, B. A., Holbrook, K. A., and Steinert, P. M. 1978. Assembly of stratum corneum, basic protein and keratin filament in macrofibrils. Nature (Lond.) 276:729.

Elias, P. M., and Friend, D. S. 1975. The permeability barrier in mammalian epidermis. J. Cell Biol. 65:180.

Elias, P. M., McNutt, N. S., and Friend, D. S. 1977. Membrane alterations during cornification of mammalian squamous epithelia: A freeze-fracture, tracer and thin section study. Anat. Rec. 189:577.

Fraser, R. D. B., MacRae, T. P., and Rogers, G. E. 1972. Keratins. Their Composition, Structure and Biosynthesis. Springfield, Ill: C. C. Thomas.

Fuchs, E., and Green, H. 1979. Multiple keratins of cultured epidermal cells are translated from different mRNA molecules. Cell 17:573.

Hayward, A. F. 1979. Membrane coating granules. Int. Rev. Cytol. 59:97.

MacKenzie, I. C. 1972. The ordered structure of mammalian epidermis, In H. I. Maibach and D. T. Rovee (eds.), Epidermal Wound Healing. Year Book Medical Publishers, p. 5.

Montagna, W., and Lobitz, W. C., Jr. (eds.). 1964. The Epidermis. New York: Academic Press.

Rice, R. H., and Green, H. 1979. Presence in human epidermal cells of a soluble protein precursor of the cross-linked envelope: Activation of the cross-linking by calcium ions. Cell 18:681.

Steinert, P. M., Cantieri, J. S., Teller, D. C., Lonsdale-Eccles, J. D., and Dale, B. A. 1981. Characterization of a class of cationic proteins that specifically interact with intermediate filaments. Proc. Natl. Acad. Sci. U.S.A. 78:4097.

Steinert, P. M., and Idler, W. W. 1975. The polypeptide composition of bovine epidermal α-keratin. Biochem. J. 151:603.

Sun, T.-T., and Green, H. 1978. Keratin filaments of cultured human epidermal cells. Formation of intermolecular disulfide bonds during terminal differentiation. J. Biol. Chem. 253:2053.

Melanocyte

Fitzpatrick, T. B., Szabo, G., Seiji, M., and Quevedo, W. C., Jr. 1979. Biology of the melanin pigmentary system. In T. B. Fizpatrick, et al. (eds.) Dermatology in General Medicine, 2nd ed. New York: McGraw-Hill, p. 131.

Langerhans Cell

Katz, S., Tamaki, K., and Sachs, D. H. 1979. Epidermal Langerhans cells are derived from cells originating in bone marrow. Nature (Lond.) 282:324.

Shelley, W. B., and Lennart, J. 1978. The Langerhans cell: Its origin, nature and function. Acta Dermatovener. (Stockholm) Suppl. 79:7.

Merkel Cell

Winkelmann, R. K. 1977. The Merkel cell system and a comparison between it and the neurosecretory or APUD cell system. J. Invest, Dermatol. 69:41.

Dermal–Epidermal Junction and Interactions

Billingham, R. E., and Silvers, W. K. 1968. Dermal–epidermal interactions and epithelial specificity. In R. Fleischmayer and R. E. Billingham (eds.), Epithelial Mesenchymal Interactions. Baltimore: Williams and Wilkins Co., p. 252.

Briggaman, R. A., and Wheeler, C. E., Jr. 1975. The epidermal–dermal junction. J. Invest. Dermatol. 65:71.

Briggaman, R. A. 1982. Biochemical composition of the epidermal–dermal junction and other basement membranes. J. Invest. Dermatol. 78:1.

McLoughlin, C. B. 1963. Mesenchymal influences in epithelial differentiation. Symp. Soc. Exp. Biol. 17:359.

Yaoita, H., Foidart, J. -M., and Katz, S. I. 1978. Localization of the collagenous component in skin basement membrane. J. Invest. Dermatol. 70:191.

Dermis

Montagna, W., Bentley, J. P., and Robson, R. L. (eds.) 1970. The Dermis. Adv. Biol. Skin 10.

Stenn, K. S. 1979. Collagen heterogeneity of skin. Am. J. Dermatopathol. 1:87.

Cutaneous Vasculature

Braverman, I. M., and Yen, A. 1977. Ultrastructure of the human dermal microcirculation. II. The capillary loops of the dermal papillae. J. Invest. Dermatol. 68:44.

Winkelmann, R. K., Scheen, S. R., Jr., Pyka, R. A., and Coventry, M. B. 1961. Cutaneous vascular patterns in studies with injection preparation and alkaline phosphatase reaction. Adv. Biol. Skin 2:1.

Cutaneous Innervation

Montagna, W., and Brookhart, J. M. (eds.). 1977. Cutaneous Innervation and Modalities of Cutaneous Sensibility. Proceedings of the 26th Annual Symposium on the Biology of the Skin. J. Invest. Dermatol. 69:3.

Winkelmann, R. K. 1960. Nerve Endings in Normal and Pathologic Skin. Springfield, Ill.: C. C. Thomas, Publisher.

Hair Follicle

Montagna, W., and Robson, R. L. (eds.) 1969. Hair Growth. Adv. Biol. Skin 9.

Orwin, D. F. G. 1979. The cytology and cytochemisty of the wool follicle. Int. Rev. Cytol. 60:331.

Sebaceous Gland

Montagna, W., Bell, M., and Strauss, J. S. (eds.) 1974. Sebaceous Glands and Acne Vulgaris. J. Invest. Dermatol. 62:119.

Strauss, J. S., Pochi, P. E., and Downing, D. T. 1976. The sebaceous glands: Twenty-five years of progress. J. Invest. Dermatol. 67:90.

Apocrine Gland

Hurley, H. J., and Shelley, W. B. 1960. The Human Apocrine Sweat Gland in Health and Disease. Springfield, Ill.: C. C. Thomas, Publisher.

Eccrine Gland

Montagna, W., Ellis, R. A., and Silver, A. P. (eds.) 1962. Eccrine Sweat Gland and Eccrine Sweating. Adv. Biol. Skin 3:1.

Nails

Zaias, N., and Alvarez, J. 1968. The formation of the primate nail plate: An autoradiographic study in squirrel monkey. J. Invest. Dermatol. 51:120.

Zaias, N., and Baden, H. 1979. Nails. In T. B. Fitzpatrick, et al. (eds.), Dermatology in General Medicine. New York: McGraw-Hill Inc., p. 418.

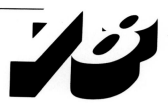

The Teeth

Hershey Warshawsky

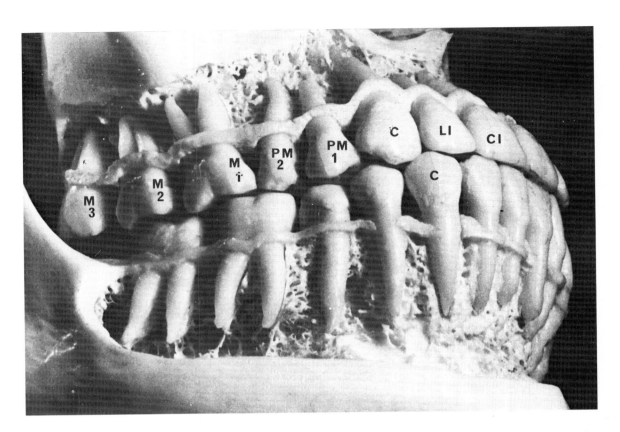

18–1 Skeletal preparation of the adult permanent dentition with the alveolar bone dissected to show the roots of the teeth. The eight teeth of the maxillary quadrant are labeled as follows: **CI**, central incisor; **LI**, lateral incisor; **C**, canine; **PM1**, first premolar; **PM2**, second premolar; **M1**, first molar; **M2**, second molar; **M3**, third molar. In the mandibular quadrant the third molar is absent.

The adult human dentition consists of 32 permanent teeth. The 16 upper teeth are embedded in the arch-shaped *alveolar processes* of the maxillae, whereas the lower teeth are embedded in the similarly shaped alveolar processes of the mandible (Fig. 18–1). The eight teeth within each half-arch, or *dental quadrant*, are differently shaped and somewhat specialized to carry out some aspect of mastication, or chewing. The central and lateral *incisors* are chisel-shaped cutting teeth. The single *canine* is a "grasping" tooth, which is highly specialized in carnivores such as lions, tigers, cats, and dogs. The two *premolars* and three *molars* have flattened occlusal surfaces that are effective in grinding the food. In

humans, the permanent dentition is preceded by a complete set of 20 *deciduous teeth*, also called *milk* or *baby* teeth (Fig. 18–2). The deciduous teeth begin to appear in the oral cavity at about 6 months of age, and the entire set of teeth is usually present by age 6 to 8 years. Beginning at about age 6, the baby teeth are shed and begin to "fall out." The deciduous dentition is replaced over a span of 10 to 12 years by the 32 permanent teeth, ending at about age 18 with the appearance of the third molar, which, because of the age of the individual, is called the wisdom tooth. Thus, in each quadrant of the deciduous dentition, which consists of five teeth, there are no baby forerunner teeth to the last three molars of the permanent dentition.

Each tooth, regardless of its external shape, consists of a *crown* and either a single or multiple *roots* (Fig. 18–3). By definition, the *anatomical crown* is covered by the highly calcified layer of *enamel*. The remainder of the crown is composed of another calcified tissue, the *dentin*, which contains a central chamber filled with the living tissue of the tooth, the *pulp*. The dentin

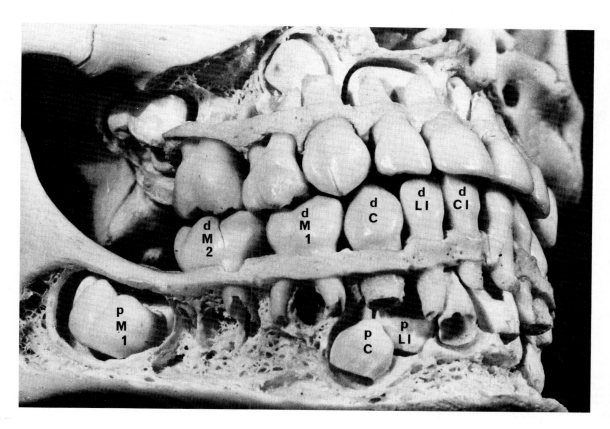

and pulp also constitute the tissues of the root. However, the outer surface of the root is covered by yet another calcified tissue called *cementum*. The enamel and cementum meet around the neck, or *cervical margin,* of the tooth and form the *cemento-enamel junction.* This junction is not normally seen on the portion of the tooth exposed to the oral cavity because the epithelial tissue covering the alveolar process, the *gingiva,* extends for a short distance onto the crown. Thus, the portion of the tooth actually seen in the mouth is called the *clinical crown* (Fig. 18–3).

18–2 Skeletal preparation of the deciduous dentition with alveolar bone removed to show the roots as well as the developing permanent teeth. The five baby teeth in the mandibular quadrant are labeled as follows: **dCI,** deciduous central incisor; **dLI,** deciduous lateral incisor; **dC,** deciduous canine; **dM1,** deciduous first molar; **dM2,** deciduous second molar. Root formation is not complete on the deciduous canine and molars. The developing permanent lateral incisor **(pLI),** permanent canine **(pC),** and permanent first molar **(pM1)** are seen in bony crypts. (Figures 18–1 and 18–2 courtesy of F. P. G. M. Van der Linden and H. S. Duterloo. *In* Development of the Human Dentition, An Atlas. Hagerstown, Md.: Harper and Row, 1976.)

Dental Nomenclature

Within the oral cavity, the surfaces of the teeth are identified by the structures that they face. Thus, in the dental quadrant, a particular tooth faces the tongue with its *lingual* surface, and the cheek or lips with its *buccal* or *labial* surface. The surface of the tooth closest to the midline is *mesial,* whereas the opposite surface is *distal* in regard to the center line of the quadrant. The surfaces that interact with the other teeth that oppose them in mastication are the *occlusal* surfaces. The tip of the roots at the opposite end of the tooth from the occlusal surface is the *apical end* because of the opening of a foramen, the *apical foramen,* which connects the *pulp canal* to the peridental tissues (Fig. 18–3).

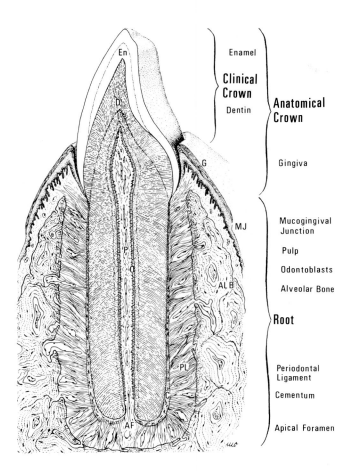

Enamel

**Clinical
Crown**

Dentin

**Anatomical
Crown**

Gingiva

Mucogingival
Junction

Pulp

Odontoblasts

Alveolar Bone

Root

Periodontal
Ligament

Cementum

Apical Foramen

18–3 Drawing of a longitudinal section through an erupted lower incisor. The arrangement into crown and root, and the relationship of the various dental tissues are shown.

History of Dental Histology

Dental histology has had a long and paradoxical history. The histological exploration of the "soft" tissues had to await the development of sophisticated embedding and sectioning methodology, whereas the "hard" tissues could easily be cut by fine saws into thin slabs that could then be ground by hand and polished into reasonably thin "sections." Because of this fortuitous situation, ground sections of teeth were among the first biological structures examined with the light microscope, as early as 1678 by Leeuwenhoeck. With the electron microscope, the use of geological replica techniques before plastic embedding methods were developed resulted in publications on tooth structure in 1944 by Gerould.

This lengthy history of scientific study, spanning three centuries, has led to a vast literature on the subject, which has caused both clarification and confusion. Consequently, we are still debating the status of various "classical" structural features. Because these doubtful features characterize ground sections of teeth, rather than decalcified or paraffin- or plastic-embedded sections, decalcified material will be described first. However, decalcification, as carried out with acids or chelating agents such as ethylenediaminotetraacetic acid (EDTA), completely removes the mature layer of enamel, and it is therefore impossible to study the structure of mature enamel in decalcified, routinely prepared sections.

Histological Structure of Dentin

Dentin forms the bulk of the tooth. It is lined on its outer aspect by enamel on the crown and by cementum on the root. Internally, the pulp occupies a *pulp chamber* in the crown and a *radicular pulp* or *root canal* in the root (Fig. 18–3). The pulp canal opens at the apical foramen, and

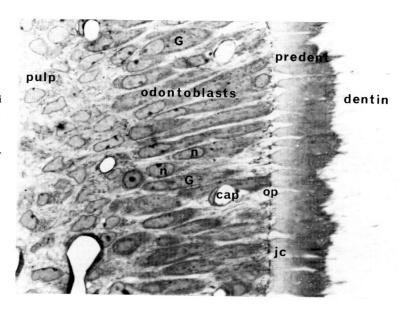

18–4 Odontoblasts at the periphery of the pulp. The columnar cells contain basal nuclei **(n)**, pale-staining Golgi regions **(G)**, and pale odontoblast processes **(op)**, which run through the predentin **(predent)** and the dentin. Junctional complexes **(jc)** delineate the cell bodies from the processes. The pulp contains undifferentiated cells and capillaries, which are also seen between odontoblast cell bodies **(cap)**. Rat incisor, × 700. (Courtesy of A. Nanci.)

the blood vessels, nerves, and lymphatics enter and leave the tooth via this opening. At the periphery of the pulp is a layer of cells that produce the dentin. They are called *odontoblasts* and are active secretory cells that synthesize and secrete the collagen and noncollagenous substances that form dentin.

Odontoblasts

These cells consist of a cell body and an elongated odontoblast process (Fig. 18–4).

Odontoblast Cell Body. The cell bodies form an irregularly columnar, epithelial-like layer on the inner aspect of the dentin. The proximal surface of the cell body is adjacent to pulp cells, and the distal extremity is tapered and embedded in *predentin*, an unmineralized layer of dentin-like material (Fig. 18–4). The process is prolonged as a narrowing, branched cytoplasmic extension enclosed within dentin in a canalicular system, the *dentinal tubule*. The large oval nucleus is contained in the proximal portion of the cell body. The level of the nucleus varies among the cell bodies, giving an irregularly staggered appearance to this layer. In certain regions, capillaries are present between the cell bodies close to the predentin (Fig. 18–4). The cytoplasm in the cell bodies is basophilic because of the abundance of rough-surfaced endoplasmic reticulum (RER), which fills the cytoplasm of the body but does

not extend into the tapered portion of the process within the predentin (Fig. 18–6). Also, a spherical region distal to the nucleus is usually devoid of RER, but it contains a well-developed Golgi apparatus. The RER is made up of parallel cisternae that are either narrow and flattened, or distended. The cisternal content is flocculent, or often irregularly filamentous, and is usually denser than the background cytoplasm (Fig. 18–5). The system of flattened *Golgi saccules* is roughly spherical. The outer surface is close to the RER and forms the *immature* or *cis face* of the apparatus. The *mature* or *trans face* of the Golgi sphere faces the center, which contains distended vacuoles and prosecretion granules (Fig. 18–5). A typical stack of Golgi saccules consists of three to five flattened saccules with distensions, particularly at the periphery of the upper two saccules. A series of stacks, placed edge to edge, forms the circular shape of the apparatus.

The distended portions of the mature saccules usually contain a tangled mass of threadlike filaments. As the distensions separate from the saccules, they become *prosecretion granules* and their content organizes into a blocklike unit in which the threads are aligned parallel to the longer axis of the block. The granules then decrease in size, and the blocklike units become condensed and acquire four to six dense beaded crossbands (Fig. 18–5). The beads along the threadlike strands resemble an abacus, and these granules were first called abacus bodies by Reith

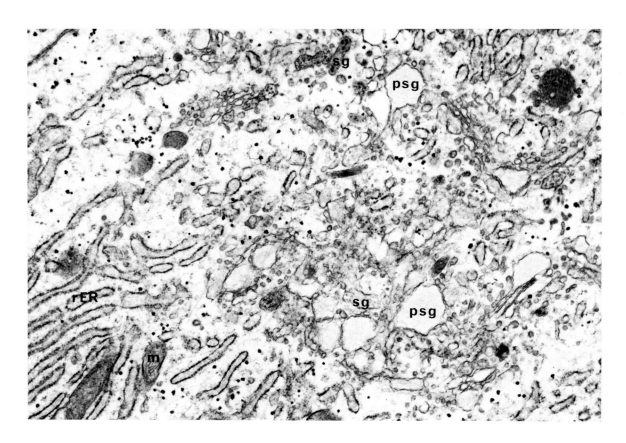

18–5 Electron micrograph of the odontoblast cell body showing the rough endoplasmic reticulum **(rER)** and the Golgi region. Mitochondria **(m)**, large prosecretion granules **(psg)**, and mature secretion granules **(sg)** are seen. Rat incisor, × 25,000.

(1968). They were then identified as secretion granules by Weinstock and Leblond (1974), using radioautography, and have been shown by immunohistochemical methods to contain procollagen (Karim et al., 1979). The mature secretion granules are found in the Golgi region as well as in the tapered odontoblast process (Fig. 18–6). Weinstock and Leblond (1974) demonstrated exocytosis of these granules along the odontoblast process. The liberated procollagen packets then undergo enzymatic cleavages at both ends to become tropocollagen macromolecules that aggregate extracellularly as banded, native dentinal collagen (see Chap. 4). The nature of the beadlike dense cross-banding material in the secretion granule has not been identified. In rare cases, bodies resembling the content of secretion granules (Fig. 18–8) have been seen in predentin and in mature dentin (Warshawsky, 1972; Weinstock, 1977). The significance of this finding, as either an artifact of preparation or an accident of nature, is unknown.

The junction of the cell body with the odontoblast process is marked by a cell web that is associated with a junctional complex (Figs. 18–4

18–6 Electron micrograph of odontoblast processes within the predentin. **jc**, junctional complexes; **m**, mitochondria; **sb**, side branches of odontoblast processes; **sg**, mature secretion granule. Rat incisor, × 15,000.

18–7 Freeze-fracture replica of odontoblast processes in the dentin. The dentinal tubules are either lined by E-face membranes or contain processes revealing their P face. The latter often show impressions of the collagenous fibrils of the tubule wall. **sb**, side branches coming off the main process. Rat incisor, × 12,000. (Courtesy of A. Nanci.)

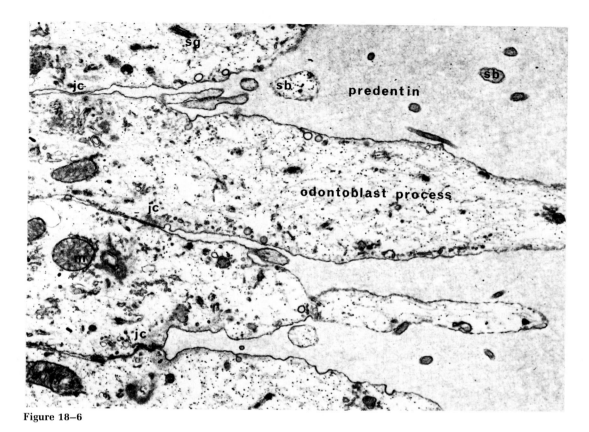

Figure 18–6

Figure 18–7

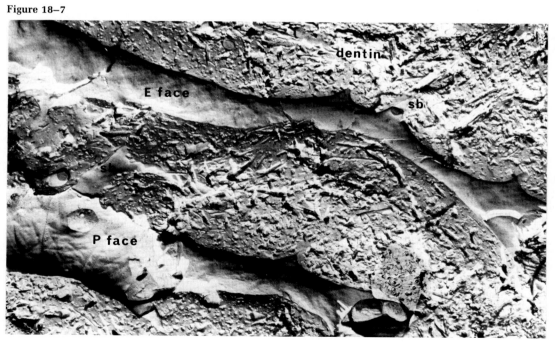

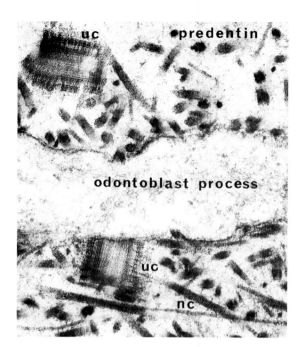

18–8 Unusual segments of fibrous long spacing collagen **(uc)** in the predentin close to an odontoblast process. Native collagen fibrils **(nc)** can be seen for comparison. Rat incisor, × 60,000.

and 18–6). In sections the complex resembles a modified zonula adherens. In freeze-fracture replicas only small circular gap junctions are found here as well as at other sites on the cell body (Weinstock, 1981).

Odontoblast Processes. These cytoplasmic, membrane-bound processes usually extend throughout the dentin, particularly in recently formed teeth (Figs. 18–6 and 18–7). However, in older teeth, some processes extend only part way toward the outer limits of the dentin, leaving empty dentinal tubules. These empty spaces may become filled with extracellular fluid and proteinaceous material, which can lead to calcification and eventual filling of the tubule.

At the origin of the odontoblast processes near the enamel or cementum, the processes are highly branched. They have been seen in ground sections to form a "granular layer," particularly in root dentin, because of the numerous sections through their branches (Ten Cate, 1972). The main process is wider toward the cell body, and the side branches are narrow and less numerous.

The cytoplasm contains microtubules, microfilaments, some small mitochondria, smooth membrane vesicular profiles, and secretion granules (Fig. 18–6). The granules may be close to the cytoplasmic membrane, and images of fusion of the granule membrane to the cell membrane can be seen (Weinstock and Leblond, 1974). There is no RER in the processes beyond the cell web (Fig. 18–6), accounting for the pale appearance in epoxy-embedded material stained with toluidine blue (Fig. 18–4).

The membrane of the process is closely associated with the dentinal collagen of the tubule wall (Fig. 18–6), and in freeze-fracture replicas the membrane is often criss-crossed by imprints of these collagenous fibril bundles (Fig. 18–7).

Predentin

The youngest layer of dentin formed at any particular time is adjacent to the junction between the odontoblast cell body and its major process (Figs. 18–4, 18–6, and 18–9). This layer of young dentin is essentially unmineralized, stains poorly with most dyes, and ends abruptly in contact with the mature dentin (Fig. 18–9). The thickness of this *predentin layer* is uniform in any tooth at a given moment of development. However, it tends to be thicker during rapid dentin formation and thinner during periods of slower dentin deposition. The predentin is an irregular meshwork of collagenous fibrils that tend to be thin closer to the cell body and somewhat larger in diameter near the mature dentin. The fibrils are faintly cross-banded and there is abundant extrafibrillar space with no formed elements. The predentin contains no glycoproteins as determined by the lack of PAS staining and no minerals, except for occasional small clusters of crystals near the dentin as seen with the electron microscope.

Dentin

The transition to mature dentin is very sudden. The demarcation is called the *frontier line,* or *mineralization front,* and is associated with the onset of PAS staining, an increased diameter of the collagenous fibrils, and a sudden and dramatic mineralization related to these fibrils (Fig. 18–9). In calcified sections, collagenous fibrils can be followed from the predentin, where they are clearly cross-banded, into the dentin, where

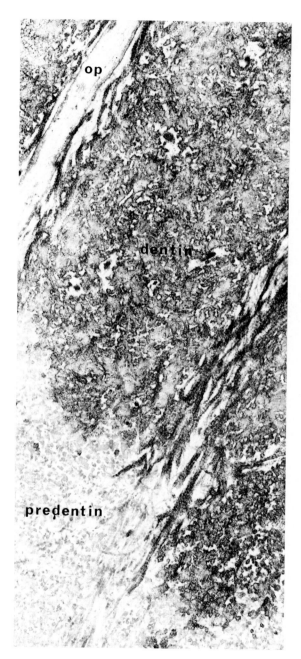

18–9 Electron micrograph of a decalcified tooth to show the difference between predentin and dentin. Electron-dense particles are associated with the collagenous fibrils of dentin, but not predentin. The collagenous fibrils lining the odontoblast process **(op)** and making up the walls of the dentinal tubule run parallel to the process, in contrast to the random arrangement elsewhere in the predentin and dentin. Rat incisor, × 18,000. (Courtesy of A. Nanci.)

they are nearly masked by the dense aggregation of small crystallites of hydroxyapatite. In demineralized sections, predentinal fibrils that can be followed into mature dentin become covered with small particles of electron-dense material, presumably organic in nature (glycoproteins or mucopolysaccharides). These particles are left on the fibrils after the crystallites are removed (Fig. 18–9) and, because they are added at the frontier line, they may be involved in the mineralization process.

The calcified collagenous fibrils of mature dentin are more or less uniform in size but larger in diameter than the uncalcified fibrils in predentin. They are heavily encrusted with hydroxyapatite crystallites. However, these fibrils remain randomly woven with no apparent organization except in relationship to the odontoblast process, where they tend to be oriented along its length (Fig. 18–9). These fibrils wrap the process lengthwise and form the actual wall of the dentinal tubule.

Occasionally, some thicker fibers, usually in bundles oriented perpendicularly to the surface of the dentin, have been described. These bundles seem to originate between odontoblasts. They are also mineralized but may have a somewhat different history from the usual collagenous fibrils. The special fibers are called *Korff's fibers*, but their significance is being questioned (see Ten Cate et al., 1970).

The layer of mature dentin is very thick in functional teeth, and, indeed, forms the bulk of the tooth.

Pulp

The most important constituent of the pulp is the layer of dentin-secreting odontoblasts (Figs. 18–3 and 18–4). The remainder of the pulp consists of a "stromal" tissue containing nerves, blood vessels, and lymphatics. The stromal tissue is composed of cells and extracellular material (Fig. 18–10). There appears to be only one type of cell, which is a rather primitive-looking cell, resembling mesenchyme but capable of producing extracellular material including collagen. Thus, the cell could be called a fibroblast, or simply a *pulpal cell*, since little agreement exists on nomenclature. The pulpal cell is irregularly stellate in shape, contains a variably placed nucleus, and has a paucity of organelles. It does, however, contain profiles of RER, Golgi saccules, and mi-

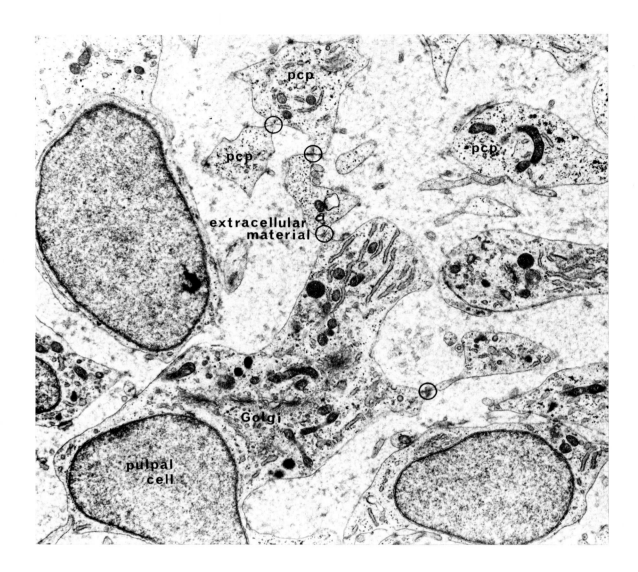

18–10 Electron micrograph of pulpal cells in the abundant extracellular material of the pulp. These cells are irregular in shape, contain some RER profiles and Golgi saccules, and show junctional contact with other pulpal cell processes (inside **circles**). **pcp**, pulpal cell process. Rat incisor, × 12,000. (Courtesy of A. Nanci.)

tochondria (Fig. 18–10). The processes of the pulpal cells contact each other as a "reticular network," and gap junctions are found at these contacts. Pulpal cells also contact odontoblast cell bodies (Fig. 18–4), but little is known about the relationship between these two cell types in a developing or functioning tooth. The intersti-

tial space between pulpal cells is filled with an amorphous material that stains with fast green, indicating the presence of collagen. This material is also metachromatic and stains with the PAS reaction. With the electron microscope (Figs. 18–10 and 18–11), the interstitial space is seen to contain small, randomly arranged fibrils, some of which are faintly cross-banded and resemble collagenous fibrils.

Blood vessels in the pulp enter through the apical foramen. They are small in diameter and resemble thin-walled arterioles. These vessels give off numerous branches that run toward the odontoblast layer and ramify as a capillary network among the odontoblast cell bodies (Fig.

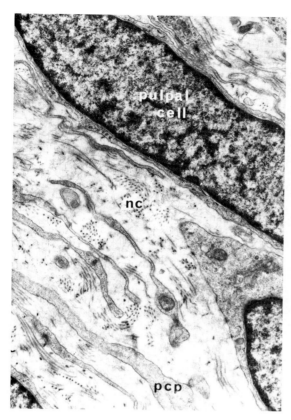

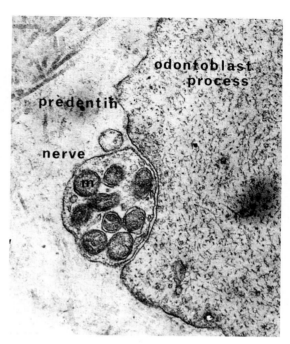

18–12 Unmyelinated nerve fiber related to an odontoblast process within the predentin. **m,** mitochondria. Human permanent premolar, × 61,000.

18–11 Electron micrograph of pulpal cells and their thin elongated processes **(pcp).** Native collagen fibrils **(nc)** are seen in the extracellular material. Human pulp, × 11,000.

18–4). Very thin-walled venules, of larger diameter than their companion arterioles, parallel the arterioles and leave the pulp at the apical foramen. Lymphatic vessels are difficult to identify, but they resemble the venules. The pulpal response to such trauma as physical damage to the vasculature at the apical foramen, or inflammation due to pathogenic invasion from tooth decay, or dental surgery is identical to the tissue response in other structures. Plasma seeping from capillaries leads to an edema in the extracellular space. In other tissues this inflammatory response causes local swelling and pain. In the pulp, because there is no room for swelling, an inflammation (pulpitis) will rapidly lead to death of the pulp by cutting off the blood supply.

Nerves are present in the pulp and supply the vessel walls and the odontoblasts. The larger nerve branches contain myelinated fibers and run along with the blood vessels. Smaller bundles of myelinated fibers can be followed to the odontoblasts, and unmyelinated nerve cell processes have been seen among odontoblast cell bodies and even along the odontoblast processes in predentin and dentin (Fig. 18–12). These free nerve endings mediate the only sensory modality from teeth: pain. Autonomic nerves, usually unmyelinated, innervate the walls of the blood vessels. Curiously, very few nerves are found in the pulp of the continuously erupting rat incisor (Bishop, 1980), and the distribution of nerves in human teeth is variable and seems to depend on the age of the tooth.

Cementum

The outer surface of the root is covered by a relatively thin layer of a bonelike mineralized tissue called cementum (Fig. 18–3). The cementum meets the enamel at a knife-edge abutment around the cervical or neck region of the tooth (Fig. 18–13). This junction is the *cemento-enamel junction* and separates the anatomical crown from the root. From this junction the ce-

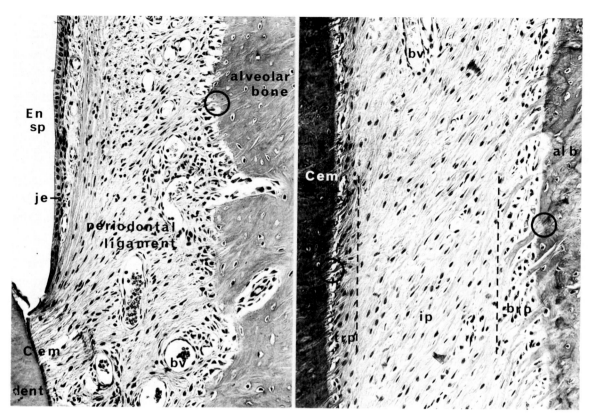

18–13 Periodontal ligament at the level of the cemento-enamel junction. Enamel occupied the enamel space **(En sp)** before decalcification. The junctional epithelium **(je)** was attached to the enamel surface. A thin layer of acellular cementum **(Cem)** covers the root dentin **(dent)**. Fibers of the periodontal ligament run from the cementum to the alveolar bone and insert as Sharpey's fibers (in the **circle**). Numerous blood vessels **(bv)** occupy spaces between bundles of ligament fibers. Monkey incisor, × 170.

18–14 Periodontal ligament at the level of the midportion of the root. Tooth-related portions of the ligament fibers **(trp)** originate from the cellular cementum. Bone-related portions of the fibers **(brp)** are inserted into the alveolar bone **(al b)**. The intermediate portion **(ip)** constitutes the major part of the ligament. Blood vessels **(bv)** are present between bundles of collagenous fibers. Sharpey's fibers, the calcified ends of collagenous fibers in cementum and bone, are seen within the **circles.** Dog molar, × 170.

mentum progressively thickens as it approaches the apical foramen and is thickest at the tip of the root. Cementum, like bone, consists of a matrix of calcified collagenous fibrils, glycoproteins, and mucopolysaccharides. The layer immediately adjacent to the dentin consists of a cementum without trapped cells (Stern, 1964). This layer of *acellular cementum* is thin, and it alone is present on the root close to the enamel. The layer of cementum thickens by adding cementum with osteocyte-like cells, the *cementocytes*, trapped in lacunae (Fig. 18–14). This *cellular cementum* resembles bone in all its structural fea-

tures. The outermost layer of cementum is an uncalcified precementum produced by the discontinuous layer of irregularly shaped *cementoblasts* (Fig. 18–15). The continuity of the cementoblast layer is disrupted by bundles of thick collagenous fibers from the *periodontal ligament*, which is the major suspensory ligament holding the teeth in the sockets of the alveolar bone. These fiber bundles run between cementoblasts and insert in the cementum layer that is actually secreted around them (Stern, 1964). This arrangement provides a firm anchoring for the tooth-related portion of these periodontal liga-

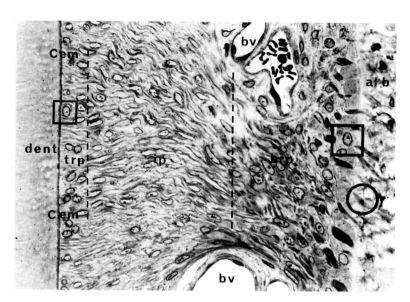

18–15 Periodontal ligament of the continuously erupting rat incisor. The three portions of the ligament fibers are well defined. Cementoblasts (in **small square**) are secreting cementum (**Cem**) adjacent to the dentin (**dent**), and osteoblasts (in **large square**) are secreting bone on the alveolar bone surface (**al b**). Within the **circle**, Sharpey's fiber; **brp**, bone-related portion; **bv**, blood vessel; **ip**, intermediate portion; **trp**, tooth-related portion. Rat incisor, × 480.

ment fibers. The fibers within the cementum usually calcify and can easily be seen in routine preparations as *Sharpey's fibers* (Fig. 18–14).

Cementum seems more resistant to resorption than bone, and normally no osteoclastic, or *cementoclastic,* activity is seen (except in root resorption during replacement of the deciduous dentition). Cementum is deposited slowly and more or less continuously.

Passive Eruption

The abrasive action of occlusion gradually causes the occlusal surfaces to wear down, thus, shortening the clinical crowns of opposing teeth. The resulting alteration in biting characteristics is manifested throughout the entire mouth and elicits a modest attempt to keep the clinical crowns a constant length. This is accomplished by a *passive eruption* caused by an increased deposition of cementum at the root tip. Because the width of the periodontal ligament space between the tooth and bone tends to remain constant, the additional cementum deposition pushes the tooth farther into the oral cavity. This phenomenon is particularly striking in such cultures as the Eskimo, where the women chew animal hides in order to soften the fur. The excessive abrasion causes the teeth to wear almost to the gingival margin. In these teeth, practically no crowns are left, and the roots consist almost entirely of cementum.

Periodontal Ligament

Human teeth are never directly fused to the bone that surrounds them. Such a fusion (ankylosis) is present in some animals, but it is not the most adaptive mechanism of anchoring teeth to bone. In humans the tooth is suspended from the bone via a complex collagenous ligament (Fig. 18–3). The fibers of this ligament are bundled together for strength, but spaces are present between bundles to allow blood vessels, nerves, and lymphatics to supply the tissues without being compressed by forces applied to the collagenous fibers. In essence, the ligament fiber bundles on the sides of the root extend from their cemental insertion in an *occlusal direction* toward a similar insertion on the alveolar bone (Figs. 18–13 to 18–15). The woven-type alveolar bone is secreted around the ends of the fiber bundles, which then calcify and are also called *Sharpey's fibers* (Fig. 18–14). The fiber bundles at the tip of the root run more or less directly to the alveolar bone nearest them. This organization provides a mechanism whereby the apically directed forces of occlusion are translated via the ligament fibers into a pull, or tension, on the alveolar bone. Thus, instead of a situation that could produce pressure on the bone near the root tip and lead to its resorption according to Wolff's law, a tension is produced on the side walls of the alveolar bone sockets. This tension favors a minimal deposition of bone on the alveolar wall and prevents the osteoclastic resorption of the bone around the root tip. The tensile strength and resilience of the ligament fibers give the teeth a certain mobility during occlusion and allow more chance for survival in cases of trauma.

Unlike other ligaments in the body, the periodontal ligament is a highly cellular, vascular, and metabolically active tissue, and its turnover rate is higher than that of other ligaments (Carneiro and de Moraes, 1965). This rapid renewal of constituents ensures a greater vitality for the tooth suspensory mechanism and provides for maintenance, repair, and a greater resistance to bacterial and pathogenic invaders from the oral cavity.

The collagenous fibers do not all extend uninterrupted between the tooth and bone. Conceptually, three divisions of ligament fibers can be drawn (Smith and Warshawsky, 1976): a tooth-related portion, a bone-related portion, and a so-called intermediate portion between them (Figs. 18–14 and 18–15). The tooth- and bone-related portions are more stable and may have a slower rate of turnover. The intermediate portion consists of younger and smaller-diameter collagenous fibers that are tentatively cross-linked, or otherwise attached to the ends of the more stable parts of the ligament. This intermediate portion is more cellular, and the fibroblasts here, as well as in the other portions, actively produce collagen. This collagen production can be demonstrated radioautographically after injection of radioactive proline (Carneiro and de Moraes, 1965), which is a prominent amino acid in collagen. In addition, the phagocytosis and degradation of collagen fibrils is evident in these fibroblasts (Ten Cate and Deporter, 1975; Beertsen and Everts, 1977; Beertsen et al., 1978). Thus, degradation of older fibrils and the formation of new ones by the same cellular population provide the mechanism for the active turnover. The fibroblasts are flattened cells, elongated in the direction of the collagenous fibers and closely associated with them. The cells contain much RER, a Golgi complex near their oval nuclei, and large phagosomes and phagolysosomes containing the ingested, clearly cross-banded collagen fibrils.

It can be imagined that newly aggregated fibrils would cross-link with older tooth- and bone-attached fibrils, whereas older attachments would be broken by some degradative mechanism (perhaps enzymes) and the liberated fibrous debris would be scavenged by fibroblasts and broken down by their lysosomal enzymes.

This dynamic making and breaking of fibrous attachment provides strength and at the same time permits turnover or minor tooth movement. This feature is utilized in orthodontic tooth movement where forces applied to the teeth favor the predominant breakdown of some fibrils and their "repair" without disrupting the general attachment of the tooth. This aspect of periodontal ligament dynamics is particularly important in the continuously erupting rodent incisor. Here, the tooth-related portions of the ligament fibers migrate with the erupting incisor, whereas the bone-related fibers remain stationary (Smith and Warshawsky, 1976). The intermediate portion makes and breaks fibrous connections continuously, thus maintaining a strong attachment and yet providing the mobility necessary to permit the tooth to erupt. Indeed, this repeated attachment, concomitant with the contraction in length that is known to occur in maturing collagenous fibers, is thought to be the mechanism responsible for the continuous eruption of rodent incisors.

Alveolar Bone

The alveolar processes of the maxillae and mandible function as the insertion for the periodontal ligament fibers (Figs. 18–3 and 18–13 to 18–15). Thus, histologically they resemble bone seen at other ligamentous insertions. The bone is made up of woven collagenous fibrils that surround and hold the ligament fibers, which also calcify and become part of the bone (Sharpey's fibers). Osteocytes (Fig. 18–16) are numerous, and vascular channels permeate the bone. The surfaces of the bone devoid of ligament insertions are lined by osteoblasts adjacent to prebone. Osteoclasts are present along some areas of the bone, indicating resorption, which is, however, balanced toward a net deposition because of the tension exerted on the ligament fibers during occlusion.

Gingiva

The lining of the oral cavity is an extension of the skin and a transition to the inner lining of the gastrointestinal tract. The stratified squamous keratinized epithelium of the face is continuous over the reddish lips. The color change is due to the loss of keratinization and heightened papillae of connective tissue, which bring capillaries closer to the surface. The lip is a region of tran-

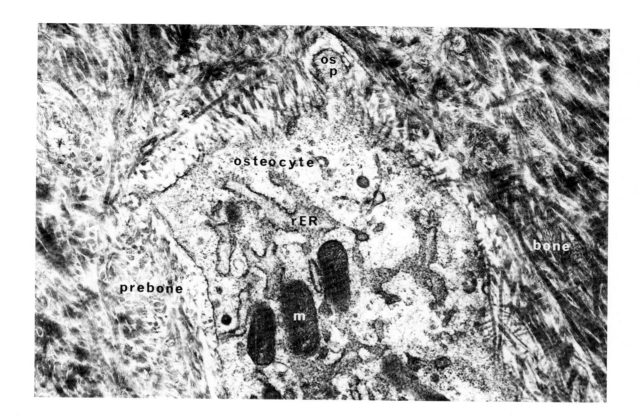

18–16 Osteocyte of the alveolar bone at the junction between prebone and bone. The osteocyte occupies the entire lacuna, and osteocyte processes **(os p)** extend from the cell into canalicules radiating from the lacuna. **m,** mitochondria; **rER,** rough endoplasmic reticulum. Rat incisor alveolar bone, × 30,000.

sition between skin and the stratified squamous nonkeratinized epithelium of the mucosa that lines the oral aspects of the lips and cheeks. This wet-surface epithelium is reflected around the vestibule onto the outer surface of the alveolar bone. As it approaches the teeth, this deep red mucosal layer meets a firm, pinkish layer at a scalloped outer *muco-gingival junction*. The firm epithelium from this line to the teeth is the *gingiva* (Fig. 18–3). It extends around each tooth, and on the mandible it covers the inner aspect of the alveolar bone and again meets the regular oral mucosa at a less well defined inner muco-gingival junction. On the maxillae, the gingiva lines the entire *hard palate* forming the roof of the mouth.

Gingiva is a stratified squamous epithelium with deep papillary projections from the underlying lamina propria (Figs. 18–17 and 18–18). The latter contains a rich capillary network that is consequently brought relatively close to the surface. The epithelium is firmly attached to the lamina propria by *hemidesmosomes* related to the basal lamina and collagenous *anchoring fibrils* that originate from the hemidesmosomes

and form loops in the lamina propria. Collagenous fibrils from the lamina propria itself pass through these loops, thus contributing to the firm attachment between the two tissues (Susi, 1969). The basal layer of the epithelium is cuboidal and shows numerous mitotic figures, which provide for the renewal of this epithelium. The cells of the stratum spinosum above the germinative layer are polyhedral. They are firmly attached to each other by many large desmosomes situated at the ends of cellular extensions that project into an extracellular space between cells (Listgarten, 1964). The innermost plaque of each desmosome provides insertion for bundles of tonofilaments that run in the cytoplasm of the cells as an extensive network. Toward the surface of the epithelium, the cells flatten to form a com-

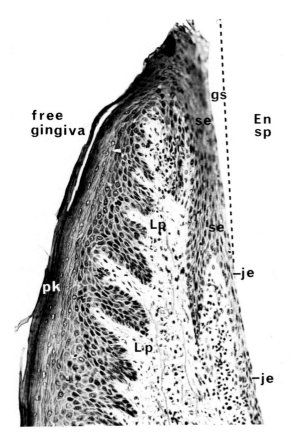

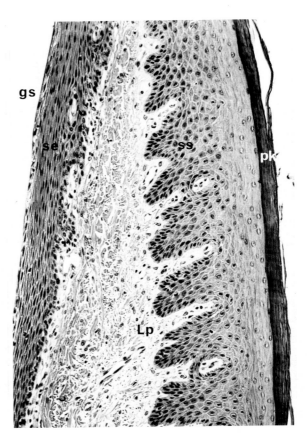

18–17 Free gingiva showing the parakeratinized stratified squamous epithelium **(pk)** on the oral surface. This epithelium is reflected over the gingival crest to become the sulcular epithelium **(se)**, which lines the gingival sulcus **(gs)** lying between the epithelium and the enamel (enamel space, **En sp**). The sulcular epithelium becomes the junctional epithelium **(je)**, which is attached to the enamel surface. Deep papillae of lamina propria **(Lp)** are seen on the oral side, but no projections are present on the tooth-related side. Chronic inflammatory cells are present in the lamina propria beneath the sulcular and junctional epithelia. Monkey, × 170.

18–18 The fully developed free gingiva consists of a thick layer of stratified squamous epithelium **(ss)**, with deep papillary projections of lamina propria **(Lp)**. The surface dozen or more layers are flattened, but they often retain their nuclei and form a deeply stained parakeratinized layer **(pk)**. No stratum granulosum is evident. The sulcular epithelium **(se)** lining the gingival sulcus **(gs)** is thinner, lacks papillary projections, and consists of many layers of loosely packed squamous cells. The lamina propria contains blood vessels and connective tissue, which is loose in the papillae but denser near the sulcular epithelium. Monkey, × 170.

pact layer in which the cells are partially filled with keratin but the nucleus and some organelles survive. Thus, the dozen or so cell layers at the surface are keratinized but not dead, and some thin, very flat nuclei remain. This layer stains with eosin and is thick and almost homogenous in appearance on the surface of the gingiva (Fig. 18–18). These half-dead, half-alive cells desquamate at the surface.

This epithelium differs from that of the skin where cells are keratinized at the level of the granulosum cells, which contain keratohyalin granules. The granulosum cells then die and the resulting layer of dead, cornified cells forms the dry surface of the skin. This "normal" state of keratinization is called *orthokeratosis*, as compared with the gingival process, which is called *parakeratosis* by contrast. Thus, the parakeratinized gingiva lacks a distinct stratum granulosum and has a thick, dense layer of flattened cells that still contain nuclei and are presumably alive. These living cells desquamate into the oral cavity. Gingiva is a strong resilient epithelium that turns over rapidly enough to withstand and heal the trauma and abrasion caused by chewing hard foods.

Relationship of the Gingiva to the Teeth

The lamina propria of the gingiva is firmly attached to the periosteum of the alveolar bone except as it approaches to within 1 or 2 mm of the crown surface. This narrow band of gingiva surrounding each tooth is called the *"free gingiva"* as opposed to the rest of the gingiva, which is *"attached"* to the alveolar bone. In a healthy mouth, the junction between the free and attached gingiva on the oral surface is marked by the shallow *free gingival groove*. The free gingiva forms the *interdental papillae* between adjacent teeth. The space (or potential space) between the free gingiva and the surface of the crown is called the *gingival sulcus* (Fig. 18–17). The epithelium lining the gingival sulcus is called *sulcular epithelium* and is thinner than the epithelium on the oral surface of the free gingiva. There are no papillary projections from the lamina propria, and the surface facing the sulcus consists of a few layers of very flattened, nonkeratinized squamous cells (Figs. 18–17 and 18–18).

The sulcular epithelium continues as the *junctional epithelium*, which is actually attached to the surface of the tooth (Figs. 18–17 and 18–19). Junctional epithelium ends by abutting on the cementum and the periodontal ligament (Fig. 18–13). The surface in contact with the tooth, which is technically the outer surface of the stratified squamous epithelium, becomes specialized. It reverts to a situation seen in the oral epithelium during tooth development (see Fig. 18–51), whereby these surface cells elaborate a layer of material that resembles a thick basal lamina both in electron-microscopic structure (Fig. 18–19) and in PAS staining. This "cuticle" is in firm contact with the enamel surface and is attached to the surface cells of the junctional epithelium by *hemidesmosomes* (Fig. 18–19). Hemidesmosomes are responsible for the attachment of the gingiva as a continuous cuff around the tooth (Listgarten, 1966; Schroeder and Listgarten, 1971). This attached cuff fulfills the essential function of sealing off the access route from the mouth to the periodontal tissues. Breakdown of this seal results in gingival infections (gingivitis) and invasion by microorganisms, leading to periodontal disease. Even in

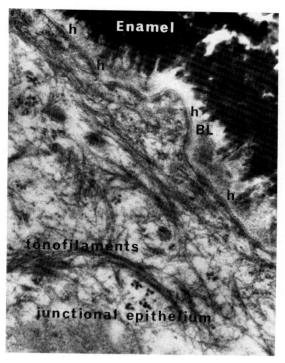

18–19 Electron micrograph of the surface cell in the junctional epithelium and its contact with the surface of the tooth. Numerous tonofilaments within the cytoplasm are associated with the hemidesmosomes **(h)** between the cell and the basal lamina like material **(BL)** on the surface of the enamel. Human tooth, × 44,000.

"normal" mouths, the chronic inflammatory potential causes large numbers of polymorphonuclear leukocytes and other defense cells to be present in the lamina propria of the gingiva (Fig. 18–17).

Tooth Development

The teeth begin to develop as early as the sixth week of gestation. The embryonic dental arch consists of a layer of stratified ectoderm separated by a basal lamina from the subepithelial connective tissue, which is presumably derived from cranial neural crest cells (Fig. 18–20a). This "neural crest mesoderm" contains neural cells believed to possess messages that initiate tooth formation (Slavkin, 1979a). Clusters of these inductive neuroectodermal cells accumulate at 10 separate sites in the arch and induce the overlying epithelial cells to proliferate locally and form swellings, the *epithelial tooth buds*, correspond-

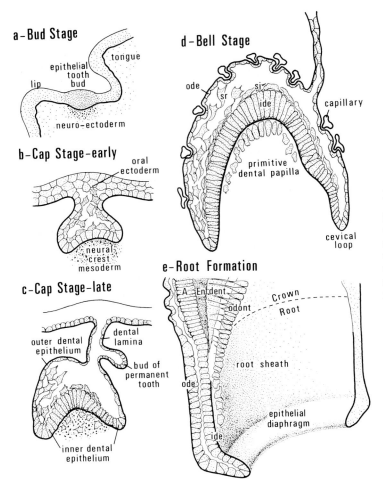

a-Bud Stage

tongue
epithelial
tooth
bud
lip
neuro-ectoderm

b-Cap Stage-early

oral
ectoderm

neural
crest
mesoderm

c-Cap Stage-late

outer dental
epithelium

dental
lamina

bud of
permanent
tooth

inner dental
epithelium

d-Bell Stage

ode
sr
si
ide
capillary

primitive
dental papilla

cevical
loop

e-Root Formation

A En dent
odont
Crown
Root

ode

root sheath

epithelial
diaphragm

ide

18–20 Drawing of various stages in tooth development. Sequence in the formation of a lower incisor is depicted. **A**, ameloblast; **dent**, dentin; **En**, enamel; **ide**, inner dental epithelium; **ode**, outer dental epithelium; **Odont**, odontoblast; **si**, stratum intermedium; **sr**, stellate reticulum. The thick **black line** represents the basal lamina.

ing to each of the 10 deciduous teeth. These buds proceed along identical developmental paths at different times of gestation so that in any particular embryo various stages of tooth development can be found. The developmental process will be described for a specific tooth, a lower central incisor.

Development from "Bud" to "Cap" Stage

Cells within the localized epithelial swelling for the tooth continue to divide and begin to invaginate into the underlying connective tissue, drawing with them the epithelial basal lamina (Fig. 18–20b). The thin cellular stalk that connects the downward-growing cells with the epithelium is called the *dental lamina*. The bulb of cells at the growing end of the dental lamina expands and flattens. At its undersurface, a shallow invagina-

tion occurs that pushes the cell layer into itself to form a caplike structure (the *cap stage*), with the stalk being attached to the outer aspect of the cap (Fig. 18–20b,c). The outer aspect is continuous around the rim of the cap with the inner aspect, which is now a concavity filled with cells of the neural crest mesoderm. The cap is the beginning of the *odontogenic organ*, which will first form the entire anatomical crown of the tooth. After the crown is completed, it will fulfill the remaining odontogenic or tooth-forming potential by forming the root of the tooth. From the thin stalk of the dental lamina, another outbudding of cells and basal lamina occurs off to one side. This *bud of the permanent tooth* (Fig. 18–20c) will remain dormant for a long time; it will then begin to develop into the crown of the permanent tooth in preparation for the replacement of the deciduous or baby tooth.

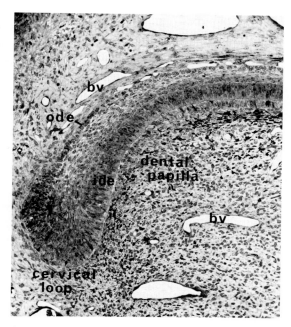

18–21 A stage in the development of the rat incisor that resembles the cap stage. The outer dental epithelium **(ode)**, outside the cap, is reflected at the cervical loop onto the inner aspect of the cap as the inner dental epithelium **(ide)**. The concavity of the cap contains the dental papilla, which differentiates into odontoblasts adjacent to the enamel organ. **bv,** blood vessel. Rat incisor, × 110.

A section through the developing cap of the baby tooth (Fig. 18–20c) shows that the basal lamina of the epithelium is continuous over the dental lamina and surrounds both surfaces of the cap. Thus, the cap consists entirely of epithelium (Figs. 18–21 and 18–22). The epithelial cells on the basal lamina are in direct continuity with the cells of the stratum germinativum of the oral epithelium. These cells maintain their mitotic potential and divide to make the cap increase in size (Fig. 18–22). The epithelium on the outer surface of the cap is the *outer dental epithelium.* The continuation of this layer on the inner aspect is called the *inner dental epithelium.* The epithelial cells that fill the interval between the two epithelial layers are poorly differentiated at this stage. The connective tissue within the concavity of the cap is separated from the epithelium by the basal lamina. The connective tissue forms the *primitive dental papilla,* which is to give rise to the odontoblasts and the pulp of the tooth.

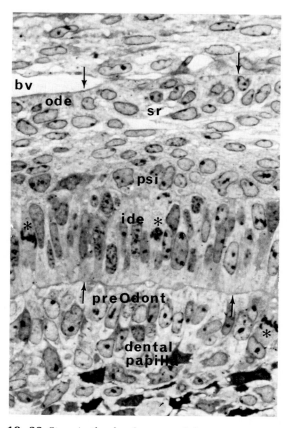

18–22 Stage in the development of the rat incisor resembling the transition from late cap to early bell stage (similar to Fig. 18–20d). The enamel organ consists of the epithelial tissue between the two sets of arrows. The continuous basal lamina is seen adjacent to the outer dental epithelium **(ode, arrows** pointing down) and adjacent to the inner dental epithelium **(ide, arrows** pointing up). The differentiating layers of cells between the dental epithelia are the provisional stratum intermedium **(psi)** and the stellate reticulum **(sr).** Preodontoblasts **(pre Odont)** are forming from cells of the dental papilla adjacent to the basal lamina of the inner dental epithelium. Numerous mitotic figures **(asterisks)** are seen. **bv,** blood vessel. Rat incisor, × 600.

Development from "Cap" to "Bell" Stage

With continued growth, by about 2 months of gestation, the cap transforms into a bell-like structure (the *bell stage*), which resembles in shape the crown of the primary tooth that is forming (Fig. 18–20d). The outer dental epithelium is a low cuboidal epithelium. It is not smooth, but is ridged by a network of capillaries that depresses its surface. The capillaries are thus brought close to the developing epithelial odontogenic organ, but they are always separated from the epithelial cells by the epithelial and endothelial basal laminae. The outer dental epithelium reflects around the rim of the bell to form the inner dental epithelium on the inner surface of the bell. The rim of the bell where the two epithelial layers reflect is called the *cervical loop* because this point will form the cervix or neck between the crown and root. It will also mark the site of the future cemento-enamel junction.

The inner dental epithelium continues to respond to the inductive stimuli of the neural crest elements and develops into a regular, simple columnar cell layer; cells in this layer are destined to become the enamel-secreting *ameloblasts*. At this time the intervening epithelial cells between the inner and outer dental epithelia begin to differentiate into two layers. One or two cell layers adjacent to the columnar inner dental epithelial cells develop into the cuboidal *provisional stratum intermedium* (Fig. 18–22). The rest of the cells are stellate in shape and form a meshwork with much intercellular space. This *stellate reticulum* is a fluid-filled intraepithelial layer that may offer a hydrostatic protective cushion to the developing inner dental epithelium.

The four epithelial layers thus defined form an organ whose main function becomes the direct formation of enamel and the indirect induction of dentin formation. The organ is therefore "odontogenic," but it is customarily called the *enamel organ* to reflect its immediate and most evident function.

Further Development of the Inner Dental Epithelium

This columnar layer of cells undergoes a remarkable series of differentiations that over a considerable length of time, are responsible for the production of enamel. The various stages in this production, called *amelogenesis*, constitute the life cycle of these cells. For convenience and for lack of consensus, these cells are known from this stage on as the *ameloblasts*, and their various stages are named by applying descriptive modifiers to the name. Strictly speaking, "ameloblast" means enamel-forming cell; however, only part of the ameloblast life cycle is occupied with the actual secretion of enamel. The cells so engaged are called *secretory ameloblasts*. Before they secrete enamel, the cells are called *presecre-*

tory ameloblasts. After the layer of enamel is secreted, the cells participate in poorly understood activities collectively called *maturation*, and the cells are called *maturative ameloblasts*.

The entire enamel organ is destroyed during the process of eruption, which pushes the fully formed crown through the enamel organ, through

---

18–23 Various stages in the development of enamel (amelogenesis) as seen in the rat incisor, **A,** ameloblast; **bv,** blood vessel; **ode,** outer dental epithelium; **Odont,** odontoblast; **psi,** provisional stratum intermedium; **si,** stratum intermedium; **sr,** stellate reticulum. × 600.

a. Presecretory ameloblasts, still referred to as inner dental epithelium **(ide)** are related to undifferentiated preodontoblasts **(pre Odont).** The embryonic base of the epithelial cells is in contact with the basal lamina **(BL).** The embryonic apex is adjacent to the provisional stratum intermedium. The stellate reticulum and outer dental epithelium are distinguishable. **Asterisk,** mitotic figure.

b. Presecretory ameloblasts showing reversed, or functional polarity. The odontoblasts have secreted the mantle predentin (predent).

c. Initial enamel **(En)** is secreted by the ameloblasts adjacent to a layer of mineralized dentin **(dent).** The ameloblasts show high- and low-level nuclei, and their functional base is adjacent to the definitive stratum intermedium. **predent,** predentin.

d. Fully functional ameloblasts have secreted a thick layer of inner enamel. These cells show Tomes' processes, a wide supranuclear region, two levels of nuclei, and mitochondria in an infranuclear position.

e. Ameloblasts that secrete outer enamel have slender Tomes' processes and are more tilted in relation to the enamel surface.

f. After secreting the final enamel layer, the ameloblasts reorganize their morphology and many cells die. The debris is seen as dark globules phagocytized by the living ameloblasts and the cells of the papillary layer.

g. Ameloblasts with a striated-like border make up 80% of the cell population in the maturation zone. Mitochondria cause the dark staining beneath the striated-like border and in the infranuclear region. The papillary layer is maximally developed. The enamel is now mature and is completely removed during decalcification leaving an enamel space.

h. Ameloblasts with smooth apexes occupy 20% of the maturation zone. They form narrow strips that alternate with wide bands of cells with striated-like borders. There is a wider intercellular space between these smooth-apex ameloblasts.

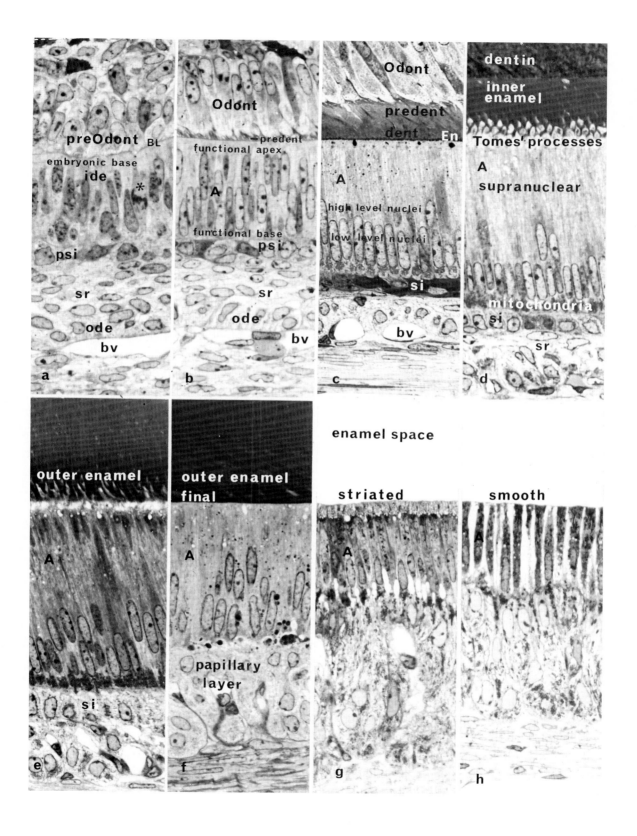

the gingiva, and into the oral cavity. Thus, a study of the ameloblast layer permits a detailed analysis of the birth-to-death life cycle of this cell type. This is possible in humans by analyzing the teeth at various stages of their development from a large number of embryos of different ages. This difficult sampling procedure leaves many gaps of information and, even if nonhuman primates are used, it does not allow for convenient experimental manipulation. Fortunately, the incisors of rodents like the common laboratory rat offer an unique system for such a study because these teeth are growing and erupting continuously while being worn down at the same rate by attrition. Thus, in each incisor at any time, the entire life history from birth to death is revealed in the ameloblast layer on the surface of the tooth. In any longitudinal section all the stages of this cycle can be analyzed (Warshawsky and Smith, 1974), and the transformations from one stage to another can be carefully documented (Fig. 18–23). By correlating these studies with the limited number of studies on developing human teeth, the exact sequence of formation of the human tooth can be deduced (Matthiessen and Rømert, 1980a,b).

Development from Presecretory to Early Secretory Stage of Amelogenesis

In the earliest stages of development, when the cells are still referred to as inner dental epithelial cells, they are a columnar layer with two or three staggered levels of elongated oval nuclei (Fig. 18–23a). The embryonic base is in contact with the basal lamina, and the opposite end, or apex, is in contact with cells of the provisional stratum intermedium (Fig. 18–23a). (The orientation of the cells in Fig. 18–23 is reversed from the orientation in Fig. 18–22. Although the orientation in Fig. 18–23 is correct for a developing lower incisor, the ameloblasts in all subsequent figures are shown as secretory cells, which by convention are depicted with their functional apexes toward the top of the figure.) The embryonic or original polarity is reversed in later differentiation because the enamel will ultimately be secreted out of the "base" of the cell, which will thus become the *functional apex* while the opposite end becomes the *functional base* (Fig. 18–23b). The reversal of polarity is manifested by the displacement of nuclei toward the functional base and a migration of the Golgi elements

into a position between the nucleus and the basal lamina. At the early stages, this *supranuclear compartment* is short; further differentiation leads to a lengthening of the cell, primarily at the supranuclear level. The cells continue to elongate up to the beginning of enamel secretion, and the organelles assume a layered distribution (Fig. 18–23c,d,e). During the period of elongation, the apical cell membrane is smooth and close to the basal lamina. Inductive messages from the ameloblasts cause the adjacent cells of the primitive dental papilla to differentiate into odontoblasts. Although derived from the neural crest cells, the odontoblasts secrete the collagen and other substances of dentin. With the presence of the first layer of predentin, the presecretory ameloblasts differentiate further toward secretory ameloblasts. As the first predentin mineralizes to become dentin, the ameloblasts begin to secrete mineralized enamel. Thus, the dentino-enamel junction is delineated by both mineralized tissues.

Once formed, the junction has its definite shape for that particular tooth. The further deposition of dentin pushes the odontoblasts into the pulp, whereas the continued deposition of enamel pushes the enamel organ outward to the connective tissue surrounding the developing tooth (Figs. 18–20e, 18–24, and 18–25).

Interaction Between the Presecretory Ameloblasts and the Cells of the Primitive Dental Papilla

Experiments using cultures of enamel organs separated from primitive dental papillae by millipore filters have demonstrated that inductive messenger molecules are produced by the ameloblasts and pass across the basal lamina (see review in Slavkin, 1979b). These molecules induce the adjacent stellate primitive-looking cells of the dental papilla to differentiate into low columnar preodontoblasts next to the basal lamina (Figs. 18–22 and 18–23a). Immediately after differentiating, the odontoblasts secrete the first layer of predentin against the epithelial basal lamina (Fig. 18–23b). The collagen fibrils are nearly perpendicular to the basal lamina and radiate like a fan from between the apexes of the odontoblasts. Concomitantly, the apexes start to elongate and form the beginning of the odontoblast processes. The presence of this first layer of

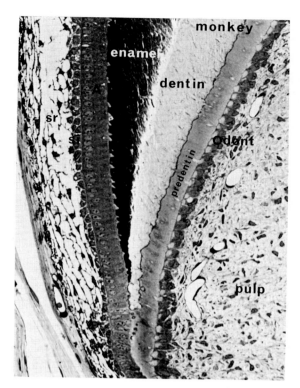

18–24 Developing crown of a monkey lower second premolar close to the cervical loop. This figure is diagrammatically depicted in the crown part of Fig. 18–20e. **A,** ameloblasts; **si,** stratum intermedium; **sr,** stellate reticulum. × 256.

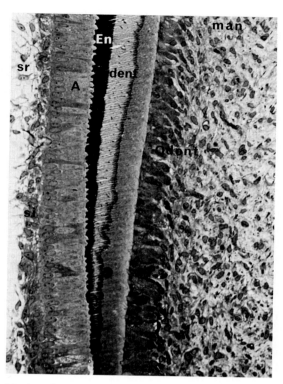

18–25 Identical region of a forming human crown as seen in Figs. 18–20e (crown) and 18–24. **A,** ameloblasts; **dent,** dentin; **En,** enamel; **si,** stratum intermedium; **sr,** stellate reticulum. × 256.

predentinal matrix triggers responses in the adjacent ameloblasts. The apical membrane becomes deeply infolded, and finger-like projections extend across the basal lamina (Kallenbach, 1976). These projections insinuate between the collagenous fibrils and many come into contact with cellular projections of the odontoblasts. Evidence also suggests that the ameloblasts endocytose and resorb the basal lamina (Kallenbach, 1976). With the rapid disappearance of the lamina, short cellular projections from the ameloblast apexes fill the spaces between the ends of the collagenous fibrils of the predentin (Fig. 18–26). This interdigitation determines the pattern for the dentino-enamel junction. As more predentin is secreted, the first-formed matrix mineralizes and becomes dentin. At the same time the ameloblast projections begin to withdraw, leaving behind secretory material resembling mineralized enamel at the scalloped dentino-enamel junction (Figs. 18–27 to 18–29).

The ameloblasts attain their maximal height during enamel secretion. In the rat incisor, two configurations of enamel are produced: the *inner enamel* is formed first (Fig. 18–23d), then the *outer enamel* (Fig. 18–23e). The tall columnar secretory cells of the rat incisor are in many respects similar to the much shorter ameloblasts in human tooth development (compare Figs. 18–30 and 18–31). In both species the cytoplasm can be divided into *infranuclear, nuclear, supranuclear,* and *apical* portions (Figs. 18–30 and 18–31). The portion of the cell between the nucleus and the cell base is the infranuclear cytoplasm (Figs. 18–23d, 18–30, 18–31, and 18–34). Because this end was formerly the cell apex, a junctional complex and cell web develop close to the base. This *proximal junctional complex* (Fig. 18–38) and the *proximal cell web* subdivide

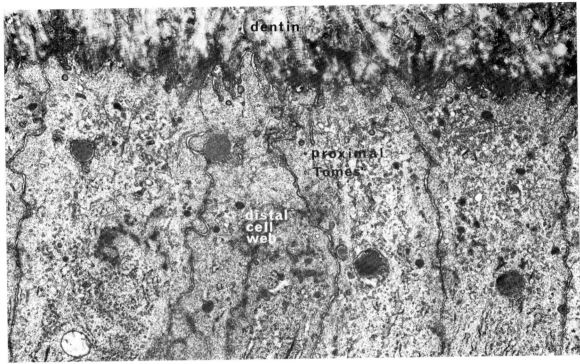

Figure 18–26

Figure 18–27

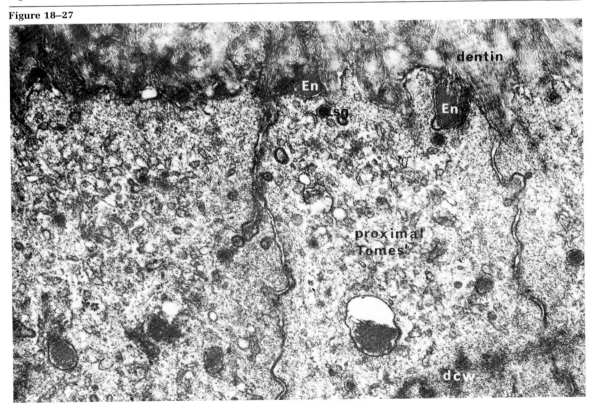

18–26 Before enamel is secreted, the presecretory ameloblasts have developed the proximal portions of Tomes' processes. The distal cell web delimits the process from the supranuclear cytoplasm. Finger-like projections of the ameloblast surface extend between the collagenous fibrils of the mantle dentin. Rat incisor, × 15,000.

18–27 At the beginning of enamel formation, small clumps of enamel **(En)** are deposited on the mineralized dentin. Some secretion granules **(sg)** are seen in the proximal portions of Tomes' processes. Rat incisor, × 30,000.

row in cells that contain nuclei further removed from the cell base, the *high-level nuclei* (Figs. 18–23c,d,e and 18–30). The supranuclear cytoplasm (Figs. 18–30, 18–31, and 18–35) contains much RER in closely packed cisternae parallel to the long axis of the cell. It also contains the extensive Golgi apparatus, which in the rat incisor ameloblast forms a central tubular-shaped structure (Kallenbach et al., 1963) with stacks of flattened saccules making the walls of the tubule (Figs. 18–30 and 18–35). The outer or cis surface is adjacent to the RER, whereas the inner or trans surface faces cytoplasm that contains few organelles except for some secretion granules, lyso-

the infranuclear cytoplasm into a small *basal bulge* and a large *mitochondrial compartment* (closer to the nucleus, Figs. 18–23d, 18–30, 18–31, and 18–34). The larger compartment houses most of the cell's mitochondria in the rat incisor (Fig. 18–34; Warshawsky, 1968), but not in the human ameloblast (Fig. 18–31; Matthiessen and Rømert, 1978). The mitochondrial compartment is short and as wide as the cell body in those cells with nuclei close to the base, the *low-level nuclei*. However, it is longer and quite nar-

18–28 With the formation of a more or less complete layer of initial enamel, large droplets of enamel-like material accumulate between the proximal portions of Tomes' processes. This material is homogeneous, rather than streaked by light clefts as is the initial enamel, and it may not be a direct precursor to enamel. However, these droplets occupy the space into which prongs of enamel will form to delineate the interdigitating portions of Tomes' processes (see Fig. 18–29). Rat incisor, × 30,000.

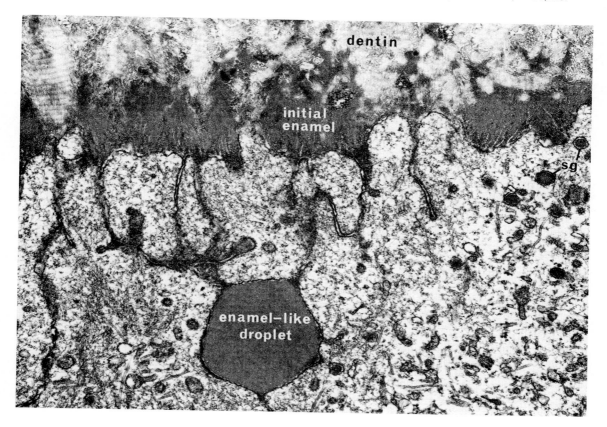

dentin

initial enamel

sg

enamel-like droplet

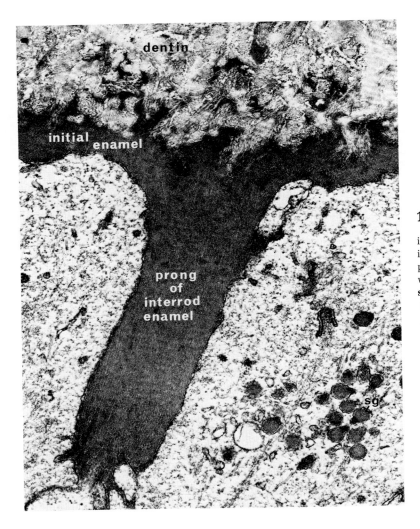

18–29 Prongs of interrod enamel are continuations of the initial enamel. They separate the interdigitating portions of Tomes' processes and create the cavity in which the processes are housed. **sg,** secretion granule. Rat incisor, × 30,000.

18–30 Fully differentiated inner enamel secretory ameloblasts. The cytoplasmic division into infranuclear, nuclear, supranuclear, and apical portions is shown. **si,** stratum intermedium. Rat incisor, × 1,000.

18–31 Ameloblasts in a region that would correspond to that of inner enamel secretion in the human enamel organ. Cytoplasmic divisions similar to those in the rat incisor ameloblasts can be defined, but the cells are much shorter, the infranuclear cytoplasm lacks mitochondria, and the tubular configuration of the Golgi apparatus is not seen. **si,** stratum intermedium. Human tooth, × 1,400.

18–32 Scanning electron micrograph of the surface of forming inner enamel in the rat incisor. The holes, arranged in rows, are occupied in life by interdigitating portions of Tomes' processes. The walls of the holes are made of interrod enamel and appear as "prongs" in sections. The walls slant in opposite directions to accommodate the similarly inclined rows of Tomes' processes as seen in Fig. 18–30. Rat incisor, × 2,800.

18–33 Surface of forming human enamel at an equivalent stage to inner enamel formation in the rat incisor. This scanning electron micrograph shows holes, arranged in less regular, but recognizable horizontal rows. The holes are occupied in life by the interdigitating portions of Tomes' processes, and the walls are interrod enamel. This configuration is conceptually similar to the situation in rat incisors. Human enamel, × 3,000.

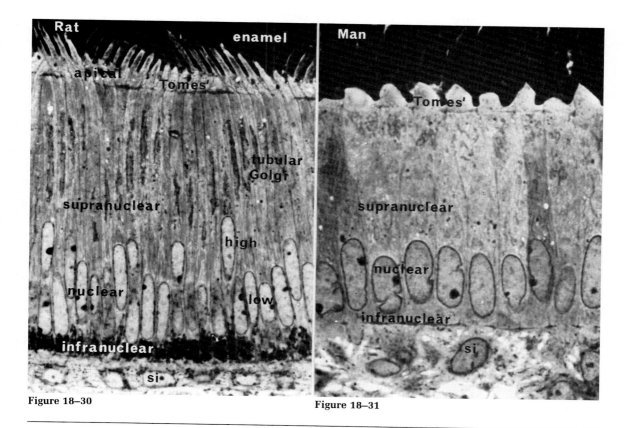

Figure 18–30

Figure 18–31

Figure 18–32

Figure 18–33

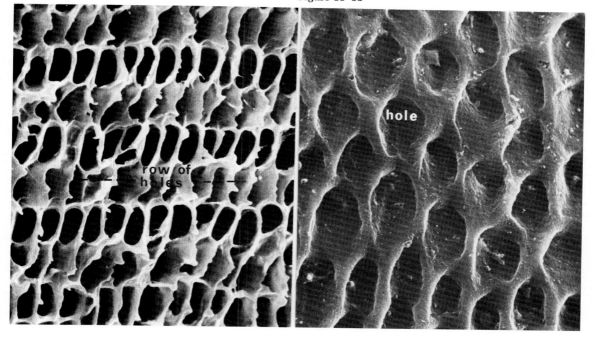

somes, and a few profiles of smooth and rough ER. Just below the functional apex (Fig. 18–30), a second, more extensive junctional complex and cell web develops. This *distal cell web* (Fig. 18–36) and *distal junctional complex* (Fig. 18–37) determine the shape of the apical end of the ameloblast and hold the cells together as a highly organized epithelium. The short projection of cytoplasm first seen on the presecretory ameloblast between the distal cell web and the basal lamina and, later, between the web and the predentin (Figs. 18–26 and 18–27) is called the *proximal portion of Tomes' process*. It is the forerunner of the *interdigitating portion of Tomes' process*, a cytoplasmic extension of the fully differentiated secretory ameloblast (Fig. 18–36). The proximal portion is devoid of RER but contains some smooth ER and, in later stages, some secretion granules (Figs. 18–26 and 18–27). The interdigitating portion develops during enamel secretion. It is also devoid of RER but contains a core of numerous secretion granules, smooth ER, multivesicular bodies, microtubules, and microfilaments (Figs. 18–29 and 18–36).

Formation of Enamel

The first-formed enamel fills the spaces between the ends of the calcified collagenous fibrils of dentin (Figs. 18–27 and 18–28) and eventually forms a continuous 4- to 6-μm-thick layer between the dentin and the apical surfaces of the ameloblasts (Figs. 18–28 and 18–29). The enamel contains thin flat ribbon-like crystallites of hydroxyapatite (Fig. 18–39) that are perpendicular to the surface of the dentin. The layer is called *initial enamel* and is produced by the *secretory ameloblasts*.

Further enamel deposition fills the intercellular spaces between the apexes of the ameloblasts (Figs. 18–29 and 18–36). This enamel is directly continuous with the initial enamel and is produced in a coordinated manner by all the secretory ameloblasts. The result is a honeycomb pattern in which the apexes of the ameloblasts fill holes outlined by thin partitions of enamel. The honeycomb pattern can be seen best with the scanning electron microscope after the ameloblast layer has been pulled off the forming surface of the tooth (Figs. 18–32 and 18–33). In most species the honeycomb pattern shows a regularity related to linear rows of holes, which in life are occupied by cytoplasmic extensions of ameloblasts (visualize Tomes' processes seen in

Figs. 18–30 and 18–31 filling the holes in Figs. 18–32 and 18–33).

Each ameloblast has one extension, Tomes' process, which by definition begins above the distal junctional complex. The proximal portion develops in presecretory ameloblasts and is present during initial enamel secretion (Figs. 18–27 and 18–28). The portion that occupies the hole in the honeycomb develops from the proximal portion and is called the interdigitating portion of Tomes' process because it "interdigitates" with walls or prongs of enamel (Figs. 18–29 and 18–36). The rows of holes reflect the linear organization of the ameloblasts themselves. Thus, in rat incisors, the cells are arranged in almost perfect rows (Fig. 18–32). In monkey and humans, the rows are less perfect but can still be distinguished; generally they run parallel to the cervical loop of the developing crown (Fig. 18–33). In thin sections, the honeycomb pattern appears as narrow partitions of enamel resembling "prongs" of equal length separating the interdigitating portions of adjacent Tomes' processes (Fig. 18–36). Each process, therefore, is surrounded by enamel on all sides except where it is continuous with the proximal portion of the process and then with the body of the ameloblast.

The end of each enamel prong is a section through the actual surface of the honeycomb and represents a growing surface onto which more enamel will be deposited to lengthen the prong. Related to this surface are irregular projections of cytoplasm from the ameloblasts in the region. The membrane of these projections is irregularly infolded, when compared with the smooth membrane of the Tomes' process within the honeycomb hole itself (Fig. 18–36). The crystallites in the initial enamel continue directly into the prongs of enamel and end in relation to the infolded membrane of the cytoplasmic projections. Thus, the initial enamel and the prongs or partitions making up the walls of the honeycomb

18–34 Electron micrograph of the infranuclear cytoplasm of the secretory ameloblasts. The proximal cell web forms the boundary between the basal bulge and the mitochondrial compartment. The cell web is associated with the proximal junctional complex **(pjc)** between ameloblasts. Numerous profiles of mitochondria **(m)** are present below the nuclei. The junction between the ameloblast base and the stratum intermedium is markedly interdigitated and irregular. **rER,** rough endoplasmic reticulum. Rat incisor, × 12,500.

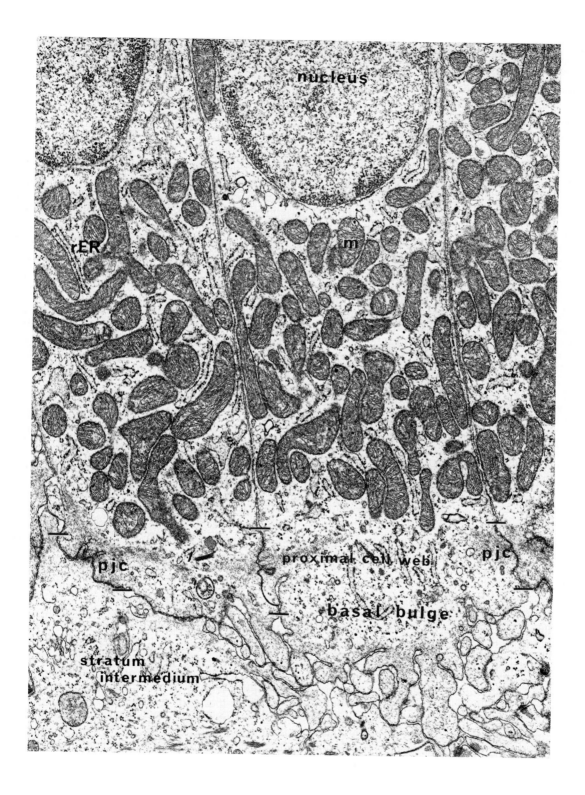

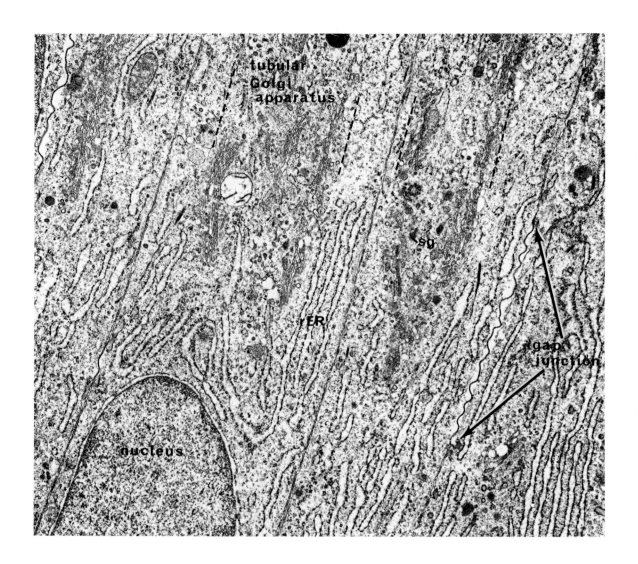

18–35 Electron micrograph of the supranuclear
△   cytoplasm of the secretory ameloblasts.
Numerous profiles of rough ER **(rER)** lie parallel to
each other and to the long axis of the cell. The Golgi
saccules make up the side walls of a tubule that fills
the central axis of the cell (between **dashed lines**).
Secretion granules **(sg)** are found in the center of the
tubule. Long wavy gap junctions are present between
the ameloblasts. Rat incisor, × 15,000.

holes are continuous and constitute the *interrod
enamel*. Because the ends of the enamel prongs
are sites where more interrod enamel is continuously being added, they are called *interrod
growth regions* (Fig. 18–36).

18–36 Electron micrograph of the apical cytoplasm
of the secretory ameloblasts. The distal cell
web delimits the supranuclear cytoplasm from the
Tomes' process. Tomes' process consists of a proximal
portion and an interdigitating portion. Proximal
portions are in contact, whereas interdigitating
portions alternate with interrod enamel prongs. The
prong tips are interrod growth regions, and the cell
membrane adjacent to this region is irregularly
infolded. The interdigitating portion is lined by a
noninfolded membrane that is very close to the
interrod enamel. Cytoplasmic microfilaments **(mf)** are
found next to the membrane, and the process core
contains secretion granules **(sg)**, microtubules **(mt)**,
and multivesicular bodies **(mvb)**. Rat incisor,
× 25,000.

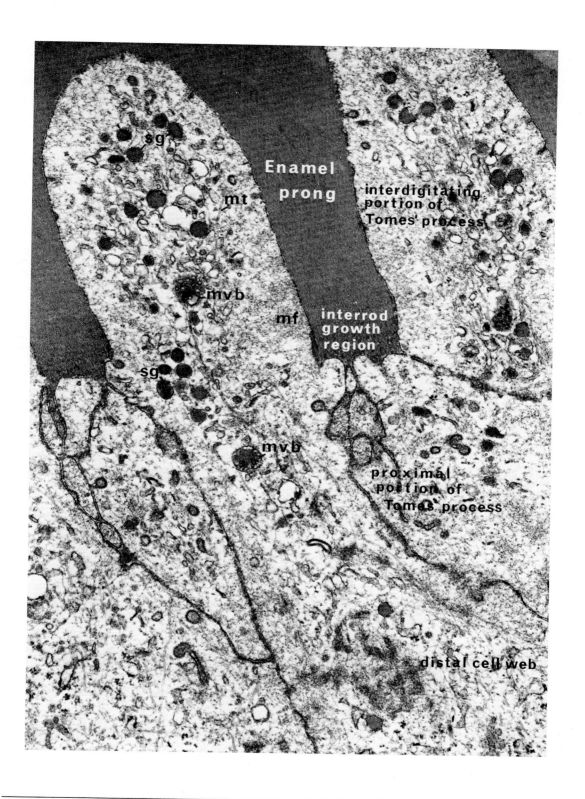

Enamel prong

interdigitating portion of Tomes' process

sg

mt

mvb

mf

interrod growth region

sg

mvb

proximal portion of Tomes process

distal cell web

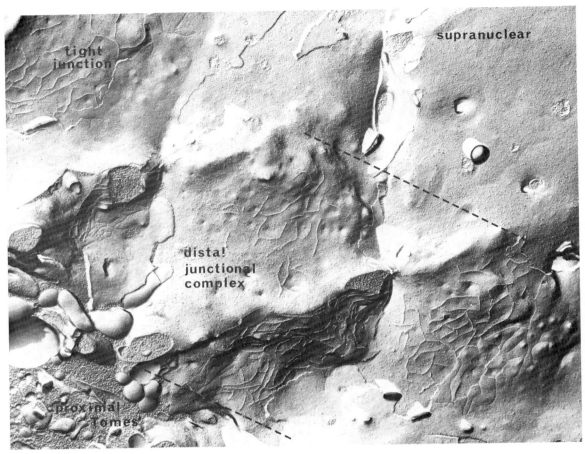

supranuclear

tight junction

distal junctional complex

proximal Tomes

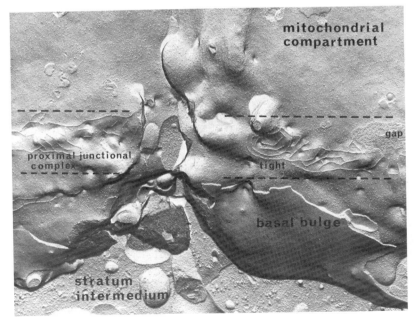

mitochondrial compartment

proximal junctional complex

tight

gap

basal bulge

stratum intermedium

18–37 ◁ Freeze-fracture replica of the distal junctional complex between rows of secretory ameloblasts. The complex, between **dashed lines** on the surface of three ameloblasts, consists of discontinuous tight junctions between the three cells of one row and three cells of the adjacent row. Rat incisor, × 25,000.

18–38 ◁ Freeze-fracture replica of the proximal junctional complex between rows of secretory ameloblasts. The complex on the surface of two ameloblasts (between **dashed lines**) separates basal bulge from mitochondrial compartment. The junction consists of incomplete tight junctions and gap junctions. Rat incisor, × 24,000.

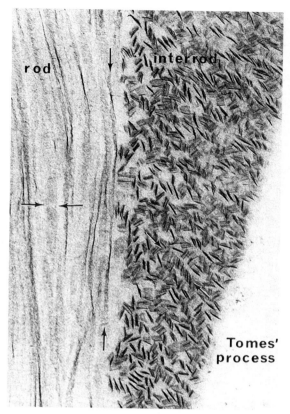

18–39 Young enamel crystallites close to Tomes'
process during inner enamel secretion.
Interrod and rod crystallites differ only in orientation
relative to the plane of section. In the rod,
longitudinally oriented crystallites appear as gray
ribbons when seen from their wide surface (between
horizontal arrows) or thin dark lines when viewed
from their edge. The twisting can be seen by following
the gray ribbon into a dark line and then into a gray
ribbon (between **vertical arrows**). Cross-sectioned
crystallites in the interrod enamel appear as short
dark lines with a gray smear on one side. The lines
tend to be stacked into linear aggregates (between
oblique arrows) but are otherwise randomly oriented.
Rat incisor, × 90,000. (Courtesy of A. C. Karim.)

The exact relationship of the interrod growth
regions to the neighboring ameloblasts is uncertain. Electron microscopy of rat incisor ameblo-
lasts shows rather isolated islands of cytoplasm
at the ends of the enamel prongs (Fig. 18–36).
These islands are at the level of the proximal
portions of Tomes' processes. Freeze-fracture replicas (Fig. 18–37) have shown that the islands

between two adjacent ameloblasts within a given
row are actually projections from the ameloblasts
in the rows in front and behind (Warshawsky,
1978). Hence, each interdigitating portion of
Tomes' process is partitioned from adjacent processes of that row by interrod enamel secreted by
projections of ameloblasts that lie in front or behind them, as well as by the ameloblasts on either side.

Once formed, the honeycomb of interrod
enamel, containing Tomes' processes in its holes,
becomes the pattern that determines the shape,
size, and orientation of the rest of the enamel
that will be secreted by Tomes' processes to fill
the holes with *enamel rods*.

Formation of Enamel Rods

The enamel rod has classically been considered
as the unit structure of enamel. However, this
view needs to be modified in light of the primary
organizing effect of interrod enamel on the arrangement, shape, and size of the rods. Rods can
now be considered as linear structures that passively conform to the shape determined by the
interrod enamel.

After the first honeycomb of interrod enamel
is formed, the interdigitating portions of Tomes'
processes (inside the holes) develop irregular infoldings on one side of their membrane. This infolded surface resembles the situation seen at interrod growth regions and, indeed, rod enamel is
secreted through this surface. The first rod
enamel formed at the *rod growth region* becomes
confluent with interrod enamel at one site on the
interrod hole (Fig. 18–40). At this site the interrod enamel is continuous with the forming
enamel rod. Because the forming rod occupies
some of the space within the hole, the cytoplasm
of Tomes' process is compressed away from the
rod growth region. As the cylindrical rod continues to grow in diameter, Tomes' process is
pushed to one side of the hole as a crescent- or
arcade-shaped projection of cytoplasm (Fig.
18–41). The continued growth of the rod
squeezes the cytoplasm of the process virtually
out of existence, and the rod enamel comes into
contact with the interrod enamel, thus filling the
entire hole (Fig. 18–41). While rods are forming,
continued formation of interrod enamel provides
a new honeycomb surface containing interdigitating portions of Tomes' processes. Thus, a
steady state exists between the formation of in-

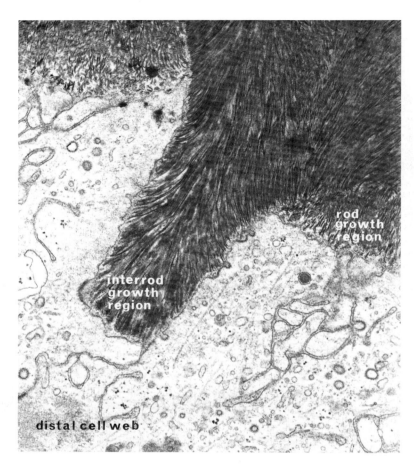

18–40 Tomes' processes of human ameloblasts showing interrod and rod growth regions. Both growth regions are associated with irregularities of the adjacent cell membrane. The orientation of crystallites in the forming rods differs from the orientation in the interrod enamel. Human tooth, × 20,000. (Courtesy of M. E. Matthiessen and P. Rømert.)

terrod enamel (honeycombs) and the filling of the interrod holes by enamel rods. Within each row of Tomes' processes the rod growth regions are on similar surfaces of the processes, and the rods begin to form at a similar site on each interrod hole.

Distinction Between Rod and Interrod Enamel

The enamel secreted by the ameloblasts, whether at the interrod or rod growth regions, is identical in all respects except that the crystallites are oriented in different directions. Hence, in a section, the distinction between the rods and the interrod enamel surrounding the rods is that crystallites will be cut along different planes (Fig. 18–39). In general, the orientation of the interrod crystallites is perpendicular to the dentino-enamel junction and to the enamel surface, whereas the crystallites in the enamel rod lie parallel to the long axis of the rod. Because the rod tends to run obliquely through the interrod enamel, its crystallites are nearly perpendicular to those of interrod enamel. At the point where each rod originates from the interrod wall, the crystallites are similarly orientated. With increasing deposition of rod material, the crystallite orientation gradually changes until it differs markedly from the orientation of the nearby interrod crystallites.

Relationship Between Tomes' Processes and Enamel Rods

The rods begin next to the initial layer of enamel, and they end close to the enamel surface. The very surface of the enamel is similar to initial enamel in that it consists of interrod enamel with

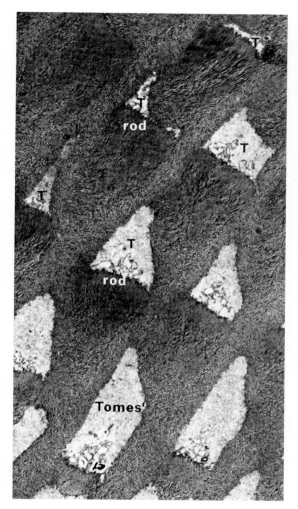

18–41 The filling of the interrod holes with enamel rods is seen progressively from the bottom to the top of this figure. As the interrod hole fills with rod enamel, the Tomes' process **(T)** is pushed to one side of the hole until only a thin rim of cytoplasm remains. Monkey tooth, × 4,000.

crystallites perpendicular to the enamel surface. This layer of *final enamel* (Fig. 18–23f) is also about 4 to 6 μm thick and provides a smooth outer surface for the enamel (Fig. 18–51). The path taken by each enamel rod, as stated above, is determined by the course of the interrod hole. That path is also followed by the "retreating" Tomes' process, which is replaced by the forming enamel rod. Controversy exists about how

that process and the cell body to which it is attached move away from the forming rod. Some investigators believe that the cell merely pulls its process out of the hole. Thus, its withdrawing membrane would slide along the walls of the hole and over the surface of the rod growth region that is in the process of forming enamel (Osborn, 1970; Kallenbach, 1973). However, there is evidence that the process remains in the hole as it is compressed by the forming rod (Warshawsky and Vugman, 1977). If this is true, then the processes must grow continuously, adding more cell substance adjacent to the cell body, while dying at their extremity where they are obliterated by the almost completed rods. This cellular growth would also push the ameloblast body away from the forming rod. The implication is that ameloblast processes are theoretically as long as the rods they form and that the ameloblast bodies trace the paths of the enamel rods. The conceptual ramifications of this type of cell movement and its implications about cell movements in the confines of an epithelial layer form a fascinating, but still poorly understood aspect of amelogenesis.

Course of the Enamel Rods

In the rat incisor, the rod can be divided into two parts (Warshawsky, 1971; Warshawsky and Smith, 1971): an inner portion, which is closer to the dentino-enamel junction, and an outer portion nearer to the final enamel (also seen in rat molars, Fig. 18–42). The inner portions of a particular row of rods are parallel to each other but take an oblique course from their origin toward the outer rod portion. The inner portions of the rods in the rows in front and behind that row are also parallel to each other, but follow an oblique course in the opposite direction. Hence, these rod portions cross each other or *decussate* (Boyde, 1969). This regular decussation of inner rod portions is characteristic of rodent incisor enamel, and the layer of enamel containing the decussating portions is called *inner enamel*. In sections, inner enamel occupies one-half to three-quarters of the total thickness of enamel. The outer portions of the rods are not aligned in rows and they do not decussate; thus, they are parallel to each other. These rod portions characterize the *outer enamel*, which in sections makes up the remaining enamel thickness. Hence, four layers of enamel can be seen: initial,

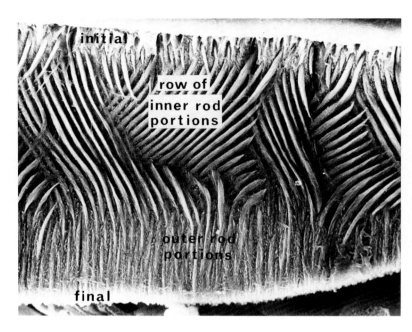

initial

row of inner rod portions

outer rod portions

final

18–42 Scanning electron micrograph of a ground section from a rat molar etched to enhance the surface features. Initial and final layers of enamel do not contain rods. Inner rod portions are arranged in rows that decussate. The inner rod portions are continuous with outer rod portions. The latter are parallel to each other and, thus, do not decussate. Rat molar, × 1,000. (Courtesy of S. Risnes.)

inner, outer, and final layers. The initial and final layers are very thin and consist of interrod enamel exclusively, whereas the inner and outer layers make up most of the enamel and contain rods surrounded by interrod enamel. The rod portions of inner enamel decussate, whereas those of outer enamel do not. This basic structure can also be seen in other types of teeth, such as rat molars (Fig.18–42 and Risnes, 1979) and monkey and human teeth (Fig. 18–43); however, the degree and regularity of the decussating pattern are the most species-variable features.

Structural Analysis of Enamel Secretion

The biochemical constituents of the organic matrix of enamel are synthetic products of the secretory ameloblasts (Frank, 1970; Weinstock and Leblond, 1971; Slavkin et al., 1976; Warshawsky and Vugman, 1977). The proteins of the matrix are synthesized on the polysomes of the RER throughout the ameloblast body. The nascent proteins are sequestered within the cisternae of the RER and are transported rapidly to the region of the Golgi apparatus. Transfer vesicles carry the proteins to the cis, or immature saccules on the outer aspect of the Golgi tubule. The proteins themselves, or perhaps the saccules containing the proteins, are moved progressively through

the stack of saccules until they reach the trans, or mature surface. The membrane-bound secretion granules, often several linked together in a common membrane (Fig. 18–44), are found free in the core of the tubule. The secretion granules are spherical, uniformly electron-dense, and surrounded by a unit membrane that is separated from the granule content by a thin halo (Fig. 18–36). These granules are then transported through the filaments of the distal cell web to occupy a position in the core of Tomes' processes (Fig. 18–36). Within the processes, groups of granules are clustered together and appear as a single dark globule with the light microscope (Fig. 18–30). The content of the secretion granules is then released to the extracellular space at either the interrod or rod growth regions. Although the mechanism of release is thought to be exocytosis, little evidence is available to document the actual fusion of granule membrane with the cell membrane. On the other hand, the cell surfaces at the rod and interrod growth regions are characterized by infoldings of the cell membrane. These incursions of membrane into the cell may contact the granules, which then empty their content into these membrane "channels" to the outside of the cell (Weinstock and Leblond, 1971). However, even this is difficult to prove because it is too infrequently seen. An alterna-

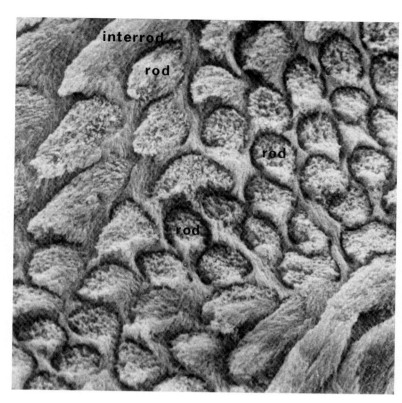

18–43 Scanning electron micrograph of a ground section from a human molar that was etched with a demineralizing agent to enhance the surface features. Three groups of rods run diagonally across this figure; in the top left corner, rods run obliquely from top to bottom; in the center, the rods are cut in cross section; and in the lower right corner, the rods are again oblique. Thus, these groups of parallel rods cross each other or decussate. Interrod enamel can be followed as a continuous phase between rod profiles. In cross-cut rods, the rod merges with the interrod enamel on the lower (cervical) surface but is clearly separated from the interrod enamel on the other surfaces. Human enamel, × 4,000. (Courtesy of O. Fejerskov and A. Thylstrup.)

tive view is that the granules remain linked together by membrane, like round sausages in a common skin (Smith, 1979). The membrane of the links of granules may momentarily fuse with the secretory surfaces at pinpoint sites and the granule contents may thus be released.

Radioautographic analysis of the secretory process in ameloblasts has shown that enamel proteins are synthesized entirely within the ameloblast cytoplasm as early as 10 min after injection of tritium-labeled proline (Fig. 18–45a). The radioactive proteins are rapidly secreted as a layer of enamel at 30 min (Fig. 18–45b), and this layer of labeled enamel increases in width at 1 and 4 h after injection (Figs. 18–45c,d). With electron-microscopic radioautography, using ^{3}H-tyrosine as a precursor, silver grains are located at 2 min over the cisternae of RER (Fig. 18–46). By 5 min, proteins labeled by incorporating the radioactive amino acids are present in the saccules of the Golgi apparatus (Fig. 18–47). By 20 min after injection, labeled secretion granules are found in the core of the Golgi apparatus and in Tomes' processes (Fig. 18–48). By 30 min, la-

beled enamel is present at the rod and interrod growth sites. Beginning at 1 or 2 h (Fig. 18–49) and progressing until 1 to 4 days after injection, the labeled enamel proteins behave in a most unusual way, which is very different from the behavior of labeled bone and dentin matrix (see below). The labeled enamel proteins progressively spread from the initial site of deposition and become homogeneously dispersed throughout the entire layer of enamel (Fig. 18–50a–d). This process in which recently formed enamel proteins intermix with previously formed matrix is called *randomization* (see review in Leblond and Warshawsky, 1979), and its significance is not known.

Using ^{3}H-fucose, a terminal sugar on the carbohydrate side chain of glycoproteins, and ^{3}H-N-acetylmannosamine, a precursor of sialic acid (which is another terminal sugar), one sees silver grains first over the Golgi region of the ameloblasts. By 1 and 4 h, the enamel matrix is weakly labeled, but Tomes' processes are strongly labeled (Warshawsky, 1979; Leblond and Warshawsky, 1979). This indicates that glycoproteins

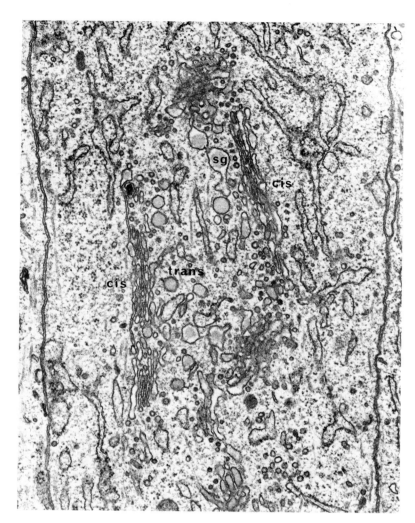

18–44 Electron micrograph of the Golgi region of a secretory ameloblast. Four or five saccules make up the stacks that form the tubular apparatus. Each stack has an immature or cis face, and a mature, or trans face. Secretion granules **(sg)** are seen in the center of the Golgi tubule, and often several granules are linked together in a common membrane. Rat incisor, × 25,000. (Courtesy of C. E. Smith.)

form a constituent of enamel (Weinstock and Leblond, 1971) but, more important, it demonstrates a turnover or addition of glycoproteins, perhaps cell-coat material, at the cell surface. These findings thus provide some evidence in support of the view that ameloblast processes continuously grow during enamel rod formation.

Nature of the Organic Matrix

Two things are known for certain about the nature of enamel matrix proteins. They are not collagen, which makes enamel unlike all other mammalian calcified tissues, and they are not keratin, which had been supposed previously because of the ectodermal origin of ameloblasts.

Enamel proteins are difficult to study because they seem to change continuously from the moment they are secreted until they are all but eliminated from the mature enamel. The original gene product of enamel protein is unknown. It may be a relatively large protein (up to 60,000 daltons; Chrispens et al., 1979) that leaves the cell and is immediately involved in the elongation of the crystallites at the growth regions. This protein has been operationally called *amelogenin* and represents the "embryonic" secretion product. Its amino acid composition is characterized by a high content of proline, glutamic acid, and histidine. The protein obtained from mature enamel has a different amino acid composition: it is much lower in glutamic acid and proline but higher in aspartic acid, serine, and glycine (Rob-

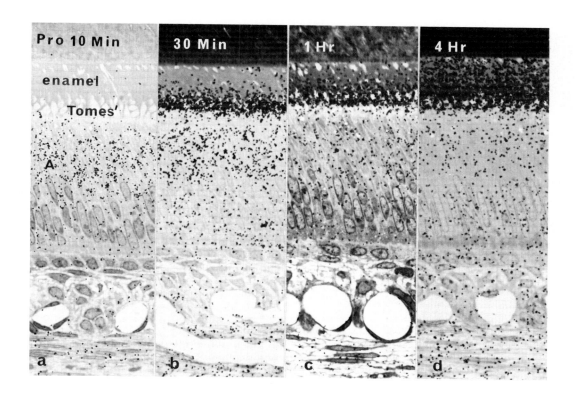

18–45 Radioautographic visualization of enamel synthesis and secretion using ³H-proline as a precursor to the enamel proteins. **a.** By 10 min after injection, the ³H-proline is incorporated into proteins synthesized mainly in the supranuclear cytoplasm of the ameloblasts **(A).** The sites of this synthesis are indicated by the location of black silver grains in the photographic emulsion overlying the section. **b.** At 30 min, labeled proteins are secreted from the cell and become part of the enamel matrix. **c.** At 1 h after injection, labeled enamel proteins spread in the enamel; **d.** by 4 h, the entire thickness of inner enamel is labeled. Radioautographs exposed 6 weeks. Rat incisor, × 560.

inson et al., 1977, 1979). The mature enamel protein is, again by operational definition, called *enamelin*. Because small amounts of enamelins are present even in the immature secretion region, both proteins may be different secretion products of the ameloblast, or they may be derived from a common protein. The enamel also contains smaller peptides that may result from the breakdown of the larger proteins. Also, small amounts of free sugars, glycoproteins (Seyer and Glimcher, 1969), phosphoproteins (Glimcher, 1979), and lipids (Odutuga and Prout, 1974) may be present. Enamel has also been reported to contain proteolytic enzymes, which could break down larger proteins into smaller, more mobile fragments (Shimizu et al., 1979).

It has been proposed that the amelogenin-type proteins are freely mobile and are not bound to the crystallites. However, the *"crystal bound"* proteins, which are solubilized only when the crystallites are dissolved, may represent the enamelins (Termine et al., 1979). This may help to explain the radioautographic observation of randomization. It is possible that the initial deposition of ³H-proline-labeled proteins at the growth regions represents amelogenin necessary for crys-

tallite elongation. Within a short time these proteins become modified, migrate throughout the enamel, and somehow participate in the process that regulates the growth of the crystallites in thickness and width. These proteins would then become the crystal-bound enamelins. With maturation, the role of amelogenin would no longer be required and these proteins would be removed, leaving only a small amount of crystal-bound enamelins as remnants of the organic matrix.

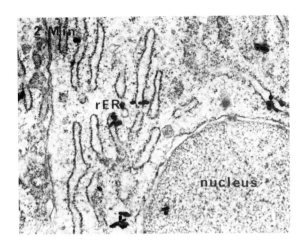

18–46 Electron microscope radioautograph 2 min after injection of ³H-tyrosine. Silver grains are located over the rER of the supranuclear region of the secretory ameloblasts. At this early time, the reactions presumably indicate the site of synthesis of proteins. Radioautograph exposed 6 months. Rat incisor, × 30,000.

18–47 Electron microscope radioautograph 5 min after ³H-tyrosine injection. Silver grains now appear over the saccules of the Golgi apparatus. Thus, within 3 min, labeled proteins first seen within the rER have migrated to the Golgi apparatus. Radioautograph exposed 6 months. Rat incisor, × 30,000.

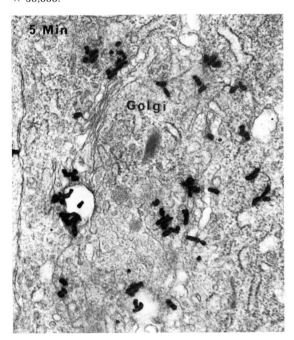

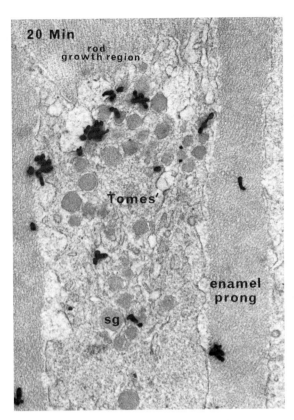

18–48 Electron microscope radioautograph 20 min after injection of ³H-tyrosine. Labeled secretion granules **(sg)** formed earlier in the Golgi apparatus are now seen in the interdigitating portion of Tomes' process near a rod growth region. Some grains are seen over the enamel prongs. Radioautograph exposed 6 months. Rat incisor, × 30,000.

Structure of the Enamel Crystallite

The hydroxyapatite crystallites are the most apparent structural feature of enamel. They have an intrinsic electron density and do not require osmium tetroxide or heavy metal stains to be visualized in thin sections with transmission electron microscopy. During secretion of the enamel, the crystallites abut against the cell membrane adjacent to the growth regions. Hence, unlike bone, dentin, and cementum, enamel has no unmineralized precursor. Since there is no preenamel, the deposition of the organic matrix and the formation of the crystallites must occur simultaneously. In general terms, mineralization is visualized as a two-step process involving *initiation* at a mineralizing site and subsequent *crys-*

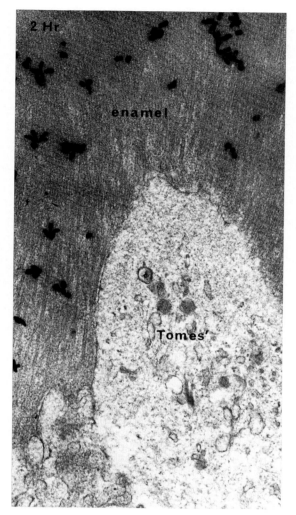

18–49 Electron microscope radioautograph 2 h after injection of ³H-tyrosine. No labeling is seen over Tomes' process, but numerous silver grains are found over the enamel matrix. Radioautograph exposed 6 months. Rat incisor, × 30,000.

are extremely long and extend from the dentino-enamel junction to the enamel surface as interrod crystallites, or along the entire length of the rods, as rod crystallites.

The individual crystallite is a long, thin, flattened ribbon of hydroxyapatite (Fig. 18–39). It has a gradual spiral course (Kerebel et al., 1979; Leblond and Warshawsky, 1979), and groups of crystallites appear in stacks that run and spiral parallel to each other. The ribbon has three dimensions: the length has been discussed above and is known as the crystalline "C" axis; the thickness is the smallest dimension and averages about 1 to 2 nm in very young crystallites; the width of the ribbon averages 30 nm. As the crystallites age, they grow in all three dimensions. The length increases at the rod or interrod growth regions, the thickness increases progressively to a maximum of about 25 nm, and the width reaches about 50 to 60 nm in the most mature enamel *crystals* (Nylen et al., 1963; Travis and Glimcher, 1964; Selvig and Halse, 1972). With high-resolution transmission electron microscopy, the periodic lattice fringes supposedly given by the repeating unit structure of the hydroxyapatite can be seen (Selvig and Halse, 1972). The fringes are about 8.2 Å apart.

There is a great deal of debate about the cell's role in pumping mineral ions (calcium and phosphate) into the enamel. Radioautographic studies using ⁴⁵Ca as a mineral tracer have shown that the ameloblasts are never labeled and therefore have no role in sequestering calcium for enamel mineralization (Munhoz and Leblond, 1974). Instead, as early as 30 sec after injection of ⁴⁵Ca, labeling is uniformly distributed over the entire enamel layer (Fig. 18–55a). The diffuse and random distribution is essentially unchanged at 5 min (Fig. 18–55b) and at 24 h after injection. This finding demonstrates that the rate of accretion of mineral ions on the surface of growing crystallites is uniform; hence, the size of a crystallite is directly related to its age.

Relationship Between the Organic Matrix and the Crystallites

The enamel formed by the secretory ameloblast is *immature enamel*. It consists of 30% organic matrix and 70% minerals by weight. *Mature enamel*, as found on the surface of the erupted tooth, consists of 99% mineral and less than 1% organic matrix by weight. Therefore, the organic matrix must be necessary for crystallite growth or orientation and is then almost completely lost,

tallite growth. Within enamel, the initiation is postulated to occur on the mineralized dentin that always precedes enamel formation (Bernard, 1972). Thus, the mineralization seen in enamel is thought to represent only crystallite growth. The consequence of this hypothesis is that crystallites initiated within the interrod or rod enamel would be constant in number throughout the entire secretory period. They would then grow in length in the growth regions, and in thickness and width in the rest of the enamel. According to this view, the enamel crystallites

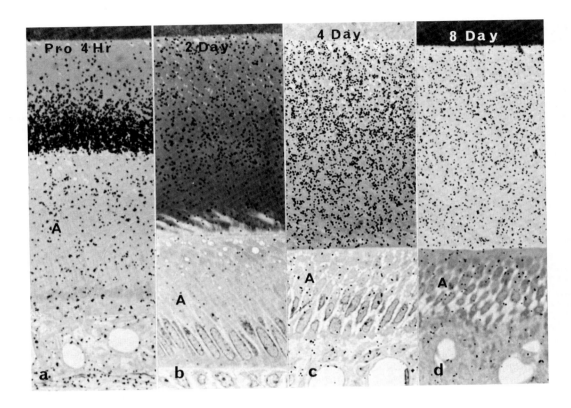

18–50 Randomization of radioactive proteins in the enamel matrix visualized by radioautography using ³H-proline as a precursor of enamel proteins. **a.** Radioactive proteins deposited by the ameloblasts (A) during the 4 h after injection of ³H-proline occupy about one-half the enamel thickness. **b.** The same region 2 days after injection shows a thicker layer of enamel, but the original radioactive proteins now occupy almost the entire thickness of enamel. **c.** The same region at 4 days shows a complete randomization of labeled proteins. **d.** At 8 days, the proteins begin to disappear as the enamel undergoes maturation and, thus, fewer silver grains overlie the enamel. Radioautographs exposed 6 weeks. Rat incisor, × 560.

leaving an enamel layer that is almost exclusively crystalline. A fundamental problem at the morphological level is to understand the relationship between the organic matrix and the crystallites. This problem is complicated by the lack of knowledge about the solubility of matrix and mineral components during fixation and histological processing. Conceptually, there are three possible locations for the matrix: between the crystallites, on the surface of the crystallites, or within the crystallites. If the proteins are not washed out during processing for electron microscopy, they ought to be seen in the spaces between crystallites. When various staining procedures that usually reveal proteins are applied, no electron-dense material is seen between the crystallites. There is some evidence that a coat of staining is found around the crystallites. This coat is seen in older crystallites, but it is difficult to visualize in the immature enamel (Nylen, 1979). There is also some evidence that an organic "ghost" is left after the minerals are dissolved (Bonucci, 1969; Frank, 1979; Leblond and Warshawsky, 1979). Thus, most evidence supports the presence of both a crystal coat and an organic stroma for the crystallites. However, the problem is still unresolved and requires further investigation.

Maturation of Enamel

When the final layer of enamel is formed, the secretory ameloblasts have completed their job. The end of enamel secretion is marked by a sudden death of ameloblasts (Smith and Warshawsky, 1977). The dead cells appear as globules of dark-staining material of nuclear and cytoplasmic origin located between and within the surviving ameloblasts (Fig. 18–23f). The remaining ameloblasts in this region of *postsecretory transition* become markedly shortened, and a massive internal reorganization of organelles occurs that typifies the change from secretion to some other function. In the rat incisor, all ameloblasts that begin the process of enamel secretion live to complete their work. Thus, every ameloblast leaves behind an entire enamel rod. However, at the end of secretion, 25% of the ameloblast population dies and the debris is phagocytized and destroyed in the lysosomal system of surviving ameloblasts. This entire phenomenon of massive cell death and removal requires only 19 h in the rat incisor out of a maximum total ameloblast life span of 32 days (Smith and Warshawsky, 1977). The rest of the population becomes organized into essentially two types of *maturative ameloblasts*. In the rat incisor, these types appear in cohorts that seem to change or *modulate* from one type to the other and back again several times along the tooth (Josephsen and Fejerskov, 1977). In the developing teeth of other species, and in rat molars, both cell types can be seen. Thus, a similar modulation might also occur in these teeth. The major cell type has a striated-like, or ruffled apical border. This *striated-like border cell* (Fig. 18–23g) occupies most of the maturation zone of the rat incisor. Alternating with these cells are short bands of cells with *smooth apical surfaces* (Fig. 18–23h). The striated-like border is associated with smooth membrane invaginations from the base of the striations and with numerous mitochondria (Fig. 18–51). These characteristics are also seen in known resorptive cells such as striated border cells of the intestine, gall bladder epithelial cells, striated duct cells in the salivary glands, and the proximal convoluted tubule cells of the kidney. Thus, it has always been assumed that these ameloblasts are responsible for the maturation changes in enamel (Reith and Cotty, 1967). These changes include resorption of enamel matrix (amelogenins) and water, and the concomitant increase in minerals (Deakins, 1942). Despite these resemblances, however, no direct evidence exists to substantiate this assumption.

In addition, the striated-like border cell shares some features with the bone-resorbing osteoclast. Both cells have striated or ruffled borders associated with subsurface mitochondria, and both show reactions for the enzyme naphthylamidase (Hammarstrom et al., 1971). They differ in that osteoclasts disrupt the physical morphology of bone, whereas the maturative ameloblasts do not alter the structure of enamel.

The only function definitely known to be performed by maturative ameloblasts is the synthesis and secretion of an electron-dense layer of material resembling a basal lamina at the surface of the enamel (Weinstock, 1970; Takano, 1979; Fig. 18–51). Related to this basal lamina, the apical surfaces of both types of ameloblasts show hemidesmosomal attachments. Interestingly, this situation is identical to the beginning of amelogenesis, in which the inner dental epithelial cells contact the original basal lamina.

In rodent incisors, one other function for the maturative cells is known. They form an iron-containing compound that is released into the enamel surface and imparts the yellow color to rodent enamel (Selvig and Halse, 1975).

Within the enamel itself, maturation involves no change in enamel morphology other than an increase in width and thickness of the enamel crystallites. However, it is during this process of maturation that most of the proteins are removed, most of the water is removed, and the full complement of minerals is added to produce the final product—the enamel on the surface of the tooth.

Formation of Dentin

The structure of dentin and the manner in which it forms, slowly but continuously during life, was discussed above. Much of what is known about dentin secretion has been demonstrated by radioautography. The intracellular steps in collagen synthesis, packaging, and secretion (see collagen, Chap. 4) can be visualized by using labeled amino acids and radioautography (Weinstock and Leblond, 1974). Similar information can be obtained on glycoprotein formation in dentin by using labeled sugars (Weinstock et al., 1972). In addition, the mineralization of dentin can also be investigated radioautographically with labeled mineral ions (Munhoz and Leblond, 1974).

Radioautography of Collagen Formation

Using ^{3}H-proline, one can localize the site of synthesis of proteins (presumably mainly collagen) as early as 2 min after injection on the polysomes

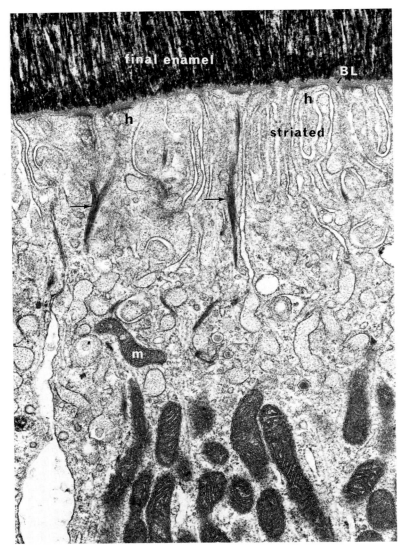

final enamel

BL

h

h

striated

m

18–51 Electron micrograph of the striated-like border of maturative ameloblasts. The border consists of irregularly but deeply infolded surface membranes associated with tubular vesicles opening into the base of the striations. Some of the processes making up the border are flattened and form hemidesmosomal attachments **(h)** with the basal lamina-like layer **(BL)** that separates the cells from the final enamel layer. Thick bundles of fibrils **(arrows)** run toward and insert in these hemidesmosomes. Numerous mitochondria **(m)** are associated with the striated-like border. Rat incisor, × 25,000. (Courtesy of C. E. Smith.)

of the RER in the body of the odontoblasts. By 10 to 30 min after injection, grains are present over the cytoplasm of the odontoblasts (Fig. 18–52a,b). With the electron microscope, these grains are localized over the Golgi saccules and some prosecretion granules. By 30 min to 1 h, labeled granules are found in the odontoblast processes, and labeling is seen over the predentin closest to the cell bodies (Fig. 18–52b,c). By 4 h after injection the entire predentin is uniformly but heavily labeled (Fig. 18–52d). After 1 day a band of heavily labeled matrix is half over predentin and half over the mineralized dentin, and a weak reaction is present between that band and the odontoblast bodies (Fig. 18–52e). By 2

18–52 Radioautographic visualization of dentin secretion using ^{3}H-proline as a precursor to dentinal proteins, presumably mainly collagen. **a.** At 10 min after injection, silver grains are found over the bodies of the odontoblasts. **b.** At 30 min, labeled proteins appear in the predentin as a decreasing gradient toward the dentin. **c.** By 1 h the entire predentin is uniformly labeled. **d.** Some labeled dentin is present by 4 h. **e.** The band of labeling is half over predentin and half over dentin by 1 day. **f.** By 2 days, the band is entirely within the dentin. Weakly labeled dentin and predentin between the labeled band and the odontoblasts were secreted in less than 2 days after injection. Radioautographs exposed 3 weeks. Rat incisor, × 560.

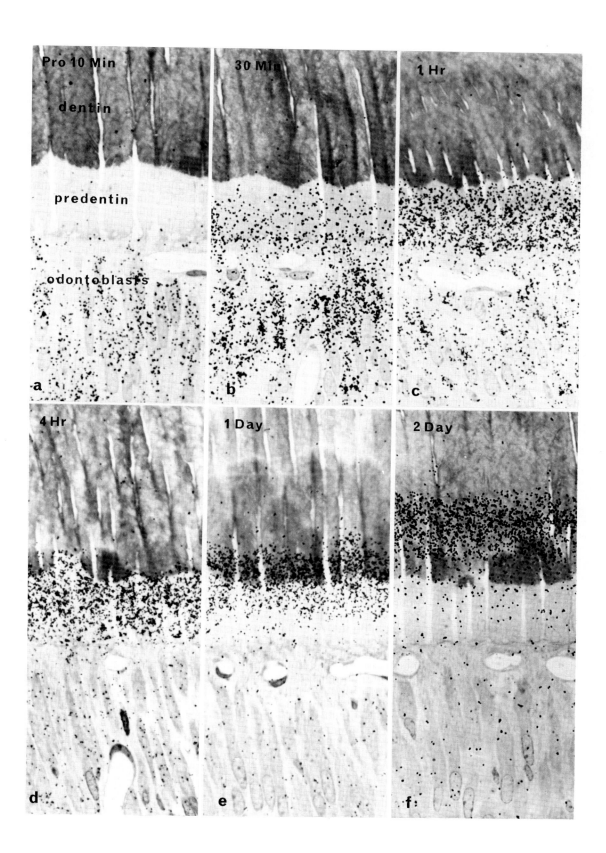

Pro 10 Min

dentin

predentin

odontoblasts

a

30 Min

b

1 Hr

c

4 Hr

d

1 Day

e

2 Day

f

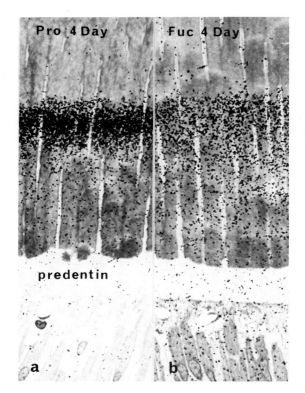

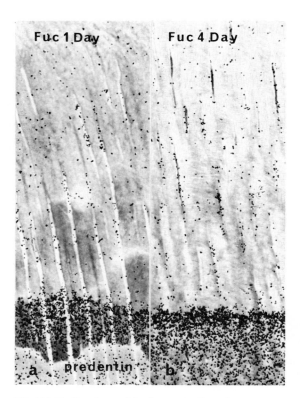

18–53 Radioautographic comparison of the uptake into dentin of ³H-proline **(a)**, presumably mainly into collagen, and ³H-fucose **(b)**, presumably into glycoproteins, at 4 days after injection. There is a discrete band of labeling with ³H-proline, but with ³H-fucose the labeling is heavy and diffuse over the entire thickness of dentin and predentin formed since the injection. Radioautographs exposed 3 weeks **(a)** and 9 months **(b)**. Rat incisor, × 560.

18–54 Radioautographic demonstration of glycoprotein addition to the odontoblast process. At 1 day **(a)**, and 4 days **(b)** after injection of ³H-fucose, silver grains are found over the odontoblast processes within the dentin that was formed before the label was injected. This indicates that material labeled with ³H-fucose, presumably glycoprotein, is being added to the odontoblast processes and reflects either turnover or growth. Radioautographs exposed 9 months. Rat incisor, × 560.

days (Fig. 18–52f) the radioactive band is located entirely within the dentin, and by 4 (Fig. 18–53a) or 8 days it is seemingly buried deeper and deeper into the dentin as new, still weakly labeled dentinal matrix continues to be added. The intensely labeled band of dentin is remarkably stable and does not turn over to any extent during the life of the tooth.

A similar intracellular sequence occurs when another labeled amino acid ³H-tyrosine, is used. However, in this case a very weak reaction is seen over predentin 1 h after injection. At 4 h, the band of labeling is still in the predentin, but the intensity of the reaction is reduced by about one-third. This decrease in radioactivity is interpreted in part as a loss of the labeled terminal peptides of procollagen (Josephsen and Warshawsky, 1982). These peptides are cleaved by procollagen peptidases in the conversion of procollagen to tropocollagen, and the removal of these fragments from the predentin can be monitored by the decrease in labeling.

Radioautography of Glycoprotein Formation

With ³H-fucose (Weinstock et al., 1972) and ³H-N-acetylmannosamine, the earliest reactions are over the saccules of the Golgi apparatus. Secretion granules are labeled at about 30 min to 1 h, and labeled predentinal glycoproteins appear within the predentin close to the cells by 4 h. Some grains tend to accumulate on the dentin side of the predentin–dentin border (Weinstock et al., 1972). The addition of glycoprotein at the mineralizing frontier line is particularly evident at 4 h and reflects the weak PAS staining in predentin but the intense staining in the dentin. With time, more labeling appears over the mineralized dentin, but not as an intense labeled band of definite width as seen with protein (cf. parts a and b of Fig. 18–53). Instead, for at least 1 to 4 days after injection, the predentin remains heavily labeled and radioactivity is progressively added to the mineralized dentin, creating a wide gradient of labeling over the newly formed dentin right up to the predentin (Fig. 18–53b). A unique feature of glycoprotein labeling is the intense reaction along the odontoblast processes by 1 to 4 days after injection of ^{3}H-fucose (Fig. 18–54a,b). This was not seen with protein tracers and suggests that the processes have an active turnover of glycoproteins, presumably the cell coat. Alternatively, the addition of labeled glycoprotein may be a reflection of the continuous growth of these processes as the cell body moves away from the newly deposited predentin (Warshawsky and Josephsen, 1981). If this is the case, then the new membrane glycoprotein, wherever it is added, is redistributed over the entire surface of the cell and its process.

Mineralization of Dentin

Initiation of mineralization in dentin begins after the first layer of predentin is deposited along the basal lamina of the enamel organ. The relatively large collagenous fibrils of the first layer of predentin (called *mantle predentin*) are oriented perpendicular to the basal lamina and radiate like a fan between the newly formed odontoblast processes. The processes are highly branched; soon after this layer is formed, the basal lamina disintegrates and projections of ameloblast cytoplasm extend between the collagenous fibrils. It is within this zone, a few micrometers from the ameloblasts, that small membrane-bound vesicles, the *matrix vesicles* (Bernard, 1972), are first seen. They usually contain one or a cluster of thin elongated electron-dense lines that have been identified as crystallites of hydroxyapatite. The crystallites are at first related to the vesicle membrane but then fill and overlap the boundaries of the vesicle. From these initiation sites crystal growth proceeds to mineralize the colla-

gen, which has by now been glycosylated, thus converting predentin to dentin. Most workers believe that enamel requires no de novo initiation, but that enamel crystallite growth is induced by mineralization sites within the dentin.

More recently, tiny amorphous mineral deposits have been seen on the plasma membrane of cells involved with mineralizing tissues. These deposits are present before obvious crystal growth occurs and may be involved with initiation in a manner similar to matrix vesicles (Almuddaris and Dougherty, 1979). Because they are seen on the surface of ameloblasts, as well as odontoblasts, it may be that each mineralizing site initiates its own crystallite growth.

Radioautography of Dentin Formation with ^{45}Ca

Radioautography has failed to reveal any incorporation of labeled calcium into the cells associated with mineralization. As early as 30 sec (Fig. 18–55a) and 5 min (Fig. 18–55b) after injection, the main reaction is present over the mineralized dentin at the frontier line adjacent to the unlabeled predentin (Munhoz and Leblond, 1974). A lower-intensity reaction is spread throughout the entire, previously formed dentin. Contrary to enamel, which acquires its mineral content gradually but immediately on being secreted, the dentin receives more than 90% of its total minerals instantly but at the mineralization front several hours after its matrix is formed. The rest of the previously mineralized dentin becomes significantly labeled presumably because of exchange with nonlabeled calcium at the crystallite surfaces. With time, the calcium-labeled band becomes buried in the dentin by the deposition of newly formed, less heavily labeled dentin.

Root Formation and Eruption

When the entire crown is complete, the tooth is ready to erupt into the oral cavity. The enamel organ overlying the completed layer of enamel is reduced to a stratified squamous epithelium with shrunken cuboidal cells (reduced ameloblasts) nearest the enamel. At the cervical loop region, the reflection of inner to outer dental epithelia turns inward toward the pulp center and forms an epithelial diaphragm (Fig. 18–20e). This diaphragm encloses much of the pulp and separates it from the connective tissue outside the crown. However, it leaves a wide opening, which is

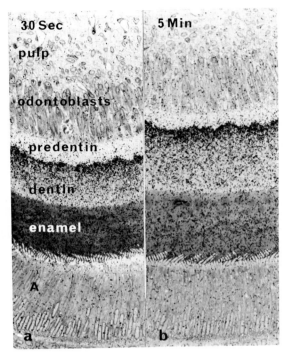

18–55 Radioautographic visualization of the distribution of ^{45}Ca at 30 sec **(a)** and 5 min **(b)** after injection. Ameloblasts **(A)** and odontoblasts show a background level of radioactivity. The enamel is uniformly labeled, indicating a uniform addition of calcium to all the growing crystallites. Thus, the older crystallites will contain more calcium and be proportionately larger. The dentin is intensely labeled at the frontier line or calcification front, and a weak diffuse reaction extends over the remaining dentin. Thus, intense mineralization occurs near the predentin, and some crystallite growth or exchange occurs on previously formed crystallites. Predentin shows a background level of labeling. Radioautographs exposed 5 days **(a)** and 2 days **(b)**. Rat incisor, × 250. (Courtesy of C. P. Leblond.)

equivalent to the future apical foramen that will eventually be the opening into the pulp. The diaphragm is lined on both surfaces by basal lamina and is known as *Hertwig's epithelial diaphragm*. At the point where this diaphragm originates from the cervical margin of the tooth, the combination of inner and outer epithelia begins to manifest its ability to induce adjacent pulpal cells to differentiate into odontoblasts. These newly differentiating odontoblasts align themselves with the preexisting cells at the cervical margin, which are already functional odontoblasts. The new odontoblasts begin to secrete

predentin, which is continuous with the predentin already formed in the crown. In time, this predentin becomes dentin that is also continuous with previously made dentin. Thus, a new rim of dentin has been added around the cervical region of the tooth, but this rim is not related to enamel. It is, therefore, the first rim of root dentin. The portion of the combined inner and outer dental epithelia that initiated the formation of this dentin is called *Hertwig's epithelial root sheath* (Fig. 18–20e). The root sheath proliferates further from the crown (in an apical direction indicating its growth toward the future root apex); it induces more pulp cells into odontoblasts as it goes and, thus, lengthens the rim of new root dentin. However, this apparent downward, or apical, proliferation is only relative to the crown if the crown is taken as a fixed point in space. In reality, the epithelial diaphragm should be taken as the fixed point, and thus the rim of new root dentin would have to jack up the crown to make room for itself. This basic principle is in fact the way in which root formation is causally linked to tooth eruption. The eruptive pathway followed by the crown seems to be genetically determined and is created by localized, programmed disintegration along the path (Cahill, 1969). As the root lengthens it pushes the crown through this path until the crown breaks through the gingiva. As it erupts further, the reduced enamel organ fuses with the gingiva, and the naked crown, with perhaps some covering of extraneous cellular debris over the basal lamina–like cuticle on the enamel, reaches the oral environment.

Development of the Periodontal Ligament Attachment

With the continued lengthening of the root, the portion of the epithelial root sheath that has performed its inductive role disintegrates. Thus, the connective tissue cells lying outside the epithelial sheath can come into contact with the outermost dentin. However, before the root sheath degenerates, the inner dental epithelial component seems to perform one last secretory function reminiscent of its ameloblastic role: it secretes a layer of enamel-like material onto the dentin (Schonfeld and Slavkin, 1977). This region is now somewhat similar to the dentino-enamel junction in the crown. After the epithelial root sheath breaks down, it is with the enamel-like material that the connective tissue cells come into contact. The fibroblast-like cells from the connective tissue surrounding the developing tooth differentiate into cementoblasts and secrete acellular cementum on the root surface. Further secretion of cementum begins to trap the ends of collagen fibrils of the developing periodontal ligament. The fibers are produced by fibroblasts differentiating between the newly forming root and the walls of the bony crypt in which the tooth developed. Collagen fibers also become anchored in the bone of the crypt, which can now be considered as alveolar bone. The oriented ligamentous nature of the periodontal connective tissue becomes evident shortly after root elongation begins. It is believed that the active remodeling of the ligament by fibroblasts may provide the force necessary for the crown to erupt, in much the same way as the ligament has been implicated in the continuous eruption of rat incisors. As the root lengthens and the crown approaches and breaks through the gingiva, the ligament fibers thicken and strengthen to provide support and attachment for the tooth. In their orientation, the fibers resemble those of the functional periodontal ligament (Figs. 18–13 and 18–14). The tooth is, therefore, ready for occlusion and function as soon as it meets its opposing teeth.

Remnants of the disintegrating epithelial root sheath are thought to persist as a network of cells among the periodontal ligament fibers even into adulthood (in the case of permanent teeth). These remnants are called *epithelial rests of Malassez*, and they may give rise to pathological conditions.

After root formation is complete, the dentin forms the apical foramen, which initially has about the same diameter as the opening in Hertwig's epithelial diaphragm. Cementum production at the apex is responsible for narrowing the foramen still further to its mature size.

Development of Permanent Teeth and Shedding of Baby Teeth

The bud of the permanent tooth, which lay dormant from its initial formation (Fig. 18–20c), is stimulated to begin developing by factors that are largely unknown. When triggered, the tooth undergoes the same developmental sequences described for the deciduous tooth and starts to enlarge within the bony crypt that encloses it. The pressure of this expansion enlarges the crypt by inducing osteoclastic resorption. The resorption of the alveolar bone that separates the crypt of the permanent tooth from the socket of the baby

tooth leads to direct pressure on the root of the baby tooth. The pressure stimulates resorption of the root by osteoclast-like cells. However, the hydrostatic cushion provided by the enamel organ over the developing crown protects the enamel from the effects of this pressure.

With the elongation of the root and the eruptive forces acting on the permanent tooth, the root of the baby tooth and the attached portion of the periodontal ligament are entirely resorbed. Concomitantly, blood and nerve supplies to the pulp are broken. Eventually, the baby tooth—consisting of only the crown—is held entirely by its attachment to the gingiva. When the crown "falls out," and is placed beneath the pillow to be exchanged for money by the tooth fairy, the occlusal tip of the permanent crown can be seen just beneath the gingival surface. It erupts into the oral cavity to take up its position as part of the permanent dentition.

References and Selected Bibliography

General

Gerould, C. H. 1944. Ultrastructures of the human tooth as revealed by the electron microscope. J. Dent. Res. 23:239.

Leeuwenhoeck, A. 1678. Microscopical observations of the structure of teeth and other bones; and, Of the grain of ivory. Phil. Trans. R. Soc. Lond. 140:1002.

Odutuga, A. A., and Prout, R. E. S. 1974. Lipid analysis of human enamel and dentine. Arch. Oral Biol. 19:729.

Reith, E. J. 1968. Collagen formation in developing molar teeth of rats. J. Ultrastruct. Res. 21:383.

Slavkin, H. C. 1979a. Developmental Craniofacial Biology. Philadelphia: Lea and Febiger.

Smith, C. E., and Warshawsky, H. 1976. Movement of entire cell populations during renewal of the rat incisor as shown by radioautography after labeling with ³H-thymidine (with an appendix on the development of the periodontal ligament). Am. J. Anat. 145:225.

Warshawsky, H., and Josephsen, K. 1981. The behavior of substances labeled with ³H-proline and ³H-fucose in the cellular processes of odontoblasts and ameloblasts. Anat. Rec. 200:1.

Calcification

Bernard, G. W. 1972. Ultrastructural observations of initial calcification in dentine and enamel. J. Ultrastruct. Res. 41:1.

Bonucci, E. 1969. Further investigation on the organic/inorganic relationships in calcifying cartilage. Calcif. Tissue Res. 3:38.

Munhoz, C. O. G., and Leblond, C. P. 1974. Deposition of calcium phosphate into dentin and enamel as shown by radioautography of sections of incisor teeth following injection of ^{45}Ca into rats. Calcif. Tissue Res. 15:221.

Nylen, M. U. 1979. Matrix-mineral relationships—A morphologist's viewpoint. J. Dent. Res. 58(B):922.

Dentin (Odontoblasts)

Almuddaris, M. F., and Dougherty, W. J. 1979. The association of amorphous mineral deposits with the plasma membrane of pre- and young odontoblasts and their relationship to the origin of dentinal matrix vesicles in rat incisor teeth. Am. J. Anat. 155:223.

Josephsen, K., and Warshawsky, H. 1982. Radioautography of rat incisor dentin as a continuous record of the incorporation of a single dose of ^{3}H-labeled proline and tyrosine. Am. J. Anat. 164:45.

Karim, A., Cournil, I., and Leblond, C. P. 1979. Immunohistochemical localization of procollagens. II. Electron microscopic distribution of procollagen I antigenicity in the odontoblasts and predentin of rat incisor teeth by a direct method using peroxidase linked antibodies. J. Histochem. Cytochem. 27:1070.

Ten Cate, A. R. 1972. An analysis of Tomes' granular layer. Anat. Rec. 172:137.

Ten Cate, A. R., Melcher, A. H., Pudy, G., and Wagner, D. 1970. The non-fibrous nature of the von Korff fibres in developing dentine. A light and electron microscope study. Anat. Rec. 168:491.

Warshawsky, H. 1972. The presence of atypical collagen fibrils in EDTA decalcified predentine and dentine of rat incisors. Arch. Oral Biol. 17:1745.

Weinstock, M. 1981. Gap junctions in the odontoblasts of the rat incisor teeth. Anat. Rec. 199:270A.

Weinstock, M. 1977. Centrosymmetrical cross-banded structures in the matrix of rat incisor predentin and dentin. J. Ultrastruct. Res. 61:218.

Weinstock, M., and Leblond, C. P. 1974. Synthesis, migration and release of precursor collagen by odontoblasts as visualized by radioautography after ^{3}H-proline administration. J. Cell Biol. 60:92.

Weinstock, A., Weinstock, M., and Leblond, C. P. 1972. Autoradiographic detection of ^{3}H-fucose incorporation into glycoprotein by odontoblasts and its deposition at the site of the calcification front in dentin. Calcif. Tissue Res. 8:181.

Development

Slavkin, H. C. 1979b. The nature and nurture of epithelial–mesenchymal interactions during tooth morphogenesis. J. Biol. Buccale 6:189.

Enamel (Ameloblasts)

Boyde, A. 1969. Electron microscopic observations relating to the nature and development of prism decussation in mammalian dental enamel. Bull. Group Int. Rech. Sci. Stomat. 12:151.

Chrispens, J., Weliky, B., Bringas, P., and Slavkin, H. 1979. "Proenamel–enamel–polypeptides": A concept. J. Dent. Res. 58(B):988.

Deakins, M. 1942. Changes in the ash, water and or-

ganic content of pig enamel during calcification. J. Dent. Res. 21:429.

Frank, R. M. 1970. Autoradiographie quantitative de l'amelogenese en microscopie electronique a l'aide de la proline tritiee chez le chat. Arch. Oral Biol. 15:569.

Frank, R. M. 1979. Tooth enamel: Current state of the art. J. Dent. Res. 58(B):684.

Glimcher, M. J. 1979. Phosphopeptides of enamel matrix. J. Dent. Res. 58(B):790.

Hammarstrom, L. E., Toverud, S. U., and Hanker, J. S. 1971. Naphthylamidase in ameloblasts during enamel maturation. Calcif. Tissue Res. 7:267.

Josephson, K., and Fejerskov, O. 1977. Ameloblast modulation in the maturation zone of the rat incisor enamel organ. A light and electron microscopic study. J. Anat. 124:45.

Kallenbach, E. 1973. The fine structure of Tomes' process of rat incisor ameloblasts and its relationship to the elaboration of enamel. Tissue Cell 5:501.

Kallenbach, E. 1976. Fine structure of differentiating ameloblasts in the kitten. Am. J. Anat. 145:283.

Kallenbach, E., Sandborn, E., and Warshawsky, H. 1963. The Golgi apparatus of the ameloblast of the rat at the stage of enamel matrix formation. J. Cell Biol. 16:629.

Kerebel, B., Daculsi, G., and Kerebel, L. M. 1979. Ultrastructural studies of enamel crystallites. J. Dent. Res. 58(B):844.

LeBlond, C. P., and Warshawsky, H. 1979. Dynamics of enamel formation in the rat incisor tooth. J. Dent. Res. 58(B):950.

Listgarten, M. A. 1966. Phase-contrast and electron microscopic study of the junction between reduced enamel epithelium and enamel in unerupted human teeth. Arch. Oral Biol. 11:999.

Matthiessen, M. E., and Rømert, P. 1978. Fine structure of the human secretory ameloblast. Scand. J. Dent. Res. 86:67.

Matthiessen, M. E., and Rømert, P. 1980a. Ultrastructure of the human enamel organ. I. External enamel epithelium, stellate reticulum and stratum intermedium. Cell Tissue Res. 205:361.

Matthiessen, M. E., and Rømert, P. 1980b. Ultrastructure of the human enamel organ. II. Internal enamel epithelium, preameloblasts and secretory ameloblasts. Cell Tissue Res. 205:371.

Nylen, M. U., Eanes, E. D., and Omnell, K. A. 1963. Crystal growth in rat enamel. J. Cell Biol. 18:109.

Osborn, J. W. 1970. The mechanism of ameloblast movement: A hypothesis. Calcif. Tissue Res. 5:344.

Reith, E. J., and Cotty, V. F. 1967. The absorptive activity of ameloblasts during the maturation of enamel. Anat. Rec. 157:577.

Risnes, S. 1979. The prism pattern of rat molar enamel. A scanning electron microscope study. Am. J. Anat. 155:245.

Robinson, C., Briggs, H. D., Atkinson, P. J., and Weatherell, J. A. 1979. Matrix and mineral changes in developing enamel. J. Dent. Res. 58(B):871.

Robinson, C., Lowe, N. R., and Weatherell, J. A. 1977.

Changes in amino acid composition of developing rat incisor enamel. Calcif. Tissue Res. 23:19.

Schonfeld, S. E., and Slavkin, H. C. 1977. Demonstration of enamel matrix proteins on root-analogue surfaces of rabbit permanent incisor teeth. Calcif. Tissue Res. 24:223.

Schroeder, H. E., and Listgarten, M. A. 1971. Fine Structure of the Developing Epithelial Attachment of Human Teeth. Monographs in Developmental Biology, vol. 2. Basel: S. Karger.

Seyer, J., and Glimcher, M. J. 1969. The content and nature of the carbohydrate components of the organic matrix of embryonic bovine enamel. Biochem. Biophys. Acta 184:509.

Selvig, K. A., and Halse, A. 1972. Crystal growth in rat incisor enamel. Anat. Rec. 173:453.

Selvig, K. A., and Halse, A. 1975. The ultrastructural localization of iron in rat incisor enamel. Scand. J. Dent. Res. 83:88.

Shimizu, M., Tanabe, T., and Fukae, M. 1979. Proteolytic enzyme in porcine immature enamel. J. Dent. Res. 58(B):782.

Slavkin, H. C., Mino, W., and Bringas, P., Jr. 1976. The biosynthesis and secretion of precursor enamel protein by ameloblasts as visualized by autoradiography after tryptophan administration. Anat. Rec. 185:289.

Smith, C. E. 1979. Ameloblasts: Secretory and resorptive functions. J. Dent. Res. 58(B):695.

Smith, C. E., and Warshawsky, H. 1977. Quantitative analysis of cell turnover in the enamel organ of the rat incisor. Evidence for ameloblast death immediately after enamel matrix secretion. Anat. Rec. 187:63.

Takano, Y. 1979. Cytochemical studies of ameloblasts and the surface layer of enamel of the rat incisor at the maturation stage. Arch. Histo. Jpn. 42:11.

Termine, J. D., Torchia, D. A., and Conn, K. M. 1979. Enamel matrix: Structural proteins. J. Dent. Res. 58(B):773.

Travis, D. F., and Glimcher, M. J. 1964. The structure and organization of, and the relationship between the organic matrix and the inorganic crystals of embryonic bovine enamel. J. Cell Biol. 23:447.

Warshawsky, H. 1968. The fine structure of secretory ameloblasts in rat incisors. Anat. Rec. 161:211.

Warshawsky, H. 1971. A light and electron microscopic study of the nearly mature enamel of rat incisors. Anat. Rec. 169:559.

Warshawsky, H. 1978. A freeze-fracture study of the topographic relationship between inner enamel-secretory ameloblasts in the rat incisor. Am. J. Anat. 152:153.

Warshawsky, H. 1979. Radioautographic studies on amelogenesis. J. Biol. Buccale 7:105.

Warhawsky, H., Josephsen, K., Thylstrup, A., and Fejerskov, O. 1981. The development of enamel structure in rat incisors as compared to the teeth of monkey and man. Anat. Rec. 200:371.

Warshawsky, H., and Smith, C. E. 1971. A three-dimensional reconstruction of the rods in rat maxillary incisor enamel. Anat. Rec. 169:585.

Warshawsky, H., and Smith, C. E. 1974. Morphological classification of rat incisor ameloblasts. Anat. Rec. 179:423.

Warshawsky, H., and Vugman, I. 1977. A comparison of the protein synthetic activity of presecretory and secretory ameloblasts in rat incisors. Anat. Rec. 188:143.

Weinstock, A. 1970. Uptake of ^{3}H-fucose and ^{3}H-galactose label by "resorptive" ameloblasts and its secretion into a periodic acid (PA)-Schiff-positive surface layer during the phase of enamel maturation. Anat. Rec. 166:395. (abstr.).

Weinstock, A., and Leblond, C. P. 1971. Elaboration of the matrix glycoprotein of enamel by the secretory ameloblasts of the rat incisor as revealed by radioautography after galactose ^{3}H-injection. J. Cell Biol. 51:26.

Gingiva

Lustgarten, M. A. 1964. The ultrastructure of human gingival epithelium. Am. J. Anat. 114:49.

Innervation

Bishop, M. A. 1981. A fine structural survey of the pulpal innervation in the rat mandibular incisor. Am. J. Anat. 160:213.

Periodontal Tissue

Beertsen, W., and Everts, V. 1977. The site of remodelling of collagen in the periodontal ligament of the mouse incisor. Anat. Rec. 189:479.

Beertsen, W., Brekelmans, M., and Everts, V. 1978. The site of collagen resorption in the periodontal ligament of the rodent molar. Anat. Rec. 192:305.

Cahill, D. R. 1969. Eruptive pathway formation in the presence of experimental tooth impaction in puppies. Anat. Rec. 164:67.

Carneiro, J., and de Moraes, F. F. 1965. Radioautographic visualization of collagen metabolism in the periodontal tissues of the mouse. Arch. Oral Biol. 10:833.

Stern, I. B. 1964. An electron microscopic study of the cementum, Sharpey's fibers and periodontal ligament in the rat incisor. Am. J. Anat. 115:377.

Susi, F. R. 1969. Anchoring fibrils in the attachment of epithelium to connective tissue in oral mucous membranes. J. Dent. Res. 48:144.

Ten Cate, A. R., and Deporter, D. A. 1975. The degradative role of the fibroblast in the remodeling and turnover of collagen in soft connective tissue. Anat. Rec. 182:1.

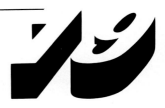

The Gastrointestinal Tract

Marian R. Neutra
and Helen A. Padykula

The microscopic structure of the digestive tract reflects the sequential functional changes that occur as food is propelled from the mouth toward the anus. The propulsion is caused primarily by waves of involuntary muscular contraction (peristalsis). The food is digested en route by enzymes secreted by the mucosae in fluids of appropriate pH and ionic composition. Current research has provided better definition of the local endocrine control mechanisms that influence this secretory and peristaltic activity; a large but diffusely distributed system of endocrine cells occurs throughout the gastrointestinal epithelia. Thus, locally produced hormones, such as gastrin, glucagon, secretin, and cholecystokinin, affect the physiological activity of the digestive tract and of the pancreas and liver as well. Certain components of the food are digested and absorbed. An important physiological action is the reabsorption of fluid that is poured into the digestive cavity as part of the salivary and gastrointestinal secretions. Undigested material is eliminated by the combined activity of involuntary and voluntary muscles. These functions occur in a well-defined progression and are reflected by distinctive gross, histological, and cellular variations along the length of the digestive tube. After the oral cavity, the hollow digestive tube is differentiated into four major organs: esophagus, stomach, small intestine, and large intestine. Grossly the organs are separated by muscular valves or *sphincters* (Greek, *sphinkter*, that which binds tight). The sphincters control the passage of contents from one organ to the next. At the junctions between organs of the digestive tube, the nature of the lining layer, the *mucous membrane* or *mucosa*, changes abruptly.

The digestion of carbohydrates begins in the oral cavity, but most of the *digestion* and *absorption* is accomplished by mucosae of the stomach and small intestine in coordination with the secretions of the pancreas and liver. Although it has long been known that lymphatic tissue occurs abundantly in the digestive tube, its participation as a *local immune system* in the body's defense mechanisms has only recently begun to be appreciated. We now know that, in response to the presence of antigens and microorganisms in the lumen, the mucosae produce antibodies, especially immunoglobulin A. The alimentary tract also serves as an avenue of *excretion*, eliminating certain waste products, some of which are secreted by the liver and carried in the bile to the duodenum. Except for the oral cavity, the histological organization of the digestive tube has a common plan throughout its length.

General Structural Plan

Layers

The digestive tube from the esophagus through the large intestine is made up of four concentric layers that exhibit considerable regularity. From the lumen outward, they are the mucosa, the submucosa, the muscularis, and the adventitia or serosa (Fig. 19–1). The mucosa, or mucous membrane, has three components: (1) a superficial epithelium; (2) an underlying stroma composed of a vascularized, loose connective tissue rich in immunocompetent cells (lamina propria); and (3) a relatively thin layer of smooth muscle (muscularis mucosae). Typically, the smooth muscle cells in the muscularis mucosae are subdivided into an inner circular and an outer longitudinal layer. Large accumulations of lymphoid cells and typical lymphatic nodules are often present in the stroma. With its abundance of plasma cells and lymphocytes, the entire lamina propria of the gut is a major site of immunological response.

The lining epithelium may invaginate to form glands that extend into the lamina propria (mucosal glands) or submucosa (submucosal glands), or ducts that lead through the wall of the tract to glands outside the tube proper (e.g., liver and pancreas). In other instances, the entire mucosa and submucosa project into the lumen as folds (plicae and rugae); the mucosa alone may evaginate into the lumen as fingers (villi). The glandular invaginations greatly enlarge secretory capacity, whereas the luminal evaginations increase its effective absorptive surface.

The *mucosa* differs considerably from segment to segment of the alimentary tract, reflect-

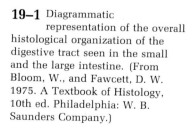

19–1 Diagrammatic representation of the overall histological organization of the digestive tract seen in the small and the large intestine. (From Bloom, W., and Fawcett, D. W. 1975. A Textbook of Histology, 10th ed. Philadelphia: W. B. Saunders Company.)

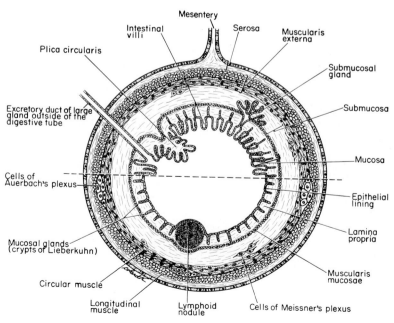

ing changing functional activity. The descriptions that follow will emphasize the distinctive epithelial cells responsible for the special secretory and absorptive functions of each segment of the tract. On the other hand, the surrounding supportive and muscular layers change relatively little, and thus only their distinctive features will be noted.

The *submucosa* is a collagenous connective tissue layer with far fewer cells than the lamina propria, but often containing accumulations of lymphatic tissue. In the esophagus and duodenum, it also contains glands that extend from the mucosa. The submucosa is a vascular service area with large blood vessels, lymphatic vessels, and nerves that send finer branches into the mucosa and muscularis.

The *muscularis* contains at least two layers of muscle. The muscle is smooth in all parts except the upper esophagus and the anal sphincter, where it is composed of skeletal muscle fibers. The fibers of the inner layers are disposed in a roughly circular fashion around the tube (circular layer), and those of the outer layer are disposed lengthwise along the tube (longitudinal layer). Contractions of the circular layer constrict the lumen; contractions of the longitudinal layer shorten the tube. At the various sphincters and valves along the tube (pharyngoesophageal, esophagogastric, pyloric, ileocecal, and anal), the layer of circular muscle is greatly thickened. Careful dissection of the muscle layers has shown that the fibers are actually disposed in a helical fashion, those in the circular layer forming a tight helix and those in the longitudinal layer an elongated one. The connective tissue fibers in the submucosa and adventitia are likewise oriented helically.

The *adventitia* of the tract is composed of several layers of loose connective tissue, alternately collagenous and elastic. Where the tract is suspended by a peritoneal fold, it is covered by a mesothelium continuous with that of the peritoneum (see Suspensory Folds, below). Wherever a mesothelial covering occurs, the adventitial layer is customarily termed a *serosa*.

Blood Vessels

At intervals, blood and lymphatic vessels and nerves enter the tract from the surrounding tissues or via the supporting peritoneal fold. The largest arteries are disposed longitudinally in the submucosa, and smaller branches also run in the serosa (Fig. 19–2). From these two sets of ves-

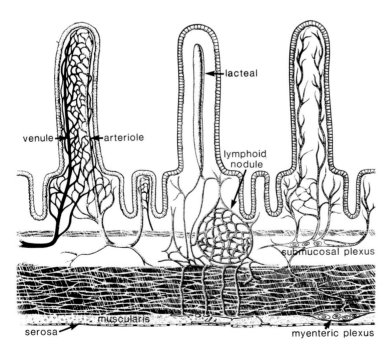

19–2 Diagram illustrating the blood circulation **(left),** lymphatic drainage **(center),** and innervation **(right)** of the small intestine. (Drawing by S. Colard-Keene; adapted from Junquiera, L. C., Carneiro, J., and Contopoulos, A., 1971, Basic Histology, 2nd ed. Los Altos, Calif.: Lange Medical Publications.)

sels, branches ramify perpendicularly to both the mucosa and the muscularis. In the latter, the capillaries run parallel with the muscle fibers. In the mucosa, the arteries supply an irregular capillary plexus around the glands and, in the small intestine, send terminal branches into the villi. The small capillaries associated with the intestinal epithelium typically have fenestrated endothelial cells.

The veins arising in the mucosa anastomose in the submucosa and pass out of the intestine beside the arteries. The muscularis mucosae has been described as forming a sphincter for the veins penetrating it. Valves are found in the larger veins only in the adventitia or serosa; they do not occur in the mesentery where these veins form the branches of the portal vein leading to the liver.

Lymphatic Vessels

The alimentary tract is richly supplied with lymphatic vessels that arise as blind tubes in the mucosa. In the small intestine, each villus usually contains a single blind-ending central lymphatic vessel known as a lacteal (Figs. 19–2 and 19–23). In some stages of digestion, the distention of these lymphatics is so great that they are easily recognized in sections. When the vessels are collapsed, their walls are difficult to distinguish from the surrounding connective tissue. Viewed at the ultrastructural level, these lymphatic vessels lack endothelial pores, thus differing from the local blood capillaries. Like blood capillaries, however, they contain many pinocytotic vesicles that shuttle macromolecules and chylomicrons from the interstitial space across the cytoplasm of the endothelial cells into the lymphatic circulation (see Transcytotic Vesicles, Chap. 9). Recent evidence obtained with tracers suggests that the endothelial cell junctions of lymphatics in the intestinal villi are not permeable to macromolecules, although they may open and become permeable when injured. The basal lamina of the lymphatic endothelium is discontinuous.

In the submucosa, the larger lymphatic vessels branch freely and have numerous valves. They cross the muscle layers, spreading in the intermuscular tissue and serosa, and leave through the mesentery. Unlike lymphatic vessels in many other parts of the body, those in the mesentery have muscular walls and are thus able to propel their contents.

Lymphatic Tissue

The lymphatic tissue of the alimentary tract occurs primarily in the lamina propria and assumes three forms: diffuse lymphatic tissue, solitary lymphatic nodules (Figs. 19–19 and 19–40), and aggregate nodules (Figs. 19–36 and 19–45). Large lymphatic masses may break through the muscularis mucosae and spread into the submucosa (Fig. 19–40). The superficial lymphatic vessels form a plexus as they pass through a nodule (Fig. 19–2). Blood vessels also form a net in the lymphatic tissue.

Diffuse lymphatic tissue occurs under the simple epithelia throughout the stomach and intestines. The cells found most abundantly are lymphocytes, macrophages, and plasma cells. Eosinophils and mast cells are also common inhabitants of the lamina propria.

Solitary nodules occur in the esophagus, in the pylorus of the stomach, and along the entire length of the small and large intestines. Aggregate nodules occur in the small intestine (Peyer's patches) and in the appendix (Figs. 19–36 and 19–45). Peyer's patches appear to the naked eye as oval bodies, usually about 1×2 cm but occasionally much larger. Microscopically, they are composed of many nodules in close contact. These patches distort and push aside the nearby glands and, immediately above the nodules, villi are largely effaced. There are approximately 30 such patches in the human intestine, principally in the lower part of the ileum on the side opposite the mesenteric attachment. A few occur in the jejunum and lower duodenum. Aggregate nodules are always present in the vermiform appendix (Fig. 19–45) but do not occur elsewhere in the large intestine.

This widely distributed tissue is part of the local immune system that responds to antigenic stimuli primarily by producing secretory immunoglobulin (IgA) and other antibodies (see Immune Defense Mechanisms, below).

Nerves

The nerves consist of both autonomic motor and sensory fibers. (At the two extremes of the tract there is, of course, voluntary innervation of the skeletal muscle fibers.) The motor fibers are both parasympathetic and sympathetic. The fibers of both types ramify in the wall of the tract as shown in Fig. 19–2, forming plexuses in each of

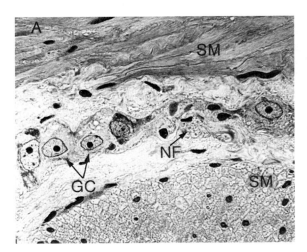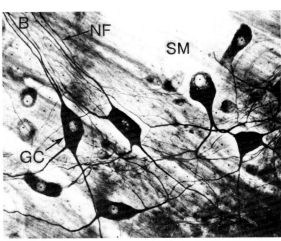

19–3 Parasympathetic ganglia of Auerbach's plexus, interposed between circular and longitudinal smooth muscle layers **(SM). A.** Histological section of a ganglion in monkey stomach with large neurons (GC, ganglion cells) and nerve fibers **(NF). B.** Whole mount of gold-impregnated ganglion cells **(GC)** viewed "en face." (Preparation of Graham C. Schofield.)

the layers. The ganglia of the sympathetic nerves are external to the gut wall, lying in the celiac plexus and in the superior and inferior mesenteric plexus. The parasympathetic ganglia are located within the wall; they are connected with nerves derived from the vagus and the sacral outflow.

The neurons of the intramural parasympathetic ganglia occur in two locations: (1) in nodes of the submucosal plexus (of Meissner) and (2) between the two layers of the muscularis, in the myenteric plexus (of Auerbach) (Fig. 19–2). The ganglia and the associated fibers form an irregular rectilinear pattern when viewed from the surface. The autonomic ganglion cells, surrounded by the usual satellite cells, possess many dendrites and have eccentrically located nuclei (Fig. 19–3). Sympathetic fibers ramify through the wall of the tube along with the parasympathetic fibers to innervate the muscularis and the blood vessels.

Recent immunocytochemical studies suggest that parasympathetic nerves of the gut wall may contain both the neurotransmitter acetylcholine and vasoactive intestinal peptide (VIP), which is generally considered a gut hormone (Fig. 19–4). Several other peptide hormones including somatostatin, gastrin, cholecystokinin, and substance P have been identified in nerve fibers of the gastrointestinal tract—fibers that also contain classic neurotransmitters (see Gastrointestinal Endocrine Cells, below). Stimulation of the parasympathetic nerves to the intestinal tract generally increases muscular activity, circulation, and secretion, whereas these activities are decreased by stimulation of the sympathetic nerves. Because the postganglionic parasympathetic fibers arise locally, their influence may be limited to a fairly short length of the tube. Postganglionic fibers of the sympathetics, however, arise from ganglia outside the gut and are much more widely distributed. Sympathetic activity is reinforced, moreover, by the concomitant release of catecholamines from the adrenal medulla.

Suspensory Folds

The esophagus runs through the thorax within the connective tissue of the superior and posterior mediastinum. The stomach and intestines are mostly supported by suspensory folds from the peritoneal wall known as the omenta and mesenteries, respectively. However, the duodenum and the ascending and descending limbs of the colon adhere to the posterior wall of the abdominal cavity and are thus considered secondarily retroperitoneal. The stomach is peculiar in that it retains a ventral suspensory fold and thus has both a dorsal (greater) and a ventral (lesser) omentum. The omenta differ from the mesenteries proper in that they are perforated.

The *peritoneum* is a closed sac lined by a

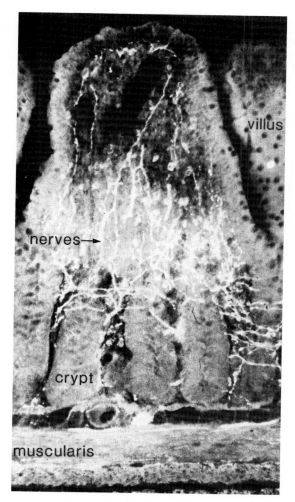

19–4 Immunocytochemical visualization of autonomic nerves in the rat small intestine; section treated with fluorescein-conjugated antibodies to VIP and viewed by fluorescence microscopy. VIP is present in a plexus of mucosal nerves and in submucosal ganglion cells. The nerves are presumably parasympathetic and may also contain acetylcholine. (From Hökfelt, T., Johansson, O., Jungdahl, A. L., Lundberg, J. M., and Schultzberg, M. 1980. Nature [Lond.] 284:515.)

moist slippery membrane that allows the suspended abdominal organs to slide freely over one another during peristaltic movements. Its entire surface is covered by a continuous single layer of flat polygonal cells, the "mesothelium." Mesothelial cells have microvilli on their free surfaces and may be capable of phagocytosis. The portion of the sac that lines the body wall is called "pa-

rietal peritoneum"; the portion that is reflected onto the suspensory folds and the digestive tube or viscera is called "visceral peritoneum."

Mesenteries and *omenta* are thin sheets of loose connective tissue covered on both surfaces by mesothelium. Through the connective tissue of the mesentery course the lymphatic vessels, blood vessels, and nerves that supply the suspended alimentary organs. The connective tissue contains elastic networks, interwoven bundles of collagen fibers, and various cells, especially mast cells, eosinophils, monocytes, lymphocytes, macrophages, and adipose cells. Dense aggregates of lymphocytes, monocytes, and macrophages are visible to the naked eye as "milky spots," especially common in the omenta and in the peritoneal lining of the diaphragm. These leukocytic cells are also found free in the peritoneal fluid.

Esophagus

The esophagus is a tubular passageway for the chewed, partly digested food received from the oral cavity. In the adult human it is about 25 cm long. It is composed of regular concentric tissue layers (Figs. 19–5 and 19–6A) that are continuous superiorly with those of the pharynx and inferiorly with those of the stomach. Because of the tonus of the circular layer of muscularis, the mucous membrane is thrown into many temporary longitudinal folds that effectively obliterate the lumen of the resting esophagus (Fig. 19–5); these folds flatten out while a bolus of food is passing.

The mucosal *epithelium* is stratified squamous (Fig. 19–6B) and extremely thick (about 300 μm). In humans, complete keratinization of the epithelium is rare unless the esophagus is subject to an unusual degree of trauma. Such keratinization occurs normally in some mammalian species, especially in herbivores.

The *lamina propria* of the esophagus is less cellular than in lower parts of the digestive tube. Lymphatic nodules occur occasionally, especially around the ducts of glands. The *muscularis mucosae* is broad, being 200 to 400 μm thick. It is unusual in that it consists of longitudinally directed fibers. It replaces the elastic layer of the pharynx at the level of the cricoid cartilage. The submucosa is thick (300–700 μm) and is characterized by abundant coarse elastic fibers, which permit distension during swallowing.

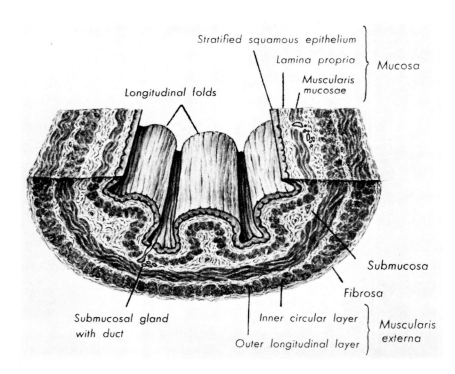

Stratified squamous epithelium
Lamina propria
Muscularis mucosae
Mucosa
Longitudinal folds
Submucosa
Fibrosa
Submucosal gland with duct
Inner circular layer
Outer longitudinal layer
Muscularis externa

19–5 Reconstruction of a segment of the dorsal half of the human esophagus. (From Copenhaver, W. M., Bunge, R. P., and Bunge, M. B. 1971. Bailey's Textbook of Histology. Baltimore: The Williams & Wilkins Company.)

The *muscularis* (0.5–2 mm thick) is composed of a circular inner layer and outer bundles of longitudinal fibers, arising at the level of the cricoid cartilage. At its upper extremity is the superior esophageal (pharyngoesophageal) sphincter, consisting of a thickened layer of circular (oblique) muscles. Because the initiation of swallowing is voluntary, the muscle fibers in the upper quarter of the tube are skeletal rather than smooth. Striated and smooth muscle fibers intermingle in the second quarter of the tube, and only smooth muscle fibers occur in the lower half. This transition marks the beginning of a continuous muscularis of smooth muscle that extends throughout the stomach and intestines to the anus.

The *adventitia* is loose connective tissue containing many longitudinally directed blood vessels, lymphatic vessels, and nerves. For 2 to 3 cm above the stomach, elastic fibers are numerous and attach the esophagus to the diaphragm.

The orifice between the esophagus and stomach is bounded by a broad band of circular smooth muscle, the inferior esophageal (esophagogastric) sphincter. At the esophageal–stomach junction, the epithelium abruptly changes from stratified squamous to the simple columnar epithelium that characterizes the stomach. Isolated mucous glands occur in the esophagus. They are described by their position, as superficial (mucosal) and deep (submucosal). The *mucosal glands* occur only in the narrow zones near the two ends of the esophagus, between the level of the cricoid cartilage and the fifth tracheal ring and again near the entrance of the stomach. The mucus formed by these superficial glands is neutral whereas that of the deep glands is acidic. Because the mucosal glands resemble those occurring at the cardiac end of the stomach, an alternative name is cardiac glands.

The *submucosal glands* are scattered tubular downgrowths that pass through the lamina propria and muscularis mucosae into the submucosa (Fig. 19–7). The secretory cells have the typical cytological characteristics of mucous cells. The smallest ducts are lined with simple columnar epithelium; the main ducts that enter the mucosa are lined with stratified epithelium. The number of deep glands varies greatly in different individ-

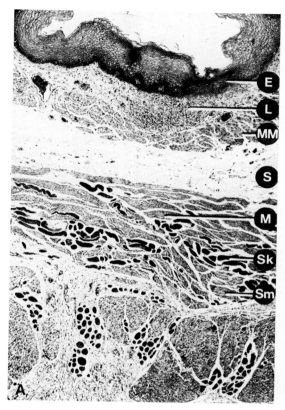

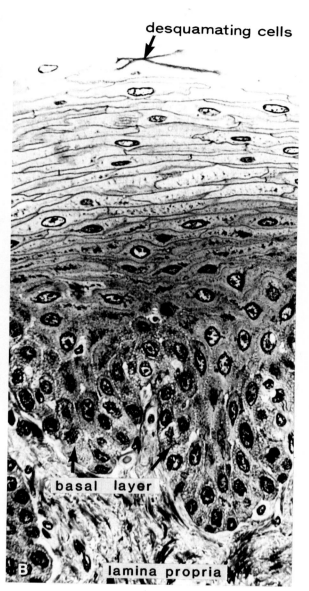

19–6 A. Midregion of the human esophagus, cross
section. At this level, the muscularis **(M)**
contains skeletal muscle fibers **(Sk)** in addition to
smooth muscle fibers **(Sm).** The muscularis mucosae
(MM) is thick. **E,** epithelium; **L,** lymphoid cells;
S, submucosa. Eosin and methylene blue. × 45.
B. Epithelium of monkey esophagus. The basal side of
the epithelium is deeply indented by extensions of the
lamina propria. The basal, proliferative cell layer is
cuboidal, but daughter cells become progressively
flattened as they are displaced upward. Nucleated
squamous cells of the superficial lay are sloughed off,
having lived about 4 weeks.

uals. They are usually more abundant in the upper half of the esophagus.

Stomach

The stomach is a remarkable exocrine secretory
organ that produces after each meal a large volume of acidic (pH 2) secretion containing the
protease pepsin. This enzyme initiates protein
digestion, a process that is continued in the intestinal lumen by pancreatic enzymes. The gastric surface is protected from its own highly
acidic secretion by a thin film of mucus that is
being constantly produced by the surface epithelial cells. Another exocrine gastric product is
"intrinsic factor," a glycoprotein that combines
with vitamin B_{12} to form a complex necessary for
the absorption of vitamin B_{12} in the ileum. The
stomach is also, in part, an endocrine gland that
produces several hormones including gastrin.
Gastrin influences the activity of the gastric
exocrine and muscle cells as well as the
physiological activity of the pancreas and small
intestine. Gastric digestion is facilitated by con-

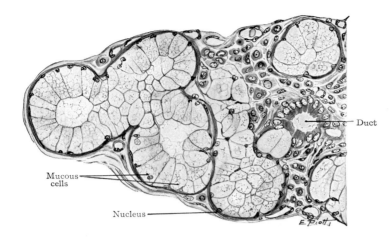

19–7 Drawing of the terminal portion of a submucosal gland in the esophagus of a child. The secretory cells produce mucus. A small duct occurs at the right. H&E.

Duct

Mucous cells

Nucleus

tractions of the heavy muscularis, which churn the food.

The opening through which the esophagus connects with the stomach is the cardiac orifice, and the opening from the stomach to the intestine is the pyloric orifice (Greek, *pyloros*, gatekeeper). The lining of the stomach is thrown into major longitudinal folds, or rugae, when the organ is contracted. They disappear when the stomach is distended with food (Fig. 19–8).

Histological Organization

The stomach of most mammals, including humans, is lined completely by a simple columnar epithelium. At the cardiac opening, the cells are continuous with the basal layer of the stratified epithelium of the esophagus. The lining of the

19–8 Drawing of the interior of a contracted human stomach showing the major regions and the internal folds or rugae. (From Gray, H., and Goss, C. M. 1966. Gray's Anatomy, 28th ed. Philadelphia: Lea & Febiger.)

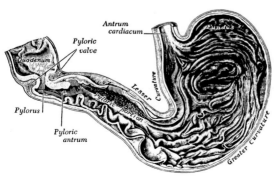

organ is indented by many pits (foveolae); at the base of each pit are the openings of several branched tubular glands. There are about 3.5 million foveolae on the stomach wall, serving about 15 million glands. All of the glands are confined to the mucosa.

The glands of the stomach are of three histologically distinct types. The *cardiac glands* occur in the first 5 to 40 mm from the cardiac orifice; the *pyloric glands* are found along the 4 cm from the pyloric vestibule to the pyloric sphincter. In the large area between these two extremities lies the most common type, the *gastric* (or erroneously, *fundic*) *glands*. The cells of the cardiac and pyloric glands are primarily mucous. The epithelium of the gastric glands is more diversified, containing enzyme- and acid-secreting cells as well as mucous cells. The cardiac and pyloric glands are conspicuously coiled (Fig. 19–9), in contrast to the gastric glands, which are relatively straight (Fig. 19–10). The pyloric region is distinguished by long pits or foveolae that occupy nearly one-half the depth of the mucosa; in the cardia and body of the organ, the pits are shorter and occupy only one-fourth the thickness of the mucosa.

The *mucous membrane* of the stomach is 0.3 to 1.5 mm thick, being thinnest in the cardiac region. Underlying the epithelium is a richly vascularized, cellular lamina propria (Fig. 19–10). Occasionally lymphatic nodules occur. As in the intestines, the gastric lamina propria contains lymphocytes and plasma cells that indicate local immunological activity. Smooth muscle fibers extend upward from the muscularis mucosae around the glands, and their shortening may help to expel secretory products.

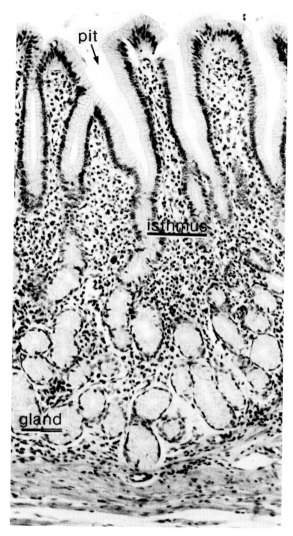

19–9 Human pyloric mucosa. Pyloric **pits** are deeper than those of the gastric mucosa, and they are lined by typical surface mucous cells. A short **isthmus** leads to coiled **glands** consisting of a separate population of mucous cells, and numerous gastrin-producing endocrine cells (G cells, not visible here). H&E.

The *submucosa* consists of coarse collagenous bundles, many elastic fibers, blood and lymphatic vessels, and the submucosal nerve plexus. Clusters of fat cells are common in older people.

The *muscularis* is composed of three primary layers: an inner oblique, a middle circular, and an outer longitudinal layer. The oblique layer is best developed at the cardiac end and in the body of the organ. The circular bundles are thickened at both ends of the stomach in the regions of the sphincters. The myenteric nerve plexus occurs in the thin connective tissue layer separating the circular from the longitudinal muscle layer. It coordinates contractions of the extensive muscle coat that churn and homogenize ingested food as gastric juices are added to it.

The *serosa*, consisting of connective tissue plus mesothelium, is continuous, via the omenta, with the peritoneum.

Cytology of the Gastric Epithelium

The entire gastric surface and the glands are lined by simple columnar epithelium. Cells of four major types are seen in routine histological sections: (1) *Surface mucous cells;* (2) *neck mucous cells;* (3) *parietal,* or *oxyntic cells;* and (4) *chief,* or *peptic cells* (Figs. 19–10 and 19–11; see here and color insert). In addition, a fifth class of cells present in the glands of the stomach is stained by certain empirical methods that use heavy metal salts, such as chromium, silver, or osmium (Figs. 19–12 and 19–19; see here and color insert). This heterogeneous population has been shown by immunocytochemical methods to be the source of a variety of peptides and complex amines that function as hormones, neurotransmitters, or both: hence, they are known collectively as (5) *enteroendocrine cells.*

The surface of the stomach is lined entirely by *surface mucous cells,* forming a uniform simple columnar epithelium that extends into the pits (foveolae) (Figs. 19–10 and 19–13). They continuously secrete carbohydrate-rich glycoproteins that make up a mucous film that protects the mucosa from the high acidity of the gastric fluid. Without this film, ulceration of the mucosa occurs. These surface cells are constantly being shed into the lumen and replaced from below. In routine preparations (Fig. 19–10) the mucus is not well preserved and is poorly stained, so that the apical cytoplasm appears pale or foamy, but the glycoprotein nature of the mucus is demonstrable by the PAS procedure, and its strong negative charge is evident by its intense staining with toluidine blue. At the ultrastructural level, the intracellular mucous droplets are dense ovoid, spherical, or discoid granules located apically and formed within the membranes of the well-developed Golgi complex (Fig. 19–13).

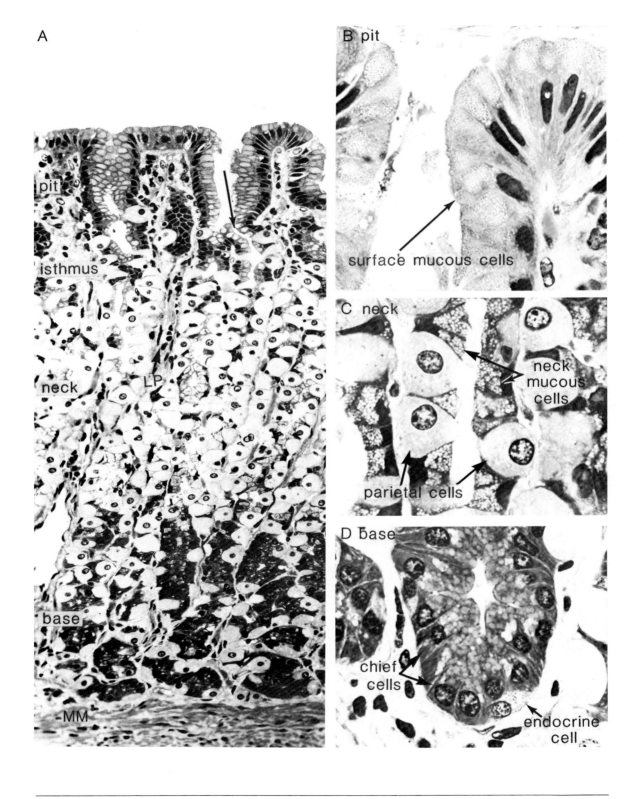

A

pit

isthmus

neck

LP

base

MM

B pit

surface mucous cells

C neck

neck mucous cells

parietal cells

D base

chief cells

endocrine cell

19–10 Gastric mucosa of a monkey, 2-μm section, H & E. **A.** At the base of each of the surface pits are the openings of several long narrow gastric glands **(arrow).** A short **isthmus** region leads to the long **neck** of the gland, and finally to its **base** just above the muscularis mucosae **(MM).** Elements of the lamina propria **(LP)** are insinuated between the crowded glands. **B.** The epithelium of the luminal surface and pits consists entirely of surface mucous cells. **C.** The neck is dominated by parietal (oxyntic) and neck mucous cells. The lumen is narrow. **D.** The base of the gland is lined primarily by chief (peptic) cells. Two endocrine cells are visible, lying next to the basal lamina with no luminal contact.

The *neck mucous cells* are located in the middle and upper parts of the gastric gland (that is, immediately below the base of the pit), where they are interspersed among parietal cells (Fig. 19–10). The neck mucous cells produce acidic glycoproteins and they differ structurally and functionally from the surface mucous cells, which produce a more neutral mucus. Neck mucous cells exhibit more cytoplasmic basophilia in light-microscopic preparations and more rough endoplasmic reticulum (ER) in electron-microscopic preparations than do the surface mucous cells. Their Golgi complex is exceptionally well developed. Their secretion granules are larger, more spherical, and less dense than those of the surface cells.

The *parietal, or oxyntic, cells* secrete 0.1 N hydrochloric acid, a remarkable secretory feat since this concentration of acid can destroy living cells. Parietal cells are located principally in the middle and upper part of the gastric gland, but they also occur in the lower half among the pepsin-producing chief cells (Fig. 19–10). They are present but fewer in the pyloric glands. At the light-microscopic level, parietal cells are easily identified by their large size and clear or acidophilic cytoplasm (Fig. 19–10C). They usually contain one nucleus but may be binucleate. The intense cytoplasmic acidophilia of the parietal cells reflects the abundance of smooth membranes and mitochondria. They contain a relatively small amount of rough ER (Fig. 19–3), and the Golgi complex is small and located basally.

The distinctive ultrastructural feature of these acid-secreting cells is the presence of intracellular (or secretory) canaliculi, which are trenchlike invaginations of the apical cell surface (Figs. 19–14 to 19–16). (These deep invaginations may also be interpreted as extensions of the glandular lumen.) The canaliculi are lined by numerous

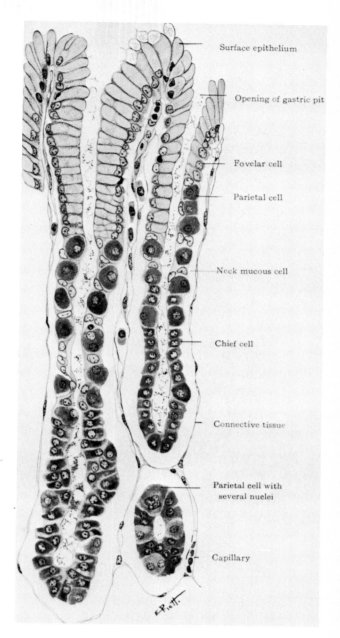

19–11 Drawing of two gastric glands of the adult human stomach. This is a black and white rendition of a color plate. See color section.

microvilli, and thus the surface area of the apical plasma membrane is greatly increased. The secretion of HCl is believed to occur along this vast internalized surface. The basolateral membrane apparently carries receptors for histamine, gastrin, and acetylcholine, all of which stimulate se-

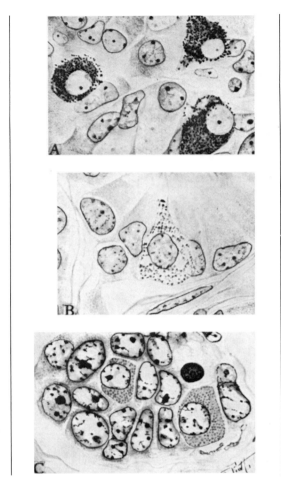

19–12 Reactions of granules in argentaffin cells from the small intestine of a pig. This is a black and white rendition of a color plate. See color section.

is evident that active acid secretion requires a large area of free surface and has a high energy requirement (oxidative metabolism). This requirement is reflected morphologically by an abundance of mitochondria that have many cristae and matrix granules (Figs. 19–15 and 19–16).

The *chief or peptic cells* are located primarily in the basal half of the gastric gland (Figs. 19–10 and 19–12; see here and color insert); they have also been called zymogenic because they are typical protein-secreting cells that resemble the pancreatic acinar cell. The basal cytoplasm contains an extensive rough ER (Fig. 19–17), which is reflected light-microscopically as a striated basophilic region. The supranuclear region is filled with acidophilic zymogen granules that are often not preserved in routine preparations. These secretory granules form in the Golgi complex and are believed to be released by exocytosis in the same manner as the zymogen granules of pancreatic acinar cells.

The chief cells synthesize and secrete pepsinogens, the precursors of the active enzymes "pepsins," which hydrolyze proteins into smaller molecules. The acid milieu of the stomach is required to convert pepsinogen to pepsin.

Enteroendocrine cells of several types occur in the glands of the stomach and are most abundant in the antrum of the pylorus. They are described in detail below.

Gastrointestinal Endocrine Cells

The enteroendocrine cells as a group resemble the peptide-synthesizing cells found in endocrine glands such as the anterior pituitary (Fig. 19–18). Because some endocrine cell types located in the gut proper occur also in the islets of Langerhans in the pancreas, the entire population is sometimes called "gastroenteropancreatic (GEP) cells." Endocrine cells are widely distributed in the epithelia of the stomach, small and large intestine, appendix, distal esophageal glands, and even in the ducts of the pancreas and liver. (Similar cells occur in the epithelia of the respiratory passages, another outgrowth of the primitive embryonic gut.) Were they grouped together, these cells would constitute the largest endocrine gland in the body.

Gut endocrine cells are small clear pyramidal cells with broad basal cytoplasm that contains dense granules (Figs. 19–12 and 19–19A; see here and color insert). They were originally identified by staining methods using heavy metal salts and, on this basis, were given various

cretion of hydrogen ions into the lumen and bicarbonate ions into the interstitium.

An extensive closed system of smooth membrane, the tubulovesicular system, occupies the cytoplasm adjacent to the canaliculi (Fig. 19–16). When acid is secreted, microvilli rapidly become more abundant in the canaliculi, whereas the tubulovesicular system diminishes (Fig. 19–15). When acid secretion is inhibited experimentally, the situation reverses: microvilli decrease and the tubulovesicular system enlarges. The tubulovesicular system may represent a membrane reserve that is translated to the surface during acid secretion. Thus, these two membrane systems are functionally interconnected. Overall, it

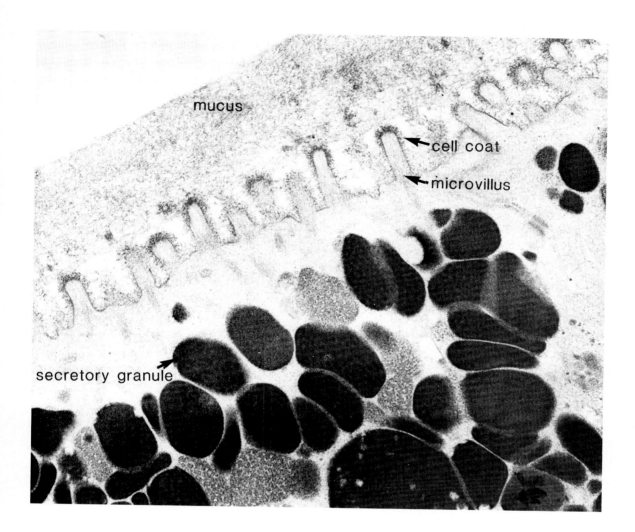

mucus

cell coat

microvillus

secretory granule

19–13 Surface mucous cell of human stomach. The apical cytoplasm of the surface mucous cell is crowded with secretion granules that contain a condensed form of mucous glycoprotein. Secreted mucus forms a hydrated gel that covers the surface of the epithelium. The cell surface has many short microvilli and a dense filamentous cell coat. (Courtesy of Susumu Ito.)

names. The granules of some of these cells precipitate silver from an ammoniacal silver nitrate solution (Figs. 19–19B and 19–12) and thus were called *argentaffin cells*. Many may also be stained by solutions of potassium dichromate; hence the name *enterochromaffin cells*. A few granules precipitate silver only when an external reducing agent is present; cells with these granules were called *argyrophylic cells*.

With the electron microscope, at least 12 different types of gut endocrine cell have been recognized by their ultrastructurally distinctive secretory granules, but more than 12 types presumably exist. Immunocytochemical methods (Fig. 19–19C) are currently being used to identify which morphological cell type is responsible for each of the more than 20 gastrointestinal hormones, candidate hormones (see below), and neurotransmitters that these cells produce. They

are now known to be crucial in the coordination and control of all gastrointestinal functions.

Ultrastructurally, the various types of enteroendocrine cell resemble each other. Some (the "open" types) have a narrow apical pole with a tuft of microvilli extending into the glandular lumen, which presumably sample the changing composition of the local environment (Fig. 19–19). Others (the "closed" types) contact only the basal lamina and not the lumen (Fig. 19–10).

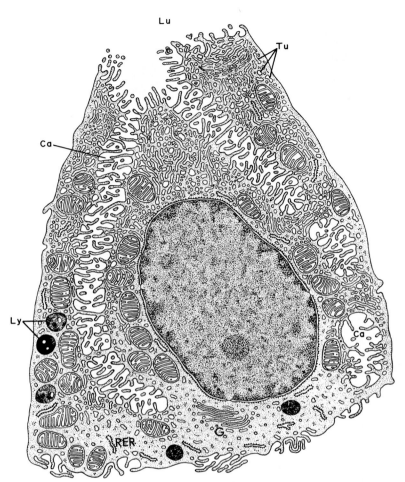

19–14 Drawing summarizing the ultrastructural features of a gastric parietal cell. The secretory canaliculus **(Ca)** is a deep, troughlike invagination of the apical cell surface. Its surface area is further increased by numerous microvilli. An extensive tubulovesicular system **(Tu)** of smooth membranes is concentrated in the cytoplasm surrounding the canaliculus. Mitochondria are abundant, but the rough ER **(RER)** and Golgi **(G)** membranes are relatively sparse. The dense bodies **(Ly)** may be derivatives of the lysosomal system. **Lu,** lumen. (From Lentz, T. L., 1971. Cell Fine Structure. Philadelphia: W. B. Saunders Company.)

The broad basal cytoplasm, which always makes extensive contact with the basal lamina, contains membrane-bound secretory granules whose contents are released into the underlying connective tissue and capillaries (Fig. 19–18). The rough ER and Golgi membranes are relatively sparse as compared with pancreatic acinar or hepatic cells.

The staining density, the size, and the shape of the secretory granules allow us to distinguish different gut endocrine cells by electron microscopy (Fig. 19–20). Although work is still in progress to correlate electron-microscopic identification with a specific peptide or amine product, several hormones and transmitters have been definitely or tentatively assigned to specific cells (Table 19–1). This list, however, is continually being revised and expanded. (For a listing that also includes GEP cells of the pancreatic islets, see Chap. 21.)

Most GEP cells are able to take up and process biogenic amines and thus may be considered members of the so-called APUD (amine precursor uptake and decarboxylate) series. This characteristic led Pearse to propose that all GEP cells are derived from the neural ectoderm in the early embryo. Indeed, several peptide hormones and an amine transmitter are secreted by GEP cells and by peripheral and central neurons (see below). On the other hand, there is convincing evidence that GEP cells are derived from embryonic endoderm. In the adult intestine, they arise from the same pool of stem cells that produces all of the intestinal epithelial cells. Furthermore, transplanted embryonic endoderm produces both gut and pancreatic endocrine cells.

Some of the substances produced by enteroendocrine cells act as true peptide hormones. For example, gastrin, secretin, and cholecystokinin are secreted into the blood stream to reach their

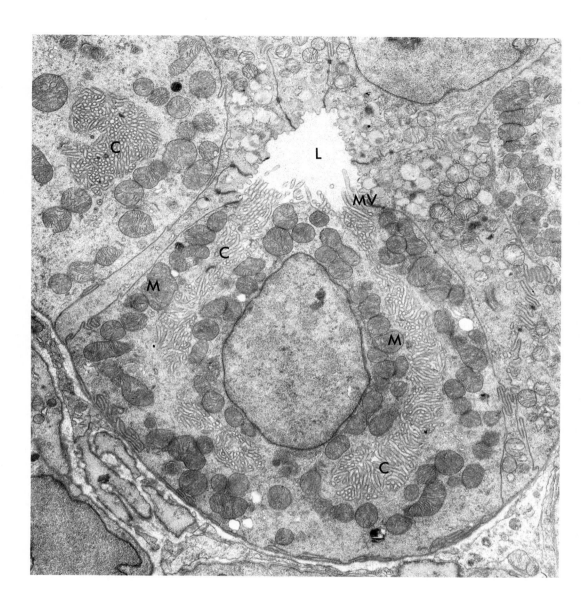

target organs (stomach, pancreas, and gallbladder), and soon after are rapidly broken down and eliminated, mainly by the kidneys. Other peptides, such as gut-type glucagon, motilin, and VIP, are currently termed "candidate hormones" because although their pharmacological actions are known, their exact physiological role is unclear. Some peptides, such as somatostatin, may be released from enteroendocrine cells into the local subepithelial connective tissue or directly onto other cell types via long basal cytoplasmic processes ("paracrine" secretion) to influence cells and tissues in the immediate vicinity. Local release of peptides may modulate the function of

19–15 Gastric gland of a bat, cross section. The electron micrograph shows one parietal cell, the narrow gland lumen **(L)**, and portions of other parietal and neck mucous cells. This stomach had been stimulated in vitro to produce hydrochloric acid. The lumens of the secretory canaliculi **(C)** are filled with numerous microvilli **(MV)**. Mitochondria **(M)** are abundant and lie near the canaliculi. (From Ito, S. 1967. *In* C. F. Code and W. Heidel [eds.], Handbook of Physiology, vol. 2, sec. 6. Washington, D.C.: American Physiological Society, chap. 41.)

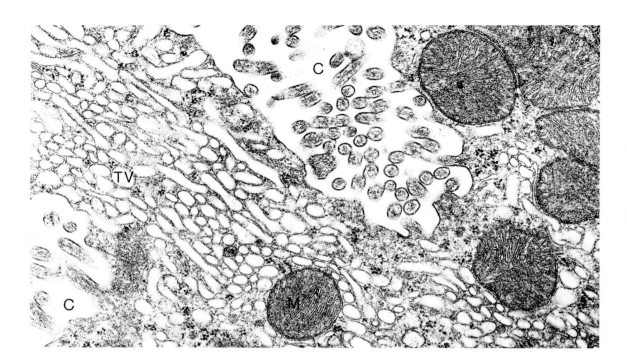

19–16 Interior of a nonsecreting parietal cell showing portions of two secretory canaliculi **(C)**, abundant smooth membranes of the tubulovesicular system **(TV)**, and mitochondria **(M)**. (Courtesy of Susumu Ito.)

nearby enteroendocrine and exocrine cells. One group of enteroendocrine cells (called entero-chromaffin or EC because of their staining properties) synthesizes and secretes serotonin (5-hydroxytryptamine) along with either substance P or motilin. EC cells exemplify the fact that some gut endocrine cells can produce both a biogenic amine and a peptide hormone, an ability that they share with nerves of the digestive tract and with cells in the central nervous system. In addition, many gastrointestinal hormones may interact with neural mechanisms and with the hypothalamic–pituitary axis to orchestrate the secretory activity and motility necessary for digestion. Finally, some gastrointestinal hormones enhance metabolic levels and promote growth of digestive tissues: for example, gastrin is trophic for much of the gastrointestinal mucosa, and cholecystokinin stimulates pancreatic growth.

The cells of "classic" endocrine glands are aggregated together; they receive stimuli from the bloodstream and nervous system and deliver their hormone products via the bloodstream to distant target organs. Gut endocrine cells, in contrast, are anatomically dispersed in a unique way that allows for local signals to be received from points along the entire length of the gastrointestinal lumen (as well as from blood and nerves) and for chemical messages to be delivered to nearby and distant target cells.

Several types of endocrine cells occur in the stomach. EC (serotonin) cells are present throughout the mucosa, A (glucagon) cells occur only in the upper third, and G (gastrin) cells predominate in the lower portion including the pyloric antrum. D (somatostatin) cells are distributed both in A-cell regions above and in G-cell regions below, but they are absent from the midportion of the stomach. G cells secrete gastrin in response to an elevated pH and to autonomic stimulation. The A cells, like their counterparts in the pancreatic islets, seem to be involved in carbohydrate metabolism. The close association of D cells with both A- and G-cell populations is consistent with the idea that somatostatin plays a local regulatory role.

Small Intestine

Macromolecular nutrients in food are digested extracellularly in the small intestine, largely by the action of pancreatic enzymes. The terminal digestion of proteins and carbohydrates occurs at

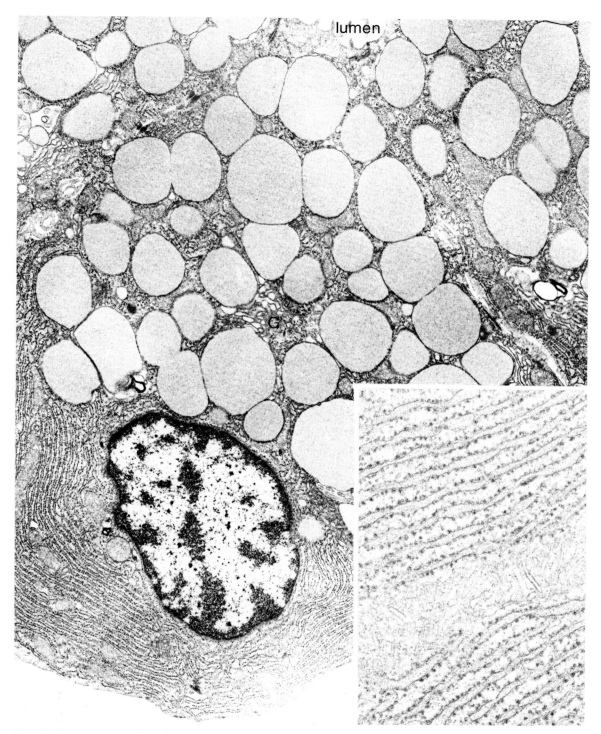

19–17 Chief (peptic) cell in the gastric gland of a monkey. The basal cytoplasm is filled with parallel cisternae of rough ER (see **inset**). The cell apex contains zymogenic secretory granules and elements of the Golgi complex. (Courtesy of Susumu Ito.)

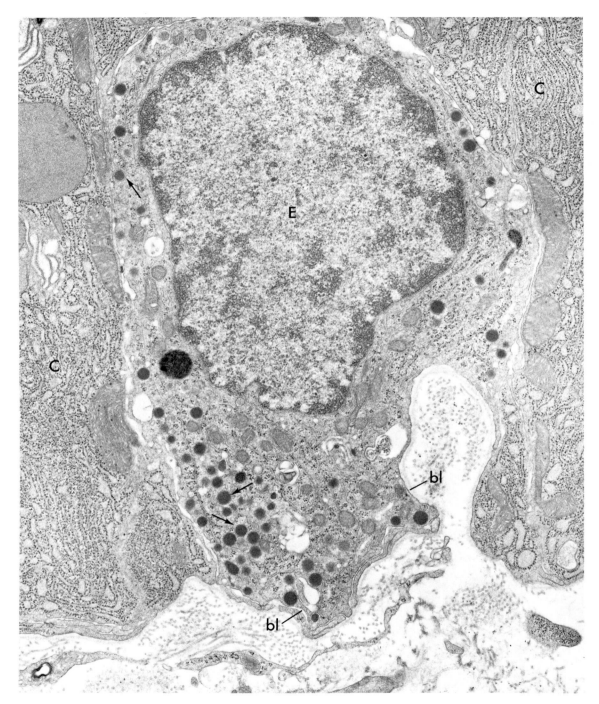

19–18 Endocrine cell **(E)** in the gastric gland of a bat, situated between two chief cells **(C)**. Its basal surface rests against the basal lamina **(bl)**, and its cytoplasm contains small, dense, membrane-limited granules **(arrows)**. × 18,000. (Courtesy of Susumu Ito.)

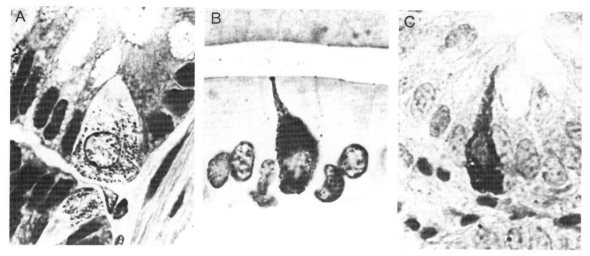

19–19 Enteroendocrine cells visualized by several staining methods. **A.** Monkey colonic crypt, 2-μm plastic section, H&E stain. Enteroendocrine cells are identified by their pyramidal shape, broad contact with the basement membrane, clear cytoplasm, and small basal granules. **B.** Guinea pig small intestine, Bodian silver stain for argentaffin cells. The narrow apical cytoplasmic contact with the lumen is clearly seen. **C.** Human colonic crypt, immunocytochemical identification of glucagon. A glucagon-containing cell makes broad contact with the basal lamina and narrow contact with the crypt lumen. (Courtesy of Pamela C. Colony.)

19–20 Electron micrographs of the basal cytoplasm of three different endocrine cells in the small intestine of a human fetus. **A.** Large irregular electron-dense granules typical of an EC cell (5-HT plus peptides). **B.** Small round granules of variable density, consistent with S-cell morphology (secretin). **C.** Round, dense granules of variable size, possibly in a D cell (somatostatin). Positive identification of these cell types would require specific cytochemistry. (Courtesy of Pamela C. Colony.)

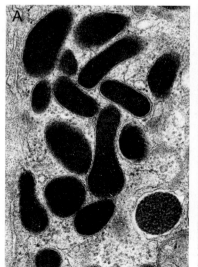
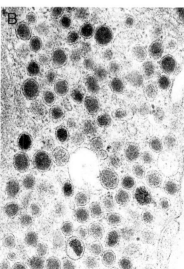
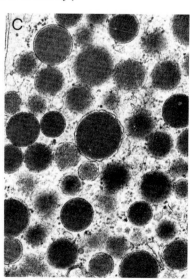

Table 19–1 Secretions of Gut Endocrine Cells

Cell name	Location	Product	Major action
A	Stomach	Pancreatic glucagon	Hepatic glycogenolysis
D	Pylorus, duodenum	Somatostatin	Local inhibition of endocrine cells (?)
D_1	Stomach, intestines	Vasoactive intestinal peptide (VIP)	Ion/water secretion, gut motility
EC	Stomach, intestine, submucosal glands, appendix, etc.	Serotonin (5-HT), motilin, substance P	Gut motility
G	Pylorus, duodenum	Gastrin	Gastric acid secretion
I	Small intestine	Cholecystokinin	Pancreatic enzyme secretion, gallbladder emptying
K	Small intestine	Gastric inhibitory peptide (GIP)	Inhibition of gastric acid secretion
L	Small intestine, colon	Gut-type glucagon, pancreatic glucagon	Hepatic glycogenolysis
N	Small intestine	Neurotensin	
S	Small intestine	Secretin	Pancreatic and biliary ion/water secretion

the mucosal surface by enzymes of intestinal origin. The resultant amino acids, monosaccharides, fatty acids, and monoglycerides are absorbed along a vast internal absorptive surface. Water and electrolytes from salivary, gastric, pancreatic, and hepatic secretions are also reabsorbed.

The human small intestine is a thin-walled tube about 4 m in length, extending from the pylorus of the stomach to the colon. At the pylorus, the smooth-surfaced gastric mucosa changes abruptly to a rough-surfaced intestinal mucosa with numerous projections (villi) (Fig. 19–21). The small intestine consists of three portions: the duodenum, jejunum, and ileum. The duodenal–jejunal junction is marked externally by the suspensory ligament of Treitz, a thickening of the mesentery. Otherwise, no definite structural landmarks distinguish the three segments, although certain distinctive histological features characterize their mucosae (see Regional Differences, below). In addition, functional differences in absorptive activities have been demonstrated along the length of the small intestine.

Histological Organization

The lining of the small intestine has gross and microscopic devices for increasing the surface area available for digestive and absorptive activities. The entire lining, including both mucosa

and submucosa, may be thrown into large folds. Relatively permanent, circularly arranged folds (plicae circulares, or valves of Kerckring) are highly developed in the jejunum and form its most conspicuous feature (Fig. 19–22). In the duodenum and ileum, they are less conspicuous, and they generally end two feet above the entrance to the colon.

The surface of the small intestine is studded with innumerable villi that give it a velvety appearance grossly. They greatly increase the absorptive surface and are unique to this segment of the adult digestive tract. At their bases are simple tubular invaginations or pits that extend to the muscularis mucosae but do not penetrate it; these pits are the intestinal glands, or *crypts of Lieberkuhn* (Fig. 19–23). The crypts have generative and secretory functions, as will be described later.

The villi are essentially fingerlike or leaflike evaginations of the mucosa (Figs. 19–23 to 19–26). They have a simple columnar epithelial cover and a core of highly cellular connective tissue (lamina propria) rich in cells of the immune system. Each villus contains an arteriole, a capillary network, a vein, and a central lymphatic vessel or lacteal (Fig. 19–23). A rich network of blood capillaries ramifies through the lamina propria and is closely apposed to the basement membrane of the absorptive epithelium (Figs. 19–2 and 19–26). The vascularity of the villi is consid-

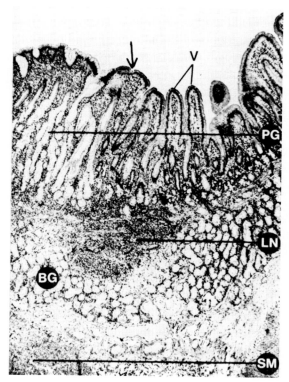

19–21 Longitudinal section between the pylorus and the duodenum of a monkey. In the epithelium, an abrupt transition occurs approximately at the **arrow. V,** villi; **PG,** pyloric gland; **BG,** Brunner's glands in the submucosa; **LN,** diffuse lymphatic nodule; **SM,** circular smooth muscle. H&E. × 50.

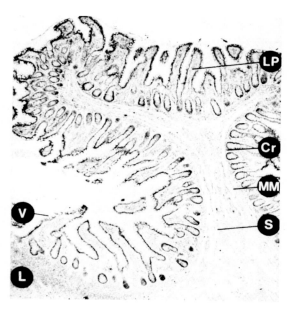

19–22 Plica circularis of the human jejunum. This permanent fold of the inner intestinal layers includes the submucosa. The isolated islands of tissue lying near the villi at upper left are sections of villi that were bent through the plane of section. **V,** villus; **L,** lymphatic tissue; **LP,** lamina propria; **Cr,** crypt; **MM,** muscularis mucosae; **S,** submucosa. H&E. × 40.

erably greater than that of the tissue around the crypts. Also, capillaries in the villus are fenestrated and are permeable to macromolecules, whereas capillaries around the crypts are not. Villi vary in height and form in different regions of the human small intestine (Fig. 19–25). They contract and shorten intermittently, owing to the activity of smooth muscle cells that extend from the muscularis mucosae into the long axis of the villi. Their contraction may serve to force lymph from the lacteal into more basal lymphatic vessels. With the electron microscope, small bundles of unmyelinated nerves have been observed in the lamina propria in association with blood vessels and smooth muscle fibers.

The simple columnar *epithelium* that lines the crypts and covers the villi is a continuous sheet that is constantly being renewed (see Epithelial Replacement, and Fig. 19–24). Most crypt epithelial cells migrate upward to become vil-

lous epithelial cells. Because crypt cells are relatively undifferentiated, the crypt epithelium is histologically different from that of the villus. In the crypt, the principal cell type is the *undifferentiated columnar cell;* this cell has a pale basophilic cytoplasm and divides frequently. Its progeny differentiate into four cell types, three of which migrate onto the villous surface. On the villus, the principal cell type is usually called the *absorptive cell,* although we now know that it also produces the enzymes necessary for terminal digestion of carbohydrates and proteins. It has a moderately basophilic cytoplasm and a conspicuous microvillous surface, the striated or brush border (Fig. 19–28A). Interspersed among the columnar absorptive cells, both in the crypts and on the villi, are mucus-secreting *goblet cells* and *enteroendocrine cells* (see Gastrointestinal Endocrine Cells, above). The bottom of the crypt is lined with a cluster of *Paneth cells,* which have the cytological characteristics of protein-secreting zymogenic cells (Fig. 19–36). These different cell types will be described in greater detail below. Migrating lymphocytes occur frequently between the epithelial cells of the vil-

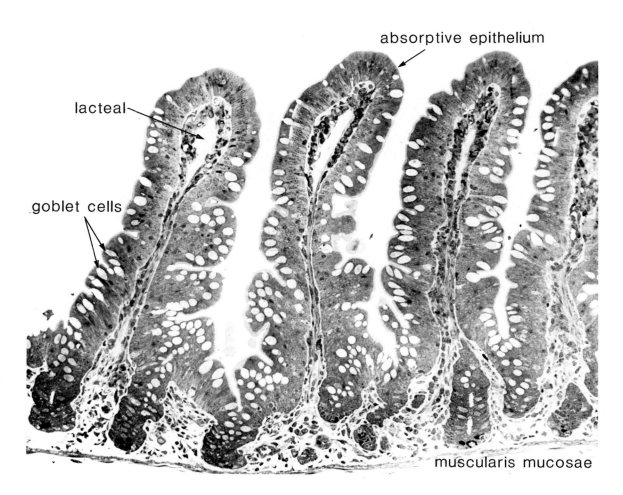

19–23 Monkey jejunal mucosa. The long villi and short crypts are supported by a well-vascularized lamina propria rich in cells. Lymphatic drainage begins with the lacteal, a lymphatic capillary located at the center of the villous core. Goblet and absorptive cells populate the epithelium. 1-μm plastic section, toluidine blue. (Courtesy of James L. Madara.)

lus (Fig. 19–28B). The epithelial cells rest on a well-defined but delicate basement membrane.

The *lamina propria* that forms the core of the villi and surrounds the glands is a highly cellular connective tissue typical of the alimentary tract. A special population of flat stellate fibroblasts lies just under the basal lamina; their interdigitating cytoplasmic processes are oriented circumferentially around the crypts and the villi. Cells of this "subepithelial fibroblast sheath" proliferate in the region of the crypt base and

migrate upwards at roughly the same rate as do the epithelial cells (see Epithelial Replacement, below). Their fate at the tip of the villus is unknown.

Lymphatic nodules and aggregates are frequent in the small intestine. The *submucosa* and *muscularis* follow the common pattern described above. The distribution of blood and lymphatic vessels and nerves in the small intestine has been described above (Fig. 19–2).

Cytology of the Small Intestinal Epithelium

The *absorptive cells* of the villi are tall and columnar, approximately 25 μm high and 8 μm wide, with oval nuclei located in the lower half of the cells. The absorptive cells of all adult mammals have a common design. Their apical striated or brush border (Fig. 19–29) consists of minute rodlike microvilli in a parallel array (Fig.

A

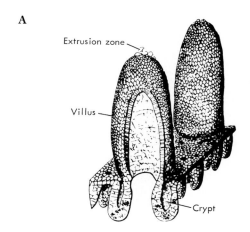

Extrusion zone

Villus

Crypt

B duodenum

jejunum

ileum

colon

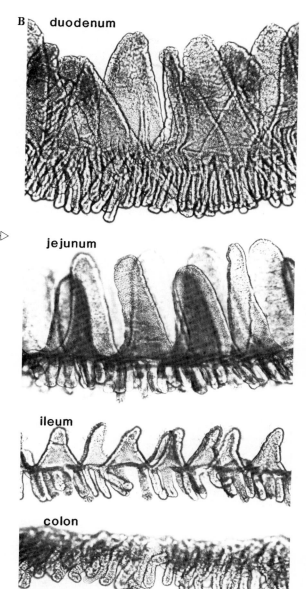

19–30). The hundreds of microvilli (each about 1.4 μm high and 0.08 μm wide on human jejunal cells) tremendously increase the cellular surface area exposed to the intestinal contents.

The brush border is PAS-positive because of a thick (0.1–0.5 μm) filamentous surface coat on the microvilli that is rich in glycoproteins (Figs. 19–30 and 19–31B). Radioautographic evidence indicates that each absorptive cell continuously synthesizes new components of the membrane and the cell surface coat and transports them, in the form of small vesicles, to the microvillous surface. The proteins and glycoproteins of the surface coat (also called the "glycocalyx") include the external, active portions of digestive enzymes such as dipeptidases and disaccharidases that cleave small peptides and sugars; these enzymes are anchored by smaller hydrophilic portions in the microvillous membrane. Several other enzymes, including enterokinase, ATPase, and alkaline phosphatase are also integral parts of the cell membrane and extend into the surface coat. They are synthesized and processed within the intracellular membrane systems of the absorptive cell before being transported to the microvillous surface, and they may be further processed by pancreatic enzymes in the glycocalyx. Thus, the so-called absorptive cell has important secretory functions. Pancreatic enzymes from the intestinal lumen are adsorbed onto the glycocalyx or surface coat. Here intestinal enterokinase cleaves and activates pancreatic trypsinogen; the product of this interaction, trypsin, in turn, cleaves and activates other pancreatic hydrolases. Because of the high concentration of active enzymes and their

19–24 A. Spatial scheme of the intestinal epithelium. The epithelium of the crypts is continuous with that covering the villi. Epithelial cells originate in the crypt of Lieberkuhn; they differentiate and migrate along the villus to its apex, where they are shed at the extrusion zone. **B.** Light micrographs of mouse intestinal epithelium, isolated by perfusion with a calcium chelator. The epithelium forms a continuous sheet. The normal size and shape of villi and crypts are preserved, even in the absence of underlying connective tissue. (Part A from Quastler and Sherman; part B from Bjerknes, M., and Cheng, H., 1981. Anat. Rec. 199:565.)

682

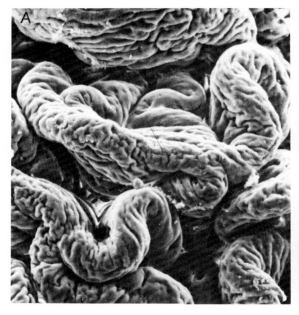

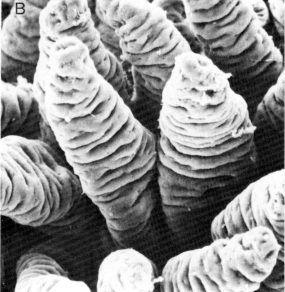

19–25 Scanning electron micrographs of the mucosal surface of monkey small intestine. **A.** Duodenal–jejunal junction. Villi are leaf-shaped. Depending on the plane of section, they may appear in histological sections either as broad (see Figs. 19–4 and 19–35) or narrow (see Fig. 19–22). **B** Ileum. Villi are finger-like. Their surfaces are wrinkled by the contraction of smooth muscle fibers in the villous core. (Courtesy of Robert Specian.)

19–26 Human jejunal mucosa. India-ink injection of a branch of the mesenteric artery within 1 h postmortem. A rich capillary network exists in the distal half of each villus; the rest of the mucosa is less vascular. (Courtesy of W. T. Cooke, G. I. Nicholson, and A. Ayres.)

19–27 Scanning electron micrograph of the surface of a small intestinal villus. The apical membranes of individual columnar cells are outlined by narrow grooves that mark the sites of apical cell junctions. Hundreds of microvilli stud the luminal surface of each cell. (Courtesy of Robert Specian.)

Villus Crypt

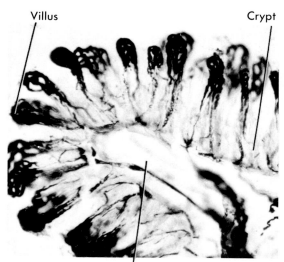

Submucosa

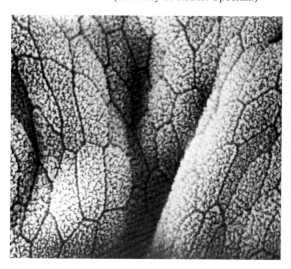

substrates in the brush border, their breakdown products (such as monosaccharides and amino acids) are efficiently delivered to transport proteins in the microvillous membrane.

The core of each microvillus contains a bundle of longitudinal filaments that merge just beneath the microvillous border with the *terminal web* (Figs. 19–30 and 19–31). The terminal web is a dense meshwork of filaments arranged in a plane parallel to the free surface of the cell; it inserts into the lateral cell membrane at the zonula adherens or "band desmosome" of the apical junctional complex. The longitudinal core filaments of the microvillus consist of actin (Figs. 19–31 and 19–32). They are anchored to the plasma membrane at the tip of the microvillus by a dense protein matrix and to the sides of the microvillus (and to each other) by cross-bridges of at least three other distinctive proteins, but no myosin is found within the microvillus. The filaments of the terminal web include both actin and myosin. Where actin filaments of the terminal web abut the lateral plasma membrane of the cell, a band of α-actinin has been detected. Although the terminal web and the microvilli can be induced to contract in vitro, it is not clear to what extent the web or the microvilli move in vivo. The rigid apex of the columnar cell, including microvilli, terminal web, and some smooth vesicles and tubules, can be separated from homogenates of intestinal mucosa and studied as "isolated brush borders."

Freeze-fractured microvillous membranes are rich in intramembrane particles (Fig. 19–31C). Membranes of villous absorptive cells actively engaged in digestion and transport contain more particles than those of immature crypt cells; however, the identity of the particles has not been determined. They are unrelated to the membrane insertion sites of the cytoskeletal filaments.

The apical cytoplasm just below the terminal web is rich in vesicles, tubules, and cisternae of smooth ER (Fig. 19–33). The rest of the supranuclear cytoplasm is rich in rough ER and free ribosomes. Immediately above the nucleus, several vertically oriented stacks of Golgi cisternae are arranged to form a short cylinder, which is demonstrable by heavy metal impregnation or by the cytochemical localization of glycoprotein or of nucleoside diphosphatase activity. Here, proteins destined for the microvilli and for other cell surfaces are glycosylated. Absorptive cells contain numerous elongate mitochondria oriented parallel to the long axis in the cell apex

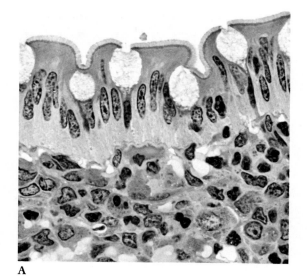

A

B

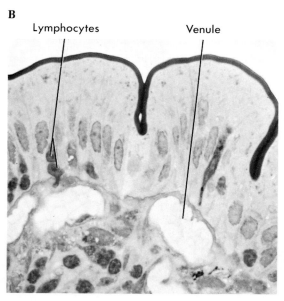

Lymphocytes   Venule

19–28 Absorptive epithelium of small intestinal villi, 1-μm plastic sections. **A.** Monkey, H&E. The apical microvillous (striated, or brush) border of the absorptive cells is distinct. Goblet cells are interspersed among them. Note the abundance of cells in the lamina propria. **B.** Human, PAS stain for glycoproteins. This specimen was obtained with an intraluminal biopsy capsule. The striated border is strongly stained, indicating the presence of carbohydrate–protein complexes. Small PAS-positive granules occur in the apical cytoplasm. Lymphocytes are migrating between epithelial cells. Note venules in the lamina propria. × 1,000. (From Padykula, H. A., Strauss, E. W., Ladman, A. J., and Gardner, F. H. 1961. Gastroenterology 40:735.)

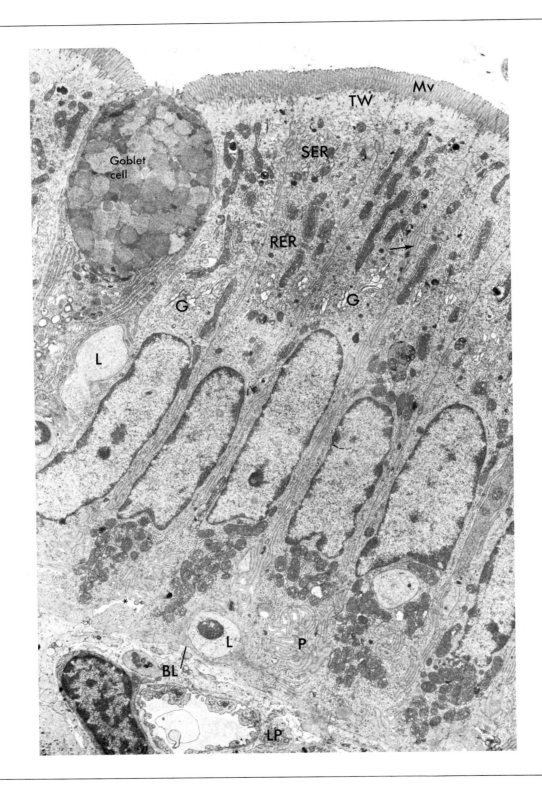

19–29 Intestinal epithelium of the villus from a starved rat. Several absorptive cells and a portion of a goblet cell are shown. The polarity of the absorptive cells is evident in structural differences between the free and attached surfaces and also in the distribution of the organelles. The luminal surface is composed of closely packed, regularly arranged microvilli **(Mv);** the subjacent cytoplasm, which is relatively free of organelles, is the region of the terminal web **(TW).** Below the terminal web the cytoplasm contains smooth ER **(SER),** whereas somewhat deeper the rough form **(RER)** occurs. The Golgi complex **(G)** occurs immediately above the nucleus. Mitochondria are widely distributed and here are heavily concentrated in the infranuclear cytoplasm. The lateral cell surfaces in the supranuclear region are closely apposed and sometimes folded **(arrow),** whereas below the nucleus the lateral surfaces form interdigitating processes **(P)** and the intercellular space is wider **(asterisk). BL,** basal lamina; **LP,** lamina propria. × 6,000. (From Cardell, R. R., Badenhausen, S., and Porter, K. R. 1967, J. Cell Biol. 34:123.)

19–30 Apical border of absorptive cells in the ileum of a cat, rapid-frozen and freeze-substituted with OsO₄ in acetone. The uniform microvilli contain bundles of actin microfilaments that extend into the terminal web cytoplasm. A thick, matlike coat, the "glycocalyx," is closely associated with the microvillous membranes and covers the apical cell surface. Portions of two absorptive cells are seen, joined by an occluding junction **(OJ)** and by interdigitating cell processes **(arrow).** (Courtesy of Susumu Ito.)

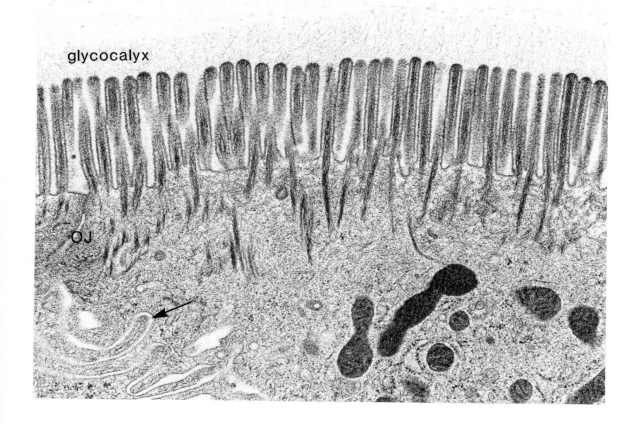

glycocalyx

OJ

A

MICROVILLI

Actin
filaments

Myosin
in the
terminal web

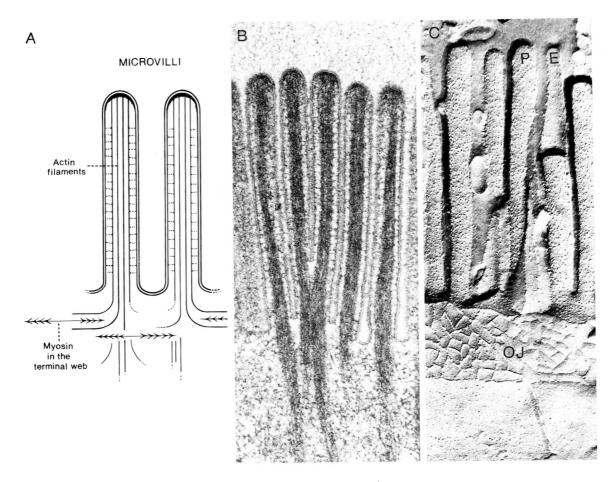

19–31 The structure of intestinal microvilli.
△ **A.** Schematic drawing. Actin filaments insert into a dense protein matrix on the cytoplasmic side of the membrane at the tip. Other proteins anchor them together and form bridges to the lateral membrane. Myosin occurs in the terminal web, but not in the core of the microvillus. (Diagram modified from Mooseker, M. S., and Tilney, L. G. 1975. J. Cell Biol. 67:725; redrawn by S. Colard-Keene; provided by Don W. Fawcett.) **B.** Rapid-frozen microvilli, as in Fig. 19–28. Note the filamentous glycocalyx, the actin bundles, and the lateral bridges extending from the actin bundle to the microvillous membrane. (Courtesy of Dr. Susumu Ito.) **C.** Freeze-fracture replica of small intestinal microvilli exposing the internal membrane faces. Intramembrane particles are abundant on the protoplasmic **(P)** face, and relatively sparse on the external **(E)** face. These microvilli were located at the lateral cell border, near the occluding junction **(OJ)** whose network of strands is seen on the P face **(left)** and whose grooves appear on the E face of the membrane of an adjacent cell **(right).** (From Madara, J. L., Trier, J. S., and Neutra, M. R. 1980. Gastroenterology 78:963.)

19–32 Intestinal microvilli cut tangential to the cell
▽ surface. More than 20 actin filaments are cross-sectioned in the core of each microvillus. Cross-bridges to the lateral unit membrane are not seen in this conventional electron-microscopic preparation.

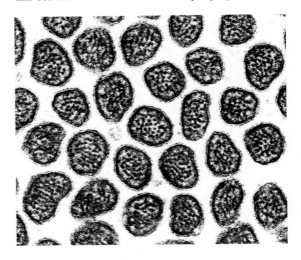

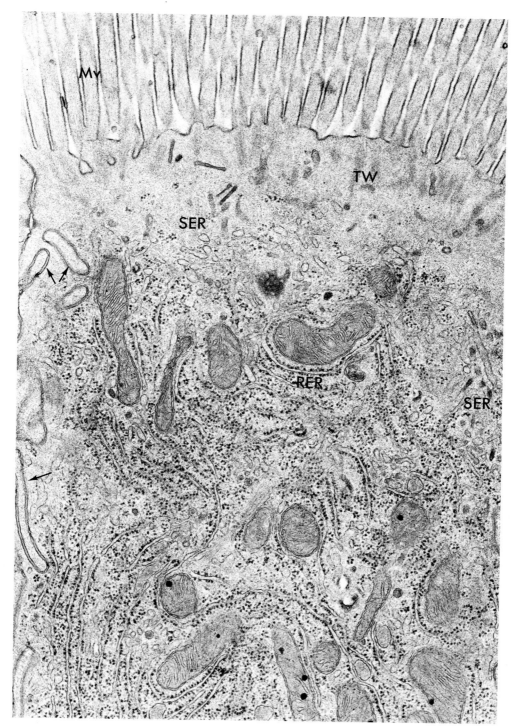

19–33 Supranuclear cytoplasm of an intestinal absorptive cell in a starved rat. The smooth ER **(SER)** occurs beneath the terminal web **(TW)**, whereas the rough ER **(RER)** is deeper. The interdigitating lateral cell surfaces are indicated by **arrows. Mv,** microvilli. × 37,800. (From Friedman, H. I., and Cardell, R. R. 1977. Anat. Rec. 88(1):77.)

and congregated at random in the cell base (Fig. 19–29).

Junctional complexes bind the apical-lateral surfaces of intestinal epithelial cells to each other (Fig. 19–31C; also described and illustrated in Chap. 3) and prevent the passage of macromolecules from the lumen into the intercellular spaces and lamina propria. Below the junctional complex, the lateral cell surfaces are plicated as tight interdigitations with the adjacent cells, and small footlike cytoplasmic processes near the cell base extend under the bases of adjacent cells. In areas of close apposition, the lateral intercellular space is uniform and narrow, but the space may be greatly dilated in the basal half of the epithelium when ions and water or lipid are being actively absorbed.

The plasma membrane covering the basolateral cell surfaces has no digestive enzymes but is rich in Na, K-dependent ATPase, a membrane-intercalated enzyme that pumps sodium (and hence passively draws water) into the lateral intercellular space. The enzyme activity of this membrane, along with the movement of ions and water between epithelial cells (the paracellular pathway), results in rapid and efficient retrieval of water from the lumen of the small intestine. Exactly how small ions and water pass between these cells, which are joined by tight junctions, is not known. It has recently been appreciated that tight junctional structure varies considerably among individual cells in a local region of the small intestinal epithelium. For example, crypt cell tight junctions tend to be more loosely organized and consist of fewer strands than do those between villus cells. The structure of the junctions suggests that the crypt epithelium may be "leakier" than that of the villus.

As crypt cells migrate onto the villus, their brush borders acquire alkaline phosphatase and digestive enzyme activity. Absorptive cells migrating toward the apex of the villus continue to differentiate as the microvilli become longer, narrower, and more numerous, and the cells' ability to absorb lipids, sugars, and amino acids increases.

The final products of digestion such as fatty acids, amino acids, and simple sugars are too small and soluble to be visualized by microscopy. Intact protein, however, can be visualized by autoradiography or by immunological labeling methods. During the neonatal suckling period, absorptive cells of the ileum (but not the proximal intestine) pinocytose intact proteins nonspecifically and degrade them intracellularly in a phagolysosome-like vacuole. In adult mammals, including humans, only trace amounts of intact protein are transported across the epithelium and most of this transport may occur over lymphoid follicles (see Immune Defense Mechanisms, below). A separate, highly specific transport system occurs transiently in the proximal intestine of neonatal rodents. Here, maternal immunoglobulin G (IgG) ingested orally by the newborn, specifically binds to Fc receptors in the microvillous membranes. Intact IgG is then endocytosed, transported, and released at the basolateral cell membrane to confer passive immunity to the suckling young.

The process of fat absorption can be partially visualized because lipid droplets and lipoprotein are fixed and stained by osmium tetroxide, a heavy metal salt routinely used in preparing tissues for electron microscopy. Tiny lipid droplets in the lumen, emulsified by interaction with bile salts, are broken down by pancreatic lipase. This process releases free fatty acids and monoglycerides that diffuse across the apical membrane and accumulate in the apical cytoplasm (Fig. 19–34). Short-chain fatty acids proceed to diffuse on through the cell and enter the blood capillaries below. Long-chain fatty acids and monoglycerides serve as substrates for triglyceride-synthesizing enzymes located in the smooth ER membranes near the cell apex. Resynthesized triglyceride, combined with cholesterol ester and phospholipid, appears as small droplets within the vesicles and labyrinthine apical network of smooth ER. A glycoprotein component (apoprotein), presumably synthesized in the rough ER and transported via structural or functional connections to smooth ER, Golgi-associated vesicles, or both, is added to the lipid to form chylomicrons. Lipid droplets of various sizes appear in the Golgi complex. Chylomicrons are transported in vesicles (whose membrane is apparently derived from the Golgi complex) to the lateral cell surfaces and are discharged by exocytosis into the intercellular space where they may accumulate (Fig. 19–34). Lipoprotein droplets devoid of membranes cross the basal lamina and gain entrance to the lacteals either by passing between endothelial cells or via a pinocytotic shuttle.

Lipid absorption is limited to villous absorptive cells and is most efficient in the jejunum (Fig. 19–35). When protein synthesis is inhibited by puromycin, lipid droplets accumulate intracellularly because of lack of apoprotein and new

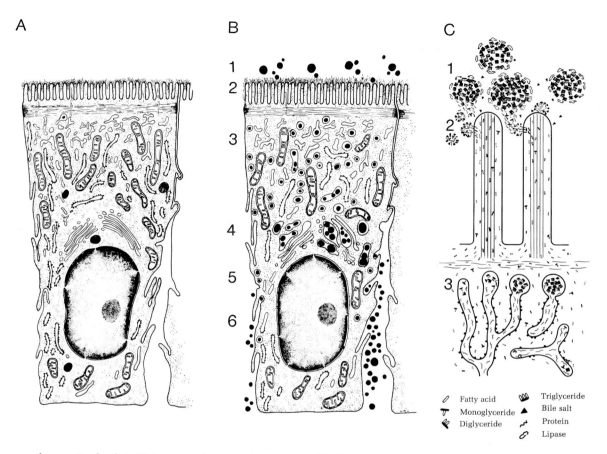

19–34 Diagrammatic drawings of the ultrastructure of small intestinal absorptive cells during fasting (**A**) and during lipid absorption (**B** and **C**).

1. Emulsified lipid droplets in lumen are digested by pancreatic lipase.
2. Free fatty acids and monoglycerides diffuse across the microvillous membrane.
3. Triglycerides are resynthesized in the apical smooth ER.
4. Cholesterol, phospholipid, and apoprotein are added to form chylomicrons.
5. Chylomicrons are transported in membrane-bound vesicles.
6. They are released by exocytosis at the basolateral cell membrane.

(Drawings by S. Colard-Keene, from Bloom, W., and Fawcett, D. W. 1975. A Textbook of Histology Philadelphia: W. B. Saunders Company. Redrawn from an original plate from Cardell, R. R., Badenhausen, S., and Porter, K. R. 1967. J. Cell Biol. 34:123.)

membrane. Lack of Ca^{++} ions results in a similar accumulation, perhaps by inhibiting the exocytosis of chylomicrons from the cell. The morphological aspects of lipid absorption were first studied in laboratory animals and later were confirmed in humans after safe intraluminal biopsy procedures had been developed.

The epithelium of the villus is covered by a protective layer of mucus lying outside the glycocalyx or surface coat of the microvilli. It is secreted by *goblet cells*, recognized in the epithelium by their dense basophilic cytoplasm, their basally located nuclei, and the accumulation of mucous secretory granules that fill and distend their apexes to give the cells their characteristic goblet shape. Goblet cells increase in frequency along the length of the small intestine, being most numerous in the lower ileum. Their apical mucous granules are poorly preserved in routine preparations so that the cells usually appear empty, but with special stains, their carbohydrate-rich, acidic glycoprotein secretory product is intensely basophilic, metachromatic, and PAS-

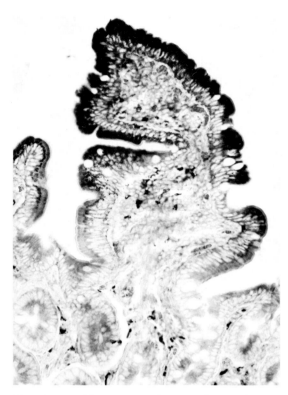

19–35 Normal human jejunal mucosa biopsied 20
min after ingestion of corn oil. Lipid droplets
have accumulated principally in the absorptive
epithelium of the upper half of the villus. Epithelial
cells at the base of the villus and in the crypt are free
of lipid droplets. Heavily sudanophilic cells in the
lamina propria are tissue eosinophils. Formalin-fixed;
frozen section stained with Sudan black. × 200.
(From Ladman, A. J., Padykula, H. A., and Strauss,
E. W. 1963. Am. J. Anat. 112:389.)

positive. Goblet cell structure and function is
further described below (see Large Intestine).

A cluster of protein-producing *Paneth cells*
occur at the base of the small intestinal crypt.
These pyramidal cells have the cytological characteristics of serous or zymogenic cells, with a
strongly basophilic basal cytoplasm, a large supranuclear Golgi complex, and large acidophilic
refractile granules in the apical cytoplasm (Fig.
19–36A). The basal cytoplasm contains well-organized cisternae of rough ER (Fig. 19–36B). The
secretory granules contain arginine-rich basic
protein, as well as glycoprotein. The presence of
the antibacterial enzyme lysozyme has been revealed by the immunocytochemical studies of

Erlandsen and co-workers (Fig. 19–37). Lysozyme is a highly cationic protein that digests certain bacterial cell walls; its strong positive
charge may explain the intense acidophilia and
high pH (10) of the granular contents. Paneth cell
granules are normally released at a low rate, but
secretion is accelerated after feeding and by exposure to acetylcholine. The precise role of Paneth cells is elusive: they are present in humans,
monkeys, and other mammals including bats, rodents, and ruminants but are absent from rabbits,
cats, and pigs. Their production of lysozyme and
their ability to phagocytose certain invading bacteria and protozoa in the crypts (Erlandsen et al.,
1976) suggest that their secretions may regulate
the flora associated with the small intestinal mucosa.

Regional Differences

Although the entire small intestine has the same
basic histological structure, gradual changes occur along its length. The three major regions—
duodenum, jejunum, and ileum—have distinctive hallmarks visible in histological sections at
low magnification.

The upper duodenum is characterized by
Brunner's glands, which lie in the submucosa
(Fig. 19–21). These branched tubuloalveolar
glands produce a neutral or alkaline mucus that
passes via small ducts through the muscularis
mucosae and into the intestinal crypts. Brunner's
glands secrete in response to vagal (parasympathetic) stimulation and also in response to
feeding, even in the absence of extrinsic innervation. Their viscous secretion probably acts as
a neutral, hydrated lubricating barrier, protecting
the mucosal surface of the duodenum from the
acidic chyme entering from the stomach. Ultrastructurally, Brunner's gland cells resemble "se-

19–36 Paneth cells. **A.** Monkey ileum, 2-μm plastic
section, H & E. A cluster of Paneth cells at
the base of a crypt are recognized by their refractile
eosinophilic apical granules, prominent supranuclear
Golgi complex (unstained), and heavily basophilic
basal cytoplasm. **B.** Mouse jejunum. Ultrastructurally,
Paneth cells resemble other zymogenic cells, with
well-organized basal rough ER and membrane-bound
apical granules. **C.** Human jejunum. Paneth cell
granules are large and electron-dense. They contain
lysozyme and other proteins. (Part B courtesy of
David Chase; part C courtesy of Jerry S. Trier.)

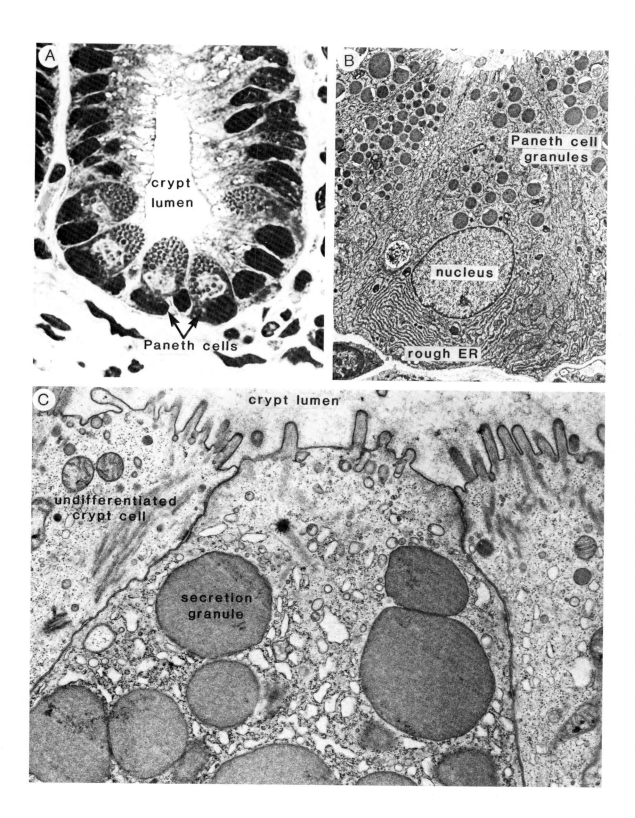

A — crypt lumen, Paneth cells

B — Paneth cell granules, nucleus, rough ER

C — crypt lumen, undifferentiated crypt cell, secretion granule

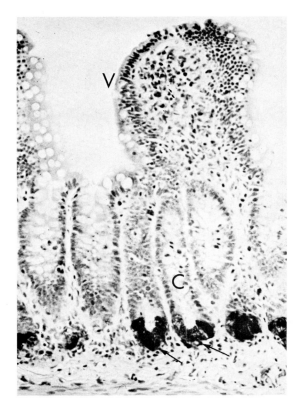

19–37 Human small intestinal mucosa; immunocytochemical localization of lysozyme, an antibacterial enzyme. Lysozyme is concentrated in the Paneth cells at the bottom of the crypts **(arrows).** The rest of the mucosa is unreactive. Ultrastructural study of this material reveals that lysozyme is localized in the secretory granules. **V,** villus; **C,** crypt. (Courtesy of Stanley Erlandsen.)

rous" or protein-secreting cell types, with well-organized rough ER, large Golgi complex, and small, dense apical secretory granules.

Plicae circulares occur in all three regions but are best developed in the jejunum (Fig. 19–20). There are species differences in the length and shape of villi along the small intestine. In the human duodenum they are leaflike folds (0.2–0.5 mm high) that may be branched (Fig. 19–25A); in the jejunum they are long, finger-like projections; in the ileum, they tend to have a shorter, clublike form (Fig. 19–25B). These differences are not easily recognized in sections. In the jejunum and ileum, the villi are 0.2 to 1.0 mm in height, standing 10 to 40 to the square millimeter; they are taller and more numerous in the je-

junum than in the ileum. Villi disappear in the region of the ileocecal valve. The number of goblet cells in the villous epithelium increases progressively from the duodenum to the ileocecal valve, so that the villous epithelium of the ileum is much richer in goblet cells than that of the duodenum. Finally, the amount of lymphatic tissue progressively increases from proximal to distal small intestine.

In summary, the three regions may be recognized in histological sections as follows:

Duodenum—Brunner's glands; few goblet cells
Jejunum—Plicae circularis (submucosal folds)
Ileum—Peyer's patches; many goblet cells

Immune Defense Mechanisms

The gastrointestinal tract presents a vast, vulnerable surface to the outside world. The lumen contains an ever-changing mixture of antigens, microorganisms, and other potentially harmful foreign substances that are separated from the mucosal blood vessels only by a simple columnar epithelium and a variable layer of mucus. It is not surprising, then, that the mucosa is heavily populated with cells of the immune system. The number of such cells is minimal in fetuses but increases rapidly after birth and greatly during enteric infections. In the normal adult, about one-quarter of the mucosa consists of lymphoid tissue; this tissue includes organized cellular aggregates such as the lymphatic nodules, dispersed lymphocytes and plasma cells in the lamina propria, as well as many wandering lymphocytes insinuated between the epithelial cells (intraepithelial lymphocytes).

We now know that this gut-associated lymphoid tissue (GALT), in cooperation with epithelial cells, is able to sample luminal antigens. Even in healthy subjects, antigens from the lumen occasionally gain access to intercellular spaces in the epithelium where they appear to be sampled and processed by the intraepithelial lymphocytes. Most of these lymphocytes are T cells, but B cells are also present. They are often in contact with the extended pseudopod of a nearby macrophage lying just under the basal lamina. Owen and his associates have shown that most efficient antigen sampling occurs in the flattened epithelium overlying lymphatic nodules such as those in Peyer's patches (Figs. 19–38 and 19–39). Here, a peculiar type of epithelial cell whose apical surface carries micro-

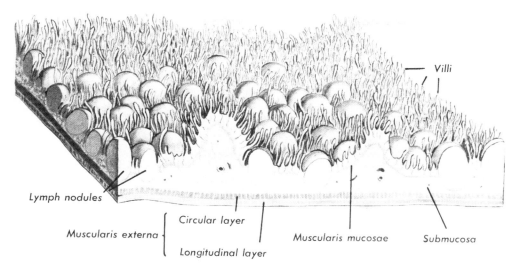

Villi

Lymph nodules

Muscularis externa { Circular layer

Longitudinal layer

Muscularis mucosae   Submucosa

folds (the "M" cell in Fig. 19–40) endocytoses macromolecules and transports them in small vesicles toward the intraepithelial lymphocytes gathered along its basolateral membrane (Fig. 19–40B, D). The next steps are not clear, but it is postulated that both B and T lymphocytes migrate out of the epithelium and toward the aggregates of lymphoid cells in the lamina propria, where helper T cells may participate in the maturation of B cells into antibody producers. These lymphocytes also appear to pass to mesenteric lymph nodes, proliferate, and enter the lymphatic and blood circulation. By this long route they eventually "home" back to the mucosal surfaces. Here, the B cells further proliferate within lymphatic nodules such as those of Peyer's patches and differentiate into sedentary, local

19–38 Drawing of a low-power magnification of a portion of one Peyer's patch. (From Copenhaver, W. M., Bunge, R. P., and Bunge, M. B. 1971. Bailey's Textbook of Histology. Baltimore: The Williams & Wilkins Company.)

19–39 A. A lymphoid nodule or follicle in the mucosa of monkey ileum. The area over the follicle is devoid of villi, but is covered by "follicle-associated epithelium" **(FAE)** rich in intraepithelial lymphocytes. Although a cluster of goblet cells occurs over the crest of this follicle, goblet cells are generally absent from the FAE. 2-μm plastic section, H & E. **B.** Human ileum, scanning electron micrograph. A lymphoid nodule covered by follicle-associated epithelium **(FAE)** and surrounded by villi. The surface of the FAE is shown at higher magnification in Fig. 19–40C. (Courtesy of Robert L. Owen.)

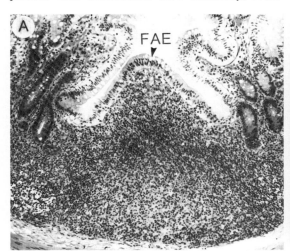

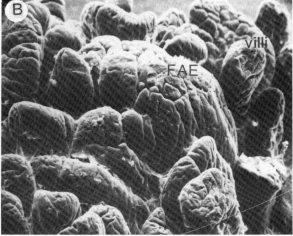

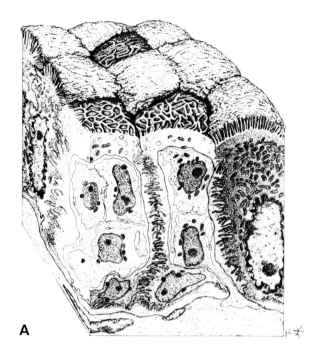

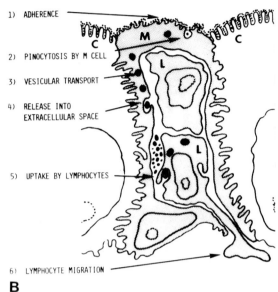

HORSERADISH PEROXIDASE TRANSPORT ACROSS LYMPHOID FOLLICLE EPITHELIUM

1) ADHERENCE

2) PINOCYTOSIS BY M CELL

3) VESICULAR TRANSPORT

4) RELEASE INTO EXTRACELLULAR SPACE

5) UPTAKE BY LYMPHOCYTES

6) LYMPHOCYTE MIGRATION

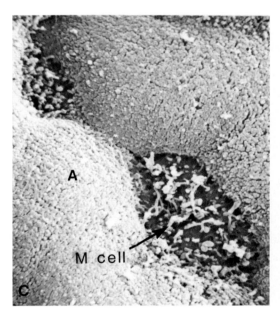

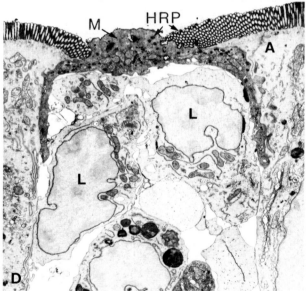

immunoglobulin-producing plasma cells. Although many of the migratory lymphoid cells committed to secretory immunoglobulin production seem to return to the intestinal mucosa, others settle in such distant secretory sites as the respiratory mucosa, genital mucosa, and glands. In the mammary gland, secretory immunoglobulins (IgA) are transported into milk where they may passively protect the suckling newborn from the intestinal antigens previously encountered by the mother.

By fluorescent labeling studies, we know that many of the plasma cells in the lamina propria throughout the oral cavity and the gastrointestinal tract (as well as in the salivary glands, respiratory passages, and mammary glands) are pro-

19–40 Microfold ("M") cells in the lymphoid follicle-associated epithelium. **A.** Drawing representing the ultrastructure of the follicle-associated epithelium in three dimensions and in section. M cells, bearing microfolds, are situated among columnar absorptive cells bearing microvilli. The M cell's basolateral surface is deeply invaginated by intraepithelial lymphocytes, which migrate in and out of the intercellular space of the epithelium. **B.** Schematic diagram summarizing the transport of exogenous horseradish peroxidase observed by Owen and Jones. They hypothesize that the M cell transports intact macromolecules from the lumen to allow efficient "sampling" of luminal antigens by lymphocytes (see text). **L,** lymphocytes; **C,** columnar absorptive cells. **C.** Scanning electron micrograph of the apical surfaces of absorptive cells **(A)** and M cells. Note the microfolds on the M cell. **D.** Electron micrograph showing the attenuated apical cytoplasm of an M cell over a cluster of intraepithelial lymphocytes **(L).** The protein tracer horseradish peroxidase **(HRP)** was introduced into the intestinal lumen 1 h before fixation. Dense reaction product reveals the presence of HRP on the microvillous border of two adjacent absorptive cells and within small vesicles in the M-cell cytoplasm. (Courtesy of Robert L. Owen. Parts A, C, and D from Owen, R. L., and Nemanic, P. 1978. *In* Scanning Electron Microscopy, Vol. II. AMF O'Hare, Ill.: SEM, Inc., p. 367; part B from Owen, R. L. 1977. Gastroenterology 72:440.)

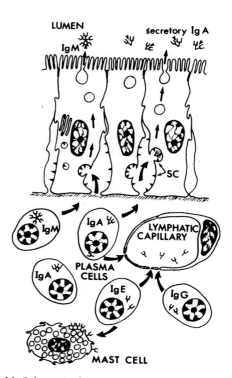

19–41 Schematic drawing summarizing the production and fate of immunoglobulins synthesized by plasma cells in the lamina propria. IgG and IgE are secreted as monomers, most of which enter the lymphatic circulation but some of which may leak between epithelial cells into the lumen. IgE also binds to receptors on mast cell surfaces. IgA-producing plasma cells secrete principally IgA dimers (linked by a peptide "J" chain). Small amounts of monomeric IgA are also secreted and enter lymphatics. Dimeric IgA binds to a glycoprotein secretory component **(SC)** displayed on the basolateral membrane of crypt columnar cells. It is endocytosed, transported in vesicles, and secreted with the secretory component into the lumen. Pentameric IgM follows a transcellular path through crypt cells similar to that of dimeric IgA. (Adapted from Tomasi, 1972; Brown, W. R., Isobe, Y., and Nakane, P. K., 1976. Gastroenterology, 71:985; and Brandtzaeg, P., and Baklein, K. 1977. *In* Immunology of the Gut, Ciba Foundation Symposium 46 [new series]. Amsterdam: Elsevier, p. 77.)

ducing the dimeric secretory immunoglobulin IgA (Fig. 19–41). Others produce IgM, a polymeric secretory immunoglobulin. Both IgA and IgM are delivered into intestinal or glandular secretions by a specific vesicular carrier system localized in the columnar epithelial cells of intestinal crypts and in exocrine glandular cells elsewhere in the body. The current hypothesis is as follows: (1) IgA dimers released from plasma cells move to the basolateral membranes of nearby epithelial cells; (2) either at the basolateral membrane or after uptake into the epithelial cells, dimers are linked to glycoprotein "secretory component"; (3) the complex is transported across the cell in vesicles and then is released by exocytosis into the lumen. Secretory IgA combines with antigens, enterotoxins, and microorganisms in the lumen to protect the epithelial surface by "immune exclusion." Immunoglobulin A monomer is also secreted by plasma cells; it enters the lymphatic and blood circulation as "serum IgA."

Smaller populations of plasma cells in the lamina propria produce the monomeric antibodies IgG and IgE. These antibodies are believed to diffuse nonspecifically, in small amounts, between epithelial cells at the tip of the villus to gain access to the intestinal lumen where they are rapidly degraded. Immunoglobulin E is also selectively bound by the plasma membranes of local mast cells in the lamina propria, sensitizing them to specific luminal antigens.

Large Intestine

The large intestine begins at the ileocecal valve and includes an initial blind pouch, the *cecum* (with a terminal narrow extension called the *vermiform appendix*); the *ascending, transverse, descending,* and *sigmoid colon;* and the *rectum,* ending at the external orifice or *anus.* Its total length is roughly 1.5 m in humans. The histological organization of the colon reflects its principal functions: reabsorption of water and elimination of undigested material, the feces. Elimination is facilitated by the secretion of mucus, which lubricates and protects the mucosa from the solid dehydrated luminal contents.

Histological Organization

The *mucosa* of the entire large intestine lacks villi: its flat surface is punctuated by the openings of straight tubular glands or crypts (Figs. 19–42 and 19–43). These crypts are about 0.5 mm long and extend to the muscularis mucosae. The lamina propria contains many solitary lymphatic nodules which are often so large that they displace the crypts and extend into the submucosa (Fig. 19–42). It also contains many lymphocytes, macrophages, and plasma cells that locally produce IgA (Fig. 19–44A). The abundance of lymphoid cells and nodules in the large intestinal mucosa reflects the presence of hundreds of bacterial species (over 500 types of anaerobe alone) that inhabit the large intestinal lumen of healthy humans. Certain bacteria are associated closely with the surface epithelium of the colon without causing ill effects. Microorganisms of the colon digest residual organic matter such as plant cell walls, and the breakdown products may be absorbed. Trace nutrients synthesized by bacteria are also absorbed. The submucosa contains the usual constituents plus large accumulations of fat cells.

The simple columnar epithelium lining the crypts and luminal surface of the colon is a continuous sheet that is constantly renewed (see Epithelial Replacement, below). The crypt epithelium consists of undifferentiated cells, immature (vacuolated) absorptive cells, goblet cells, and enteroendocrine cells (Fig. 19–44B). On the luminal surface, mature absorptive cells predominate, with goblet cells interspersed among them. As in the small intestine, a "subepithelial fibroblast sheath" encircles the crypts. These flat, stellate fibroblasts arise by mitosis near the crypt base and migrate toward the mucosal surface. They seem to participate in the synthesis of the "collagen table," a thick layer of collagen and glycosaminoglycans immediately under the basal lamina of the luminal surface epithelium. The cell bodies of subepithelial fibroblasts lie on the underside of the collagen table and send octopus-like cytoplasmic processes toward the basal lamina.

The *muscularis* of the colon and cecum has a characteristic arrangement not found in the vermiform appendix, rectum, or the more proximal

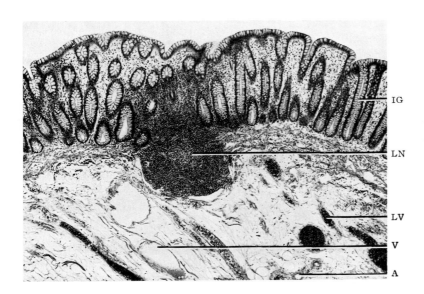

19–42 Longitudinal section of mucosa and submucosa of the human colon. **IG,** intestinal gland; **LN,** lymphatic nodule, which extends through the muscularis mucosae into the submucosa; **LV,** lymphatic vessel filled with lymphocytes; **V,** vein; **A;** artery. × 50.

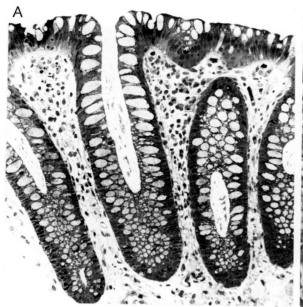

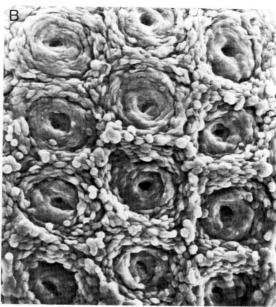

portions of the alimentary tract. The longitudinal smooth muscle fibers of the outer layer gather into three equidistant longitudinal bundles known as taeniae (Greek: bands). Between them, the longitudinal fibers form a thinner, sometimes interrupted layer. Because of the tonus of the taeniae, the wall of the colon bulges outward as sacculations or haustra (Latin: buckets). Between these sacculations, the wall is thrown into crescentic folds, "plicae semilunares," that project into the lumen. The ileocecal valve consists of two such folds. A peculiarity of the colon is that the fascicles of longitudinal fibers from the taeniae frequently join the circular layer. This arrangement interrupts the continuity of the circular layer, and different intertaenial areas may contract independently.

The *serosa* is incomplete, since the ascending and descending limbs of the colon are retroperitoneal. It may contain lobules of fat that form pendulous projections (appendices epiploicae).

Cytology of the Large Intestinal Epithelium

The undifferentiated cells in the lower half of the large intestinal crypts closely resemble their counterparts in the small intestine. Most (at least 80%) of the cells lining the middle and upper crypt are young *columnar absorptive cells*, whose apical surfaces carry variable numbers of

19–43 **A.** Human rectal mucosa. Biopsy obtained from a healthy volunteer. The straight tubular glands are regularly spaced. 1-μm plastic section, iron hematoxylin stain. × 405. **B.** Monkey colonic mucosa viewed from the lumen by scanning electron microscopy. The regular placement of crypt openings is similar to that seen in human large intestine. (Courtesy of Robert D. Specian.)

well-formed but relatively short microvilli, and whose terminal web is poorly developed. While in the crypt, columnar cells synthesize, store, and release a glycoprotein-containing secretory product held in large, clear membrane-bound vesicles in the apical cytoplasm (Fig. 19–44). Because the vesicle content appears fibrillar in electron-microscopic sections, some investigators think that it consists of glycocalyx material destined for the brush border, but autoradiographic evidence suggests that this cell may also secrete glycoprotein directly into the lumen. In any case, vesicles disappear as the cell emerges onto the mucosal surface. As the columnar cells approach the crypt opening, alkaline phosphatase activity appears in the brush border and the microvilli increase in number and elongate. The filamentous, glycoprotein-containing glycocalyx on large intestinal columnar cells is continuously renewed (turnover time, 16–24 hr

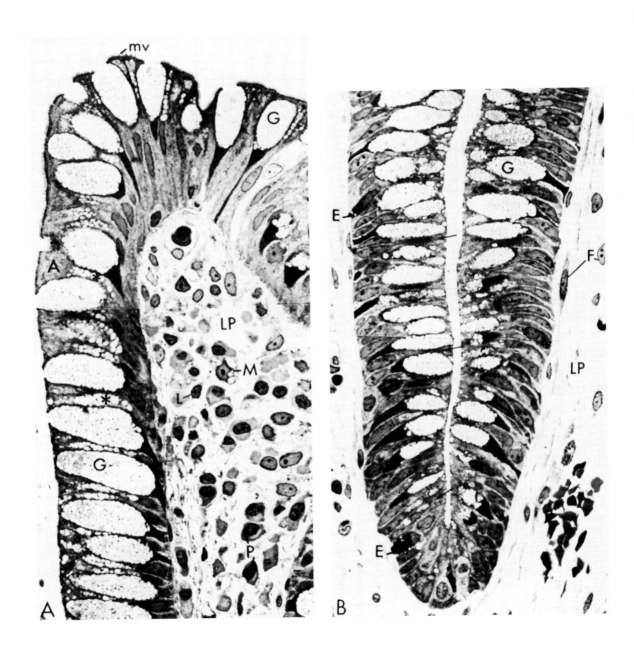

19–44 Mucosa of the human large intestine.

　　A. Luminal surface, including a portion of a mucosal gland (left margin) and the lamina propria **(LP).** The luminal epithelium consists of absorptive cells **(A)** with microvilli **(mv)** and interspersed goblet cells **(G).** These same cell types are evident in the glandular epithelium (left margin) where vacuolization **(*)** is conspicuous in the absorptive cells. In the lamina propria, macrophages **(M),** plasma cells **(P),** and lymphocytes **(L)** are present. **B.** Mucosal gland and surrounding lamina propria **(LP).** Goblet cells **(G)** are numerous and are interspersed with tall columnar cells **(arrows)** in the upper part of the gland; the base of the gland contains undifferentiated precursor cells. Endocrine cells **(E)** with aggregates of infranuclear granules are infrequent. **F,** fibroblast. 1-μm section, iron hematoxylin stain. × 840.

in humans) even though digestive enzymes are generally absent.

Normally, dietary fats are completely digested and absorbed in the small intestine, but if absorption is incomplete, lipids enter the colon. Surface epithelial cells of the colon (especially the ascending segment) may absorb fatty acids, resynthesize triglyceride, form chylomicrons, and release them into the lamina propria, although the process is not as efficient as in the small intestine. A principal function of surface cells throughout the colon is the final absorption of water and salt from the feces; thus their basolateral membranes are rich in Na, K-dependent ATPase. Sodium and chloride are absorbed with water following passively, whereas potassium and bicarbonate are released into the lumen.

Goblet cells are numerous in the crypt epithelium (up to one goblet for every four columnar cells). Their broad shape creates the false impression that they constitute a majority (Fig. 19–44A). They differentiate deep in the crypts and become progressively filled with mucous granules as they migrate upward (Fig. 19–44B), so that mid- and upper-crypt goblet cells are distended with granules, and the nucleus is confined to a small dense basal region (Fig. 19–44A). As the cell migrates onto the surface of the mucosa, its mucous store is reduced and the cell elongates, maintaining contact with the basal lamina via its long narrow basal cytoplasm. Autoradiographic studies have established that both synthesis and secretion of mucus occur continuously throughout the life span of the cell. Secretion is accelerated on the mucosal surface so that mucous stores diminish in spite of active synthesis.

The glycoproteins in mucus are large (up to 2×10^6 daltons), carbohydrate-rich (80% dry weight), and negatively charged. The peptides of mucus are synthesized in the basal and lateral cisternae of rough ER, glycosylated and sulfated by membrane-bound transferases located primarily in the Golgi cisternae, and "packaged" in Golgi-derived membrane (Fig. 19–45). Membrane-bound granules of mucus migrate slowly (4–8 h in rat, 12–24 h in humans) to the apical membrane where they are released by conventional exocytosis. Secreted mucus forms a highly hydrated gel that binds macromolecules, coats bacteria, and cushions particulate matter.

Mucous secretion is accelerated by chemical or physical irritation of the mucosa. Parasym-

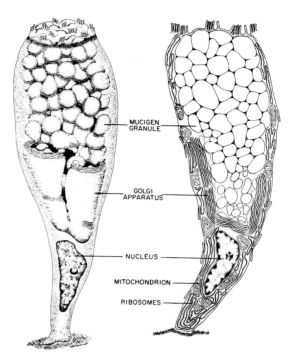

19–45 Schematic drawings of a goblet cell as imagined in three dimensions **(left)** and in electron-microscopic section **(right)**. Elements of the Golgi apparatus are arranged roughly as a cup above the nucleus. The membranes and content of Golgi saccules give rise to mucus-filled secretory granules that move slowly toward the apical membrane and are secreted by exocytosis. (From Neutra, M. R., and Leblond, C. P., 1966, J. Cell Biol., 30:119.)

pathetic stimulation induces secretion of mucus from crypt goblet cells, but not from those on the mucosal surface (Fig. 19–46). Rapid secretion occurs through the sequential exocytosis of large numbers of intracellular mucous granules, called compound exocytosis, and results in deep cavitation of the apical cell surface (Fig. 19–46B). During secretion, the plasma membrane remains intact, and the cell can rapidly replenish its stores of mucus.

Cecum and Vermiform Appendix

The cecum is a blind pouch at the proximal end of the colon, and its terminal thin tip is known as the vermiform appendix. The structure of the cecum resembles that of the rest of the colon, and the vermiform appendix has a similar struc-

700

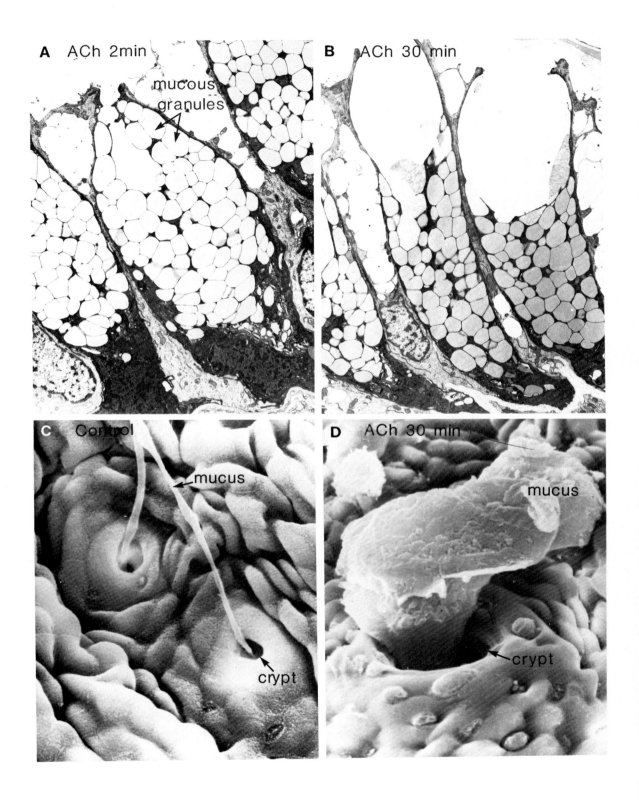

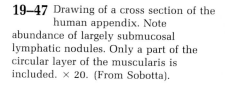

19–46 Mucous secretion in rabbit colon viewed by transmission (**A** and **B**) and by scanning electron microscopy (**C** and **D**). **A.** A goblet cell in a crypt after a 2-min exposure to acetylcholine. The contents of several apical mucous granules have been secreted by compound exocytosis. **B.** After a 30-min exposure to acetylcholine, the compound exocytosis of many granules leaves the cell deeply cavitated; the apical plasma membrane is intact but is greatly amplified. **C.** Without stimulation, a thin wisp of mucus emerges from each crypt opening. **D.** After a 30-min exposure to acetylcholine, mucus secreted from crypt goblet cells flows from a dilated crypt opening. (From Specian, R. D., and Neutra, M. R., 1980, J. Cell Biol., 85:626.)

ture in miniature (Fig. 19–47) except that taeniae are absent. The glands of the appendix are simple tubes, sometimes forked; the epithelium is rich in mucous cells and contains many endocrine cells, mainly of the EC type. The surface epithelium consists of columnar cells with few mucous cells. Lymphatic nodules are abundant and more or less confluent. The wealth of lymphatic vessels and lymphatic tissues is a most conspicuous histological feature of the appendix.

The lumen of the normal appendix in the adult, when empty, is thrown into folds separated by deep pockets. However, this normal condition is found in scarcely 50% of individuals over 40 years of age because of a history of subclinical appendicitis. Often the lumen is narrowed or even obliterated. The epithelium and the underlying lymphatic tissue then disappear and are replaced by an axial mass of fibrous tissue.

Rectum and Anus

The rectum is divided into two parts, an upper part that extends from the third sacral vertebra to the pelvic diaphragm, and a lower part, or anal canal, that continues down to the anus. The lining of the first part is thrown into several large, semilunar, circular folds, the *plicae transversales recti*. For most of its length the anal canal has on its inner wall a number of longitudinal folds, the anal columns.

The mucosa in the first part of the rectum is similar to that of the colon, but its glands are somewhat longer (0.7 mm). Solitary lymphatic nodules are common. A continuous layer of longitudinal muscle with no taeniae is present. The rectum has no mesentery, and the serosa is replaced by adventitial connective tissue.

The lower portion of the rectum, or anal canal, is 2 to 3 cm in length and roughly elliptical in cross section. It ends at the anus, where its lining becomes continuous with the external skin. In the anal canal, the epithelium changes abruptly from simple columnar to stratified cuboidal at the pectinate line (Fig. 19–48), which

19–47 Drawing of a cross section of the human appendix. Note abundance of largely submucosal lymphatic nodules. Only a part of the circular layer of the muscularis is included. × 20. (From Sobotta).

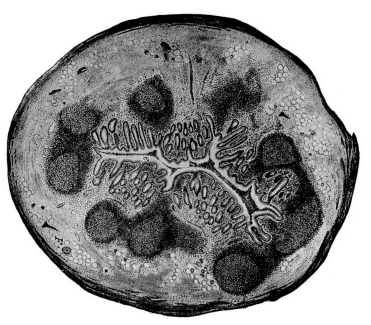

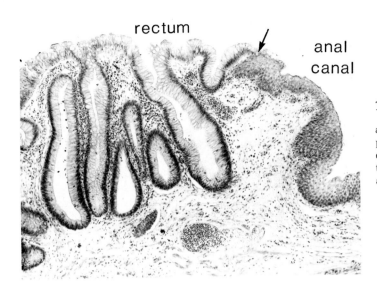

rectum

anal canal

19–48 Longitudinal section through the junction of the human rectum and anal canal. The **arrow** indicates the pectinate line, where the simple columnar epithelium of the rectum is converted to the stratified squamous epithelium of the anal canal.

is about 2 cm above the anal opening. The anal columns join one another somewhat below this line, creating pocket-like anal valves. Above each valve is a recess called an anal sinus. At this level the muscularis mucosae disappears. The nonkeratinized epithelium of the canal changes into typical keratinized, stratified squamous epithelium at the anus proper. In the lower part of the anal canal there are a few isolated sebaceous glands.

The skin immediately around the anus forms the "zona cutanea." Sweat glands are absent from the region immediately bordering the anus, but at a distance of 1.0 to 1.5 cm there is an elliptical zone 1.5 cm wide, containing simple tubular glands, the circumanal glands. These glands are apocrine sweat glands that secrete an oily fluid related, in lower mammals, to sexual activity.

The outer layers of the anal canal include a very vascular submucosa that contains blood vessels, numerous nerves, and Pacinian corpuscles. The veins form the large hemorrhoid plexus and are especially susceptible to varicosities. The circular layer of the muscularis becomes thickened at its termination, forming the internal anal sphincter. Beyond this, striated muscle fibers surround the orifice and form the external anal sphincter.

Epithelial Replacement

The *epithelial cells* lining the surface of the entire gastrointestinal tract are continuously lost by being sloughed into the lumen and replaced by new cells proliferating and migrating from the glands or crypts. The production of new cells depends on the mitotic activity of undifferentiated "stem" cells. Replacement is precisely balanced with loss to ensure the maintenance of a healthy, optimally functioning epithelium. The dynamics of this steady state have been elucidated over the past 30 years, largely through the radioautographic studies of Leblond and his associates. Dividing cells can be "tagged" in the living animal by injection or infusion of ^{3}H-thymidine, a DNA precursor that is specifically incorporated into the replicating genome before mitosis. In tissues fixed shortly after exposure to ^{3}H-thymidine, proliferative cells are identified in situ by the presence of silver grains over their nuclei as seen in radioautographs of histological sections. If the same tissues are fixed at progressively later times, such as 12 h or 1 to 30 days, the daughter cells carrying the radioactive tag can be followed as they migrate and differentiate (Fig. 19–49).

Stomach

In the gastric glands of the stomach, mitotic activity is confined to cells of the isthmus and neck. Most of the new cells produced are destined to differentiate into surface mucous cells. They migrate upward into the pits and onto the surface, secreting mucus continuously as they go. They are finally sloughed into the lumen, having lived only about 4 to 6 days in humans or 3 days in the mouse. Other daughter cells remain in the neck of the gland and develop into

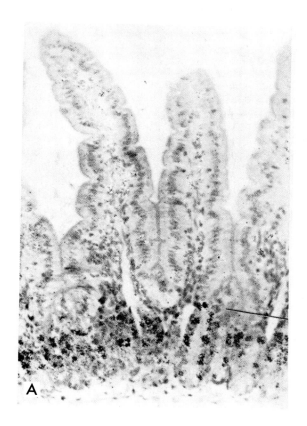

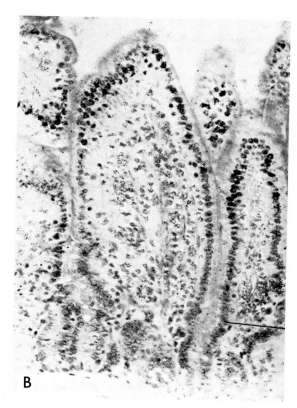

mucous neck cells, a population that is turned over somewhat more slowly than the surface mucous cells. Finally, some new cells migrate downward into the glands and differentiate into parietal, chief, or enteroendocrine cells. These cell types are renewed at a relatively slow rate.

The regeneration of the stomach epithelium over areas denuded by mechanical trauma or by treatment with alcohol has been carefully studied. Cells in the neck and pit divide and migrate out from the edges of the wound to cover the exposed connective tissue, and then new pits and glands form. Within them, the specialized cells differentiate in a manner reminiscent of the process seen during fetal development.

In the pyloric region, long surface pits are joined to short coiled mucous glands by a short transition region called the isthmus. As in the gastric glands throughout the stomach, the isthmic region of the pyloric glands is a site of cell proliferation. It produces surface mucous cells that migrate upward and are short-lived (about 3 days in the mouse; unmeasured in humans), gland mucous cells that migrate downward and seem to have varying survival times,

19–49 Radioautographs of mouse jejunum 8 h **(A)** and 72 h **(B)** after injection of tritiated thymidine. The horizontal marker indicates the approximate junction of the crypt and villus. At 8 h, radioactivity is limited to the upper crypts, whereas by 72 h it is located in the surface epithelium of the upper third of the villus. (From Leblond, C. P., and Messier, B. 1958. Anat. Rec. 132:247.)

and enteroendocrine cells whose exact life span is unknown.

Small Intestine

A zone of intense mitotic activity is located in the lower half of the crypts of Lieberkuhn, a site rich in undifferentiated stem cells. Most of the progeny of these stem cells are destined to become columnar absorptive cells; a few differentiate into mucus-secreting goblet cells, and a few become various enteroendocrine cells. All three types migrate upward together and as they pass through the mid-crypt level, columnar and goblet cells continue to divide. They further differentiate but no longer divide as they move up onto the villus. After a lifetime of 5 to 6 days in humans (2 days in the rat, 3 days in the mouse), all three cell types are extruded and lost from the villus tip. The Paneth cells in the base of the crypt are turned over much more slowly; each lives for about 4 weeks before dying and being replaced by the differentiation of a nearby committed crypt cell. Once visibly differentiated, Paneth cells do not divide.

The extrusion zone at the apex of the villus is marked by a distinct cleft in the epithelium that contains shortened degenerating cells; the emerging cells become round as they are shed into the intestinal lumen. Under normal conditions, cell proliferation in the crypts exactly balances this loss, but the rates of both production and loss are lower without normal bacterial flora in the lumen (as in germfree animals) and when dietary protein and calories are greatly reduced (as in severe malnutrition). Conversely, both the proliferation and loss of cells may be accelerated in certain intestinal infections. Under these conditions, the process of cellular differentiation is not speeded up proportionally, and the crypts become elongated, apparently to accommodate the back-up of young differentiating cells.

Large Intestine

In the large intestinal epithelium, dividing cells are located in the lower half of the crypts. As in the small intestine, undifferentiated stem cells give rise to daughter cells committed to differentiate into columnar, goblet, and enteroendocrine cells as well as a rarer cell type of unknown function, the caveolated "tuft" cell. Columnar, goblet, and tuft cells migrate together up the crypt wall and onto the flat mucosal surface. They are sloughed from the luminal surface at extrusion zones located approximately midway between crypt openings, after a lifetime of about 6 days. The enteroendocrine cells located in the lower crypts are joined to their neighbors by tight junctions, but those located in the upper crypts and on the surface have usually lost contact with the lumen and lie close to the basal lamina. Because the average life span of these endocrine cells is relatively long (over 3 weeks in the mouse), they must migrate independently. The exact turnover times of individual enteroendocrine cell subtypes have not been determined.

Implications of Epithelial Renewal

Epithelial cells of other organs are known to synthesize type IV collagen and glycosaminoglycans for their own basal laminae. We presume that intestinal epithelial cells do likewise and that the fibroblasts of the lamina propria synthesize the underlying network of collagen fibers and the thick "collagen table" that supports the surface epithelium of the large intestine. Whether the basal lamina moves along with the migrating epithelium or remains stationary is unresolved. Nor is the mechanism of epithelial movement understood. Furthermore, radioautographic studies have revealed that the flattened subepithelial fibroblasts, which form a sheath around small and large intestinal crypts, proliferate near the crypt bases and migrate upward in synchrony with the epithelial cells. During fetal life, when mucosal architecture is being established, epithelial cells and fibroblasts make frequent direct contacts across the basal lamina via cytoplasmic processes. How and why the migration of the two cell populations is coordinated in the adult mucosa are not known.

Irradiation treatment and antimitotic compounds (i.e., chemotherapy), commonly used therapeutically to destroy rapidly dividing cancer cells, also affect the normal, rapidly renewing epithelial cells of the gastrointestinal tract. Normal cell sloughing continues in spite of the death of proliferating cells, and the mucosa atrophies. Because mature functional epithelial cells are not being replaced, malabsorption and diarrhea develop after irradiation or chemotherapy. Fortunately, enough quiescent stem cells remain to repopulate and reconstruct the mucosa when treatment is discontinued.

References and Selected Bibliography

Esophagus

Hopwood, D., Logan, K. R., and Bouchier, I. A. D. 1978. The electron microscopy of normal human esophageal epithelium. Virchows Arch. B. Cell Pathol. 26:345.

Parakkal, P. 1967. An electron microscopic study of the esophageal epithelium in the newborn and adult mouse. Am. J. Anat. 121:175.

Stomach

Bensley, R. R. 1932. The gastric glands. In E. V. Cowdry (ed.), Special Cytology, 2nd ed., Vol. 1. New York: Paul B. Hoeber, Inc.

Dibona, R., Ito, S., Berglindh, T., and Sachs, G. 1979. Cellular site of gastric acid secretion. Proc. Natl. Acad. Sci. U.S.A. 76:6689.

Grossman, M. I., and Marks, I. N. 1960. Secretion of pepsinogen by the pyloric glands of the dog, with some observations on the histology of the gastric mucosa. Gastroenterology 38:343.

Ito, S. 1981. Functional gastric morphology. In L. R. Johnson (ed.), Physiology of the Gastrointestinal Tract, Vol. 1. New York: Raven Press, chap. 17.

Ito, S., and Schofield, G. C. 1974. Studies on the depletion and accumulation of microvilli and changes in the tubulovesicular compartment of mouse parietal cells in relation to gastric acid secretion. J. Cell Biol. 63:364.

Kramer, M. F., and Geuze, J. J. 1977. Glycoprotein transport in the surface mucous cells of the rat stomach. J. Cell Biol. 73:533.

Plenk, H. 1932. Der Magen. In W. von Mollendorff and W. Bargmann (eds.), Handbuch der mikroskopischen Anatomie der Menschen, Vol. 5, Part 2. Berlin: Springer-Verlag OHG.

Rubin, W., Ross, L. L., Sleisenger, M. H., and Jeffries, F. H. 1968. The normal human gastric epithelia. A fine structural study. Lab. Invest. 19:598.

Schofield, G. C., Ito, S., and Bolender, R. P. 1979. Changes in membrane surface areas in mouse parietal cells in relation to high levels of acid secretion. J. Anat. 128:669.

Spicer, S. S., Katsuyama, T., and Sannes, P. L. 1978. Ultrastructural carbohydrate cytochemistry of gastric epithelium. Histochem. J. 10:309.

Enteroendocrine Cells

Grube, D., and Forssmann, W. G. 1979. Morphology and function of the entero-endocrine cells. Horm. Metab. Res. 11:603.

Helmstaedter, V., Feurle, G. E., Forssmann, W. G. 1977. Relationship of glucagon-somatostatin and gastrin-somatostatin cells in the stomach of the monkey. Cell Tissue Res. 177:29.

Hökfelt, T., Johansson, O., Jungdahl, A. L., Lundberg, J. M., and Schultzberg, M. 1980. Peptidergic neurones. Nature (Lond.), 284:515.

Johnson, L. R. 1976. The trophic action of gastrointestinal hormones. Gastroenterology 70:278.

Makhlouf, G. M. 1974. The neuroendocrine design of the gut. The play of chemicals in a chemical background. Gastroenterology 67:159.

Pearse, A. G. E., Polak, J. M. and Bloom, S. R. 1977. The newer gut hormones. Cellular sources, physiology, pathology, and clinical aspects. Gastroenterology 72:746.

Small Intestine

Bennett, G., and Leblond, C. P. 1970. Formation of cell coat material for the whole surface of columnar cells in the rat small intestine, as visualized by radioautography with L-fucose-³H. J. Cell Biol. 46:409.

Bretscher, A., and Weber, K. 1978. Localization of actin and microfilament-associated proteins in the microvilli and terminal web of the intestinal brush border by immunofluorescence microscopy. J. Cell Biol. 79:839.

Brunser, O., and Luft, J. H. 1970. Fine structure of the apex of absorptive cells from rat small intestine. J. Ultrastruct. Res. 31:291.

Cardell, R. R., Badenhausen, S., and Porter, K. R. 1967. Intestinal absorption in the rat. An electron microscopical study. J. Cell Biol. 34:123.

Clementi, F., and Palade, G. E. 1969. Intestinal capillaries. I. Permeability to peroxidase and ferritin. J. Cell Biol. 41:33.

Crane, R. K. 1975. A digestive-absorptive surface as illustrated by the intestinal cell brush border. Trans. Am. Microsc. Soc. 94:529.

Erlandsen, S. L., Parsons, J. A., and Taylor, T. D. 1974. Ultrastructural immunocytochemical localization of lysozyme in the Paneth cells of man. J. Histochem. Cytochem. 22:401.

Friedman, H. I., and Cardell, R. R. 1977. Alterations in the endoplasmic reticulum and Golgi complex of intestinal epithelial cells during fat absorption and after termination of this process: A morphological and morphometric study. Anat. Rec. 188:77.

Friend, D. S. 1965. The fine structure of Brunner's glands in the mouse. J. Cell Biol. 25:563.

Isselbacher, K. J. 1975. The intestinal cell surface: Properties of normal, undifferentiated, and malignant cells. Harvey Lect. 69:197.

Ito, S. 1974. Form and function of the glycocalyx on free cell surfaces. Philos. Trans. R. Soc. Lond. (Biol.) 268:55.

Ladman, A. J., Padykula, H. A., and Strauss, E. W. 1963. A morphological study of fat transport in the normal human jejunum. Am. J. Anat. 112:389.

Madara, J. L., Trier, J. S. and Neutra, M. R. 1980. Structural changes in the plasma membrane accompanying differentiation of epithelial cells in human and monkey small intestine. Gastroenterology 78:963.

Moog, F. 1979. The differentiation and redifferentiation of the intestinal epithelium and its brush border membrane. In K. Elliott and J. Whelan (eds.), Development of Mammalian Absorptive Processes, Ciba Foundation Series 70. Amsterdam: Elsevier, p. 31.

Mooseker, M. S., and Tilney, L. G. 1975. Organization of an actin filament-membrane complex. Filament polarity and membrane attachment in the microvilli of intestinal epithelial cells. J. Cell Biol. 67:725.

Ockner, R. K., and Isselbacher, K. J. 1974. Recent concepts of intestinal fat absorption. Rev. Physiol. Biochem. Pharmacol. 71:107.

Padykula, H. A., Strauss, E. W., Ladman, A. J., and Gardner, F. H. 1961. A morphologic and histochemical analysis of the human jejunal epithelium in nontropical sprue. Gastroenterology 40:735.

Rodewald, R. 1980. Distribution of immunoglobulin G receptors in the small intestine of the young rat. J. Cell Biol. 85:18.

Schonfeld, G., Bell, E., and Alpers, D. H. 1978. Intestinal apoproteins during fat absorption. J. Clin. Invest. 61:1539.

Trier, J. S., and Madara, J. L. 1981. Functional morphology of the mucosa of the small intestine. *In* L. R. Johnson (ed.), Physiology of the Gastrointestinal Tract, Vol. 2. New York: Raven Press, chap. 35.

Immune Defense Mechanisms

Brandtzaeg, P., and Baklein, K. 1977. Intestinal secretion of IgA and IgM: A hypothetical model. *In* R. Porter and J. Knight (eds), Immunology of the Gut, Ciba Foundation Symposium 46 (new series). Amsterdam: Elsevier, p. 77.

Brown, W. R., Isobe, Y., and Nakane, P. K. 1976. Studies on translocation of immunoglobulins across intestinal epithelium. Gastroenterology 71:985.

Douglas, A. P., and Weetman, A. P. 1975. Lymphocytes and the gut. Digestion 13:344.

Erlandsen, S. L., Rodning, C. B., Montero, C., Parsons, J. A., Lewis, C. A., and Wilson, I. D. 1976. Immunocytochemical identification and localization of immunoglobulin A within Paneth cells of the rat small intestine. J. Histochem. Cytochem. 24:1085.

Kagnoff, M. F. 1981. Immunology of the digestive system. *In* L. R. Johnson (ed.), Physiology of the Gastrointestinal Tract, Vol. 2. New York: Raven Press, chap. 54.

Owen, R. L. 1977. Sequential uptake of horseradish peroxidase by lymphoid follicle epithelium of Peyer's patches in the normal unobstructed mouse intestine: An ultrastructural study. Gastroenterology 72:440.

Owen, R. L., and Jones, A. L. 1974. Epithelial cell specialization with human Peyer's patches: An ultrastructural study of intestinal lymphoid follicles. Gastroenterology 66:189.

Owen, R. L., and Nemanic, P. 1978. Antigen processing structures of the mammalian intestinal tract: An SEM study of lymphoepithelial organs. *In* Scanning Electron Microscopy, Vol. II. AMF O'Hare, Ill.: SEM, Inc., p. 367.

Large Intestine

Essner, E., Schreiber, J., and Griewski, R. A. 1978. Localization of carbohydrate components in rat colon with fluoresceinated lectins. J. Histochem. Cytochem. 26:452.

Lineback, P. E. 1925. Studies on the musculature of the human colon, with special reference to the taeniae. Am. J. Anat. 36:357.

Lorenzonn, V., and Trier, J. S. 1968. The fine structure of human rectal mucosa. The epithelial lining at the base of the crypt. Gastroenterology 55:88.

Martin, B. F. 1961. The goblet cell pattern of the large intestine. Anat. Rec. 140:1.

Neutra, M. R., Grand, R. J., and Trier, J. S. 1977. Glycoprotein synthesis, transport and secretion by epithelial cells of human rectal mucosa: Normal and cystic fibrosis. Lab. Invest. 36:535.

Neutra, M. R., and Leblond, C. P. 1966. Synthesis of the carbohydrate of mucus in the Golgi complex as shown by electron microscope radioautography of goblet cells from rats injected with glucose-H^3. J. Cell Biol. 30:119.

Specian, R. D., and Neutra, M. R. 1980. Acceleration of secretion in colonic goblet cells by acetylcholine. J. Cell Biol. 85:626.

Epithelial Renewal

Chang, W. W. L., and Leblond, C. P. 1971. Renewal of the epithelium in the descending colon of the mouse. Parts I, II and III. Am. J. Anat. 131:73, 101, and 111.

Cheng, H., and Leblond, C. P. 1974. Origin, differentiation and renewal of the four main epithelial cell types in the mouse small intestine. Parts I–V. Am. J. Anat. 141:461–562.

Eastwood, G. L. 1977. Gastrointestinal epithelial renewal. Gastroenterology 72:962.

Leblond, C. P., and Messier, B. 1958. Renewal of chief cells and goblet cells in the small intestine as shown by radioautography after injection of thymidine-H^3 into mice. Anat. Rec. 132:247.

Lipkin, M. 1981. Proliferation and differentiation of gastrointestinal cells in normal and disease states. *In* L. R. Johnson (ed.), Physiology of the Gastrointestinal Tract, Vol. 1. New York: Raven Press, chap. 4.

MacDonald, W. C., Trier, J. S., and Everett, N. B. 1964. Cell proliferation and migration in the stomach, duodenum and rectum of man: Radioautographic studies. Gastroenterology 46:405.

Parker, F. G., Barnes, E. N., and Kaye, G. I. 1974. The pericryptal fibroblast sheath. IV. Replication, migration and differentiation of the subepithelial fibroblasts of the crypts and villus of rabbit jejunum. Gastroenterology 67:607.

Pascal, R. R., Kaye, G. I., and Lane, N. 1968. Colonic pericryptal fibroblast sheath: Replication, migration, and cytodifferentiation of a mesenchymal cell system in adult tissue. I. Autoradiographic studies of normal rabbit colon. Gastroenterology 54:835.

Tsubouchi, S., and Leblond, C. P. 1979. Migration and turnover of entero-endocrine cells in the epithelium of the descending colon, as shown by radioautography after continuous infusion of ^{3}H-thymidine into mice. Am. J. Anat. 156:431.

Williamson, R. C. N. 1978. Intestinal adaptation. Parts I and II. N. Engl. J. Med. 298:1393 and 1444.

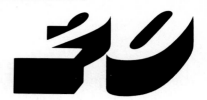

The Liver and Gallbladder

Albert L. Jones
and Elinor Spring-Mills

General Morphology and Function

The liver is the largest *gland* in the human body, constituting approximately one-twentieth of the body weight in the neonate and one-fiftieth in the adult. It lies in the right upper quadrant of the abdominal cavity, beneath and attached to the diaphragm. It is made up of four incompletely separated *lobes*. A thin connective tissue *capsule* (Glisson's capsule), usually covered by reflected peritoneum, lines the external surface of the liver. A definite hilus, the *porta hepatis*, is present where vessels enter and ducts leave the liver, and the surface capsule becomes continuous with the internal stroma. Right and left *hepatic bile* ducts emerging from the gland unite in the porta hepatis to form the *hepatic duct* proper. A short distance outside the liver, the hepatic duct joins the *cystic duct,* or *ductus choledochus,* which enters the duodenum about 10 cm below the pyloric–duodenal junction.

The liver has a dual blood supply. The *portal vein,* carrying blood that has already passed through the capillary beds of the alimentary tract, spleen, and pancreas, brings approximately 75% of the afferent blood volume to the liver. This blood is rich in nutrients and other absorbed substances but relatively poor in oxygen. The *hepatic artery,* a branch of the celiac trunk, carrying well-oxygenated blood, supplies the remaining blood to the liver. Blood from branches of these two vessels mixes in passing to and

20–1 Liver lobule. Schematic view. The central vein lies in the center of the figure, surrounded by anastomosing cords of blocklike hepatocytes. Around the periphery of the schema are six "triads," evenly spaced from one another, lying at an angle in the polyhedron lobule. Each triad consists of branches of the portal vein, hepatic artery, and bile duct. See text.

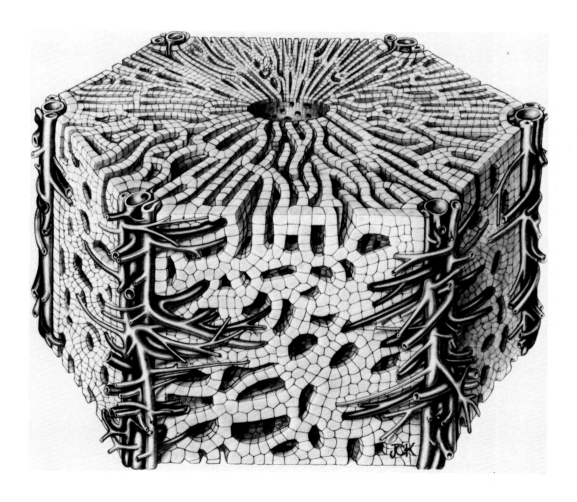

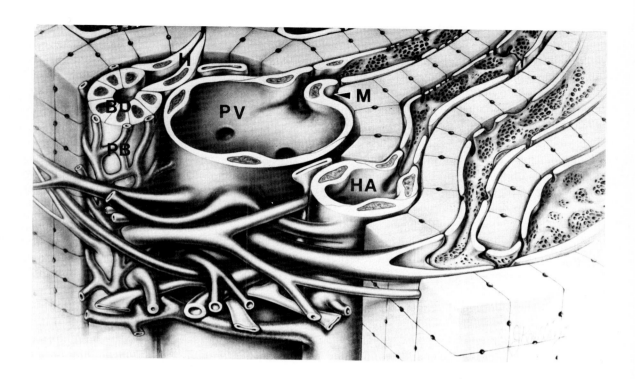

20–2 Liver lobule. Schematic view, higher power of Fig. 20–1. The relationship of branches of the portal vein **(PV)**, hepatic artery **(HA)**, and bile duct **(BD)** are shown. **H**, canal of Hering; **PB**, peribiliary plexus; **M**, space of Mall. See text.

through the liver lobules (Figs. 20–1 and 20–2). Sinusoidal blood flows toward the center of each lobule and is collected by the *central vein* (terminal hepatic venule). After leaving the lobules, the central veins unite to form the larger *sublobular* or *intercalated* veins, which finally join the large *hepatic veins*. Blood returns to the heart via the *inferior vena cava*.

The classic structural unit of the organ is the *hepatic lobule*, a polyhedral prism of tissue, approximately 2 mm long and 0.7 mm wide, containing anastomosing plates of parenchymal cells and a labyrinthine system of blood sinusoids. Branches of the afferent blood vessels and bile ducts run along the edges of the polyhedron, and the central vein runs throughout its center. *Bile*, produced by the parenchymal cells, is secreted into minute *bile capillaries* or *canaliculi* between the glandular epithelial cells. At the periphery of the lobule, bile flows into small *bile ductules*, or *canals of Hering*, and eventually into the larger *bile ducts*. The liver is composed of approximately 1 million lobular units.

The liver is essential for life; mammals survive subtotal hepatectomy mainly because the cells have extraordinary regenerative powers and the capacity to tolerate the increased metabolic demands. The functional diversity and complex-

ity of the liver are rivaled only by the central nervous system. The liver functions both as an *exocrine* and *endocrine gland*. It secretes bile, which flows into the duodenum and contains, among other constituents, *bile salts* that emulsify dietary fats prior to digestion. The liver takes up digested foodstuffs from the afferent blood and stores carbohydrate (glycogen), proteins, vitamins, and some lipids. Stored substances not used by the hepatocyte can be released into the blood unbound (for example, glucose) or in association with a carrier (for example, triglyceride molecules complexed in a lipoprotein). The liver also synthesizes many substances in response to the body's demands: albumin and other plasma proteins, glucose, fatty acids for triglyceride synthesis, cholesterol, and phospholipids. The liver metabolizes, detoxifies, and inactivates exogenous compounds, such as drugs and insecticides, endogenous compounds, such as steroids, and probably most other hormones. In addition, it has the ability to convert substances into more active forms, for example, T_4 to T_3. It also plays a major role in the intestinal immune system by sequestering dimeric IgA and secreting it into the intestinal lumen via the biliary tree. By virtue of its large vascular capacity, it serves as a major storehouse for blood. During embryogenesis and certain diseases of the adult, it is a site of hematopoiesis. Finally, its abundance of phagocytes makes the liver one of the principal filters for foreign particulate matter, especially for bacteria coming from the gut.

Histological Organization of the Human Liver

Stroma

Most of the liver's free surface, except for a small area within its diaphragmatic attachment, is covered by a single layer of flattened *peritoneal mesothelial cells*. Beneath the mesothelium lies a thin *surface capsule* (Glisson's capsule) composed of regularly arranged collagen fibers, scattered fibroblasts, and small blood vessels. The capsule surrounds the four lobes and is thickest around the inferior vena cava and the hilus or porta hepatis. The capsule is reflected inwardly at the porta, where its fibers merge with the denser connective tissue surrounding the vascular and biliary branches. Inside the organ, the connective tissue arborizes to such an extent that no segment of the parenchyma is more than a few millimeters away from one of its branches. Examination of liver sections that have been stained selectively for connective tissue and preparations of isolated hepatic stroma reveals that despite its size, the large, bulky human liver normally contains relatively little connective tissue. Nevertheless, the connective tissue (1) provides an internal supporting framework for the hepatic parenchyma; (2) ensheaths most of the vessels, bile ducts, and nerves; and (3) subdivides the parenchyma into *lobules*. The only connective tissue within the lobule is the *reticular network* between the sinusoidal endothelium and plates of parenchymal cells. The reticular fibers presumably support the liver parenchyma and also may keep the sinusoids open (see Fig. 20–3 for size and arrangement of reticular fibers). When this reticular framework survives hepatic injury, the parenchyma regenerates more rapidly and in a more orderly fashion (Rappa-

port, 1969). Electron microscopic observations and autoradiographic studies have shown that normal livers contain a few true fibroblasts within the perisinusoidal space of Disse. In addition, it has been suggested that a fat-containing perisinusoidal cell (that is, the so-called Ito cell, or lipocyte) may be the progenitor of the perisinusoidal fibroblast, since fat cells in other tissues can be transformed into fibroblasts (Popper and Udenfriend, 1970).

At the periphery of the lobule, the reticular meshwork of the sinusoids becomes continuous with the *interlobular connective tissue*. The term *Glisson's capsule* is sometimes applied to both the surface capsule and the internal connective tissue. However, because the interlobular tissue is not composed exclusively of fibrous tissue and in any one site usually serves two or more contiguous lobules, the broader terms *portal canal, area, space, radicle,* and *tract* are more commonly used to designate the tissue in these regions. The stroma forms the bed of a portal canal. It ensheaths and carries the so-called portal triad (that is, branches of the hepatic artery, portal vein, and bile duct), the lymphatic vessels, and the nerves throughout the interior of the liver (Fig. 20–4). The size of a portal canal depends on its position in the branching connective tissue stroma. Large portal canals in the thicker branches of connective tissue may contain both large and small vessels derived from the portal vein and hepatic artery. The larger vessels carry blood to more distant sites, whereas the small vessels are usually terminal branches of the vein and artery carrying blood into the adjacent lobules. The smallest portal canals contain only terminal branches of the blood and biliary vessels. Sections through these regions usually reveal no more than four tubular structures (for example, venule from the portal vein, arteriole from the hepatic artery, lymphatic, and bile duct) embedded in a tiny isolated patch of loose connective tissue.

Alterations in the Stroma

Hepatic fibrosis, or excess connective tissue, is an early histological sign of chronic liver disease; it is important to be able to recognize this phenomenon in liver sections. Fibrosis occurs primarily at four sites: (1) in the portal canals, (2) around central veins, (3) around hepatocytes, and (4) around proliferating bile ductules that extend from the portal canals into the paren-

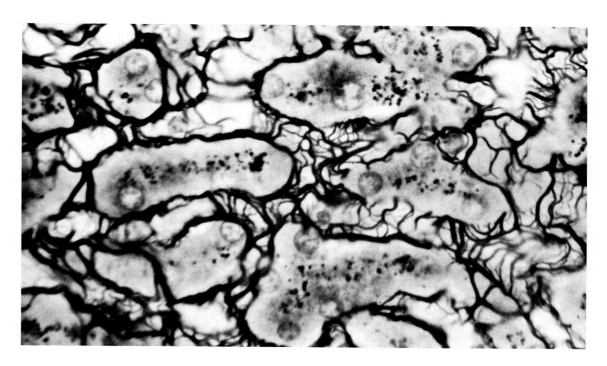

chyma. Parenchymal cell injury or degeneration is probably one of the primary stimuli for the formation of excess connective tissue. The connective tissue under these conditions often forms new, irregular septa around nodules of regenerating parenchymal cells, preventing these cells from making appropriate connections with blood

20–3 Photomicrograph of the human liver showing the close meshwork of reticular fibers (collagen type III) in the perisinusoidal space between the parenchymal cells and the sinusoidal lining. A few perisinusoidal cell nuclei can be seen within the meshes of the reticulum. Silver, gold, hematoxylin, and Van Gieson's stains.

20–4 Photomicrograph of a portal canal from human liver. Branches of the portal vein, hepatic artery, bile duct **(B)**, and lymphatic vessel can be found within the connective tissue. Note the large lumen in the portal vein and the cuboidal epithelium that lines the bile duct. Mallory-Azan. × 200.

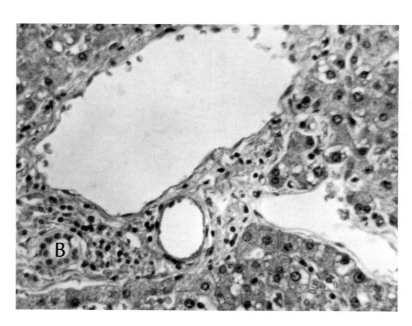

and biliary vessels, while the inelastic septa ultimately compress the nodules and restrict their growth. As a result, the flow of blood and bile through the liver is impeded, cellular nutrition is impaired, and the organ is often unable to restore its normal architecture. Factors responsible for stimulating fibroblasts, deposition, and catabolism of fibers are being investigated with the hope that the insidious fibrotic and cirrhotic changes associated with many liver diseases can be treated and controlled (Rojkind and Dunn, 1979).

Lobulation

The presence of small *histological units*, or *lobules*, within the mammalian liver has been generally accepted since the pioneering observations of Wepfer (1664) and Malpighi (1666), but the validity and usefulness of the traditional definition of a hepatic lobule, based primarily on the disposition of structural boundaries such as connective tissue septa and vessels within the liver lobes, have been questioned. As a result, three primary schemata have been developed to describe the histological and functional units of the liver. The names *classic lobule*, *portal lobule*, and *liver acinus* have been assigned to the three interpretations. Each concept was formulated under different circumstances, yet they are not mutually conflicting. They represent different ways to interpret particular aspects of liver structure and function and thus facilitate our understanding of this organ (see Table 20–1).

The *classic lobule* was described above; it is a polyhedral prism of hepatic tissue about 0.7 × 2 mm, the boundaries of which are demarcated by connective tissue septa (portal canals) or the regular distribution of biliary and vascular vessels (portal triad), or both. In cross section, the lobule is roughly hexagonal, but adjacent lobules are not perfectly aligned or precisely the same size. In the angles of the hexagon are the portal areas containing connective tissue stroma and the portal triad or terminal branches of the hepatic artery, portal vein, and bile duct. The center of the lobule contains the *central vein* or *terminal hepatic venule* (the smallest subdivision of the hepatic veins) surrounded by a minute amount of connective tissue (Fig. 20–5). *Parenchymal* or *glandular epithelial cells* (hepatocytes) separated on either side by narrow vascular spaces, the *sinusoids*, radiate from the central vein to the portal areas at the periphery

of the lobule (Figs. 20–1, 20–2, and 20–6). The lobules are composed of a continuous system of parenchymal *cell plates*, or laminae, and not single strands or columns of cells (Elias, 1949). The parenchymal cells throughout an entire lobule are interconnected and subdivided by spaces or lacunae into anatomosing plates one cell thick. The sinusoids run within the center, and the perisinusoidal *space of Disse* occupies the periphery of each lacuna. The lacunae form a continuous labyrinth within each lobule. Stereograms of a liver lobule show that each lacuna opens directly into a *central space* containing the central vein. At the periphery of the lobule, a *limiting plate* of hepatic cells surrounds the circumference of the lobule, forming a nearly continuous wall between the interior of the lobule and the space occupied by the portal canals. Only tiny terminal branches of the hepatic artery, portal vein, and bile duct can penetrate the liver parenchyma via the occasional fenestrations in the limiting plate (see Figs. 20–1 and 20–2).

The classic lobule is best seen in species (for example, pig, racoon, camel, and polar bear) in which relatively thick bands of interlobular connective tissue encircle each lobule (see Fig. 20–7, here and color insert). In humans, lobulation is incomplete and poorly defined. The sparse perilobular connective tissue does not form a continuous boundary between contiguous lobules, and the parenchyma often appears to be coextensive between adjacent lobules. Nevertheless, the approximate boundaries of a human classic lobule can be visualized by first locating a central vein and then following the successive, regularly placed portal triads that encircle the periphery of each lobule (see Fig. 20–8, here and color insert).

Blood flows from the portal canals (hepatic artery and portal vein) into the lobule, passes along the sinusoids, and is removed from the lobule by the central vein. Bile, however, flows in the opposite direction, from the parenchymal cells where it is formed to the interlobular bile ducts in the portal canals.

Although the classic lobule is regarded primarily as a structural unit, certain changes that are physiological (for example, fat and glycogen deposition after a meal) or pathologic (for example, necrosis) often seem confined to specific areas within the lobule. Such changes may originate and spread through the territory of the classic lobule from either the peripheral (portal)

Table 20–1 Important Features of Three Concepts of Liver Lobulation

	Classic lobule	Portal lobule	Liver acinus
Cross-sectional appearance of three types of hepatic units. Classic lobules (hexagons) outlined in each diagram. Shaded regions show amount of tissue included in each unit and its relationship to classic lobules.	Central vein / Portal canals	Central vein / Portal canals	Central vein / Portal canals
Shape	Polygonal or hexagonal	Roughly triangular or wedge-shaped	Irregular, sometimes oval or diamond-shaped
Morphological axis	Central vein	Portal area, especially interlobular bile duct	Terminal branches of portal triad lying along border of two adjacent classic lobules
Peripheral landmarks	Approximately six portal areas	Three (or more) central veins	Two (or more) central veins
Relationship to classic lobule		Encompasses those portions of all classic lobules that secrete bile into a common interlobular bile duct	Small sectors of two adjacent classic lobules
Direction of blood flow	From periphery (portal areas) to center (central vein)	From center (portal area) to periphery (central veins)	From center (portal area and edges of two adjacent classic lobules) to periphery
Direction of bile flow	From center toward periphery	From periphery to center	From periphery toward center
Advantages of concept	1. Emphasizes endocrine function of liver 2. Useful in understanding histological changes associated with centrolobular necrosis (for example, CCl_4 poisoning)	1. Emphasizes exocrine function of liver (that is, bile secretion) 2. Makes histological organization of a hepatic lobule comparable to those of most exocrine glands	1. Offers best explanation for gradient of metabolic activity or zonation within liver, that is, direct correlation between blood supply and metabolism 2. Helps to explain pattern of regeneration 3. Useful in understanding development of cirrhosis
Principal developers of concept	Wepfer; Malpighi; Mascagni; Kiernan; Müller	Theile; Brissaud and Sabourin; Mall; Arey	Rappaport and co-workers; Novikoff and Essner

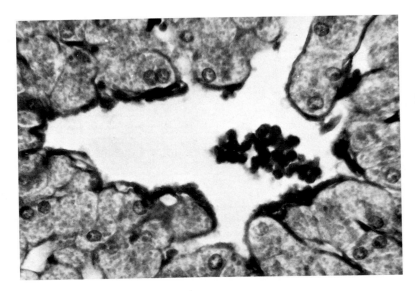

20–5 Several sinusoids empty into the central vein shown in this photomicrograph. Note that the central vein is larger than the sinusoids. It has extremely thin walls and is surrounded by sparse connective tissue. Human liver. Mallory-Azan. × 400.

areas or the central areas (central vein), producing an unusual circular gradient in which similar microscopic alterations appear in concentric bands or zones around the central vein (Table 20–1). Because of this, some histologists believe that the classic lobule can and should be re-

garded as both a structural and a functional unit of the liver.

The concept of the *portal lobule* is seldom used in modern hepatology. It emerged during the mid-nineteenth century as histologists discovered that liver lobules are not well-defined

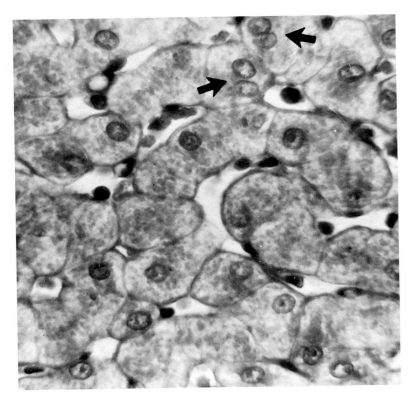

20–6 Liver parenchymal cells are shown at higher magnification in this photomicrograph. The cells are polyhedral, yet adjacent cells may vary in size and shape. The hepatic cells form branching and anastomosing single-cell-thick plates that are separated by the sinusoids (light areas). **Arrows** point to binuclear cells. Human liver. Mallory-Azan. × 600.

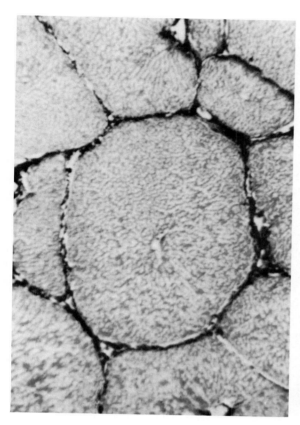

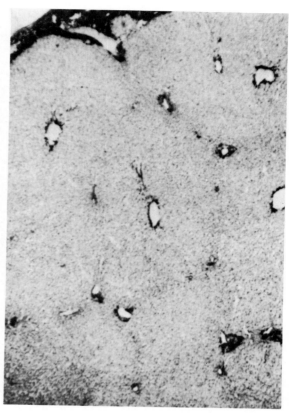

20–7 Low-power photomicrograph of a section of pig liver, showing a classic lobule. This is a black and white rendition of a color plate. See color section.

20–8 Low-power photomicrograph of a section of human liver. This is a black and white rendition of a color plate. See color section.

anatomical units in most mammals and that in many exocrine glands it is more convenient to consider a lobule as a *functional unit* rather than a segment of tissue enclosed by fissures or septa.

The portal lobule is a roughly triangular or wedge-shaped prism of hepatic tissue (Table 20–1). The morphological axis of the portal lobule is the interlobular bile duct in the portal space, and its peripheral limits are formed by three different "central" veins. According to this schema, bile flows from the periphery to the centrally located bile duct, and blood flows from the center of the lobule to the periphery. Hence, the pathways for bile drainage and blood flow are similar to most exocrine glands. Those who oppose the recognition and use of this concept often argue that it unduly emphasizes the liver's role as an exocrine gland, but since no valid judgment can be made about the relative impor-

tance of the exocrine and endocrine activities of the liver, each schema is useful to explain the myriad functions of the liver.

Rappaport (1969) introduced the concept of the *liver acinus*, described as the smallest functional unit within the liver. Observations of hepatic circulation in vivo and preparations of specially injected human liver casts revealed that the tissue around each central vein is derived from different sources, suggesting that this tissue is not one unit but a series of units or liver acini. The *simple liver acinus* is defined as a small, irregular mass of unencapsulated parenchymal tissue lying between two (or more) terminal hepatic venules ("central veins"). Its axis is a small radicle of the main portal canal containing a terminal portal venule, hepatic arteriole, bile ductule, lymph vessel, and nerves. In histological sections, it includes only small segments of two

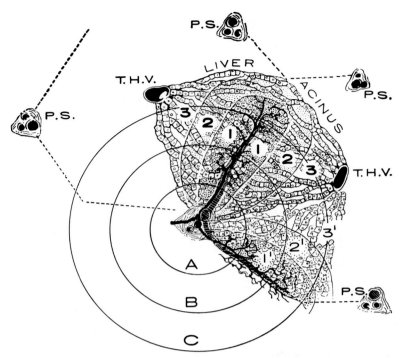

20–9 Blood supply of the simple liver acinus. The oxygen tension and nutrient level of the blood in sinusoids decrease from zone 1 through zone 3. Zones 1', 2', and 3' indicate corresponding volumes in a portion of an adjacent acinar unit. Circle A encloses the area commonly designated as periportal; B and C represent the areas more peripheral to the portal space (PS). THV, terminal hepatic venules (central veins). (From Rappaport, A. M., Borowy, Z. J., Laugheed, W. M., and Lotto, W. N. 1954. Anat. Rec. 119:11, Fig. 1.)

adjacent classic lobules. The acini extend at right angles from the preterminal branches of the portal veins (at the edges of the classic lobules) to the central veins (see Figs. 20–1, 20–9, and 20–10 and Table 20–1). The parenchyma is continuous between the classic lobules, and blood flows toward both central veins from the terminal branches of the portal veins. Although there is extensive communication among sinusoids, the tissue within each acinus is supplied mainly by its parent vessels. Moreover, the cells within each acinus appear to be grouped into concentric zones around the axis of the acinus. Cells close to the axis and the terminal afferent vessels (for example, zone 1) are the first to receive blood and nutrients, the last to die, and the first to regenerate. Cells in more distant regions receive blood of poorer quality and also appear less resistant to damage. The concept of acinar circulatory zones has been extended by Rappaport to provide an explanation for the histological appearance of many pathological changes in the liver.

Parenchymal Cells

The hepatic plates are composed of large, polyhedral parenchymal cells approximately 30 μm long and 20 μm wide (see Fig. 20–6). These cells make up approximately 80% of the cell population in the human liver (Gates et al., 1961). They are different sizes: The smallest ones border perforations in the liver plate, and the largest ones are either polyploid or located in the corners where three cell plates meet. The six or more surfaces on each parenchymal cell are of three different types: (1) those abutting other parenchymal cells, (2) those bordering bile canaliculi, and (3) those touching the perisinusoidal space (space of Disse). The latter surface constitutes a limiting plate. In addition, cells bordering the portal zone have a surface in contact with the portal connective tissue. The cell membrane undergoes characteristic modifications in each of these three sites. In optimal routine histological preparations or after special procedures (for example, indigo blue staining, silver impregnation, or staining for adenosine triphosphatase), bile canaliculi are seen on surfaces between contiguous cells. These tiny channels follow an incomplete chicken-wire pattern along contiguous surfaces of parenchymal cells (Figs. 20–2, 20–11, and 20–12).

The nuclei are large, round, and usually centrally located. They contain one or more nucleoli and scattered clumps of chromatin. Generally the nuclei of parenchymal cells stain less intensely than the smaller nuclei of other cells in the liver.

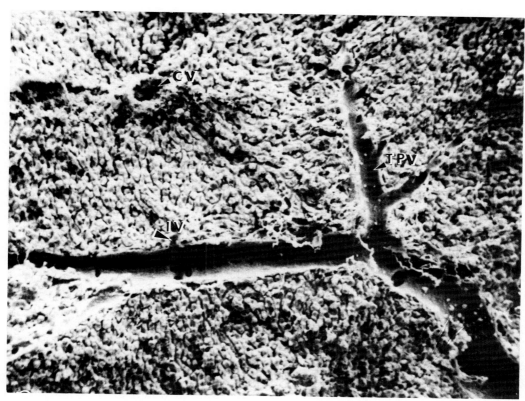

20–10 A low-magnification scanning electron micrograph depicting a portion of a liver lobule from rat liver. Images like this lend credence to Rappaport's concept of the liver acinus. Compare with Fig. 20–9. **CV,** central vein (terminal hepatic venule); **TPV,** terminal portal venule (perilobular); **IV,** inlet venules. Approximately × 400. (From Jones, A. L., and Schmucker, D. L. 1977. Gastroenterology 73:833.)

Moreover, in the adult liver, parenchymal cell nuclei can be subdivided into several nuclear-sized groups or classes (Doljanski, 1960). Polyploid nuclei and binucleated and multinucleated cells are easily found. Adult mammalian livers contain 30 to 80% polyploid cells, and there appears to be good correlation between nuclear size and ploidy, that is, doubling of DNA content being accompanied by an approximate doubling of nuclear volume. The two nuclei of binuclear cells have roughly the same size and staining properties. Both nuclei divide simultaneously and are thought to arise from mononuclear cells through endomitosis. Binuclear cells can account for as much as 25% of the parenchymal cell population. The factors influencing the formation of polyploid and binuclear liver cells and the physiological consequences of these phenomena are not understood. The work of Carriere (1969) and

20–11 Drawing of a network of bile canaliculi in dog liver, showing the entrance of canaliculi into a terminal bile ductule at the edge of a lobule. Silver preparation. (From Elias, H. 1949. Am. J. Anat. 85:379.)

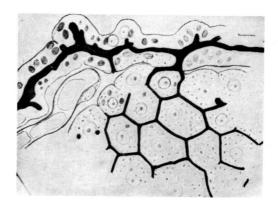

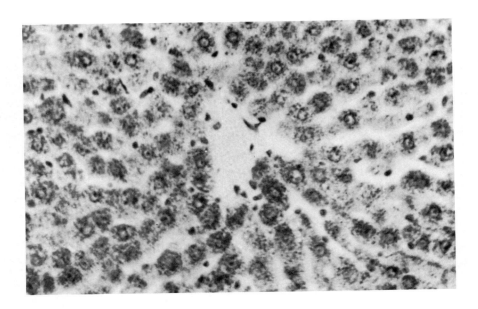

20–12 Glycogen deposits within the parenchymal cells are stained by Best's carmine. This is a black and white rendition of a color plate. See color section.

others suggests that certain hormones regulate both the liver's mitotic index and the formation of the polyploid and binuclear cells. Mitotic activity, however, is rare in the intact normal adult liver (1 mitosis per 10,000–20,000 cells), and the minimum average life span of a parenchymal cell is about 150 days. It is hoped that eventually new techniques will reveal more about the submicroscopic organization of these nuclei and their relation to ploidy, cell renewal, regeneration, and nuclear–cytoplasmic interactions.

The cytoplasm of the parenchymal cell is usually granular; however, it can vary widely in appearance, often reflecting the functional and nutritional state of the cell. Usually large clumps of basophilic *ribonucleoprotein* and abundant mitochondria can be demonstrated throughout the cytoplasm. However, after a prolonged fast, the basophilic bodies decrease and the cytoplasm becomes predominantly eosinophilic. The Golgi complex is ordinarily located near a bile canaliculus, and there is usually more than one Golgi area per section. Stored materials such as glycogen and fat are usually not preserved in conventional histological sections, but empty round vacuoles in the cytoplasm normally indicate the

sites occupied by fat, and irregular empty spaces or flocculent, grainy cytoplasmic regions mark areas that were rich in glycogen.

It is generally assumed that all parenchymal cells can store or secrete any of the substances demonstrable histochemically (see Fig. 20–13, here and color insert). Disparities in the appearance and contents of the cytoplasm are thought to depend on the position of the cell within the lobule and the nutritional status of the individual. However, in our opinion, these problems have not been resolved and require additional work to determine how much uniformity exists among liver cells in metabolic capacity, nutritional requirements, and disease susceptibility (Table 20–2).

Blood Vessels and Sinusoids

The liver is highly vascularized, and its function is intimately related to the distribution and histology of its blood vessels. Blood is brought to the liver via the *portal vein* and *hepatic artery*. The livers of the dog, cat, and human being receive a total blood flow of 100 to 130 ml per min per 100 g tissue; of this, 70 to 75% is supplied by the portal vein and the remainder by the hepatic artery. Total hepatic blood flow is about one-quarter of the cardiac output.

The afferent blood vessels enter the organ at the *porta* and promptly form several large branches that initially course between the lobes

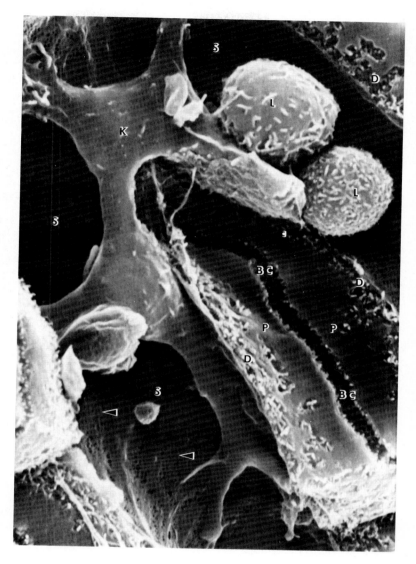

20–13 Scanning electron micrograph of guinea pig liver. Note the centrally located hemibile canaliculus **(BC)** between adjacent parenchymal cells **(P)** and the fenestrae within the endothelial lining cells **(arrowheads)** of the sinusoids **(S)**. A large Kupffer cell **(K)** reaches into sinusoids through a lacuna in the hepatic plates. **D,** space of Disse; **L,** lymphocytes. × 5,000. (Courtesy of Pamela Williams.)

ensheathed in the largest trabeculae of connective tissue and then follow the successive, graduated branchings of the stroma. The gross intrahepatic vascular anatomy has been studied by combined radiological and injection-corrosion techniques. Specially injected plastic casts of adult human livers reveal that the liver can be divided into segments on the basis of its internal vasculature. Each branch of the afferent vessels entering the liver is essential for proper function, because each one supplies blood to a specific area. Usually there are no anastomoses between the major branches and no accessory or additional portal veins or hepatic arteries that could provide the segment with an adequate blood supply should the major branches be impaired (Healey, 1970).

The incoming portal vein contains no valves, and its lumen is much larger than the lumen of the accompanying hepatic artery. It bifurcates into two trunks in the porta that, in turn, divide into large branches or *rami venae portae,* which are usually *interlobar* vessels. In humans, branches of the portal vein with a diameter of 400 μm or more are called *conducting veins.* They are visible to the unaided eye and include the rami venae portae, their largest branches, and subbranches. These vessels are *large-* and *me-*

Table 20–2 Cytochemical and Ultrastructural Evidence of Metabolic Heterogeneity in Liver Parenchymal Cells

Substance or organelles	Experimental conditions	
	Animal	Method[a]
Glycogen deposits	Fed	LM: PAS or Best's carmine EM: Lead stain
	Fasted 21 + h	LM: PAS or Best's carmine EM: Lead stain
Fat droplets	Fed	LM: Sudan stains; oil red O; osmium impregnation
	Ethanol-treated	LM: Sudan stains; oil red O; osmium impregnation
	Starved	LM: Sudan stains; oil red O; osmium impregnation
	Choline deficient	LM: Sudan stains; oil red O; osmium impregnation
Bile acids	Fed	LM: barium chloride precipitation and acid fuchsin
Acid phosphatase	Fed	LM, EM: modified Gomori lead salt technique
Lysosomes (all categories)	Fed	EM: quantitative stereology
Krebs' cycle enzymes	Fed	LM, EM: tetrazolium salt techniques
Mitochondria	Fed	EM: quantitative stereology
Pentose shunt enzymes	Fed	LM, EM: tetrazolium salt techniques
Peroxisomes	Fed	EM: quantitative stereology
Albumin	Fed	Fluorescent antibody techniques
Rough endoplasmic reticulum	Fed	EM: quantitative stereology
Smooth endoplasmic reticulum	Fed	EM: quantitative stereology
Golgi complex	Fed	EM: quantitative stereology

[a]LM, light microscope; EM, microscope.

dium-size branches of the portal vein. The histological organization of the large conducting veins is like that of other large veins, except that the portal vein contains no valves. The smaller branches of the conducting veins often lack a longitudinal layer of smooth muscle and are usually interlobular.

In humans, the smallest branches of the portal vein (terminal portal venules or perilobular veins) have a diameter of 280 μm or less and are essentially endothelial tubes surrounded by a thin layer of smooth muscle fibers. They are found in the smallest portal canals and form the axis of the simple liver acinus. At intervals, they

Distribution		
Cytoplasm	Lobule	References
Throughout; often in close association with SER	Appears first in periphery of classic lobule or zone 1 of liver acinus	Deane, 1944; Novikoff and Essner, 1960
Low or absent	Depends upon maximal hepatic glycogen level	Babcock and Cardell, 1974; Deane, 1944
Random, throughout	Appear transiently after meal in central cells (zone 3)	Deane, 1944
Increased number of droplets; random, throughout	Most numerous in central (zone 3)	Elias and Sherrick, 1969
Increased after 24 h; random, throughout	Depot fat appears as droplets in peripheral cells (zone 1)	Rappaport, 1969
Increased; random, throughout	Accumulate first in central cells (zone 3)	Rappaport, 1969
Random, throughout	Most concentrated in peripheral cells (zone 1)	Deane, 1944
In lysosomes, especially peribiliary dense bodies	Activity highest in peripheral cells (zone 1)	Novikoff and Essner, 1960
Peribiliary	Most in central cells (zone 3)	Loud, 1968
In mitochondria	Activity highest in peripheral cells (zone 1)	Novikoff and Essner, 1960
Random, throughout	Smaller and more numerous in central cells (zone 3), approximately 800 per cell	Loud, 1968
Random, throughout	Activity highest in central cells (zone 3)	Isselbacher and Jones, 1964; Wachstein, 1959
Random, throughout	Most numerous in central cells (zone 3), approximately 200 per cell	Loud, 1968
Variable	No evidence of zonation; pronounced variation among adjacent cells	Hamashima et al., 1964
Random, throughout	No zonation; about 25,000 μm^2 membrane area per cell	Loud, 1968
Throughout; often in association with glycogen	Membrane area in square micrometers per cell periphery 15,700 midzonal 16,900 central 21,600	Loud, 1968
Peribiliary	Largest in peripheral cells (zone 1)	Jones et al., 1975

produce short branches (*inlet venules*) that pass through the limiting plate at the periphery of the lobule. Inlet venules arise perpendicularly from the axial perilobular vein (see Figs. 20–10 and 20–14). The extreme ends of the inlet venules (terminal twigs) lead directly into the sinusoids; these terminal segments lack a muscle coat. In certain species, inlet venules may contain contractile endothelial cells, showing sphincter activity that regulates the portal blood flow into the sinusoids.

The largest intrahepatic branches of the hepatic artery are thick walled. As the arteries branch and form smaller vessels, the muscle coat

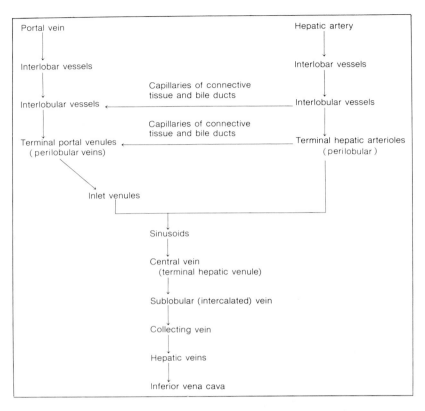

20–14 Overview of hepatic circulation.

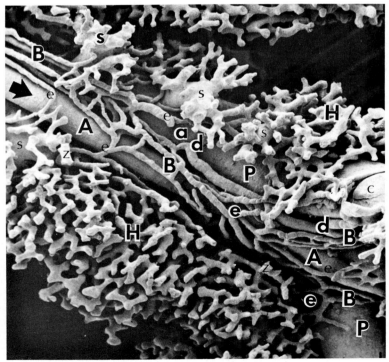

20–15 Methyl methacrylate casts of a small peribiliary plexus and its connecting vessels from a crab-eating monkey are shown after dissection in the scanning electron micrograph. This and similar preparations clearly demonstrate that the afferent vessels supplying the peribiliary blood vascular plexus come from the hepatic artery. In contrast to human beings and rats, in this species the efferent vessels draining the peribiliary plexus empty directly into the hepatic sinusoids. **A,** hepatic artery branch; **B,** peribiliary plexus; **H,** hepatic sinusoids; **P,** portal vein branch; **a,** afferent vessels of the peribiliary plexus; **c,** cut edges of the portal vein; **d,** collateral branches of the hepatic artery; **e,** efferent vessels of the peribiliary plexus; **s,** side branches of the portal vein; **arrow** is directed distally. Approximately × 121. (From Murakami, T., Itoshima, T., and Shimada, Y. 1974. Arch. Histol. Jpn. 37:245.)

is reduced. Terminal branches contain only endothelium surrounded by a thin adventitia. Most of the blood within the hepatic arteries is distributed to the stroma, extrahepatic bile ducts, and gallbladder, so that only a very small volume enters the sinusoids directly. Blood from terminal branches of the hepatic artery usually enters the peribiliary or periductal capillary plexus within the portal canals. Small bile ducts are surrounded by one subepithelial capillary plexus, whereas larger bile ducts have a subepithelial and a submucosal plexus. These plexi, in turn, are usually drained by small branches of the portal vein. As a result, most arterial blood reaches the hepatic sinusoids via an indirect route (see Figs. 20–2, 20–15, and 20–16 for additional details).

The sinusoids, forming the rich intralobular vascular network, anastomose and converge toward the central vein. They differ from conventional capillaries in several aspects: they are larger and more variable in caliber (9–12 μm wide), their cell boundaries do not blacken with silver nitrate, and many of their cells are phagocytic. The sinusoid contains two types of cells: typical, flattened endothelial cells; and large, fixed macrophages, or Kupffer cells. The endothelial cell contains a small compact nucleus, many micropinocytotic vesicles, small mitochondria, and only scattered short profiles of rough ER. The stellate-shaped Kupffer cells occur at various points along the sinusoidal lumen (Figs. 20–13, 20–17, and 20–18). They contain larger, oval nuclei, more mitochondria, and more rough ER than the endothelial cells. They are active phagocytes. Their cytoplasm usually contains phagocytic vacuoles with amorphous debris, engulfed blood cells, or iron, or all three.

20–16 Terminal branches of the hepatic artery in the rat. Arterioles **(HA)** and terminal arterioles **(ha)** give rise to capillaries **(c)**, which surround bile ducts **(BD)**. Capillaries arising from arterioles **(pc)** have well-developed sphincters. The periductal capillaries terminate by joining portal veins or sinusoids **(s)**, or both. A few capillaries join larger interlobular veins **(PV)**, and some join terminal distributing veins **(pv)**. Endothelial cell nuclei **(EN)** are usually located at or near the junctions of capillaries with other vessels. Sinusoids arising from capillaries are identical in structure to those arising from portal veins. At the periphery of the lobule all sinusoids resemble capillaries, having a complete basement membrane **(BM)** and unfenestrated endothelium. A short distance into the parenchyma they lose their basement membrane, become fenestrated, and are true sinusoids. There are numerous lymphatic vessels **(L)** and unmyelinated nerves **(N, n)** in the portal tissue. The nerves supply the smooth muscle of arterioles and precapillary sphincters. Occasionally small nerve fibers **(n)** are found in close relation to endothelial cells. (From Burkel, W. E. 1970. Anat. Rec. 167:333.)

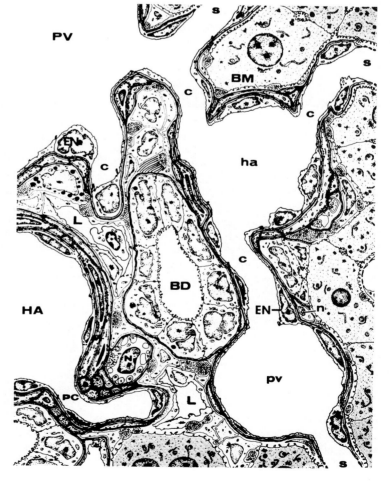

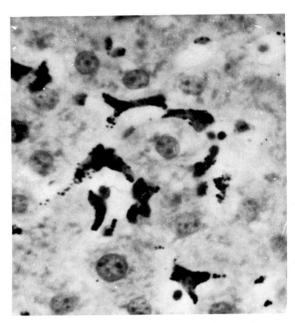

20–17 Kupffer cells within the sinusoid linings are phagocytic and belong to the reticuloendothelial system. They stand out as dark bodies in this photomicrograph because they have ingested carbon particles from the India ink that was injected intravenously before the animal was sacrificed. Rat liver India ink vascular injection. Formol. H&E. × 700.

The perisinusoidal space of Disse, surrounding the sinusoid wall, lies between the sinusoids and the parenchymal cells. Numerous parenchymal cell microvilli project into this space. Bundles of collagen can be seen in this region, but never in the abundance suggested by reticular fiber stains at the light microscopic level (Fig. 20–19). Fat-laden lipocytes are found occasionally. Their function is not understood, although they have been implicated in vitamin A storage and the production of fibroblasts. Although hematopoietic cells are numerous in this region during fetal life, they are seldom seen in the adult except during chronic anemia.

The structure of the sinusoids is important for understanding how materials are exchanged between the blood and hepatic cells. It is thought that in most mammals the sinusoid wall and the cells and fibers within the perisinusoidal space of Disse pose no significant morphological barrier between the fluid phase of blood and the parenchymal cells. This assumption is based on the following observations: (1) Gaps may be present between the attenuated processes of adjacent endothelial cells; (2) small fenestrae in the endothelial cells of most mammals (except ruminants) contain no diaphragm (see Figs. 20–13 and 20–18 to 20–20); (3) the sinusoid endothelium of most mammals (except ruminants) does not have a continuous basal lamina; and (4) the cells and reticular fibers in the perisinusoidal space do not form a continuous boundary. Because the fluid phase bathes the microvilli projecting into the space of Disse, this region may be a site for exchange of materials between the fluid and the parenchymal cells.

Blood leaves the lobule via the central vein, or *terminal hepatic venule* that runs longitudinally through the middle of the lobule in the so-called central space. Central veins are lined by a simple endothelium covered by an external adventitia composed of a few spirally arranged connective tissue fibers. They are larger than sinusoids (45 μm in diameter), they travel alone, and their extremely thin walls contain numerous pores that communicate directly with the sinusoids. Several sinusoids can be seen opening into the central vein in Fig. 20–5. Note that there is no limiting plate of parenchymal cells as there is around the portal canal. At the periphery of the lobule, the central vein connects at right angles with *sublobular* or *intercalated veins*. These vessels are larger than central veins (90–200 μm in diameter), lined by endothelium, and surrounded by a distinct inner circular and outer longitudinal layer of connective tissue fibers. Elastic fibers are numerous and arranged irregularly in nets throughout the walls. These veins run along the base of the lobules and enter the stromal trabeculae where they follow a solitary, isolated course, unaccompanied by other blood vessels or ducts. Several sublobular veins join to form larger collecting veins, which subsequently join to form the *hepatic veins* (Fig. 20–21).

The hepatic veins lack valves and have numerous anastomoses among their branches. The larger branches have a moderately well-developed tunica media and vasa vasorum. They usually travel alone and are surrounded by considerable amounts of connective tissue. Hepatic veins eventually join the *inferior vena cava*.

Lymphatics, Tissue Space of Mall, and the Perisinusoidal Space of Disse

The liver's capsule and stroma contain numerous lymphatic vessels. Just beneath the capsule, *superficial lymphatic vessels* form loose plexuses that connect at intervals with the *deep lym-*

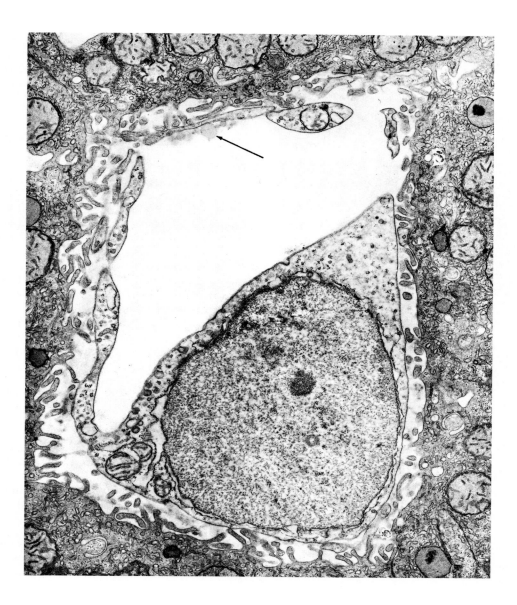

phatic vessels within the portal canals (Fig. 20–22). Lymphatic capillary plexuses, coursing within the connective tissue trabeculae, follow and surround branches of the portal vein, hepatic artery, and bile duct to their finest ramifications at the edge of the lobules. Because lymphatic capillaries have not been found between parenchymal cells, the origin and transport of liver lymph have been the subject of extensive investigation and controversy. The most widely accepted theory at present contends that the perisinusoidal space of Disse is the primary site for formation of liver lymph. From there, the fluid enters the *periportal tissue space of Mall*,

20–18 Rat liver sinusoid. Note the large Kupffer cell filling half of the lumen and the discontinuity of the sinusoidal lining. A chylomicron is observed within the vascular space **(arrow).** Approximately × 10,000.

which lies between the portal connective tissue and the limiting plate (see Fig. 20–2). Subsequently, the fluid diffuses from the space of Mall through the connective tissue and is collected by the lymphatic capillaries within the portal canal. Lymph is then conveyed by progressively larger lymphatic vessels to the collecting vessels that leave the liver at the hilus. On leaving the hilus,

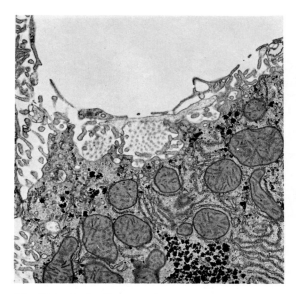

20–19 Reticular fibers can be seen in this electron micrograph within the perisinusoidal space of Disse between a sinusoid and the vascular surface of a rat hepatocyte. Small bundles of reticular fibers presumably serve as cables supporting the liver parenchyma. × 6,165.

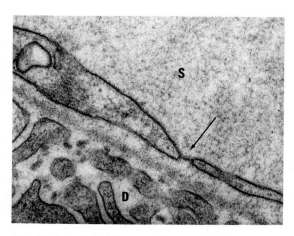

20–20 Endothelial lining of the sinusoid from sheep liver. Note the diaphragm covering one fenestra **(arrow)** and basal lamina. **S,** sinusoidal space; **D,** space of Disse. (From Grubb, D. J., and Jones, A. L. 1971. Anat. Rec. 170:75).

approximately 80% of the liver lymph flows into hilar lymph channels and then to the thoracic duct. The remaining lymph presumably originates directly from blood in the large branches of the hepatic veins. These vessels are surrounded by small networks of lymphatics, and their vasa vasorum often contains lymph vessels. Lymph formed in these vessels leaves the liver and enters retrosternal collecting lymphatics that ascend to the neck along the internal thoracic artery.

Nerves

In humans, nerves enter at the hilus. The fibers are mainly unmyelinated and from the autonomic nervous system. A few bundles of unmyelinated fibers and parasympathetic ganglion cells are found in the larger portal canals, gallbladder,

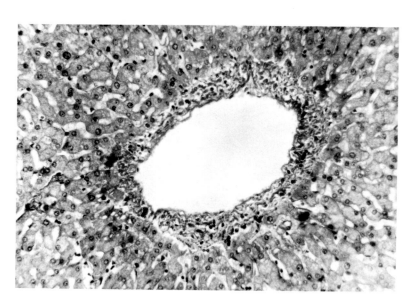

20–21 A branch of the hepatic vein is shown surrounded by a considerable amount of connective tissue. These vessels usually travel alone. Human liver. Zenker formol in H&E.

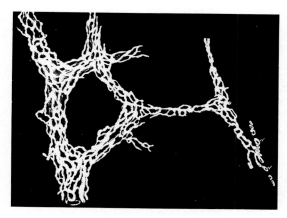

20–22 Network of lymphatic vessels. The vessels, shown in white, surround branches of the portal vein (to the left), connecting with superficial lymphatics in Glisson's capsule (to the right). × 25. (Courtesy of Teichmann.)

and capsule. Parasympathetic innervation of the liver comes from preganglionic fibers in the dorsal efferent nucleus of the vagus. Sympathetic innervation is derived from preganglionic fibers (with cells originating in T_5 to T_9 of the thoracic cord), which synapse in the celiac ganglion. Postganglionic sympathetic fibers from cells in the celiac ganglion are distributed to the hepatic arteries within the liver and the smooth muscle of the gallbladder. The arteries are thought to be innervated by sympathetic fibers only, whereas the bile ducts are innervated by sympathetic and parasympathetic fibers. Some fibers follow the vessels and ducts into the smallest portal canals. The principal influence of the nervous system is thought to be exerted on the blood and biliary vessels. However, unmyelinated nerve fibers have been observed within the perisinusoidal space in human and nonhuman primate livers (Ito and Shibashaki, 1968; Forssman and Ito, 1977). Forssman and Ito found nerve endings on hepatocytes and categorized them as efferent adrenergic nerves.

Ultrastructural and Functional Aspects of the Parenchymal Cells

Endoplasmic Reticulum and Golgi Complex

Structure. Unlike most cells, both smooth and rough ER are well developed in hepatic parenchymal cells, although their relative quanti-

ties, precise postion, and arrangement vary from cell to cell and may be significantly altered during different physiological and experimental conditions. In addition to the membrane-bound ribosomes of the rough ER, the liver cell contains many free ribosomes and polyribosomes that fluctuate in response to various conditions (see Fig. 20–23).

The rough ER usually forms aggregates of parallel, flattened cisternae scattered randomly throughout the cytoplasm. They correspond to the *basophilic bodies*, or *ergastoplasm*, seen in specially stained histological sections (Figs. 20–23 and 20–24). In the rat, the surface area of the rough and smooth membranes is equal in cells surrounding the central vein but in the peripheral and midzonal cells, the rough ER has approximately 50% more surface area than the smooth (Loud, 1968) (see Table 20–2).

The smooth ER is composed of a complex meshwork of twisting, branching, and anastomosing tubules that frequently communicate with the rough ER and Golgi apparatus but never with the nuclear envelope. These tubules follow a highly tortuous course and often exhibit variations in caliber. Smooth ER in the liver often shows local specializations and almost invariably is associated with *glycogen*, although the functional significance of this relationship is unclear. In the rat, the surface area of the smooth ER is significantly higher in central (21,600 μm^2 per cell) and midzonal (16,900 μm^2 per cell) cells than in the peripheral cells (15,700 μm^2 per cell) of the classic lobule (Loud, 1968).

The Golgi complex consists of three to five closely packed, parallel smooth-surfaced cisternae, a variable number of associated vesicles (large and small), and, occasionally, lysosomal elements (see Fig. 20–23). These structures and the associated cytosol constitute up to 5% of the parenchymal cells in the periportal zones and approximately 2% in the centrolobular areas. Claude (1970) speculated that each hepatocyte may contain as many as 50 such complexes; however, they may be interrelated, representing a single complex with multiple branching. Early in fetal life, the Golgi complex is paranuclear but migrates into the peribiliary cytoplasm early in the second trimester when bile secretion begins (Koga, 1971). In the rat, Jones et al. have found significantly more Golgi area in the periportal cells. The fine structure of the Golgi complex is similar, but not identical, to that in other cell types. The bulbous ends of the cisternae and their associated large vesicles are often filled

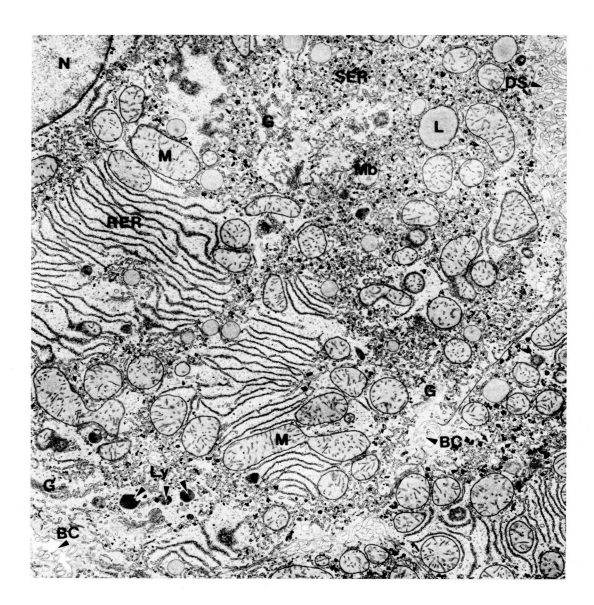

20–23 A transmission electron micrograph showing portions of three rat liver parenchymal cells (hepatocytes) demonstrating the appearance and relationships of organelles and inclusions. **N,** nucleus; **M,** mitochondria; **G,** Golgi; **L,** lipid; **Mb,** microbodies; **Ly,** lysosomes; **SER,** smooth surfaced endoplasmic reticulum; **RER,** rough surfaced endoplasmic reticulum; **BC,** bile canaliculi; **DS,** space of Disse. Approximately × 10,000. (From Jones, A. L. and Schmucker, D. L. 1977. Gastroenterology 73:833–851.)

with electron-dense particles, 250 to 800 Å in diameter. These particles are thought to be the triglyceride-rich *very low density lipoproteins* (VLDL), which play an important role in the transport of lipids within the plasma (Jones et al., 1967; Hamilton et al., 1967; Mahley et al., 1969).

Function. The liver microsomal fraction (ER) is known to participate in (1) the synthesis of albumin, fibrinogen, and other plasma proteins; (2) the synthesis of cholesterol for export and bile-salt formation; (3) glucuronide conjugation of

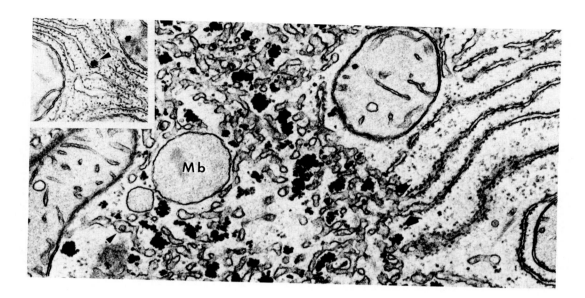

bilirubin, drugs, and steroids; (4) metabolism of drugs and steroids; (5) esterification of free fatty acids to triglycerides; (6) the breakdown of glycogen; and (7) deiodination of T_4 to T_3.

Most studies of protein synthesis for export (for example, albumin and other plasma proteins) show that protein synthesis is a function of the rough ER. The product is thought to leave the rough ER and migrate via the smooth ER to the Golgi complex and finally to the cell's vascular surface for release. However, a study by Lin and Chang (1975) does not support this theory. Instead, these investigators observed that albumin molecules, synthesized on polysomes bound to the rough ER and nuclear envelope, were discharged into the cytosol, and then into the extracellular spaces.

Cholesterol biosynthesis seems to be a function of the smooth ER. Evidence for this function came from the discovery that after phenobarbital was administerd and smooth ER hypertrophied, liver cells were four times more active in cholesterol biosynthesis than cells in control livers (Jones and Armstrong, 1965) (Fig. 20–25).

Most lipid-soluble drugs and steroids are metabolized by the liver microsomal fraction. The microsomal *mixed-function oxidase system*, a chain of enzymes such as NADPH cytochrome *c* reductase and cytochrome P_{450}, is thought to perform these functions. Although there is evidence that this functional chain occurs in both categories of ER, the principal activity of the chain probably resides in the membranes of the smooth

20–24 The continuity between rough and smooth surfaced endoplasmic reticulum membranes is shown in this micrograph **(large arrows)**. Note the association between the large **(Mb)** and small microbody **(arrowhead)** and the association of glycogen with the SER. **Inset:** A very low density lipoprotein (VLDL) is seen forming within the cisternae of the smooth surfaced endoplasmic reticulum **(arrowhead)**. Approximately × 45,000. (From Jones, A. L., and Schmucker, D. L. 1977. Gastroenterology 73:833–851.)

ER (Jones and Fawcett, 1966). Most lipid-soluble compounds with diverse chemical structure (for example, phenobarbital as against DDT) are metabolized by the microsomes and also promote a marked hypertrophy of the smooth ER and many of its enzymes. This adaptive response enables the liver to metabolize more effectively the inducing substances and is obviously valuable in the detoxification of drugs, certain carcinogens, and insecticides. Progesterone and certain anabolic steroids are also inducers of liver smooth ER, its associated cytochrome P_{450}, and the mitochondrial enzyme Δ-aminolevulinic acid synthetase (ALA syn) (Jones and Emans, 1969). Increased ALA syn activity results in increased heme production and stimulates the formation of cytochrome P_{450} (Fig. 20–26). Interference with the terminal steps of heme synthesis produces an abnormal accumulation of porphyrin and the clinical condition of porphyria (Marver and Schmid, 1972). As a result, it is currently as-

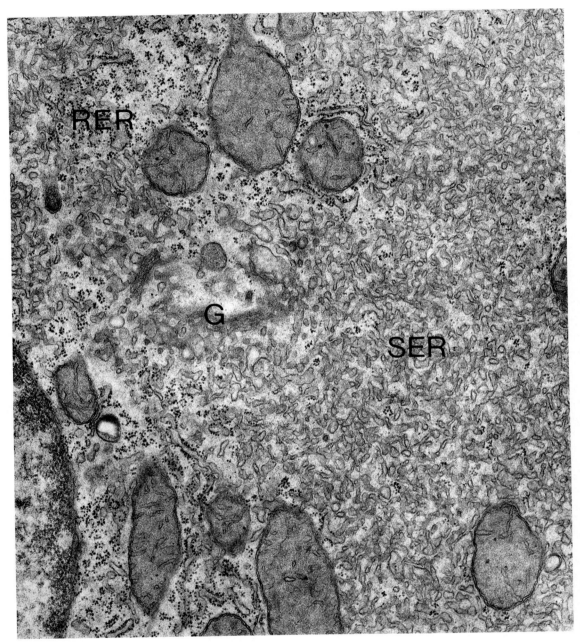

20–25 Liver cell from a phenobarbital-treated animal showing an extraordinary hypertrophy of the smooth-surfaced endoplasmic reticulum **(SER).** Because of its abundance, the smooth-membraned elements appear to crowd the profiles of rough-surfaced endoplasmic reticulum **(RER)** into localized areas. The tangential section through the Golgi complex **(G)** shows several areas of communication between this organelle and the SER. Approximately × 40,000. (From Jones, A. L., and Fawcett, D. W. 1966. J. Histochem. Cytochem. 14:215.)

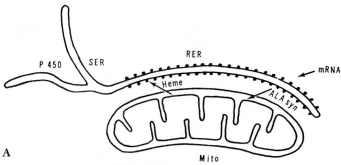

A

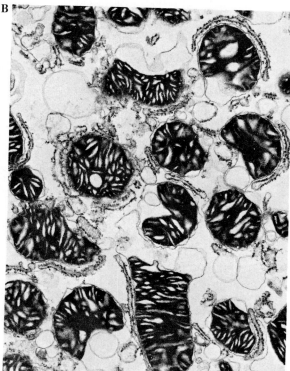

B

20–26 A. The close association of the rough-surfaced reticulum with mitochondria seen in electron micrographs of intact hepatocytes is diagrammatically represented here. This relationship may be necessary for the production of smooth reticulum and cytochromes. Under the influence of messenger RNA **(mRNA)**, the rough-surfaced endoplasmic reticulum **(RER)** synthesizes the enzyme Δ-aminolevulinic acid synthetase **(ALA syn)**, which is transferred to the mitochondria. This results in an increased production of heme. Some heme is transferred back to the endoplasmic reticulum and utilized for the production of the microsomal heme protein P450. (From Jones, A. L., and Emans, J. B. 1969. *In* H. A. Salhanick, D. Kipnes, and R. L. Van de Wiele (eds.), Metabolic Effects of Gonadal Hormones and Contraceptive Steroids. New York: Plenum Press, Plenum Publishing Corporation.) **B.** Using special techniques, it is now possible to isolate a mitochondrial-RER complex from liver homogenates. Early studies indicate that this may be a functional unit essential for microsomal hemoprotein synthesis. Approximately × 20,000. (Courtesy of U. A. Meyer, P. J. Meier, and M. A. Spycker.)

sumed that sex steroids in some way influence the normal quantities of smooth ER and hence certain functional activities within the liver cells. The induction of liver ER and its subsequent effect on porphyrin and drug metabolism should be considered by the physician when administering gonadal hormones for contraceptive purposes.

Deliberate induction of microsomal enzymes, to increase glucuronyl transferase activity, has been found beneficial in certain cases of hyperbilirubinemia. However, inducing liver microsomal enzymes is *not* always beneficial. First, the ER induction following the initial exposure to an inducing compound can alter the individual's subsequent response to the same or another therapeutic agent: the additional enzymes may metabolize a drug at a new rate. Second, some compounds metabolized by the ER are more dangerous than the parent compound. One example is 3,4-benzpyrene, a relatively innocuous component of cigarette smoke, which on hydroxylation becomes a potent carcinogen. Another example is carbon tetrachloride: The centrolobular necrosis associated with carbon tetrachloride poisoning is not caused by the parent compound but by a free radical formed during its metabolism.

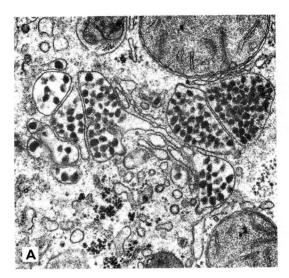
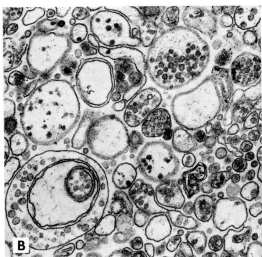

20–27 Electron micrographs of very low-density lipoprotein particles within the Golgi complex of an intact liver cell **(A)** and within the membranes of the isolated Golgi-rich fraction **(B)** of rat liver. The lipoprotein particles can be further isolated from the Golgi membranes for analysis. Approximately × 25,000. (Courtesy of R. L. Hamilton.)

Fat metabolism is another important liver function associated with the ER. In the parenchymal cell, free fatty acids not used for energy or membrane synthesis are reesterified into triglycerides. A small amount of triglyceride is stored in cytoplasmic fat droplets and the rest is released into the blood as VLDL (Figs. 20–27 and 20–28). The VLDL particle is a lipid–protein complex. Its triglyceride, or fatty core, is encompassed by a surface apoprotein and a mixture of cholesterol and phospholipid. Presumably, the particle is synthesized in the ER, the smooth ER forming the lipid and the rough ER synthesizing the protein. The mechanism of complexing the two components is not understood (see Fig. 20–24).

After synthesis, the lipoprotein is transferred through the smooth ER and is released from the cells. This appears to be accomplished in two ways: (1) smooth vesicles containing lipoproteins may bud off the smooth ER, migrate to the surface, and be released by exocytosis, or (2) the lipoproteins within the smooth ER may be sequestered in Golgi vesicles, which in turn are released at the cell surface in a packet (see Figs. 20–27 and 20–28). This latter mode of transport

is similar to that used by the pancreatic acinar cells for protein secretion. The recent intracellular localization of sugar nucleotide glycoprotein glycosyltransferases in Golgi-rich fractions from liver strongly suggests that the Golgi complex may be involved generally in producing glycoproteins and in adding a carbohydrate component to the lipoprotein (see Fig. 20–28). Recently Novikoff and Yam (1978) noted that a population of Golgi secretory vesicles containing nascent VLDL particles reacted positively for acid phosphatase. These observations suggested that certain secretory vesicles undergo a catabolic transition to secondary lysosomes (Fig. 20–28).

Membrane Synthesis and Turnover. A number of important relationships between the subcellular structure and function of hepatic ER have been derived from the elegant studies of fetal and newborn rat livers by Dallner and his colleagues (1966). Three days before delivery, glycogen markedly increases in the parenchymal cells. Although parenchymal cell rough ER is essentially fully developed, the activity of certain microsomal enzymes (for example, mixed-function oxidases and glucose-6-phosphatase) is nearly unmeasurable. Furthermore, there is little or no smooth ER in these cells. After birth, glycogen falls and smooth ER increases in the cells, while the activity of the enzymes mentioned above begins to rise (although not at the same rate for all enzymes) and the liver acquires the ability to metabolize certain drugs.

After ER is formed within the hepatocyte, the

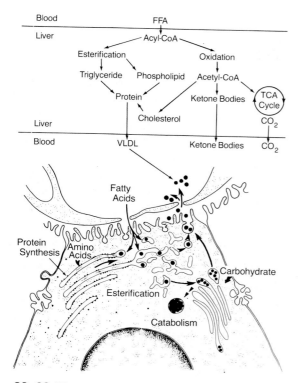

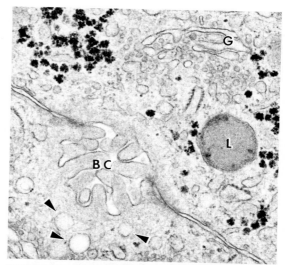

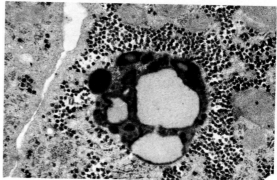

20–28 Diagrammatic representation of the possible steps in lipoprotein production and release. (Modified from Jones, A. L., Ruderman, N. B., and Herrera, M. G. 1967. J. Lipid Res. 8:429.)

ER membranes undergo constant renewal or turnover. The half-life of adult liver ER has been calculated to be 2 to 2.5 days (Schimke et al., 1968). It is becoming clear, however, that not all components within these membranes turn over at the same rate. Moreover, studies of lipoprotein synthesis show that lipoproteins can be synthesized and transported out of the liver cell within 5 min. Because each particle or packet of particles is surrounded by a portion of smooth ER or Golgi membrane, or both, which accompanies the particle to the plasmalemma, it appears likely that membrane turnover might take minutes rather than days or hours, as previously thought.

Lysosomes

Structure. Liver parenchymal cells contain many lysosomes (Fig. 20–29). They can be found almost invariably within the cytoplasm bordering each bile canaliculus and Golgi complex. Ly-

20–29 Normal human liver. **(top)** A characteristic lysosome **(L)** is found near the bile canaliculus **(BC).** Note the vesicles in the pericanalicular cytoplasm **(arrowheads).** In the rat, similar vesicles have been found to carry IgA and insulin destined for secretion into the biliary space. **G,** Golgi. Approximately × 20,000. **(bottom)** This membrane-bounded structure in a human hepatocyte is a lipofuscin pigment granule. These pigment deposits are thought to be undigestible residues of lysosomal activity and are common in livers from older humans and animals. (Bottom micrograph courtesy of H. I. Friedman.)

sosomes in these sites correspond to the so-called peribiliary dense bodies described by early histologists. These highly pleomorphic organelles vary in size, number, and position during different conditions. Because no two lysosomes look alike, their positive identification in electron micrographs requires that the intracellular particle be bounded by a single membrane and exhibit a positive staining reaction for acid phosphatase. Their contents may be homogenous, heterogeneous, dense, or finely granular and may include myelin figures, pigment, intact or partially digested organelles, or inclusions, or all four. Cytochemistry can be used to identify the Golgi cisternae from an adjacent specialized region of smooth ER that is rich in acid phosphatase. The acronym GERL (Golgi, Endoplasmic Reticulum, Lysosomes) has been given to this region in the Golgi complex because it seems to be important in producing various types of lysosomes (Novikoff, 1976).

Function. Lysosomes perform a number of digestive and lytic functions for the parenchymal cells. Under normal conditions, they catabolize certain unwanted exogenous substances, effete organelles, and inclusions. The last two processes are especially important for maintaining and rejuvenating the parenchymal cells, since some products of digestion may be utilized by the cells for energy and repair. Loss of liver mass and the presence of increased numbers of lysosomes in livers of starved animals are associated with the mobilization and release of stored energy-producing substances needed to maintain the entire body. Hepatic lysosomes also seem to participate in the storage of iron. They normally contain ferritin-like substances and accumulate large quantities of them in iron-storage diseases, for example, hemochromatosis and hemosiderosis.

There is now considerable evidence that lysosomes have an important role in cellular pathology. Hepatic lysosomes increase in viral hepatitis, cholestasis, and cell injury following anoxia. The livers of children with type 2 glycogenosis (Pompe's disease) lack the enzyme α-glucosidase and contain large glycogen deposits within their lysosomes (see Weissman, 1969, for review).

Microbodies (Peroxisomes)

Structure. The microbody is a single membrane-bounded particle (approximately 0.2–1 μm in diameter) with a fine granular matrix. Each parenchymal cell has approximately 200 microbodies, or one microbody per four mitochondria. They vary greatly in size within the same cell, but there appears to be no difference in enzymatic composition between small and large microbodies having the same structure. He-

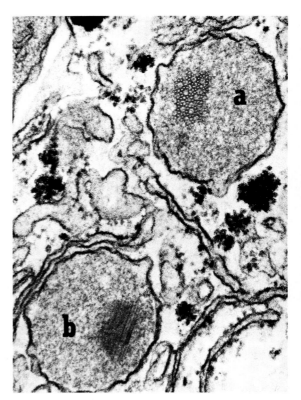

20–30 Microbodies. In the rat, these single-membrane-bounded structures contain a crystalloid enmeshed in a homogenous matrix. Both a cross section **(a)** and longitudinal section **(b)** of the crystalloid are observed in this micrograph. (See text.) Approximately × 100,000.

patic microbodies in many mammals contain a crystalloid, laminated core or nucleoid, which distinguishes them from the denser peribiliary bodies, the lysosomes. The structure of the core varies greatly from species to species. In the rat, it is made up of tubules of two different sizes: small ones, approximately 45 Å in diameter, and large ones, 95 to 115 Å in diameter (see Figs. 20–24 and 20–30). The two types of tubules, in longitudinal section, produce the laminated appearance of the crystalloid. The core is thought to contain urate oxidase whereas catalase and D-amino acid oxidase presumably are present in the matrix. The livers of uricotelic animals, anthropoid primates, and human beings usually contain anucleoid microbodies deficient in urate oxidase. In some species, the liver contains a mixture of nucleoid and anucleoid microbodies.

Function. The physiological significance of hepatic microbodies is not known, although it is speculated that they may participate in any one or all of the following: disposal of hydrogen peroxide; metabolism of purines, lipids, and alcohols; oxidation of reduced NAD; and gluconeogenesis. Recently Lazarow (1978) presented data indicating that rat liver peroxisomes were specialized for the β-oxidation of long-chain fatty acids.

Hepatic microbodies proliferate during embryological development and early postnatal life, during recovery from partial hepatectomy, and after the administration of salicylates and the lipid-lowering agent ethyl-α-p-chlorophenoxyisobutyrate (CPIB, or clofibrate).

Mitochondria

Parenchymal cells contain numerous well-developed mitochondria (approximately 800 per cell) (see Fig. 20–23). In rat and human livers the mitochondria are usually round or oblong (for example, 0.5–1.5 μm in diameter, 1.5–4.5 μm in length) and appear to be randomly distributed throughout the cytoplasm. However, there is good evidence that the number, size, shape, and enzymatic properties of liver mitochondria are related to the position of the cell within the lobule (Novikoff and Essner, 1960; Loud, 1968).

Liver mitochondria are thought to be self-replicating bodies with a half-life of about 10.5 days. The presence of mitochondria within lysosomes has fostered the idea that the lysosomes destroy effete mitochondria. The speed with which the mitochondria are thought to turn over, in comparison with the life-span of the cell, presumably accounts for the presence of a few atypical or abnormal mitochondria in otherwise healthy cells. The genesis of the liver mitochondrion, however, is still subject to conjecture. Budding or dividing mitochondria are not readily found in normal liver, but they are commonplace during recovery from simple riboflavin (Tandler et al., 1969) or dietary iron (Dallman and Goodman, 1971) deficiency. The giant mitochondria formed during the course of these diseases are restored to normal dimensions by means of division after replacement therapy has begun.

Intramitochondrial inclusions have been described in hepatic mitochondria in a number of human diseases; however, their significance remains obscure.

Aging

Although very little is known about the structural changes with aging in human liver, several studies indicate that aging leads to significant structural alterations in rat liver. In this species, the number of hepatocytes per unit volume of tissue decreases with age whereas the cell size and incidence of polyploidy increase (Wheatley, 1972).

Previous investigators have also suggested that the number of mitochondria and microbodies changes with age, but recent quantitative studies do not support this idea. Instead, these investigations show that lysosomes increase and smooth ER decreases with age in rat liver (Schmucker et al., 1978). Smooth ER membrane, however, may suffer from age-related changes, because the animal's microsomal drug-metabolizing capabilities per mg of protein decrease with age. The accumulation of nondigestible materials such as lipofuscin pigment in lysosomes or residual bodies of otherwise healthy liver cells occurs even in young animals, but the number of lysosomes with residue increases as the individual ages.

The Biliary Space

Bile Canaliculi

The bile canaliculi are the smallest biliary spaces, ranging from 0.5 to 1.5 μm in diameter. They are usually centrally located between adjacent parenchymal cells (see Figs. 20–2, 20–11, 20–13, 20–29, 20–31, and 20–36). Microvilli of the parenchymal cells protrude into the lumen of the canaliculi (see Fig. 20–29A), and fine actin-containing cytoplasmic filaments circumscribe the area beneath the canaliculi. They insert into desmosomes and extend into the core of the microvilli. Histochemical preparations, such as ATPase and alkaline phosphatase stains, have enabled investigators to observe the biliary network clearly with the light microscope. The finding of ATPase activity in this area suggests that bile secretion is an energy-requiring process.

The biliary space is separated from the other intercellular spaces by junctional complexes between the parenchymal cells (Figs. 20–32 and 20–33). Immediately adjacent to the canalicular lumen is a tight junction (Fig. 20–32). Lanthanum injected into the portal vein or retrograde up the common bile duct will not normally

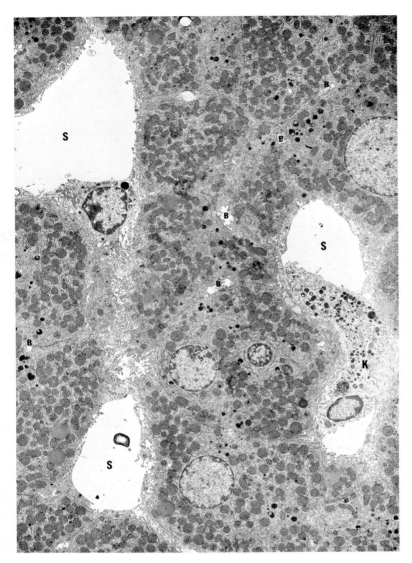

20–31 This low-power electron micrograph of rat liver shows hepatocytes disposed between sinusoids **(S)**, the blood vascular channels within the lobule. Bile canaliculi **(B)** are centrally located between adjacent parenchymal cells. At this magnification one can appreciate the random distribution of the organelles. Golgi complexes, however, are almost always located between the nucleus and bile canaliculus. A large Kupffer cell **(K)** extends across part of a sinusoid. Approximately × 2,520. (From Jones, A. L., and Spring-Mills, E. 1974. Am. J. Drug Alcohol Abuse 1:111; micrograph courtesy of D. L. Schmucker.)

pass across this junction (Matter et al., 1969). Because of this, it is speculated that certain components of bile, such as conjugated bilirubin, may gain access to the intercellular space by this route during times of chronic biliary obstruction. Another cellular attachment near the canaliculus is the nexus or gap junction. The membranes in this junction are parallel to one another with a 20-Å gap, which normally will admit lanthanum. The function of the junction is still not clear; it may provide an electrical communication between cells. The nexus occurs along any part of the plasmalemma between adjacent liver cells. Desmosomes appear near the canaliculi.

Terminal Ductules

Bile flows in the canaliculi to the periphery of the classic lobule and enters small terminal bile ductules or canals of Hering. These canals form short channels that convey bile from the canaliculi through the limiting plate and into the interlobular bile duct of the portal canals.

At first, one or two fusiform-shaped ductular cells share a canalicular lumen with a hepatocyte (Figs. 20–2 and 20–34). Subsequently, they are lined by two to four cells that become cuboidal as the ductule nears the portal canal. The terminal ductules are smaller than the interlobular

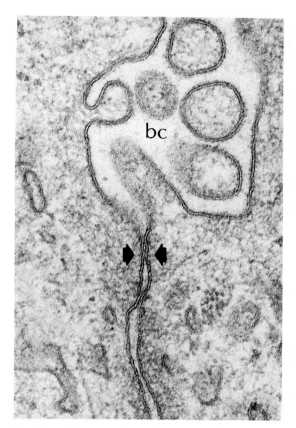

20–32 Tight junction adjacent to a bile canaliculus **(bc)** in rat liver. Note the local merging of the two outer leaflets of the plasma membrane of the parenchymal cells **(arrowheads).** Approximately × 100,000. (Courtesy of D. Friend.)

ducts, having diameters usually less than 15 μm. Many blunt microvilli project from their lumenal borders. The nuclei are elongated and the mitochondria are smaller than those of neighboring hepatocytes. Endoplasmic reticulum is sparse, but the Golgi complex and pinocytotic vesicles are well developed, suggesting that the ductules are metabolically active. A basal lamina completely encompasses the ductules except at the point of contact between the hepatocytes and ductule cells.

The origin of the terminal ductule cell is a matter of debate. Some investigators believe that it is derived from cells of the larger interlobular ducts, whereas others claim it is of parenchymal origin. During chronic extrahepatic cholestasis, the ductule cells proliferate and almost completely replace the liver cells (Steiner et al.,

1962). Wilson believes they are primitive cells capable of differentiating into either parenchymal or bile epithelium. Whatever their source or potentials, the epithelial cells of the terminal ductules are very unusual.

Intrahepatic Bile Ducts

Bile in the terminal ductules empties into *interlobular bile ducts* (30–40 μm in diameter) in the portal canals (see Fig. 20–4). These ducts form a continuous network of passageways whose size increases as they near the porta. They are lined by a single layer of cuboidal or columnar epithelial cells which have microvilli on their lumenal surface (see Figs. 20–35 and 20–36). The epithelium is surrounded by a basal lamina. The basal nuclei are round and contain considerable chromatin often arranged like cartwheel spokes. These cells, like those of the ductules, contain a prominent Golgi complex and vesicles considered to be pinocytotic. Cholesterol crystals have been observed in the cytoplasm. Occasionally, areas of mucus-secreting epithelium surrounded by a vascular plexus have been seen in the larger ducts. The walls of the intrahepatic bile ducts are made up of dense fibrous tissue containing many elastic fibers. Smooth muscle fibers in the walls of the ducts near the hilus of the liver form the morphological basis for the narrowing of the ducts in this location often seen in cholangiograms (Rappaport, 1969).

Extrahepatic Bile Ducts

The extrahepatic ducts are enclosed by tall columnar cells. Their walls possess the same layers as the intestine, that is, mucosa, submucosa, muscularis, and adventitia. Tubular glands containing cells rich in mucopolysaccharides are occasionally noted at regular intervals in the submucosa. The wall of the extrahepatic ducts receives its blood supply from small branches of the hepatic and gastroduodenal arteries.

The *common hepatic duct* is approximately 3 cm long. It arises at the porta from the confluence of the right and left hepatic lobular ducts. It is joined by the *cystic duct* from the gallbladder to form the *common bile duct* (ductus choledochus), which is approximately 7 cm long and empties into the duodenum. Tubular glands containing PAS-positive cells are scattered along the length of the common duct. These glands are more extensive in mammals lacking a gallbladder, such as the rat.

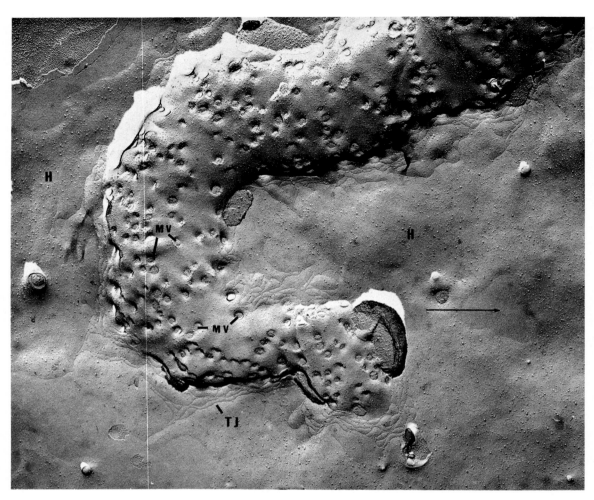

20–33 Electron micrograph of a replica of a frozen-fractured membrane from a hepatocyte **(H)** showing the origin of a bile canaliculus. The tight junctions **(TJ)** appear as anastomosing, thin, linear grooves surrounding the bile canaliculus. The **arrow** points to a gap junction. The large pits or indentations in the surface are bases of the microvilli **(MV)**. (Courtesy of N. Scott McNutt.)

Gallbladder

Located on the undersurface of the right liver lobe and connected to the relatively rigid ducts of the biliary tree is a readily distensible bag: the gallbladder. In humans, it is large enough to hold 30 to 50 ml of bile. The surface of the filled gallbladder is stretched evenly, but in the empty contracted gallbladder it forms numerous elongated, decussating folds or rugae. The wall contains a surface epithelium, lamina propria, muscularis, and a serosa (Fig. 20–37).

The musosa contains an inner layer of simple columnar epithelium. The apex of each cell con-

20–34 Adjacent to a portal canal a junction is seen between a terminal ductule cell and three hepatic parenchymal cells **(arrow)** by both light (upper left figure, × 1,100) and electron microscopy (lower figure, × 8,000). Note the fusiform shape of the ductule cell and its basal lamina. **pv,** portal vein; **c,** capillaries; **bd,** bile duct; **D,** ductule cell. (Courtesy of R. L. Wood). The scanning electron micrograph (upper right figure, approximately × 5,300) shows three bile canaliculi converging to form a canal of Hering. (From Layden, T. J., Schwartz, J., and Boyer, J. L. 1975. Gastroenterology 69:724.)

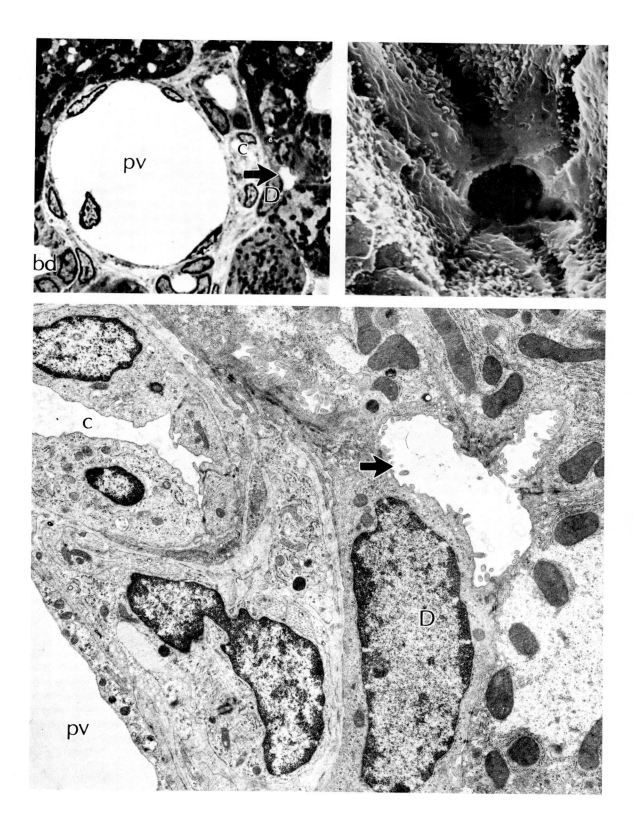

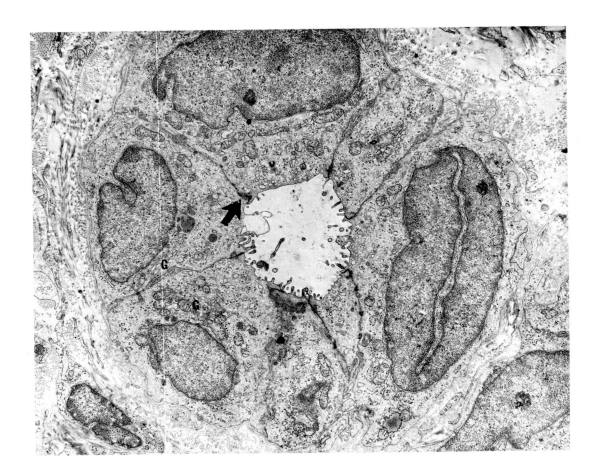

20–35 Small interlobular bile duct. These ducts are encompassed by a thin basal lamina. The cuboidal cells contain few organelles although pinocytotic vesicles are abundant and the Golgi complex **(G)**, when included in the plane of section, is well developed. Note the microvilli on their luminal surface and the apical zones of adhesion **(arrow)**. Approximately × 12,000.

tains numerous microvilli (Fig. 20–38), lateral junctional complexes, and associated tonofilaments. Desmosomes occur at frequent intervals along the entire length of the lateral cell membranes. The Golgi complex is usually supranuclear and well developed. Rough ER and membrane-bounded granular inclusions are especially prominent in humans. Mitochondria are numerous but relatively small.

The lamina propria is rich in blood vessels and connective tissue fibers. The muscularis consists of a number of layers of smooth muscle separated by a fairly extensive network of elastic fibers. The serosal coat is a broad layer of connective tissue containing numerous collagen fibers and the blood vessels and lymphatics that supply the organ. Numerous nerves from the autonomic nervous system can also be noted on the serosal surface. Glands can be found occasionally in the lamina propria of the human gallbladder, especially near the neck. These glands contain goblet cells and a few cells that are identical to the argentaffin cells in the intestine. These so-called mucous glands, sparse in normal tissue, are moderately abundant in people who have had chronic inflammation of the gallbladder. However, it is difficult to tell whether a common pathological factor promotes inflammation and stimulates the development of the glands or whether there is a secondary causal relationship between the development of cholecystitis and the presence of these glands.

Rokitansky-Aschoff crypts, or *diverticula,* are invaginations of the surface epithelium. Some of these crypts, or sinuses, extend through

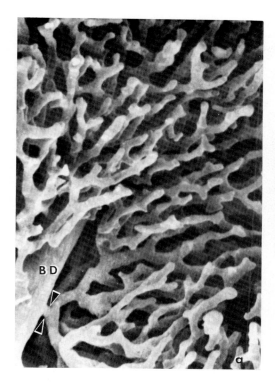

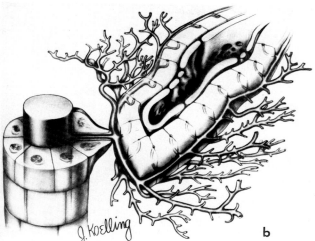

20–36 A. A scanning electron micrograph of a corrosion cast of a branch of the biliary tree demonstrating the interlobular bile ducts within a portal canal **(BD)** and a canal of Hering **(arrowheads)**, as well as an anastomosing network of periportal bile canaliculi. × 330. **B.** A three-dimensional artist's conception of the biliary tree as it is related to bile duct, ductule, and parenchymal cells. (Courtesy of T. Murakami and A. L. Jones.)

the entire width of the muscular layer. They favor bacterial retention and inflammation and are usually regarded as antecedents to pathological changes.

Luschka's bile ducts are seen occasionally in some gallbladders. Serial sections reveal that these bile ducts, located along the hepatic surface of the gallbladder, open directly into the liver. The epithelium has a variable morphology but is generally similar to normal intrahepatic ducts.

The arterial supply of the gallbladder is via the *cystic artery*, which usually arises from the right hepatic artery. At the gallbladder it divides into a superficial branch supplying the free or serosal surface and a deep branch that arborizes throughout the deeper, interior layers of the wall. These branches anastomose freely and may send twigs into the adjacent liver substance. Venous drainage from the gallbladder and cystic duct is via the *cystic vein*, which ends in the right branch of the portal vein. Occasionally, some small venous branches may pass directly into the hepatic parenchyma and join the sinusoids. The lymph vessels of the gallbladder are reportedly intimately connected with lymph vessels of Glisson's capsule.

The neck of the gallbladder is continuous with the *cystic duct*. This duct retains all the layers of the wall of the gallbladder, is about 4 cm long, and joins the common hepatic duct. Its mucous membrane is thrown into a series of folds arranged in a spiral fashion around the tube (spiral valve) (Fig. 20–39). Many nerve cells are found in the fibromuscular layer of the cystic duct.

Choledochoduodenal Junction

The junction of the common bile duct, pancreatic duct, and the duodenum is an anatomic area of medical and physiological importance. It regulates the flow of bile and pancreatic enzymes into the duodenum and governs the filling of the gallbladder. Occlusion of the choledochoduodenal junction by small gallstones or tumors results in cholestasis (and various sequelae).

In the human embryo, the ventral pancreatic and common bile duct arise from the hepatic diverticulum of the foregut. In the adult, the associated bile and pancreatic ducts pass obliquely through an opening in the circular musculature of the duodenum. The ducts empty their contents into a duodenal ampulla, the *ampulla of*

742

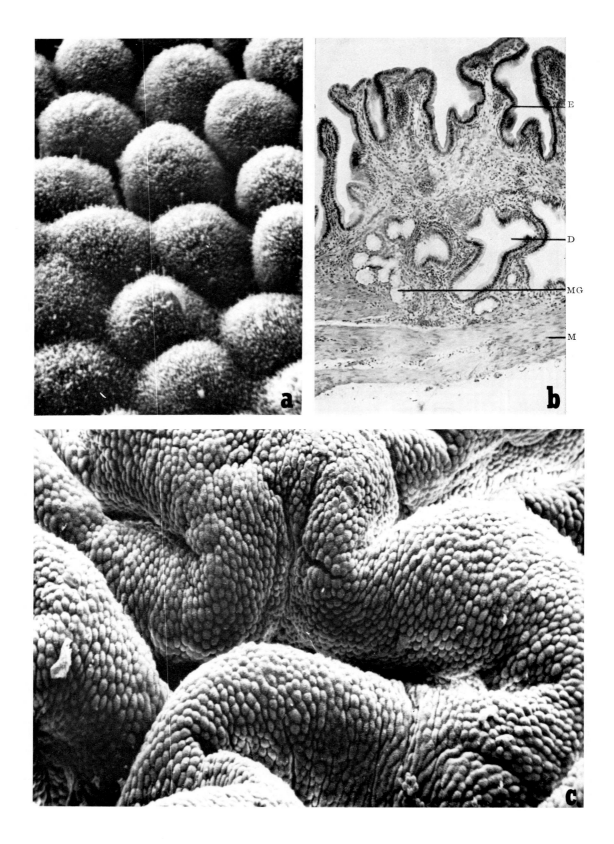

20–37 Contracted gallbladder. Parts **a** (× 3000) and
c (× 350) are scanning electron micrographs
of the inner surface of guinea pig gallbladder. Part **c**
shows the pronounced folding of the gallbladder
mucosa. In **a** the bulging individual epithelial cells
are covered with bristlelike microvilli. Compare with
Fig. 19–38. Part **b** (× 90) is a light micrograph of
contracted human gallbladder. Note the diverticula **(D)**
into the wall and the mucous gland **(MG).** The
muscularis **(M)** is present but the serosa has been
stripped off. Fixed in Zenker's fluid; H&E. (a and c
from Mueller, J. C., and Jones, A. L., and Long, L. A.
1972. Gastroenterology 62.)

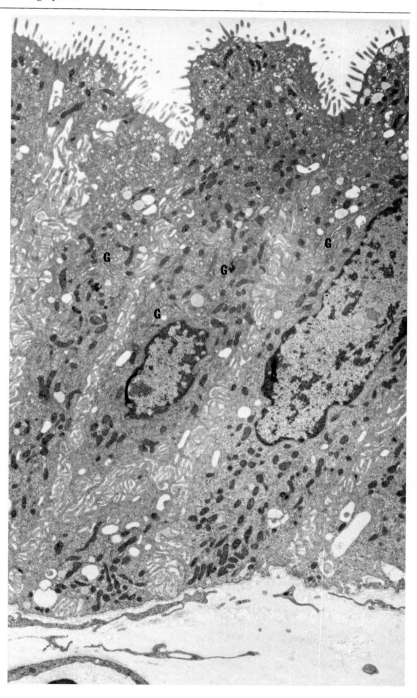

20–38 Epithelial cells from a
normal guinea pig
gallbladder. Note the long
microvilli and the characteristic
bulging of the apical region of
the cell into the gallbladder
lumen. The Golgi **(G)** apparatus
is supranuclear, and the small
mitochondria are distributed at
random in the cytoplasm.
Numerous pinocytotic vesicles
and larger PAS-positive
granules are in the apical
cytoplasm. The lateral cell
borders are markedly
interdigitated, and a basal
lamina encompasses the basal
region of the cells. × 7000.
(From Mueller, J. C., Jones,
A. L., and Long, L. A. 1972.
Gastroenterology 62.)

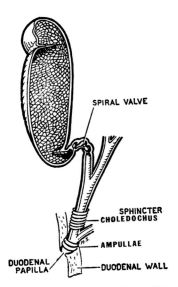

SPIRAL VALVE

SPHINCTER CHOLEDOCHUS

AMPULLAE

DUODENAL PAPILLA

DUODENAL WALL

20-39 The mucous membrane of the gallbladder and extrahepatic bile passages. The two sphincters are shown diagrammatically. (From Grant's Method of Anatomy. 1965. Baltimore: The Williams & Wilkins Co.)

Vater. The bile and pancreatic enzymes pass through the orifice in the ampulla into the lumen of the duodenum (Fig. 20–39).

During passage through the intestinal wall, the associated bile and pancreatic ducts are invested by a common musculus proprius, termed the *sphincter of Oddi.* This structure varies greatly among individuals but usually contains four subdivisions: (1) the *sphincter choledochus,* a strong annular sheath surrounding the common bile duct before its junction with the pancreatic duct; (2) the *fasciculi longitudinales,* consisting of longitudinal muscle bundles that span the intervals between the two ducts from the margins of the fenestrae to the ampulla; (3) the *sphincter ampullae,* or terminal musculature surrounding the ampulla of Vater; and (4) the *sphincter pancreaticus,* surrounding the intraduodenal segment of the pancreatic duct, before its junction with the ampulla.

Contraction of the sphincter choledochus prevents the flow of bile, whereas contraction of the fasciculi longitudinales shortens the ducts and facilitates the flow of bile into the duodenum. When both the pancreatic and common bile duct end in the ampulla, contraction of the sphincter ampullae may promote reflux of bile into the pancreatic duct, which, in turn, may result in pancreatitis.

Bile Production and Transport

The bile is an aqueous solution containing various organic and inorganic solutes. Bile salts, phospholipid, cholesterol, and bile pigments are the major organic solutes. Lecithin, the chief phospholipid, and cholesterol are insoluble in water but remain in solution even when the bile is concentrated in the gallbladder, presumably because they form mixed micelles with the bile salts.

Although bile is secreted continuously from the hepatic parenchymal cells into the bile canaliculi, the organelles that produce bile, except for certain vesicles, have not been positively identified. Renston et al. (1980), utilizing cytochemistry and electron-microscopic autoradiography, demonstrated that two biliary proteins, insulin and dimeric immunoglobulin A, travel transcellularly from plasma to bile inside 1,000-Å vesicles. Other organelles possibly involved in bile secretion include the microvilli of the canalicular membrane, junctional complexes, microfilaments, cytoplasmic and pericanalicular vesicles, the Golgi complex including GERL, and multivesicular bodies (see Jones et al., 1980, for review).

When the flow of bile is impeded (cholestasis), the canaliculi dilate with subsequent flattening of the microvilli. The rough ER partially degranulates and there is a reduction in the amount of Golgi, rough ER, and smooth ER membrane (Jones et al., 1975).

Adult human livers daily produce 15 ml of bile per kg body weight. Bile is secreted at a rate of approximately 0.6 ml per min in a 60-kg adult. The rate of synthesis and secretion depends largely on the blood flow to the liver. Bile is produced at a pressure of 200 to 300 mm H_2O. This pressure is regulated by the rate of secretion and viscosity of the bile, the contractility of the gallbladder, and the resistance of the sphincter of Oddi.

It has been suggested that there is some fluid reabsorption in the intrahepatic bile ducts (Fig. 20–40). This is a well-established phenomenon in the gallbladder, but direct studies are difficult in intrahepatic bile ducts. Certain gastrointestinal hormones, such as secretin, cholecystokinin (CCK), and gastrin, increase bile flow and bicarbonate concentration. Cholecystokinin reportedly encourages the flow of bile into the intestinal lumen by inducing contraction of the gallbladder and relaxation of the sphincter of Oddi. The parasympathetic vagus nerve is

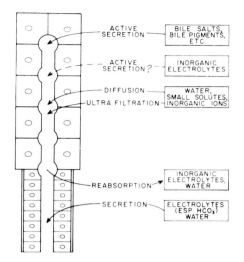

20–40 Diagrammatic summary of some of the mechanisms involved in bile formation. The larger cells represent liver parenchymal cells and the smaller ones the bile duct system. (From Wheeler, H. O. 1965. *In* L. Schiff (ed.), Diseases of the Liver, 3d ed. Philadelphia: J. B. Lippincott Company.)

thought to contract the sphincter of Oddi between fatty meals.

The constituents in the bile that reach the intestine are not completely lost. Many are reabsorbed and transported by the portal blood to the liver for reexcretion (enterohepatic circulation). Most bile salts and the fatty acids from the phospholipid and cholesterol in the bile are reabsorbed.

In addition to providing a pool of bile for digestion of fat, the gallbladder also plays a role in concentrating the bile. Absorption in the normal gallbladder is confined largely to water and inorganic ions, especially sodium, calcium, chloride, and bicarbonate. In the dog, water is reabsorbed at a rate of 3 to 6 cm³ an hour. This concentrates the bile 4 to 10 times (Cameron, 1970).

The Development of the Liver and Gallbladder

Origin of the Hepatic Diverticulum

The liver primordium appears in human embryos (2.5 mm) during the middle of the third week of gestation. It begins as a thickening of the endodermal epithelium lining the cranioventral wall of the foregut near its junction with the yolk sac (that is, the anterior intestinal portal). The thickening rapidly develops into a ventral outgrowth, which becomes hollow and lined by columnar epithelium. The cavity of the diverticulum is continuous with the region of the intestine destined to become the duodenum. As the diverticulum enlarges, it grows into the mesenchyme of the *septum transversum* and separates into (1) a cranial, hepatic portion that eventually forms the liver and intrahepatic bile ducts; (2) a smaller caudal, cystic portion that becomes the gallbladder, common bile duct, and cystic duct; and (3) a ventral portion that evolves into a segment of the head of the pancreas.

The Hepatic Parenchyma, Sinusoids, and Ligaments

As the hepatic diverticulum invades the septum transversum, the irregularly shaped endodermal cells migrate forward from the original invagination in the form of solid strands or cords. The cords grow between the two *vitelline veins* into the capillary network of the septum transversum that arises from these vessels. In so doing, the hepatic cords subdivide the capillaries in the plexus and become surrounded by them. This process ultimately leads to the development of the complicated adult pattern of the *parenchyma* and *sinusoids*, as the cell cords become hepatic plates and the capillaries become liver sinusoids. The hepatic plates at this stage are three to five cells thick and remain this way until several years after birth. Once the plates are formed, the liver cells become more regular in shape and are usually cuboidal. There are no binucleated cells until after birth, and the cell volume increases as the cells undergo terminal differentiation. In the 10-mm, 6-week embryo, the liver is bilobed. Mesenchymal tissue from the septum transversum forms the *stroma, capsule,* and *mesothelium* of the liver. Reflections of peritoneum off the diaphragm onto the liver's surface will form the triangular and coronary ligaments, whereas the area of original contact with the septum transversum, which is not covered by peritoneum, forms the *bare area* of the liver.

Hematopoiesis

By the tenth week, the liver constitutes approximately 10% of the body weight. Hematopoiesis in the liver commences at the 10-mm stage (6 weeks) and contributes much of this weight. For a short time the liver is the primary site for fetal blood formation, predominantly erythroblastic. The hematopoietic cells are extravascular and in close contact with the parenchymal cells. The ratio of liver to body weight decreases during the last trimester when most hematopoietic sites within the liver disappear (see Chap. 12).

Intrahepatic Biliary Tree and Bile Canaliculi

The first bile canaliculi appear as small vesicles between parenchymal cells of the 6-week embryo, far in advance of bile secretion. During the sixth to ninth weeks, the remainder of the intrahepatic biliary tree begins to form and apparently is derived from limiting plate hepatocyes abutting the edges of the portal canals. It is thought that certain limiting plate hepatocytes, surrounding lumina or vesicles in the wall, are transformed into ductal epithelium as the mesenchyme penetrates the limiting plate. In later stages, connective tissue separates the transforming cells from the liver parenchyma. Bile production begins at 4 months of gestation. The bile flows into the gallbladder and then to the duodenum, producing the characteristic dark color of the meconium.

Extrahepatic Biliary Tract and Gallbladder

Little is known about the early development of the extrahepatic biliary tract and gallbladder in humans. However, as the originally hollow pars cystica elongates, its lumen is obliterated by the migration of cells into the original lumen. Hence, in the 6- to 7-mm embryo, the future gallbladder and common bile duct form a solid epithelial cord in the septum transversum just below the developing liver. Vacuolization of the solid cord produces a lumen in the common bile duct at 7.5 mm, the hepatic duct at 10 mm, the cystic duct at 16 mm, and the gallbladder at 18 mm. However, the gallbladder is not completely hollow until the third month. The mucosa, muscularis, and serosa of the gallbladder are established in the 29-mm embryo, but the mucosal folds are not formed until the very end of gestation.

Congenital atresia of the bile ducts can cause cholestasis and jaundice in the newborn. Untreated infants develop cirrhosis, liver failure, and portal hypertension and usually do not live longer than 2 years.

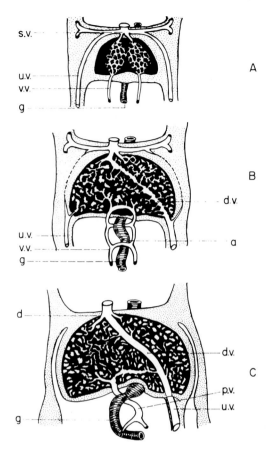

20–41 Diagram showing development of liver veins. **sv,** sinus venosus; **uv,** umbilical veins; **vv,** vitelline veins; **g,** gut; **dv,** ductus venosus; **a,** caudal anastomosis of distal vitelline veins; **d,** diaphragm. (From DuBois, A. M. 1963. The Embryonic Liver. *In* C. Rouiller (ed.), The Liver, vol. 1. New York: Academic Press, Inc.)

Development of the Hepatic Venous System

The vasculature undergoes drastic changes during fetal life. In the 4.5-mm human embryo (5 weeks), the hepatic diverticulum and its associated capillaries (derived from the vitelline veins) lie between the right and left *umbilical veins* (Fig. 20–41A). During the 5-mm stage, the caudal segments of the vitelline veins begin to form three anastomoses. The anterior anastomosis occurs within the liver, whereas the middle and posterior are outside the liver, dorsal and ventral to the duodenum (Fig. 20–41B). As a result, two venous rings are formed. The right half of the upper ring and the left half of the bottom ring disappear by the 9-mm stage, and a new **S**-shaped vessel, composed of segments from the cross-connected vitelline veins, is formed. This vessel is the portal vein (Fig. 20–41C).

The efferent hepatic veins, which drain the liver, are derived from the vitelline veins proximal to the vitelline capillary plexus. In Fig. 20–41A, the vitelline veins are shown entering into the sinus venosus anterior to the liver. The stem of the right vitelline vein enlarges, and by the 9-mm stage it forms the termination of the inferior vena cava.

Except for very early stages, all maternal blood in the placenta flows through the umbilical veins. In the 5-mm embryo, the umbilical veins send ramifications into the liver (Fig. 20–41B). The right umbilical vein and proximal portions of the left umbilical vein disappear during the 6- to 7-mm stage. The remaining distal portion of the left umbilical vein supplies the liver with oxygenated blood from the maternal circulation (Fig. 20–41B).

The ductus venosus, which shunts blood directly from the left umbilical vein to the inferior vena cava, develops within the hepatic diverticulum during the 5- to 6-mm stage (Fig. 20–41B and C). The ductus venosus persists until birth, when it collapses and begins to atrophy. Eventually it forms a connective tissue remnant, the *ligamentum venosum*. Concomitantly, the left umbilical vein atrophies, forming the *ligamentum teres*, which extends from the liver to the umbilicus.

References and Selected Bibliography

General

DuBois, A. M. 1963. The embryonic liver. *In* C. Rouiller (ed.) The Liver, Vol. 1. New York: Academic Press, p. 1.

Elias, H. 1949. A re-examination of the structure of the mammalian liver. I. Parenchymal architecture: II. The hepatic lobule and its relation to the vascular and biliary systems. Am. J. Anat. 84:311 and 85:379.

Elias, J., and Sherrick, J. C. 1969. Morphology of the liver. New York: Academic Press, Inc.

Gates, G. A., Henley, K. S., Pollard, H. M., Schmidt, E., and Schmidt, F. W. 1961. The cell population of human liver. J. Lab. Clin. Med. 57:182.

Jones, A. L., Schmucker,D. L., Renston, R. H., and Murakami, T. 1980. The architecture of bile secretion. Digest. Dis. Sci. 25:609.

Mall, F. P. 1906. A study of the structural unit of the liver. Am. J. Anat. 5:227.

Weissman, G. 1969. Lysosomes. N. Engl. J. Med. 273:1084.

Wilson, J. W., and LeDuc, E. H. 1950. Movement of macrophages studied with the use of thortrast. J. Natl. Cancer Inst. 10:1348.

Biliary System and Gall Bladder

Boyden, E. A. 1957. The anatomy of the choledochoduodenal junction in man. Surg. Gynecol. Obstet. 104:641.

Chapman, G. B., Chiarodo, A. J., Coffey, R. J., and Wieneke, K. 1966. The fine structure of mucosal epithelial cells of a pathological human gallbladder. Anat. Rec. 154:579.

Elying, G. 1960. Crypts and ducts in the gallbladder wall. Acta Pathol. Microbiol. Scand. 49 (Suppl. 135).

Matter, A., Orci, K., and Rouiller, C. 1969. A study on the permeability barriers between Disse's space and the bile canaliculus. J. Ultrastruct. Res. 11 (Suppl.).

Mueller, J. C., Jones, A. L., and Long, A. J. 1972. Topographical and subcellular anatomy of the guinea pig gallbladder. Gastroenterology 63:856.

Growth and Regeneration

Bucher, N. L. R. 1967. Experimental aspects of hepatic regeneration. N. Engl. J. Med. 277:686.

Cameron, I. L. 1970. Cell renewal in the organs and tissues of the nongrowing adult mouse. Tex. Rep. Biol. Med. 28:3.

Carriere, R. 1969. The growth of the liver parenchymal nuclei and its endocrine regulation. Int. Rev. Cytol. 25:201.

Doljanski, F. 1960. The growth of the liver with special reference to mammals. Int. Rev. Cytol. 10:217.

Hepatocytes

Babcock, M. B., and Cardell, R. R., Jr. 1974. Hepatic glycogen patterns in fasted and fed rats. Am. J. Anat. 140:299.

Claude, A. 1970. Growth and differentiation of cytoplasmic membranes in the course of lipoprotein granule synthesis in the hepatic cell. I. Elaboration of the elements of the Golgi complex. J. Cell Biol. 47:745.

Dallman, P. R., and Goodman, J. R. 1971. The effects of iron deficiency on the hepatocyte: A biochemical and ultrastructural study. J. Cell Biol. 48:79.

Dallner, G., Siekevitz, P., and Palade, G. E. 1966. Biogenesis of endoplasmic reticulum membranes. I. Structural and chemical differentiation in developing rat hepatocyte. J. Cell Biol. 30.

Dallner, G., Siekevitz, P., and Palade, G. E. 1966. Biogenesis of endoplasmic reticulum membranes. II. Synthesis of constitutive microsomal enzymes in developing rat hepatocyte. J. Cell Biol. 30.

Deane, H. W. 1942. The cytology of the mouse liver in a controlled diurnal cycle. Anat. Rec. 84:477.

Deane, H. W. 1944. A cytological study of the diurnal cycle of the liver of the mouse in relation to storage and secretion. Anat. Rec. 88:39.

Fawcett, D. W. 1955. Observations on the cytology and electron microscopy of hepatic cells. J. Natl. Cancer Inst. 15:1475.

Lin, C., and Chang, J. P. 1975. Electron microscopy of albumin synthesis. Science (Wash., D.C.) 190:465.

Loud, A. V. 1968. Quantitative stereological description of the ultrastructure of normal rat liver parenchymal cells. J. Cell Biol. 37:27.

Mahley, R. W., Hamilton, R. L., and LeQuire, V. S. 1969. Characterization of lipoprotein particles isolated from the Golgi apparatus of rat liver. J. Lipid Res. 10:433.

Wheatley, D. N. 1972. Binucleation in mammalian liver. Exp. Cell Res. 74:455.

Innervation

Forssmann, W. G., and Ito, S. 1977. Hepatocyte innervation in primates. J. Cell Biol. 74:299.

Pathology

Marver, H. S., and Schmid, R. 1972. The porphyrias. In J. B. Stanbury, J. B. Wyngarden, and D. S. Frederickson (eds.), Metabolic Basis of Inherited Disease, 3rd ed. New York: McGraw-Hill Book Co., Inc., p. 1087.

Tandler, B., Erlandson, R. A., Smith, A. L., and Wynder, E. L. 1969. Riboflavin and mouse hepatic cell structure and function. II. Division of mitochondria during recovery from simple deficiency. J. Cell Biol. 41:477.

Wheeler, H. O. 1969. Secretion of bile. In S. Schiff (ed.), Diseases of the Liver, 3rd ed. Philadelphia: J. B. Lippincott Co., p. 84.

Vasculature

Brauer, R. W. 1963. Liver circulation and function. Physiol. Rev. 43:115.

Burkel, W. E. 1970. The fine structure of the terminal branches of the hepatic arterial system of the rat. Anat. Rec. 167:329.

Grubb, D. J., and Jones, A. L. 1971. Ultrastructure of hepataic sinusoids in sheep. Anat. Rec. 170:75.

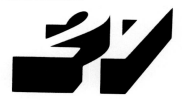

The Exocrine Pancreas and Salivary Glands

James D. Jamieson

Both the major salivary glands and the exocrine pancreas are derived from evaginations of the endodermal lining of the embryonic gut that arise during the fourth week of gestation in humans. In the case of the pancreas, two outpocketings arise from the dorsal and ventral aspects of the small intestine at the level of the bile duct, but they eventually fuse to form the head, uncinate process, body, and tail of the adult pancreas (Fig. 21–1). The ventral portion of the adult pancreas can still be recognized by the relatively high concentrations of pancreatic polypeptide in its islets of Langerhans (see Chap. 22). These blind-ended tubes, lined by undifferentiated simple columnar epithelial cells, undergo sequential branching (Fig. 21–2). With this branching the epithelial rudiment begins to organize into acini, lobules, and eventually lobes characteristic of these organs. During the course of branching, the epithelial cells come into contact with a blanket of mesenchymal tissue that not only is responsible for overall gland morphogenesis but that also, through poorly understood mechanisms, induces the epithelial cells to differentiate structurally and functionally into acinar (serous), mucus, and duct cells. These adult characteristics are first discernible at the third or fourth month of gestation (Fig. 21–3). In the case of the pancreas, endocrine islets bud from the epithelial mass as discussed in Chap. 22. In the adult, the epithelial lining of the ducts of the salivary gland and exocrine pancreas is continuous with that of the oral cavity and duodenum, respectively, the ducts themselves having penetrated the muscularis,

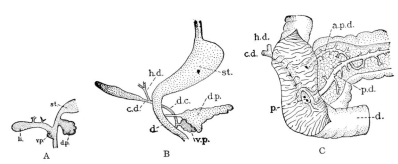

21–1 A and **B.** Diagram of the pancreas of human embryos, 10 and 15 mm. **C.** Dissection of duodenum and pancreas of adult human. **a.p.d.**, accessory pancreatic duct; **c.d.**, cyst duct; **d.**, duodenum; **d.c.**, ductus choledochus; **d.p.** dorsal pancreas; **h.d.**, hepatic duct; **li.**, liver; **p.**, duodenal papilla; **p.d.**, pancreatic duct; **st.**, stomach; **v.p.**, ventral pancreas.

21–2 Schematic diagram of pancreatic morphogenesis. In **1**, the embryonic human gut is shown at about 2 weeks of gestation and consists of a simple elliptical tube lined by columnar epithelial cells. Between the third and fourth weeks of gestation **(2)**, the embryonic foregut evaginates as a pair of blind-ended tubes constituting the dorsal and ventral pancreatic primordia, respectively. The tubes invade the surrounding mesenchyme, indicated by stellate cells and strands of connective tissue. These diverticula undergo branching **(3)** and by about the seventh week of gestation **(4)**, recognizable simple acinar structures can be seen. At this time the dorsal and ventral pancreatic primordia fuse. Beginning at about 3 weeks of gestation, endocrine A cells producing glucagon are present **(dark regions)** and become organized into islet-like structures external to the epithelial bud **(4)**. (Reproduced from Pictet, R., and Rutter, W. J., 1972, *In* D. Steiner and N. Freinkel [eds.], Handbook of Physiology, Vol. I. Baltimore: The Williams and Wilkins Co., p. 25; with permission of the authors.)

submucosa, and mucosa. Minor glands of the gut, secreting mostly mucus, are found in the lamina propria and submucosa throughout the gut and presumably arise in a manner similar to that of the major salivary glands.

The Exocrine Pancreas

Anatomic Relationships

In human adults, the pancreas is a large (90–100 g) organ located retroperitoneally at the level of L1–L3. It is enclosed on its right by the duodenal loop. It overlies the inferior vena cava and abdominal aorta and extends left to the hilus of the kidney, making contact anteriorly on the left with the spleen. Anteriorly, the pancreas is overlain by the stomach. It is divided grossly into the head and uncinate process, which are enclosed by the duodenal loop, and the body and tail,

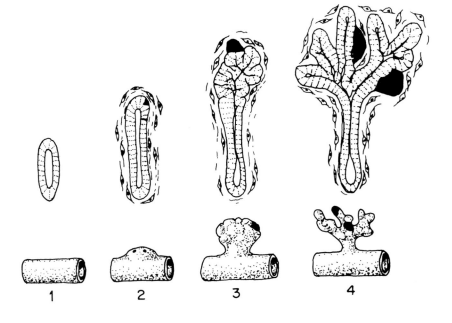

1   2   3   4

21–3 Light micrographs of plastic sections from rat pancreatic rudiments at days 15 **(1a)**, 17 **(1b)**, and 19 **(1c)** of gestation corresponding to human gestational ages of 7, 10, and 20 weeks. In **1a** (corresponding to parts 3 and 4 in Fig. 21–2), undifferentiated epithelial cells of the pancreatic diverticulum, outlined by **arrows,** invade the surrounding mesenchyme (m). Note the apparent absence of an open acinar lumen. At this stage (termed the protodifferentiated state), rapid cell division takes place and the cells synthesize low but detectable amounts of exocrine and endocrine secretory proteins. **1b** shows the presence of a well-demarcated centroacinar lumen **(asterisk)** and appearance of a few zymogen granules in the apical poles of acinar cells undergoing cytodifferentiation **(arrowheads).** At this stage, the rudiment enters the secondary transition state characterized by an exponential increase in the synthesis of secretory proteins and of organelles involved in their intracellular processing. In **lc,** the rudiment enters the differentiated state in which acinar cells, distinguished by abundant zymogen granules, are grouped in characteristic acini whose centroacinar lumina are continuous with small collecting ductules lined proximally by centroacinar cells **(c).** Numerous mitotic figures, some in cells containing zymogen granules **(arrow),** are seen. × 620. (Reproduced from Maylié-Pfenninger, M. F., and Jamieson, J. D., 1980, J. Cell Biol., 86:96; with permission of the publishers.)

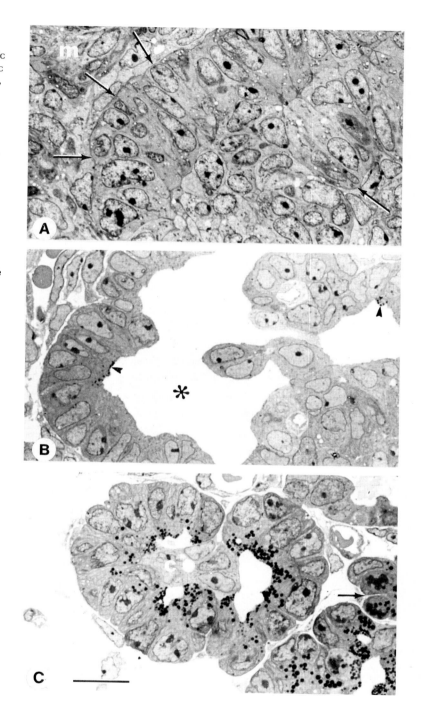

which extend to the left. The head, body, and tail of the pancreas are drained horizontally from the left by the main pancreatic duct, derived from the embryonic ventral anlage. This duct enters the duodenum through the ampulla of Vater. An accessory pancreatic duct, derived from the em-

bryonic dorsal pancreas, is found in about 10% of individuals and enters the duodenum rostral to the ampulla; it drains the head of the pancreas.

In general, the blood supply, lymphatics, and nerves accompany the duct system to its finest

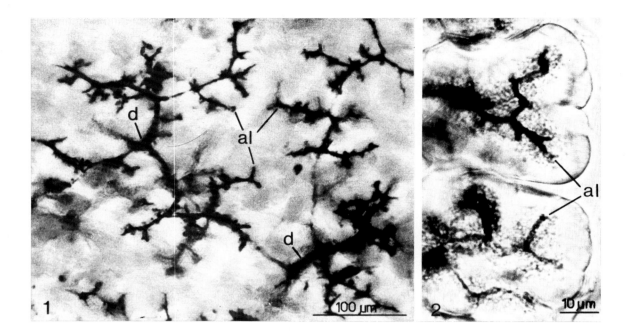

21–4 Light micrographs of rat pancreas in which
India ink **(1)** or horeseradish peroxidase **(2)** has
been infused up the pancreatic duct. In **1**, India ink
marks small collecting ducts **(d)** and delineates the
centroacinar lumen **(al)**. In **2**, the reaction product of
horseradish peroxidase is seen clearly in the
centroacinar lumina (al) adjacent to fields of zymogen
granules in the apical poles of acinar cells. Part 1,
× 270; part 2, × 1,100. (Micrographs courtesy of V.
Herzog and H. Reggio. 1980. Eur. J. Cell Biol. 21:141;
with permission of the publishers.)

termini in the acini (Fig. 21–4). The pancreas is
innervated both by parasympathetic (cholinergic)
fibers from the vagus nerve and by sympathetic
fibers arising from the celiac, superior mesenteric, and hepatic plexus. Their function in regulating secretion of the gland is discussed below.
As noted in the following chapter, part of the arterial blood supply of the acinar tissue of the
exocrine pancreas comes from capillaries that
have first perfused the islets; thus, local high
concentrations of islet hormones come into contact with the exocrine secretory units.

Secretory Proteins of the Exocrine Pancreas

Pancreatic juice from the stimulated gland consists of a protein-rich fluid whose ionic composition is given in Table 21–1. This slightly alkaline fluid is thought to be elaborated by the

centroacinar and epithelial cells of smaller ducts.
The final ionic composition probably reflects
modification of the fluid as it courses to the intestine through the duct system of the gland.

The proteins in pancreatic juice consist of a
group of 15 or more enzymes and proenzymes
(zymogens) capable of digesting the main components of ingested food in the small intestine,
i.e., carbohydrates, lipids and phospholipids,
proteins, and nucleic acids. These pancreatic
proteins range in mass from about 13,000 to
55,000 daltons, have isoelectric points ranging
from about 4.5 to 9, and in some species are
partly glycoproteins. As indicated in Table 21–2,
except for lipase, amylase, RNase, and DNase,
most of the secretory proteins are in the form of
proenzymes in the pancreatic juice. They must
therefore be activated by tryptic cleavage in the
intestine, trypsinogen first being converted to
trypsin by enterokinase, an enzyme of the intes-

Table 21–1 Ionic Composition of
Pancreatic Juice

Ion	Concentration (mM)
HCO_3^-	120
K^+	5
Na^+	140
Ca^{++}	2.3
pH 7.2–7.4	

Table 21–2 Secretory Proteins Produced by Pancreatic Acinar Cells

	Mass (daltons, approximate)	IEP[a]	Mass proportion (%)
Zymogens			
Trypsin(ogen) (3)[b]	30,000	4.4–6.4	~40
Chymotrypsin(ogen)	29,000	7.2	~2
(Pro)carboxypeptidase (4)	47,000	4.6–6.7	~32
(Pro)elastase (2)	29,700	7.5	~4
(Pro)phospholipase A_2	17,500	7.5	?
Enzymes			
α-amylase	54,800	6.3	~5
Triacylglycerol lipase	50,500	6.5	~1
Ribonuclease	13,600	8.7	?
Deoxyribonuclease	~30,000	~5.0(?)	?
Other			
Colipase (2)	10,000	7.3	?
Secretory trypsin inhibitor	~5,000	acid	?
Acid proteoglycan	large	3.5	?

Modified in part from data of G.A. Scheele; reproduced with permission.
[a]Isoelectric point
[b]Number of forms found is given in parentheses.

tinal brush border. (This process is considered in detail below, under Physiological Regulation of Pancreatic Function.) The secretion of enzymes as inactive proenzymes serves to protect the gland from autodigestion. An additional safeguard against premature activation is a trypsin inhibitor that is cosecreted by the acinar cell in amounts sufficient to block any active trypsin that may be formed.

Histological Organization of the Exocrine Pancreas

The pancreas is a mixed endocrine and exocrine gland with acinar (i.e., exocrine) cells forming most of the gland's volume (Table 21–3). The main functional pancreatic unit, responsible for synthesizing and secreting enzymes and proenzymes, is the acinus (Latin for berry). At the

Table 21–3 Volume of Cellular Elements in Pancreas

Cell type	Volume occupied (%)
Acinar	82.0
Duct	3.9
Endocrine	1.8
Blood vessels	3.7
Extracellular space	9.4

Modified from Bolender (1974).

light-microscopic level (Fig. 21–5) each acinus comprises about 50 acinar cells. These cells surround the beginning of the duct system of the gland, which is called the centroacinar lumen. In routine histological preparations stained with hematoxylin and eosin, the individual acinar cells can be seen as pyramidal-shaped cells whose apical cytoplasm is packed with numerous orange-red (acidophilic), spherical zymogen granules. The basal cytoplasm of the acinar cell contains the nucleus and is highly basophilic, reflecting the distribution of rough-surfaced endoplasmic reticulum (RER) in the cell. In favorably preserved specimens (Fig. 21–6) embedded in plastic, a paler-staining cytoplasmic zone can be recognized between the apical and basal poles of the cell in a supranuclear location. This zone corresponds to the Golgi complex, whose structure and function are discussed in detail below.

In occasional sections, one or two pale-staining cells can be seen in the hilus of the acinus in continuity with the epithelium. They mark the beginning of duct systems of the gland. These cells, called centroacinar cells, are believed to be responsible for producing the bicarbonate-rich fluid of pancreatic juice. They are characterized by an abundance of mitochondria, which is typical of cells actively involved in fluid and electrolyte transport (see Fig. 21–7). Their proximity to the centroacinar lumen probably reflects their role in solubilizing the content of the zymogen granules during exocytosis.

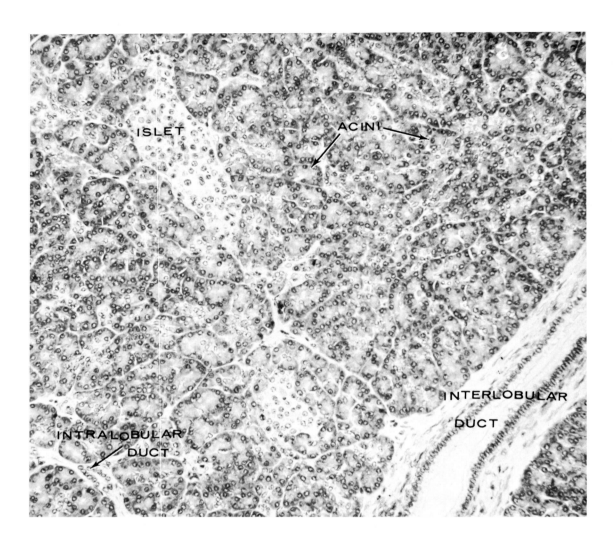

21–5 Photomicrograph of human pancreas. Two islets of Langerhans and a number of small intralobular ducts are present in the acinar tissue. An interlobular duct is shown at the lower right. × 160.

epithelium; near the ampulla of Vater, occasional goblet cells occur in the lining epithelium of the duct.

Each acinus is surrounded by a basal lamina continuous with that investing the ductules, and the entire unit is supported by a loose connective tissue matrix. Groups of acini, whose ductules converge on an increasingly large intralobular duct, form primary lobules, and each lobule is separated from adjacent lobules by a thicker layer of interlobular connective tissue. Groups of lobules, in turn, are segregated into lobes by connective tissue septa, where interlobular ducts are frequently seen. These ducts and the larger main collecting ducts are lined with a simple cuboidal

Intracellular Organization of Acinar and Centroacinar Cells

At the electron microscope level, the distribution of organelles in the acinar cell is highly polarized (Fig. 21–7). The basal pole of the cell is packed with abundant parallel cisternae of the RER, each cisterna bounded by a thin membrane (about 6 nm) studded with many attached ribosomes (polysomes) (Fig. 21–8). Between adjacent RER cisternae, the cytoplasm contains free ribosomes and numerous mitochondria that are strategically placed to supply energy required for protein syn-

21–6 Light micrograph of a section of plastic-embedded mammalian pancreas. A single acinus, including a centroacinar cell **(CAC)** is outlined by the **solid line;** individual acinar cells surrounding the centroacinar lumen **(L)** are indicated by **dashed lines.** The acinar cell in the top left of the acinus is divided into a basal **(B)** zone containing the basophilic elements of the RER (termed ergastoplasm in older literature); a centrally located paler-staining region comprising elements of the Golgi complex **(G),** and the apical zone **(A)** packed with zymogen granules **(ZG).** Note the typical polarized arrangement of subcellular organelles in this cell type, which reflects their temporal and functional interrelationships in the secretory pathway. A small collecting duct **(D)** and blood vessel **(V)** are indicated. Other symbols point out mitochondria **(m)** in an acinar cell, a nucleus **(N),** and a nucleolus **(n).** × 1,700.

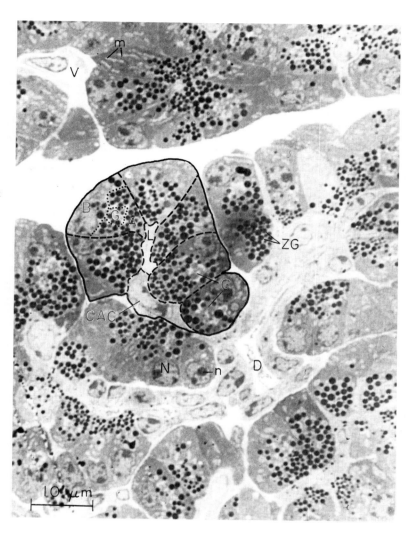

thesis. Reflecting the intense specialization of the acinar cell for producing exportable proteins, the RER occupies approximately 20% of the cytoplasmic volume, and its membranes account for approximately 60% (about 8,000 μm^2/cell) of the total surface area of the cell's membranes. The portions of the RER adjacent to the Golgi complex extend out as smooth-surfaced membranous evaginations termed transitional elements (see Fig. 21–9). Their function in transporting secretory proteins from the RER to the Golgi complex is discussed below.

The Golgi complex, which occupies about 8% of the cytoplasmic volume and about 10% of the membrane area of the cell, consists of a series of compartments whose membranes are smooth-surfaced and somewhat thicker (approximately 10 nm) than those of the RER. The membranous elements of the Golgi complex consist of (1) sets of stacked cisternae, whose usually concave or trans surface faces the apical pole of the cell; (2) numerous small smooth-surfaced vesicles located primarily between the transitional elements of the RER and the convex or cis face of the stacked cisternae; and (3) forming secretory granules, termed condensing vacuoles, found budding from and adjacent to the trans side of the stacked cisternae. In addition to membrane-bounded compartments, microtubules, microfilaments, and mitochondria are found in the cytoplasmic matrix of the Golgi complex.

Finally, in the resting acinar cell, the apical

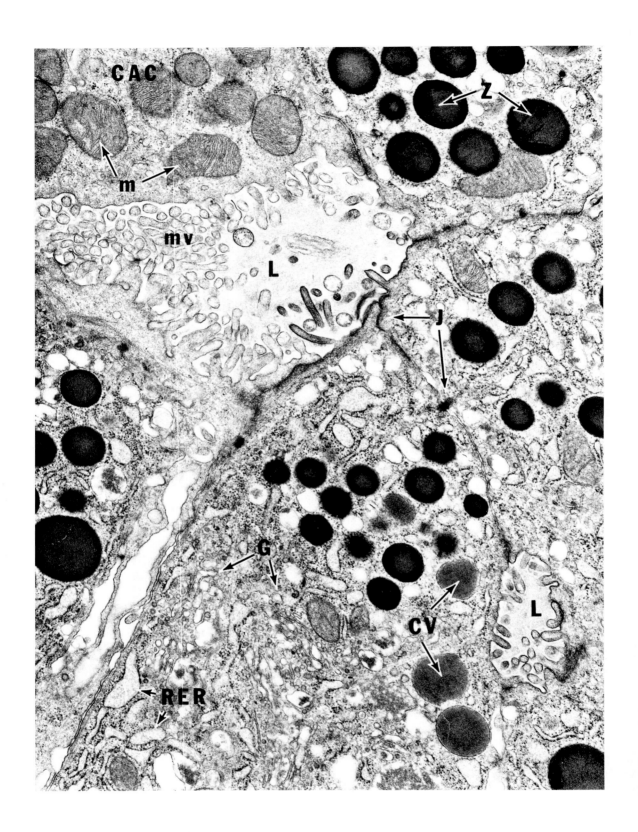

21–7 Electron micrograph of a thin section through the apical region of a mammalian pancreatic acinus. Note that the apical surface of the acinar cells and the centroacinar cell are provided with numerous stubby microvilli (mv), which protrude into the centroacinar lumen (L). Typical junctional complexes (J) join adjacent acinar and centroacinar cells and effectively seal off the lumen space from that of the lateral intercellular space. **RER**, rough-surfaced endoplasmic reticulum; **G**, elements of the Golgi complex; **CV**, condensing vacuoles; **Z**, zymogen granules. Note the numerous mitochondria (m) in the centroacinar cell (CAC). × 19,000. (Micrograph courtesy of B.E. Hull.)

cytoplasm is packed with numerous storage or zymogen granules that are bounded by a smooth bilayer and have a homogenous electron-opaque content. Zymogen granules occupy about 20% of the cytoplasmic volume and account for about 3% of the cell's membrane area.

The basolateral plasmalemma of adjacent acinar cells is relatively smooth, lacking the extensive interdigitations found in the salivary gland acinar cells. The apical plasmalemma of the acinar cell is invested with numerous stubby microvilli, each containing a core of actin filaments. These filaments course into the apical cytoplasm to intermingle with a mat of microfilaments that separates the zymogen granule population from the cell surface. The apical plasmalemma is segregated from the basolateral plasmalemma by typical junctional complexes. The tight-junctional elements in these complexes form a gasket or seal around the apical zone of adjacent acinar cells and prevent the egress of secretory proteins from the centroacinar lumen into the extracellular space. When the tight-junctional continuity is disrupted, secretory proteins are able to enter the extracellular space and eventually the circulation. Because, lipase is active as secreted, entry of secretory proteins into the extracellular space leads to damage of the plasmalemma and to further leakage of secretory proteins, which eventually results in the common and life-threatening disease acute pancreatitis. Adhering zonules and desmosomes of the junctional complex are involved in cell-to-cell adhesion. Typical gap junctions (zonulae communicantes), located on the lateral plasmalemma of adjacent acinar cells, are responsible for electrical and metabolic coupling of cells within one or more acini.

The structural features of the acinar cell discussed above are diagrammed in Fig. 21–9. In

the following discussion of the function of the acinar cells, one should keep in mind two points: (1) the cell is basically divided into two regions. The cytoplasmic matrix contains the protein synthetic machinery of the cell (free and attached ribosomes), and the enzymes, coenzymes, and substrates of intermediary metabolism. This region is separated from a series of functionally (and structurally) interconnected compartments or cisternae enclosed by membranes of the rough and smooth variety. (2) The arrangement of the membrane-bounded compartments of the cell reflects the functional and temporal interrelationships of these compartments during the synthesis and secretion of exportable proteins.

Functional Aspects of the Acinar Cell in Processing Exportable Proteins

For nearly 100 years, the pancreatic acinar cell has provided a model system for studying the basic aspects of protein synthesis and secretion. For convenience (see Fig. 21–9 and Table 21–4) the life history of secretory proteins can be arbitrarily divided into six steps, which will be discussed individually below; it is important to remember, however, that these steps are functionally continuous.

Steps 1 and 2: Synthesis and Segregation of Exportable Proteins. Synthesis of exportable proteins occurs according to the scheme outlined in Fig. 21–10. After large and small ribosomal subunits associate in the cytosol with messenger RNA (mRNA) for the synthesis of secretory proteins, a special nucleotide sequence on the 3′ side of the AUG initiation codon is translated as an amino terminal extension or signal sequence of 20 to 40 amino acids that precedes the bulk of the peptide chain. As protein synthesis proceeds, the signal peptide is extruded from the large ribosomal subunit and interacts with the membrane of the RER. This interaction presumably creates a pore or channel in the membrane through which the signal peptide and the following portion of the growing protein is threaded. As a consequence of this interaction, ribosomes become attached to the membrane of the RER and remain so until reading of the mRNA is completed. Because mRNAs for nonexportable proteins lack a signal codon, these proteins cannot gain access to the cisternal space of the RER.

758

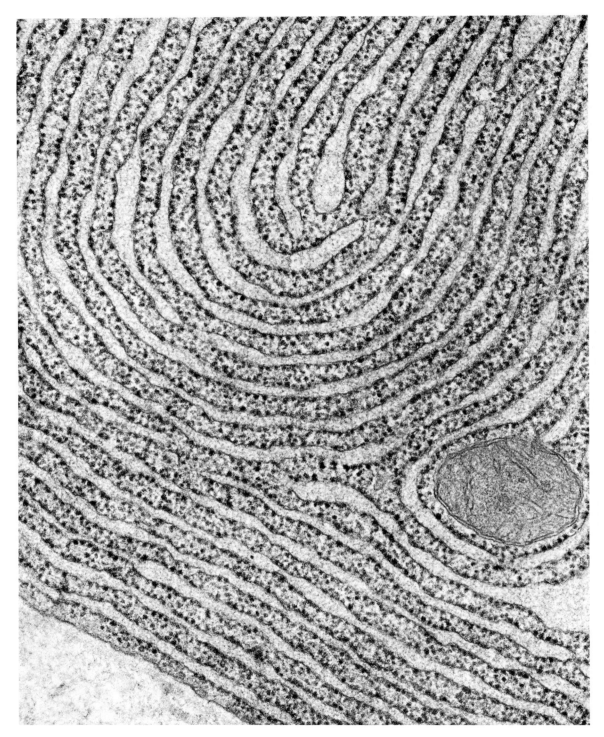

21–8 Electron micrograph of the basal cytoplasm of a human pancreatic acinar cell. Extensive lamellar arrays of ribosome-studded endoplasmic reticulum are characteristic features of these cells. The cisternae are filled with a flocculent precipitate of newly synthesized protein. A profile of a mitochondrion is included in the cytoplasm. × 65,000.

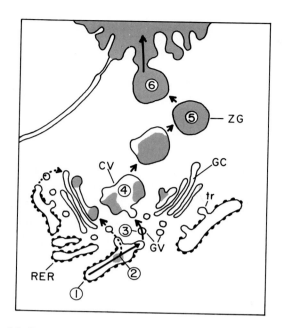

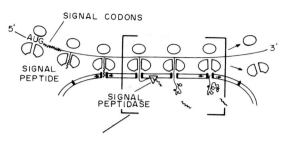

Cotranslational modifications of secretory proteins

1) Cleavage of signal peptides
2) Core glycosylation of asparagine residues in glycoproteins
3) Formation of disulfide bonds and assumption of tertiary and quarternary structure

21–10 Summary of initial events occurring during the synthesis and segregation of secretory proteins in the RER (Steps 1 and 2 of Fig. 21–9). See text for details. Cotranslational modifications are indicated in **brackets.** (Modified with permission from Blobel, G., Walter, P., Chang, C. N., Goldman, B. M., Erickson, A. H., and Lingappa, V. R. 1979. *In* Secretory Mechanisms, Symposia of the Society for Experimental Biology, Vol. 33. Cambridge: Cambridge University Press, p. 9.)

21–9 Diagrammatic representation of a pancreatic acinar cell representative of a variety of polarized epithelial cells specialized in the synthesis and packaging of exportable proteins. The numbers refer to steps in the secretory pathway discussed in the text. The **solid arrows** in step 3 refer to the transport route from the RER to condensing vacuoles **(CV)** found in the pancreas; the more typical situation in other cells is indicated by the dashed **arrow,** where forming secretory granules bud from the distal ends of trans Golgi cisternae. **RER,** rough-surfaced endoplasmic reticulum; **tr,** transitional elements of the RER facing the cis side of the Golgi complex; **GV,** smooth surfaced transporting vesicles of the Golgi complex; **GC,** Golgi cisternae; **CV,** condensing vacuoles on the trans side of the Golgi complex; **ZG,** zymogen granules.

As the polypeptide chain traverses the membrane of the RER, a number of important cotranslational modifications occur. The first of these modifications (see Fig. 21–10) is the removal of the signal peptide by a membrane-associated endopeptidase. In the case of insulin biosynthesis, cotranslational proteolysis converts preproinsulin to proinsulin; for exocrine pancreatic secretory proteins, excision of the signal peptide converts, for example, pretrypsinogen to trypsinogen. For secretory proteins that will be secreted as glycoproteins, a second cotranslational modification is the addition of the core oligosaccharide to asparagine residues in the nascent poly-

Table 21–4 Summary of Cellular Events in Pancreatic Secretory Protein Processing

Operation	Effector	Compartment	Requirements	
			Protein synthesis	Energy
1. Protein synthesis	Attached polysomes	Cytoplasmic matrix	+	+
2. Segregation	Ribosome–RER junction	Cisternal space of RER	+	−
3. Intracellular transport	Transitional elements and transporting vesicles of Golgi	Cisternal spaces of RER and Golgi	−	+
4. Concentration	Condensing vacuoles	Cisternal space of Golgi	−	−
5. Storage	Zymogen granules	Cisternal space of zymogen granule	−	−
6. Exocytosis	Secretory granules, apical plasmalemma junction	Extracellular space	−	+

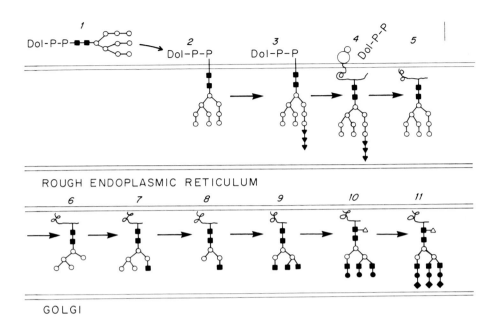

21–11 Summary of biosynthetic steps that are believed to occur in the glycosylation of asparagine-linked glycoproteins. In the upper portion of the diagram, core glycosylation is shown to occur in the RER by the bulk transfer of a mannose- and glucose-rich oligosaccharide from a lipid carrier, dolichol-P-P, to asparagine residues on the growing polypeptide chain. Dolichol-P-P-oligosaccharide is thought to be synthesized in the cytosol and transferred to the cisternal side of the RER by the lipid-soluble dolichol molecule. The precise location of dolichol in the ER membrane is unknown. In the Golgi complex (lower part of the diagram), a mannosidase, activated by addition of an N-acetylglucosamine group, trims the mannose core back to three residues preparatory to step-wise addition of further N-acetylglucosaminyl residues and of galactosyl, sialyl, and fucosyl residues from nucleotide sugars by glycosyl transferases associated with the inner surface of the membranes of the Golgi complex. **Squares,** N-acetylglucosamine; **open circles,** mannose; **solid triangles,** glucose; **solid circles,** galactose; **diamonds,** sialic acid; **open triangles,** fucose. (Modified with permission from Kornfeld, R., and Kornfeld, S., 1980. In W. J. Lennarz [ed.], The Biochemistry of Glycoproteins and Proteoglycans. New York: Plenum Press, p. 1.)

peptide. This core oligosaccharide, which consists of two N-acetylglucosamine residues and up to nine mannose and three glucose residues, is added in part by bulk transfer of the oligosaccharide from a lipid donor molecule termed dolichol (Fig. 21–11). All of the glucose and most of the mannose groups are subsequently removed by specific glycosidases in the RER and Golgi complex before modification of the terminal of the oligosaccharide in the Golgi, as discussed below. Finally, disulfide bonds are formed within peptides by an enzyme located in the RER that converts the linear polypeptide into a globular form, ensuring irreversible segregation in the RER cisternae. With the exception of energy required to drive protein synthesis and other covalent modifications, transit of the secretory protein from attached ribosomes across the RER membrane is energy-independent; propulsion is effected by the elongation of the peptide chain.

Step 3: Intracellular Transport. After synthesis and segregation in the RER cisternae, the newly synthesized secretory protein diffuses toward the transitional elements of the RER, which pinch off and transfer a small bolus of secretory proteins to the Golgi complex by smooth-surfaced transporting vesicles. These vesicles are believed to deliver their content into the Golgi cisternae by membrane fusion and fission; the exact site of docking is unknown but is thought, in some cases, to be the cis side of the Golgi complex. Available evidence indicates that a mixture of all secretory proteins, both glycosylated and unglycosylated, is transported in this manner. However, acidic hydrolyses (lysosomal enzymes) may be sorted from bona fide secretory proteins and routed to lysosomes at the level of the RER–Golgi zone. It is now believed that phosphorylated mannose residues on the oligosaccharide side chains of lysosomal enzymes interact with membrane receptors located on the cisternal side of the elements of the Golgi complex. The membrane containing these receptors ultimately pinches off the vesicles that enclose the lysosome enzymes and thereby form primary lysosomes. Patients with I-cell (I, inclusion) disease appear to synthesize lysosomal enzymes that lack the phosphomannosyl recognition markers. Thus, their lysosomal enzymes enter the general secretory pathway and are secreted, leading to a deficiency of intracellular lysosomal enzymes, consequent accumulation of undigested debris in autophagosomes, and eventual cell death.

Transport of secretory proteins from the RER to the Golgi complex is independent of further protein synthesis; but it does require energy in the form of ATP, which presumably serves to open a lock or valve that allows the two intracellular compartments, the RER and the Golgi complex, to be functionally interconnected. The energy requirements for this and subsequent steps in the secretory pathway are shown diagram-

matically in Fig. 21–12 and summarized in Table 21–4.

Step 4: Processing of Secretory Proteins in the Golgi Complex. After secretory-proteins enter the cisternae of the Golgi complex, they un-

21–12 Diagram of movement of secretory proteins in the acinar cell from the RER to the acinar lumen in the normal state, following inhibition of protein synthesis by the antibiotic cycloheximide, and during block of production of ATP by respiratory inhibitors. In all cases, a short "pulse" of radioactively labeled proteins is introduced biosynthetically into the RER cisternae (indicated by **open circles**) by application of radioactive amino acids; its subsequent fate is followed under experimental conditions. Secretory proteins previously synthesized by the cell are indicated by **solid circles.** In the normal state, the wave of labeled proteins passes sequentially from base to apex of the cell, being replaced by "cold" proteins synthesized after the radioactive amino acid precursors are removed. If protein synthesis is inhibited **(dashed lines)**, secretory proteins move as usual through the cell but the intracellular pool is depleted. Addition of respiratory inhibitors blocks movement of secretory proteins from the RER to the Golgi complex **(GC)** and blocks exocytosis (lower panel 1 and 2) but does not inhibit conversion of condensing vacuoles **(CV)** to zymogen granules **(ZG)** (lower panel, 3).

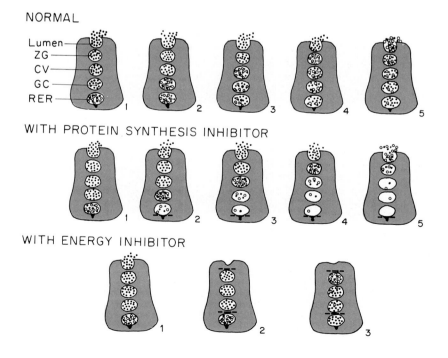

NORMAL

Lumen — ZG — CV — GC — RER

WITH PROTEIN SYNTHESIS INHIBITOR

WITH ENERGY INHIBITOR

dergo a number of posttranslational modifications. Most obviously, the initially dilute solution of proteins entering from the RER becomes highly concentrated, leading to the formation of mature zymogen granules. This modification takes place in condensing vacuoles. Condensing vacuoles are limited by a smooth-surfaced bilayer; depending on species and cell type, they are asscoiated with the rims or trans side of the Golgi stacks, but they are, in effect, part of the Golgi system. Although the mechanism of concentration is not fully understood in the pancreatic acinar cell, it probably involves ionic interactions both among secretory proteins of differing charge and between basic secretory proteins and a large anionic proteoglycan that is sulfated in the Golgi complex. The net result of concentration is the flow of water (and probably electrolytes) into the cell sap and the formation of an osmotically inactive mass of secretory proteins, which are reflected morphologically as spherical, electron-opaque zymogen granules. Because concentration requires neither additional protein synthesis nor ATP, the condensing vacuole can be regarded as a passive sink for incoming secretory proteins that leads to their irreversible energy-independent sequestration.

During accumulation and concentration in the Golgi complex, secretory proteins undergo a variety of covalent modifications. As mentioned above, glycoproteins are synthesized in the RER as mannose- and glucose-rich precursors; upon arrival in the Golgi complex, residual mannose residues not removed in the RER are cleaved off preparatory to final processing of the oligosaccharide (Fig. 21–11). This processing involves the sequential addition, from nucleotide sugar intermediates of the terminal sugars, of what will become complex oligosaccharides, i.e., N-acetylglucosamine, galactose, sialic acid, and fucose. The sugar transferases mediating this process are integral membrane proteins of the Golgi complex. In addition, SO_4 groups are covalently added to a large proteoglycan in the Golgi complex, thus converting it to an acidic polyanion whose postulated role in concentrating secretory proteins in condensing vacuoles is mentioned above. In the endocrine pancreas, proteolytic cleavage of prohormones to biologically active hormones occurs in the Golgi complex. In the case of exocrine pancreatic secretory proteins, proteolysis of proenzymes to active enzymes (e.g., conversion of trypsinogen to trypsin or of procarboxypeptidase to carboxypeptidase) occurs extracellularly in the gut lumen.

Unlike endocrine glands, where individual peptide hormones are synthesized by separate cell types, each pancreatic acinar cell not only synthesizes the full complement of secretory proteins but transports and packages them together.

Steps 5 and 6: Storage and Discharge of Zymogen Granules. The total time for synthesis, intracellular transport, and packaging of secretory proteins into zymogen granules is approximately 45 to 60 min. Thereafter, the zymogen granules are temporarily stored in the acinar cell until their release is triggered by the appropriate neural or hormonal stimulus. The physiological regulation of pancreatic secretion is discussed below; here we shall consider the cellular aspects of exocytosis.

Exocytosis involves three cellular events (Fig. 21–13): (1) movement of the zymogen granule from its site of formation in the Golgi complex to the apical pole of the cell; (2) specific recognition of the secretory granule membrane by that of the apical plasmalemma; and (3) fusion of the zymogen granule membrane and the apical plasmalemma, with elimination of the bilayer at the point of fusion. As a result, continuity is established between the two membranes and the content of the zymogen granule is exposed to the centroacinar lumen. Importantly, at no time during the exocytosis is the selective permeability of the plasmalemma compromised. Although the molecular events involved in this sequence remain unknown, we do know that, like step 3 in intracellular transport, it is independent of protein synthesis but requires metabolic energy. In

21–13 Diagram of steps involved in exocytosis. See text for details.

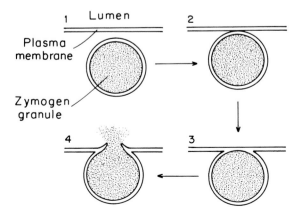

this case, the energy is needed to connect an intracellular compartment (that of the zymogen granule) with the extracellular space.

In the resting acinar cell the membrane area of the zymogen granule population is about 900 μm^2/cell. This membrane area would be potentially inserted into and become part of the cell's apical plasmalemma if complete degranulation of the cell were to occur during intense stimulation of exocytosis. We might therefore expect the surface area of the acinar cell to increase approximately twofold with an attendant loss of intracellular membrane under such conditions. In fact, during the course of exocytosis, only a transient increase in the surface area of the apical plasmalemma is observed and the intracellular membrane balance is maintained. Recent studies indicate that the excess membrane is retrieved from the cell surface as vesicles and is recycled in part back to the Golgi complex to participate in successive rounds of secretory protein processing.

General Conclusions

On the basis of the above discussion, we can summarize the function of the acinar cell as follows (refer to Fig. 21–9 and Table 21–4):

1. During their intracellular history, secretory proteins cross a membrane bilayer only once, i.e., at the time of synthesis, and thereafter are transported and processed within membrane-enclosed compartments up to the point of exocytosis.

2. Intracelluar transport of secretory proteins is vectorial: it proceeds in a basal–apical direction determined both by the structural orientation of intracellular membrane-bound compartments and the functional interactions between them.

3. Intracellular transport is discontinuous and quantal at two stages in the pathway: during movement of secretory proteins from the RER to the Golgi complex mediated by transporting vesicles, and during delivery of secretory proteins from the Golgi complex to the extracellular space, which is carried out by zymogen granules.

4. Transport involves specific interactions between membranes of interacting compartments (i.e., at steps 3, 5, and 6 in the pathway). These interactions are accompanied by nonrandom recycling of membranes of the transport containers, which preserves the specific biochemical and functional properties of the donor and recipient compartments.

5. In general, the scheme outlined for the pancreatic acinar cell pertains to a variety of exocrine and endocrine cells that temporarily store their exportable products in secretory granules. Such cells are usually under neural or hormonal control and are required to secrete large amounts of exportable product over short times at rates faster than could be maintained by biosynthesis. In other cell types (such as fibroblasts and plasma cells) that do not normally contain storage granules, it is now clear that the RER–Golgi portion of the secretory pathway pertains as described for acinar cells. Synthesis and discharge of secretory products in these cells is usually continuous and not subject to neural or hormonal regulation, and hence temporary storage of secretory products is not required. Nonetheless, more recent evidence indicates that discharge in these cells is effected by small, Golgi-derived vesicles that move to and fuse with the plasmalemma as in the case of classic exocytosis.

Physiological Regulation of Pancreatic Function

The overall function of the pancreas in digestion is shown schematically in Fig. 21–14. Five main peptide hormones—cholecystokinin, secretin, pancreatic polypeptide, gastric inhibitory polypeptide, and vasoactive intestinal polypeptide—regulate this process. The properties and actions of these hormones are indicated in Table 21–5.

The classic regulatory hormones of the exocrine pancreas are cholecystokinin and secretin. These two hormones are synthesized and stored in endocrine cells located in the base of the crypts of Lieberkühn. In response to the acid gastric contents (chyme) entering the duodenum, they are released into the circulation. Cholecystokinin is liberated principally by fatty acids and L-amino acids in the chyme, whereas release of secretin is stimulated by acid pH.

Upon reaching acinar cells via the circulation, cholecystokinin induces exocytosis of enzymes and proenzymes into the acinar lumen. Cholecystokinin also causes the gallbladder to contract, releasing bile salts into the gut lumen that emulsify lipids and render them more susceptible to hydrolysis by pancreatic lipase. At the same time, secretin stimulates centroacinar and

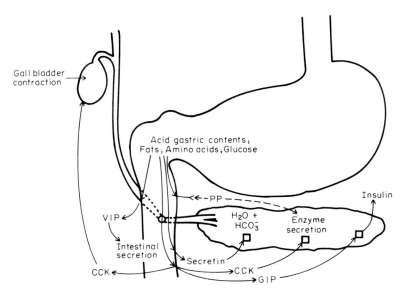

21–14 Diagram of physiological effects of gut endocrine system in the intestinal phase of digestion. **CCK**, cholecystokinin; **VIP**, vasoactive intestinal polypeptide; **GIP**, gastric inhibitory polypeptide; **PP**, pancreatic polypeptide. The names VIP and GIP describe pharmacological effects initially observed for these hormones and do not accurately reflect their physiological function.

duct cells to secrete the fluid portion of pancreatic juice at a high flow rate and with an alkaline pH of 8.4 accounted for by HCO^-_3. The alkaline pancreatic juice, rich in enzymes and proenzymes, reaches the duodenum where it neutralizes the gastric products and provides the correct pH for pancreatic enzyme activity. To initiate this process, trypsinogen is converted to trypsin by enterokinase, a proteolytic enzyme present on the brush border of enterocytes. Trypsin, in turn, converts all of the other proenzymes (including trypsinogen itself) to their active forms by proteolytic cleavage. When the gastric contents in the duodenum are neutralized, release of cholecystokinin and secretin subsides. Concurrently, the gastric contents cause nerve reflexes to release pancreatic polypeptide from the islets of Langerhans. This event is thought to oppose locally the action of cholecystokinin on the acinar cell via the endocrine–acinar portal system discussed in Chapter 22. As a consequence of these negative feedback loops, the pancreas returns to its resting state as digestion and absorption proceed in the small intestine. In addition, release of gastric inhibitory polypeptide into the circulation from gut endocrine cells,

Table 21–5 Hormones Regulating Exocrine Pancreatic Function

Hormone	Mass (daltons)	Stimuli for release	Main actions
Cholecystokinin (CCK)	3,920	L-amino acids; fatty acids	Exocytosis stimulation in acinar cell; gallbladder contraction
Secretin	3,070	Acid pH in duodenum	Secretion of H_2O and electrolytes in pancreatic juice
Pancreatic polypeptide (PP)	4,270	Nerve reflexes stimulated by amino acids and fatty acids in gut	Opposes action of CCK
Vasoactive intestinal polypeptide (VIP)	3,300	Unknown but probably nerve reflexes	Stimulates H_2O and electrolyte secretion by small intestine; peptidergic neurotransmitter
Gastric inhibitory polypeptide (GIP)	5,160	Glucose and fatty acids	Postprandial stimulation of insulin release

in response to glucose and fatty acids in the duodenum, stimulates insulin release from endocrine B cells of the islets. The increased insulin is necessary to regulate the surge of blood glucose that will occur during intestinal absorption. Finally, vasoactive intestinal polypeptide is released locally, possibly by nerve reflexes, and causes water and electrolytes to be secreted from the intestinal epithelium into the gut lumen.

Major Salivary Glands

The parotid, submandibular (formerly submaxillary), and sublingual glands elaborate a major portion of the saliva. These compound tubuloacinar glands secrete proteins, glycoproteins, proteoglycans, electrolytes, and water into the oral cavity. This secretory activity is controlled almost entirely by the autonomic nervous system. The average daily output of saliva in humans is about 750 to 1,000 ml. Saliva is a dilute aqueous fluid; it is not an ultrafiltrate of the blood, as it differs in the concentration of hydrogen ions, chloride ions, glucose, proteins, and other constituents as well. The principal function of saliva is to moisten, lubricate, and initiate digestion of food. This last activity is carried out by the major secretory enzyme, salivary α-amylase, which digests carbohydrates in the oral cavity. Pancreatic α-amylase in the duodenum completes carbohydrate digestion. Smaller amounts

of RNase and DNase are found in the saliva. Saliva solubilizes molecules in food and conveys them to the taste buds, where taste recognition is initiated (Fig. 21–15). Finally, saliva contains gamma-globulins, the predominant one being immunoglobulin A (IgA). Peroxidase has also been recently identified as a component of saliva; this enzyme, along with IgA, is part of a salivary antibacterial system.

From this brief physiological introduction, it should be evident that the histological–cytological organization of these exocrine glands reflects mechanisms for protein and glycoprotein synthesis and transport, as well as mechanisms related to the transport of water and electrolytes. Among different mammals there is considerable morphological variation in these glands, variation probably related primarily to dietary differences (carnivores versus herbivores).

These exocrine glands are organized around a branching duct system that carries the secretion to the oral cavity. The secretory cells are arranged as *acini* around the smallest branches of

21–15 ATPase activity in the taste buds of circumvallate papillae (rat). **A.** Normal papilla. Note the intense ATPase activity in the numerous taste buds in the epithelium that lines the trench. **B.** Papilla 2 weeks after denervation. The taste buds have disappeared. × 70. (From Zalewski, A. A. 1971. Exp. Neurol. 30:510.)

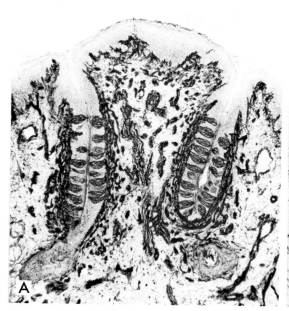

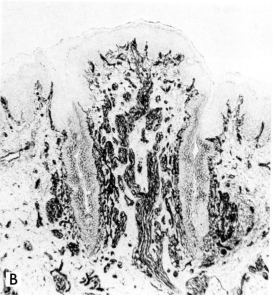

the duct system to form many individual lobules that may be viewed as secretory units (Fig. 21–16), as in the case of the pancreas. Each acinus is limited by a distinct basement membrane, and two types of secretory cells occur in the acinar epithelium, the *serous cells* and the *mucous cells*. The parotid gland of most species is composed entirely of serous acini (Fig. 21–17), whereas the submandibular and sublingual glands contain both (Figs. 21–18 and 21–19; see here and color insert). In the submandibular gland of humans, serous cells outnumber the mucous cells, whereas the opposite is true for the sublingual gland.

At the light-microscopic level, the *serous cells* are pyramidal in shape, their nuclei are basal, cell boundaries are indistinct, the basal and perinuclear cytoplasm are basophilic (Fig. 21–17), and the apical cytoplasm contains secretory granules that vary in number according to functional state.

At the ultrastructural level, the organization of the serous cells of the salivary glands (Fig. 21–20) is similar to that of the pancreatic acinar cell and, as expected, the processing of secretory proteins follows the scheme discussed in detail for the pancreatic acinar cell. In addition, ultrastructural variations occur that may be related particularly to the secretion of saliva. For example, the serous cells of the human submandibular gland possess numerous slender basal projections that extend beyond the lateral margins as radiating foot processes that interdigitate with adjacent cells. This device increases surface area directed toward the vascular pole by at least 60-

21–16 Reconstruction of the acinus and intralobular ducts of the submandibular gland. **D,** demilune composed of serous cells; **M,** mucous cells; **My,** myoepithelial cells; **SC,** secretory capillaries in a serous acinus; **ID,** intercalated duct; **SD,** striated duct. **A.** Cross section through the striated duct. **B.** Cross section through the intercalated duct. **C.** Cross section through a mucous acinus. **D.** Cross section through a serous acinus. (From Braus, H. 1924. Anatomie der Menschen. Berlin: Springer-Verlag OHG.)

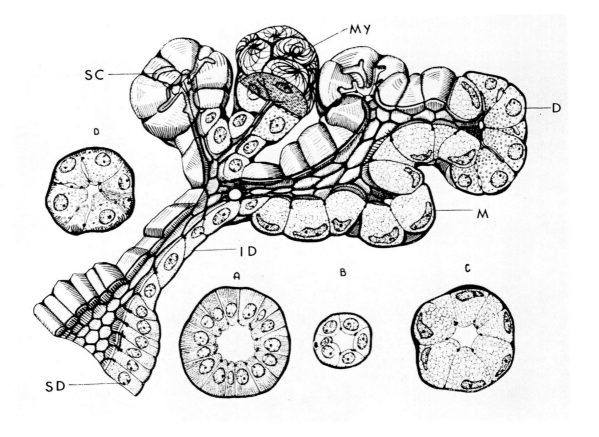

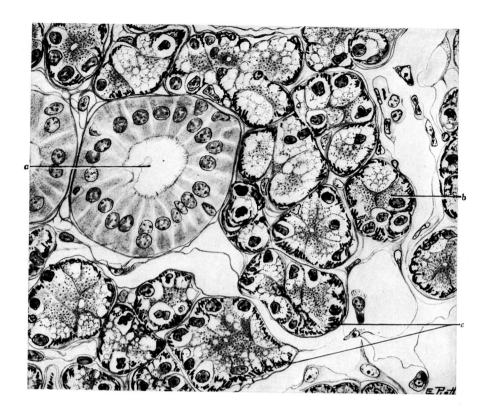

21–17 Section of a human parotid gland. *a*, Section of a striated duct; *b*, serous cell; *c*, basal striations of serous cells. Zenker fixation; methylene blue and eosin.

fold and may be a specialization for transport of electrolytes and water into the primary secretion that enters the acinar lumen. Amylase, peroxidase, DNase, and RNase are produced by the serous cells of the parotid gland.

The *mucous cells* of the salivary glands may be viewed as variations of the intestinal goblet cell, which has been the subject of considerable ultrastructural and analytic interpretation (see Chap. 19). When fresh, the cytoplasm may be filled with numerous droplets of mucus; in routine preparations these droplets are usually dissolved out and the cytoplasm assumes an empty or vacuolated appearance (Figs. 21–18 and 21–19, see here and color insert). The mucous droplets are intensely reactive in the periodic acid Schiff (PAS) procedure, since they contain neutral glycoproteins and mucosubstances, such as sulfated and sialated polysaccharides. Some mucous cells produce sulfomucin (for example, most acini of the human sublingual) whereas others produce sialomucin or mixtures of the two (human submandibular). When the acid mucosubstances are preserved in a tissue section, the droplets are strongly basophilic. In a fully

laden cell, the nucleus is basal and appears to be compressed by the accumulated secretion. The ultrastructure of the mucous cell is essentially similar to that of the goblet cell; that is, most of the supranuclear cytoplasm is filled with secretory droplets that have been derived from the large central supranuclear Golgi complex. As secretion accumulates, the mitochondria and RER are relegated to the lateral and basal cytoplasm.

A secretory structure or acinus may be composed entirely of serous cells or mucous cells or may contain both cell types. In the latter situation, the serous cells occupy the fundus of the acinar sac, and the mucous cells are located closer to the opening to the initial duct segment (intercalated duct). Thus the serous cells form basophilic crescent-shaped groups that are called *demilunes* (Figs. 21–16 and 21–18). The cells of the demilune seem to be separated from the aci-

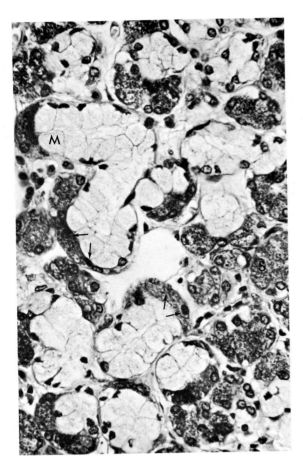

21–18 Human submandibular gland showing demilunes **(arrows)** of the mixed acini. **M,** mucous cells; **S,** serous cells.

nar lumen by the mucous cells, but actually they are directly connected by the secretory capillaries, which are extensions of the acinar lumen that may penetrate deeply between serous cells (Fig. 21–16). Microvilli occur along these secretory capillaries and thereby increase free surface area.

Another component of the acinus is the *myoepithelial cell*, which, as the name suggests, has generally been regarded as a contractile element. Myoepithelial cells have a distinctive form and occupy a unique position; they are flat cells with long cytoplasmic processes that extend over the outer surface of the acinus in a basket-like configuration (Fig. 21–16). They are located between the secretory cells and the basal lamina (Fig.

21–20). Their stellate form is difficult to discern in routine light-microscopic preparations because usually only their nuclear regions are recognizable. The ultrastructure of the myoepithelial cells resembles that of smooth muscle cells; in particular, there are numerous parallel fine filaments that occupy large areas of the cytoplasm. The geometry and arrangement of the myoepithelial cells, as well as their ultrastructural features, suggest a role in expelling the primary secretion.

The primary secretion is most likely modified during its passage through the branching duct system, since certain cytological features, especially those of the striated ducts, suggest participation in transport activities. The first two segments, the *intercalated duct* and the *striated duct*, are intralobular (Fig. 21–16). The secretion first enters the intercalated ducts, which have a low cuboidal epithelium (Fig. 21–23A) and also have associated myoepithelial cells. Then it moves into the larger striated ducts, which are lined by a tall columnar epithelium that is distinctly acidophilic. This segment derives its name from the light-microscopic appearance of the basal cytoplasm of the columnar cells; parallel striations are created by the vertical orientation of mitochondria within numerous slender cytoplasmic compartments that are outlined by deep infoldings of the basal plasma membrane (Fig. 21–21). These basal cytoplasmic compartments represent interdigitating processes of adjacent cells, similar to those that occur in the distal tubule of the nephron. This specialization, which creates a vast basal surface area and associates it closely with energy-producing mitochondria (Fig. 21–22), is characteristic of other epithelia known to be involved in rapid transport of ions and water. Larger ducts, known as *interlobular ducts*, course through the stroma, become progressively larger, and finally join the primary duct that leads into the oral cavity. The interlobular ducts are initially simple columnar and then pseudostratified columnar with occasional goblet cells. The largest ducts are lined by stratified columnar epithelia (Fig. 21–23B), and those near the orifice usually consist of stratified squamous epithelium.

The salivary glands differ in the extent to which the intralobular ducts are developed. The intercalated ducts are longest in the parotid, and the striated ducts are best developed in the submandibular gland. Both types of intralobular

21–19 Section of the sublingual gland of a 30-year-old man. This is a black and white rendition of a color plate. Please see color section.

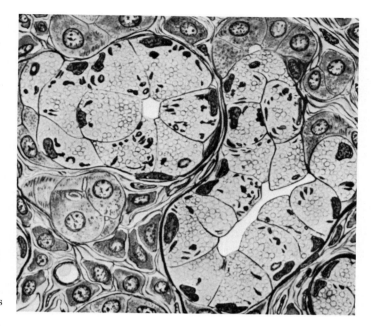

21–20 Human submandibular gland, serous cell, electron micrograph. Rough endoplasmic reticulum **(ER)** occurs in the basal cytoplasm. Secretory granules **(SG)** occupy most of the cell. A process of a myoepithelial cell **(M)** occurs between the serous cell and the basal lamina **(arrow). N,** nucleus. × 9,000. (Courtesy of Bernard Tandler.)

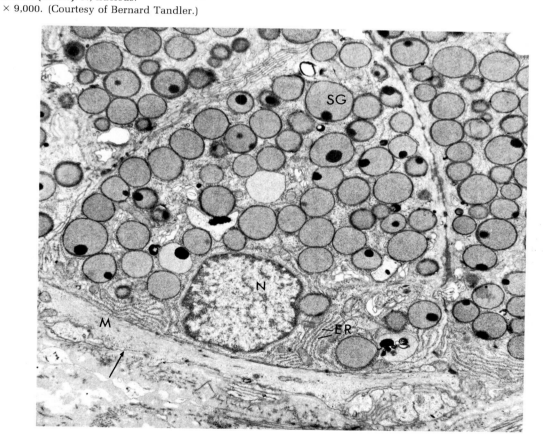

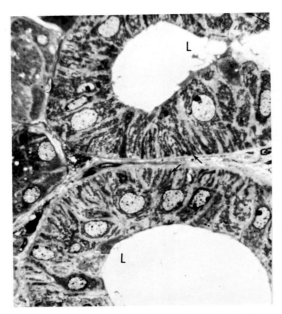

21-21 Human submandibular gland. Portions of two
striated ducts are shown. The basal striations
(arrows) created by parallel alignment of
mitochondria are evident. **L,** lumen. Toluidine blue;
1-μm section. × 1,300. (Courtesy of Bernard Tandler.)

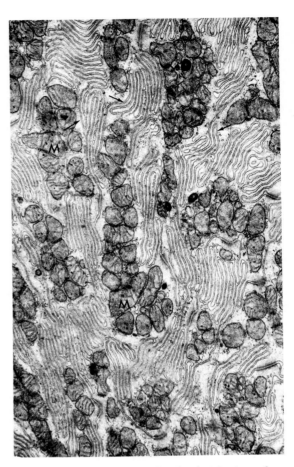

21-22 Human submandibular gland. A horizontal
section through the base of the striated duct
reveals the close association of mitochondria **(M)** with
infoldings of basal plasma membrane **(arrows).**
Electron micrograph. × 17,000. (Courtesy of Bernard
Tandler.)

ducts are quite inconspicuous in the sublingual
gland.

The connective tissue among the acini of the
salivary glands is a reticular connective tissue
that contains many plasma cells, some small
lymphocytes, and the usual stromal cells and fibers. In 1965, Tomasi and his associates demonstrated the presence of IgA in most of the plasma
cells in the interstitium of the human parotid
gland (via the fluorescent antibody technique).
Further work led to the following hypothesis:
IgA is produced in local plasma cells; it combines with a unique protein called the *secretory
piece,* which is believed to be produced by the
acinar epithelial cells; and then it is released
into the secretion as *secretory IgA,* which is resistant to proteolysis. Secretory IgA probably
plays an important role in the oral cavity in defense against pathogens. See Chap. 19 for a discussion of secretory immunoglobin.

The major blood vessels course through the
connective tissue, following the route of the large
branching ducts. Within the lobules, some arteries form rich capillary networks around the intralobular ducts, whereas other arterial branches

continue to create capillary plexuses around the
acini. The venous drainage retraces the arterial
pathway. An extensive system of lymphatic
drainage follows the course of the duct system.

Each major salivary gland is innervated by
both the parasympathetic and sympathetic divisions of the autonomic nervous system, and it is
generally agreed that secretory activity is mainly
under neural control. Stimulation of either the
sympathetic or parasympathetic innervation produces qualitatively different salivas. Parasympathetic stimulation produces a more voluminous saliva than does sympathetic (β-adrenergic)
activation, which causes secretion of a viscous

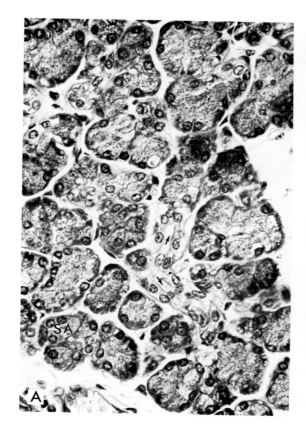

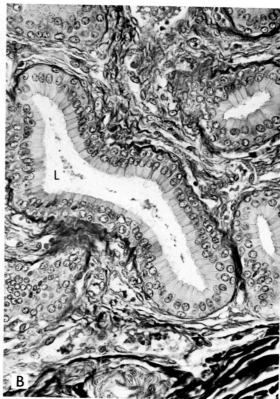

21–23 Portions of the duct system of salivary glands. **A.** The intercalated duct of the human parotid with a flattened simple epithelium. The **arrows** are within the lumen of the duct. **B.** A large excretory duct of the human sublingual lined with a two-layered stratified columnar epithelium. **L,** lumen.

protein-rich fluid. Ultrastructural observations on the cat submandibular gland indicate that terminations of both sympathetic and parasympathetic fibers are associated with the surface of one acinar cell (Hand, 1970). As illustrated in Fig. 21–24, autonomic nerve fibers penetrate the acinar basal lamina and acquire an intraepithelial position. A 20-nm space separates the surfaces of the neuronal and epithelial cells, as is typical of nerve terminals.

Summary of the Major Features of Human Salivary Glands

The parotid gland is almost purely serous (Figs. 21–17 and 21–23A). The secretory granules are PAS-positive, indicating that they contain a carbohydrate–protein polymer. The intercalated ducts are long and abundant, whereas the striated ducts are less elaborate.

The submandibular[1] gland (Fig. 21–18) is a mixed gland with seromucous acini and demilunes predominating over the purely mucous acini. The secretory granules of the serous cells are PAS-positive; they are rich in sialoglycoproteins although some cells contain sulfated polysaccharides. The mucous cells contain either sialomucin or sulfomucin or a mixture of both. The striated ducts are best developed in the submandibular gland; the intercalated ducts are present but less conspicuous.

The sublingual gland[1] is a mixed gland composed mainly of mucous acini, although there may be considerable variation in the proportion

---

[1]Portions of the human submandibular and sublingual glands intermingle in a manner that constitutes a gross submandibular sublingual complex (Leppi, 1967).

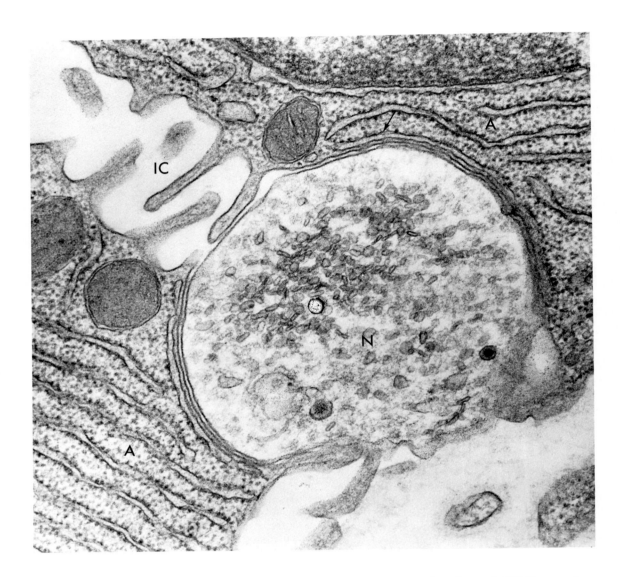

21–24 Intraepithelial autonomic nerve terminal **(N)** between two acinar cells **(A)** of the rat parotid gland. Note regions of close apposition between the surfaces of the nerve fiber and the secretory cells. A cisterna of endoplasmic reticulum **(arrows)** parallels the apposed surfaces. **IC,** intercellular space. × 57,000. (From Hand, A. R. 1970. J. Cell Biol. 47:540.)

of mucous to serous acini and demilunes in different regions of the gland (Fig. 21–19, see here and color insert). Sulfated polysaccharides are the major components of the abundant mucous secretion. The serous cells are rich in sulfated glycoproteins. Both segments (intercalated and striated ducts) of the intralobular duct system are poorly developed.

References and Selected Bibliography

The Exocrine Pancreas

Blobel, G., Walter, P., Chang, C. N., Goldman, B. M., Erickson, A. H., and Lingappa, V. R. 1979. Translocation of proteins across membranes: The signal hypothesis and beyond. *In* Secretory Mechanisms, Symposia of the Society for Experimental Biology, Vol. 33. Cambridge: Cambridge University Press, p. 9.

Herzog, V., and Farquhar, M. G. 1977. Luminal membrane retrieved after exocytosis reaches most Golgi cisternae. Proc. Natl. Acad. Sci. U.S.A. 74:5073.

Herzog, V., and Reggio. H. 1980. Pathways of endocytosis from luminal plasma membrane in rat exocrine pancreas. Eur. J. Cell Biol. 21:141.

Jamieson, J. D. 1975. Membranes and secretion. *In* G. Weissman and R. Claiborne, (eds.), Cell Membranes. H. P. Publishing Co., Inc., p. 143.

Jamieson, J. D., and Palade, G. E. Production of secretory proteins in animal cells. *In* R. B. Brinkley and K. R. Porter (eds.), International Cell Biology, 1976–1977. New York: The Rockefeller University Press, p. 308.

Kornfeld, R., and Kornfeld, S. 1980. Structure of glycoproteins and their oligosaccharide units. *In* W. J. Lennarz (ed.), The Biochemistry of Glycoproteins and Proteoglycans. New York: Plenum Press, p. 1.

LeBlond, C. P., and Bennett, G. 1977. Role of the Golgi apparatus in terminal glycosylation. *In* R. B. Brinkley and K. R. Porter (eds.), International Cell Biology, 1976–1977. New York: The Rockefeller University Press, p. 326.

Maylié-Pfenninger, M. F., and Jamieson, J. D. 1980. Development of cell surface saccharides on embryonic pancreatic cells. J. Cell Biol. 86:96.

Palade, G. E. 1975. Intracellular aspects of the process of protein secretion. Science (Wash., D. C.) 189:347.

Pictet, R., and Rutter, W. J. 1972. Development of the embryonic endocrine pancreas. *In* D. Steiner and N. Freinkel (eds.), Handbook of Physiology, Vol. 1. Baltimore: The Williams and Wilkins Company, p. 25.

Reggio, H. A., and Palade, G. E. 1978. Sulfated compounds in the zymogen granules of the guinea pig pancreas. J. Cell Biol. 77:288.

Struck, D. K., and Lennarz, W. J. 1980. The function of saccharide-lipids in synthesis of glycoproteins. *In* W. J. Lennarz (ed.), The Biochemistry of Glycoproteins and Proteoglycans. New York: Plenum Press, p. 35.

Salivary Glands

Amsterdam, A., Ohad, I., and Schramm, M. 1969. Dynamic changes in the ultrastructure of the acinar cell of the rat parotid gland during the secretory cycle. J. Cell Biol. 41:753.

Castle, J. D., Jamieson, J. D., and Palade, G. E. 1972. Radioautographic analysis of the secretory process in the parotid acinar cell of the rabbit. J. Cell Biol. 53:290.

Hand, A. R. 1970. Nerve–acinar cell relationships in the rat parotid gland. J. Cell Biol. 47:540.

Leeson, C. R. 1967. Structure of salivary glands. *In* C. F. Code and W. Heidel (eds.), Handbook of Physiology, Vol. 2, Sec. 6. Washington, D. C.: American Physiological Society, chap. 1.

Leppi, T. J. 1967. Gross anatomical relationships between primate submandibular and sublingual salivary glands. J. Dent. Res. 46:359.

Leppi, T. J., and Spicer, S. S. 1966. The histochemistry of mucins in certain primate salivary glands. Am. J. Anat. 118:833.

Munger, B. L. 1964. Histochemical studies on seromucous- and mucous-secreting cells of human salivary glands. Am. J. Anat. 115:411.

Strum, J. M., and Karnovsky, M. J. 1970. Ultrastructural localization of peroxidase in submaxillary acinar cells. J. Ultrastruct. Res. 31:323.

Tamarin, A. 1966. Myoepithelium of the rat submaxillary gland. J. Ultrastruct. Res. 16:320.

Tandler, B. 1962. Ultrastructure of the human submaxillary gland. I. Architecture and histological relationships of the secretory cell. Am. J. Anat. 111:287.

Islets of Langerhans

G. Eric Bauer

Gross Structure

The endocrine tissue of the pancreas is scattered throughout the gland in ovoid clusters of cells called the islets of Langerhans. Each pancreatic islet is composed of a few to several hundred hormone-producing cells and is demarcated from the surrounding acini by a delicate investment of reticular fibers. Most of the islets are between 100 and 200 μm in diameter. Although the distribution of islets is nearly random, the lobules of the tail (splenic portion) of the gland tend to have the highest islet concentration.

There is an average of 500,000 islets in the adult human pancreas, and collectively they make up 1 to 2% of the gland by volume. In routinely stained sections, the islets are paler and their cells smaller than the acinar cells. The islet parenchyma itself is arranged in irregular cords of polyhedral endocrine cells that follow the tortuous course of an abundant capillary bed.

The major cell types of the islets of Langerhans were described originally on the basis of special staining procedures and differential solubilities of stored components (Fig. 22–1, see here and color insert). Three endocrine cells were named: A (alpha), B (beta), and D (delta) cells. However, more recent studies based on hormone content have shown the presence of additional endocrine cell types. A small number of nongranulated clear (C) cells also were described within islets, but their significance remains unknown.

The B cells are the most numerous of the islet cells and, although their numbers vary widely

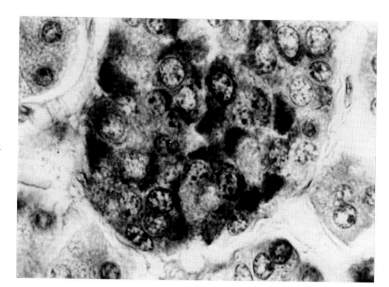

22–1 Photomicrograph of a human pancreatic islet. This is a black and white rendition of a color plate. See color section.

among individual islets, they usually constitute about 70% of the total endocrine tissue. The A cell in humans represents 15 to 20% and the D cell, 5 to 10% of the tissue. The other islet endocrine cells collectively total about 5% of the endocrine tissue. In humans and rodents, the B cells tend to be located centrally in the islet, whereas the other cells lie in a peripheral mantle, or cortex, two or three cell layers in thickness. In human islets, large vascular channels often penetrate the central mass of B cells, bringing with them a sleeve of A and D cells (Fig. 22–2). In some animals, like the horse and monkey, the A and D cells occupy the central core of the islet, and in others, like the dog and several teleost fish, the A, B, and D cells are fairly randomly

distributed within the islet. In addition to hormone-producing cells, the islets contain small numbers of fibroblasts, pericytes, and other connective tissue cells related to the capillaries; these supporting tissues occupy about 10% of the islet volume. Autonomic nerve fibers enter the islets to innervate the parenchyma and its vasculature. Lymphatics of the islet tissue have not been described.

Histogenesis of Pancreatic Islets

The pancreas arises in the human embryo at about the fourth week of gestation as two separate evaginations of the foregut entoderm. During rotation of the gut, the ventral and dorsal pancreatic primordia, with their surrounding mesoderm, fuse to form the head, body, and tail of the pancreas. The primary ducts, which are extensions of the duodenal epithelium, continue to elongate and produce numerous secondary branches of decreasing caliber. The larger ducts persist as the pancreatic excretory ducts, whereas the smaller ones give rise to acinar and islet cells. These cells arise by differentiating from progenitor cells within the ductular epithelium. The definitive A cells first appear at about 9 weeks, whereas D and B cells are observed at the tenth to eleventh week of development. The adult arrangement of islet cells appears soon after their emergence. Many islets detach from the ductules; others maintain their connections throughout life.

22–2 Drawing of the arrangement of endocrine cells typical of rat **(left)** and human islets **(right)**. Large vascular septa invaginate the central core of B cells **(stippled)** in many human islets. A cells, **filled circles**; D cells, **triangles**; PP cells, **open circles**. (Courtesy of S. L. Erlandsen.)

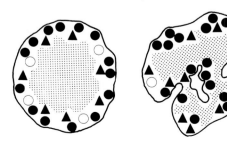

Islet cells possess a definite but limited capacity to regenerate, but the mechanism involved in this regeneration is unknown. Because some islets remain attached to the ductules from which they sprang, it may be that some of the ductule cells in the adult differentiate into islet cells (a process called nesidioblastosis) in response to stimuli such as prolonged hyperglycemia. Another possible source of islet regeneration is from differentiated islet cells themselves. Although cell division is rare in adult islet tissue, stressful stimuli such as chemical injury or prolonged hyperglycemia reportedly increase mitotic activity in the islets. Finally, hybrid cells containing both B-cell secretory vesicles and zymogen granules sometimes occur in areas where islet and acinar cells adjoin. These acinar-islet cells also are extremely rare; it is not known if they contribute substantially to the renewal of islet endocrine tissue.

An entirely different origin for islet endocrine cells has been proposed on the basis of the observation that epithelial cells, presumably of neural crest derivation, migrate into the pancreatic primordia and reside in the entodermal epithelium during development of the pancreas. These neuroectodermal progenitor cells, rather than entodermal cells, may later differentiate into the islet endocrine cells. This proposed mechanism accounts for several similarities among secretory cells of diverse origins and sites throughout the organism. For example, islet cells and other peptide-secreting endocrine cells as well as neurosecretory cells in the central and peripheral nervous systems accumulate, metabolize, and secrete biogenic amines (such as serotonin and dopamine), which places them all in the APUD (amine precursor uptake and decarboxylation) system of cells (see Chap. 29). Despite the appeal of this unifying theory, however, experiments to demonstrate directly the origin of islet cells from the neuroectoderm have not supported the concept. Until such support is obtained, the islet cells are considered to be entodermally derived.

Regional variations may occur in the cellular composition of islets from different areas of the pancreas. In the human, for example, the islets in the body and tail have the usual ratios of B, A, and D cells, and they are relatively poor in PP cells.[1] The ratios may be described as B > A >

D >> PP. However, islets in the posterior half of the head have fewer B and D cells, few or no A cells, and numerous PP cells (B > PP >> D > A). These regional differences in composition probably reflect the origin of the islets: The PP-rich islets are derived from the ventral pancreatic primordium, whereas the ordinary islets originate from the dorsal primordium.

Islet Cell Morphology

The endocrine cells of the islets of Langerhans can be differentiated most readily by the comparative morphology and hormone contents of their secretory vesicles. The most powerful tool for identifying them is electron microscopy correlated with immunocytochemistry.

Histologically, the B cell is identified by its affinity for selective stains such as aldehyde fuchsin and pseudoisocyanin (which are believed to bind to insulin stored within the secretory vesicles) and by its reactivity with anti-insulin serum (Fig. 22–1, see here and color insert, and Fig. 22–3). Ultrastructurally, the B cell is characterized by its numerous secretory vesicles (about 300 nm in diameter) containing a moderately electron-dense core that in humans is composed of rhomboidal or polygonal crystalloids (Fig. 22–4); this core has a subunit crystal periodicity believed to represent insoluble insulin. A finer granular material fills the space between the core and the limiting unit membrane of the vesicle. Other insulin secretory vesicles, sometimes within the same B cell, may contain a homogeneous spherical core exhibiting no subunit structure. These two types of granules are thought to be different stages in the maturation of insulin secretory vesicles. In pancreata of other vertebrates, the central cores vary in apparent shape as spheres, plates, rosettes, or rhomboidal crystalloids depending on the species. The reality and functional significance of high concentrations of zinc in insulin secretory vesicles, originally identified by histochemical procedures, have been questioned recently (see Figlewicz et al., 1980).

The nucleus, rough endoplasmic reticulum (RER), free polysomes, and other cytoplasmic details are not readily distinguishable from similar components of other islet endocrine cells. However, the mitochondria of the B cell are said to be nearly spherical and more numerous than those of the A cell, and the Golgi apparatus is more extensive in the B cell. The RER is sparse in islet cells compared with the rich RER in aci-

---

[1]These distinctive endocrine cells contain a pancreatic peptide (PP). They are described in the section on Islet Cell Morphology.

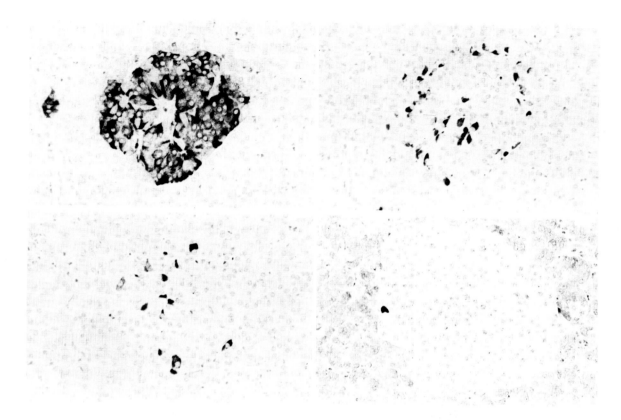

22–3 Semiadjacent sections of islet of Langerhans from adult human pancreas stained with antisera against insulin **(upper left)**, glucagon **(upper right)**, somatostatin **(lower left)**, and, in an adjacent islet, pancreatic polypeptide **(lower right)**. The antibody–antigen complexes in each section were visualized by coupling to peroxidase–antiperoxidase (PAP) and subsequent reaction with 3,3′-diaminobenzidine (DAB). Hematoxylin counterstain. × 250. (Courtesy of S. L. Erlandsen.)

nar cells. When suitably fixed for electron microscopy, the islet cells display microtubules and microfilaments within the cytoplasm, especially near the capillary pole of the cell. In the B cell, a submembranous web of microfilaments can be observed; microtubules are arrayed in association with the insulin secretory vesicles. Both cytoplasmic components are believed to participate in hormone exocytosis.

The A cell is identified by its affinity for phosphotungstic acid, argyrophilia by the Grimelius technique (staining by silver impregnation), and reactivity with antiglucagon serum. Recent immunocytochemical studies suggest that, in addition to glucagon, the A cell may produce other peptides such as gastric inhibitory peptide (GIP), cholecystokinin-pancreozymin (CCK), and ACTH–endorphin. Filamentous mitochondria, a small Golgi apparatus, and the RER are evident. The nucleus of the A cell often appears indented or lobulated. Closely packed secretory vesicles of generally uniform diameter (about 250 nm) also characterize the A cell. These vesicles have an eccentrically placed core of high electron density embedded in a matrix of less dense material, closely surrounded, in turn, by the limiting vesi-

cle membrane. Of the staining procedures used to demonstrate A cells at the ultrastructural level, phosphotungstic acid has been localized to the dense core, whereas silver salts precipitate in the paler matrix. Also, the dense-core granule binds glucagon antibodies, indicating that it is the site of stored glucagon (Figs. 22–3 and 22–5).

In humans, the D (type III) cells are somewhat larger than A cells and usually are located in the vicinity of A cells. The D cell was formerly believed to represent a stage in the maturation or degeneration of other islet cells, but its existence as an independent hormone-producing cell is now established. Histologically, secretory vesicles of the D cell stain blue with the Mallory

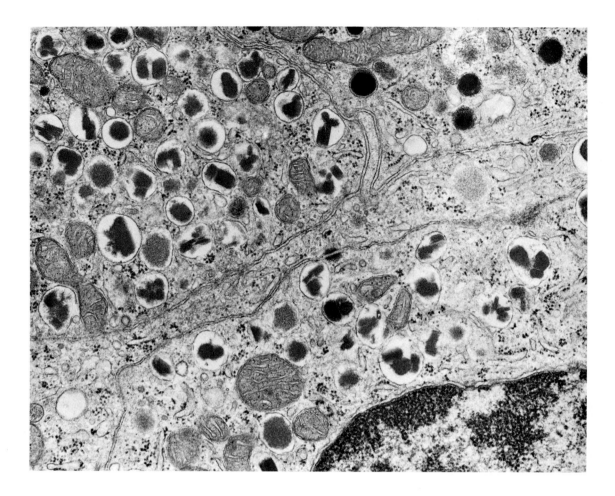

22–4 Electron micrograph of portions of several endocrine cells from adult human islet. Two B cells containing membrane-bound secretory vesicles with crystalline cores, and a few with amorphous cores, are illustrated. A portion of an A cell is present in the upper right. A desmosome, one of the cell junctions between islet cells, is seen near the center of the figure. × 30,000. (Courtesy of A. A. Like.)

azan stain. Ultrastructurally, the secretory vesicles are variable in size, but they are usually larger than A and B vesicles and show a fine granular matrix of low or medium electron density. The granular matrix is homogeneous and almost completely fills the vesicle. These vesicles are the intracellular storage site of somatostatin (Figs. 22–3 and 22–6).

A subpopulation of D cells (exhibiting argyrophilia by Grimelius's silver technique), named the D_1 or type IV cell, contains relatively small (150–200 nm) secretory vesicles with a homogeneous granular interior and narrow electron-lucent space. Immunoreactive vasoactive intestinal peptide (VIP) has been localized to the secretory vesicles of this cell. The D_1 cells are smaller than D cells, are ovoid or comma-shaped, and often have thin cytoplasmic processes. They occur as single cells scattered throughout the islet and are found occasionally among the exocrine cells.

Recently, the PP or F cell (Figs. 22–3 and 22–7) has been described in human islets and in

22–6 Electron micrograph of portion of a D cell from fetal human islet, showing membrane-bound secretory vesicles with homogeneous matrix of low or medium electron density. Profiles of Golgi apparatus are seen. The relative sizes of D vesicles can be compared with vesicles of A cell at the right of the figure. × 25,000. (Courtesy of A. A. Like.)

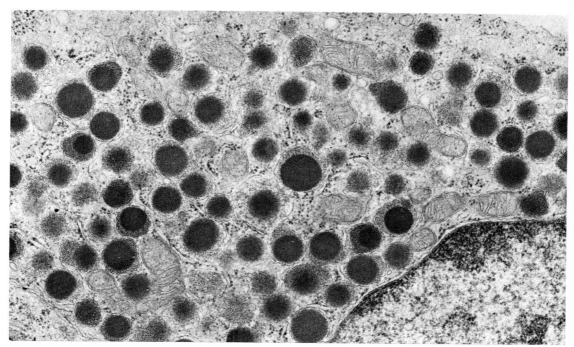

22–5 Electron micrograph of portion of an A cell from adult human islet. The membrane-bound secretory vesicles contain an eccentric dense core embedded in a moderately dense matrix. × 31,000. (Courtesy of A. A. Like.)

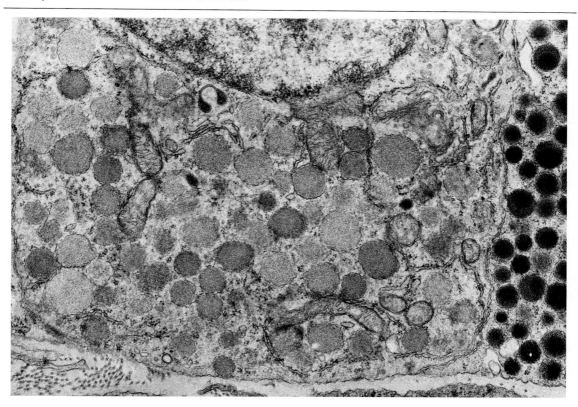

780

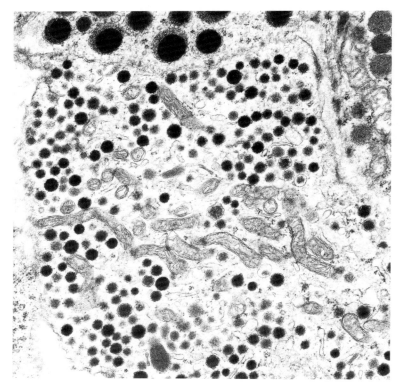

22–7 Electron micrograph of portion of a PP cell from adult human islet, showing small membrane-bound secretory vesicles with homogeneous matrix of variable density. Compare size of PP vesicles with those of adjoining A cell at top of figure. × 20,000. (Courtesy of A. A. Like, 1980, *In* J. Rassan, R. Girard, and E. B. Marliss [eds.], Diabetes Mellitus: A Pathophysiologic Approach to Clinical Practice. New York: John Wiley & Sons.)

Table 22–1 Cell Types and Characteristics of Islets of Langerhans

Islet endocrine cell name with synonyms	Staining affinities	Structure of secretory vesicle	Hormone localization by immunocytochemistry[a]
A, alpha, α_2	Argyrophilic,[b] red (Mallory azan)	Dense, eccentric, spherical core in paler matrix; about 250 nm diameter	*Glucagon* gastric inhibitory peptide (GIP) Cholecystokinin (CCK) ACTH–endorphin
B, beta	Magenta (aldehyde fuchsin), brownish orange (Mallory azan)	Moderately dense, polyhedral core in paler matrix; about 300 nm diameter	*Insulin*
D, delta, type III, α_1	Blue (Mallory azan)	Pale homogeneous matrix of variable density, 300–350 nm diameter	*Somatostatin* (SRIF)
D_1, type IV	Argyrophilic[b]	Pale homogeneous matrix, 150–200 nm diameter	Vasoactive intestinal peptide (VIP)
EC, enterochromaffin	Argentaffinic[c]	Markedly pleomorphic vesicles, 175–400 nm	5-HT (serotonin), motilin, substance P
PP, F, X	—	Slightly pleomorphic, pale homogeneous matrix of variable density; 150–200 nm diameter	*Pancreatic polypeptide* (PP)

[a]Italicized hormones are known to be secreted by the cells, whereas others have been identified in cells by immunocytochemistry alone. Peptide hormones such as secretin and thyroid releasing factor (TRF) have been detected in islet extracts by immunoassay but not localized to an endocrine cell.

[b]Argyrophilic by Grimelius's silver impregnation.

[c]Silver staining without reduction of tissue.

islets from fish, birds, and other mammals. It is identified by its content of small-diameter (140–200 nm) secretory vesicles, with homogeneous granular cores that react with antibodies to human pancreatic polypeptide (PP). Unlike the other endocrine cells that generally are confined to the islet parenchyma, the PP cell often is associated with acinar cells and also is found within epithelia of small- and medium-sized pancreatic ducts.

An intraislet source of gastrin has been documented by some investigators but denied by others. Although immunoreactive gastrin has been extracted from islets, and gastrin-secreting tumors of human pancreatic islet tissue occur in the Zollinger-Ellison syndrome, no unequivocal evidence exists for the presence of gastrin-producing (G) cells in adult human islets. Therefore, the major site of G cells in humans is considered to be in the stomach and small intestine.

The enterochromaffin (EC) cells, which occur infrequently in the islet parenchyma, are more

typical of the gut endocrine system and are described in Chap. 19.

The cell types of the pancreatic islets are summarized in Table 22–1. Considerable diversity exists in the naming of the endocrine cells of the pancreatic islet and gastrointestinal mucosa because uniform criteria have not always been applied in describing them. The identity of the various cells in this system and their hormonal products will undoubtedly be modified after further evaluation by modern immunocytochemical and electron-microscopic methods.

Blood Supply and Innervation of the Pancreatic Islets

The arterial blood supply of the pancreatic islets is derived from the celiac and superior mesenteric arteries. Branches of these vessels form interlobular and intralobular arteries within the pancreas (Fig. 22–8). The intralobular arteries

22–8 Drawing of pancreatic A cell **(left)** and B cells **(right)** adjoining a capillary **(CAP)**, illustrating the relationship of the endocrine cells to one another and to their blood supply. Both the fenestrated endothelium and islet cells possess basal laminae, through which nutrients (e.g., glucose) and hormonal products (e.g., insulin) pass. The islet cells have specialized cell junctions, such as desmosomes **(MA)** and gap junctions **(GJ).** This A cell is innervated by an unmyelinated nerve fiber. Also illustrated are the events in the secretory cycle of the B cell. A nutrient stimulus (blood glucose) binds to hypothetical glucoreceptor in the B-cell membrane, which leads to increased flux of calcium ions and increased synthesis of cyclic AMP by membrane-bound adenylate cyclase.

These events activate the microtubule-dependent migration of secretory vesicles from the Golgi apparatus **(GA)** and facilitate the fusion of secretory vesicle membranes with the plasma membrane. Micropinocytotic vesicles **(MV)** return membrane to the lysosomes **(LYS)** and Golgi apparatus for recycling. Preproinsulin synthesis in the RER is stimulated also by glucose. The signal peptide **(SP)** is cleaved in the RER, and the resulting proinsulin (A + B + C) is taken by transport vesicles **(TV)** to the Golgi apparatus, where cleavage of proinsulin to insulin begins. The secretory vesicles store the insulin (A + B) and C-peptide **(C)** prior to exocytosis. Occasional crinophagy **(CR)** of secretory vesicles occurs (center cell). **MF,** microfilamentous web.

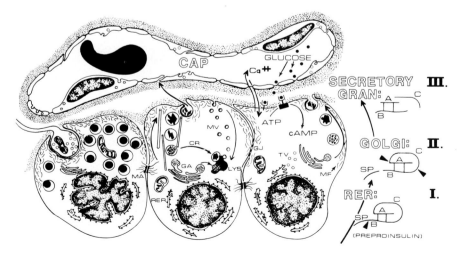

contribute one or more arterioles (the vas afferens) to each islet. This vessel enters the mantle and supplies first the A and D cells and then the centrally located B cells via an extensive capillary network. The endothelium of the islet capillary wall is continuous, but the endothelial cells contain numerous fenestrations 50 nm in diameter that facilitate exchange of materials between the endocrine cells and the blood. Several capillaries (vasa efferentia) radiate from the islet to supply the periacinar capillary network of the exocrine pancreas. Thus a large fraction of the arterial blood to the pancreas first supplies the islet parenchyma. By this arrangement, islet hormones may interact with other islet cells and then be distributed to the acinar tissue in very high concentrations.

Unmyelinated efferent nerve terminals of both the sympathetic and the parasympathetic division of the autonomic nervous system have been observed in close association with islet endocrine cells. Because only 10% or fewer of the islet endocrine cells seem to receive direct innervation, it is assumed that cell junctions between islet cells serve to spread the ionic changes resulting from autonomic nerve stimuli from innervated to noninnervated cells. Innervation of blood vessels in the islet also has been documented, and this nerve input may function in controlling the rate of perfusion of the capillary bed.

Hormones of the Islets of Langerhans

Hormone Identities

Because of both the growing number of recognized peptide hormones localized to the islet cells and the complexity of the biological effects of these peptides, a brief description of them is offered here. As shown in Table 22–2, many islet cells have structural and functional counterparts in the gastrointestinal endocrine system, which has led to their being grouped into a so-called gastroenteropancreatic endocrine system. The interrelationship of these endocrine cells extends to their origin and development. Phylogenetically, the islet cells seem to be derived from epithelial cells of the gut mucosa; embryologically, the islet cells differentiate from the foregut entoderm by way of the dorsal and ventral pancreatic primordia. Table 22–2 also shows that all islet cells are represented somewhere in the gut mucosa with the exception of the B cell, which resides only in the pancreatic islets. Recently, the existence of two forms of glucagon (pancreatic glucagon, and gut glucagon or enteroglucagon) has been established. These closely related peptides, which can be differentiated immunologically, are synthesized and secreted by two different cell types. Pancreatic glucagon-producing A cells are found in the gastric antrum and

Table 22–2 Distribution and Hormone Products of Human Gastroenteropancreatic (GEP) Endocrine Cells[a]

| Islets of Langerhans[b] | Stomach[b] | Intestines[b] | | Hormone |
		Small	Large	
A	A			Glucagon (and GIP, CCK, ACTH–endorphin in islet A cell)
B				Insulin
D	D	D	D	Somatostatin (SRIF)
D_1	D_1	D_1	D_1	Vasoactive intestinal peptide (VIP)
EC	EC	EC	EC	5-HT, substance P (EC_1), motilin (EC_2)
PP	(PP)	(PP)	(PP)	Pancreatic polypeptide (PP)
(G)	G	G		Gastrin
		I		Cholecystokinin (CCK)
		K		Gastric inhibitory peptide (GIP)
		L	L	Enteroglucagon (gut glucagon)
		N		Neurotensin
(P)	P	P		Bombesin
		S		Secretin

[a]Modified from Lausanne, 1977 classification; see Bloom, S. R. (ed.), 1978, Gut Hormones. New York: Churchill Livingston.
[b]Parentheses denote that cell is normally found in this organ only in human fetuses or in some animals.

the pancreatic islets, whereas enteroglucagon-producing L cells are found only in the intestines.

The B cell produces insulin; quantitatively and functionally it is the major hormone synthesized and secreted by the islet tissue. Insulin stimulates the uptake and utilization of sugars by target tissues (e.g., liver, adipose tissue, and skeletal muscle). One of its primary actions is at the cell membrane, where it enhances the transport of glucose into the cell and stimulates phosphorylation of glucose by glucokinase. Insulin also selectively activates glycogen synthase and other glucose metabolic enzymes. Its overall effect is to lower blood sugar by favoring the storage and utilization of energy substrates. Also, it is regarded as an anabolic hormone because it stimulates protein and triglyceride synthesis in some target tissues.

The major A-cell hormone is glucagon, a linear polypeptide of 29 amino acids (MW 3,500) that opposes the overall effects of insulin. In the liver it stimulates glycogenolysis by initiating the cascade of events leading to activation of glycogen phosphorylase. Glucagon is both a catabolic hormone, in that it affects proteolysis, and a gluconeogenic hormone in that it stimulates the synthesis of glucose. It also stimulates hepatic lipase activity and fat mobilization in adipose tissue.

The other recently identified peptides in the islet A cell have hormonal activities, but their secretion and roles in A-cell physiology have not been clearly demonstrated. The presence of ACTH–endorphin immunoreactivity, originally described in the central nervous system, is puzzling. The exact nature of this peptide antigen is not revealed by its immunocytochemical reactivity, because both ACTH (corticotropin) and endorphin are synthesized (e.g., in the hypophyseal B_1 basophil) as part of a common precursor called proACTH/LPH or propiocortin. It is known that during posttranslational processing in the hypophysis this precursor protein is cleaved to yield several biologically active peptides, including ACTH and endorphin. It is possible that in the islet A cell, also, a similar large precursor is synthesized that accounts for the ACTH and endorphin activities.

Apparently, the major hormone of the islet D cell is somatostatin, a peptide of 14 amino acids that is identical to hypothalamic somatostatin. It was first described as a somatotropic hormone release-inhibiting factor (SRIF), but in the islet it is believed to inhibit the secretion of insulin and glucagon.

The D_1 cell produces VIP, a linear peptide containing 28 amino acids. Vasoactive intestinal peptide resembles glucagon in its hyperglycemic and glycogenolytic properties, but it also participates in the regulation of motor tone, motility, and secretory activity of the gastrointestinal tract.

The PP cell produces pancreatic polypeptide, a 36-amino-acid linear peptide of molecular weight 4,200. This newly characterized hormone stimulates gastric enzyme secretion but inhibits bile secretion and intestinal motility.

Many islet hormones may directly or indirectly influence the activity of pancreatic acinar cells. Insulin, CCK, and VIP have stimulatory effects, whereas glucagon, pancreatic polypeptide, and somatostatin inhibit pancreatic exocrine secretion.

Secretion of Islet Hormones

The secretion (biosynthesis, intracellular transport, and release) of islet hormones resembles in major respects the mechanisms described for proteins in the acinar pancreas. Although we have some information on these events for glucagon and somatostatin, more is known about insulin secretion (see Fig. 22–8).

The insulin molecule (MW 6,000) consists of two polypeptides (the A and B chains), which are joined by disulfide bridges between cysteine residues of the two chains. Insulin is synthesized on polysomes of the RER by way of a polypeptide intermediate called preproinsulin, which is considerably larger (MW 12,000) than insulin. The initial portion of this precursor (an N-terminal sequence of about 25 amino acids) serves as a signal for directing the transport of the growing polypeptide from the polysome across the membrane and into the cisternal space of the endoplasmic reticulum. While the signal sequence is transversing the membrane it is removed by an enzyme called signal peptidase. The resulting polypeptide, proinsulin (MW 9,000), accumulates in the RER and then is carried within small transport vesicles to the region of the Golgi apparatus, where it is packaged into the larger secretory vesicles. A connecting (or C) peptide of 35 amino acids, which extends from the C-terminus of the B chain (30 amino acids) to the N-terminus of the A chain (21 amino acids), is cleaved by a cathepsin-like enzyme within the Golgi apparatus and maturing secretory vesicles. Most of the insulin within the B cell is stored in these secretory vesicles before release by exocytosis. Crinophagy, whereby lysosomes fuse with secretory vesicles and destroy their contents, is the occasional alternate fate of some secretory vesicles.

The connecting peptide of proinsulin, which undergoes limited proteolysis after its removal from insulin, also is stored within the secretory vesicles in concentrations equimolar to insulin. A small amount of proinsulin, which apparently escapes cleavage to insulin, accumulates within secretory vesicles and subsequently is secreted into the blood with insulin (and C peptide) during exocytosis. During exocytosis in the B cell, the secretory vesicle membrane fuses with the plasma membrane and the vesicle contents are consequently released.

The discharge or release of islet hormones appears to be stringently regulated by various stimuli (see below). Although probably all the islet endocrine cells adjoin a capillary wall, the secreted peptide hormones must traverse several barriers on their way to the capillary lumen. These barriers include the islet cell basal lamina, a pericapillary space, and the capillary basal lamina. However, no barrier extends between neighboring islet cells, a situation that allows the various endocrine cells to establish cell junctions (tight junctions, gap junctions, and desmosomes). The gap junctions observed between islet cells may interconnect them into a functional syncitium whereby chemical information is quickly transmitted from one cell to another.

The Control of Islet Hormone Secretion

All of the hormones known to be secreted by the pancreatic islet act in some capacity on the uptake, distribution, and utilization of nutrients. The factors regulating the secretion of islet hormones are (1) the concentrations of nutrients (e.g., sugars, fatty acids, and amino acids) in the blood, (2) the activity of the autonomic nervous system, and (3) other islet and gastrointestinal hormones that, beyond their effects on the nutrient metabolism of target cells throughout the body, have profound effects on the secretory activity of neighboring endocrine cells. The interaction of these regulatory factors with the islet cells provides the organism with a highly responsive mechanism for controlling the release of its hormones.

A catalog of the regulatory factors in islet hormone secretion will not be presented here, but we shall instead provide examples of how the secretion of insulin and glucagon are regulated. The rate and magnitude of insulin and glucagon release are sensitive to the concentrations of nutrients in the blood. That nutrients exert their effects directly on the A and B cells is shown by in vitro experiments using either an isolated pancreas, or isolated islets incubated in perfusion chambers or maintained in organ culture. For example, when the glucose concentration is raised above the normal blood levels (about 70 mg/100 ml), the secretion of insulin by the B cell is stimulated. High levels of glucose have an opposite, inhibitory, effect on glucagon secretion by the A cell. Fatty acids also shown reciprocal effects on the release of these hormones. The effects of amino acids may seem paradoxical, since both hormones are secreted in response to amino acids such as arginine and leucine.

The autonomic nervous system helps to regulate insulin and glucagon secretion, as shown by nerve-stimulation and extirpation experiments and by studies using drugs that mimic or inhibit the effects of neurotransmitters. A and B cells have parasympathetic (cholinergic) and sympathetic (adrenergic) receptors. Stimulation of the vagus (parasympathetic) nerve apparently elicits secretion of both insulin and glucagon, whereas splanchnic (sympathetic) nerve impulses result in the inhibition of insulin release and in augmentation of glucagon release. Insulin release is augmented by parasympathetic input during vegetative activities such as feeding. During stress (when the sympathetic nervous system is activated) the release of glucagon is maximally stimulated, where insulin release is suppressed.

The hormones of islet tissue are thought to exert short-range (paracrine) control over their own secretion. Insulin inhibits the release of glucagon from the A cell, whereas glucagon stimulates the secretion of insulin from the B cell. Somatostatin inhibits the release of both insulin and glucagon.

Specific receptors for the factors controlling insulin secretion are thought to be present on the plasma membrane of the B cell. A glucoreceptor, leucine receptor, and cholinergic and adrenergic receptors all have been postulated as the binding sites for chemical signals that serve to activate the insulin secretory response. The receptor theory proposes that a specific regulatory agent (glucose) binds to a specific B-cell receptor, an event that triggers a generalized response mechanism culminating in the exocytotic release of insulin. Alternatively, a metabolite theory proposes that glucose itself, or one of its metabolites, controls insulin release. Whatever the specific signal, the exocytosis of insulin involves: (1) a cytoplasmic system of mictotubules that, when activated, propels the secretory vesicle toward the plasma membrane; (2) a calcium transport system involved in the vesicle marginalization process; (3) an adenylate cyclase–phosphodiesterase enzyme system to generate and destroy cyclic AMP, which also may mediate vesicle movement by activating protein phosphorylation reactions; and (4) a subplasma membrane barrier of microfilaments that, when signalled to disperse, allows secretory vesicle–plasma membrane fusion.

Glucose, the most potent of the physiological nutrient regulators of insulin secretion, controls many other metabolic processes in the B cell. For example, the synthesis of insulin is stimulated by glucose at the transcriptional level (mRNA synthesis) and at the site of mRNA translation (the initiation step in the reading of mRNA by the polysomes). Glucose also enhances tubulin synthesis and turnover in the B cell. How the glucose signal is transduced to control these nuclear and cytoplasmic events is not yet known.

Histopathology of the Islets of Langerhans

Diabetes Mellitus

Several metabolic disorders result from disturbances in islet cell function; of them, diabetes mellitus is the most severe and epidemiologically important. About 10 million people suffer from this disorder in the United States alone. Diabetes mellitus is a family of diseases that result from the improper uptake of sugar from the blood and its subsequent utilization by the cells of the body, usually because of a deficiency in the level of circulating insulin. The islet B cells are almost always involved, by being functionally deficient, numerically reduced, or, in severe cases, totally absent. The remaining islet endocrine cells often proliferate in the diabetic state, thus exacerbating the condition. Other less common conditions that result in diabetes mellitus are (1) resistance of peripheral (target) cells to circulating insulin and (2) production of abnormal insulin or proinsulin by the B cell.

Variations in onset, severity, and complications of diabetes have led to the recognition of at least two different diseases. Growth-onset (insulin-dependent) diabetes is life-threatening, strikes suddenly during childhood or early adulthood, and requires insulin injection therapy. Few, if any, B cells survive the acute initial phase of the disease. Maturity-onset (noninsulin-dependent) diabetes, on the other hand, may be a less severe disorder; it is manageable by diet, drugs, and exercise, and may go undetected clinically.

Although definite genetic susceptibilities to diabetes exist, the inheritance of the trait still is poorly understood. Certainly, environmental factors sometimes trigger the onset of symptoms. For example, some infections caused by mumps, rubella, and Coxsackie viruses are thought to precipitate diabetes in genetically susceptible individuals by causing B-cell necrosis.

Primary diabetes mellitus was a grave and often fatal disease until insulin was successfully isolated from animal pancreata by Banting and Best in 1922. With the subsequent introduction of insulin injection therapy, diabetic coma and death are now preventable, but the secondary complications of diabetes, which are largely related to blood vessel diseases, remain. Among the complications of small blood vessels (microangiopathies) in long-standing diabetes is diabetic retinopathy, currently a leading cause of blindness. Another such complication is diabetic nephropathy, a specific renal disease involving destruction of nephrons, the treatment of which ultimately requires renal dialysis or kidney transplantation to sustain life. The macroangiopathies associated with diabetes are the greater tendencies to develop atherosclerosis, heart attacks, stroke, and peripheral vascular disease leading to gangrene.

Experimental Studies. Current research on the causes, management, and treatment of diabetes and its complications is extremely active and varied, and we shall mention only several examples here.

The genetic etiology of diabetes is being studied in human populations and in animal models in which diabetes either develops spontaneously or is induced by diabetogenic drugs such as alloxan or streptozotocin. Environmental factors, such as viral infections, stress, and hormonal imbalances are being evaluated to find methods for preventing the disease in genetically susceptible individuals. The pathology of blood vessels and the nervous tissue in diabetes is under investigation in attempts to understand and perhaps prevent the debilitating sequelae of the disorder. Because the wide fluctuations in blood sugar that inevitably occur even in diabetics under careful control with insulin therapy are thought to lead to the secondary complications of diabetes, many investigators are working to develop treatments that supply insulin in response to ambient blood sugar levels. Two current approaches offering some hope of success are the artificial pancreas, a device that monitors the patient's blood sugar and mechanically delivers appropriate infusions of insulin as required, and pancreatic or islet transplantation, in which cadaver islet tissue is introduced into the immunosuppressed patient. Finally, much work is being done on the structure, cytochemistry, and physiology of normal pancreatic islets, work that will provide a fuller understanding of this complex organ.

References and Selected Bibliography

General References on the Pancreatic Islets

Bloom, S. R. (ed.). 1978. Gut Hormones. New York: Churchill-Livingstone.

Cooperstein, S. J., and Watkins, D. T. (eds.). 1981. The Islets of Langerhans. New York: Academic Press.

Falkmer, S., Hellman, B., and Taljedal, I. B. (eds.). 1970. The Structure and Metabolism of the Pancreatic Islets. New York: Pergamon Press.

Fujita, T. (ed.). 1976. Endocrine Gut and Pancreas. New York: American Elsevier Publishing Company.

Polypeptide Hormones: Molecular and Cellular Aspects. 1976. Ciba Foundation Symposium 41.

Steiner, D. F., and Freinkel, N. (eds.). 1972. Handbook of Physiology, Sec. 7: Endocrinology I. Endocrine Pancreas. Washington, D. C.: American Physiological Society.

Histogenesis of Pancreatic Islets

Andrew, A. 1976. An experimental investigation into the possible neural crest origin of pancreatic APUD (islet) cells. J. Embryol. Exp. Morphol. 35:577.

Bensley, R. R. 1911. Studies on the pancreas of the guinea pig. Am. J. Anat. 12:297.

Fujita, T., and Kobayashi, S. 1977. Structure and function of gut endocrine cells. Int. Rev. Cytol. 44 (Suppl. 6):187.

Like, A. A., and Orci, L. 1972. Embryogenesis of the human pancreatic islets: A light and electron microscopic study. Diabetes 21 (Suppl. 2):511.

Melmed, R. N., Benitez, C. J., and Holt, S. J. 1972. Intermediate cells of the pancreas I. Ultrastructural characterization. J. Cell Sci. 11:449.

Orci, L., Stefan, Y., Malaisse-Lagae, R., and Perrelet, A. 1978. Instability of pancreatic endocrine cell populations throughout life. Lancet ii:1200.

Pearse, A. G. E., Polak, J. M., and Bloom, S. R. 1977. The newer gut hormones. Gastroenterology 72:746.

Pictet, R., and Rutter, W. J. 1976. Development of the embryonic endocrine pancreas. In D. F. Steiner and N. Freinkel (eds.), Handbook of Physiology, Sec. 7: Endocrinology I. Endocrine Pancreas. Washington, D.C.: American Physiological Society, p. 25.

Pancreatic Islet Morphology and Immunocytochemistry

Baetens, D., DeMey, J., and Gepts, W. 1977. Immunohistochemical and ultrastructural identification of the pancreatic polypeptide-producing cell (PP-cell) in the human pancreas. Cell Tissue Res. 185:239.

Erlandsen, S. L. 1980. Types of pancreatic islet cells and their immunocytochemical identification. Int. Acad. Pathol. 21:140.

Erlandsen, S. L., Hegre, O. D., Parsons, J. A., McEvoy, R. C., and Elde, R. P. 1976. Pancreatic islet cell hormones: Distribution of cell types in the islet and evidence for the presence of somatostatin and gastrin within the D cell. J. Histochem. Cytochem. 24:872.

Grube, D., Voigt, K. H., and Weber, E. 1978. Pancreatic glucagon cells contain endorphin-like immunoreactivity. Histochemistry 59:75.

Like, A. A. 1967. The ultrastructure of the secretory cells of the islets of Langerhans in man. Lab. Invest. 16:937.

Munger, B. L., Caramia, F., and Lacy, P. E. 1965. The ultrastructural basis for the identification of cell types in pancreatic islets, II. Rabbit, dog and opossum. Z. Zellforsch. 67:776.

Orci, L., Malaisse-Lagae, F., Amherdt, M., Ravazzola, M., Weisswang, A., Dobbs, R., Perrelet, A., and Unger, R. 1975. Cell contacts in human islets of Langerhans. J. Clin. Endocrinol. Metab. 41:841.

Smith, P. H., Merchant, F. W., Johnson, D. G., Fujimoto, W. Y., and Williams, R. H. 1977. Immunocytochemical localization of a gastric inhibitory polypeptide-like material within A-cells of the endocrine pancreas. Am. J. Anat. 149:585.

Blood Supply and Innervation

Fujita, T., Yanatori, Y., and Murakami, R. 1976. Insuloacinar axis, its vascular basis and its functional and morphological changes caused by CCK-PZ and caerulein. In T. Fujita (ed.), Endocrine Gut and Pancreas. New York: American Elsevier Publishing Company, Inc., p. 347.

Legg, P. G. 1967. The fine structure and innervation of the beta and delta cells in the islets of Langerhans of the rat. Zellforsch. 80:307.

Lifson, N., Kramlinger, K. G., Mayrand, R. R., and Lender, E. J. 1980. Blood flow to the rabbit pancreas with special reference to the islet of Langerhans. Gastroenterology 79:466.

Samols, E., and Weir, G. C. 1979. Adrenergic modulation of pancreatic A, B, and D Cells. J. Clin. Invest. 63:230.

Smith, P. H., and Porte, D., Jr. 1976. Neuropharmacology of the pancreatic islets. Annu. Rev. Med. :269.

Islet Cell Biochemistry and Physiology

Ashcroft, S. J. H. 1976. The control of insulin release by sugars. In Polypeptide Hormones: Molecular and Cellular Aspects. Ciba Foundation Symposium 41, p. 117.

Bloom, S. R. 1977. Gastrointestinal hormones. Rev. Physiol. 12:71.

Figlewicz, D. P., Formby, B., Hodgson, A. T., Schmid, F. G., and Grodsky, G. M. 1980. Kinetics of ^{65}zinc uptake from cultured rat islets of Langerhans. Diabetes 29:767.

Fletcher, D. J., Quigley, J. P., Bauer, G. E., and Noe, B. D. 1981. Characterization of proinsulin and proglucagon converting activities in isolated islet secretory granules. J. Cell Biol. 90:312.

Gerich, J. E., Raptis, S., and Rosenthal, J. (eds.) 1978. Somatostatin Symposium. Metabolism 27 (Suppl. 1):1129.

Lacy, P. E. 1975. Endocrine secretory mechanisms. J. Pathol. 79:170.

Lacy, P. E., Finke, E. H., and Codilla, R. C. 1975. Cinemicrographic studies on B granule movement in monolayer culture of islet cells. Lab. Invest. 33:570.

Noe, B. D., Baste, C. A., and Bauer, G. E. 1977. Studies on proinsulin and proglucagon biosynthesis and conversion at the subcellular level. J. Cell Biol. 74:589.

Permutt, M. A., and Kipnis, D. M. 1975. Insulin biosynthesis and secretion. Fed. Proc. 34:1549.

Sorenson, R. L., Elde, R. P., and Seybold, V. 1979. Effect of norepinephrine on insulin, glucagon, and somatostatin secretion in isolated perifused rat islets. Diabetes 28:899.

Steiner, D. F., Cunningham, D., Spiegelman, L., and Aten, B. 1967. Insulin biosynthesis: Evidence for a precursor. Science (Wash., D.C.) 157:697.

Unger, R. H., Dobbs, R. E., and Orci, L. 1978. Insulin, glucagon, and somatostatin secretion in the regulation of metabolism. Annu. Rev. Physiol. 40:307.

Zühlke, H., Steiner, D. F., Lernmark, A., and Lipsey, C. 1976. Carboxypeptidase B-like and trypsin-like activities in isolated rat pancreatic islets. In Polypeptide Hormones: Molecular and Cellular Aspects. Ciba Foundation Symposium 41:183.

Histopathology and Experimental Studies

Banting, F. G., and Best, C. H. 1922. The internal secretion of the pancreas. J. Lab. Clin. Med. 7:251.

Dixit, P. K., and Lazarow, A. 1969. Effect of alloxan on the enzyme activity of microdissected mammalian pancreatic islets. Diabetes 18:589.

Gomori, G. 1943. Pathology of the pancreatic islets. Arch. Pathol. 36:217.

Lazarow, A., Wells, L. J., Carpenter, A.-M., Hegre, O. D., Leonard, R. J., and McEvoy, R. C. 1973. Islet differentiation, organ culture, and transplantation. Diabetes 22:877.

Volk, B. W., and Wellmann, K. F. (eds.) 1977. The Diabetic Pancreas. New York: Plenum Press.

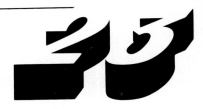

The Respiratory System

Sergei P. Sorokin

The respiratory system consists of the lungs and a number of associated structures whose primary functions are to provide the living organism with oxygen from the air and to remove excess carbon dioxide from the bloodstream. The system is composed of three functional parts: a conducting portion, a respiratory region, and a ventilating mechanism. The *conducting portion* of the system includes the nasal cavity and associated sinuses, the nasopharynx, the larynx, the trachea, and the branching bronchial passages of the lungs. Collectively they warm, moisten, and filter the inspired air before it reaches the expansive *respiratory region* of the lungs, located distal to the bronchial tubes. There the cellular barrier between inspired air and blood stream is sufficiently thin to promote rapid exchange of gases. An efficient musculoelastic mechanism moves air over the respiratory surface and forms a third functional part of the system. The components of this *ventilating mechanism* include the thoracic cage and its intercostal muscles, the muscular diaphragm, and the elastic connective tissue of the lungs. During inspiration, contraction of the muscles raises the ribs and lowers the floor of the thoracic cavity to increase its volume and to expand the lungs. During expiration, the muscles relax; elastic recoil of the expanded pulmonary tissue causes the thorax to contract. In forced expiration the natural recoil is abetted by contraction of the abdominal and external intercostal muscles, which decreases the volume of the thoracic cavity and lungs beyond their normal resting levels.

Nasal Cavity and Sinuses

The surfaces of the nasal cavity are covered by two types of lining: a *respiratory mucosa* that warms and moistens the air, and an *olfactory mucosa* that houses the receptors of smell. As the first segment of the conducting portion of the respiratory tract, the cavity is most fully developed in warm-blooded animals, where it is well separated from the oral cavity by the hard palate. The olfactory mucosa occupies a large proportion of the nasal lining of keen-scented animals such as carnivores and rooting ungulates; it is greatly restricted in primates and other forms that have a poor sense of smell. The respiratory mucosa is well developed in both the keen- and the feebly scented. In the former, the mucosa is both more highly folded and more extensive in area; moistening the air enhances olfaction.

Respiratory Mucosa

The nasal cavity is divided into symmetric halves by the nasal septum (Fig. 23-1), which contains hyaline cartilage. Stratified squamous epithelium of the facial skin continues through the nostrils into the *vestibule,* beneath the projecting cartilaginous portion of the nose. Large hairs and associated sebaceous glands form the first defense there against the entry of particulate matter. Posteriorly the hair and glands become sparse, and the epithelium thins as it approaches the paired openings to the principal nasal chambers, located within the skull. These chambers are smooth-sided along the septum but are convoluted laterally by turbinate projections from the underlying ethmoid and inferior turbinated bones, and each forms a narrow, ribbon-like passage for air. Their surfaces total about 160 cm² in humans and are coated with a mucous film. These anatomic arrangements help to promote

23-1 Section through the nasal septum of a monkey, showing hyaline cartilage on the left and the richly glandular nasal mucosa on the right. Masson's trichrome stain. × 100.

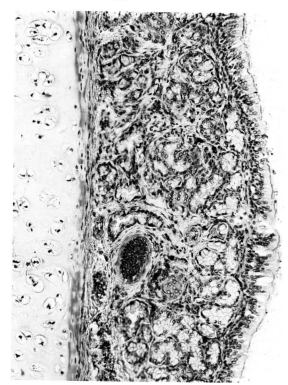

turbulence in air flow, which ensures the mucous film effective contact with the airstream. The epithelium beneath is pseudostratified, ciliated, and columnar. Goblet cells are abundantly but unevenly distributed within it, since they concentrate in sheltered regions. More exposed portions of the epithelium, such as that over the turbinates, may have small areas of transition to a stratified squamous lining. In fine structure, this epithelium resembles the epithelium of the trachea and bronchi, described later.

Numerous branched, tubuloalveolar glands extend into the underlying connective tissues as invaginations of the epithelium. They resemble minor salivary glands, having short ducts and acini both lined by secretory cells. These glands vary widely in type within a mucous to serous range, and the cellular makeup of a typical gland varies with the species. In general, mucous cells occur nearer the openings of the glands along the ducts and acini, whereas serous cells occur more peripherally in the acini or in demilunes beyond them. The larger ducts occasionally contain a distinct columnar epithelium that separates the secretory cells from the surface lining of the nasal cavity, but the columnar cells lack basal striations and give no indication of participating in the secretory process.

Beneath the epithelium, the connective tissue is of fairly uniform composition until it blends into the periosteal and perichondrial layers of the nasal skeleton. Epithelium and glands are enveloped in a richly collagenous connective tissue. Mononuclear leukocytes may infiltrate the tissue freely or may occur as nodular aggregations.

Vascular Supply. The vascular supply to the nose is rich and has several unusual features. Although some differences in distributional pattern exist among mammals, the respiratory and olfactory mucosae usually have separate arterial supplies: the sphenopalatine and the ethmoidal arteries, respectively. Both vessels and their branches anastomose rather freely throughout their subdivisions. The main vessels to the respiratory mucosa lie next to the periosteum in a latticework pattern that becomes a close-meshed net as they run either obliquely or horizontally forward across the nasal septum and lateral walls. In contrast, arteries to the olfactory region spread out in a radial array. The main respiratory arteries send out superficial arcading branches; from them, other vessels run perpendicularly to-

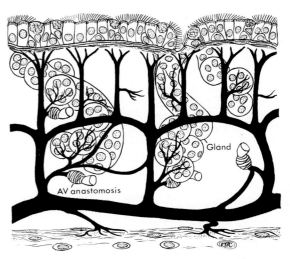

23–2 Arterial supply to the nasal mucosa. (After Dawes, J. D. K., and Prichard, M. M. L. 1953. J. Anat. 87:311.)

ward the surface, where they divide into arterioles. Some of these arterioles supply a network of capillaries just beneath the epithelium, and others supply the glands and the submucosal tissues. Arteriovenous anastomoses are common, particularly where the vasculature is richest, as in the path of the inspiratory stream and in the swell bodies described below (Fig. 23–2). These communicating vessels are tortuous; in their thick walls the medial smooth muscle has an epithelioid appearance, and the intima lacks an internal elastic membrane. As befits a secretory mucosa, the subepithelial and periglandular capillaries are fenestrated whereas the deeper ones are not. The veins are rather more conspicuous than the arteries, particularly where they lie over the arteries, as they do in humans, dogs, cats, and rabbits. There they exist as a superficial, fine-meshed plexus of small vessels and a deeper, coarser latticework of thick-walled tubes. These drain into larger veins at the anterior and posterior ends of the nasal cavity. In addition, a well-developed lymphatic system is present.

Over the middle and inferior turbinates the superficial venous plexus consists of cavernous, thin-walled vessels that lack muscular septa but otherwise resemble erectile tissue (Chap. 28). This is the region of the *swell bodies*. In humans and in other animals, blood flow is so regulated there that hourly periods of swelling occur alternately on the two sides of the nasal cavity, causing a reduction in air flow on the affected side and an upward deflection of the airstream on inspiration. Most of the respired air passes through the neighboring passage, giving the mucosa on the occluded side time to recover from desiccation and assisting the narial muscles in directing air to the olfactory region. This physiological cycle is regulated autonomically. Engorgement results from constriction of the deeper veins and dilatation of the arterioles that feed the plexus through capillaries. Adrenergic fibers from the superior cervical ganglion form rich networks not only over the arteries and arterioles, as in other vascular beds, but over the veins as well, particularly in the swell bodies. They exert a tonic, vasoconstrictive action. Cholinergic nerves from the pterygopalatine ganglion promote vasodilatation and secretion by the glands. In the olfactory region, on the other hand, blood flow is not clearly affected by either sympatho- or parasympathomimetic agents.

Histophysiology. From the rear of the nasal cavity forward, the numerous circulatory loops each receive fresh arterial blood; but blood flow in the superficial vessels of each loop generally counters the flow of inspired air, and the whole forms a compound countercurrent system. Viewed from the surface, the small vessels are set in rows as in a heat exchanger. These are ranked most closely under surfaces most exposed to the inspiratory stream, where glands are particularly abundant as well. In an engineer's terms, the nose is said to function like a scrubbing tower supplied with fresh fluid at successive levels. Despite a fractional-second contact time with the nasal mucosa, the inspired air is efficiently cleared of ozone, sulfur dioxide, and other water-soluble pollutant gases far better than it is cleared by the oropharynx. These gases are dissolved in the mucous carpet overlying the epithelium. They are partially absorbed and partially carried off to the pharynx by ciliary action.

Olfactory Mucosa

The olfactory mucosa of humans is limited to an area that covers approximately 500 mm^2 of the roof of the nasal cavity and upper portions of the nasal septum. Compared with the respiratory mucosa, its pseudostratified columnar lining is taller, and the glands beneath are of a serous rather than mixed type (Fig. 23–3). The mucosa produces an ample fluid secretion in which

odored substances are dissolved before being detected by cells of the epithelium. Three cell types predominate: *olfactory cells, sustentacular cells,* and *basal cells.* Olfactory cells are bipolar neurons. The others combine characteristics of epithelial and Schwann cells. The tall sustentacular cell is differentiated along secretory lines, whereas the short basal cell is undifferentiated and remains able to divide and to transform into either of the mature types. Special methods, such as silver impregnation or staining with methylene blue, are needed to distinguish the cells clearly by light microscopy. In routine sections identification is aided by a tendency for the round nuclei of olfactory cells to be concentrated at a level between those of the basal cells and the ovoid nuclei of the supporting cells. The olfactory cells also occur at the base of the epithelium, particularly in keen-scented species like rats and mice, where cell bodies of the receptors are crowded together and appear stacked in columns (Fig. 23–3).

Individual olfactory cells within the epithelium may respond differently to various odors; nonetheless, these receptor cells all look alike. They are widest around the nucleus and from there taper into two processes, an apically directed *dendrite* and a centrally directed *axon.* Unlike many neurons, the cell body contains little ergastoplasm, but a supranuclear Golgi apparatus and other organelles are present in moderation. The dendrite, approximately 1 μm in thickness, is filled with microtubules that run along its length in parallel courses. Its apical end extends above the surface of the epithelium as a bulbous *olfactory knob,* which contains basal bodies, mitochondria, and profiles of agranular reticulum and bears a tuft of cilia. Among different vertebrates the shape of this knob and the number of cilia present are highly variable characteristics of the olfactory cell. Frequently the knob measures about 4 μm high by 1.5 μm thick, and the cilia number 12 or more (Fig. 23–5). These cilia have the dimensions and "9 + 2" axial structure of typical cilia for a few micrometers; then they abruptly narrow to half the usual diameter for the rest of their length. Ciliary tubules within the distal segment change in configuration from doublets to singlets and gradually diminish in number. The shafts may be as long as 80 μm in cats, and the distal segment may be four or five times longer than the proximal segment in frogs. These measurements differ in other species. Olfactory cilia rarely exhibit motil-

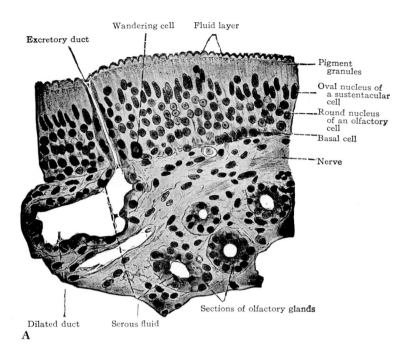

Excretory duct

Wandering cell   Fluid layer

Pigment granules

Oval nucleus of a sustentacular cell

Round nucleus of an olfactory cell

Basal cell

Nerve

Dilated duct   Serous fluid

Sections of olfactory glands

A

23–3 A. Vertical section through the olfactory region of an adult human being. × 400. **B.** Olfactory epithelium in a neonatal rat. Dark cells are the receptors. × 750.

B

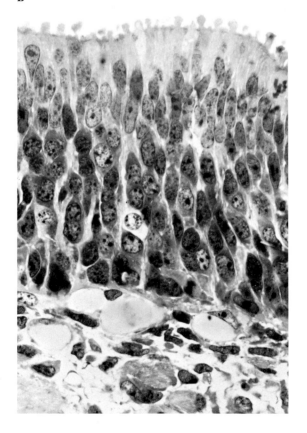

ity. Their distal segments are too thoroughly enmeshed with other cilia and microvilli in the surface fluid to beat effectively. More certainly, they greatly increase the exposure of the receptor cell to odorate substances.

Below the nucleus, the olfactory cell becomes drawn into a threadlike axon. The process, whose diameter is about 0.2 μm, is just visible with the light microscope. It extends below the basal lamina to join axons from adjacent cells in forming small fascicles, which become invested by Schwann cells but remain unmyelinated. The fascicles penetrate the cribriform plate of the ethmoid bone and become grouped into *fila olfactoria*. These lead into the ipsilateral member of the paired *olfactory bulbs*, where the axons synapse.

Among cells of the olfactory epithelium, the sustentacular cells are the most conspicuous even though outnumbered by the receptor cells. They differ in histochemical attributes from olfactory cells, but they share some attributes, such as a capacity for reducing NADP, with basal cells and those of the glands beneath (Fig. 23–4). This property provides them with the reductive potential needed to synthesize complex molecules from simpler ones and is a characteristic of many secretory cells. Sustentacular cells are rich in organelles, notably a supranuclear Golgi apparatus and a tightly compacted agranular reticulum. To-

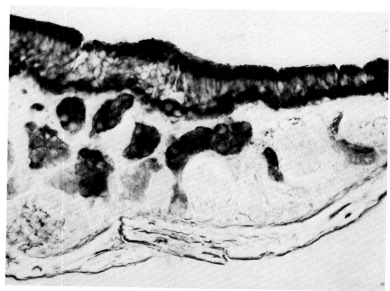

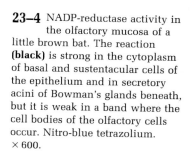

23-4 NADP-reductase activity in the olfactory mucosa of a little brown bat. The reaction **(black)** is strong in the cytoplasm of basal and sustentacular cells of the epithelium and in secretory acini of Bowman's glands beneath, but it is weak in a band where the cell bodies of the olfactory cells occur. Nitro-blue tetrazolium. × 600.

gether with numerous lipid-rich granules, the reticulum may fill the apical cytoplasm. In addition to lysosomes, other membrane-bounded granules are present, although they differ in appearance from one species to another. Along the apical surface, microvilli are prominent. Laterally the cells form the usual variety of junctional contacts with adjacent olfactory and sustentacular cells; gap junctions have occasionally been observed. As a rule, these cells are spaced so as to separate adjacent olfactory cells. Moreover, they ensheathe the dendritic and axonal processes of those neurons in mesaxons, and in this respect they resemble gliocytes. Metabolic exchanges evidently occur along the sustentacular–olfactory interfaces. Accordingly, the supportive function of these cells can be understood broadly. Toward the base of the epithelium, olfactory axons become ensheathed in processes from basal cells, but these processes are finger-like rather than sheetlike and the wrapping is discontinuous (Fig. 23–5).

Beneath the olfactory epithelium the connective tissue contains the branched tubuloalveolar glands of Bowman and myelinated fibers of the trigeminal nerve, in addition to unmyelinated olfactory axons, Schwann cells, and the usual elements of connective tissue. Cuboidal cells of Bowman's glands contain secretory granules and discharge a serous fluid onto the olfactory surface by way of excretory ducts, which are lined by flattened cells (Fig. 23–3). The glands secrete

continuously and provide fresh solvent for odored substances. The fibers of the trigeminal nerve terminate in slender processes that extend into the epithelium. Some of them synapse with nonciliated brush cells sparsely distributed there (Fig. 23–5) and elsewhere in the nasal and pulmonary linings. These intraepithelial trigeminal receptors conceivably play a small role in olfaction, because impulses from the ethmoidal division of the nerve travel out from the brain to influence electrical activity in the olfactory bulbs. The brush cells may also provide sensory input for the sneeze reflex. Blood vessels to the olfactory region supply a rich subepithelial capillary plexus and a deeper one of veins. Lymphatics run among the veins, and the tissue blends into the subjacent perichondrium and periosteum.

Histophysiology. The olfactory cell is recognized as the primary receptor for smell, because only this cell type degenerates after the olfactory nerves are sectioned. Moreover, it resembles known sensory cells of the eye and ear in such details as the presence of some type of cilia at the apex, the microtubular arrays between the apex and main body of the cell, and the sheathing of its processes by other elements of the epithelium. If an odored substance is added to the surface fluid, a change occurs in the electrical potential recorded along the nerve. The change in potential is probably a summation of several activating and inhibitory discharges, including a

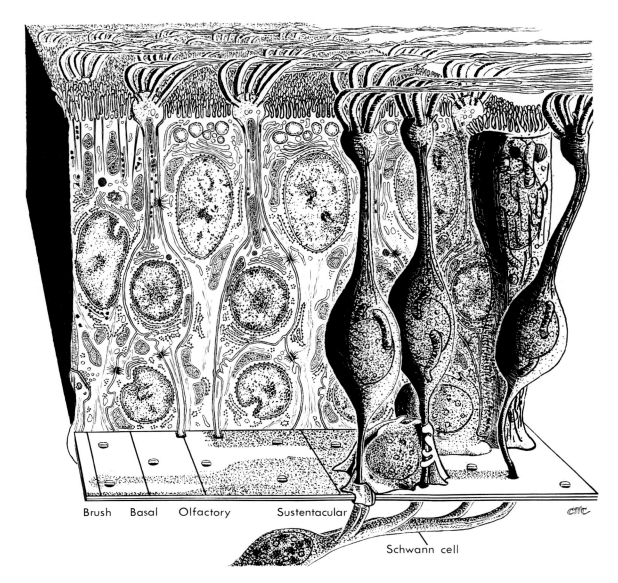

Brush   Basal   Olfactory   Sustentacular

Schwann cell

23–5 Olfactory epithelium, showing three-dimensional and ultrastructural aspects.

negative potential representing the olfactory cell's initial response to stimulation and a positive potential associated with secretion by neighboring cells. Stimulation apparently results from depolarization of the plasma membrane covering exposed portions of the olfactory cells. It is not known whether the knobs or the cilia are the main receptor sites even though ciliary processes make earlier contact with the stimulating sub-

stance. In exceptional instances, olfactory cells are not provided with cilia, but then the coating overlying the epithelium is thin and depolarization occurs on the microvilli.

Precisely how olfactory cells discriminate among a vast number of odors is not known. Over a broad phylogenetic range, however, the olfactory organ is organized much as described here, consisting of an epithelial sheet that contains many individual receptors. These receptors respond to odorous substances dissolved in the fluid that passes over them. Several receptors must fire to provide sufficient signal strength for detection of odor, but they can be mustered from among the many present, and the particular combination of units firing conveys information about the quality of the odor. Thus, the raw data for olfactory discrimination are garnered by receptors in the epithelium, but they are modified at more central levels until they become subjectively recognized in the various divisions of the olfactory cortex.

Recordings made from single olfactory cells in the frog have indicated that these cells differ markedly in selectivity for odor. Exposed to a range of odors, some cells respond to none, others to only one or two, and most to a fairly wide range. This behavior is too unselective to support the idea that discrimination of odor depends solely on the presence of highly specific receptor sites on individual olfactory cells, so modified from cell to cell that, although each responds to only a narrow range of stereochemically similar molecules, the whole sheet of receptors detects the full range. Other factors evidently affect the process.

In aquatic animals the olfactory receptors monitor the fluid environment, but in terrestrial animals the fluid is secreted and forms a layer of appreciable thickness. To judge from the latency of response after an odorous substance is introduced into the airstream, the substance must first pass into this layer before being detected. This provides an opportunity for *spatiotemporal patterning* of an extrinsic sort to be imposed on the olfactory epithelium, for upon entering the fluid layer different odorants migrate differentially, both vertically past the cilia and toward the olfactory knobs and horizontally toward other olfactory cells. Shortly after being introduced, different substances will have spread out for different distances and have reached or passed many olfactory cells, some of which will respond to the stimulus. Even odorous substances that bind strongly to components in the fluid and migrate slowly might behave in this manner because they are moved over the receptor surface as a result of continuous secretion by the epithelium and glands. Thus, the access of different receptors to an odorant is affected by the physical properties of both the particular odorant and the fluid layer, and possibly by secretory dynamics as well.

In higher terrestrial vertebrates the olfactory epithelium is usually sheltered from the respiratory airstream traversing the nose, but it can be reached by sniffing. Air flow is then channeled over the receptor sheet so that new odors arrive from one direction; this arrangement also favors spatiotemporal patterning. A third factor is that olfactory cells responsive to similar odors seem to be grouped together so as to create an intrinsic patterning within the epithelial sheet.

Experimental support for the existence of intrinsic patterning has been obtained by comparing the electrical activity at different points on the frog's olfactory epithelial surface elicited by various odorants. The region of maximal excitation for one substance usually differs from that for another, although they sometimes overlap. In mammals a similar concept has arisen from studies carried out on second-order neurons in the olfactory bulbs, to which olfactory cells project. Nevertheless it is not certain if this patterning results because cells with inherently similar odor specificity are really grouped together or because cells responding to a given odor can influence nearby receptors of low specificity into firing with them. Against this, the case for extrinsic patterning includes evidence showing that when certain odors are introduced at the internal naris and the usual direction of air flow is reversed, the pattern of firing in the olfactory epithelium is reversed. These results may raise more questions than they answer, but they are grounds for suspicion that both extrinsic and intrinsic patterning affect the response of the epithelium through action on receptors with relatively low odor specificity.

If cells with low or similar odor specificity are grouped together, they are at least in a position to interact and possibly modify the signals they send to the brain. Histologically, groupings of olfactory cells are frequently seen, as exemplified in mice where the receptors are segregated in close-packed columns stacked many cell bodies high. The odor specificity of these cells and the extent of their interactions are unknown. Nevertheless, electrophysiological studies suggest that olfactory cells receive signals from neighboring cells in the epithelium and partially integrate them with other input in the cell bodies before transmitting an impulse along the axon. Furthermore, axons from adjacent neurons tend to reach similar destinations in the olfactory bulb; hence, a number of associated cells will act on a more centrally located common pathway. These olfactory axons at first run in parallel but become intermixed as they enter the outermost layer of the bulb. They end by projecting topographically, although less precisely so than projections of the retina or cochlea on nuclei of the brain.

In the olfactory bulbs, axons from the olfactory cells branch and synapse with dendrites of second-order neurons, called *mitral* or *tufted* cells, within spherical tangles of neuropil called *olfactory glomeruli*. Signals from about 1,000 olfactory cells converge on each second-order cell. In mammals each second-order cell sends its one main dendrite to a single glomerulus so that a given glomerular system represents a specific group of olfactory cells. In the bulb, numerous subsidiary circuits connect neurons of the mitral series with smaller *granule* cells, as evidenced by the presence of dendrodendritic, dendroaxonal, and somatodendritic synapses between them. These circuits serve to inhibit incoming signals and are abetted by feedback to the granule cells from higher centers. By suppressing extraneous electrical activity, they enhance the clarity of the signal being sent inward along the olfactory tract. In addition, inhibitory feedback from the cortex largely accounts for the phenomenon of *olfactory adaptation*, whereby odors first noticed on entering a room are soon forgotten.

Recordings made from olfactory bulbs of human subjects seem to show that at this level odor quality is coded as patterns of frequency components, whereas odor detection is dependent on adequate signal strength and its characterization, on still greater amplitude. From the bulbs, incoming signals are passed to third-order neurons in the olfactory cortex and nearby subcortical regions at the base of the forebrain. These higher centers and the olfactory bulbs interact directly or indirectly with more caudal parts of the brain, including the thalamus and hypothalamus, although the hypothalamus is not well connected. The topographical representation of olfactory cells so evident in the olfactory bulb does not extend more centrally, however, for signals from a given olfactory neuron are not confined to a discrete area of olfactory cortex. Olfactory sensations are represented bilaterally, owing to the presence of interbulbar fibers and cross-connections at higher levels.

Cell Turnover. The question of regeneration in the olfactory epithelium is of special interest because this is the only tissue in mammals where neurons are known to be formed during adult life. Experimental studies have been performed on several mammalian species but have been more extensive in amphibians. In both orders the olfactory cells normally turn over after a comparatively short life span for neurons of 1 to 2 months in frogs and about a month in mice. When the olfactory nerve is unilaterally resected, the affected olfactory cells degenerate but are replaced by new cells formed from dividing basal cells. These cells differentiate into neurons, reestablish synaptic connections with cells in the bulb, and restore the epithelium to a normal appearance within a few weeks. In the event of more complete destruction of the epithelium by chemical or mechanical means, both the remaining basal cells and the epithelial cells in the underlying glands seem capable of replacing the damaged tissue, although a disfiguring and permanent metaplasia sometimes results. The presence of gap junctions between cells may be more significant as a provision for metabolic interaction during regeneration than a requirement for olfaction. Retention of a capacity to form neurons can be seen as an adaptation to permit continued neuronal function within a tissue chronically assailed by air-borne gases, pathogens, and dust; it also raises the question of how consistency in response to odors is maintained within a shifting population of receptors.

Vomeronasal Organs

The vomeronasal (Jacobson's) organs are paired tubular structures located in the floor of the nasal cavity along each side of the septum. Their cavities are lined in part by an *accessory olfactory epithelium* and open by ducts either to the nasal or oral cavities. They are well developed in many mammals but in primates exist only during embryonic life. The accessory epithelium and the glands beneath resemble their counterparts in the olfactory mucosa, but accessory olfactory cells often lack cilia and their axons lead to small *accessory olfactory bulbs*, located one to a side on the dorsomedial aspects of the main bulbs. These accessory bulbs are like olfactory bulbs of amphibians, which are simple in structure and do not possess segregated glomerular systems, as do the mammalian bulbs. The vomeronasal system has separate connections to the brain from the olfactory system; in particular, the region of the amygdala it joins has direct access to the hypothalamus, where interaction with the endocrine system may occur.

Sensory specificities of accessory olfactory neurons have not been directly established, but the anatomical relations of the organs make it possible for them to sample substances of relatively low volatility, such as may be obtained by licking as well as after inhalation. Probably they are more concerned than the olfactory mucosa with behavioral responses related to specific odors. Indeed, physiological experiments in hamsters implicate the system in the recognition of a pheromonal substance released by females as an incitement to mating.

Paranasal Sinuses

The paranasal sinuses are blind pockets that reach the nasal cavity through narrow openings. Their linings are continuous with the nasal mucosa and are similar in type, although less highly developed. Much of the epithelium is simple, ciliated, and columnar; the glands are smaller; and the connective tissue is reduced in amount. The sinuses contribute to the humidification of the nasal cavity. In keen-scented carnivores, portions of the sphenoidal and frontal sinuses may be occupied by ethmoturbinal bodies and serve as extensions of the olfactory area.

Nasopharynx

The pseudostratified ciliated columnar lining and glands of the nasal mucosa continue into the upper or nasal portion of the pharynx. With some interruption by stratified epithelium as the oropharynx and larynx are crossed, a similar covering is found in the remaining major conducting portions of the respiratory tract. In the pharynx, however, the mucosa becomes thinner and generally rests directly on skeletal muscle, being separated from it by a broad elastic layer. Below the *fornix*, or roof of the pharynx, a zone of stratified columnar epithelium may extend for short distances as the lining undergoes transition to the noncornified, stratified squamous epithelium typical of the oral cavity and oropharynx. Ventrally, stratified squamous epithelium covers most of the nasal surface of the soft palate; laterally the ciliated epithelium extends downward around the openings of the eustachian tubes, which are similarly lined. The midline *pharyngeal tonsil* is located on the dorsal wall of the nasopharynx. Patches of stratified squamous epithelium are common on its surface, but pseudostratified columnar cells predominate. Ordinarily small, the tonsil may become quite large in childhood and together with lymphoid tissue

near the auditory orifices constitutes the *adenoids*. Stratified squamous epithelium is continued below the oropharynx into the laryngeal pharynx, where the respiratory tract becomes separated from the alimentary tract at the entrance to the larynx. During swallowing movements, food is excluded from the nasopharynx by the contraction of the pharyngopalatine muscles and the retraction of the uvula between them.

Larynx

The larynx is a hollow, bilaterally symmetric structure framed by cartilages, bound together by ligaments and muscles, and located between the pharynx and the trachea. It acts primarily as a valve to prevent swallowed food from entering the lower respiratory tract, but it is a tone-producing instrument as well, and in humans it has important additional functions in the production of speech. The anatomic valve itself is termed the *glottis* and consists of a pair of lateral mucosal folds, the *vocal folds*, located partway inside the larynx. The size of the glottal aperture changes with circumstance. Partly open during quiet breathing, it widens to permit deep inspiration but closes prior to swallowing and before intrathoracic or intraabdominal pressures are raised. During phonation the aperture fluctuates between slightly open and fully closed positions.

General Structure

The larynx (Fig. 23–6) is based on a ring-shaped *cricoid* cartilage that rests upon the trachea. Above, the ventral and lateral walls of the larynx are framed largely by a shieldlike *thyroid* cartilage, which articulates with the side of the cricoid by means of two *inferior cornua* and with the hyoid bone by means of two *superior cornua*. A pair of pyramidal, *arytenoid* cartilages arise from the dorsocranial surface of the cricoid cartilage and delimit the dorsal wall. The summit of each is capped by a small *corniculate* cartilage. A midline *epiglottis* extends cranially from within the thyroid to define the ventral border of the laryngeal entrance, becomes attached to the hyoid bone, and thereafter ends as a clublike protuberance in the pharynx. These framing cartilages are additionally linked to one another and to the hyoid bone by dense connective tissue, notably a sheetlike cricothyroid membrane that

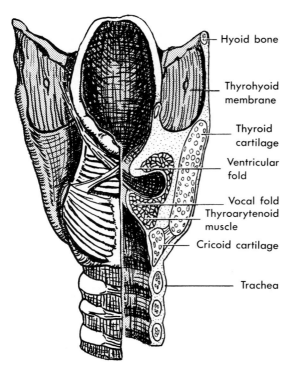

Hyoid bone

Thyrohyoid membrane

Thyroid cartilage

Ventricular fold

Vocal fold

Thyroarytenoid muscle

Cricoid cartilage

Trachea

23–6 Diagram of the human larynx showing the dorsal aspect on the left and a cutaway view of ventricular and vocal folds on the right. Approximately × 1.5.

extends below the thyroid cartilage and is thickened ventrally (conus elasticus) and a thyrohyoid membrane that extends from the cranial edge of the thyroid cartilage to the hyoid bone and becomes ligamentous at the ventral midline and at the sides. These interconnections bind framing elements into a unit and yet permit some freedom for moving the cartilages relative to one another. The movements are effected by intrinsic muscles, whose origins and insertions are confined to laryngeal structures. Extrinsic muscles join the laryngeal framework to adjacent structures. In effect, the larynx is suspended from the hyoid bone and slides up and down within a sleeve of connective tissue whenever the hyoid is raised or lowered.

Within the larynx the mucosa is thrown into three pairs of lateral folds as a result of being reflected over three paired bands of ligamentous connective tissue that extend from the arytenoid cartilages across the laryngeal cavity to insert respectively on the epiglottis and on two midline points not far apart on the inside of the thyroid

cartilage and just caudal to the attachment of the epiglottis. The most cranial of these folds, the aryepiglottic folds, extend from the tips of the arytenoids around the sides of the epiglottis to define the laryngeal inlet. They incorporate the corniculate cartilages and frequently are stiffened by small cuneiform cartilages as well. The ventricular folds, or false vocal folds, are next in order, and the true vocal folds are last. Both the ventricular and vocal folds may contain bits of cartilage, especially near the dorsal attachments of their supporting ligaments, which join, respectively, the ventricular and vocal processes of the arytenoids. As both of these folds come to the midline ventrally, they divide the laryngeal cavity into several compartments. Above the ventricular folds, the laryngeal space (vestibule) is roughly triangular in cross section but increases gradually in cross-sectional area as it ascends. Between vocal and ventricular folds the side walls recess to form the laryngeal ventricles, which are extended ventrally into a pair of appendixes. These appendixes extend caudalward for some distance, separating the ventricular fold and the thyroid cartilage. Below the vocal folds the lumen (atrium) gradually becomes cylindrical.

The Glottis. The glottal aperture (rima glottidis) is located at the level of the paired vocal ligaments (Fig. 23–8). Beginning ventrally it is bordered on each side for the initial three-fifths of its length by mucosa of the vocal fold; for the remaining distance it is bordered by the mucosa covering the vocal process and base of the arytenoid cartilage. Lateral to the ligaments, the vocal folds contain striated muscle of the thyroarytenoid group, which extends between the thyroid and arytenoid cartilages. Being suspended between these two cartilages, both of which articulate with the cricoid, each vocal fold is affected whenever the cartilages are moved. Because the intrinsic muscles interconnect the laryngeal cartilages, they serve to regulate the glottis by their actions. By the same token, they also move the ventricular folds, although to a lesser extent. The principal actions to affect the glottal aperture are those that rock the arytenoids on the cricoid and those that rock and glide the thyroid on the cricoid. When the arytenoids are rotated outward (action of the posterior cricoarytenoid muscles), the glottis opens. Conversely, when they are rotated inward (lateral cricoarytenoids), or when they are approximated in a

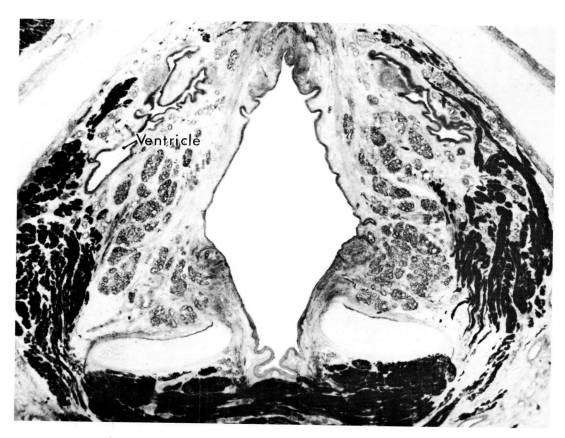

Ventricle

gliding motion (transverse arytenoid), it closes. When the thyroid is tilted forward (cricothyroids) or the cricoid is pulled backward (lateral cricothyroids and extrinsic cricopharyngeus), the vocal folds stretch; and when the thyroid is tilted backward (thyroarytenoids) they relax. Such muscular actions are related primarily to the valvular function of the glottis, for not all are essential to phonation. In phases of deglutition the larynx is moved principally by the extrinsic muscles. The intrinsic muscles nevertheless contribute to this process by drawing the arytenoid cartilages forward against the epiglottis to help close off the larynx (thyroarytenoids, aryepiglottics, and arytenoid).

Histology

Epithelium and Glands. The mucosa of the larynx is continuous with that of the pharynx and the trachea and exhibits features of both. Stratified squamous epithelium from above extends partway into the larynx, over the aryepiglottic folds laterally and somewhat farther ven-

23–7 Cross section of the human larynx at the level of the ventricular folds. Muscles (arytenoideus and ventricularis portion of thyroarytenoideus) and glands are revealed by their reaction for succinic dehydrogenase. The ventricular appendixes extend between the folds and the thyroid cartilage (top of picture). × 10.

trally, where it covers the entire lingual side of the epiglottis and the upper half of its laryngeal aspect. It is also present at other points of wear, such as over the vocal folds and the arytenoid cartilages. Elsewhere this stratified squamous epithelium gives way to a pseudostratified, ciliated, columnar lining after a transitional zone of stratified columnar epithelium. The pseudostratified epithelium and its associated glands resemble those of the trachea and bronchi and function similarly in conditioning the inspired air and in adding to the protective coating of mucus spread over the epithelial surface. Much of this mucus reaches the larynx from the lower respiratory tract either after coughing or by ciliary action and, in turn, is driven into the pharynx.

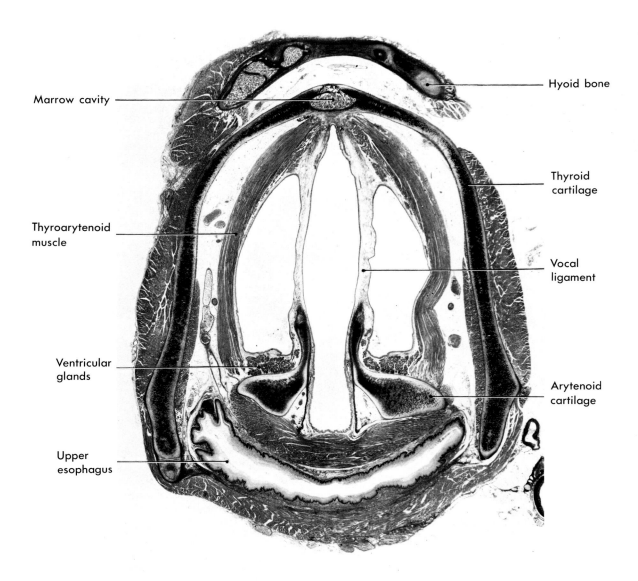

Marrow cavity

Hyoid bone

Thyroid cartilage

Thyroarytenoid muscle

Vocal ligament

Ventricular glands

Arytenoid cartilage

Upper esophagus

23–8 Cross section of the human larynx at the level of the true vocal folds. The vocal ligaments are elevated above part of the laryngeal ventricles on each side. × 8.

The laryngeal glands are small, branching, tubuloalveolar invaginations of the epithelium. They occur in groups and generally remain confined to the lamina propria. Exceptionally, they may penetrate parts of the framing cartilages. Most frequently, as in humans, these deep excursions occur only in relation to the epiglottis and give that cartilage a uniquely pockmarked appearance. The glands are especially abundant along the rim of the aryepiglottic fold; these are *arytenoid glands*. Many occur as well in the ventricular folds, in the dorsal wall of the laryngeal ventricles, and in the laryngeal appendixes (Fig. 23–7) where the secretion is expressed onto the surface of the vocal folds by muscular contraction. Glands are absent from the vocal ligaments and only gradually reappear toward the base of the vocal folds, where they increase and eventually encircle the laryngeal space at the level of the cricoid cartilage. Most of the glands produce a mucous secretion that stains less brilliantly with PAS than goblet cell mucus and is contained in fairly uniform-sized droplets that resist a tendency to coalesce within the cells. Accord-

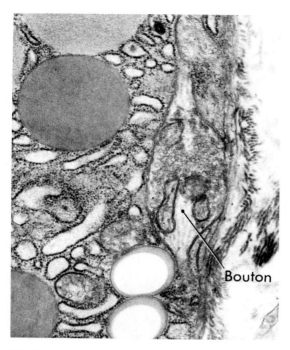

Bouton

23–9 Part of a seromucous acinus in the epiglottis of the little brown bat, showing an intraepithelial nerve ending with synaptic vesicles. × 12,000.

ingly, they can be considered *seromucous* glands. Like their counterparts in the nose and in conducting airways of the lungs, the laryngeal glands are regulated by unmyelinated secretomotor nerves. These frequently penetrate the basal laminae of acini and ramify among the secretory cells as threadlike processes each bearing one or more swellings charged with predominantly clear (cholinergic) synaptic vesicles (Fig. 23–9). In addition to glands, a few taste buds occur at the base of the epiglottis.

Connective Tissue. Within the larynx the usual elements of connective tissue are combined in a great variety of textures. Beneath the epithelium this tissue is a rather loose lamina propria, but it becomes denser around solid structures and so is not everywhere distinct from the encircling submucosa. Elastic fibers are unusually abundant. These are heaviest in the glottis where they are bundled in parallel arrays to make up the vocal ligaments, which may be regarded as thickenings of the submucous cricothyroid membrane. The fibers of this membrane diminish in size and number in caudal parts of the vocal folds; and in the lamina propria above,

the tissue becomes particularly loose so as to offer little resistance to edematous swelling. In humans the laryngeal connective tissue is unusually rich in *mast cells*, which release histamine and other edema-producing agents during immediate-type hypersensitivity reactions. The laryngeal reaction often can be life-threatening, as are laryngeal infections, because both can lead to occlusion of the airway.

Small lymphoid nodules and migratory leukocytes frequently occur here as in all connective tissues close to the outside environment. Such nodules are rarely found near the glottis but become prominent below, in the atrial part of the larynx. In capillaries supplying the epithelium and glands, fenestrated plaques appear in the endothelium at points where the vessels closely approach the basal laminae. The capillaries drain into venous plexuses situated more deeply. The lymphatic system is similarly arranged with a superficial network leading to a deeper plexus of larger vessels.

Cartilage. The laryngeal cartilages, not only furnish examples of all the main histological types of cartilage but illustrate some of the variations to be found within each type. Early in life, all are hyaline cartilages. Later on, most of the cuneiforms and corniculates, part of the epiglottis, and the apexes and vocal processes of the arytenoids become converted to elastic cartilage, and smaller portions of the epiglottis and the arytenoids become fibrocartilage. In sum, the larger structural cartilages remain hyaline, whereas the smaller ones become elastic. The fiber-containing cartilages of the larynx differ from each other most conspicuously in the patterns made by their fibrous networks, which follow lines of stress and may be curved and interlacing in the epiglottis but are straight and parallel where the vocal ligaments join the arytenoids. Certain differences are seen as well among the hyaline cartilages. For example, the capsular matrix is often more basophilic in the thyroid cartilage than in the others. However, any of the hyaline cartilages may ossify with age, and a marrow cavity may form inside the bone (Fig. 23–8). Among these variant cartilages the epiglottis stands out, for even though its cells unquestionably are chondrocytes, its matrix is sparse, variously admixed with other connective tissue cells and fibers, and closely intruded on by adjacent tissues. In some species it resembles *chondroid tissue* of lower vertebrates more than typical mammalian cartilage.

Muscle and Nerves. All the laryngeal muscle is cross-striated muscle, an unusual tissue to find in tubular viscera of vertebrates but present there as well as in adjacent portions of the esophagus. Functionally this muscle enables the larynx to carry out its specialized tasks. Phylogenetically it reflects the development of this region from the visceral skeletal system derived from splanchnic mesoblast and formed into cartilages and muscles of the mandibular, hyoid, and branchial arches. At first intended to expand and contract the pharynx for purposes of feeding and respiration, the muscles were later put to new uses as the branchial arches became transformed into the skeleton of the larynx. The intrinsic muscles seem to be composed of fiber types in the intermediate to red range, judging from criteria discussed in Chapter 7. The fibers are small and strongly reactive for the mitochondrial enzyme succinic dehydrogenase. Furthermore, electron micrographs of these muscles show that the mitochondria frequently occur in subsarcolemmal and interfibrillar chains. In bats, cricothyroid fibers additionally possess a highly developed sarcoplasmic reticulum. Such visible features might well help these muscles to achieve short refractory periods and rapid contractility, but alone they are an inadequate basis for predicting muscular performance. More certainly, physiological characteristics of skeletal muscles are greatly influenced by their innervation.

The larynx is extensively represented in both sensory and motor cortex, and the muscles are under fine control. Impulses are projected through the pyramidal system to motor neurons in the *nucleus ambiguus*, and signals reach the larynx through branches of the vagus nerve. One of these, the superior laryngeal nerve, innervates the cricothyroid muscle through its external branch. Other intrinsic muscles are controlled by the recurrent laryngeal nerve. Afferent impulses from the larynx initiate the cough reflex, mediate a general chemical sense, and influence reflex activity in swallowing. Sensory and secretomotor impulses are carried predominantly by the internal branch of the superior laryngeal nerve. It represents most of the region above the glottis and the subglottal region as well through communication with the recurrent nerve. Sensory input travels this path to cell bodies in the *nodose ganglion*. Sensation from part of the area of the epiglottis is carried to the *petrous ganglion* of the glossopharyngeal nerve, whose domain is in the vicinity of the nasopharynx. Sympathetic innervation to the larynx is much as described in the section on the trachea. Owing to the small size of laryngeal motor units as well as to the widespread autonomic and sensory innervation of the region, laryngeal tissues are richly supplied with nerves. These are arranged in superficial and deep plexuses.

Role of the Larynx in Phonation

Speaking and singing are characteristic human activities controlled by large segments of the brain and effected principally by means of the larynx, other parts of the respiratory system, and structures in the mouth. In these activities, the mouth is relatively more important to speech and the larynx to singing. In both cases the glottis is the usual source of *voiced sound*, which is produced by the passage of air driven by elevated subglottic pressure through the closed vocal folds. These part intermittently to emit puffs of air, and this alternately compressed and rarefied air is delivered to the airways above, which act as resonating cavities. Voiced sound has a fundamental frequency determined by the mass of the vocal ligaments, their length, and their tension. This acoustic system has been likened to that of a reed organ pipe, where air is passed from a wind chest through the reed and into the organ pipe. In humans, however, the driving pressure, the pitch of the reed (glottis), and the size of the resonant cavity all are variable and not fixed. In singing, the larynx is called on to produce fundamental tones of greatly varied pitch, whereas for speech only a limited range is called for, centering around 125 cycles per sec for men and around 225 for women. Moreover, certain sounds of speech, such as the *f* in fast, are not voiced but produced with an open glottis, whereas others, such as the *h* in hat, are produced by gradual closure, or aspiration. The resonant cavities are of importance because, depending on their size and shape, they reinforce the fundamental tone and tones of higher pitch derived from the overtone series, beginning with a frequency of about 400 cycles per sec. With vocal training the laryngeal vestibule can be shaped into an exponential horn, which provides efficient accoustical coupling for sound produced at the glottis, while both the vestibule and the nasopharynx constitute a resonant cavity in the neck that automatically tunes itself to the frequency sung; as the pitch is raised the larynx slides upward and shortens the cavity. The nasal cavity and sinuses are tuned to certain frequencies only, as their dimensions are fixed. The oral cavity is formed into a very finely tunable resonator regulated by movements of the tongue, the jaws, the soft palate, and the lips. It can be seen that speech sounds are generated principally in the mouth and not in the larynx; for spoken sounds can be whispered, and this is done with a partially open glottis. Generally, vowel sounds are steady-state sounds and consonants are transient ones, exceptions being the nasal sounds *m* and *n*, the rolled *r*, and the sustained *s*. Each vowel sound is characterized by a set of fixed pitches to which the oral resonator is tuned. This sound is excited by a laryngeal tone of equal or lower pitch. It is precisely when words are sung to high tones that the different requirements of singing and speech become clear; if the laryngeal tone is higher than those needed to excite a certain vowel sound, the vowel cannot be pronounced correctly.

Glottic Actions During Phonation. It is believed that during phonation the edges of the closed glottis are driven apart by subglottic pressure but are drawn together again by a Bernoulli force and by *elastic recoil* of the vocal folds. This is the summation of the tension in stretched elastic fibers of the vocal ligaments and the tension exerted between antagonistic pairs of intrinsic muscles, principally the cricothyroids acting against the thyroarytenoids. Certain other muscles are involved as well, such as those acting to hold the folds together. The loudness of sound emitted from the larynx increases as the vocal folds are approximated, and when the glottis is closed, further increases result largely from increases in subglottic pressure. It has been argued that the *vocalis* muscle, the part of the thyroarytenoid group that lies adjacent to the vocal ligament, influences both character and volume of laryngeal sound by helping to open the vocal folds during phonation. This argument is based on claims that some of the vocalis fibers insert on the vocal ligaments instead of on the cartilages. Such claims have been disputed convincingly in the case of humans, although it is true that some vocalis fibers insert into the cricothyroid membrane below the glottis. The argument remains vital in relation to the larynx of certain bats that use bursts of intense laryngeal ultrasound for purposes of echolocation.

On the whole, laryngeal muscles act more to alter the pitch and mode of vibration of the vocal folds than to initiate phonation or to amplify its intensity. Characteristically, these results can be achieved in more than one way. For example, the pitch of the laryngeal sound can be changed either by altering the tension, the length, or the mass of the vocal ligaments, or by causing only part of their length to vibrate. Similarly, by thinning out the edges of the glottal aperture and locking the arytenoid cartilages together so that only the ventral three-fifths of the glottis can permit air to pass, the mode of vibration is altered from that of the *chest voice* to the *falsetto*. All these changes require complex muscle action. In trained singers they seem to involve the intrinsic muscles more and extrinsic muscles less than they do in the case of vocal amateurs.

Because the anatomical relations of human vocal and ventricular folds are similar, both folds tend to operate in parallel. Being pervaded by glands, however, the latter are not well suited to phonation and usually remain partly open while this is occurring. They close over the closed glottis before coughing. Old-time singers made use of this action to initiate their vocal attack in a maneuver known as *coup de glotte*. In echolocating bats, however, these folds may be as thin and flexible as the true vocal folds.

Trachea

The trachea, or windpipe, is a hollow tube originating at the base of the larynx and ending below at the *carina*, where it bifurcates to form the main airway, or *primary bronchus*, of each lung. Like the other conducting portions of the respiratory system, the trachea conditions the air as it passes to the lungs and provides protection from dust and air-borne infection. It runs close to the ventral surface of the neck largely unstrengthened by neighboring tissues. Consequently, it would collapse during forceful inspiration, or on inspiration against a closed glottis, were it not reinforced by a skeleton of cartilage embedded in its wall. This represents a part of the visceral skeleton of vertebrates, homologous to the fifth branchial arch of fish, and, like the laryngeal cartilages, adapted to new uses by terrestrial forms. To some extent, tracheal structures seem to reflect divergent *branchial* and *pulmonary* influences exerted on them during development. Although retaining a midline position and in large measure the bilateral symmetry associated with it, the trachea acquires a more radial plan of or-

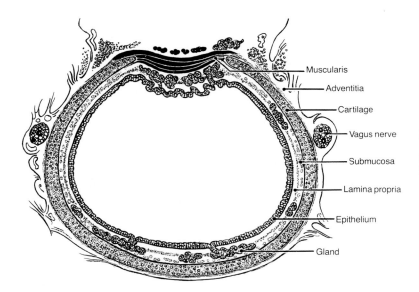

Muscularis

Adventitia

Cartilage

Vagus nerve

Submucosa

Lamina propria

Epithelium

Gland

23–10 Cross section of a generalized mammalian trachea showing salient histological features.

ganization than that of the larynx, and the tissues become arranged in concentric layers of mucosa, submucosa, an incomplete muscularis, and adventitia (Fig. 23–10). This radial plan becomes fully developed in the bronchi and serves as the organizational basis for succeeding intrapulmonary airways.

Histology

Epithelium and Glands. The tracheal mucosa closely resembles that of the nose and nasopharynx and is virtually identical to that in the lower part of the larynx and in the pulmonary bronchi. It is secretory, harboring many exocrine glands and being lined by a pseudostratified columnar epithelium in which *ciliated* and *mucous* cells predominate. This epithelium is taller in large mammals than in small ones. It may vary in appearance even among individuals of the same species, because it is sensitive to irritation and responds by increasing in height while its mucous cells and the glands beneath undergo hypertrophy. With more intense or prolonged irritation, portions of the epithelium may assume a stratified squamous form through a process of change termed *squamous metaplasia* by pathologists. This change is arguably within the epithelium's normal expressive range, since islands of stratified squamous cells normally occur in exposed parts of the pseudostratified lining of the upper airway and remain stable for a lifetime. In addition to ciliated and mucous cells, *basal* (short) cells stand out because their nuclei form a row close to the basement lamina, making the epithelium appear stratified. These cells do not extend to the free surface and evidently function as a reserve population for the epithelium. Other types of cells have minority representation but often escape notice completely because their distinguishing features are poorly resolved by light microscopy.

As seen by electron microscopy, at least six different cell types make up the mature laryngobronchial epithelium. Ultrastructural characteristics of these cells are illustrated in Fig. 23–11. The epithelium exhibits moderately high levels of activity for mitochondrial enzymes associated with oxidative phosphorylation and for lysosomal enzymes. Much of this activity is attributable to the ciliated and mucous cells. In ciliated cells the mitochondria tend to concentrate just below the apical cytoplasm, which contains the ciliary basal bodies. The basal bodies are ranged in a single layer and number about 300 per cell. Each is a centriole that has produced a cilium; these cilia extend from the basal bodies through the surface microvillous layer and into the lumen of the airway. At the base of these cells one sometimes sees one or two centrioles unassociated with cilia. The supranuclear region is occupied by the Golgi apparatus and various lysosomal elements, including a few large residual bodies. Ciliated cells have only moderate num-

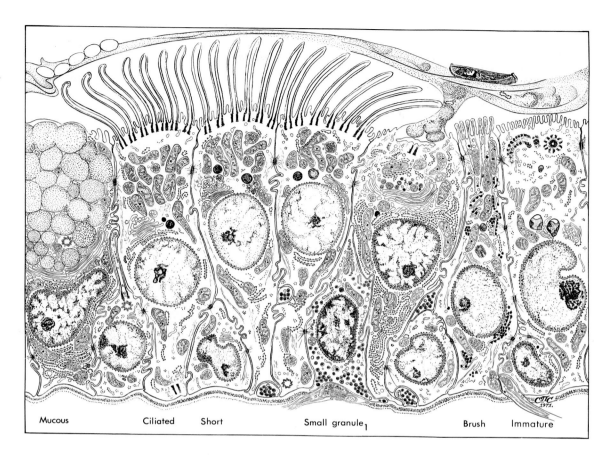

Mucous   Ciliated   Short   Small granule₁   Brush   Immature

23–11 Diagram showing ultrastructural characteristics of cells in the laryngobronchial epithelium.

bers of ribosomes, either free or attached to membranes of the endoplasmic reticulum, so that the appreciable cytoplasmic basophilia of this epithelium is ascribable in larger measure to the mucous cells. These resemble goblet cells of the small intestine and exhibit characteristics of protein-secreting cells: an extensive, cisternal ergastoplasm housed in the lower part of the cell; a supranuclear Golgi apparatus; and an apical cytoplasm charged with membrane-bound but often coalescing mucous droplets. In these cells the centrioles usually are seen amidst the secretory material in the apical cytoplasm. When secretion occurs, the droplets are shed along with some of the cytoplasmic threads separating them. Thereafter the centrioles seem to become active in reconstituting the apical plasmalemma. A cell that has just released its secretion no longer is identifiable by light microscopy as a mucous cell and becomes another nonciliated cell in the epithelium.

Among the heterogeneous group of nonciliated epithelial cells, a few are distinguished by

the presence of unusually long, straight microvilli and epitheliodendritic (afferent) synapses with nerve processes that reach in from the connective tissue. These are *brush cells*, which evidently are counterparts to similar cells in the nasal lining. They are not easily seen in all mammalian species but are conspicuous in the tracheas of rats (Fig. 23–13, see here and color insert) where they have been shown to possess glycogen granules as well as a preponderance of agranular reticulum in the cytoplasm. Other nonciliated columnar cells may contain precursors of basal bodies or intermediates in some other differentiative process, indicating that these cells are immature and have recently replaced cells that have been cast off from the epithelium (Fig. 23–11, *immature*). After trauma severe enough to destroy a region of the epithelium, neighboring

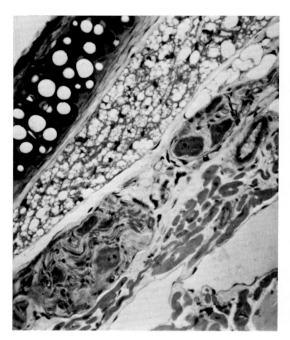

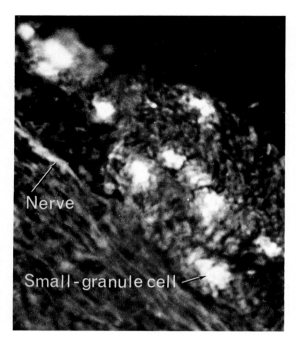

23–12 Ganglion cells of the pulmonary plexus near the tracheal bifurcation of a hamster. This is a black-and-white rendition of a color plate. See color section.

23–14 Fluorescence resulting from uptake of L-dopa by small granule cells of the upper tracheal epithelium of the rat. The section passes obliquely through the epithelium; an adrenergic nerve fiber fluoresces in the lamina propria beneath. × 364. (Work of R. Hoyt, Jr., A-W. El-Bermani, and S. Sorokin.)

23–13 Tracheal mucosa of a rat showing a brush cell **(arrowhead)** in the epithelium. This is a black-and-white rendition of a color plate. See color section.

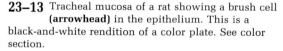

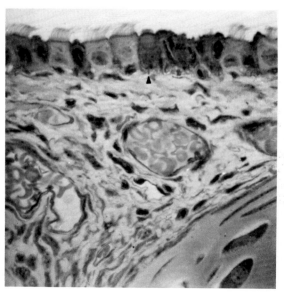

mucous and short cells apparently migrate to cover the denuded area. They then lose their distinguishing characteristics, divide, and form a population of immature columnar cells, called *indifferent cells,* which in turn divide and redifferentiate into mucous and ciliated cells.

Small-granule cells are rare cells characterized by a cytoplasm filled with small (1,000–3,000 Å) dense-core granules. Taken together with similar cells occurring elsewhere in the respiratory system, they constitute a heterogeneous population of neuroendocrine cells generally characterized by the ability to take up amine precursors and store the amines in cytoplasmic granules (Figs. 23–14 and 23–15), frequently characterized by argyrophilia, and occasionally by direct connection to pulmonary nerves. Throughout most of the tracheal epithelium these cells are solitary and sparsely distributed, but they sometimes occur more abundantly near the laryngotracheal junction (Fig. 23–14). They usually lie in the basal part of the epithelium along with short cells but sometimes reach the free surface. This class of cell is further described in the section on neuroendocrine cells of

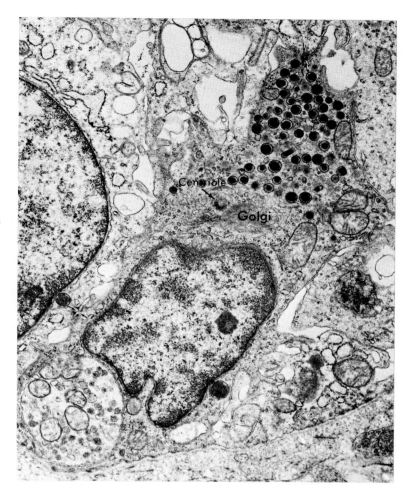

23–15 Endocrine small-granule cell in the laryngobronchial epithelium of *Myotis*. It is linked to other epithelial cells by conventional desmosomes **(arrows)** and passes over a process from a *second* type of small-granule cell. × 11,700.

the conducting airways (see also the discussion of the APUD system in Chaps. 19, 22, and 29).

The conducting airways also contain intraepithelial nerves. They are typical nervous processes containing parallel microtubular arrays along much of their length. They ramify throughout the lower part of the epithelium in potential spaces between the lateral surfaces of the cells. These spaces (Figs. 23–34 and 23–35) open up somewhat when the cells become distended with fluid. More frequently they are obliterated, and adjacent cell membranes appear tightly interlocked. Epithelial elements including the small-granule cells are joined to each other on the sides by desmosomes and, where the cells reach the surface, by junctional complexes as well.

Tracheal glands share essential features and a certain variability as to cell type with the glands of the larynx and pulmonary bronchi (Fig.

23–16, see here and color insert). In humans they are mixed mucous glands with serous crescents. Around the tracheal lumen the glands generally extend into the submucosa. They are more highly developed dorsally where they may penetrate the muscularis to enter the adventitia. A more detailed discussion of the cell types of these glands will be found in the section on bronchi.

Connective Tissue. The connective tissue compartments of the trachea are not as well defined as they are in the walls of the alimentary tract (Chap. 19). This is especially true of small mammals where the total thickness of the tracheal wall is meager. In humans, one distinguishes a lamina propria, a submucosa, and an adventitia (Fig. 23–10). The lamina propria of the mucosa is a loose tissue containing inter-

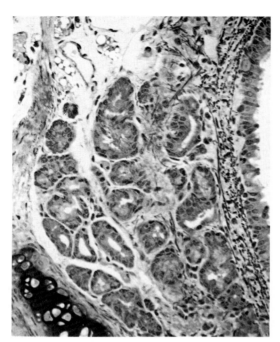

23–16 Epithelium, fiber systems, and glands on the dorsal aspect of the trachea in a mouse. This is a black-and-white rendition of a color plate. See color section.

woven collagenous and elastic fibers, many small vascular channels, and the usual fixed and wandering cells of connective tissue. The elastic fibers are joined into a continuous network in which the heavier fibers run in a predominantly longitudinal direction but are interconnected by slender fibrils (Figs. 23–16 and 23–17, see here and color insert). Peripherally these fibers become condensed into an *elastic membrane* that demarcates the lamina propria from the submucosa (Fig. 23–17), which contains the distributing vessels and larger lymphatics of the tracheal wall. The submucosa has relatively fewer elastic fibers and more collagen than the propria; these fibers run in bundles among the glands and serve to bind the elastic network of the propria to the enveloping cartilaginous skeleton. The submucosa ends by blending into the perichondrium of the cartilages.

Cartilage. The tracheal cartilages are irregular, crescentic rings embedded in a fibrous connective tissue that forms a tube about the submucosa. There are 16 to 20 cartilages in humans.

They are evenly spaced within the fibrous membrane, which normally is not fully stretched and so permits some tracheal movement. They sometimes branch, and adjacent cartilages sometimes fuse with one another, but all are incomplete dorsally where the trachea contacts the esophagus. These gaps are bridged by fibrous tissue and bands of smooth muscle joining the ends of the cartilages. Near the tracheal bifurcation a few longitudinal muscle fibers run outside the transverse bands to link a number of the cartilages with the dorsal portion of the carinal ridge. This area receives additional support from the last cartilage, which extends under the bifurcation as well as around the sides of the trachea. In animals subject to unusually high transtracheal pressures, the tracheal skeleton may be modified in different ways. In seals the tracheal rings are supplemented by smaller cartilages embedded in the fibrous membrane, and the whole structure is stiffened; in bats the cartilages overlap each other like roofing tiles and provide additional buttressing at little cost in flexibility. Topographically, the tracheal skeleton occupies the innermost portion of the adventitia, but over the dorsum the muscularis takes up the corresponding part of the wall. Developmentally, the cartilage layer is distinct from the rest of the adventitia; the cartilages appear as independent chondrifications within a continuous, crescentic, cartilage-forming rudiment, which persists in adult life as the fibrous membrane. The cartilages are hyaline but become fibrous with age. The perichondrium is virtually inseparable from the fibrous membrane and is thicker on the outer than on the inner surface of the rings. External to this region the adventitia becomes an areolar tissue rich in fat cells (Fig. 23–12, see here and color insert). It carries nerves and blood vessels to the trachea, receives its lymphatic drainage, and blends into tissues of the neck and of the mediastinum.

Nerves, Blood Vessels, and Lymphatics

The nervous, vascular, and lymphatic supplies to the trachea are independent of those to the lungs, although they resemble their counterparts in the walls of the larger pulmonary airways and function in concert with them. The trachea receives visceral afferent fibers and sympathetic and parasympathetic efferents. In its innervation it differs from the pharynx or larynx principally in lacking a branchial motor component. The courses of individual fibers are all but impossible

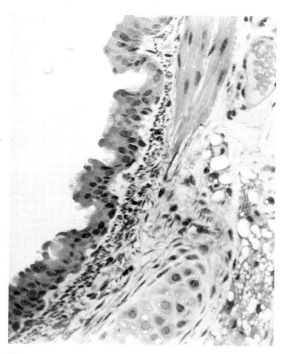

23–17 Tracheal smooth muscle of a mouse inserting on the elastic fiber skeleton. This is a black-and-white rendition of a color plate. See color section.

to trace because the sensory and autonomic nerves all contribute to plexuses formed around the viscera and, while crossing them, frequently exchange fibers. Rostral to the trachea such a plexus occurs in the lateral and dorsal walls of the pharynx, and caudally another *(pulmonary plexus)* occurs around the tracheal bifurcation. Some of the fibers in these networks end in the trachea. *Visceral afferent* fibers leave the trachea and adjacent structures through branches of the vagus nerve and travel to the nodose ganglion, or else they separate in the pharyngeal plexus and pass through the sympathetic trunk to reach cell bodies in the dorsal root ganglia of cervical and upper thoracic nerves. Cell bodies of preganglionic *sympathetic* efferents occur at upper thoracic levels of the spinal cord. Postganglionic fibers are said to originate from the three cervical ganglia and form the upper thoracic portion of the sympathetic trunk. Preganglionic *parasympathetic* fibers originate in the dorsal motor nucleus of the vagus and synapse with second-order neurons located in small tracheal ganglia embedded in the adventitia and submucosa

(Fig. 23–12, see here and color insert). Fibers of all the foregoing types reach the tracheal wall chiefly from the left side through the left recurrent nerve, but some reach it from the right through the vagus and its right recurrent branch.

Tracheal tissues receive systemic blood through branches of the inferior thyroid arteries. These ramify in the submucosa and near the carina anastomose with bronchial arteries, which supply the walls of bronchi. Venous blood drains through the thyroid venous plexus and returns to the systemic circuit via the middle and inferior thyroid veins. Tracheal lymphatics lead out laterally to a few paratracheal nodes located beside the recurrent nerves, as well as to nodes of the superior deep cervical chain.

The Lungs

External Form

The primary bronchi of the right and left lungs arise in the mediastinum from the bifurcation of the trachea. They follow a short extrapulmonary course and together with the main pulmonary vessels and nerves enter the hilum of their respective lungs (Fig. 23–23). The lungs occupy the thoracic cavity, which is smaller on the left than on the right owing to the position of the heart. Consequently, the right lung is always larger than the left and almost always subdivided into a greater number of *lobes*. The lobes are separated from each other to varying degrees among different animal species but are confluent medially in the vicinity of the main bronchus. In humans there are three on the right and two on the left, but in many mammals the right lung has a fourth, infracardiac lobe extending between the heart and the diaphragm. Where the heart strongly inclines to the left, as in the insectivores, the left lung has but one lobe. Just as the lungs can be subdivided into lobes, the lobes can be subdivided into smaller units, termed *bronchopulmonary segments, subsegments,* and *lobules;* these are demarcated to varying degrees by fissures on the lobar surfaces. For all its varied appearance, the outward form of the lung imperfectly reflects its underlying structure, for a sheet of visceral pleura covers the surfaces. In providing an airtight capsule the pleura effectively conceals the system of airways together with associated respiratory tissue and vascular supplies that from the structural basis of the organ.

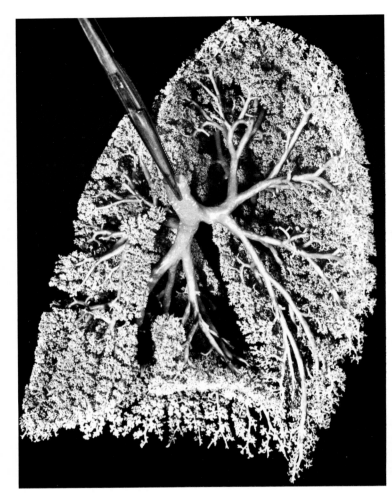

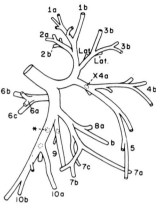

23–18 Cast of the left bronchial tree of a child, age 7 years, 10 months, in mediastinal view. **1-10,** segmental bronchi; **X4a,** displaced subsegmental branch; **asterisk,** subsuperior bronchus of lower lobe. ×0.8. (Courtesy of E. A. Boyden and D. H. Tompsett.)

Internal Structure

The lungs of birds and mammals are structurally the most complex of vertebrate lungs. Each is marvelously adapted to supply the large amounts of oxygen that these animals use; avian and mammalian lungs nevertheless differ basically from each other in the organization of conducting and respiratory regions. This chapter is concerned only with mammalian lungs, which share a single structural plan among all their prototherian, metatherian, and eutherian representatives. Wide variations on this plan nevertheless occur in some mammalian groups, especially among the marine mammals.

Each lung is organized fundamentally around its system of airways, metaphorically termed the *bronchial tree*. In this system the primary bronchus is a trunk that divides into a number of branches. These subdivide into smaller branches, and so on until tiny, thin-walled spaces are reached, where respiratory exchange takes place. In such an arrangement a given branch of the bronchial tree will ventilate a definite part of the respiratory surface. As a system of air conduits, the bronchial tree is best visualized in casts prepared by filling all but the last few generations of branches with latex or plastic casting materials, for then the branching pattern can be studied to advantage (Fig. 23–18). If the entire bronchial tree is cast, it takes on the form of the intact lung and appears solid.

The three-dimensional structure of the lungs is fully achieved by superimposing additional branching systems on the basic bronchial tree. The most important of these is the pulmonary

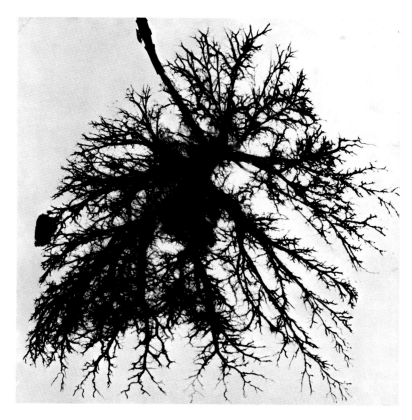

23–19 X-ray of autopsied left human lung showing pulmonary arterial tree as revealed after injection of contrast material. Compare pattern with that of the left bronchial tree (Fig. 23–18).

vascular circuit consisting of the pulmonary arteries, capillaries, and veins (Figs. 23–19, 23–20, and 23–73, see here and color insert). The arteries spread over the dorsolateral surfaces of the bronchial tree and follow its divisions precisely until in the respiratory region the vessels divide into capillaries. The bronchial arteries, pulmonary lymphatics, and nerves all follow the bronchial tree as closely as the pulmonary artery does; they also ramify along the pulmonary vessels and extend into the pleura. Pulmonary veins form at the boundaries between regions ventilated by adjacent bronchi and run within interfacial connective tissue to the main pulmonary veins, which are suspended from the ventral surfaces of the bronchi. A common adventitia of connective tissue invests the bronchial tree and associated blood vessels. It continues outward along the veins where it blends in with the surrounding septal tissue. At the surface this tissue becomes confluent with the connective tissue of the visceral pleura. The branching systems in the lungs thereby become bound together and

linked through septa to capsular tissue at the surface. The larger of these septa run out to the lobar fissures and hence are *interlobar septa*. Others follow planes of separation between the segments of a lobe and are *intersegmental septa;* still others less regularly subdivide smaller parts of the lung.

Bronchopulmonary Segments. Clinical interest in the branching pattern of the human lungs usually extends to the level of bronchopulmonary segments. These segments are supplied by branches of the lobar bronchi or by branches that immediately follow them; consequently, segmental bronchi are third- or fourth-order branches. There are three segments in the right upper lobe, two in the middle, and five in the lower lobe. On the left there are five altogether in both divisions of the upper lobe and five in the lower lobe. From the preceding it can be seen that the segments carry their own arterial supply, which branches with the bronchi, and that they are bounded by connective tissue septa. At this level the bronchial tree rarely exhibits an unu-

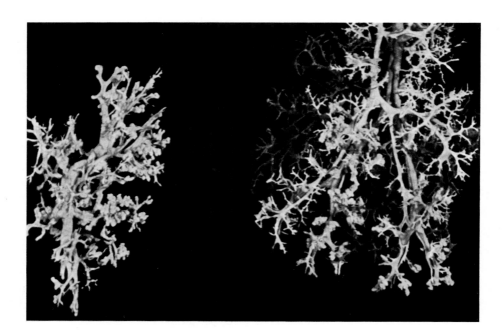

23–20 The peripheral airway with its accompanying pulmonary artery on the left, and together with the pulmonary vein on the right, as these structures appear in casts. This is a black-and-white rendition of a color plate. See color section. (From Lauweryns, J. 1962. De Longvaten. Brussels: Ed. Arscia.)

sual branching pattern. When anomalies occur, they do so at predictable sites, and the segmental artery is displaced along with the bronchus. This makes it feasible for surgeons to perform successful partial resections of the lungs in cases of serious pulmonary disease.

The Pattern of Bronchial Branching. The most typical mammalian lungs are adapted to fit comfortably within long, narrow, and deep thoracic cavities such as many quadrupeds possess. In these cavities the primary bronchi run caudally from the hilum toward the dorsomedial inferior angle of each lung. Secondary bronchi arise predominantly as outwardly directed lateral branches of the primary bronchi. They also form a dorsal and a less complete ventral series and, rarely, an internal lateral one as well. The primary bronchus thereby serves as an axis for each lung. The secondary branches are largest cranially and smallest caudally. They are given

off fairly regularly, the lateral branches in alteration with the dorsoventral sets. In humans the lungs are squeezed into a short, broad, and shallow thorax; accordingly, the pattern of bronchial branching is atypical. Informed opinion holds that the primary bronchi of humans are not true axial structures but give rise to three secondary bronchi in the right lung and two in the left. These become the lobar bronchi, and each develops its own pattern of branching.

Like the trachea, many of the subsidiary bronchi branch by unequal dichotomy, whereby the smaller of two diverging bronchi veers more from the path of its parent than the other. From this viewpoint, the bronchial tree consists of a sequence of unequal branchings that vary in number, depending on whether counts are made in long or in short segments. In humans as many as 25 generations can be counted in the longest segmental bronchi, making the maximum number of divisions 27 or 28 starting from the primary bronchus. Nevertheless, because both the caliber of bronchi belonging to the same branching order and the number of generations between the trachea and the respiratory zone will very depending on which branching path is followed, the bronchial tree must also be considered from other standpoints before one can picture it adequately. These are discussed below.

The caliber of the airways and the angles of branching have been measured in bronchial trees of human and canine lungs. These data enable one to estimate patterns of air flow and the completeness of ventilation in various parts of the lung more accurately than is possible when calculations are based on abstract models. In these species the distance from the carina to the respiratory surface (the *bronchial path length*) varies considerably in different parts of the lung. This inequality represents an accommodation of the bronchial tree to available space and is smaller in humans than in the long-chested dog, where the paths range from 2 mm to 12 cm, beginning with the base of the lobar bronchus. Other things being equal, bronchi of equal caliber have about the same number of terminal airways, and they lead to an approximately equal area of respiratory surface. Nevertheless, where the bronchial path is longer, its airways are of larger caliber than where the path is shorter; a lowered airway resistance is compensation for the long path. The main defect in this arrangement is that the respiratory surface at the end of these long pathways is exposed to a disproportionately large volume of residual air in the bronchial tree (the *anatomical dead space*), and under certain circumstances this may lead to unequal ventilation of ambient air in different regions of the lung.

As the bronchi bifurcate, the total cross-sectional area of the airway increases by a factor of about 1.3 in the first five generations and by somewhat more thereafter. If the total cross-sectional area is measured at successive distances from the carina, it is seen to reach a peak and then to decline. At first the increments due to branching predominate over the decrements due to termination of the smaller bronchial paths. Subsequently the terminations predominate. The effect of these anatomic arrangements is to make the conducting portions of the lungs as small as possible. In living specimens the airway is flexible and changes its configuration with each breathing cycle. It has been likened to a gradually expanding funnel on inspiration but to a cylinder during expiration, owing to changes in the diameters of distal bronchi (Fig. 23–21.)

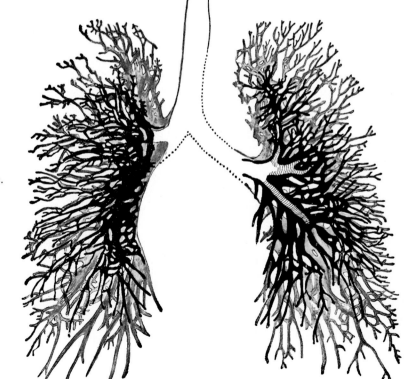

23–21 Bronchial tree. Tracings made from x-ray shadows. **Gray,** inspiration; **black,** expiration. (Work of C. C. Macklin.)

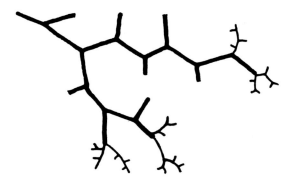

23–22 Centimeter and millimeter branching patterns in the peripheral airway. The end branches are terminal bronchioles. About natural size. (After Reid, L., and Simon, G. 1958. Thorax 13:103.)

Along the distal half of a bronchial pathway the airways divide at regular intervals, often forking obtusely and always decreasing in caliber after branching. Farther along, a fairly abrupt transition leads to a region where branching is frequent and the branches are short and slender. In humans these patterns can be seen in bronchograms made after instilling radiopaque material in the bronchial tree. The coarser branching occurs at 0.5- to 1-cm intervals along an axial path of several centimeters; the finer branching occurs at intervals of 2 to 3 mm and extends about 1 cm farther (Fig. 23–22). The fine-meshed pattern is found in the distal part of all bronchial pathways whether they end deep in the lungs or near the pleural surface. By means of correlated histological study it has been established that the final branches of this network are terminal conducting airways. The respiratory portion of the lung begins immediately afterward, the region ventilated by one terminal radiating from the outlet for a distance of 2 to 5 mm.

Histology of the Conducting Airways

The larger airways of the lungs are called *bronchi* and the smaller ones are called *bronchioles*. These are essentially anatomical terms but a fairly characteristic histological appearance is associated with each. In humans the bronchi comprise some 9 to 12 generations, beginning with the primary bronchus and ending with airways having a caliber of approximately 1 mm. The bronchioles begin as branches of the smallest bronchi and in humans continue for up to 12 generations

before ending as terminal bronchioles. A range is given because the number of bronchial and bronchiolar divisions varies, depending on the segment counted. Histologically, bronchi cannot be distinguished from bronchioles on the basis of a single characteristic. For example, it is often stated that bronchi contain cartilage in their walls whereas bronchioles do not. With such definitions one soon runs into difficulty with terminology: In the howling monkey, in mice, and in many microchiropteran bats there is virtually no intrapulmonary cartilage (Fig. 23–23). On the other hand, in whales the cartilage extends to well beyond the conducting airways. In humans it is continued for varying distances along the part of the bronchial tree having the centimeter-branching pattern; the millimeter-branching airways are safely termed bronchioles.

Bronchi. For a short distance beyond their origin, extrapulmonary bronchi retain the structural organization of the trachea and a similar histological appearance in the mucosa, submucosa, muscularis, and adventitia (Fig 23–24, see here and color insert). Gradually, two major changes become manifest: (1) the cartilaginous rings become less regular and (2) the muscularis develops into a complete ring of smooth muscle located between the submucosa and the cartilage. At first the bronchial cartilages only become shorter and narrower than those of the trachea, but not far beyond the hilum they become highly irregular in shape. Viewed in cross sections of the bronchi, the cartilages often seem isolated (Fig. 23–25), but viewed in three dimensions they remain part of a comprehensive skeletal framework. At bronchial bifurcations they are often saddle-shaped. Farther along the airway they become reduced to solitary fragments. As in the trachea, the cartilages are hyaline, although parts of them are infiltrated with elastic fibers, especially in the smaller bronchi. The muscularis becomes a more prominent layer as the cartilages decline. It is made up of numerous fascicles of approximately 20 to 30 cells each (Fig. 23–23 and 23–26). These fascicles can be identified as separate entities, but in the bronchi they are closely packed together and they all follow fairly similar circular or spiral courses about the airway. In the bronchi as in the trachea, the muscle fibers attach to each other as well as to the fibrous framework of the airway (Fig. 23–17; see here and color insert). Some muscle fibers in the outer part of the muscularis are joined to the fi-

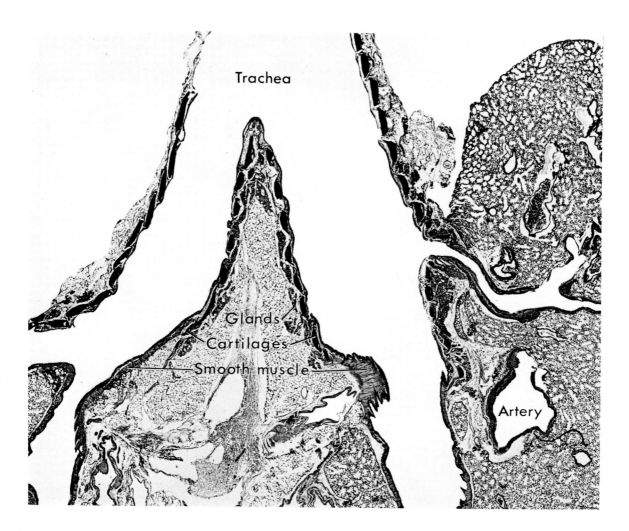

Trachea

Glands

Cartilages

Smooth muscle

Artery

brous membrane that envelops the cartilages. This membrane also serves as an attachment for numerous fine elastic and collagenous fibers that cross the muscularis to join heavier fibrous networks in the connective tissue beneath the epithelium.

As the bronchial generations are traced, the airway gradually undergoes a change from a histological appearance typical of bronchi (Fig. 23–25) toward one typical of bronchioles. With continued branching, the bronchial wall decreases in thickness, but all layers of the wall are not decreased proportionately. The disproportion alone accounts for most of the change in appearance. As the bronchi become smaller, the pseudostratified epithelium becomes lower. Connective tissue compartments internal to the muscularis become reduced in width. In small bron-

23–23 Section of a bat's lung near the hilum showing the trachea and primary bronchi and part of the right lung. Glands are coextensive with the cartilage of the bronchial wall and in this species occur largely in the adventitia. Iron hematoxylin. × 30.

chi the lamina propria becomes so thin that the fibers of its elastic membrane lie immediately beneath the epithelium. The submucosa remains appreciably thick where it houses the acini of the bronchial glands. It contains branches of the bronchial arteries, which supply nutrient capillary beds for the airway. Near the hilum it contains the bronchial veins as well.

If the cells and collagenous fibers of an inflated lung are digested away, a skeleton of elastic tissue remains, perfect in its preservation of

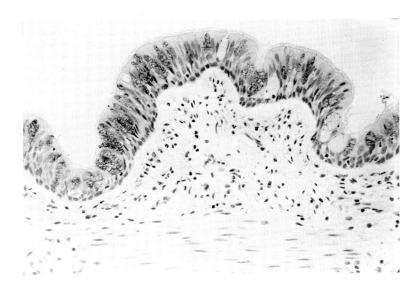

23–24 Bronchial epithelium of the human lung. × 250. This is a black-and-white rendition of a color plate. See color section.

the outlines of the bronchial tree, the pulmonary alveoli, and the blood vessels (Fig. 23–28). In the airways the elastic skeleton comprises mainly the longitudinally oriented proprial fibers and elastic fibers in the fibrocartilaginous membrane of the inner adventitia (Fig. 23–16 and 23–17, see here and color insert, and 23–27). Submu-

cosal fibers serve to suspend the mucosa from the outer layers of the airway and to support the blood vessels and glands within the submucosa. Consequently, these fibers take a more radial course overall than the proprial fibers. In the muscularis the fibers run in various, often circular, directions. Reticular fibers are distributed with the elastic fibers. They lie just beneath the epithelial basement lamina and form a delicate tracery around individual stromal cells. The coarser collagenous fibers are everywhere pres-

23–25 Cross section of a bronchus in a kitten. Mallory azan stain. × 85.

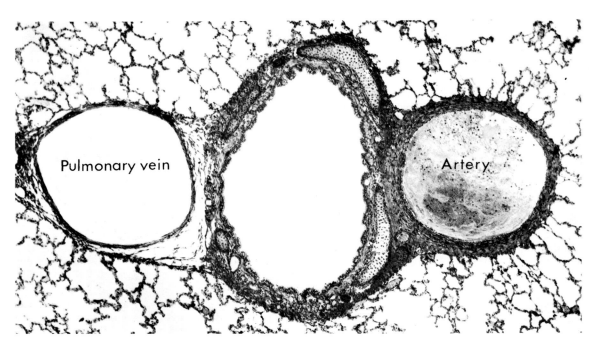

Pulmonary vein

Artery

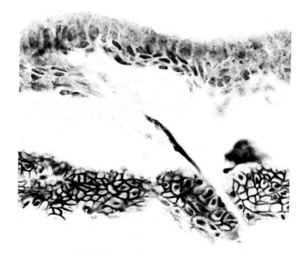

23–26 Adenosine triphosphatase activity in the lung of a beaver. The bronchial smooth muscle is strongly reactive at the cell margin (**black**) as is a small blood vessel in the space above. Gomori method, pH 9.4. × 350.

23–27 Cross section of a child's bronchus stained for elastic fibers. These are formed into an elastic membrane between the epithelium and muscularis, into a circular pattern in the muscularis, and into a longitudinal adventitial network. The cartilage is partly elastic. × 150.

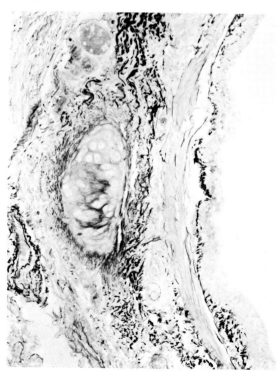

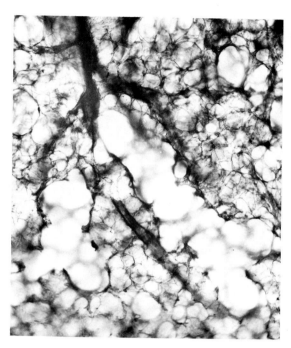

23–28 Thick section of a rat lung prepared to show the elastic fiber skeleton. Resorcin-fuchsin stain. × 80.

ent in the connective tissues but are densest in the common investments of the major pulmonary septa, vessels, and bronchi.

Bronchial Glands. The bronchial glands closely resemble the numerous small glands located in the upper air passages. They are coextensive with the cartilaginous skeleton. Accordingly, along certain bronchial paths in humans they come as close as 2 to 3 cm from the pleura but approach less closely in other paths. In bats they scarcely extend beyond the hilum (Fig. 23–23). As glands disappear from the airway, the surface mucous cells often increase in number. They are carried farther into the bronchial tree than the glands and end in the bronchioles. The glands are supplied by bronchial vascular beds furnished with fenestrated capillaries (Fig. 23–72). As in the larynx, glandular acini are penetrated by both sensory and secretomotor nerve endings. In contrast, the overlying pseudostratified epithelium has sensory but few motor endings. This difference may explain why the glands readily secrete after stimulation of parasympathetic nerves, whereas the surface cells respond more clearly to local irritation.

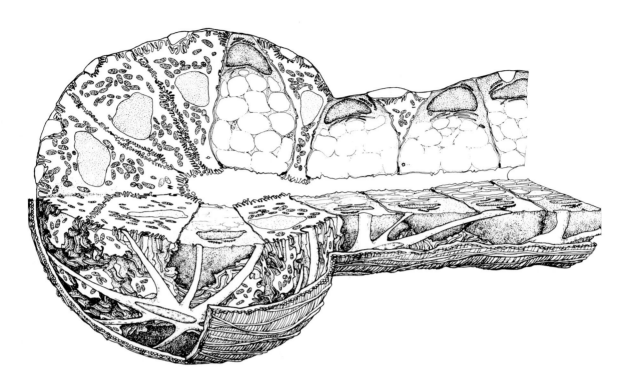

23–29 Diagram showing a three-dimensional view of
the acinus and duct of a bronchial gland.
(Drawing by G. Pederson-Krag in Sorokin, S. 1965.
Am. J. Anat. 117:311.)

The major constituents of the glands are both
mucous and serous epithelial cells and the myoepithelium. Minor constituents include small-
granule cells generically related to those in
the surface epithelium and a number of unusual
cell types that are inconspicuous in paraffin sections and, lacking mucous droplets, have sometimes been classified among serous cells. The secretory cells are concentrated in tubules or acini
located at the terminations of the branching
ductwork (Fig. 23–29), but mucous cells often
occur at all levels of branching. The main duct
leading in from the bronchial surface is lined by
typical laryngobronchial epithelium, which in
many cases directly joins small branches possessing secretory cells but without ciliated ones.
In the larger bronchial glands a transition zone
consisting of a collecting duct or ducts must first
be crossed. In human lungs this usually single
intermediate duct is lined by large, acidophil
cells unusually rich in mitochondria and apparently endowed with ion-segregating capacity
(Fig. 23–30, see here and color insert). These

cells have been called *oncocytes* because neoplastic counterparts form tumors easily recognizable by their pale-stained appearance. Oncocytes
normally may function like striated duct cells of
salivary glands (Chap. 18), acting to modify the
salinity of secretions as they pass en route to the
bronchial surface. In contrast, another ion-segregating cell type, the *hydrotic cell* of opossum
bronchial glands, occurs among mucous cells in
the terminal acini rather than in the collecting
ducts, which are lined by unspecialized cuboidal
cells. Stellate *myoepithelial cells* are found in
the acini and partway up the secretory branches.
They possess ultrastructural features of smooth
muscle and by their contraction help to force secretions onto the bronchial surface (Figs. 23–29
and 23–30, see here and color insert).

Typical mucous cells in these glands (Fig.
23–30, see here and color insert) differ little from
those of the surface epithelium, which have been
described above (Fig. 23–24, see here and color
insert). The term *serous* is a broad one applicable
to any cells producing a watery and sometimes
protein-containing secretion that might or might
not have enzymic activity. As protein-secreting
cells, they are relatively rich in granular reticulum and poor in agranular reticulum; such serous cells are the predominant ones in mamma-

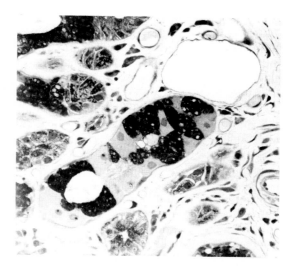

23–30 Secretory acini and intermediate duct of a human bronchial gland, showing the principal cell types present. × 420. This is a black-and-white rendition of a color plate. See color section.

lian bronchial glands, where they occur in the most peripheral regions either in acini or in demilunes attached to mucous acini. Their secretory droplets generally range from about 0.3 to 1 μm in diameter are are more electron-dense than droplets of mucus. These are released individually from the apical surface or into intercellular canaliculi that extend between the cells for a short distance.

The secretions of the glands complement those released by cells on the laryngobronchial surface. Together they make up *bronchial fluid*, which contains water admixed with a variety of mucins, serum proteins filtered from the blood, secretory immunoglobulin, some immunoglobulin M, the bacteriostatic protein lactoferrin, and a number of largely uncharacterized muco- and glycoproteins derived from serous or seromucous cells present in the glands, to which are added secretions from bronchiolar cells located deeper within the lungs. Mucins of the respiratory tract are acid glycoproteins consisting of a polypeptide core and side chains of high molecular-weight mucopolysaccharides predominantly grouped into two classes. The first contains side chains made up of repeating units or sulfated amino sugar or uronic acid (sulfomucins) and the other, a structure rich in sialic acid residues (sialomucins); of these the sialomucins

generally are more viscous. The mucous cells that produce these substances nearly all look alike ultrastructurally, but their secretions are distinguished from one another by histochemical staining. Exceptionally, in some species bronchial glands possess still other mucoid cells; these have small secretory droplets like those in surface mucous cells of the stomach (Chap. 18) instead of the large and sometimes coalescing droplets of the more typical cells.

Mucous acini of human glands contain predominantly four acid glycoproteins, two sialomucins and two sulfomucins. All are stainable with alcian blue, but the sulfomucins continue to stain at a lower pH than the sialomucins (Chap. 2). In individual cells some staining is abolished after sections are treated with sialidase (neuraminidase); one class of sialomucin is easily digested whereas the other is relatively resistant. Sulfomucins are recognized by their retention of alcian blue stainability despite prolonged sialidase digestion, and they are also divisible into two classes. The first incorporates radioactive sulfate but fails to stain for sulfate groups, whereas the second contains sufficient accessible sulfate to stain. Any given human mucous cell might contain one or more of these mucins. When only one kind is present, it tends to be either the sialidase-susceptible sialomucin or the sulfomucin stainable for sulfate groups. Mixtures of both sulfomucins may occur in one cell and mixtures of both sialomucins in another, whereas in still other cells the sialidase-resistant sialomucin may be combined with one or both sulfomucins. To a fair extent this variability in mucin content can be understood to reflect a ripening process occurring while the secretion builds up in the cytoplasm. The types of mucins present in surface mucous cells are highly species-variable, but cells in the larger airways of humans produce sulfomucin and those in the periphery, sialomucin.

Human serous cell secretions stain by periodic acid Schiff (PAS) and only faintly with alcian blue, which indicates that mucopolysaccharides are present, although neutral kinds predominate over the acid kinds present in mucus. Other histochemical evidence indicates that sulfate and sialic acid groups are nonetheless present in this polysaccharide but are incorporated differently from mucus. The secretions therefore are of a seromucous character (Fig. 23–30, see here and color insert).

A few serous cells may occur in the surface

epithelium, but far more are confined to the glands. The relative proportion of surface to glandular mucous cells is decidedly species-variable, but it is also affected by such factors as stress and chronic infection. Any irritation to the bronchial tree generally calls forth an increase in mucus production. The number of mucous cells increase and the glands enlarge. For example, tracheal and bronchial glands are far more numerous in humans than in the otherwise similar regions of the great apes, which has been attributed to the need for greater air flow in human lungs to meet requirements for phonation above that needed for respiration.

Bronchioles. At some point along any given bronchial path the airway, having lost its bronchial characteristics, gradually acquires new ones; the airway is then called a bronchiole (Fig.

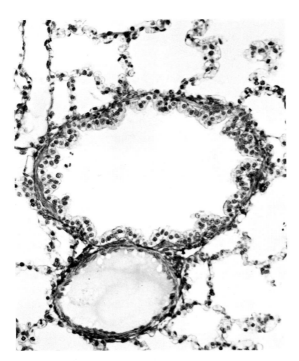

23–31 Bronchiole and small pulmonary artery in a
  △   kitten's lung. Mallory azan stain. × 125.

23–32 Longitudinal section of a large bronchiole in
  ▽   a rat. At this level the ciliated cells always outnumber the bronchiolar cells. Beneath the epithelium, bundles of smooth muscle are separated by connective tissue. Toluidine blue. × 1,440.

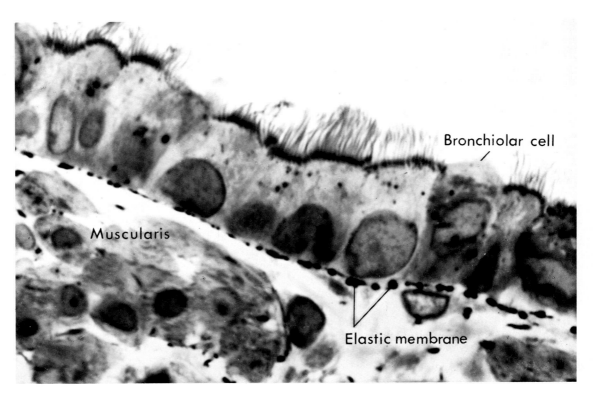

Bronchiolar cell

Muscularis

Elastic membrane

23–31). It retains the radial organization of preceding passages but no longer is lined by a laryngobronchial type of epithelium, nor does it have cartilage, glands, or a continuous muscularis. New features are (1) a columnar epithelium in which a unique type of secretory cell displaces the mucous cell; (2) a proportional increase, compared with large bronchi, in the thickness of the muscularis; and (3) a separation of smooth muscle fascicles by connective tissue (Figs. 23–32 and 23–33). All connective tissue compartments of the bronchiolar wall are united into one investing mass.

Two major cell types, ciliated and nonciliated, line the bronchioles (Fig. 23–34). In the larger branches, most cells are ciliated, but the nonciliated cells usually dominate the smaller branches (Fig. 23–37, see here and color insert). The ciliated cells are similar to those in the bronchi except that they are shorter. The nonciliated *bronchiolar* cells give the epithelium its special character. They are tall, dome-shaped, and protrude into the bronchiolar lumen to the tips of the cilia. Accordingly, in sections of bronchioles the epithelium has a scalloped contour.

As in many water-permeable epithelia, cytoplasmic leaflets extend from the lateral surfaces of both ciliated and nonciliated cells to intermingle with those from adjacent cells (Figs. 23–34 and 23–35). Moreover, capillary loops close to the basement lamina have discrete, fenestrated areas facing the epithelium. These features occur elsewhere along the conducting airways and in the body. They are a part of a mechanism to provide regulated water transport across the epithelium.

Reconstructions of the bronchiolar wall have shown the smooth muscle to be formed into a geodesic network. The separate fascicles of muscle branch and anastomose so that some fibers run circularly and others obliquely. Through this arrangement the force of contraction is exerted perpendicular to the wall. Owing to the comparative strength of the muscularis in the bronchioles, contractions are felt there more strongly than in the bronchi. Like muscles of the alimentary tract, those of the airway are activated primarily by parasympathetic fibers and are known to undergo peristaltic movements. They participate in the cough reflex and increase bronchial tone in cold weather. They also relax during inspiration and contract at the end of expiration, thereby helping bronchial fiber systems to return distended airways to resting dimensions.

Bronchiolar Epithelial Cells. The basic organization of bronchiolar cells (Clara cells) gives them an unmistakable identity in the lungs of many mammals, even though striking interspecies differences may still be present in one or more of the cytoplasmic organelles. With a basal ergastoplasm and apical, membrane-bounded droplets, these cells can be classified as serous cells, but they contrast with others of this class in possessing an unusual abundance of agranular reticulum in the supranuclear and apical cytoplasm (Fig. 23–35). This predominates over the Golgi lamellae, the lysosomal particulates, the apical centrioles, and other normal features of the region. A granular reticulum, Golgi apparatus, and secretory granules are typical features of all cells manufacturing proteins for export. In bronchiolar cells of mice, radioactively labeled leucine becomes incorporated into the granules after first passing through these organelles, which suggests that proteins are included in the secretory product. Bronchiolar cells are among the more metabolically active cells in the lungs (Figs. 23–45 and 23–58). They have also been shown to incorporate into the granules both tritiated acetate and galactose, plausible precursors of lipid and polysaccharide, respectively. In several species the secretory droplets are like zymogen granules of other cells (Fig. 23–35); in rats they have a crystalline substructure; but in mice they appear electron-lucent (Fig. 23–36), as if rich in lipid. Mature granules in rats are said to be inactive for acid phosphatase and esterase, enzymes reactive in the bronchiolar cells' lysosomes, but very little positive information has been obtained about specific granule contents. Any full explanation of the functions of bronchiolar cells must account for the extensive agranular reticulum so frequently present. This organelle is well developed in cells substantially engaged in either cholesterol or carbohydrate synthesis, and experimental evidence rather confirms that the agranular reticulum of bronchiolar cells actively synthesizes both classes of compounds. In mice, both acetate and galactose appear in this cytoplasmic compartment; and in bats, glycogen accumulates against its cytoplasmic face (Fig. 23–36). An extensive agranular reticulum may also appear in cells engaged in ion-segregation or detoxification reactions. Although there is little evidence that bronchiolar cells act in ion-segregation, those of rats and mice possess a mixed-function oxidase system that may detoxify certain atmospheric contami-

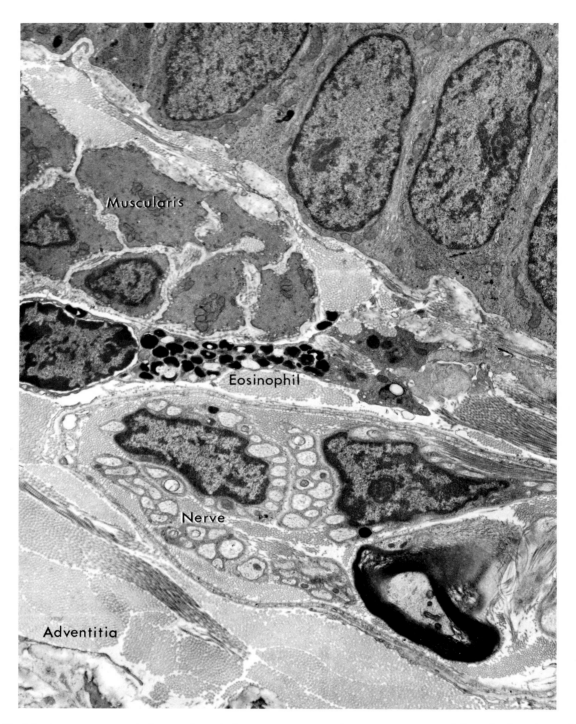

23–33 Electron micrograph showing bronchiolar connective tissue. A peribronchial nerve bundle carries a single myelinated axon and several small unmyelinated fibers wrapped in Schwann cell mesaxons. × 8,000.

nants. In any case, material from both Golgi and agranular membranes is pinched off into the secretory granules, and they are slowly and individually released from the cells into the bronchiolar lumen (Fig. 23–35, inset). The surface

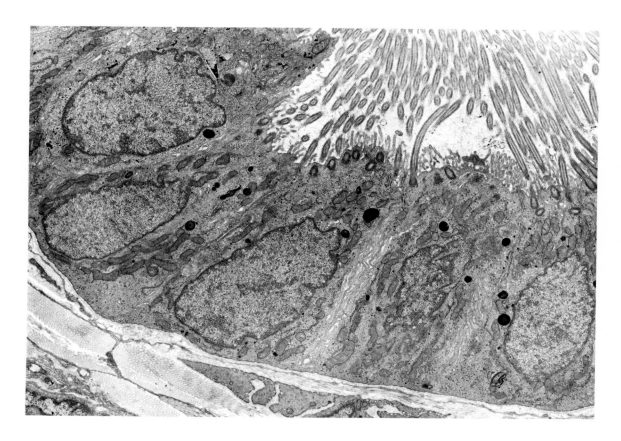

fluid is rich in protein and also contains muco-polysaccharides and cholesterol, substances similarly present in secretions released in pulmonary alveoli (discussed under great alveolar cells). To what extent alveolar and bronchiolar fluids are similar cannot be answered precisely, but it seems that surface tension-reducing lipid, abundant in alveoli, is relatively scarce in bronchioles.

Bronchiolar cells have been studied in at least 18 kinds of mammals, including common representative chiropterans (Fig. 23–35), primates, rodents (Figs. 23–36 and 23–37; see here and color insert), lagomorphs, carnivores, perissodactyls, and artiodactyls, so that the range of variability in their cytoplasmic makeup is fairly well appreciated. Cellular peculiarities shared by all include their lack of cilia, their position in small airways of the lungs, and their formation of lateral channels with adjacent epithelial cells (Fig. 23–35). Secretory granules are common to cells from all groups, but within any lung only a minority of cells have many of them at a given time. Unusual development of agranular reticulum is prominent in bronchiolar cells of most groups,

23–34 Electron micrograph of bronchiolar epithelium of a bat, showing bronchiolar (upper left) and ciliated cells and the lateral interdigitations between cells. × 7,000.

but it is less remarkable in carnivores and appears to be absent in primates. Two other features of these cells in some species are the presence of unusually large globose mitochondria with voluminous matrix and few cristae and the presence of glycogen, already described as forming in relationship to the agranular reticulum (Fig. 23–36). These features occur in no apparent relationship to the natural order of species. The unusual mitochondria are characteristic of cats and mice but are absent or variable in other species; tritiated acetate incorporation into such mitochondria is also high. The glycogen is conspicuous in mature bronchiolar cells of chiropterans, carnivores, and bovines but is variable in the rest. Overall, these variations mainly reflect different balances in the expressed activity of lipid and carbohydrate metabolism seen in bronchiolar cells of different species as they go about elaborating their secretory products.

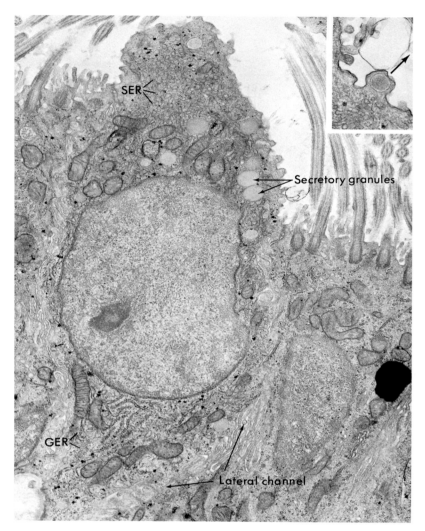

SER

Secretory granules

GER

Lateral channel

23–35 Typical features of *bronchiolar cells* are a basal granular endoplasmic reticulum **(GER)**, apical smooth reticulum **(SER)**, and secretory granules, which are released at the free surface **(inset)**. Intercellular channels and a large residual body **(black)** in a ciliated cell are also shown. Vampire bat. × 9,450.

◁

23–36 Detail of apical cytoplasm in bronchiolar cells of a mouse **(left)** and a bat **(right)**. × 30,000. ▽

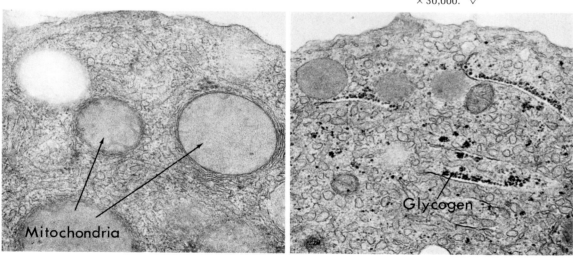

Mitochondria

Glycogen

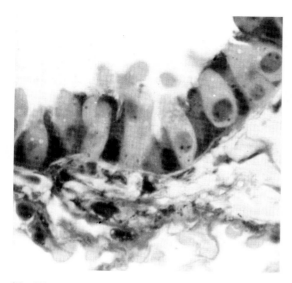

23–37 Hamster bronchiole showing predominance of nonciliated bronchiolar cells. × 1,200. This is a black-and-white rendition of a color plate. See color section.

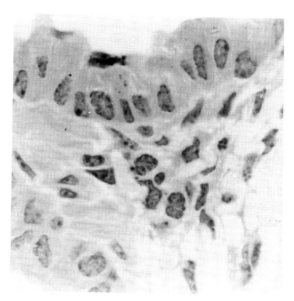

23–38 Prussian blue–stained iron particles in the bronchus of a mouse. Basic fuchsin. × 1,100. This is a black-and-white rendition of a color plate. See color section.

Bronchiolar cells are present in a greater part of the bronchial tree of small as compared with large animals, probably because most of the branches are of small caliber. That is to say, bronchiolar cells will occur in airways if they are somewhat smaller than a millimeter in diameter. In chronic bronchitis the bronchioles are the main sites of obstruction by cellular debris and mucus; keeping this in mind, one might guess that secretions of bronchiolar cells serve to prevent this in normal subjects by providing proteo- or mucolytic enzymes and possibly nonenzymic substances to alter the stickiness of the secretions released higher up in the bronchial tree. These cells lie *distal* to the mucus-producing areas of the lungs just as serous cells generally are distal to mucous cells in glands, perhaps for a similar reason.

Compared with the nonciliated bronchiolar cells, the ciliated cells have longer microvilli, somewhat obscured by the cilia, the rudiments of a system of (ca. 600-Å) tubular invaginations extending in from the apical surface, and rather large, sometimes extremely electron-dense lysosomal residual bodies (Fig. 23–35). These features arguably endow the ciliated better than the bronchiolar cells with whatever endocytotic capacity the epithelium has for both dissolved and finely particulate matter. This capacity normally is small but experimentally demonstrable; the

tubules comprise a significant channel for uptake of air-borne material deposited in the bronchi or bronchioles under conditions where mucociliary clearance becomes impeded and material remains for some time on the surface (Fig. 23–38, see here and color insert). Some of this material is shunted into the lateral channels between cells and some reaches the connective tissue beneath.

The bronchiolar epithelium also contains one or more kinds of neuroendocrine cells, to be described in the following section, as well as a presumably sensory brush cell like that described in the trachea (Figs. 23–11, *brush*; and 23–13, see here and color insert).

Neuroendocrine Cells of the Conducting Airways. Neuroendocrine *small-granule cells* of the respiratory system are members of the diffuse endocrine system of the body that includes the polypeptide hormone-secreting cells of the gastrointestinal tract and the endocrine pancreas, the parafollicular cells of the thyroid gland and ultimobranchial body, and the adrenocorticotrophs and melanotrophs of the adenohypophysis. These cells share a capacity for converting exogenously administered amine precursors like deoxyphenylalanine or 5-hydroxytryptophan by decarboxylation into dopamine or serotonin, re-

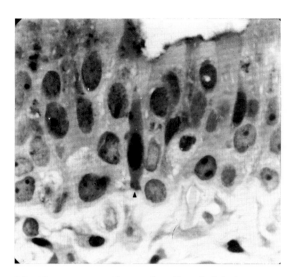

23–39 Human small-granule cell and globule leukocyte. This is a black-and-white rendition of a color plate. See color section.

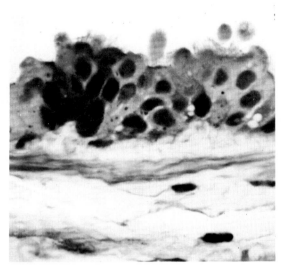

23–40 Small-granule cells (left of center) in the bronchial epithelium of a hamster. (From Sorokin, S., and Hoyt, R. F., Jr. 1978. Anat. Rec. 192:245.) This is a black-and-white rendition of a color plate. See color section.

spectively, and storing these amines in characteristic small (1,000–3,000 Å), dense-core endocrine granules; from this the general term *APUD cells* (Amine Precursor Uptake and Decarboxylation) has been derived. Chromaffin cells of the adrenal medulla, the paraganglia, and the carotid body are also classified among APUD cells, which therefore comprise a diverse and widespread group. Some occur as solitary cells within an epithelium, whereas others are gathered into rather loose clusters, and still others are arranged in distinct organoids. Within this class, a number of cell types are not innervated, although many of them are, synapsing either with autonomic efferents or visceral afferents, or both. The types of small-granule cells present in the respiratory system and their distribution are not as well codified as in the gut (Chap. 19) or islets of Langerhans (Chap. 22). It is abundantly clear, however, that they occur in many species, including commonly studied laboratory animals and the primates as well as less frequently examined mammals such as lions, pigs, hedgehogs, and rock-badgers. In the larynx or trachea these cells tend to occur singly or in small clusters, but in the lungs they frequently occur also in somewhat more highly organized aggregations termed *neuroepithelial bodies*. As is true for APUD cells in general, some small-granule cells of the respiratory tract are innervated and some are not.

Within the lung, individual small-granule cells and cell clusters are difficult to see in routine microscopic slides, although some of them can be revealed in paraffin sections by the argyrophilia of their granules. A number contain an intrinsic store of serotonin and so can be demonstrated in freeze-dried sections of lung exposed to formaldehyde vapor or plastic-embedded sections fixed in formaldehyde and examined with the ultraviolet microscope; the cells give off a yellow fluorescence from the condensation product formed between formaldehyde and the serotonin stored in the granules. Still more cells can be made to fluoresce if experimental animals are first administered the amine precursor (Fig. 23–14). Permanent light-microscopic slides are best made by staining plastic-embedded sections with PAS-lead hematoxylin (Figs. 23–39 and 23–40, see here and color insert), in which the cells or cell clusters stand out by their differential affinity for these dyes. Small-granule cells are also revealed in electron micrographs by their dense-core granules (Fig. 23–41). At the ultrastructural level the cells are seen to interdigitate with adjacent cells in a complex manner and frequently to send cytoplasmic processes beyond the cell body. These cells, and in many species particularly those cells organized into neuroepithelial bodies, are sometimes con-

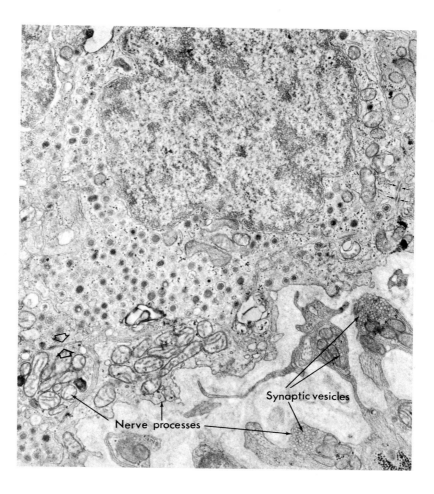

23–41 Small-granule cells of a bronchiolar neuroepithelial body. Various unmyelinated nerves approach from below, and a mitochondria-rich process closely contacts one of the cells **(open arrows)**, which join adjacent epithelial cells by desmosomes **(paired arrows).** Vampire bat. × 12,000.

Synaptic vesicles

Nerve processes

tacted by unmyelinated nerve fibers bearing clear synaptic vesicles. An efferent synapse can be said to occur at a point of close apposition where the vesicles are abundant, but other nerve processes contacting small-granule cells contain many mitochondria and only a few vesicles and may be epitheliodendritic or sensory (Fig. 23–41). Deeper in the neuroepithelial body, sections frequently pass through unsheathed nerve fibers, suggesting that cells of a cluster are individually innervated, whether by motor or sensory fibers.

The intralobar distribution of these cells has been described in great detail in hamster lungs. Approximately 30% of the cells preferentially occur in the epithelium near points of bronchial division and another 30% at *bronchiolo-alveolar portals*, or regions of transition in peripheral airways between the cuboidal bronchiolar epithelium and the flattened alveolar epithelium (de-

scribed in the following section). The remaining small-granule cells are scattered in-between. In rabbits the distribution is similar, but these endocrine cells have a strong tendency to occur in neuroepithelial bodies, and these bodies to occur along the ring of juncture between parent and daughter bronchi. In this species the bodies are especially well developed, consisting of an orderly group of tall cells perhaps 10 cells wide at the base and curved inward towards the apex somewhat like a taste bud.

Both the variability of staining observed in these cells (Fig. 23–40, see here and color insert) and differences in the ultrastructural appearance of the granules in different cells (Fig. 23–15) indicate that more than one kind of endocrine cell exists in many lungs. On this basis, three distinct cell types have been distinguished in humans, three in bats, and five in hamsters; and a specific polypeptide, *bombesin*, has been associated

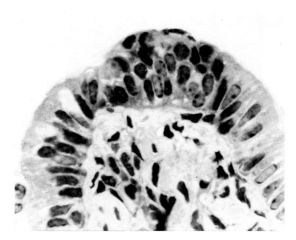

23–42 Heterophil leukocytes in migration through the epithelium at the origins of right and left bronchi in a hamster lung. This is a black-and-white rendition of a color plate. See color section.

lining of the larger airways (Fig. 23–39, see here and color insert). Globule leukocytes contain large, metachromatic granules somewhat similar to those in mast cells, which occur nearby in the subepithelial connective tissue. These granules are often less well preserved than in mast cells, giving some reason to believe that the cells represent a later stage in the life cycle of mast cells. During a pulmonic infection, or whenever particles with a chemotactic attraction for granulocytes are present in the airway, heterophils and sometimes eosinophils may be seen passing between cells of the epithelium (Fig. 23–42, see here and color insert); but these polymorphonuclear cells appear there in number only in frankly pathological states. In contrast, mononuclear phagocytes, like monocytes and alveolar macrophages (described in a later section), are almost never seen crossing the airway epithelium, although they frequently cross the thinner epithelial barrier in the respiratory zone.

with some of the endocrine cells in fetal human lungs. Some experimental evidence indicates that small-granule cells of rabbits respond to hypoxia in the airway by releasing granules at the cell base. It is also possible that innervated cells degranulate after stimulation by the central nervous system, or that the dense-core granules contain neurotransmitters to stimulate afferent nerves. Consequently, a number of regulatory roles may be envisaged for different pulmonary cells of this class. From the information gained by mapping them in the lung, it appears that most small-granule cells have a local action in that they are widely distributed throughout the bronchial tree; there they are close to the smooth muscle of the airway as well as to adjacent cells in the epithelium. At the portals, on the other hand, the association of small-granule cells with pulmonary capillaries is greater than in the airway, and secretions from these cells could more readily gain the circulation.

Migratory Cells in the Airway Epithelium. Under normal conditions, the epithelium of the trachea, bronchi, and bronchioles contains a small number of hematopoietic cells. Most often they are lymphocytes and another kind of mononuclear cell called a *globule leukocyte*, both of which participate in immunological reactions within pulmonary tissues as well as on the bronchial surface. The latter prevail in the

The Respiratory Zone

Respiratory Bronchioles and Subdivisions. In a typical branching sequence within mammalian lungs, each terminal bronchiole divides into two daughter branches called *respiratory bronchioles*. They resemble the terminal bronchiole in all but one respect: here and there the walls are interrupted by saccular outpocketings called *alveoli*, where respiratory gas exchange takes place (Figs. 23–43 to 23–45). At once possessing a respiratory surface and a bronchiolar structure, respiratory bronchioles are aptly named. Subsequently the number of alveoli increase with each branching of the airway, and after up to six divisions from the terminal bronchiole, the pathway ends in grapelike clusters of alveoli (Fig. 23–46). As these branches are traversed, the fraction of the wall taken up by alveoli increases, until the wall becomes little more than a series of openings into the alveoli. At that point the branches still retain the appearance of the conduit and are called alveolar ducts (Fig. 23–47). Farther on, the tubular sense is lost, and the remaining spaces are called, successively, atria, alveolar sacs, and alveoli (Fig. 23–48). The respiratory surface aerated by one terminal bronchiole is partitioned among the alveoli located all along the succeeding branches.

In adult humans there are normally three orders of respiratory bronchioles, and where they are not interrupted by alveoli, the walls are lined

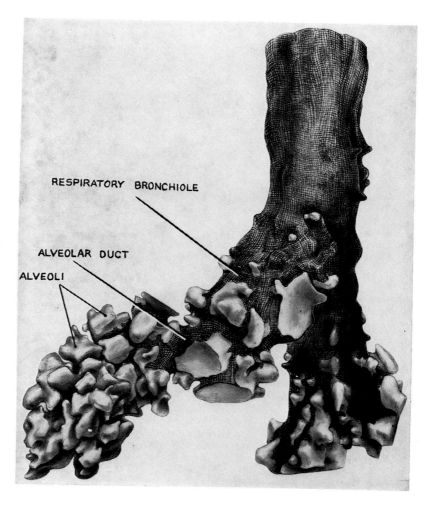

23-43 Cast model of a respiratory bronchiole with its subdivisions. Several alveolar ducts have been removed. The gradual onset of alveolarization along the bronchial path is clearly shown, although individual alveoli appear partly collapsed. The cross-hatching represents the approximate extent of the muscular coat in the airway. (From Bremer, J. L. 1935. Carnegie Institute Contrib. Embryol.)

RESPIRATORY BRONCHIOLE

ALVEOLAR DUCT

ALVEOLI

by a low columnar epithelium containing ciliated and bronchiolar cells. At the alveolar rim these cells become continuous with the thin alveolar lining. Beneath the epithelium the muscularis remains prominent within an investment of connective tissue that contains vascular beds and pulmonary nerves (Fig. 23-33) and is carried into the alveolar walls. The respiratory bronchioles are followed by about two generations of *alveolar ducts*. Along their highly alveolated walls the ducts exhibit bronchiolar characteristics only in the few places where a group of cuboidal epithelial cells cover underlying bands of muscle and connective tissue. The muscle forms a terminal sphincter at the outlet of the last alveolar duct and almost always ends there (Figs. 23-48 and 23-49). Evidently because the bronchiolar and alveolar epithelia are closely re-

lated biologically, alveolar epithelial cells sometimes are admixed in the lining of the respiratory bronchioles or ducts. The alveolar ducts open into *atria*, which are vestibules communicating with the multilocular *alveolar sacs*. Occasionally one but usually two or more sacs arise from each atrium, since they open out in all directions from it. These atria are irregular cavities surrounded by pulmonary *alveoli*, which are the individual locules of the sacs. The alveoli are the smallest subdivisions of the respiratory tree (Fig. 23-50). Within a given lung they are of fairly uniform size, but their dimensions are proportioned to the metabolic rate of the animal, being smallest (30 μm) in shrews and bats and largest (1,100 μm) in the large and sluggish Sirenia. In human beings, a total of some 300 million alveoli is divided between the lungs, and individual alveoli

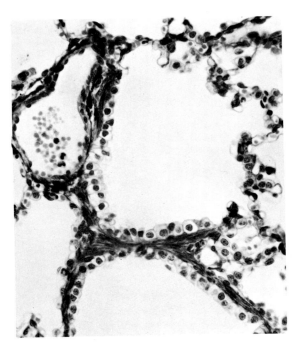

23–44 Respiratory bronchiole of a kitten. Note the low columnar epithelium on the left and the alveoli on the right. Mallory azan stain. × 125.

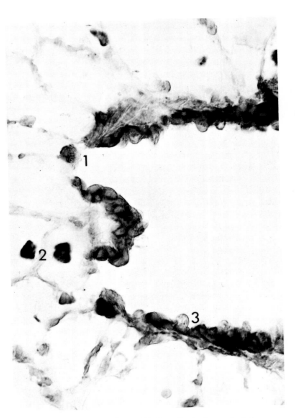

23–45 Respiratory bronchiole of a bat reacted for acid phosphatase. Ciliated cells and alveolar macrophages **(2)** are strongly reactive; great alveolar cells **(1)** and bronchiolar cells **(3),** less so. Burstone's method. × 200.

measure about 200 μm in diameter. Beyond the alveolar ducts the elastic fibers abandon their predominantly longitudinal course along the airway and form a complex network of fibers that come together to encircle the successive openings of atria, alveolar sacs, and alveoli.

Functional Respiratory Units. Those interested in pulmonary function have long sought to define functional subdivisions within the respiratory surface, aiming for an ideal unit that is at the same time modular and well defined anatomically. Such is the nonuniformity of the lungs that the ideal is unattainable, for it is one thing to find structurally similar units in this region, and it is another to find them uniform in size and shape. Moreover, the *average* size of these units is scaled up or down, depending on the animal possessing them. Among a wide range of mammals the size of such units is roughly commensurate with lung volume, which is proportional to body weight, and with respiratory surface area, which varies linearly and directly with basal oxygen consumption. The best anatomic unit is the *acinus*, which is simply the terminal

bronchiole and all its branches. In humans it has dimensions of millimeter size and is divided by its first-order respiratory bronchioles into two hemiacini. These differ in size and shape from each other and from those of other acini, the free variations on a simple pattern arising from a competition among branches for available space. A larger peripheral unit is the (secondary) *lobule*, supposedly formed by connective tissue septa passing into the lung from the pleura. Unfortunately, such septa are well defined only near the pleura and not deep within the lungs, and they do not demarcate equal volumes of lung. Consequently, this lobule has been redefined for the human lung in terms of the branching pattern in the peripheral airway (Fig. 23–22). It consists of a cluster of three to five acini whose terminal bronchioles arise close by one another

23–46 Terminal bronchial pathway in a kitten's lung. The two last bronchiolar orders **(1, 2)**, a short respiratory bronchiole, its pulmonary artery **(Art.)**, and subsequent respiratory structures are shown. The alveolated passages may vary in overall proportions among different species. Mallory azan. × 76. ▷

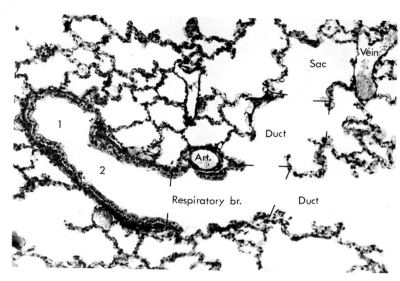

23–47 Looking down a human alveolar duct. The openings of the attached alveoli are guarded by entrance rings framed of connective tissue fibers and covered by attenuated epithelium. The pulmonary capillary bed gives the alveolar surface a rugose appearance, and interalveolar pores of Kohn **(right)** connect adjacent chambers. × 320. (From Gehr, P., Bachofen, M., and Weibel, E. R. 1978. Resp. Physiol. 32:121.) ▽

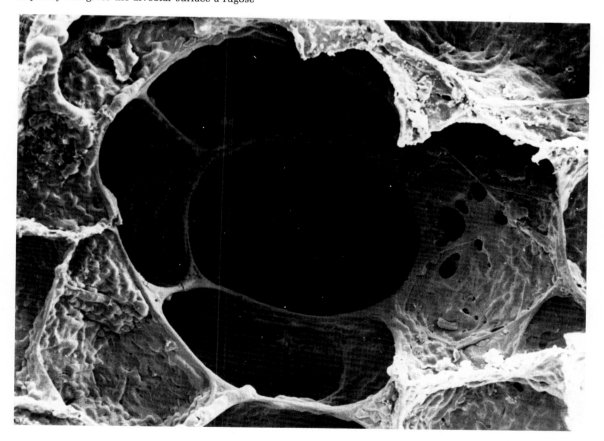

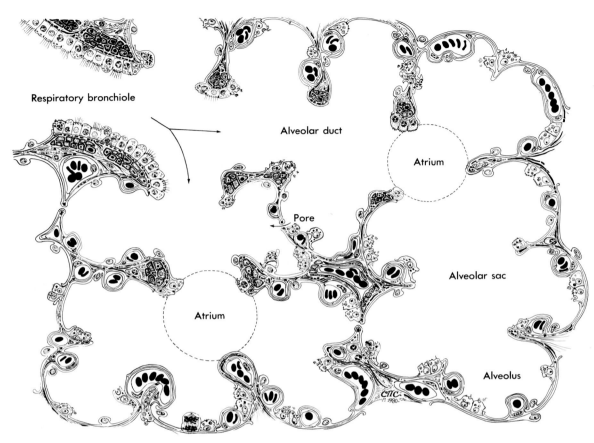

Respiratory bronchiole

Alveolar duct

Atrium

Pore

Atrium

Alveolar sac

Alveolus

23–48 Diagram of the respiratory subdivisions in the
△   lung, showing a respiratory bronchiole,
alveolar ducts, and subdivisions. Smooth muscle
(dark cells) ends in the alveolar ducts. The atria

(circled) are spaces bounded by the termination of the
alveolar duct on one end, and the openings of the
alveolar sacs on the other. In addition, major features
of the alveolar walls are presented.

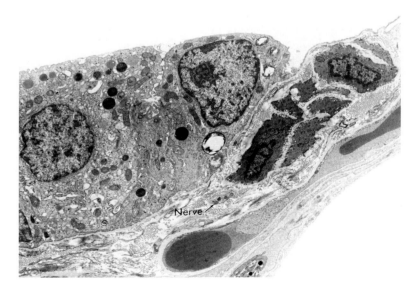

Nerve

23–49 A bronchiolo-alveolar
portal, transition from the
low columnar epithelium lining
terminal and respiratory
bronchioles to the attenuated
epithelium lining the alveoli.
Bronchiolar cells, a great alveolar
cell, and a squamous alveolar cell
are in continuity. At other portals
the exact sequence of epithelial
cells may differ; some contain
small-granule cells. The terminal
muscle sphincter lies beneath.
× 3,800.

◁

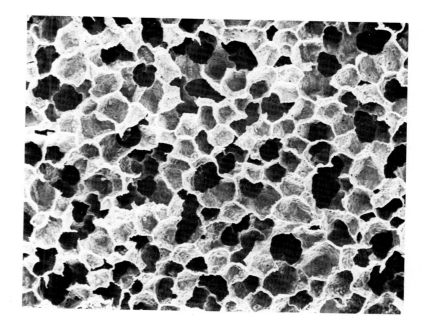

23–50 Scanning electron micrograph of the respiratory parenchyma from a horse's lung. × 175. (Courtesy of P. Gehr.)

at the end of a given centimeter-branching bronchial path. Such a unit measures 1 to 2 cm² in volume and is of a convenient size for use in radiological studies on patients.

If the acinus is a natural anatomical unit in the human lung, it is because the dichotomous branching down to terminal bronchioles is fairly regular and not excessively unequal. In many truly small animals like hamsters and mice, branching may be very unequal, commencing with the lobar bronchi, which are small tubes measuring a millimeter or less in diameter. Some of their subsidiary divisions fork off at obtuse angles, quickly diminishing in diameter and rapidly reaching the respiratory surface. Along such a branching system, the beginning of alveolarization may be marked by the appearance of an alveolar cluster that seems to protrude from the wall of an airway perhaps three generations removed from the lobar bronchus, but this can be understood as easily to result from extremely unequal branching. In a lung like this it is very difficult to find standardized respiratory units.

Structure of the Alveolar Wall. The alveolar wall is specialized toward promoting diffusion between external and internal environments (Table 23–1). As at any exposed surface, an epithelium covers a vascularized connective tissue space, but in the alveolar wall the epithelial and connective tissue layers are both very thin, and the blood vessels form the richest capillary network in the body (Fig. 23–51). In details of organization these walls are similar in most mammalian lungs. Between adjacent alveoli a framework of elastic and collagenous fibers supports a meshwork of anastomosing pulmonary capillaries. The vessels are woven through the framework much as vines are woven through a trellis. In marine mammals, alveolar capillaries run in two beds, one on each of two adjacent alveolar surfaces, being separated from each other by a central connective tissue septum rich in cells and fibers, and from the alveolar air by a

Table 23–1 Dimensions of the Human Respiratory Surface[a]

Lung volume	4,100–4,600 ml[b]
Alveolar surface area	143 m²[c]
Capillary surface area	126 m²
Capillary blood volume	213 ml
Thickness of air–blood barrier	
Arithmetic mean	2.2 μm
Harmonic mean	0.6 μm

[a]Reported by Gehr, P., Bachofen, M., and Weibel, E. R. 1978. Resp. Physiol. 32:121.

[b]Body weight approximately 74 kg.

[c]Based on measurements in electron micrographs, which yield a figure 75% higher than measurements in light micrographs, because more nooks and crannies are revealed. Functional dimensions are lower because many of these crannies are covered over by alveolar surface fluid and because alveoli and capillaries partially fold and unfold with each breathing cycle. The problem is to estimate the internal surface area of an accordion in performance!

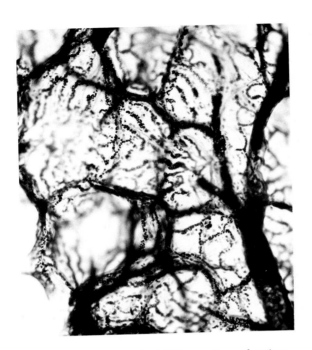

layer of epithelium. Through reduction in the connective tissue and through formation of extensive anastomoses, these capillary beds are rationalized by most other mammals into one system that serves adjacent alveoli. The connective tissue septum, having become thin and pliant, no longer occupies a distinctly central position but fills the interstices between the capillaries (Figs. 23–48 and 23–52). When alveoli abut against the pleura, the septa, an airway wall, or large blood vessels instead of against each other, the alveolar connective tissue blends in with the tissue of the adjacent structure. At such points only do alveoli contact lymphatic capillaries (Fig. 23–76, see here and color insert; and Fig. 23–79), for these vessels do not penetrate interalveolar septa except when the septa are rather thick, as in whales.

The alveolar epithelium is inhomogeneous, consisting primarily of attenuated *squamous alveolar cells* and pleomorphic *great alveolar cells* (Fig. 23–48). A brush cell of unknown function as well as a nonciliated cuboidal cell that ap-

23–51 Thick section of adult human lung, showing
△   the distribution of small blood vessels within
the alveolar walls. × 125.

23–52 Interalveolar wall in the lungs, showing the
central connective tissue space in continuity
with a pulmonary venule. × 7,000. ▽

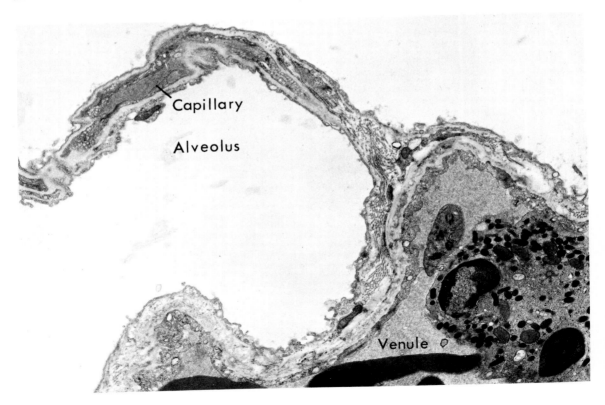

Capillary

Alveolus

Venule

pears immature are minor constituents. The endothelium consists of flattened cells of the nonfenestrated type found in muscle capillaries. By light microscopy, they are scarcely distinguishable from the squamous alveolar cells because both are thin and elongated and have small nuclei (Figs. 23–53 and 23–64, see here and color insert). Cells in the connective tissue interstitium are inconspicuous because the cytoplasm is often drawn out into fine branching processes that run in among the elastic and collagenous fibers of the alveolar wall. A thin coating of fluid on the alveolar surface completes the *air–blood barrier* that is crossed by air in the alveoli or carbon dioxide in the blood during respiratory gas exchange. It otherwise consists of alveolar epithelium, interstitial space, and capillary endothelium. The connective tissue beneath the epithelium makes up about a third of the total thickness of this barrier, which in rats averages about 1.5 μm with a range from 0.1 to several micrometers. Where capillary loops press against the epithelium, however, the connective tissue is excluded, and epithelium and endothelium are

separated by only a submicroscopic basement membrane (Fig. 23–54). These *thin-walled areas* are especially favorable to gas exchange, and along the alveolar surface they alternate with *thick-walled areas* where supporting fibers, extracellular matrix, and cells of the alveolar framework separate the epithelium from the capillaries (Fig. 23–52).

On the basis of morphometric estimates, the alveolar cell population consists of about 42% endothelial cells, 11% squamous alveolar cells, 13% great alveolar cells, and 35% interstitial cells. Because the alveolar surface area of typical lungs is approximately equal to the surface area of the pulmonary capillaries (Table 23–1), and the squamous alveolar cells cover most of the alveolar surface, it can be seen that they are much larger than the endothelial cells. They have about twice the volume of the endothelial cells

23–53 Light micrograph of a rat's lung showing bronchiolar epithelium **(above)** and respiratory tissue **(below)**. Toluidine blue. × 400.

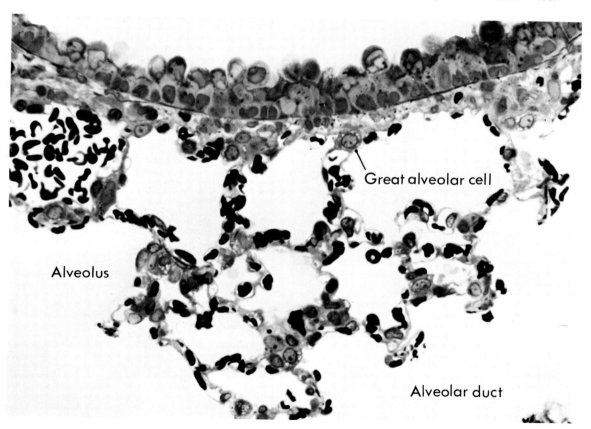

Great alveolar cell

Alveolus

Alveolar duct

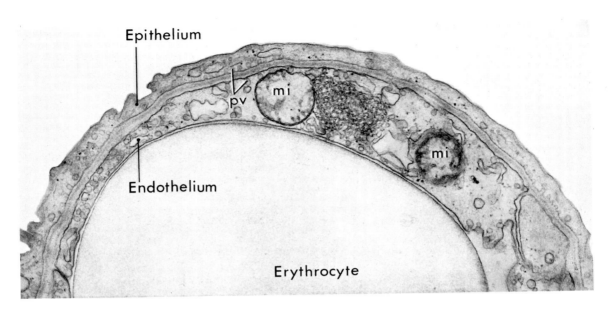

Epithelium

pv

mi

mi

Endothelium

Erythrocyte

23–54 Electron micrograph of the alveolar membrane of a rat. The barrier between alveolar air and blood consists of a thin alveolar epithelium, a basement lamina, and the capillary endothelium. Within the endothelial cell a network of fine-caliber agranular reticulum occupies the space between two mitochondria **(mi)**. Pinocytotic vesicles **(pv)** are seen in both epithelium and endothelium. × 15,000.

and four times the area. Great alveolar cells look larger than the squamous cells because most of their cytoplasm is concentrated around the nucleus, but they compare in volume only to the endothelial cells and occupy merely 2 to 3% of the alveolar surface.

Cells in the alveolar interstitium include fibrocytes, pericytes surrounding alveolar capillaries, a resident macrophage population, some plasma cells, and a few other leukocytes. Both the pericytes, which resemble smooth muscle, and the branching processes of the fibrocytes contain actomyosin. Being attached to the fibrous skeleton, both serve as contractile elements in the alveolar wall. This compartment normally is not threatened by invasion because it is kept clear of pathogens by a population of scavenging *alveolar macrophages*, which move through alveolar fluid on the epithelial surface.

A balance of hemodynamic forces in the respiratory zone normally keeps the interstitium compact and relatively dry (Fig. 23–78). The pulmonary capillaries are only relatively water-tight because their intercellular junctions are macular rather than continuous. They therefore do not

form a complete seal to prevent fluid and small proteins from escaping when the filtration pressure rises in the vessels. After severe challenge by acute or chronic infection, the integrity of the capillary wall is compromised, and then fluid and inflammatory cells enter and considerably enlarge this connective tissue space. Even so, excessive leakage into the alveoli is often prevented by the alveolar epithelium because the cells possess continuous tight junctions and remain relatively impermeable unless the cells themselves are seriously damaged.

Mast cells usually remain confined to the connective tissue surrounding the airways and blood vessels and follow the intrapulmonary course of these structures for varying distances according to the species; hence the respiratory zone is free from these edema-promoting agents. In rats these cells accompany the vessels through many generations of branching and occur in the visceral pleura as well, closely approaching but remaining outside the respiratory tissue. In guinea pigs, however, they follow the vessels further and occasionally penetrate the interalveolar walls; this fact helps to explain why anaphylaxis in these animals is centered in the lungs (Fig. 23–81, see here and color insert).

Between the capillaries one or more small, slitlike *alveolar pores* can be seen in thick sections that have been fixed and dried in an expanded state (Figs. 23–47 and 23–55). These pores connect adjacent alveoli and are fully open in expanded lungs. They are then as large as 10 to 15 μm in diameter and are encircled by a few

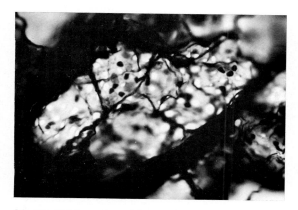

23–55 Thick section of human lung prepared to demonstrate pores between adjacent alveoli. The pores are seen as light spots and alveolar cell nuclei as dark spots on the walls. × 250.

elastic and reticular fibers. These pores are the best known among several kinds of accessory communications between adjacent air spaces. Others exist at the levels of respiratory bronchioles and alveolar ducts, where short circuits can occur between the airway and alveoli of the same or of adjacent acini. Still others come into being as a result of aberrant branching within the acini, and they interconnect airways of adjacent bronchial paths either directly or indirectly. The latter provide relatively major intercommunications, perhaps through passages as large as 0.5 mm in diameter. The extent to which these ac-

cessory channels are present varies greatly with the species. They are demonstrated physiologically by excising a fresh lung, inserting a cannula into a segmental bronchus, inflating it, and seeing if more than one segment inflates. Canine lungs have many accessory channels and good collateral ventilation; accessory channels are also apparent in human lungs both anatomically and physiologically but are very difficult to demonstrate in coatis and pigs. When a terminal bronchiole is obstructed, the alveoli connected to it can be ventilated through the larger of these channels. Because many of the smaller alveolar pores normally are filled with alveolar surface fluid, they probably do not contribute to collateral ventilation. Like the larger accessory channels, however, these pores are often used by alveolar macrophages in crossing from one alveolus to another, and they also serve as routes for the spread of pneumonia or neoplasm.

Squamous Alveolar Epithelial Cells. Squamous alveolar epithelial cells (membranous pneumonocytes, type I cells, small alveolar cells, or pulmonary epithelial cells) appear widely separated from each other because the cytoplasm is abruptly attenuated beyond the perinuclear region (Fig. 23–56). Thereafter it extends over the

23–56 Squamous alveolar epithelial and neighboring cells in the alveolar wall. (Courtesy of E. Schneeberger.)

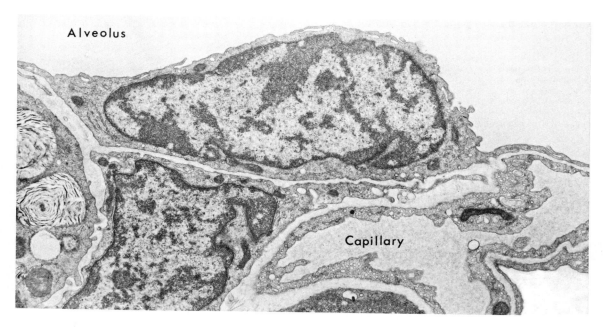

Alveolus

Capillary

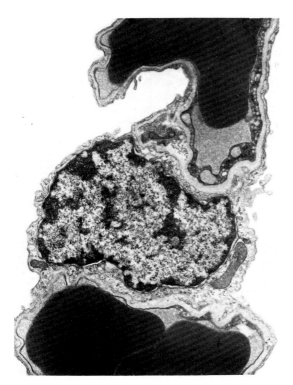

23–57 Squamous alveolar epithelial cell of the vampire bat's lung. The cell body lies in the interalveolar wall and sends sheets of cytoplasm to cover the alveolar surface on either side.

basement lamina as a thin sheet and joins other epithelial cells making up the continuous alveolar lining. In moderate-sized mammals these cells usually are simple squamous cells producing a single sheet of cytoplasm to help cover the pulmonary capillaries on one side of the interalveolar wall, but on occasion more than one sheet of attenuated cytoplasm branches off the cell body. This occurs more often in very small mammals because among them the connective tissue in interalveolar septa is reduced to a minimum, bringing epithelial sheets that line adjacent alveoli close together and so increasing the opportunities for contact. In these lungs the squamous cells not infrequently have several alternative dispositions: (1) cells lining adjacent alveoli may lie back to back, separated from each other only by a common basement lamina; (2) the body of the squamous cell may rest on one alveolar surface but a part of the cytoplasm may extend through a gap between capillary loops to reach

the alveolus opposite and so contribute to its lining; or (3) the body itself may occupy this intercapillary gap and give off sheets of cytoplasm of both alveoli (Fig. 23–57).

Among both large and small animals the attenuated cytoplasm of squamous alveolar cells usually falls below the resolving limit of the optical microscope (0.2 μm), but it is thinnest in the smallest mammals. In bats the layer may approach 250 Å, a thickness of little more than apical and basal plasmalemmae combined. For this reason a controversy raged for years about whether or not a complete alveolar epithelium existed, but the question was resolved by electron microscopy. Squamous alveolar cells have inconspicuous metabolic activity as revealed histochemically (Fig. 23–58), and much of it must be directed toward maintaining surfaces so extensively exposed to alveolar air. These cells are rather deficient in ergastoplasm and other cytoplasmic organelles, but those present are distributed fairly evenly among perinuclear and peripheral regions. Micropinocytotic vesicles occur in small numbers at both basal and apical surfaces; and from the latter, short microvilli here and there extend into the alveolar space. Squamous cells are capable of using pinocytotic action to take up small amounts of protein from the alveoli; exceptionally they store protein aggregates within the cytoplasm. These cells are also able to ingest small amounts of inhaled particulate matter that reaches the alveolar surface, and they convey some of it across the epithelium by vesicular transport. Their main role is to provide an intact surface of minimum thickness readily permeable to gases. The plasmalemmae of cells are the main barriers to diffusion in any multilayered biological membrane, but they are freely permeable to gases, which dissolve in lipids.

Great Alveolar Cells. Great alveolar cells (granular pneumonocytes, type II cells, large alveolar cells, alveolar cells, or septal cells) are exocrine secretory elements. These pleomorphic cells are roughly cuboidal as seen in tissue sections and, in three-dimensional views of alveoli, are easily recognized because they stand above the other epithelial cells, presenting an apical surface well supplied with short microvilli (Fig. 23–63). Frequently these form a tonsure about the apical rim leaving the center entirely smooth or sometimes encrusted with patches of material that had been released from the cell. Great alveolar cells are identifiable in paraffin sections of

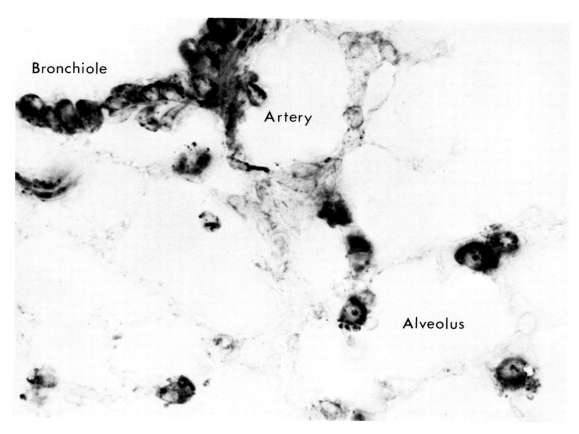

Bronchiole

Artery

Alveolus

lung because their nuclei are vesicular and relatively large and their cytoplasm appears vacuolated. At the light-microscopic level they stand out much better in 1-μm plastic sections, and then the vacuoles are seen to be characteristic inclusions known as *multilamellar bodies* or *cytosomes* (Fig. 23–53). The cells rest on the epithelial basement lamina, sometimes occupying niches between capillary loops and sometimes standing upright in twos and threes along the alveolar surface (Fig. 23–48). However they are mixed in the epithelium, they are joined to their neighbors by the same type of continuous tight junctions that bind all the epithelial cells together (Fig. 23–59). Like the squamous alveolar cells, these cells also seem able to extend through the interalveolar septum and join the epithelium on the opposite side, but this is very rarely observed. Great alveolar cells are able to divide, and in some instances one or both daughter cells appear to become transformed into squamous alveolar cells; hence, many investigators regard them as the main resource for cell renewal in the alveolar epithelium.

23–58 Frozen section of alveolar walls in a bat's lung reacted for diphosphopyridine nucleotide reductase. Great alveolar cells and the phagocytes are the most reactive cells present; they compare in reactivity with the epithelial cells of the airways. × 600.

Great alveolar cells have considerable metabolic capacity (Fig. 23–58) at a level equaled in alveolar regions only by alveolar macrophages. Within the cytoplasm this capacity is reflected by the presence of well-developed mitochondria, but a secretory function is indicated even more strongly by the presence of a loosely ordered granular endoplasmic reticulum, an extensive and widely dispersed Golgi apparatus, numerous multivesicular bodies, and the multilamellar bodies (Fig. 23–59). The latter range in size up to 1 μm and occur among forms transitional in appearance between multivesicular bodies and the cytosomes (Fig. 23–60). Multilamellar bodies give histochemical reactions for phospholipids, mucopolysaccharides, and proteins, including

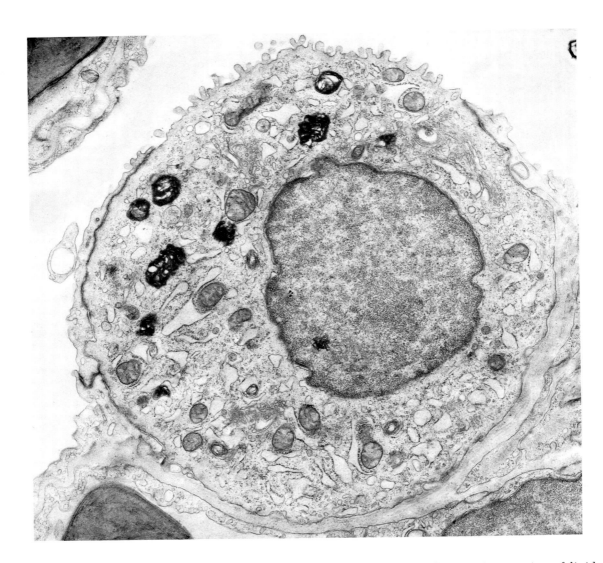

23–59 Great alveolar cell in the lungs of an opossum. (From Sorokin, S. 1966. J. Histochem. Cytochem. 14:884.)

reaction for several lysosomal hydrolases which are also found in the Golgi lamellae and in the multivesicular bodies. The cytosomes are therefore synthetic products of great alveolar cells. By their appearance and retention of some lysosomal enzyme activity, they can be considered as homologs of residual bodies present in other cells, but unlike them they differ in content and in being secreted and not retained in the cytoplasm. Synthesis and release occur continuously, the bodies being extruded singly from the apical surface of the cell.

The alveolar surface coating consists of lipid and aqueous phases and contains a detergent substance called *surfactant*. The purified substance contains 66% phosphatidylcholine, of which nearly two-third is the species dipalmitoyl phosphatidylcholine, as well as phosphoglycerol, cholesterol, and a specific protein, together with small amounts of other substances; its marked surface activity is attributable to phosphatidylcholine. In great alveolar cells, autoradiographic studies have shown that tritium-labeled leucine, galactose, and choline become incorporated in the cytosomes after first traversing synthetic centers in the cytoplasm. These cells are the only pulmonary cells to incorporate considerable amounts of choline, a specific precursor of phosphatidylcholine. Furthermore, bio-

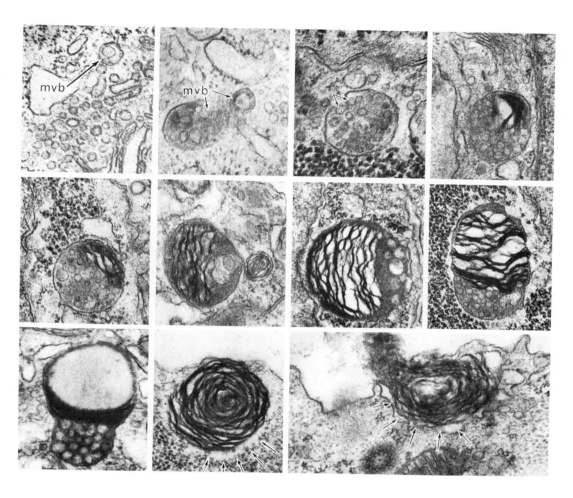

chemical analysis of purified multilamellar body fractions has shown that the lipid species present are very similar in kind and proportion to those present in surfactant. The specific surfactant protein has also been localized immunocytochemically to great alveolar cells, appearing in the endoplasmic reticulum, Golgi apparatus, and multivesicular bodies on the synthetic pathway to the cytosomes. Consequently, it is abundantly clear that the multilamellar bodies are the source of surfactant in the lungs.

After release from the great alveolar cells, the secretion spreads over the epithelial surface and endows the extracellular coating with unusual surface activity. Surfactant is interspersed with water molecules, thereby reducing their mutual cohesiveness and consequently reducing the surface tension at the air-fluid interface. In the presence of surfactant, the work of breathing is reduced because the alveolar surface tension that tends to collapse alveoli is reduced, and this re-

23–60 Sequence showing the development of cytosomes from small multivesicular bodies (**mvb**) through larger forms and on to secretion from the great alveolar cell. (From Sorokin, S., 1966. J. Histochem. Cytochem., 14:884.)

quires a lessened inspiratory force to oppose it. Alveolar diameters are stabilized as well, since the surface tension is greater in small alveoli than in large ones, because of the greater curvature of the wall. Where two such alveoli are interconnected, the larger would expand at the expense of the smaller unless surface tensions were reduced. These are the problems faced by infants suffering from respiratory distress syndrome, frequently brought on by a deficiency in the great alveolar cells.

Although the presence of a surface-active alveolar coating is not doubted, it has been difficult to present good images of the material in electron micrographs because it is often washed

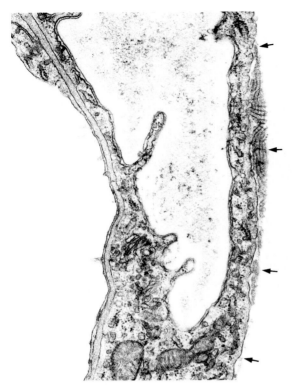

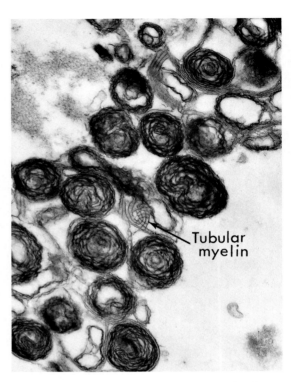

Tubular
myelin

23–61 Interalveolar wall of a hamster's lung showing a capillary space on the left, a squamous alveolar cell in the center, and the alveolar surface covered by a surfactant containing film **(arrows)** on the right.

23–62 Accumulated secretions from great alveolar cells in a culture of rat lungs. Cytosomes are the source of tubular myelin present in alveolar surfactant.

away during fixation. The most successful images to date have been made in lungs fixed by intravascular rather than intratracheal perfusion. In the former technique the extracellular lining is preserved as a coating of lipid crystals (tubular myelin) sometimes underlain by a basal aqueous layer of variable thickness containing proteins and mucopolysaccharides (Fig. 23–61). When the upper layer is distinct, it consists of several lamellae each about 100 to 400 Å thick and resembles the crystalline phase of a polar lipid–water system. Tubular myelin fortuitously can be seen in continuity with released cytosomes (Fig. 23–62), providing visual confirmation that it is derived from these bodies. The substances dissolved in the basal layer may possess properties more broadly related to defense postures than to surface activity.

So much surfactant is produced that large amounts must be broken down or removed, lest the alveoli fill up with the material. Turnover

seems to occur every few hours. Surfactant protein has been identified in endocytotic vesicles of alveolar macrophages as well as in those on the surface of squamous alveolar cells, but neither the protein nor traces of the lipids are found deeper in the tissues. Too little has been collected in the trachea for the airway to be considered an important avenue for elimination, and too few macrophages seem to be on hand to remove enough material by phagocytosis. Breakdown is thought to result mainly from the action of extracellular enzymes. Because great alveolar cells do not engage in bulk uptake of lipid, any surfactant components recycled must be taken up as small molecules.

Alveolar Macrophages. Alveolar macrophages (alveolar phagocytes, or dust cells) are preeminent among cells defending the respiratory region from contamination by microorganisms and inhaled particulate matter (Figs. 23–63 and 23–64, see here and color insert).

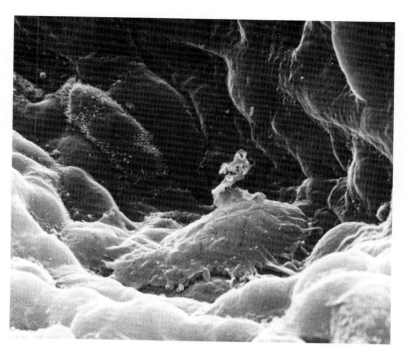

23–63 Scanning electron micrograph of a human alveolar macrophage with its advancing edge forward and numerous filopodia contacting the surface to the sides and rear. The pulmonary capillaries are formed into a close-knit meshwork, and a tonsured great alveolar cell is highlighted in the background. × 2,700. (From Gehr, P., Bachofen, M., and Weibel, E. R. 1978. Resp. Physiol. 32:121.)

23–64 Alveolar macrophages ingesting inhaled iron oxide particles deposited in alveoli of a mouse's lung. (From Sorokin, S., and Brain, J. 1975. Anat. Rec. 181:581.) This is a black-and-white rendition of a color plate. See color section.

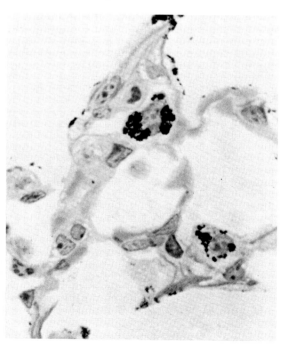

They have long been distinguished by their vigorous phagocytic activity, which is in strong contrast to the virtual absence of such activity by other alveolar cells. They are most unusual, however, because they regularly scavenge the *surface* of the epithelium. In general, macrophages rarely migrate over epithelial surfaces and almost never do so in the absence of significant inflammation in the connective tissue beneath. The metabolic capacity of these cells is considerable and diverse. This is well documented because alveolar macrophages can be washed out from the lungs through irrigation of the airway, and the resulting cell suspensions contain them in a high state of purity. In addition to possessing formidable aerobic oxidative capacity and a powerful intracellular digestive system (Fig. 23–45). these cells have a reserve synthetic capability that enables them to adapt their response to changing conditions.

In most respects, alveolar macrophages resemble macrophages from other parts of the body. A peripheral ectoplasm free of organelles and inclusions is filled with contractile myofilaments. A less fibrillar endoplasm within houses a euchromatic nucleus, the cytoplasmic organelles, and a great variety of dense bodies representing ingested matter enclosed within phagolysosomes (Fig. 23–65).

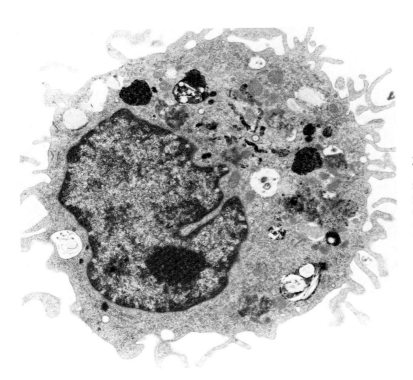

23–65 Typical, moderately stimulated mouse alveolar macrophage showing acid phosphatase activity **(black deposits)** in large rounded digestion vacuoles and smaller wormlike lysosomes. × 7,300.

Macrophages in motion are triangular with a broad and thin advancing edge that undulates as the cell feels its way along and a trailing end firmed up into a tail that helps to give it purchase. Numerous pseudopodia extend down from the sides and contact the epithelial cells beneath, holding much of the cell body up above the surface (Fig. 23–63). Contractile filaments within each pseudopod give it independent motility, and the peripheral cytoplasm is able to shear; this allows the cell to advance by a kind of walking motion, when pseudopod action is well coordinated, or to lunge forward by sliding one portion of the ectoplasm past the other, when a rift has separated it into two layers. The same contractile machinery is used in another mode to direct pseudopods around solid particles or to encircle a drop of liquid in the macroendocytotic processes of phagocytosis and pinocytosis. In addition, coated vesicles (acanthosomes) form at various points along the surface, particularly along the advancing edge, indicating that alveolar macrophages take in solids or dissolved matter by microendocytosis as well. In this respect the cells differ from heterophil granulocytes, which engage only in macroendocytosis. Although alveolar macrophages are very active in ingesting a great variety of particulate substances (Fig. 23–64, see here and color insert), they are slower than other phagocytes in moving about; a walking pace evidently aids their scavenging. Ingestion is triggered by a signal from the cell surface that recognizes the foreignness of the particle touching the plasmalemma. Mammalian alveolar macrophages have surface receptors both for immunoglobulin G and for a derivative of serum complement; if these substances bind to particles, uptake is enhanced (immune phagocytosis). Uncoated particles, such as those that might have just been breathed in, are also ingested on contact, although more slowly (nonimmune phagocytosis).

Within the cytoplasm the organelles may vary in number and disposition, giving some alveolar macrophages a quiescent appearance and others a very truculent look. This heterogeneity is apparent if one examines different cells in a suspension obtained by washing out the lungs. The Golgi apparatus may be compact and juxtanuclear but often extends throughout the perinuclear region and surrounds a distinct, fibrillar centrosome, in which the centrioles reside. From them microtubules radiate into the cytoplasm and organize the surrounding organelles about the centrosome. The endoplasmic reticulum varies in extent with different phases of cellular ac-

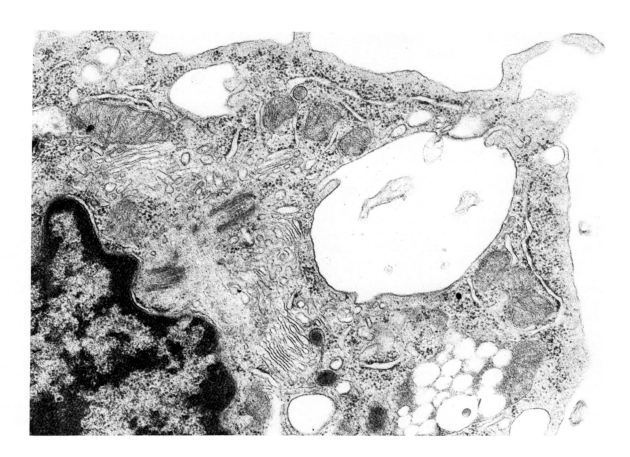

tivity. In quiescent cells the agranular reticulum predominates over the granular, but the latter increases dramatically in volume shortly after the cells have become stimulated to produce lysosomal enzymes for intracellular digestion as well as to make nonspecific antibacterial agents like lysozyme and interferon for secretion. The number of free polysomes present also varies from cell to cell. Mitochondria are abundant, rodlike, and well endowed with cristae. Pinocytotic and coated vesicles, phagosomes, a few multivesicular bodies, primary lysosomes, and phagolysosomes of great variety of sizes and shapes take up much of the space and give the cytoplasm a pronounced "digestive" character (Fig. 23–66). The varying appearance of alveolar macrophages can be understood to reflect the functional state then predominant. Unlike heterophils, which help to defend the lung under conditions of acute infection, the alveolar macrophages have an extended period of activity during which lysosome production is continued at a low level but periodically can be increased to furnish a

23–66 Cytoplasmic appearance of an activated mouse alveolar macrophage. Numerous profiles of granular endoplasmic reticulum appear in the more peripheral cytoplasm, and the Golgi region is more expanded than in quiescent cells. It is closely bordered by a large phagosome, from which a tubular passage extends toward the cell surface. An old digestion vacuole occupies the lower right, and, to its left, two dense bodies outside the Golgi region probably are lysosomes. × 21,000.

large crop of primary lysosomes in a single burst of synthesis. The contents of the primary lysosomes are transferred to phagosomes, converting them into digestion vacuoles that can be maintained active for long periods through the addition of freshly synthesized hydrolases. Eventually, many alveolar macrophages settle down like other macrophages to become *epithelioid cells*. They may also combine into multinucleate *giant cells* in responses related either to an attempt by the cells to engulf foreign bodies larger than themselves, or else to material released by infectious organisms.

Notwithstanding the alveolar macrophage functions as the primary phagocyte of the lungs, many fundamental facts about the cell and its life cycle remain unknown. The origin of the cell, the dynamics of its entrance and exit from the lungs, and the duration of its residence in alveolar walls and on the surface are imperfectly understood. Alveolar macrophages are able to divide, but their normal disinclination to do so has confounded many attempts to trace their comings and goings by means of labeling experiments using tritiated thymidine or other chromosome markers. Several sources for these cells have been proposed, including hematopoietic tissues outside the lungs and hematopoietic or connective tissues within the lungs. Some pulmonary macrophages undoubtedly are derived from hematopoietic cells outside the lungs. After indentifiable bone marrow cells are seeded into donor animals exposed to high doses of total body irradiation, it has been shown that all macrophages appearing in the alveoli can originate from donor cells. Such seeding of the lungs is usually done by cells with characteristics of monocytes, but in exceptional circumstances the seeded cells have proved to be morphologically indistinguishable from lymphocytes. In experiments that made use of total body irradiation, actively dividing populations of pulmonary cells would have been compromised by the irradiation, and consequently any intrapulmonary source of the macrophages would be suppressed. Such qualified evidence for an extrapulmonary source of pulmonary macrophages must be reconciled with knowledge that alveolar macrophages exist in the fetus and that they divide. Thus, there is an intrapulmonary reserve in the lungs from very early times whose cells derive from hematopoietic stem cells of the embryonic body wall or the yolk sac. This original macrophage pool is probably renewed from time to time not only by replication of the initial cells but by seeding of mitotically capable cells from the blood stream. Thus, the intrapulmonary pool, while remaining able to replicate itself, eventually becomes mixed in origin. In the adult organism, the main extrapulmonary source of macrophages is the bone marrow. Like heterophils and other leukocytes, monocytes are easily induced to cross the pulmonary capillaries to enter interstitial tissues and the alveoli. Having arrived in the tissues, they undergo transformation into macrophages, adding to the population. Whatever the origins of alveolar macrophages present in adult lungs, they differ in enzyme content and in levels of reactivity from blood-borne peritoneal macrophages and heterophils in relying on oxidative phosphorylation to supply energy consumed during phagocytosis.

Dust-laden macrophages leave the alveolar surface by migrating or being slowly washed to the bronchial passages, where they are carried out to the pharynx and swallowed. While in transit, a number of them continue to pursue normal activities, such as scavenging the bronchial surface and dividing; others die and release their contents, some of which is cleared or reingested by other cells, and some of which may return to the lungs by passage through the bronchial epithelium (Fig. 23–38, see here and color insert).

Pulmonary connective tissue macrophages reside beneath the airway, around blood vessels, and in the pleura. Functionally they are distinct from alveolar macrophages, perhaps only because they are sheltered from direct exposure to air-borne dusts and bacteria and not because of differences in metabolism; their position limits their mobility in any case, and they are the ultimate repository of uncleared particulate matter in the lungs (Fig. 23–80, see here and color insert). They have access to lymphatic pathways in the connective tissue and filter out material coming that way, as well as material entering the lungs from the bronchial arteries. A small part of the particulate matter deposited in the alveoli reaches these macrophages after it has crossed the intact or damaged alveolar epithelium to reach para-alveolar lymphatics (discussed under lymphatics), for it has not been demonstrated that sizable numbers of alveolar macrophages reenter the tissues after they have appeared on the alveolar surface.

Pulmonary Circulation

The main blood supply to the lungs is furnished by *pulmonary arteries*, one for each lung. They carry high volumes of blood at low pressures ($^{25}/_5$mm Hg) from the right side of the heart to pulmonary capillaries in the alveolar walls. These capillaries are drained by *pulmonary veins*, which carry oxygenated blood to the left side of the heart. *Bronchial arteries* are small derivatives of the thoracic descending aorta that carry blood at systemic pressure ($^{120}/_{80}$ mm Hg) to

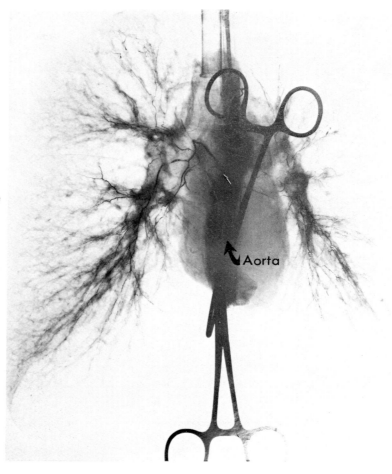

23-67 X-ray of autopsied human heart and lungs injected with contrast material to reveal the bronchial arterial system. The heart shadow overlies the descending thoracic aorta; from there the right bronchial artery **(arrow)** passes to the right bronchial tree; and on both right and left, the arteries branch with the bronchi.

the walls of most of the airways (Fig. 23–67). *Bronchial veins* are present only near the hilum and provide only accessory drainage from the bronchial wall. Consequently, most of the blood from the two arterial systems drains into the pulmonary veins, and the three vascular systems form one integrated circuit. As described in the section on the internal structure of the lungs, the arteries branch with the bronchial tree and hence alternate with the veins, which run in the septa between adjacent bronchi (Figs. 23–20 and 23–73, see here and color insert).

Pulmonary Vessels. From distributing vessels of the *pulmonary arterial system*, branches are sent to airway tissues beginning at the level of the respiratory bronchioles. Distal to the alveolar duct the artery branches; and from the level of the atrium, twigs are given off to the atria and a branch is sent to each alveolar sac. This branch

divides into two, and the newly formed branches join the pulmonary capillary network (Fig. 23–51), whose mesh can be finer than the diameters of the capillaries forming it. Other features of this capillary bed have been described in the section on alveolar organization.

Venules drain the distal ends of the alveolar sacs. Pulmonary veins have four origins: from capillaries of the pleura, from alveolar ducts, from alveoli, and from the peribronchial venous plexus (Fig. 23–73, see here and color insert). The veins draining the airway frequently occur at points where bronchi or bronchioles divide and are called *bronchopulmonary veins*. They provide the main channels for drainage of the bronchial arteries and consequently are the primary elements tying the pulmonary and bronchial circuits together. From these various origins, small vessels come together into veins that cross the respiratory tissue to enter larger-caliber

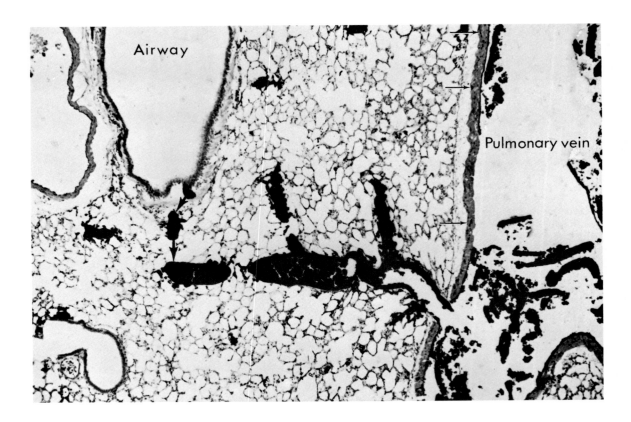

23–68 India-ink injection of bronchial arteries and pulmonary veins in the lungs of a vampire bat. A bronchopulmonary communication **(large arrows)** and injected vasa vasorum in the wall of the large vein **(small arrows)** are indicated. × 80.

pulmonary veins situated in connective tissue septa (Fig. 23–68); this explains why in histological sections the smaller veins, in contrast to arteries, appear surrounded by alveoli and are separated by varying distances from the airway (Fig. 23–46). Occupying the boundary between regions supplied by adjacent bronchi—and hence adjacent arteries—the interfacial veins receive the drainage from both. Stated another way, the venous drainage of pulmonary segments or subsegments is always by more than one vein. Such medium-to-large vessels follow connective tissue planes of the lung. They gather into still larger veins, but continue to receive small tributaries along the way. Eventually one trunk is formed for each lobe, and it comes into relation with the artery and bronchus, usually lying ventromedial to the bronchus while the artery lies dorsolateral.

In human beings, the veins to the middle and upper lobes of the right lung usually combine into one vessel, so that two veins leave the lungs on either side of the heart. Exceptionally, the three right lobar veins may enter the left atrium separately, whereas the pair from the left may enter by a single opening.

Bronchial Vessels. Usually two bronchial arteries are given off to the left lung and one is formed for the right. The left ones usually arise from the ventral aspect of the thoracic descending aorta, the cranial one just opposite the fifth thoracic vertebra in human beings, and the lower one just caudal to the left bronchus, which crosses ventral to the descending aorta. The right bronchial artery sometimes arises from the cranial left bronchial artery and sometimes from the first aortic intercostal, but the number and exact origins of all the bronchial arteries may vary, as may their intercommunication with nearby esophageal, pericardial, and even coronary circulations. On each side, the bronchial arteries run in the adventitia over the dorsal aspect of the bronchi, to end at the level of respiratory bronchioles. Along their course they send branches through the muscularis of the airway, giving off a capillary bed for the smooth muscle and another for the lamina propria. Deep to the latter, venous plexuses are formed on both sides of the muscularis. The outer one contains larger vessels that combine to form the bronchopulmonary veins. Beyond the respiratory bronchioles this system becomes supplied by branches of the pulmonary artery. Bronchial arteries also furnish blood to vasa vasorum of pulmonary arteries and veins (Fig. 23–68) and extend along interlobular septa to supply these areas as well as capillaries of the visceral pleura.

Bronchial veins are seen on the dorsal surface of the extrapulmonary bronchi where they lie next to the bronchial arteries. They drain these structures as well as the visceral pleura and lymph nodes at the hilum. They become a single vessel on each side; the right one empties into the azygous vein near its junction with the superior vena cava, and the left one joins either the highest left intercostal or accessory hemiazygous vein.

Histology. Owing to reduced pressure in the circuit, pulmonary arteries and veins resemble each other more closely than do corresponding pairs of systemic vessels. The pulmonary vessels retain histological features of arteries and veins, but among different species considerable variation occurs on both sides of the capillaries. The arteries have relatively more smooth muscle and elastic fibers than the veins and to their smallest divisions possess an internal elastic membrane. The veins contain a meshwork of predominantly longitudinally oriented elastic fibers at the intimal margin, moderate numbers of elastic fibers in the muscularis when this layer is occupied by smooth muscle, and variable amounts of them just external to it.

For some distance after they leave the heart, the pulmonary arteries remain elastic arteries, histologically comparable to the aorta and provided with elastic membranes encircling the intima and layered throughout the muscularis. Such vessels accompany major intrapulmonary bronchi of large mammals. In them the intima is multilayered and consists of an endothelium resting on a subendothelial connective tissue containing fibrocytes and relatively fine, longitudinally oriented fibers embedded in an abundant matrix. Just outside the circularly oriented muscularis, a number of smooth muscle bundles

run longitudinally in the adventitia, which elsewhere contains fine, unmyelinated nerve processes and the vasa vasorum and is densely collagenous in texture. With branching of the arteries, intimal thickness and the number of elastic lamellae become reduced; a vessel with lamellae occupying the inner third of an otherwise well-elasticized muscularis might accompany a medium-sized bronchus. These vessels are succeeded by vessels histologically closer to muscular arteries. In smaller màmmals, the arteries accompanying large bronchi have an intima composed only of endothelium and a single internal elastic membrane inside a muscularis richly layered with elastic fibers. These fibers form a meshwork rather than fenestrated lamellae (Fig. 23–69); they generally separate the smooth muscle fibers into layers, but they interconnect with each other and with an often denser meshwork of fibers at the boundary between muscularis and adventitia. The progressive thinning out of the arterial wall can be followed in the illustrations of kitten lung, beginning with a large bronchus and passing through bronchioles to respiratory bronchioles (Figs. 23–25, 23–31, 23–44, and 23–46). In small mammals the arteries throughout most of their length are relatively thin-walled musculoelastic arteries. The endothelium of pulmonary arteries is composed of elongated cells that form overlapping junctions with one another and contain rather many smooth-surfaced micropinocytotic vesicles. The cytoplasm occasionally contains membrane-bounded secretory or absorptive granules, but these are more abundant in the endothelium of small pulmonary veins (Figs. 23–69 and 23–70). In contrast, the endothelial cytoplasm of certain bronchial arteries contains approximately 50-Å filaments in a dense matting sandwiched in between the apical and basal rows of pinocytotic vesicles. Histologically, bronchial vessels otherwise resemble other systemic blood vessels of comparable dimensions (Fig. 23–30, see here and color insert.)

Pulmonary capillaries are of the muscular, nonfenestrated type throughout, whereas bronchial capillaries are fenestrated, particularly in relation to the vascular beds supplying the glands, but also in relation to the airway epithelium, and especially to the bronchioles (Figs. 23–71 and 23–72). Here and there *pericytes* encircle both types of capillaries. For the most part they lie outside the endothelial basement membrane, but they extend processes inside, and

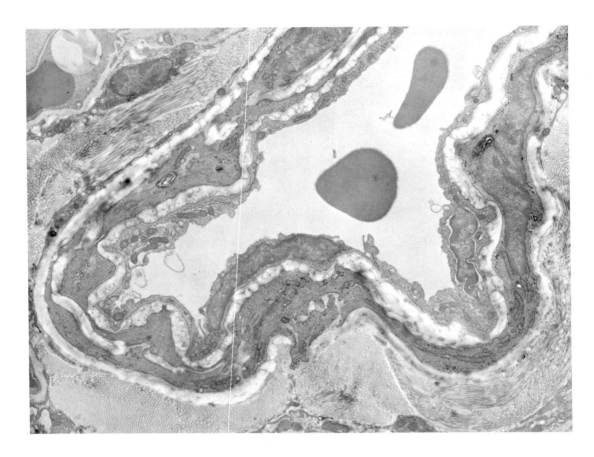

23–69 Pulmonary artery adjacent to a small
intrapulmonary bronchus in a bat. The
endothelium rests on an internal elastic membrane;
the muscularis is only one cell layer thick but is
infiltrated by (clear) elastic fibers, whereas the
adventitia is collagenous. × 7,200.

these contact the endothelial cells for short distances (Fig. 23–71). The cytoplasm of these pericytes is filamentous in texture, and the cells are
believed to function like smooth muscle; other
pericapillary processes may belong to connective
tissue macrophages.

Pulmonary veins of large animals sometimes
prove difficult to identify in histological sections
not only because the media contains considerable smooth muscle, but especially because sufficient elastic fibers are present to give the vein
a crenelated appearance reminiscent of arteries
seen in slides of material prepared with coagulating fixatives. Side by side, the vessels are
easily distinguished (Fig. 23–25). It should be

remembered that the venous adventitia is relatively thicker than the arterial, and it is always
helpful to keep the anatomical course of these
vessels in mind.

For short distances beyond their junction with
the left atrium, the pulmonary veins of human
beings have an adventitial coating of *cardiac
muscle*. This muscle spreads to the hilum in
dogs, whereas in smaller mammals the muscle
extends along intrapulmonary veins for varying
distances to reach small veins less than 100 μm
in diameter in the smallest mammals. In these
intrapulmonary vessels the cardiac muscle occupies the media sometimes together with
smooth muscle as in rats, and sometimes alone
as in shrews and bats (Fig. 23–70); when this
muscle occurs alone, the elastic fibers are heaviest beneath the intima, where they are formed
into a coarsely porous lamella. The cardiac muscle is single-layered in small veins but multilayered in larger ones, and the cells resemble myocytes of the atrium (Chap. 10). The intercalated
discs separating the cells usually follow a less

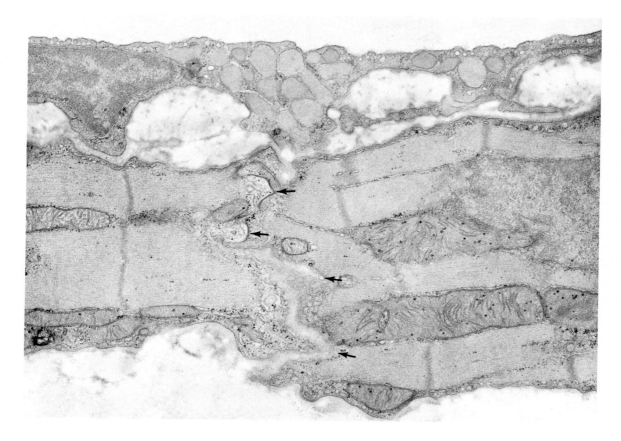

23–70 Granule-rich endothelium and cardiac-muscle investment of a small pulmonary vein of the vampire bat. A simply folded intercalated disc **(arrows)** incorporating a close-gapped junction between cells **(upper two arrows)** is shown at the center of the field. × 21,200.

staggered course across the muscle fiber than they do in the heart, and at these sites the apposed ends of the myocytes are joined with rather less interdigitation, allowing one to see gap junctions between the cells clearly. These are believed to be sites of electrical coupling between individual cells of the muscle coat. During its development the muscle first appears in venous walls next to the heart and later spreads peripherally. It contracts slightly ahead of the heart and presumably functions as a dynamic valve in facilitating venous return.

Pulmonary venules have an endothelium like the endothelium of pulmonary capillaries, and the vessels have no muscularis (Fig. 23–52). It is thought that many exchanges taking place at the capillary level also occur in the venules. As in many capillaries, the endothelium of pulmonary capillaries and venules exhibits surface adenosine triphosphatase activity possibly associated with an active transmembrane transport mechanism. Hydrolytic conversion of angiotensin I to angiotensin II as well as the inactivation of bra-

dykinin may also occur on the endothelial surface, but in other respects these cells are not conspicuous metabolically (Fig. 23–58). Near the point where smooth or cardiac muscle joins the vessel wall and the venules become small veins, the endothelium rests on a single mesh of elastic fibers supported by adventitial plies of dense collagenous connective tissue. The addition of muscle displaces the collagenous layer peripherally although a few threads of cytoplasm from fibrocytes remain interposed here and there between the elastic mesh and muscle.

Functional Interrelationships. Several types of vascular anastomoses are found in the lungs. True anastomoses between bronchial and pul-

852

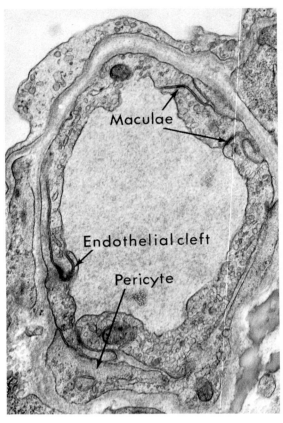

23–71 Alveolar capillary in an opossum's lung.
△ × 12,180.

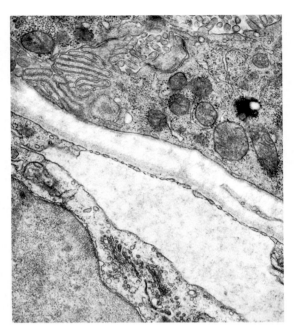

23–72 Endothelial fenestrations in a glandular
△ capillary in the bronchial wall of an opossum.
× 12,000.

23–73 Diagram showing the interrelationships
▽ among the airways, the vascular systems, and
the lymphatic networks of the lung. (After diagrams
of W. S. Miller and J. Lauweryns.) This is a black-and-
white rendition of a color plate. See color section.

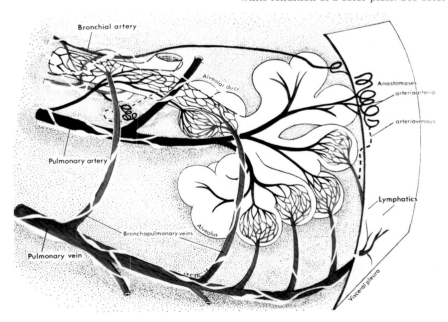

monary arteries (Fig. 23–73, green in color insert) are found in the peribronchial tissue near small peripheral bronchi and in the pleura. These vessels are small and have well-developed muscular walls. From them bronchial arteriovenous shuts (Fig. 23–73, green stripes in color insert) branch off to the pulmonary veins, reaching them by way of the bronchopulmonary veins or by small peripheral pulmonary branches. These then are secondary anastomoses. Shortcuts are also found between parallel branches of bronchial arteries, and bronchial veins intercommunicate through the bronchial plexus. In healthy lungs the blood flow through these shunts is of small magnitude, and it passes from the bronchial to the pulmonary circuit.

No proven chemoreceptors are known to exist in blood vessels of the lungs, but a glomus associated with the pulmonary trunk has been described. Histologically, it resembles the carotid body. It contains nests of epithelioid cells bound in connective tissue and richly supplied with blood from the pulmonary artery. Vagal and sympathetic fibers from the deep cardiac plexus provide innervation, but attempts to investigate glomar function have not given positive results.

Lymphatics

The lymphatics of the lung are abundant and are formed into two sets. A superficial set lies in the visceral pleura; a deep one accompanies the bronchi and pulmonary vessels (Fig. 23–73, see here and color insert). The sets interconnect at the hilum, where both enter the tracheobronchial lymph nodes. They also communicate near the origins of the pulmonary veins in the pleura and in the interlobar septa, which arise from the pleura (Fig. 23–74).

The lymphatic vessels may be compared to thin-walled veins. They exhibit abrupt changes in diameter and near the hilum frequently have valves (Fig. 23–75, see here and color insert). The walls of the larger vessels have three layers, the smaller have no media (Figs. 23–76 and 23–77, see here and color insert), and the capil-

23–74 Injected specimen of adult human lung, showing the intercommunication between superficial and deep pulmonary lymphatics. (From Lauweryns, J. 1971. *In* S. C. Sommers [ed.], Pathology Annual, vol. 6. New York: Appleton-Century-Crofts, p. 365.)

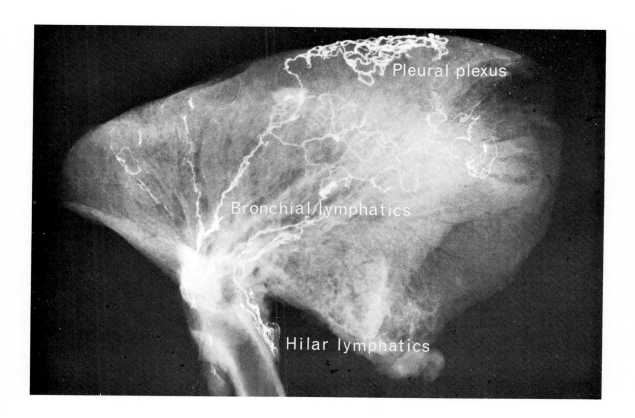

Pleural plexus

Bronchial lymphatics

Hilar lymphatics

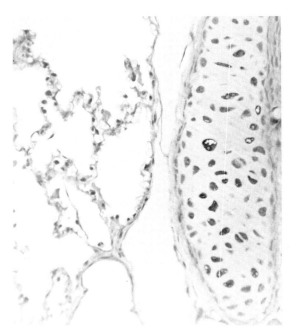

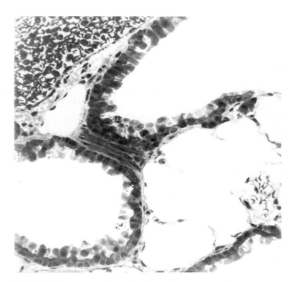

23-77 Cross section of a lymphatic vessel (upper left) near a branching point of the airway in a mouse. Prussian blue and iron hematoxylin. This is a black-and-white rendition of a color plate. See color section.

23-75 Lymphatic collecting vessel with funnel-shaped valve alongside the bronchus of a cat. This is a black-and-white rendition of a color plate. See color section.

23-76 Pleural lymphatic vessel and prominent brush border of mesothelial cells in a cat's lung. PAS-lead hematoxylin. This is a black-and-white rendition of a color plate. See color section.

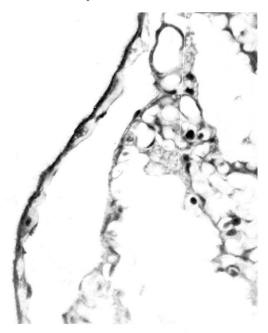

laries lack a continuous basement lamina but possess numerous anchoring filaments that tie into interstitial fibers. Lymphatic capillaries accompanying pulmonary arterioles and venules, as well as others present in pulmonary septa and bronchi, may closely approach adjacent alveoli; collectively they comprise the *paraalveolar lymphatics*, which drain their immediate surroundings as well as wick-away the more distant alveolar interstitium (Fig. 23-78). In humans and common domestic and laboratory mammals there are no lymphatic capillaries in interalveolar walls. Because the capillaries run along alveolar ducts, however, the alveoli there have more direct access to them than alveoli in most other locations.

Within the lung, lymph flows centripetally through lymphatics of the bronchial tree and the pulmonary arteries and veins, being milked along by contraction of lymphatic smooth muscle, by inspiratory movements, and by pulsations of the blood vessels they entwine. At the bifurcations of bronchi, the fluid passes through lymphoid tissue, which is scarce in neonatal animals but gradually builds up in postnatal life. Pleural lymph reaches the hilar lymphatics either through the well-developed superficial channels (Fig. 23-79) or by way of the deep lymphatics (Fig. 23-80).

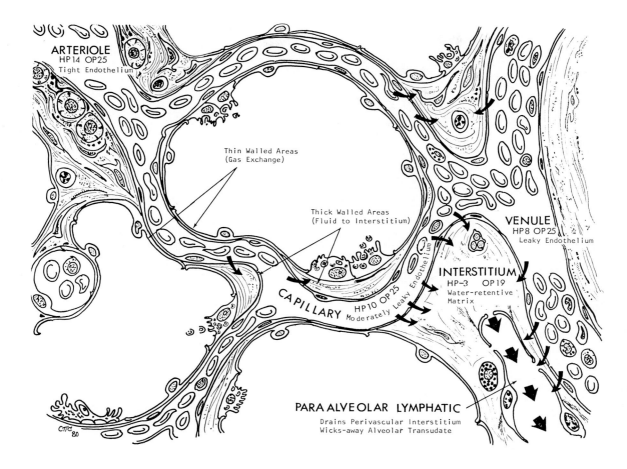

ARTERIOLE
HP 14 OP 25
Tight Endothelium

Thin Walled Areas
(Gas Exchange)

Thick Walled Areas
(Fluid to Interstitium)

VENULE
HP 8 OP 25
Leaky Endothelium

INTERSTITIUM
HP -3   OP 19
Water-retentive
Matrix

Leaky Endothelium

CAPILLARY Moderately Leaky Endothelium   HP 10 OP 25

PARA ALVEOLAR LYMPHATIC
Drains Perivascular Interstitium
Wicks-away Alveolar Transudate

23–78 Interrelationships among blood vessels, lymphatics, and interstitium in pulmonary alveoli under resting conditions. Values for hydrostatic pressure (**HP**) and colloid osmotic pressure (**OP**) are given in mm Hg. Capillaries of interalveolar walls may lose fluid to the interstitium, which has significant osmotic pressure and negative hydrostatic pressure, but is virtually absent from sites of alveolar gas exchange. A tight epithelium impedes water loss to alveoli, but some water is available to secretory great alveolar cells. Venules may also lose water despite a low hydrostatic pressure within, for their endothelial cell junctions are apt to be more leaky than those of capillaries. The interstitium holds water like a gel, but it eventually drains into para-alveolar lymphatics.

Nerves

The lungs are innervated mainly by sympathetic and parasympathetic fibers of the autonomic nervous system and by general visceral afferent nerves. They mediate various reflex actions initiated from within the lungs as well as from outside. In addition, provision is made for a poorly localized sense of pain. Within the lungs, parasympathetic fibers are exclusively distributed through branches of the vagus nerve, which also carries the greater number of general visceral afferent fibers. In general, sympathetic fibers are less prevalent, but marked interspecies variation occurs in the makeup and exact course of intrapulmonary nerves, particularly in the size of the sympathetic component. Both excitatory and inhibitory motor nerves are present, and there is evidence that neurons interact locally inside the lungs as well. Acetylcholine at endings of preganglionic nerves and postganglionic parasympathetic fibers acts as the principal neurohumoral agent; norepinephrine is released by postganglionic sympathetic nerves. In addition, a nonadrenergic, noncholinergic system participates in the regulation of airway tone, although its neurotransmitter has not been identified. Among other substances active as neurohumors in other parts of the nervous system, serotonin is

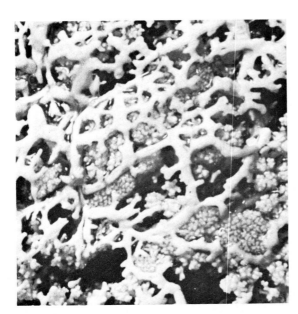

23–79 Injected specimen showing well-developed superficial lymphatic channels on the visceral pleura. (From Lauweryns, J. 1971. *In* S. C. Sommers [ed.], Pathology Annual, Vol. 6. New York: Appleton-Century-Crofts, p. 365.)

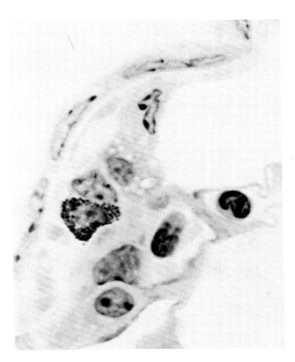

23–81 Mast cell beneath pleura in a guinea pig's lung. Leukocytes within blood vessels, a great alveolar cell (foamy cytoplasm), and the squamous pleural mesothelium are nearby. Toluidine blue. This is a black-and-white rendition of a color plate. See color section.

23–80 Subepithelial lymphoid tissue along the deep lymphatic pathway at a branching of the main bronchus in a mouse's lung. This is a black-and-white rendition of a color plate. See color section.

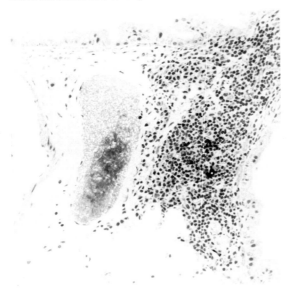

present in some of the small-granule cells as well as in mast cells of rodents, while epinephrine and various neuroendocrine agents reach the lungs through the circulation. Pharmacologically, airway nerves and smooth muscle behave comparably to their counterparts in the gastrointestinal tract (Chap. 19), and their association with an endodermal epithelium is similar.

Origins. Outside of the lungs, pulmonary nerves originate from cell bodies located close to the central nervous system: (1) *preganglionic parasympathetic efferents* from the dorsal nucleus of the vagus nerve, located in the medulla oblongata; (2) *postganglionic sympathetic efferents* from cell bodies located in thoracic ganglia #2–5 of the sympathetic chain; (3) *general visceral afferent fibers* from cell bodies located both in vagal ganglia (superior and inferior) at the base of the skull and in dorsal root ganglia at thoracic levels #2–5, where they occur together

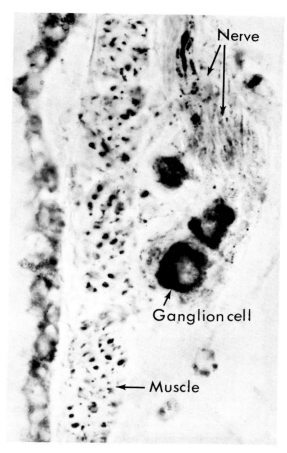

23–82 Frozen section of bat lung showing succinic dehydrogenase activity **(dark gray)** in tissues of the bronchial wall. Neurons of an adventitial ganglion are especially reactive. Left, bronchial epithelium; far right, alveoli including two reactive great alveolar cells. × 364.

with the cell bodies of somatic sensory neurons. Within the lungs, neuronal cell bodies occur in ganglia located in the adventitia of axial structures (Fig. 23–82).

Pulmonary Plexuses. Fibers from each side meet and intermingle to form plexuses located in the mediastinum over the bronchi and great vessels at the roots of the left and right lungs. From there the nerves pass internally to supply the lungs. In humans, a large *posterior pulmonary plexion* receives most of the fibers including those from the deep cardiac plexus; on the left, the recurrent laryngeal nerve contributes some fibers as well. The smaller *anterior pulmonary plex-*

uses consist of two or three branches of the vagus joined with sympathetic filaments and some from the deep cardiac plexus; the left anterior plexus also receives fibers from the superficial cardiac plexus. Some crossing-over apparently occurs at this level, so that each lung receives branches from both homolateral and contralateral vagus nerves. The extent of intermingling is species-variable; in the dog, considerable admixture of cardiac and pulmonary fibers complicates anatomical and physiological work on the system.

Intrapulmonary Course. As a whole, the intrapulmonary nerve network closely resembles the bronchial arterial system in its pattern of branching. It mainly follows the bronchial tree, yet it also accompanies the bronchial vessels as they diverge to supply the walls of the pulmonary arteries and veins. Entering the pulmonary septa along with the veins, it ultimately reaches the visceral pleura, which also receives fibers directly from the hilum. Most of the nerves are destined for axial structures, for it will be seen that relatively few fibers remain for the respiratory zone after the bronchi and vessels are supplied.

Nerves entering the lungs may at once become associated with the bronchi and blood vessels, as in the rat, or they may enter independently and join axial structures shortly afterward, as in primates. In entering the lungs they occupy a space surrounded by the bronchus, the pulmonary artery, and the veins. Interspecies variation is also found in the exact intrapulmonary course of the nerves, although it generally conforms to the following pattern.

The main nerves to the bronchial tree travel together in bundles that run in the connective tissue outside the cartilages in rats, but in primates they run both superficial and deep to the cartilages. After the cartilages disappear, superficial and deep nerve bundles come together to form a single plexus deep in the adventitia, and this extends to the respiratory bronchioles. Ganglion cells are associated with this system, being grouped into larger clusters in the hilar areas and into smaller ones or even solitary cells more peripherally (Fig. 23–12, see here and color insert; and Fig. 23–82). These ganglion cells tend to occur near points of bundle branching. The nerves contain mixed fibers, both myelinated ones with diameters in the range of 2 to 4 μm and unmyelinated ones in the range of 0.1 to 0.9

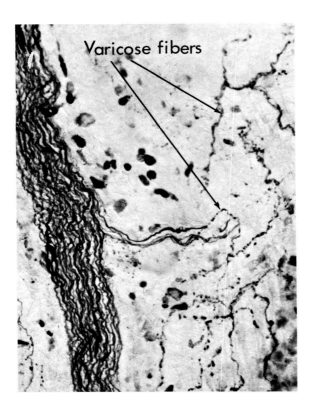

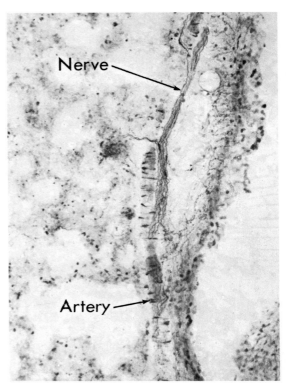

23–83 Left. Hilar peribronchial nerve bundle in a rat's lung containing thick and thin fibers. Some extend toward the bronchial wall (right) where they join a plexus of varicose fibers. Methylene blue. × 259. **Right.** Periarterial nerve bundle spiraling about a bronchial artery and giving off fibers en route. The varicose plexus lies nearer the bronchiolar lumen (right). Methylene blue. × 122. (From El-Bermani, A-W. 1973. Am. J. Anat. 137:19.)

μm, corresponding to dimensions frequently associated with autonomic pre- and postganglionic fibers, respectively. Perhaps one-third of these fibers are myelinated at the hilar level, but this proportion decreases as the bronchi are followed, because many of the myelinated nerves end in basketlike terminations on the ganglion cells. Each of these contributes a single unmyelinated axon to the nerve bundle. Peribronchial nerves in rats and primates are reactive for acetylcholinesterase and none exhibits fluorescence for catecholamines.

Along its course the *peribronchial system* gives off fibers that ramify in a layer extending throughout the thickness of the bronchial smooth muscle (Fig. 23–83). It also gives off others that do not communicate with the intramuscular layer but pass between muscle bundles to reach the submucosa. The intramuscular layer is largely derived from ganglion cells within the peribronchial bundles and consists of a tight-meshed plexus of unmyelinated, varicose fibers that are acetylcholinesterase-positive (Fig. 23–84). It is densest at bifurcations of bronchioles where contributions are received from nearby ganglion cells. The varicosities represent terminations to the bronchial smooth muscle; and where all of these motor endings contain clear synaptic vesicles, as in rats, humans, and rhesus monkeys, the muscle can be considered to be cholinergically innervated. This kind of innervation predominates in the airways of many animals, including dogs, cats, and rabbits. Although sympathetic fibers also reach the muscularis in some species, they never pervade this layer as completely as the cholinergic fibers. At the varicose terminations, the axons emerge from the Schwann cell wrapping and become exposed to the intracellular space, into which they release their neurotransmitters (Figs. 23–85 and 23–87). When many varicosities are present, the nearest myocytes are separated from them by about 2000 Å; but once depolarization has occurred on the sarcolemma, it rapidly spreads throughout the muscularis because the cells are interconnected by gap junctions (Fig. 23–85). Nerve–muscle interaction in the airway is further discussed in the section on histophysiology.

A second system of nerves to the bronchial tree runs in close association with the bronchial arteries (Fig. 23–83). In rodents this *periarterial system* contains all the adrenergic fibers destined for the lung and only a few cholinergic fibers; in primates it also contains adrenergic fibers, but nearly half its fibers are cholinergic, and these largely branch off to join the intramuscular plexus. The adrenergic fibers form a plexus that invests the bronchial artery and extends to other pulmonary vessels.

Superficial to the intramuscular plexus the submucosa is traversed by nerves having a number of different origins. Most exhibit varicosities along some part of their length and accordingly can be said to be terminal nerves of one kind or another. Those originating from the intramuscular plexus run radially into the mucosa and serve

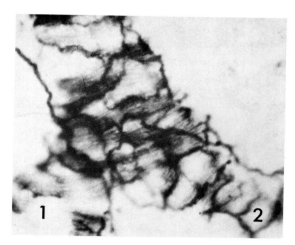

23–84 Acetylcholinesterase activity in varicose nerves of the intramuscular plexus of a rat's lung. The bronchiole branches into two (1, 2), and bands of smooth muscle are faintly discernible in the background. × 250. (From El-Bermani, A-W. 1973. Am. J. Anat. 137:19.)

23–85 Bronchial smooth muscle and portions of the intramuscular plexus. The nerves extend along the lower part of the micrograph and at several points have become free of their Schwann cell wrapping, enabling them to release the contents of their predominantly clear synaptic vesicles into the surrounding connective tissue. The muscles are coupled to one another by means of gap junctions (**arrowheads**). × 15,000.

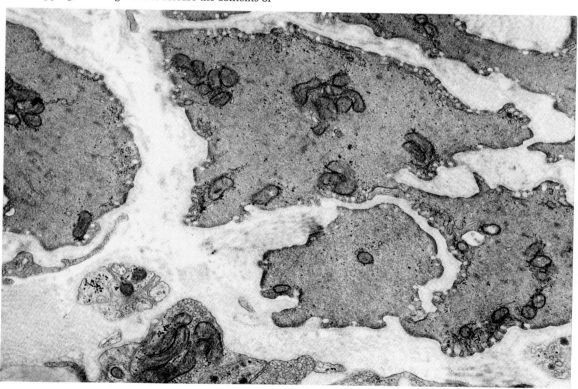

as postganglionic parasympathetic efferents. Other fibers originate from the peribronchial plexus, do not communicate with the intramuscular nerves, and extend in both longitudinal and circumferential directions in the submucosa. These unmyelinated fibers are cholinesterase-positive and are thought to be afferent terminals possibly associated with stretch receptors. The circumferential submucosal fibers eventually become single, at which point they lose their Schwann cell sheath and continue as naked processes beneath the epithelium. In monkeys, a few myelinated fibers also run in the submucosa. The larger ones are acetylcholinesterase-negative and accordingly are deemed sensory, whereas the smaller ones are cholinergic and possibly preganglionic nerves to the neuroepithelial bodies. Sensory terminals have also been described in the smooth muscle layer and in intrapulmonary connective tissue septa; these are connected to large medullated fibers that run to the nodose ganglia of the vagus nerves.

Bronchial and pulmonary arteries and the pulmonary veins are predominantly innervated by sympathetic fibers, and for this reason the plexuses about them contain no ganglia. Where cardiac muscle is present in the veins, however (Fig. 23–70), ganglia may occur in the adventitia in order to provide postganglionic parasympathetic fibers to the myocardium. In the rat, the larger pulmonary arteries receive their adrenergic supply from branches of the plexus that surrounds the bronchial arteries; these branches are carried in with the vasa vasorum. The nerves are especially concentrated around bifurcations of the pulmonary arteries; and in the vessel walls, they ramify in a plexus located at the boundary between media and adventitia, from which a few branches penetrate the media. This plexus extends to the capillaries. Venules and the smallest veins of rats also receive adrenergic fibers derived from the distribution around the bronchial arteries; but in still smaller mammals, cardiac muscle displaces the smooth muscle in the corresponding veins, and a cholinergic plexus replaces the adrenergic. Where only one layer of muscle occurs, this plexus lies just deep to it: but where the muscularis is multilayered in larger veins, the nerves run in among the cells.

Intraepithelial Nerves. Intraepithelial nerves have been briefly described in the sections on the laryngeal epithelium and glands and the bronchial glands. The range of presumptive sensory receptors in the epithelium of the respiratory tract extends from simple nerve endings through multicellular receptors associated with a nerve, like the taste buds of the epiglottis. It can be safely said that the sensory modality served in most other instances is not reliably known. In the simplest receptors, individual nerve fibers emerge from their Schwann cell investments in the submucosa or lamina propria and enter the epithelium as 0.2- to 0.4-µm, naked nerve processes. In classic silvered light-optical preparations, these are seen to extend between the cells or in grooves within them, frequently penetrating as far as the apical cytoplasm. In electron micrographs, such finger-like processes contain an array of longitudinally directed microtubules and a few mitochondria in an electron-lucent cytoplasm. They are often surrounded by interdigitating cytoplasmic leaflets from neighboring cells (Fig. 23–86). Other presumptively sensory fibers have a similar structure, except that the pro-

23–86 Intraepithelial neuronal process in the intrapulmonary airway of a vampire bat. Along its course, the nerve contacts numerous protoplasmic leaflets produced from the sides of adjacent epithelial cells. A mitochondria-rich portion of another nerve occurs at the lower left. × 22,000.

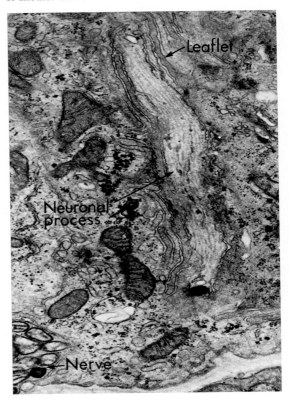

cesses contain varicosities without synaptic vesicles and may end in a bulbous swelling. Still others closely appose cells at the base of the epithelium and are filled with small mitochondria (Fig. 23–41). Intraepithelial nerves have been described in the trachea and extrapulmonary airways of rats, but in other species they are known to occur deeper inside the lungs as well. In having a sensory innervation, brush cells and certain of the small-granule cells may also qualify for inclusion among the more elaborate sensory receptors.

Motor endings in the epithelium are confined to specific sites, notably to the glands, which are richly supplied by cholinergic motor neurons in most species examined. The unmyelinated nerves originate as radial fibers from the intramuscular plexus and concentrate in the connective tissue outside of glandular acini before crossing the basement lamina to ramify among the secretory and myoepithelial cells. There the fibers enlarge at intervals into *boutons de passage* (Chap. 8) containing mitochondria and clear synaptic vesicles (Fig. 23–9). The extent to which nerve processes cross the basement lamina nonetheless varies with the species and the location of the glands in the respiratory system. In all cases, a certain number of varicosities occur below the basement lamina where synaptic vesicles are directly exposed to the intercellular space, much as in the intramuscular plexus.

Nerves in the Respiratory Zone. The extent and character of innervation beyond the respiratory bronchioles has been estimated very differently by investigators and for that reason remains controversial. Claims of an extensive innervation of alveolar ducts are based primarily on studies using silver impregnation to reveal nerve bundles, but these methods have the disadvantage that the fine collagenous fibers in these regions are likely to stain as well and so appear as nerves. In any case, conclusions based on this approach have not been confirmed by critical studies that identify nerves on the basis of acetylcholinesterase histochemistry or catecholamine fluorescence. Nerves enter the respiratory zone from the peribronchial plexus or its subsidiary branches in the muscularis and submucosa of the bronchial tree as well as along the course of the blood vessels. An extensive innervation of the respiratory tissue requires relatively large nerve bundles to supply it, and because the nerves come in with the axial structures, a rough assessment of the magnitude of innervation be-

yond can be made by examining the nerves surrounding the terminal bronchioles and the arteries and veins nearby. Compared with the size of the nerve bundles at the hilum, those at the bronchiolar level are greatly diminished, and so it is evident at once that most of the pulmonary nerves are directed to axial structures. Along bronchioles of bats, for example, peribronchial bundles typically consist of one myelinated axon and perhaps 50 to 60 unmyelinated fibers enveloped by cytoplasmic leaflets from two or more Schwann cells; the whole is embedded in a collagenous matrix and is surrounded by endoneurium (Fig. 23–33). These bundles and the myelinated nerve disappear before the airway loses its bronchiole-like wall structure and cuboidal epithelium, leaving the intramuscular plexus to send a few unmyelinated fibers on toward the terminal sphincter of smooth muscle (Fig. 23–49). Just deep to the sphincter, very few processes remain after the others enlarge into nerve terminals and begin to emerge from the single Schwann cell that at this level is sufficient to enclose all fibers present (Fig. 23–87). In other species as well, only tiny unmyelinated nerve fascicles continue to run in the walls of respiratory bronchioles and alveolar ducts. The subtended alveoli may be closely approached by the fibers present, but more peripheral alveoli are neither extensively nor evenly innervated. In other words, few nerves are left for alveolar structures after all smooth muscle in a given acinus has been provided for. The remaining fibers, which continue to follow the course of the airway, are too few to provide direct innervation for more than a small number of alveolar cells. In rats, small bundles, each containing less than 10 unmyelinated fibers, are distributed around the circumference of the alveolar ducts, and in the alveolar walls rare bundles with still fewer fibers and persisting Schwann cells are found only after concerted effort. Presumptively sensory nerves, characterized by an enlarged termination filled with mitochondria, occur among them; and, apart from very few cholinergic varicosities reported from this region, close contact has been observed between a great alveolar cell and a nerve process containing large (1,200 Å) granular vesicles. Neither adrenergic nor cholinergic, these vesicles resemble those occurring together with clear synaptic vesicles near autonomic terminals (Fig. 23–88).

It is not yet certain whether the pericytes of pulmonary capillaries are innervated or whether their responses are mediated through electrical

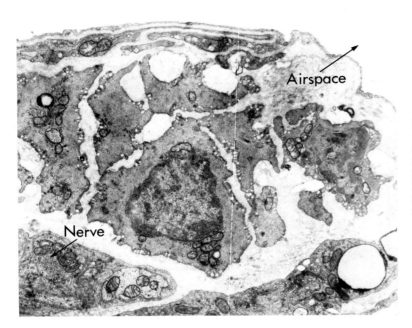

23–87 Nerve supply to a terminal muscle sphincter of an alveolated air passage. The nerve continues from the intramuscular plexus and is shown as it widens into a varicosity beneath the muscle cells. Compare with Fig. 23–49. × 6700.

contact with the capillary endothelium, or possibly the vascular smooth muscle.

Histophysiology. Within the lungs, the response of smooth muscle to nervous stimulation or to naturally occurring pharmacological agents differs according to its location in the bronchial tree or in the pulmonary arteries or pulmonary veins. For example, norepinephrine or epinephrine constricts the arteries but not the veins or the bronchi, whereas acetylcholine constricts the bronchial musculature but not the vessels, and serotonin or histamine constricts muscle at all sites. On the basis of experiments in which the autonomic inputs to the lungs are stimulated electrically, it appears that in the airway, stimulation of the vagus brings about transient vasoconstriction, but stimulation of the sympathetic nerves has no effect unless the bronchial tone is first increased, when the result is bronchodilatation. Thus, the sympathetic action is inhibitory to the parasympathetic fibers carried in the vagus, and fine control over bronchial tone can be achieved by interaction of excitatory and inhibitory stimuli. It is thought that the parasympathetic ganglion cells mediating secretion by the glands may interact with noncholinergic fibers less than those involved with regulation of airway tone. In any case, some cells in large ganglia located away from the glands are contacted by sympathetic nerves, whereas those in smaller ganglia nearer the glands are not. The nerves form synapses on the soma, and their adrenergic nature has been confirmed by catecholamine fluorescence in ganglia of rabbits, cats, and dogs. Although the extent of sympathetic innervation in the airway varies considerably with the species, it usually is more extensive in extrapulmonary than in intrapulmonary bronchi and, as in rats, may be present in the trachea (Fig. 23–14) and absent from the lungs. A nonadrenergic inhibitory circuit might be expected to occur in the lungs of such animals. Indeed, it occurs even in cats, which are well endowed with airway sympathetics: If serotonin or histamine is used to induce bronchoconstriction and the vagi are then electrically stimulated, an added bronchoconstrictive effect of short duration is followed by a slower and more prolonged dilatation. Administration of atropine abolishes only the transient increase in tone but not the relaxation, and repetition of the experiments using adrenergic blocking agents does not change the result. These findings indicate that a nonadrenergic, noncholinergic inhibitory circuit affects bronchomotor tone. It has also been detected in human airways where sympathetic fibers are not prevalent and where its dysfunction may help to bring on bronchial asthma. The system appears similar to one found operating in the myenteric plexuses of the small intestine (Chap. 19); hence, both have been considered part of a "purinergic

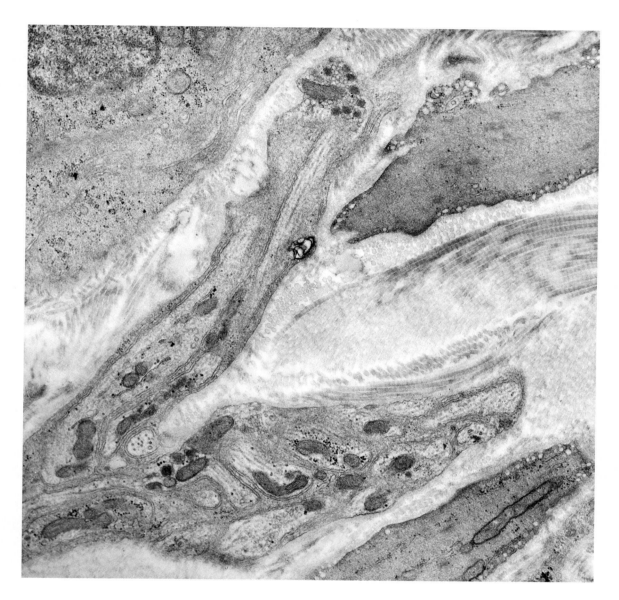

nervous system" whose neurotransmitter may be adenosine triphosphate and whose action in the gut affects the relaxation phase of peristalsis. In the lungs, the identity of the nonadrenergic, noncholinergic transmitter is unknown, but its relatively slow action may suggest that the agent must diffuse a longer distance to reach the muscle than is required for acetylcholine released at varicosities of the intramuscular plexus. Inasmuch as fetal lungs when explanted to organ culture sometimes exhibit peristaltic movements over a number of days, it would seem likely that pulmonary innervation includes an intrinsic seg-

23–88 A small unmyelinated nerve sheathed by Schwann cell cytoplasm penetrates in between smooth muscle cells to enter the bronchiolar submucosa in a bat's lung. At this level a few processes branch off to run close to the base of the epithelium; one of them expands into a varicosity containing both clear and dense synaptic vesicles. × 11,600.

ment with excitatory and inhibitory circuits, of which the nonadrenergic noncholinergic component may be a part.

It is widely known that pulmonary vessels do not respond to autonomic nerve stimulation in a manner comparable to systemic vessels. With low distending pressures in them, less constrictive effort and fewer muscles are needed to regulate flow. On the other hand, because the vessels are lightly constructed and located amidst tissues that incessantly undergo distension and compression, blood pressure of pulmonary vessels is more profoundly influenced by mechanical factors and by gravity than in most other parts of the body. Sympathetic stimulation, either by direct or reflex action, produces a small increase in arterial tone and in adults becomes large only under chronic pathological conditions when the smooth muscle has undergone hypertrophy; acetylcholine has a relaxing action on constricted vessels. Perhaps the most significant factor affecting pulmonary vascular pressure is hypoxia, which causes a rise in arterial pressure attributable to vasoconstriction; small vessels in the locality of poorly oxygenated alveoli close down in favor of those nearer a better oxygen supply. Although chemoreceptors in the aortic and carotid bodies respond to hypoxia and may stimulate pulmonary sympathetics reflexly, the same pressor effect observed in intact animals is also seen in isolated lung preparations, making it evident that the response to hypoxia can be mediated entirely within the lung. It may be expressed through release of vasoconstrictive agents like histamine and serotonin that are stored in the lung, through others like angiotensin that are activated there, or possibly through release of norepinephrine or other neurotransmitters from an intrinsic nervous segment that survives lung isolation.

Most of the sensory input from the lungs serves a number of reflexes and is not consciously felt. Physiologists currently recognize three kinds of pulmonary vagal sensory receptors. They are viewed as mechanoreceptors because use is usually made of a distending stimulus to elicit their response: (1) *Slowly adapting stretch receptors* mediated by medullated fibers from intrapulmonary walls and increasingly active until cessation of inspiration; (2) *rapidly adapting mechano- and irritant receptors* carried by medullated fibers mainly from extrapulmonary airways and active in the cough reflex; and (3) *juxtapulmonary capillary or J receptors* carried by unmyelinated fibers from the respiratory zone. The latter responds to alveolar interstitial congestion and certain other kinds of irritation by promoting rapid, shallow breathing. The morphological form of all these receptors is still uncertain. Mechanical or chemical stimulation to the airway sometimes reaches consciousness and brings on coughing, but most of the sharply localized sense of pain subjectively associated with the lungs in reality is pleuritic, detected by pain fibers in the parietal pleura. Strong stimulation to the dorsum of the trachea or to the right or left main bronchi nevertheless brings on substernal pain or pain localized to the anterior chest and neck, a little to the right or left, accordingly. On the other hand, the site of receptors associated with the pain from acute or chronic disease of pulmonary vessels is unknown, and the areas of referral are poorly localized.

Pleura

The *visceral pleura* is closely applied to each lung (Figs. 23–76 and 23–81, see here and color insert). It is covered by a simple mesothelium whose cells are notable for the complexity of their junctions and the luxuriance of their brush border, which is better developed in cells covering the ventral, caudal, and mediastinal surfaces than in those facing the ribs. They rest on a thin layer of dense fibrous tissue. Beneath lies the relatively thick connective tissue, rich in elastic fibers and sometimes rich in mast cells, that continues into the interlobar and interlobular septa of the lung. The dense pleural sheet effectively prevents leakage of air into the thoracic cavity. Pleural folds in the mediastinum may have several white patches (Kampmeier foci) where the pleural mesothelium is invaded by lymphocytes and macrophages. These may serve as windows on the thoracic cavity for immunologically competent lymphoid cells as well as points of embarkation for macrophages crossing onto the pleural surface. The *parietal pleura*, a thicker and less elastic membrane than the visceral pleura, contains fat cells. The vascular supply to the visceral pleura is derived from both pulmonary and bronchial circuits; the parietal supply is entirely systemic from vessels of the body wall.

Development of the Lungs

The airways of the lungs develop from a midline endodermal bud, the *laryngotracheal groove*, located on the floor of the pharynx between the sixth branchial arches. It branches to form the two primary bronchi and their arboreous subdivisions. The larynx develops from adjacent pharyngeal structures. The endodermal epithelium is accompanied by a sparse coating of undifferentiated mesodermal cells originally located next to the laryngotracheal groove. These tissues enter the thorax and expand by rapid growth and division of their cells. They advance amid a relatively acellular mesenchyma derived from the body wall; this gives rise to the blood vessels and lymphatics, interlobar septa, visceral pleura, cartilage, and adventitia of the bronchial wall. Bronchial branching patterns characteristic of the species are established very early, indicating that a genetic influence is exerted during development.

In the early *pseudoglandular period,* so named because the lungs then have a glandlike structure, attention is concentrated on the bronchial tree. In this system, two functionally distinct regions are recognized, that of the *terminal buds* and that of the airway previously laid down. Airway formation is a centrifugally directed process centered in the terminal buds, whose epithelial cell multiply more rapidly than cells in the invaded tissue, apparently because of an inductive interaction taking place between the endoderm and the encircling mesoderm. Cell division declines somewhat and branching normally ceases to occur in the epithelium previously laid down because the inductive interaction is no longer felt. The epithelial cells at first are morphologically unspecialized and derive much of the energy needed for growth from anaerobic glycolysis. The cytoplasm contains abundant stores of glycogen, which is most concentrated in cells of the terminal buds (Fig. 23–89). As epithelial cells begin to differentiate, they lose much of this glycogen but gain in mitochondrial enzyme activity associated with aerobic oxidative pathways. These and later morphological developments like the appearance of mucus droplets and ciliogenesis first occur in cells of the trachea and main bronchi. They gradually spread distally, so that a gradient of maturity extends between the trachea and the terminal buds. Small-granule cells are among the first differentiated cells to appear.

The surrounding mesenchyma also becomes differentiated centrifugally, as marked first by a condensation of primitive connective tissue about the epithelium and later by the differentiation of cartilage, smooth muscle, and extracellular fibers. Consequently, the operation of one continuous morphogenetic process serves to establish the fundamental structure of the trachea, bronchi, and bronchioles.

In its development, the pulmonary circulation is dependent on the lead taken by the expanding

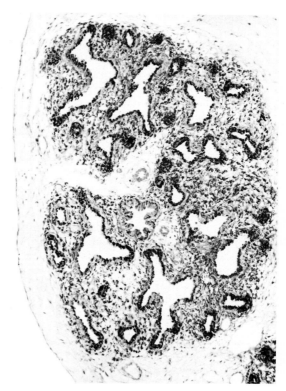

23–89 Section of a lobule from a 3.5-month fetal human lung, demonstrating glycogen **(black).** A central bronchiole is surrounded by tissue containing budding bronchial branches. These have cuboidal epithelium. Connective tissue surrounds the lobule; the visceral pleura is at the left. PAS method. × 125.

pulmonary endoderm. The pulmonary vessels are developed mainly from an irregular capillary plexus that surrounds the head gut of the embryo and serves both the esophagus and pulmonary anlagen. Rudiments of the pulmonary arteries and veins are formed early, the arteries joining the plexus as mesial outgrowths of the left pulmonary arch, and the veins growing out from the dorsal mesocardium. With expansion of the bronchial tree, a single pulmonary artery comes to be associated with the main bronchus of each lung, lying against the dorsal surface, whereas the vein lies against the ventral surface. The main arterial branches develop alongside the bronchial tree, but smaller branches leave them at right angles and later become part of the supply to alveolar capillaries. Bronchial arteries form relatively late as de novo branches of the thoracic aorta and posterior intercostals and grow down the bronchial tree to join the peribronchial plexus.

As development proceeds, newly laid down peripheral bronchial branches fail to enlarge as much as the more proximal branches did subsequent to their function, and their walls remain relatively thin. At the same time, growth of the vasculature becomes stimulated, and the fetal lung enters its *canalicular period* of development. The terminal buds become less spherical and even baggy; networks of pulmonary capillaries are developed and press against the cuboidal lining cells of the distal airways, stretching them and so helping to bring about a flattening of the epithelium. Subsequently, in the *terminal sac period*, these primitive respiratory channels become changed into thin-walled saccules suited for gas exchange in which shallow outpocketings, or primitive alveoli, begin to appear. Great alveolar cells begin to secrete surfactant; the lungs look as if they are partially expanded, and they are easily able to sustain life.

At birth, lungs of various species differ greatly in histological and histochemical maturity. The lungs of rats are yet canalicular, whereas human lungs have developed a respiratory zone containing acini approximately one cubic millimeter in volume, each subdivided into about 8 generations of short branches and 176 saccules. It is not the presence of a thin respiratory epithelium so much as the development of an adequate pulmonary vasculature that is critical to the survival of premature infants. On this basis, the extreme limit of viability has been placed at 4.5 months when the lungs are midway through the canalicular period, but the chances of survival increase sharply once surfactant and alveoli appear.

Within a few hours after birth the lungs fill with air. At that time proprioceptive and other chemically mediated mechanisms produce a decrease in pulmonary vascular resistance and increase in blood flow. These effects are enhanced by the opening of new circulatory routes on expansion of the lungs. Some time later the *ductus arteriosus* closes, and the definitive pulmonary circuit comes into being.

In humans few nonrespiratory branches are added to the bronchial tree after birth; in dogs their number may decrease. This is because alveolar formation is essentially a centripetal process superimposed on the centrifugal process that resulted in the laying down of the bronchial tree. The shallow alveoli in neonatal human lungs enlarge in the immediate postnatal period

as the terminal region is remodeled; septa grow in from the walls of the saccules, deepen the alveoli, and increase the respiratory surface. This is followed by the onset of retrograde alveolarization. As development proceeds, respiratory bronchioles become transformed into alveolar ducts, and bronchioles become respiratory bronchioles. The number of alveoli continue to increase until early adolescence, but the shorter bronchial pathways complete their development before then. The formation of accessory respiratory pathways at acinar and bronchiolar levels evidently is a by-product of this postnatal reorganization.

References and Selected Bibliography

General

Comroe, J. H., Jr. 1974. Physiology of Respiration. Chicago: Year Book Medical Publishers, Inc.

Goodrich, E. S. 1958. Studies on the Structure and Development of Vertebrates. New York: Dover Publications, Inc.

Jeffrey, P. K., and Reid, L. M. 1977. The respiratory mucous membrane. In J. D. Brain, D. F. Proctor, and L. Reid (eds.), Respiratory Defense Mechanisms. New York: Marcel Dekker, Inc., p. 193.

Lenfant, C. (ed.). 1976–1981. Lung Biology in Health and Disease, Vols. 1–18. New York: Marcel Dekker, Inc.

Macklem, P. T. 1971. Airway obstruction and collateral ventilation. Physiol. Rev. 51:368.

Miller, W. S. 1947. The Lung, 2nd ed. Springfield, Ill.: Charles G. Thomas, Publisher.

Proctor, D. F. 1980. Breathing, Speech, and Song. Vienna: Springer-Verlag.

Ross, R. B. 1957. Influence of bronchial tree structure on ventilation in the dog's lungs as inferred from measurements of a plastic cast. J. Appl. Physiol. 10:1

Sorokin, S., and Brain, J. D. 1975. Pathways of clearance in mouse lungs exposed to iron oxide aerosols. Anat. Rec. 181:581.

Upper Respiratory Tract: Nose, Pharynx, Larynx

Cauna, N., and Hinderer, K. H. 1969. Fine structure of blood vessels of the human nasal respiratory mucosa. Ann. Otol. 78:865.

Dawes, J. D. K., and Prichard, M. M. L. 1953. Studies of the vascular arrangements of the nose. J. Anat. 87:311.

Fink, B. R. 1975. The Human Larynx, A Functional Study. New York: Raven Books, Abelard-Schuman Ltd.

Negus, V. 1958. The Comparative Anatomy and Physiology of the Nose and Paranasal Sinuses. Edinburgh: E. & S. Livingstone.

Schaeffer, J. P. 1932. The mucous membrane of the nasal cavity and the paransal sinuses. In E. V. Cowdry (ed.), Special Cytology, Vol. 1. New York: Paul B. Hoeber, Inc.

Olfactory System

Allison, A. C. 1953. The morphology of the olfactory system in the vertebrates. Biol. Rev. 28:195.

Moulton, D. G. 1976. Spatial patterning of response to odors in the peripheral olfactory system. Physiol. Rev. 56:578.

Pfaffmann, C. (ed.). 1969. Olfaction and Taste. Proceedings of the Third International Symposium. New York: Rockefeller University Press.

Wolstenholme, G. E. W., and Knight, J. (eds.). 1970. Taste and Smell in Vertebrates. London: J & A Churchill.

Conducting Airways: Trachea, Bronchi, Bronchioles

Boyd, M. R. 1977. Evidence for the Clara cell as a site of cytochrome P450-dependent mixed-function oxidase activity in lung. Nature (Lond.) 269:713.

Kuhn, C., III, Callaway, L. A., and Askin, F. B. 1974. The formation of granules in the bronchiolar Clara cells of the rat. I. Electron microscopy. J. Ultrastruct. Res. 49:387.

Kuhn, C., III, and Callaway, L. A. 1975. The formation of granules in the bronchiolar Clara cells of the Rat. II. Enzyme cytochemistry. J. Ultrastruct. Res. 53:66.

McDowell E. M., Becci, P. J., Schürch, W., and Trump, B. F. 1979. The respiratory epithelium. VII. Epidermoid metaplasia of hamster tracheal epithelium during regeneration following mechanical injury. J. Natl. Cancer Inst. 62:995.

Petrik, P., and Collet, A. J. 1974. Quantitative electron microscopic autoradiography of in vivo incorporation of ³H-choline, ³H-leucine, ³H-acetate and ³H-galactose in non-ciliated bronchiolar (Clara) cells of mice. Am. J. Anat. 139:519.

Plopper. C. G., Mariassy, A. T., and Hill, L. H. 1980. Ultrastructure of the nonciliated bronchiolar epithelial (Clara) cell of mammalian lung: I. A comparison of rabbit, guinea pig, rat, hamster, and mouse; II. A comparison of horse, steer, sheep, dog, and cat. Exp. Lung Res. 1:139 and 155.

Plopper, C. G., Hill, L. H., and Mariassy, A. T. 1980. Ultrastructure of the nonciliated bronchiolar epithelial (Clara) cell of mammalian lung. III. A study of man with comparison of 15 mammalian species. Exp. Lung Res. 1:171.

Reid, L. 1958. The secondary lobule in the adult human lung with special reference to its appearance in bronchograms. Thorax 13:110.

Reid, L., and Simon, G. 1958. The peripheral pattern in the normal bronchogram and its relation to peripheral pulmonary anatomy. Thorax 13:103.

Neuroendocrine Cells

Hoyt, R. F., Jr., Sorokin, S. P., and Feldman, H. 1982. Number, subtypes and distribution of small-granule (neuro)endocrine cells in the infracardiac lobe of a hamster lung. Exp. Lung Res. 3:273.

Lauweryns, J. M., Cokelaere, M., Theunynck, P., and Deleersnyder. M. 1974. Neuroepithelial bodies in mammalian respiratory mucosa: Light optical, histochemical and ultrastructural studies. Chest 65 (Suppl.):22S.

The Respiratory Zone

Boyden, E. A. 1971. The structure of the pulmonary acinus in a child of 6 2/3 years. Anat. Rec. 169:282.

Chevalier, G., and Collet, A. J. 1972. In vivo incorporation of choline-³H, leucine-³H and galactose-³H in alveolar type II pneumocytes in relation to surfactant synthesis. A quantitative radioautographic study in mouse by electron microscopy. Anat. Rec. 174:289.

Gehr, P., Bachofen, M., and Weibel, E. R. 1978. The normal human lung: Ultrastructure and morphometric estimation of diffusion capacity. Resp. Physiol. 32:121.

Macklin, C. C. 1935. Pulmonic alveolar vents. J. Anat. 69:188.

Schneeberger, E. 1977. The integrity of the air-blood barrier. In J. D. Brain, D. F. Proctor, and L. Reid (eds.), Respiratory Defense Mechanisms. New York: Marcel Dekker, p. 68.

Sorokin, S. 1966. A morphologic and cytochemical study on the great alveolar cell. J. Histochem. Cytochem. 14:884.

Tenney, S. M., and Remmers, J. E. 1963. Comparative quantitative morphology of the mammalian lung: Diffusing area. Nature (Lond.) 197:54.

Weibel, E. R. 1973. Morphological basis of alveolar-capillary gas exchange. Physiol. Rev. 53:419.

Weibel, E. R., and Gil, J. 1968. Electron microscopic demonstration of an extracellular duplex lining layer of alveoli. Resp. Physiol. 4:42.

Williams, M. C. 1977. Conversion of lamellar body membranes into tubular myelin in alveoli of fetal rat lungs. J. Cell Biol. 72:260.

Pulmonary Macrophages

Brain, J. D., Godleski, J. J., and Sorokin, S. P. 1977. Quantification, origin, and fate of pulmonary macrophages. In J. D. Brain, D. F. Proctor, and L. Reid (eds.), Respiratory Defense Mechanisms. New York: Marcel Dekker, p. 849.

Godleski, J. J., and Brain, J. D. 1972. The origin of alveolar macrophages in mouse radiation chimeras. J. Exp. Med. 136:630.

Sorokin, S. 1977. Phagocytes in the lungs: Incidence, general behavior, and phylogeny. In. J. D. Brain, D. F. Proctor, and L. Reid (eds.), Respiratory Defense Mechanisms. New York: Marcel Dekker, Inc., p. 711.

Blood and Lymphatic Vessels

Krahl, V. E. 1962. The glomus pulmonale: Its location and microscopic anatomy. In A. V. S. de Reuck and

M. O'Connor (eds.), Pulmonary Structure and Function, Ciba Foundation Symposium. Boston: Little, Brown, and Company.

Lauweryns, J. 1971. The blood and lymphatic microcirculation of the lung. *In* S. C. Sommers (ed.), Pathology Annual, Vol. 6. New York: Appleton Century Crofts, p. 365.

Leak, L. V. 1977. Pulmonary lymphatics and their role in the removal of interstitial fluids and particulate matter. *In* J. D. Brain, D. F. Proctor, and L. Reid (eds.), Respiratory Defense Mechanisms. New York: Marcel Dekker, p. 631.

Innervation

Diamond, L., and O'Donnell, M. 1980. A nonadrenergic vagal inhibitory pathway to feline airways. Science (Wash., D.C.) 108:185.

El-Bermani, A. -W. 1973. The innervation of the rat lung. Acetylcholinesterase-containing nerves of the bronchial tree. Am. J. Anat. 137:19.

El-Bermani, A. -W., and Grant, M. 1975. Acetycholinesterase-positive nerves of the rhesus monkey bronchial tree. Thorax 30:162.

Honjin, R. 1956. Experimental degeneration of the vagus, and its relation to the nerve supply of lung of the mouse, with special reference to the crossing innervation of the lung by the vagi. J. Comp. Neurol. 106:1.

Honjin, R. 1956. On the nerve supply of the lung of the mouse, with special reference to the structure of the peripheral vegetative nervous system. J. Comp. Neurol. 105:587.

Hung, K. -S., Hertweck, M. S., Hardy, J. D., and Loosli, C. G. 1972. Innervation of pulmonary alveoli of the mouse lung: An electron microscopic study. Am J. Anat. 135:477.

Richardson, J. B. 1979. Nerve supply to the lungs. Am. Rev. Resp. Dis. 119:785.

Pleura

Wang, N.-S. 1974. The regional difference of pleural mesothelial cells in rabbits. Am. Rev. Resp. Dis. 110:623.

Development

Boyden, E. A. 1971. Development of the human lung. *In* V. C. Kelley (ed.), Brennemann's Practice of Pediatrics, Vol. 4. New York: Harper & Row Publishers, Inc., chap. 64.

Boyden, E. A., and Tompsett, D. H. 1961. The postnatal growth of the lung in the dog. Acta Anat. 47:185.

Burri, P. 1974. The postnatal growth of the rat lung. III. Morphology. Anat. Rec. 180:77.

Ham, A. W., and Baldwin, K. W. 1941. A histological study of the development of the lung, with particular reference to the nature of alveoli. Anat. Rec. 81:363.

Hislop, A., and Reid, L. M. 1977. Formation of the pulmonary vasculature. *In* W. A. Hodson (ed.), Development of the Lung. New York: Marcel Dekker, p. 37.

Sorokin, S., Padykula, H. A., and Herman, E. 1959. Comparative histochemical patterns in developing mammalian lungs. Dev. Biol. 1:125.

Sorokin, S., Hoyt, R. F., Jr., and Grant, M. M. 1982. Development of neuroepithelial bodies in fetal rabbits. I. Appearance and functional maturation as demonstrated by high-resolution light microscopy and formaldehyde-induced fluorescence. Exp. Lung Res. 3:237.

The Urinary System

Ruth Ellen Bulger

Introduction

Components of the Urinary System

The normal human urinary system consists of two kidneys, two ureters, a bladder, and a urethra. The kidneys elaborate a fluid product called urine; the ureters, two fibromuscular tubes, conduct the urine to a single urinary bladder where the fluid accumulates for periodic evacuation via the single urethra that connects the bladder to the exterior.

Kidney Function

The kidneys make significant and sometimes vital contributions to several important functions:

1. The excretion of waste products of metabolism
2. The elimination of foreign substances and their breakdown products
3. The regulation of total body water
4. The maintenance of the extracellular fluid volume
5. The regulation of various salts to be retained or excreted by the body
6. The control of acid-base balance

The kidneys carry out these various functions because of their architecture: gross, histological, cytological, and chemical. Three separate kidneys have developed during evolution: the pronephros, the mesonephros, and the metanephros. This evolutionary experience is repeated in each human embryo with the serial development of three separate kidneys and the subsequent degeneration of the first two during early embryonic life. In each of these kidneys there are filtering devices capable of developing a fluid that the distinctive tubules then modify. The filter has become more efficient and the tubule more complex during evolution.

Three separate physiological processes are involved in the formation of urine by the adult metanephric kidney: (1) filtration, (2) secretion, and (3) reabsorption. The first step in the formation of urine is a *filtration* process in which an ultrafiltrate of plasma is created. The filtering membrane retains most large proteins within the blood, but a small amount of albumin (MW approximately 70,000) passes into the filtrate. As it passes down the tubule, the filtrate is altered by *secretion*, in which additional substances are moved by the lining cells of the tubule from the surrounding renal interstitium into the filtrate within the tubular lumen, and *reabsorption*, whereby substances are moved from the intratubular filtrate across the tubular cells back into the renal interstitium. The fluid that emerges at the end of the tubule is the net result of these three processes and is called *urine.*

In humans, every 24 h 180 liters of fluid are filtered into the tubular lumens of the kidney, but normally only 1 or 2 liters of urine are produced. The remainder of the filtered fluid is reabsorbed across the tubular epithelium to reenter the blood vascular system. This process requires a large expenditure of energy.

The Kidney

The human kidneys are paired, bean-shaped organs that lie in the retroperitoneal space on the posterior aspect of the abdominal cavity. The lateral border on each kidney is convex, and the medial border is concave. Normally one kidney is found on either side of the vertebral column; their upper margins are near the upper region of the twelfth thoracic vertebra. The upper poles lie closer to the vertebral column than the lower poles, and so the long axis of the kidney is parallel with the psoas muscles. The kidney is surrounded by a fibrous capsule and situated within a mass of fatty tissue.

The medial concave border is penetrated by a vertical slit called the *renal hilus.* Branches of the renal artery, vein, lymphatics, and nerves, as well as an expanded part of the ureter (called the

pelvis), pass through the hilus to the renal parenchyma. The renal hilus communicates with a flattened cavity within the kidney called the *renal sinus.* Within the sinus, the expanded pelvis of the ureter branches into three or four major calyxes, which in turn branch to form seven to 14 minor calyxes. In addition, evaginations of the minor calyxes (called fornices) penetrate outward into the kidney parenchyma to increase the area of interface between pelvic urine and renal parenchyma. Loose connective tissue and fat tissue in the sinus provide a region through which the vessels and nerves pass.

When the kidney is bisected into dorsal and ventral portions (Fig. 24–1), it can be seen to be divided into a cortex and a medulla. The cortex consists of a broad outer zone of dark red substance and projections that extend toward the renal sinus (called the *renal columns* because of their columnar profile in a section of kidney). The medulla is composed of a variable number of conical structures of lighter, striated appearance called *medullary pyramids.* They are situated with their bases adjacent to the outer zone of cortex, and their apexes project into the renal sinus. The apex of each medullary pyramid is capped by a funnel-shaped minor *calyx.* Urine produced by the kidney exits at the medullary apex and is funneled by a minor calyx into the remainder of the extrarenal collecting system.

The kidney is divided into units called *lobes.* One lobe consists of a conical medullary pyramid and the cortical substance that surrounds it like the cap of an acorn. The kidneys of some animals, such as rodents, consist of only one lobe (unilobar). Multilobar human kidneys contain from six to 18 lobes. During human fetal life, the lobes develop separately and are demarcated by deep clefts between them (Fig. 24–2). In postnatal life, however, these clefts are generally obliterated and the organ appears to have a smooth surface, although the lobes still exist within the kidney.

At intervals along the base of each medullary pyramid, striated elements called *medullary rays* penetrate into the cortex. Although they resemble the medullary substance because of their striated appearance, the medullary rays are considered part of the cortex. Each medullary ray forms the center of a small cone of renal parenchyma called a *lobule.*

An additional zonation can be seen in the gross structure of the medulla, which is divided into an *outer zone* adjacent to the cortex and an

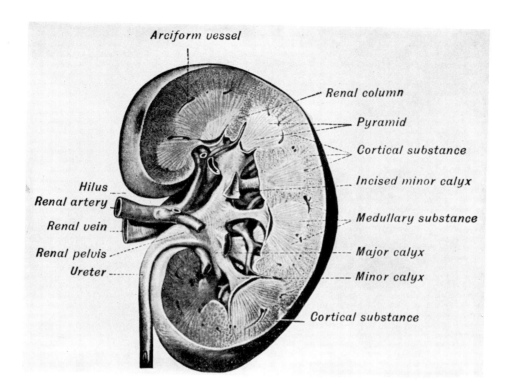

Arciform vessel

Renal column

Pyramid

Cortical substance

Incised minor calyx

Hilus

Renal artery

Renal vein

Medullary substance

Renal pelvis

Major calyx

Ureter

Minor calyx

Cortical substance

24–1 Gross anatomic appearance of a human kidney, at three-fifths its natural size. The tissue has been bisected to reveal elements of the internal structure. (From Braus, H. 1924. Anatomie des Menschen. Berlin: Springer-Verlag OHG.)

inner zone including the medullary tip (which is called the *papilla*). The outer zone, in turn, consists of an outer and inner stripe. The zones seen grossly are a reflection of the differing morphologies of the regions of the renal secretory units and of their orientation in the kidney (Figs. 24–3 and 24–4).

Functional Anatomy of the Uriniferous Tubule

The functional unit of the kidney is the uriniferous tubule. Each human kidney contains approximately one million of these units. The uriniferous tubule is composed of a long convoluted portion called the *nephron* and a system of *intrarenal collecting ducts*. Each of these segments was derived from a different embryological primordium. The nephron developed from the metanephrogenic blastema (tissue from the caudal region of the urogenital ridge) whereas the collecting ducts were derived from the ureteric bud (a diverticulum of the mesonephric duct).

Nephron. The nephron is composed of several regions of diversified morphology, but all of them are characterized by cells that have an elab-

orate shape with numerous lateral interdigitating processes. The blind end of the nephron is indented by a network of capillaries and supporting cells to form a filtering body called the *renal corpuscle*. In addition, the nephron consists of the following: (1) a neck, (2) a proximal convoluted tubule, (3) a straight region of the proximal tubule, (4) a thin limb, (5) a straight region of the distal tubule, (6) a macula densa region of the distal tubule, and (7) a distal convoluted tubule.

Nephrons are situated within the kidney in a characteristic position (Figs. 24–2 to 24–4) with the renal corpuscles and proximal convoluted tubules located in the cortex. The straight portion of the proximal tubule, the thin limb segment, and the straight portion of the distal tubule form a looping structure called the *loop of Henle*, which enters into the medullary pyramid by way of a medullary ray, forms a hairpin loop within the medulla, and returns to the cortex via

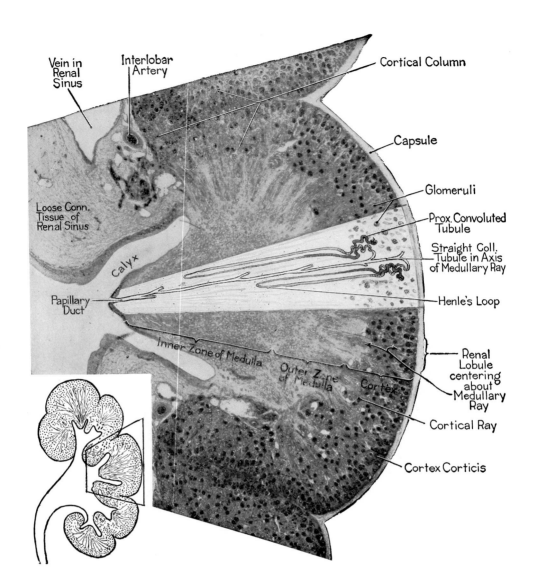

24–2 Photomicrograph showing one lobe of a metanephric kidney from a 6-month-old human fetus. The **inset** outlines the part of the kidney that appears in the photograph. The schematic diagram in the center of the lobe shows the position and arrangement of the renal tubules around a straight collecting tubule. × 18. (From Patten, B. M. 1968. Human Embryology, 3rd ed. New York: McGraw-Hill Book Company.)

the same medullary ray. As the straight portion of each distal tubule enters the cortex, it passes adjacent to its originating renal corpuscle, forming the macula densa of the distal tubule, and then continues as the distal convoluted segment.

Even though the nephron segments differ in length, each region of all nephrons tends to occupy a certain position in the kidney as a whole, causing the gross zonation described earlier (Fig. 24–3). For example, the thin limbs are seen in the inner stripe of the outer zone of the medulla and in the inner zone of the medulla, whereas the proximal and distal convoluted tubules are located only in the cortex (Fig. 24–4).

Nephrons are classified as superficial, midcortical, or juxtamedullary by the position of their renal corpuscles within the superficial, midcortical, or juxtamedullary region of the cortex. Nephrons are also classified by the region where their loops of Henle turn. Short-looped

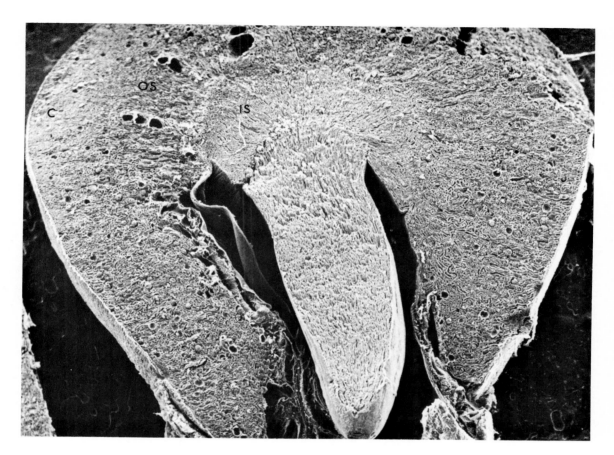

nephrons have Henle loops that turn within the outer medulla and have a short thin limb segment, whereas the loops of long-looped nephrons turn within the inner medulla and are characterized by long thin limb segments. The proportion of long- to short-looped nephrons varies with each species.

The nephrons empty into a complex system of collecting ducts. In human kidneys, the cortical nephrons tend to empty singly into a terminal collecting duct, whereas several juxtamedullary nephrons empty into an arched collecting duct that courses peripherally in the cortex and then enters the medullary ray. These cortical collecting ducts merge while traversing the medullary ray and medullary pyramid to empty as several large collecting ducts at the apex of the medullary pyramid.

RENAL CORPUSCLE. The nephron begins with a renal corpuscle located in the cortex and is roughly oval in shape (Figs. 24–5 to 24–11). Estimates of their diameter in humans range from 150 to 250 μm. Each renal corpuscle consists of

24–3 Scanning electron micrograph of a cross section from a rat kidney. The kidney can be divided into four radial zones: cortex **(C)**; outer stripe of the medullary outer zone **(OS)**; inner stripe of the medullary outer zone **(IS)**; and inner zone of medulla with its papillary tip. × 30.

tufts of capillaries and their supporting cells, which have developed within a double-walled capsule formed by half of the **S**-shaped bend in one end of the developing renal tubule. A renal corpuscle therefore has some resemblance to a balloon (the capsule) with a fist (the capillaries) punched into it. The outer wall of the capsule is called the *parietal layer;* the inner wall is the *visceral (podocyte)* layer. The space between the two walls of the capsule is called *Bowman's space.* The epithelium of this visceral wall covers the tufts of capillaries much like a glove covers each finger of a hand. Between the epithelium and the capillaries is an extracellular layer, the glomerular *basement membrane (basal lamina).*

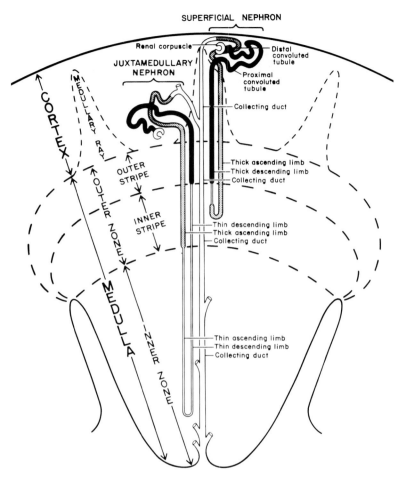

SUPERFICIAL NEPHRON

Renal corpuscle

JUXTAMEDULLARY NEPHRON

Distal convoluted tubule

Proximal convoluted tubule

Collecting duct

Thick ascending limb
Thick descending limb
Collecting duct

Thin descending limb
Thick ascending limb
Collecting duct

Thin ascending limb
Thin descending limb
Collecting duct

CORTEX
MEDULLARY RAY
OUTER STRIPE
OUTER ZONE
INNER STRIPE
MEDULLA
INNER ZONE

24–4 Schematic diagram of superficial and juxtamedullary nephrons, showing the relationship of segments of the nephron to the zones of the kidney, which can be seen grossly. ◁

24–5 Light micrograph of renal cortex showing renal corpuscles and renal tubules. Paraffin embedded. × 300. ▽

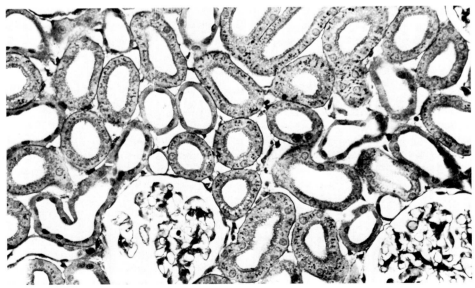

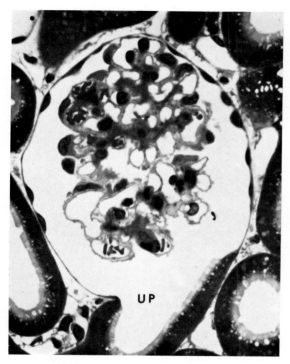

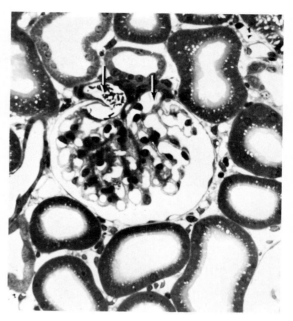

24-7 Renal corpuscle of an epoxy resin section from a rat kidney, showing the afferent and efferent vessels **(arrows)** at the vascular pole. × 320.

24-6 Renal corpuscle of an epoxy resin section from a rat kidney, showing that Bowman's space is confluent with the proximal tubule lumen at the urinary pole **(UP)**. Toluidine blue. × 520.

At one region of the renal corpuscle, called the *urinary pole*, the parietal layer of capsular epithelium is continuous with the epithelium of the neck of the tubule (Fig. 24–6). Bowman's space is therefore continuous with the lumen of the remaining nephron, so that fluid formed by filtration within the renal corpuscle enters the lumen of the proximal convoluted tubule. Another region of the renal corpuscle located roughly opposite the urinary pole is called the *vascular pole* (Fig. 24–7). It is marked by the point of entrance of the afferent arteriole and the exit of the efferent arteriole. The afferent arteriole enters the renal corpuscle and divides into four or more primary branches. Each of these branches becomes a network of anastomosing capillaries that forms a lobule. The lobule has a stalk or supporting region called the *mesangial region*. The capillaries within the lobules reunite to form the efferent arteriole, which exits from the vascular pole. Because the efferent arteriole again breaks up to form a second capillary net-

work, such an arrangement constitutes a portal system—an arterial portal system, in contrast to the venous portal system in the liver. The second capillary network surrounds the tubules and is therefore called the *peritubular capillary network*. Some authors describe a differing morphology at the vascular pole of juxtamedullary nephrons (Ljungqvist, 1964). In their descriptions, the afferent arteriole is continuous with the efferent arteriole, and the capillaries to the renal corpuscle exit from the side of this arteriolar shunt. Because of the anatomy of the arterioles in the juxtamedullary region, if the renal corpuscle dies, an aglomerular vessel can form. These vessels have been called the *vasa rectae vera*.

The renal corpuscle therefore consists of the following parts: (1) the parietal epithelium of the capsule, (2) the visceral epithelium of the capsule, (3) the glomerular basement membrane (basal lamina), (4) the endothelium of the glomerulus, and (5) the intraglomerular mesangial region (Figs. 24–6 to 24–8). These parts will be considered in order.

The Parietal Epithelium of Bowman's Capsule. The parietal epithelium consists of a layer

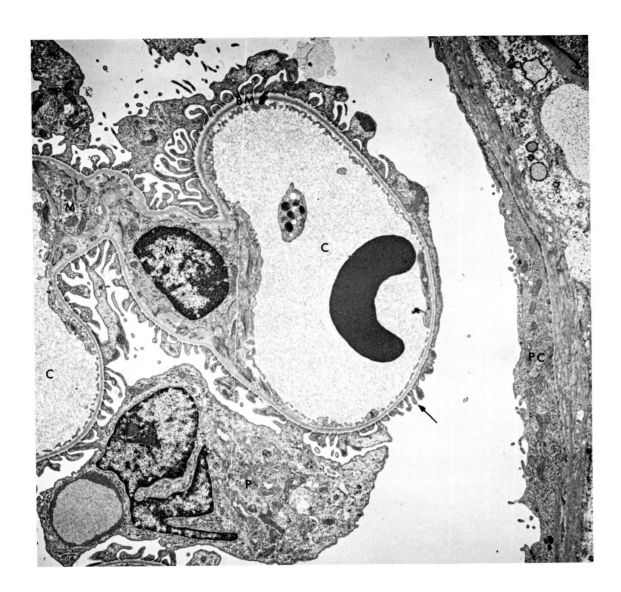

24–8 Electron micrograph from a renal corpuscle, showing capillaries **(C)**, glomerular podocytes **(P)**, with their small processes called pedicels **(arrow)**, mesangial cells **(M)**, and the glomerular basement membrane **(BM)**. A portion of a parietal cell **(PC)** can be seen at the right. × 6,100.

of simple squamous cells that bulge into Bowman's space in the region of their nuclei. They are polygonal in outline and rest on a thick basement membrane, which in some cases appears to be multilayered. At the vascular pole, the parietal epithelium is reflected to form the visceral layer.

The Visceral Epithelium of Bowman's Capsule. The visceral epithelium closely embraces the entire network of glomerular capillaries and consists of cells that have a complex shape. The cells, which are frequently called *podocytes*, do not rest on the basement membrane for long regions but tend to sit somewhat removed in Bowman's space. The cells have long primary processes called *trabeculae*. The trabeculae in turn branch to form secondary and tertiary processes. All three of these kinds of processes again branch to form thin, club-shaped terminal processes called *pedicels* (little feet), which interdigitate in a complicated manner with similar

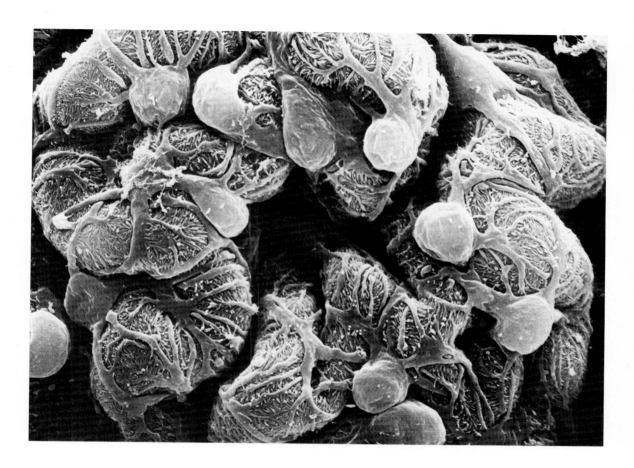

processes from adjacent cells. This is well demonstrated by scanning electron microscopy (Fig.
24–9). The pedicels form a layer along the glomerular basement membrane. This elaborate interdigitation results in an extensive pattern of
narrow slits between the pedicels. In electron
micrographs, these slits seem to be bridged by a
thin layer of material of unknown composition
called the *filtration-slit membrane,* which is
thinner than a cell membrane and appears to be
similar to the diaphragms seen across the pores
of fenestrated capillaries. The podocytes have
nuclei that are large and irregular in shape and
tend to be indented on one side in the region of
the Golgi apparatus. They contain abundant protein secretory organelles, numerous fine filaments, and microtubules (Fig. 24–8). A mucopolysaccharide containing sialic acid forms a cell
coat about 120 Å thick over the cell membrane
of the podocyte (Rambourg and Leblond, 1967).
A decrease in the amount of this cell coat has
been noted in humans with proteinuria or glo-

24–9 Scanning electron micrograph of capillary
loops from a normal kidney glomerulus,
showing the processes of podocytes interdigitating
along the surface of the capillary walls.

merulonephritis (Blau and Haas, 1973). Vascular
perfusion of polycations in rats to neutralize the
anionic charge on the sialoprotein coat causes a
loss in number of foot processes similar to that
seen in human proteinuria (Seiler et al., 1975).

*Glomerular Basement Membrane (Basal Lam-
ina).* In adult human beings, the basement membrane is thick, with a mean diameter of approximately 320 to 340 nm (Jorgensen, 1966). It is
thinner in very young children and in most experimental animals. The basement membrane
stains with periodic acid Schiff (PAS) reagent
(Fig. 24–17). It contains type IV collagen and a
glycosaminoglycan that is rich in heparin sulfate.
In addition, components that contain sialic acid

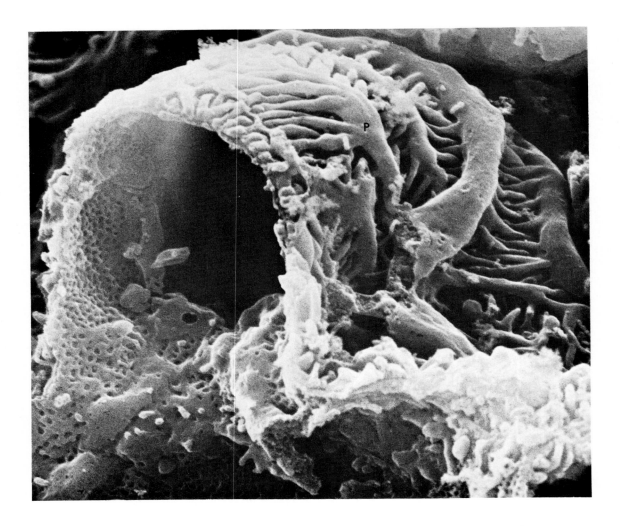

24–10 Scanning electron micrograph showing a transected capillary loop. The podocytes **(P)** interdigitate along the capillary surface. Capillary fenestra are seen on the endothelial cell surface. × 17,200.

and are sensitive to neuraminidase are involved in attachment of the epithelial and endothelial cells. These molecules seem to be related to fine filaments emanating from the glomerular basement membrane (Kanwar and Farquhar, 1980).

The basement membrane is composed of three layers: an electron-dense central layer, the lamina densa; a less dense layer on either side, the lamina rara externa (adjacent to the glomerular podocytes); and a lamina rara interna (adjacent to the capillary endothelium). In the stalk region

of each capillary loop, the basement membrane does not surround the entire endothelium but instead appears to be reflected with the glomerular epithelial cells from which it is presumably largely derived (Fig. 24–8).

Endothelium. The endothelium consists of a simple squamous layer of fenestrated cells. The cells are extremely thin, except at the stalk region of the capillary where their nuclei bulge into the lumen. In this region the cells can have complex processes extending into the capillary lumen. The fenestrae of this particular endothelium differ from those found in the more typical fenestrated endothelium of the peritubular capillaries and of other regions of the body in that the pores appear to be more irregular in shape and larger in size (approximately 50 to 100 nm

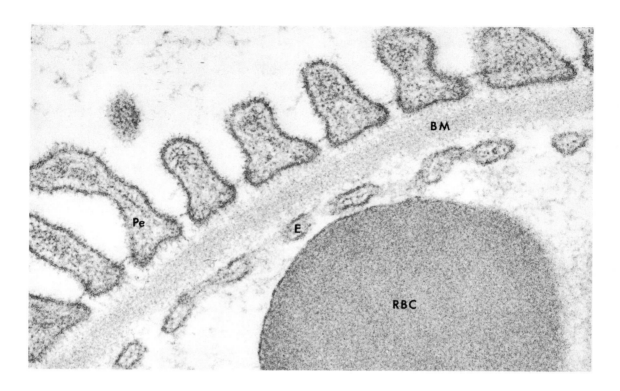

in diameter) (Figs. 24–10 and 24–11). Although pores in fenestrated endothelium are generally bridged by a thin diaphragm, only a few of the fenestrae of the glomerulus are bridged by diaphragms. Both of these modifications (large-sized pores and few diaphragms) would increase the permeability of this endothelium.

Intraglomerular Mesangial Region. The mesangial or stalk region of the capillary tuft consists of a population of cells and the matrix material in which they are embedded. The cells appear similar to pericytes seen adjacent to vessels elsewhere in the body. Each cell contains a small, densely staining nucleus, fine filaments especially abundant along the cell membranes, and dense cytoplasmic plaques located along the cell membrane. The cells have long processes, some of which can penetrate the mesangial matrix underlying the capillary endothelium to come into contact with the endothelial cell. In some cases, these processes seem to project through the endothelium into the lumen of the capillary. The function of these mesangial cell projections is unknown. Mesangial cells are of particular importance because they have a propensity to divide in certain kidney diseases. The mesangial

24–11 Electron micrograph of the filtration barrier from a rat renal corpuscle, showing a red blood cell **(RBC)** within a capillary lumen, an endothelial cell **(E)** with fenestrations, a basement membrane **(BM)**, and a layer of interdigitating pedicels **(Pe)**. × 71,700.

matrix appears to be an amorphous substance with less electron density than the lamina densa of the basement membrane. It appears to be continuous with the lamina rara interna. The mesangial cells seem to function by clearing the basement membrane of large proteins that have become lodged during filtration. It has been postulated that mesangial cells can contract when stimulated by angiotensin and thereby decrease capillary blood flow (Ausiello et al., 1979).

The intraglomerular mesangial region is continuous with the extraglomerular mesangial region (part of the juxtaglomerular apparatus) and in certain experimental circumstances can be seen to contain granulated cells like those of the extraglomerular mesangium.

Function of the Renal Corpuscle. Because of its morphology, the renal corpuscle behaves as a filtering device that allows water and ions to pass but retains large objects such as cells and even large protein molecules. Because a small amount of albumin penetrates the filter, that protein appears to be near the effective pore size of the filtration barrier. The barrier is complex and, as can be seen in Fig. 24–11, consists of three morphological structures: (1) the fenestrated endothelium, (2) the glomerular basement membrane, and (3) the slits between pedicels, which are bridged by the filtration-slit membrane.

Each of these morphological structures can provide a component of the filtration barrier depending on the particle size. The endothelial pores limit the passage of red blood cells and other formed elements of the blood, whereas the lamina densa of the basal lumina and the filtration-slit membrane provide finer filtration barriers.

Particle size is not the only factor involved in glomerular permeability. The fixed negative charges associated with the glycosaminoglycan components of the filtration surface exert profound effects on glomerular permeability (Chang et al., 1975; Rennke et al., 1975).

In addition, it has been proposed that a functional barrier exists near the endothelial fenestra and that this barrier depends on the maintenance of normal hemodynamics to maintain normal permeability (Ryan and Karnovsky, 1976).

Several morphological features favor the production of a large volume of glomerular filtrate. The kidney has a large renal blood flow (approximately 20–25% of the cardiac output), and because of the vascular arrangement of the kidney, almost all the blood must pass through a renal corpuscle. In addition, a contractile efferent arteriole helps to maintain a high filtration pressure along the glomerular capillary bed. Also, as has been mentioned earlier, the endothelial pores are larger and most seem to lack a diaphragm. The complex shape of the podocytes increases the area of the intercellular channels through which the filtrate can pass to gain access to Bowman's space, and these channels are limited only by a thin diaphragm.

The pressure relationships of the renal corpuscle also favor filtration. Indirect techniques indicate that the hydrostatic pressure in the glomerular capillaries is nearly 90 mm Hg, whereas the opposing hydrostatic pressure of Bowman's space is only 15 mm Hg. The oncotic pressure within the capillaries is approximately 30 mm Hg, but almost no oncotic pressure is present within Bowman's space. The resulting glomerular filtration pressure is therefore equal to (90 − 15) − (30 − 0), or 45 mm Hg.

Direct measurements of pressures can be taken using a mutant Wistar rat that has renal corpuscles visible on the surface. These measurements indicate that the glomerular pressures are lower than previously believed (Brenner et al., 1971); however, no evidence exists to show that the mutant glomeruli have normal pressures. In either case, the pressure results in an average of 180 liters of glomerular filtrate being formed each 24 h in a normal human adult.

NECK SEGMENT. The transition region connecting the renal corpuscle with the proximal tubule is called the *neck segment*. It is not well developed in mammalian kidneys. The neck shows variation in structure and even in its presence in different species. In rat kidneys, no neck segments are seen (Fig. 24–6), whereas in mouse kidneys, cells like those lining the proximal convoluted tubule have been observed to line the wall of Bowman's capsule. In human beings, however, certain nephrons have a short neck segment lined with simple squamous epithelium like the lining of the parietal wall of Bowman's capsule (Fig. 24–41). In cystinosis (a relatively rare inherited metabolic disease), these flattened epithelial cells extend for a greater length and constitute the Swan neck deformity (Darmady and Stranack, 1957).

PROXIMAL TUBULE. The proximal tubule is composed of segments differing somewhat in their morphology, histochemical reactions, and vulnerability to various toxins. Two of these segments are most frequently distinguished: a *proximal convoluted portion*, which constitutes the longest tubule in the cortex and hence the one most frequently seen in a random section; and a *straight portion (pars recta)* of the proximal tubule, which enters an adjacent medullary ray and turns toward the renal sinus to form the first part of the loop of Henle that penetrates into the medulla.

The lumen of the functioning proximal tubule is wide open in life because of the blood pressure. Anything that interrupts the blood supply to the organ will allow the proximal tubular lumens to collapse. To preserve the morphology of the living animal, an adequate filtration pressure must be maintained during fixation. This can be done by dripping the fixative on the kidney surface, by rapid freezing procedures, by microperfusion of single tubules, or by intravascular perfusion of fixative solutions.

Proximal Convoluted Tubule. The proximal convoluted tubule is the longest and largest segment of the mammalian nephron, averaging approximately 14 mm in length and 30 to 60 μm in diameter. It is lined by a single layer of cells that have an elaborate shape, a well-developed microvillus (or brush) border along the lumen, an active endocytotic apparatus, and an abundant acidophilic cytoplasm containing numerous mitochondria (Figs. 24–12 to 24–21).

The cells exhibit an extensive system of lateral extensions that interdigitate with corresponding lateral processes from adjacent cells. Large ridges extend the full height of the cell. More extensive but smaller interdigitating processes are also present in the apical region, and an especially prominent and elaborate system of primary and secondary interdigitations exists in the basal half of the cell (Fig. 24–16). These lateral interdigitating processes greatly increase the area of lateral cell membrane and form an extensive labyrinth of lateral intercellular spaces. The lateral processes are generally wide enough to contain one layer of large mitochondria, which are oriented with their long axes from cell apex to cell base; this orientation causes the pattern of basal striations seen in the basal cytoplasm of well-fixed kidneys.

One of the major functions of the proximal tubule is to reduce the volume of glomerular filtrate by approximately 80% of its original volume, accomplished partly by active transport of sodium ions out of the proximal convoluted tubular cells into the lateral intercellular spaces by a Mg^+-dependent Na^+-K^+ activated ATPase pump presumably located within the lateral cell membrane. The abundant mitochondria located next to the lateral cell membranes provide the ATP for this transport. Because of the electric charge of the sodium ions pumped into the lateral space, chloride ions follow passively, and this accumulation of ions causes an osmotic movement of water into this labyrinthine system. The increased hydrostatic pressure thus created in the lateral spaces in turn forces fluid out through the porous basement membrane into the renal interstitium.

The brush border lining the luminal surface of the cells consists of long, closely packed microvilli, which are covered by the apical cell membrane. An extracellular mucopolysaccharide

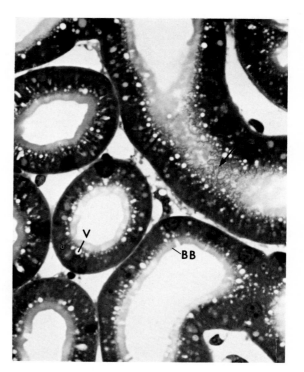

24–12 Profiles of proximal convoluted tubules in the cortex of a rat kidney embedded in epoxy resin. Note the brush border **(BB)** lining the lumen and the vacuoles **(V)** of the apical endocytotic apparatus. In the upper right-hand corner of the picture, the section cuts parallel to the surface of the cell in such a way that one can see the elaborate apical interdigitations of these cells **(arrow)**. × 570.

coats these microvilli (Fig. 24–17). The microvilli of the proximal tubule appear to reabsorb amino acids and D-glucose across the cell membrane together with sodium ions in a positively charged carrier complex. Isolated segments from rabbit renal cortex that are rich in brush border membrane contain a high concentration of two disaccharides and several ATPases (Berger and Sacktor, 1970).

Although the glomerular filtrate contains only a low concentration of protein, the volume of filtrate is so large that several grams of protein are filtered each day (Fig. 24–18). The proximal tubule reabsorbs this filtered protein. The cell therefore contains a prominent endocytotic apparatus that includes the following components. (1) Tubular invaginations of the apical cell membrane are located between the bases of the microvilli and extend down into the apical cytoplasm.

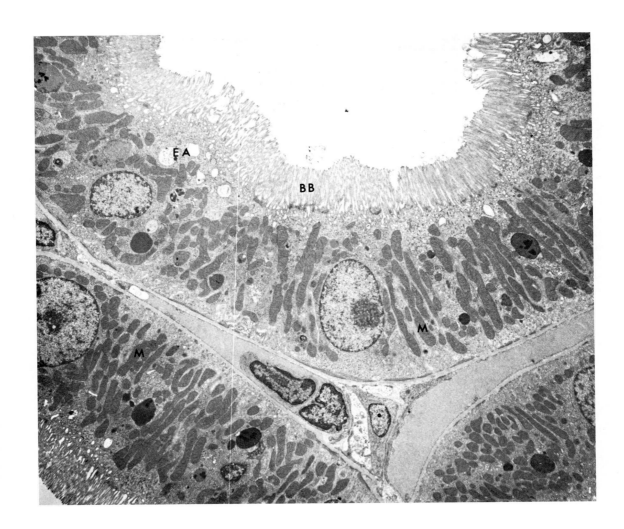

24–13 Electron micrograph of portions of three proximal convoluted tubules, showing the microvillous brush border (BB), the adundant endocytotic apparatus **(EA)**, and the numerous elongated mitochondria **(M)** oriented perpendicular to the tubular basement membrane. × 3,100.

The protein appears to be bound to the layer of fuzz (glycocalyx) radiating from the cell membrane (Fig. 24–19). (2) A series of small vesicles are thought to bud from the bases of the tubular invaginations and presumably to ferry the trapped protein molecules to the next component of the endocytotic apparatus. (3) Large apical vacuoles form by the fusion of the small vesicles (Fig. 24–20). (4) Condensing vacuoles condense the proteins. When tracer proteins such as horseradish peroxidase are injected into the vessels of a mammal, they are seen first within the lumen of the tubular invagination, second in the vesicles, third in the apical vacuoles, fourth within the condensing vacuoles, and finally within lysosomes. Studies simultaneously using horseradish peroxidase as a molecular tracer and the histochemical reaction for acid phosphatase as a lysosomal tracer (Straus, 1964) have shown that within 60 min both the acid hydrolases and the absorbed protein can be seen within the same bodies. This presumably occurs by means of the fusion of primary or secondary lysosomes with elements of the endocytotic apparatus (Fig 24–21). In general, proteins sequestered within lysosomes appear to be destined for breakdown into amino acids. In the kidney, undigested residues in lysosomes can be released from the cell by fusion of the lysosomal membrane with the cell membrane at the luminal surface.

The proximal tubular cells contain a large, round, centrally located nucleus with a prominent nucleolus. The Golgi apparatus lies in a supranuclear position and appears to consist of a large number of vesicles and membrane cisterns. Proximal tubular cells also contain microbodies (peroxisomes) that have a dense matrix substance, often a corelike nucleoid, and in some species including humans platelike structures (marginal plates) along the surface (Fig. 24–22). The bodies are frequently surrounded by smooth endoplasmic reticulum (ER). Microbodies have been called peroxisomes (De Duve and Baudhuin, 1966) because they contain enzymes concerned with cellular metabolism of hydrogen peroxide. In addition, they may function in gluconeogenesis since it is well known that proxi-

mal tubular cells utilize fatty acids as an energy source.

The proximal tubular cells are bound together by shallow, beltlike tight junctions adjacent to the lumen and deeper beltlike intermediate junctions. Desmosomes are seen only infrequently. Because of the shallow tight junction in this region, only a low transepithelial resistance can be maintained across the proximal tubule.

In addition to the functions discussed above, the proximal tubule reabsorbs bicarbonate. A number of exogenous organic acids (such as pen-

24–14 Electon micrograph of a proximal convoluted tubule, showing details of the microvillous brush border **(BB)**, the endocytotic apparatus **(EA)**, the numerous mitochondria **(M)** seen in the basal part of the cell, and the compartments formed by the lateral interdigitating processes from adjacent cells. × 9,600.

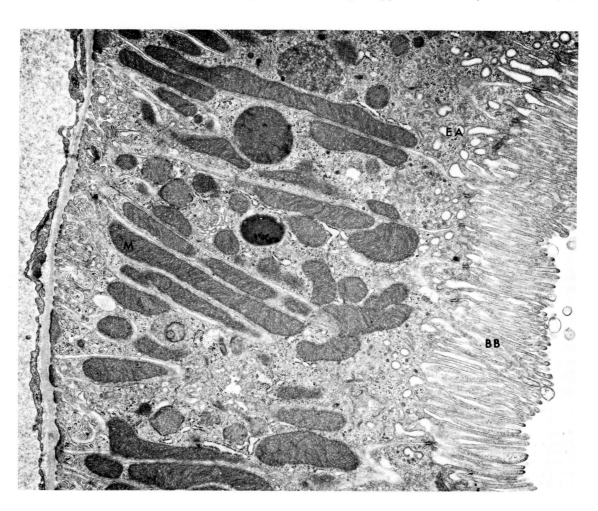

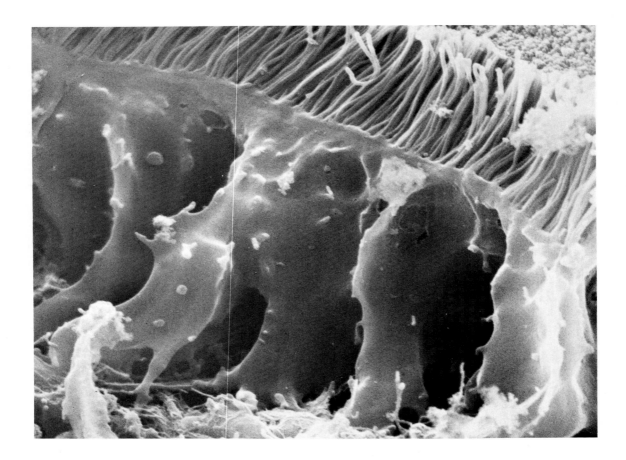

24–15 Scanning electron micrograph of a proximal convoluted tubule. Note the apical brush border of microvilli and the elaborate lateral projections of cytoplasm. × 14,900.

icillin) and organic bases are actively secreted into the tubular fluid by the proximal tubule.

Straight Part of the Proximal Tubule. The straight part of the proximal tubule begins in the medullary ray and penetrates into the medulla for varying lengths, depending on whether the nephron is of the superficial, midcortical, or juxtamedullary type. The straight part ends near the lower border of the outer stripe of the outer zone of the medulla where it abruptly changes into the cells of the thin limb of Henle's loop (Fig. 24–4).

The cells in the straight part of the proximal tubule are similar to those of the convoluted segment, but they appear to be lower in height and have a less elaborate shape (Fig. 24–23). The mi-

tochondria, although still abundant, are smaller and more randomly distributed throughout the cell. The brush border is frequently well developed and stains with the PAS procedure. The cells contain fewer lysosomes and a less well-developed endocytotic apparatus. However, microbodies are more prominent in this region of the tubule.

THIN LIMB OF THE LOOP OF HENLE. The thin limb segment can be short or absent in short-looped nephrons and occurs largely on the descending limb, or it can be long, reaching far into the inner medulla in long-looped nephrons, with both descending and ascending thin limb segments. In humans, approximately 14% of the nephrons have long loops of Henle. The tubule is approximately 20 to 40 μ in diameter. The thin limb segment is lined by a thin squamous epithelium whose wall is approximately 1 to 2 μm in height (Fig. 24–24). Although the epithelium is therefore thicker than the endothelium, it is some-

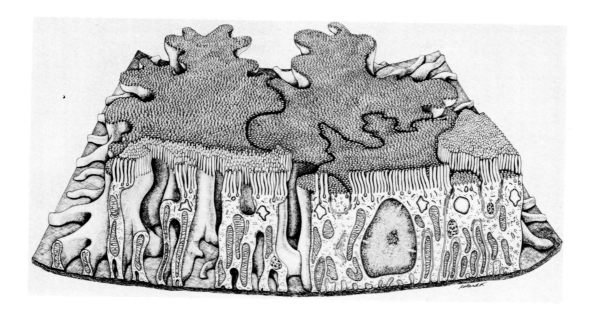

24–16 Diagram of a proximal convoluted tubular
△   cell to show the elaborate interdigitations that
occur between adjacent cells. Some interdigitating
processes extend the full height of the cells, whereas
smaller elaborate interdigitations occur in the basal
and apical regions.   (From Bulger, R. 1965. Am. J.
Anat. 116:237, Fig. 5.)

24–17 PAS reaction in mouse kidney. A positive
▽   reaction is seen in the brush border of the
proximal tubules and in the basement membranes of
the tubules and of the renal corpuscle. × 300.
(Courtesy of H. W. Deane.)

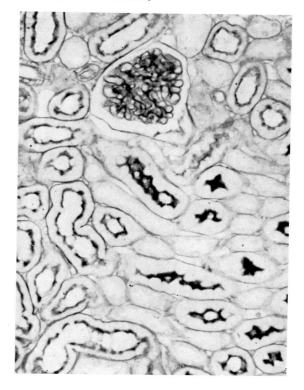

what difficult to distinguish from endothelium in
paraffin sections. In the region of the nucleus,
the cell bulges into the lumen.

The thin limb segment varies with respect to
the depth of its tight junction, the cell shape, the
species studied and the number of organelles
such as mitochondria that are contained. Four
regions with differing morphology have been
identified: the thin descending limb of short-
looped nephrons, the outer medullary descending thin limb of long-looped nephrons, the inner
medullary descending thin limb of long-looped
nephrons, and the ascending thin limb of long-
looped nephrons (Schwartz and Venkatachalam,
1974; Kaissling and Kriz, 1979).

It was noted early that birds and mammals
were the only two classes whose nephrons had
loops of Henle and that they were the only animals that could produce hypertonic urine. It was
also noted that the fluid in the cortex was isosmotic with plasma, whereas there was an increasing osmotic concentration in the medulla as

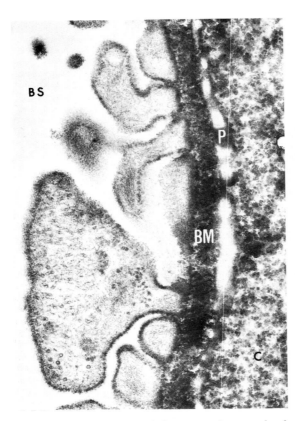

24–18 Electron micrograph from a renal corpuscle of an animal that had received horseradish peroxidase prior to fixation. The dense reaction product can be seen in the capillary lumen **(C)** within the pores **(P)** of the endothelium and within the basement membrane **(BM)**. The material is filtered into Bowman's space **(BS)**. × 30,000.

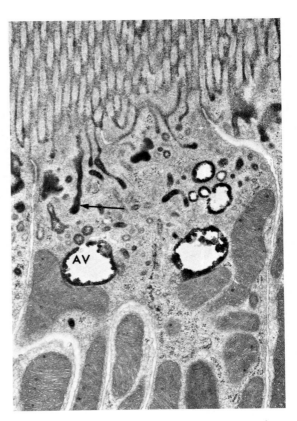

24–19 Electron micrograph of the apical region of a proximal convoluted tubular cell that was in the process of taking up horseradish peroxidase. The reaction product can be seen within the apical invaginations **(arrow)** formed by the apical plasma membrane and in apical vacuoles **(AV)**. × 17,100.

one approached the papillary tip. It was therefore postulated that the loop of Henle plays an important role in concentrating urine by serving as a countercurrent multiplier system.

The loop of Henle is believed to function in the following manner. The ascending thick limb actively pumps ions from the tubular fluid into the extracellular space. In vitro work using rabbit kidney tubules indicates that chloride is the ion moving against its electrochemical gradient. In this region the permeability to water appears to be low, so with the exit of the ions, the luminal fluid becomes hypotonic and sodium chloride is trapped in the medullary interstitium. This hypothesis will be further discussed in the section on Function of the Distal Nephron.

DISTAL TUBULE. The distal tubule is composed of three regions: a thick medullary straight part, a thinner cortical straight part including the macula densa and extending a short distance beyond it, and a distal convoluted tubule (Figs. 24–25 to 24–29) (Kaissling and Kriz, 1979).

Straight Part of the Distal Tubule. The straight part of the distal tubule begins near the border of the inner and outer medulla in a transition from the thin ascending limb. The straight part of the distal tubule forms the third component of the loop of Henle and completes the looping structure by returning through the medulla and the medullary ray to the renal corpuscle from which the tubule arose. The straight part of the distal tubule that lies in the medulla

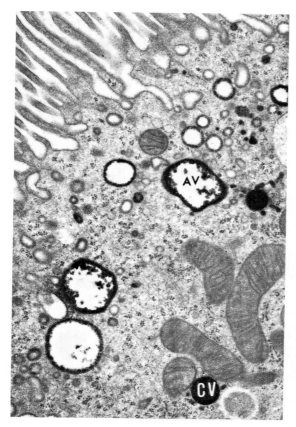

24-20 Electron micrograph of the apical region of a proximal tubular cell that was in the process of taking up horseradish peroxidase. The reaction product can be seen in apical vacuoles **(AV)** and in condensing vacuoles **(CV)** within the apical cytoplasm. × 13,700.

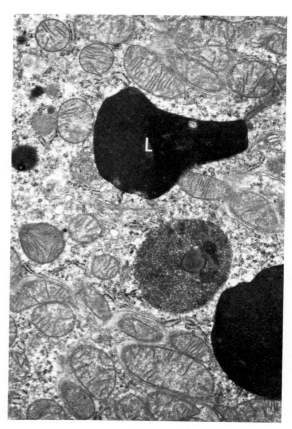

24-21 Electron micrograph of the basal region of a proximal convoluted tubular cell that had taken up horseradish peroxidase 3 days prior to fixation. The reaction product can be seen within lysosomes **(L)** in the basal cytoplasm. × 11,500.

is lined by a thicker cell layer than the straight part located within the cortex. The cells of the ascending thick limb are extremely irregular in shape, with many of their interdigitations extending from the lumen to the basal region of the cell (Fig. 24–25). Although this straight part resembles the convoluted part of the distal tubule, the cells of the cortical straight part are shorter and therefore their nuclei bulge into the lumen. A few microvilli are seen along the cell surface. The lateral interdigitating processes contain numerous mitochondria, which appear to be involved with the lateral cell membrane in the active transport of ions from the tubular luminal fluid that is present in this region. The permeability of the tubule to water is low in this region

and therefore water does not become osmotically equilibrated and the luminal contents remain hypotonic to blood.

Macula Densa. As the distal tubule returns to the renal corpuscle of its origin, it runs adjacent to the efferent arteriole, the extraglomerular mesangium, and the afferent arteriole. In this region, the cells in the wall of the distal tubule are narrow and their nuclei are close together. In stained sections the nuclear accumulation causes a dense region; hence the name *macula densa* (Fig. 24–42). This association of the distal tubule with the two arterioles and the extraglomerular mesangium is called the *juxtaglomerular apparatus*, which will be discussed under that heading later in the chapter. A short segment of the

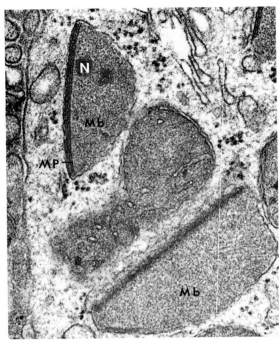

24–22 Electron micrograph showing microbodies **(Mb)** from a proximal convoluted tubular cell of a primate (Galago). The microbody is characterized by a single membrane surrounding it, a dense homogeneous matrix, dense bodies within the matrix, called nucleoids **(N),** and, in certain species, platelike structures along the edge of the body, called marginal plates **(MP).** × 50,400. ◁

24–23 Electron micrograph of the straight part of the proximal tubule from a normal human kidney. The cells are of less elaborate shape, and the mitochondria are more circular in profile than in the convoluted portion. The brush border **(BB)** and lysomes **(L)** can be seen. × 16,000. ▽

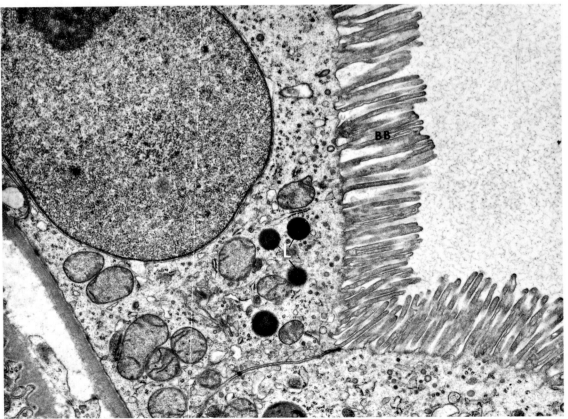

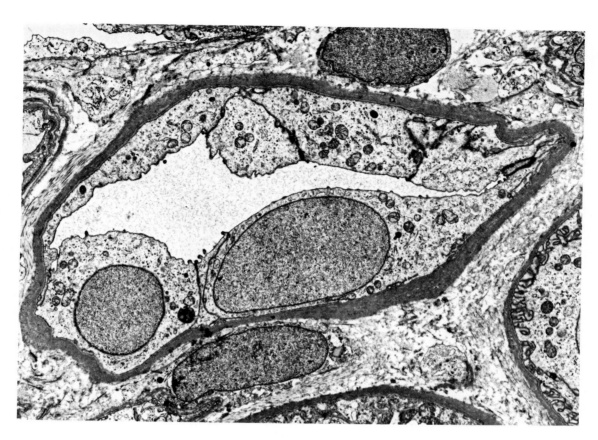

straight part of the distal tubule extends beyond the macula densa.

Distal Convoluted Tubule. The distal convoluted tubule is shorter (approximately 5 mm) than the proximal tubule and hence fewer profiles are seen in a random section of the cortex. The diameter of this tubule is somewhat variable, being approximately 20 to 50 μm. The cells appear to be lower, and more nuclei are seen in a cross-sectional profile than in the proximal tubule (Figs. 24–26 and 24–27), because, in part anyway, many cells are binucleate. Because the cells are short, distal tubules frequently have a larger luminal diameter than proximal tubules. The cells do not have a brush border, but a few luminal microvilli are seen. The endocytotic apparatus is not well developed; however, a few vacuoles and lysosomes can be seen within the cells. The cytoplasm appears somewhat less acidophilic than in the proximal tubule. In the basal region of the cytoplasm, lateral processes interdigitate with those from adjacent cells, forming an extensive lateral intercellular labyrinthine

24–24 Electron micrograph of the thin limb segment from a normal human kidney. The number of processes seen indicates that the cells are elaborate in shape; however, human beings have a much simpler cell shape in this region than most experimental animals. ×9,600.

space like that seen in the proximal tubule (Fig. 24–28). The processes contain large mitochondria and form a pattern of basal striations similar to that seen in the proximal tubule. The active transport of sodium ions from the tubular filtrate can continue in this segment of the nephron. The nuclei appear to lie in the apical cytoplasm near the lumen. A continuous basement membrane surrounds the tubule.

Intrarenal Collecting Ducts. CONNECTING TUBULE. In superficial nephrons, the connecting tubule empties directly into a cortical collecting duct. In midcortical and juxtamedullary nephrons, the connecting tubules join together to constitute the arcades and then empty into the cor-

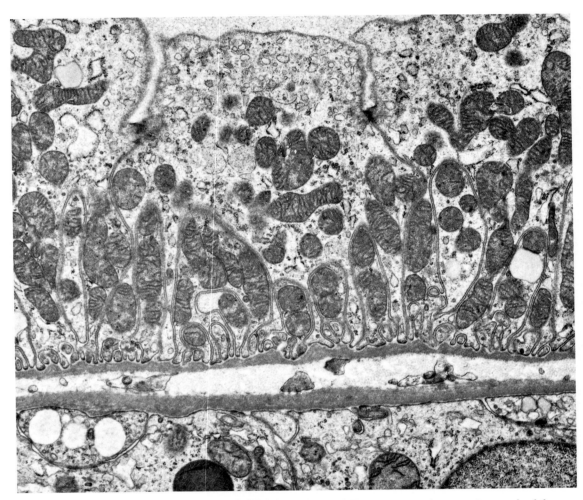

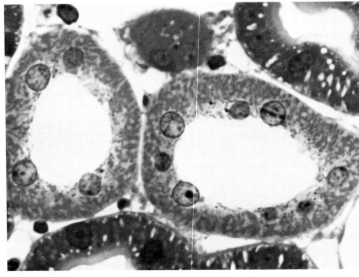

24–25 Electron micrograph of the △ ascending thick part of the distal tubule from a normal human kidney. The cells are highly interdigitated, and the lateral processes contain large mitochondria. × 12,800.

◁

24–26 Light micrograph of two distal convoluted tubules from a rat kidney embedded in epoxy resin. The cells contain large mitochondria but lack a brush border. × 1,000.

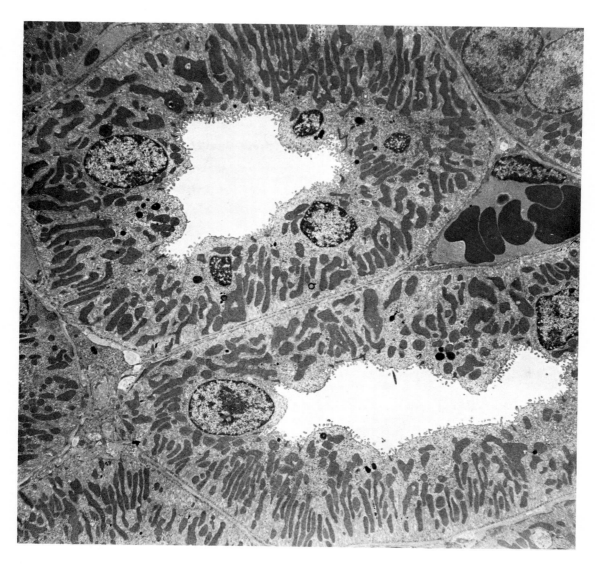

tical collecting ducts. The arcades begin deep in the cortex, ascend, and then turn to descend within a medullary ray. The number of nephrons that empty into arched collecting ducts before entering a terminal collecting duct versus those entering singly varies with the species. In humans both types occur. The connecting tubule is lined by two epithelial cell types (Figs. 24–30 to 24–35). The connecting tubule cell is characterized by true basal cell membrane infoldings (not interdigitations) that penetrate throughout the cell, including into the apical cytoplasm. The mitochondria are found between the infoldings and are not mainly apical to the infoldings as in true collecting duct light cells. The second cell is

24–27 Electron micrograph of two distal convoluted tubular profiles, showing the large number of mitochondria contained in these cells and the few small microvilli that line the lumen but do not form a brush border. The nuclei lie in an apical position. × 2,800.

a typical *intercalated (dark) cell* as seen in the collecting duct proper.

CORTICAL COLLECTING DUCTS. The cortical collecting tubule is found primarily within the medullary ray. The principal (light) cells are low cuboidal cells with well-defined cell margins; round, centrally placed nuclei; a fairly pale-

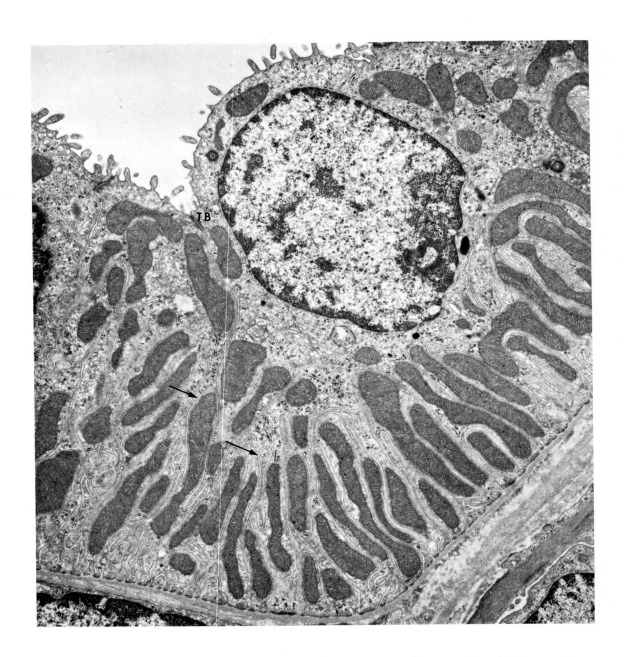

24–28 Electron micrograph of a distal convoluted tubule, showing the lateral intercellular labyrinth **(arrows)** formed by the interdigitation of lateral processes in the basal region of the distal tubular cells. The large elongate mitochondria occupy these processes. The cell nucleus occupies an apical position. The cell surfaces are joined apical-laterally by prominent terminal bars **(TB),** and the apical cell membrane has only small microvilli. × 10,300.

staining cytoplasm; and multiple, small, randomly oriented mitochondria. In electron micrographs, these cells are seen to have a few small microvilli and a basal cell region that contains some small, short, interdigitating processes as well as some tortuous infoldings of the basal cell membrane.

Interspersed between the principal cells are intercalated (dark) cells, which have a more intensely staining cytoplasm and contain more mi-

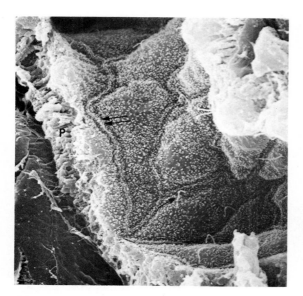

24–29 Scanning electron micrograph of a distal tubule. This tubule is characterized by position in the kidney, lateral projections **(P)** which interdigitate with those from adjacent cells, and luminal microvilli and cilia **(arrow)**. The microvilli appear to be most numerous along the cell borders **(double arrow)**. × 2,100.

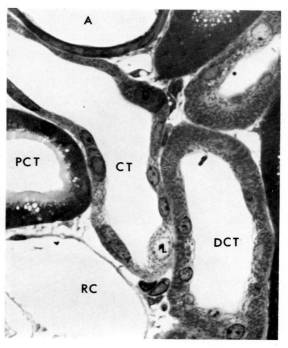

24–30 Light micrograph of a cortical collecting tubule **(CT)** from a rat kidney embedded in epoxy resin. Light **(L)** and dark **(D)** cells lining this tubule can be identified. Profiles of proximal **(PCT)** and distal **(DCT)** convoluted tubules, an arteriole **(A)**, and a renal corpuscle **(RC)** can be seen. × 670.

tochondria located all around the nucleus. The cell surface of intercalated cells is frequently covered by folds called microplicae (Fig. 24–34). The number of folds can vary. Their apical cytoplasm contains a large number of vesicles. Dark cells are seen throughout the cortex and in some of the medulla but not in the papillary region.

MEDULLARY COLLECTING DUCTS. The medullary collecting ducts are similar in structure to the cortical ones, although the cells gradually increase in height (Fig. 24–36). They do not branch as they traverse the outer medulla.

PAPILLARY DUCTS. The convergence of the collecting tubules within the kidney leads to the formation of several large straight collecting ducts called *papillary ducts (or ducts of Bellini)* (Fig. 24–36). These large collecting ducts have a diameter of 200 to 300 μm. They empty their contents into the minor calyxes through small holes on the surface of the papillary apex. This surface is called the *area cribrosa* (Figs. 24–37 and 24–38). Figure 24–39 summarizes the morphology of the various nephron segments.

FUNCTION OF THE DISTAL NEPHRON. Because it is difficult to separate the functions of the distal tubule and collecting duct, the two regions are often referred to as the distal nephron and are discussed together.

Concentration and Dilution of Urine. The mammalian kidney can rid the body of water by producing a copious volume of dilute urine or conserve water by producing a small amount of concentrated urine (Fig. 24–40). It manages this because it contains a countercurrent multiplier (the loop of Henle) and two countercurrent exchangers: the first, the descending and ascending limbs of the looping medullary vessels and the second, the large collecting ducts passing through the medullary interstitium.

The ultrafiltrate formed in the renal corpuscle is isosmotic with the blood. While the filtrate traverses the proximal tubule, sodium ions are actively reabsorbed across the proximal tubular cells. In order to maintain electrical equilibrium,

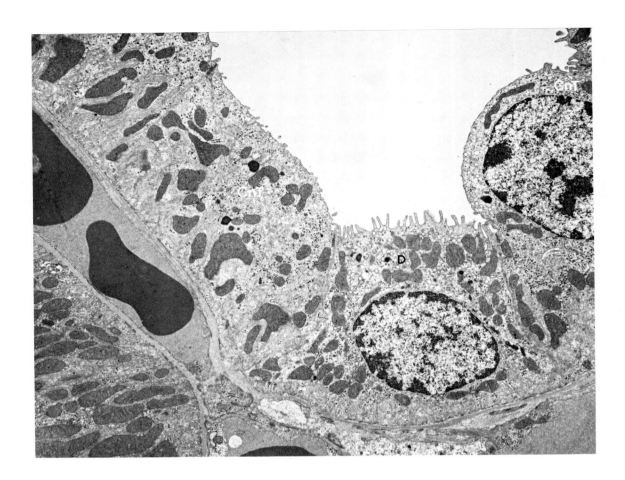

24–31 Electron micrograph of a cortical connecting tubule from a rat kidney, showing connecting tubule cells **(CnT)** and a dark cell **(D).** The dark cell is characterized by numerous mitochondria and an elaborate pattern of the apical cell membrane forming folds and microvilli. Abundant apical vesicles are also seen in the dark cell. × 5,600.

chloride ions follow passively. This movement of ions disrupts the osmotic equilibrium allowing water to follow passively. Therefore, although 70 to 80% of the filtered sodium chloride is reabsorbed by the cortical proximal tubule, the remaining filtrate is still isosmotic with the blood.

The ascending limb of the loop of Henle lying in the medulla actively moves chloride ions into the medullary interstitium from the tubular lumen. This active transport occurs largely if not entirely within the ascending thick region in most species. In this case, sodium follows to re-

establish electrical equilibrium. The water permeability of this epithelium is low, and therefore water does not equilibrate. Because of the looping shape of the nephrons and because the medullary vessels also form a looping countercurrent exchanger, many of these ions are trapped within the medullary interstitium, forming a hypertonic environment. Since sodium chloride has been removed from the filtrate in the ascending thick limb of Henle's loop and water permeability of this segment is low, the filtrate entering the distal tubule within the cortex will be hypotonic to the blood. Continued active reabsorption of sodium ions can occur in the distal tubule (with passive reabsorption of chloride ions). If the tubular cells of the remaining regions of the nephron still retain a relative impermeability to water, an extremely dilute filtrate will be formed that can be excreted as a copious volume of dilute urine.

When water is being conserved, a smaller vol-

24–32 Electron micrograph of a cortical collecting duct with dark cells **(D)** and light cells **(L)**. × 2,300. ▷

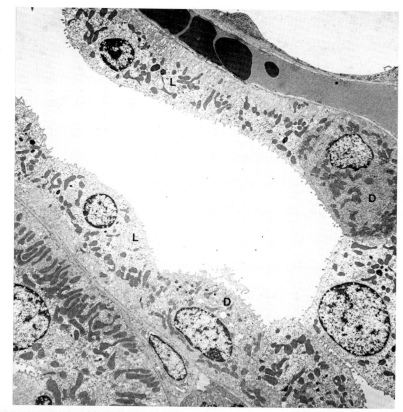

24–33 Scanning electron micrograph of two collecting ducts. The light cells **(LC)** have apical microvilli and a single cilium. The dark cells **(DC)** are characterized by branching irregular apical flaps and no cilia. × 1,420. ▽

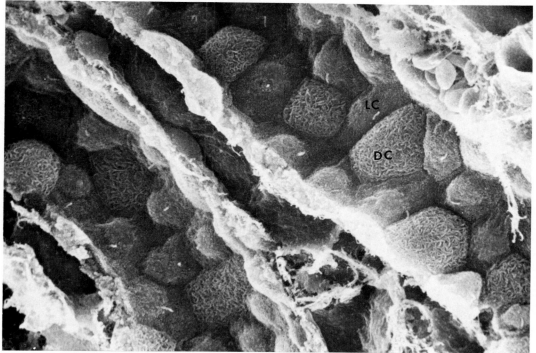

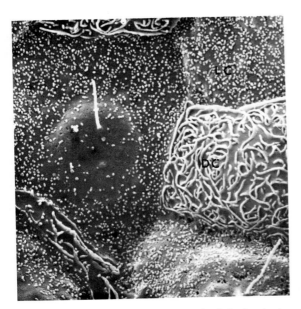

ume of concentrated urine is formed. In this case, the ultrafiltrate produced by the renal corpuscle is still isosmotic with blood. This isosmoticity is retained throughout the cortical proximal tubule, while 70 to 80% of the filtrate is reabsorbed. The cells of the ascending thick limb of Henle's loop function similarly when producing a concentrated urine as when producing a dilute urine, trapping sodium chloride in the medullary interstitium while forming a hypotonic filtrate. In human beings, the osmolality of the interstitium may be 1,200 mOsm/liter at the papillary tip. When a concentrated urine is being produced, a hormone called antidiuretic hormone (ADH) is released from the posterior lobe of the pituitary gland. When blood levels of this hormone are high, the permeability of the collecting duct to water is increased. The filtrate within cortical collecting ducts equilibrates with

24–34 Scanning electron micrograph of the luminal △ surface of a cortical collecting duct. The dark cells (**DC**) and light cells (**LC**) can be identified by the type of surface specializations present. × 5,000.

24–35 Electron micrograph of light cells from a ▽ human collecting tubule. These cells have a somewhat less elaborate contour to their cell membranes than do those of the rat. × 7,700.

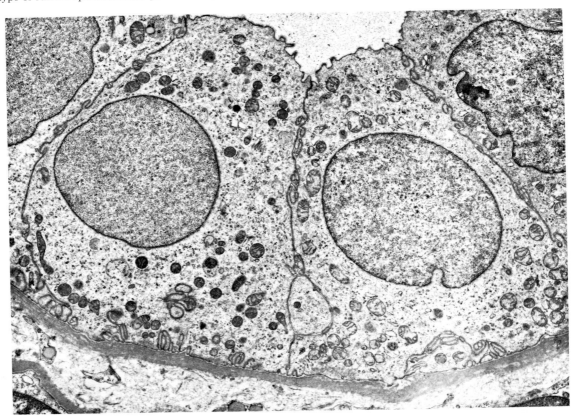

the blood, again becoming isosmotic. Finally, the medullary collecting ducts course through the hypertonic medullary interstitium to empty at the apex of the papilla. When ADH is present, these ducts are also permeable to water. Therefore, the hypertonic environment of the renal medulla becomes a driving force to remove water from the tubular lumens by osmosis, producing a highly concentrated urine.

Kokko and Rector (1972) have suggested a model for the production of concentrated urine in which the papilla plays only a passive role. In this model, the concentrating process in the inner medulla is driven by gradients created by the presence of high urea concentrations within the medullary interstitium as well as the high solute levels. Urea osmotically extracts water from the descending limb of Henle's loop, thereby concentrating sodium chloride in the descending limb fluid. When the fluid rich in sodium chloride enters the thin ascending limb, which is permeable to sodium chloride but impermeable to water, sodium chloride moves passively out of the ascending thin limb.

FUNCTION OF THE MEDULLARY VESSELS. The blood vessels that serve the renal medulla have a looping form (Fig. 24–48). The vessels enter the medulla from the cortex, they run toward the papilla and form a loop within the medulla, then finally exit back into the cortex. The two limbs of the vessel loop (descending and ascending) function as a countercurrent exchanger preventing excessive loss of osmotically active solute from the medullary interstitium. Both limbs of

24–36 Electron micrograph of a medullary collecting tubule from a normal human kidney.
Medullary collecting cells are taller than cortical ones but still contain some basal membranous infoldings and oval mitochondrial profiles. × 30,700.

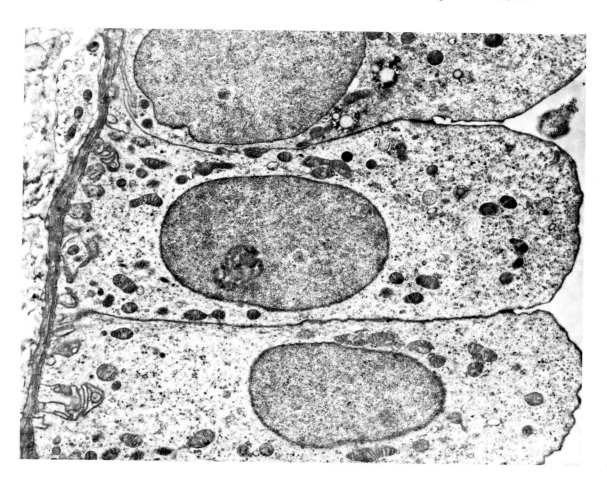

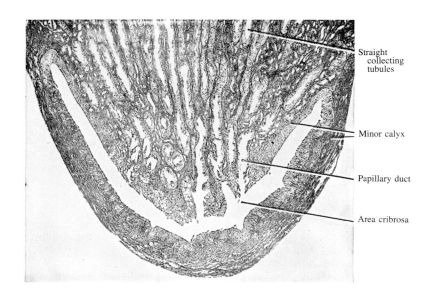

Straight
collecting
tubules

Minor calyx

Papillary duct

Area cribrosa

24–37 Longitudinal section of the kidney papilla of a rhesus monkey, showing the area cribrosa and the wall of the minor calyx. × 40.

the vessel loop are permeable to solute and water. Blood entering the loop becomes increasingly hyperosmotic as the vessels descend into the medulla, but as the looping vessels return to the cortex the process is reversed. This unique

24–38 Scanning electron micrograph of the papillary tip of a rat kidney. The large collecting ducts open onto this surface. × 300.

looping form allows the blood to provide oxygen to the tissue and to remove absorbed water and solutes while preserving the hypertonic environment of the medulla.

Acidification of Urine. Although about half the bicarbonate ion is reabsorbed in the proximal tubule, the distal nephron still plays an important role in acid-base balance. It is the site of

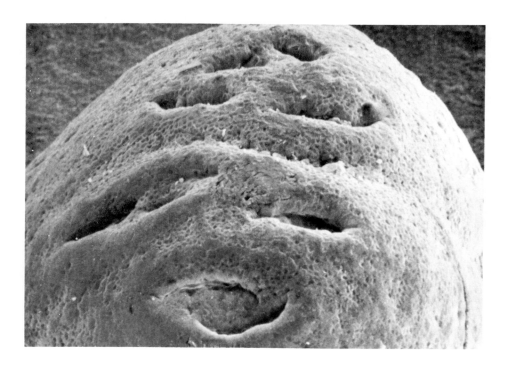

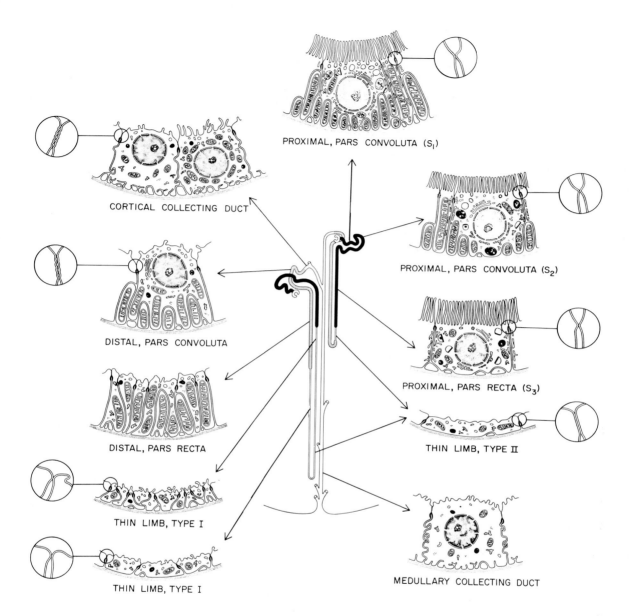

PROXIMAL, PARS CONVOLUTA (S₁)

CORTICAL COLLECTING DUCT

PROXIMAL, PARS CONVOLUTA (S₂)

DISTAL, PARS CONVOLUTA

PROXIMAL, PARS RECTA (S₃)

DISTAL, PARS RECTA

THIN LIMB, TYPE II

THIN LIMB, TYPE I

THIN LIMB, TYPE I

MEDULLARY COLLECTING DUCT

continued reabsorption of bicarbonate with resulting secretion of hydrogen ions, it is the site of secretion of hydrogen ion into the tubular lumen for buffering with anions of weak acids and of the acidification of the urine, and it is the site of conversion of ammonia to ammonium ions (although the ammonia might be produced elsewhere in the kidney).

Sodium Ion–Potassium Ion Exchange. The distal nephron is also the site at which the hormone aldosterone stimulates sodium ion reabsorption and potassium ion secretion.

24–39 Diagram showing ultrastructural characteristics of the nephron segments from the rat nephron. (From Kidney Disease—Present Status, IAP Monograph #20. 1979. Baltimore: Williams and Wilkins Co.)

The Juxtaglomerular Apparatus

At the vascular pole of the renal corpuscle, a specialized portion of the distal tubule, the macula densa, comes into an intimate relationship with the afferent and efferent arterioles of a glomerulus as well as with a pad of cells called

DIURESIS   ANTIDIURESIS

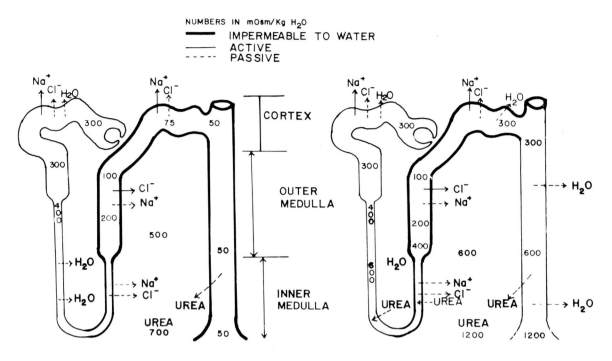

24–40 Summary of water and ion exchanges in the nephron during diuresis and antidiuresis.

the *extraglomerular mesangium* (Barajas, 1970; Barajas and Latta, 1967). Unmyelinated nerve endings are associated with these structures. These four entities (the afferent arteriole, the efferent arteriole, the macula densa of the distal tubule, and the extraglomerular mesangium) constitute the juxtaglomerular apparatus (Figs. 24–41 and 24–42).

Modified smooth muscle cells in the wall of the afferent (and sometimes the efferent) arteriole in this region produce granules that can be identified by their staining properties and have been shown to contain the hormone renin (pronounced as in renal). These modified smooth muscle cells are called *juxtaglomerular cells*. Although the modified cells still contain intracellular filaments and dense bodies like other smooth muscle cells, they have more rough ER, a large Golgi apparatus, and a number of membrane-bounded secretory granules in various states of production, condensation, and storage (Fig. 24–43).

The *macula densa* comprises the cells lining the wall of the distal tubule where the ascending straight portion returns to the glomerulus of its nephron. The macula densa appears as a dense spot because the cells of this region are narrower than in adjacent portions of the tubule, and so the nuclei are closer together, hence staining more densely. In addition, the interdigitations generally seen in the basal cytoplasm of distal tubular cells are oriented parallel to the basement membrane instead of perpendicular to it. Some basal processes extend close to the juxtaglomerular cells and to the cells of the extraglomerular mesangium. The macula densa cells have mitochondria that appear shorter and more randomly oriented. The cells appear to be polarized toward the basal surface, and the Golgi apparatus is found lateral or basal to the nucleus. Because of its unique location, this region could be a sensing device of some parameter in the distal tubular fluid content and could affect the granulated cells in the arteriolar wall. The cells of *extraglomerular mesangium* (sometimes called *Polkissen, Lacis cells,* or *polar cushion*) form a cushion of cells between the walls of the afferent and efferent arterioles. These cells re-

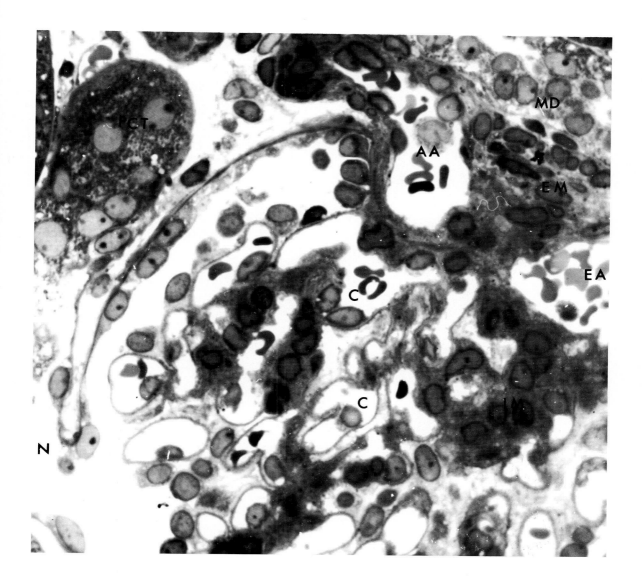

semble the intraglomerular mesangial cells with which they are contiguous. Although some of the cells contain granules, most are filled with fine intracytoplasmic filaments, dense attachment bodies at the cell membrane, and the usual organelles.

In response to a decrease in the extracellular fluid volume in an animal, the juxtaglomerular apparatus releases the enzyme renin, which acts on a plasma α_2-globulin, called *angiotensinogen*, and releases an inactive decapeptide known as *angiotensin I*. A converting enzyme, presumably located in the lung, converts angiotensin I to the octapeptide angiotensin II, which

24–41 Light micrograph of a juxtaglomerular apparatus from a human renal corpuscle showing the macula densa **(MD)**, the afferent arteriole **(AA)**, the efferent arteriole **(EA)**, the extraglomerular mesangium **(EM)**, the intraglomerular mesangium **(IM)**, the capillaray loops **(C)**, a neck region **(N)**, and a proximal convoluted tubule **(PCT)**. × 760.

is the trophic hormone for the zona glomerulosa of the adrenal cortex and causes the release of aldosterone. Aldosterone then stimulates the distal nephron to reabsorb sodium ions in exchange for hydrogen or potassium ions. Since sodium is

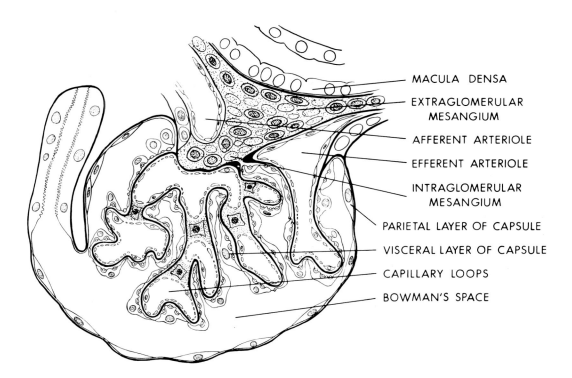

MACULA DENSA

EXTRAGLOMERULAR MESANGIUM

AFFERENT ARTERIOLE

EFFERENT ARTERIOLE

INTRAGLOMERULAR MESANGIUM

PARIETAL LAYER OF CAPSULE

VISCERAL LAYER OF CAPSULE

CAPILLARY LOOPS

BOWMAN'S SPACE

24–42 Diagram of the juxtaglomerular apparatus redrawn and simplified from Fig. 24–41 to show the four elements of the juxtaglomerular apparatus as well as the position of the capillaries, mesangial cells, and epithelial cells of the renal corpuscle.

the major extracellular ion, its renal retention leads to an increase in the extracellular fluid volume of the animal. Angiotensin II is also a potent vasoconstrictor.

A local action for the renin–angiotension system also has been proposed in which the juxtaglomerular apparatus provides feedback control of the glomerular filtration rate at the level of individual nephrons. This feedback mechanism could be related to renal autoregulation of blood flow (Thurau and Levine, 1971).

Renal Interstitium

The cortical interstitium is small in normal animals. However, in a variety of disease processes the interstitium increases in volume and becomes fibrotic. Around the vessels, the interstitium is abundant (Swann and Norman, 1970). Two main cell types are seen within the cortical interstitium. The most frequently seen is the fi-

broblast. The second is a cell in the mononuclear series which, under certain circumstances, can be seen to contain a large number of phagocytic vacuoles and lysosomes. Fine collagen bundles traverse the cortical interstitium. Under normal circumstances, the interstitium also contains a fluid reabsorbate, which is in transit from the lumen of the tubules to the capillaries.

In contrast, the interstitium of the medulla is much more abundant; it contains a population of elongate interstitial cells whose long axes lie perpendicular to the long axes of the tubules in that region (Fig. 24–44). The cells are characterized by long, branching processes that come close to vessels and tubules and in some circumstances appear to encircle them. The unique feature of these cells is that they contain a variable number of lipid droplets within their cytoplasm. In addition, the cytoplasm contains fine intracellular filaments, rough ER, numerous lysosomes, and other organelles. The cells appear to be partially surrounded by a layer of material that resembles basement membrane (external lamina), and this material also extends into the intercellular space around the cells, forming a network. Small bundles of collagen, flocculent material, and fine filaments (approximately 13 nm in diameter with an electron-lucent core) are seen within the in-

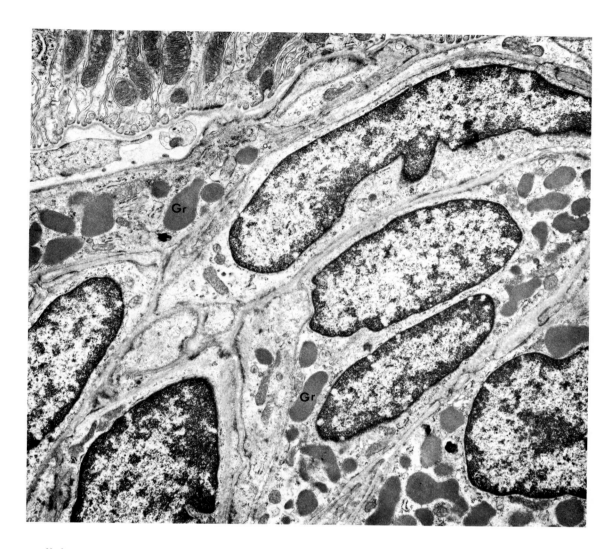

24–43 Electron micrograph showing juxtaglomerular cells from a rat kidney. The juxtaglomerular granules **(Gr)** can be seen within the cytoplasm of the modified smooth muscle cells. × 9,300.

tercellular matrix. Several functions have been proposed for these unique interstitial cells: (1) they elaborate the interstitial matrix; (2) they are contractile and presumably by contraction play a role in the concentration or urine; (3) they are phagocytic; and (4) they produce the vasodepressor substances that have been isolated from the renal interstitium in certain animals, which are most likely prostaglandins E_2 and A_2 and neutral lipids (Westura et al., 1970: McGiff et al., 1970: Muehrcke et al., 1970).

Blood Vessels

Arteries. The *renal arteries* generally arise from the lateral region of the abdominal aorta at the level of the first and second lumbar verte-

brae. Each artery runs downward and laterally and then usually divides into an *anterior* and *posterior division* before it reaches the renal hilus. The anterior division runs in front of the renal pelvis; the posterior division enters the renal sinus behind the renal pelvis. Although there seems to be variation in the next branching, five *segmental* branches are generally described. The anterior division branches into the upper, middle, and lower segmental arteries, and the posterior division becomes a posterior segmental artery. The fifth, or apical, segment can arise

Collecting duct   Thin segment   Interstitial cells

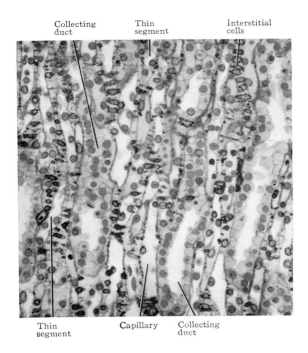

Interstitial cells   Collecting duct

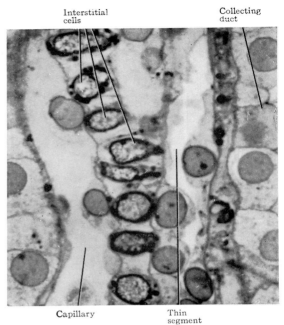

Thin segment   Capillary   Collecting duct

Capillary   Thin segment

24–44 Light micrograph of sections taken of the renal pyramid from a rat kidney, showing the horizontal, ladder-like array of interstitial cells located in this region. Epoxy resin section, toluidine blue. **Left,** × 275; **Right,** × 1,100.

from either the anterior or posterior or from branches of both divisions. While in the renal sinus, the segmental arteries branch to form interlobar arteries that enter the renal columns adjacent to the renal pyramids. At the base of the renal pyramid, the *interlobar* artery branches into many *arcuate arteries* that run across the base of the medullary pyramid near the corticomedullary junction (Fig. 24–45). The arcuate arteries give off branches called *interlobular* arteries that course peripherally in the cortex midway between medullary rays (hence between renal lobules). As the interlobular arteries ascend, they give off *afferent arterioles* which can serve one or more renal corpuscles. The afferent arteriole enters the renal corpuscle and forms several lobules of capillary networks. Anastomosis occurs between the capillaries in any lobule, but not between capillaries of adjacent lobules. The capillaries then converge to form the efferent arteriole which exits from the renal corpuscle at the vascular pole.

Postglomerular Capillary Circulation. The efferent arterioles leave the renal corpuscle and divide into a second capillary network. The morphology of these capillaries differs, depending on whether the renal corpuscle is of the cortical or juxtamedullary type. The efferent arterioles from cortical nephrons are short and divide to form a tortuous *peritubular capillary network* supplying the associated convoluted tubules (Fig. 24–45). It appears that the blood in this capillary network flows rapidly in the direction opposite to that of the fluid in the tubular lumen (Steinhausen et al., 1970).

The majority of efferent arterioles from juxtamedullary nephrons divide to form several parallel unbranched vessels called the *arteriolae rectae spuriae*. These vessels descend into the medullary pyramid, where they give rise to capillaries and ascend again in the region adjacent to the descending limb forming a vascular countercurrent exchanger (Figs. 24–45 to 24–48). The descending limbs are called arteriolae rectae, and the ascending limbs are called venae rectae. The walls of the arteriolar vessels in the outer medulla have a thicker endothelium (2–4 μm) than the walls of the ascending venous vessels. The vessels form capillary plexuses lined by fenestrated endothelium at various levels throughout

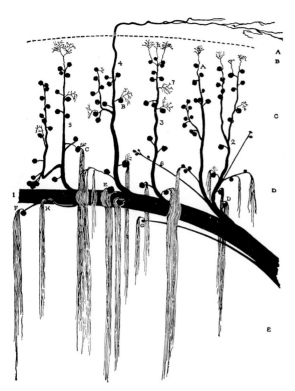

24–45 Diagram to represent the finer arterial distribution of the kidney. **A,** capsule; **B,** subcapsular zone; **C,** cortex; **D,** juxtamedullary zone; **E,** medulla. The arcuate artery (1) gives off numerous interlobular arteries. The long, straight arteriolae rectae can be seen passing down into the medulla.

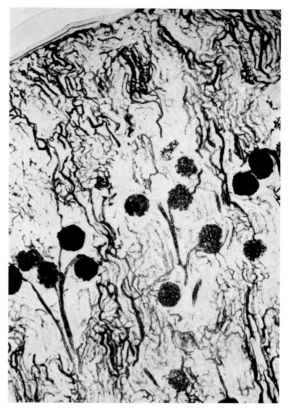

24–46 Arteries of the dog kidney were infused with a gelatin solution to make visible the interlobular arteries, the afferent arterioles, the glomerulus, the efferent arterioles, and the peritubular capillary anastomoses around the tubules. × 46.

the medullary pyramid. Blood flow through the medulla is much lesser in volume and slower than that in the cortex, so that the inner medulla has a lower oxygen supply and derives most of its energy from glycolysis. The looping form of the vessels allows the osmotic gradient of the papilla to be maintained.

Veins. The venous supply in the kidney is quite irregular, and anastomoses occur between its vessels. Near the renal capsule, small venules drain in a starlike pattern, forming the stellate veins which, in turn, form the interlobular veins that course adjacent to the interlobular arteries and receive numerous tributaries from the cortical peritubular capillary network. The interlobular veins empty into the arcuate veins, which extend across at the level of the corticomedullary junction. The arcuate veins also receive blood

from the venous branches of the vasae rectae. Interlobar veins are formed by the confluence of arcuate veins; they course adjacent to the medullary pyramid in company with the corresponding artery. The confluence of these vessels forms the renal vein. On the right side of the body, the renal vein is short, but on the left side of the body it is longer and receives blood from the gonadal, suprarenal, and inferior phrenic veins.

Lymphatics. Lymphatic vessels have been identified accompanying the larger renal vessels and appear to be more prominent around the arteries than around the veins. They have been identified along the interlobular, arcuate, interlobar, segmental, and renal arteries and veins (Kriz and Dieterich, 1970). In the region of the renal sinus, they converge into several large

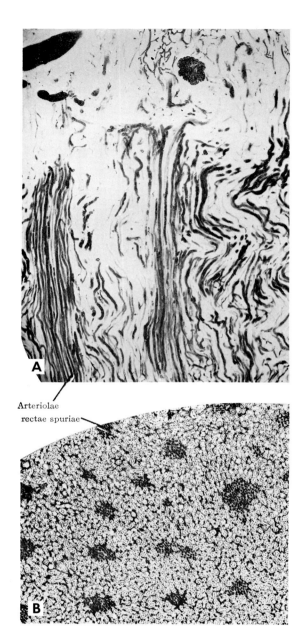

Arteriolae
rectae spuriae

24–47 Arteriolae rectae spuriae of a dog. Arteries
were infused with colored gelatin. **A.** Radial
section through the base of a renal pyramid, showing
origin of tassels of arterioles at the junction of cortex
and medulla. × 45. **B.** Transverse section of pyramid
showing islands of arteriolae rectae spuriae. × 42.
(Courtesy of D. Fawcett.)

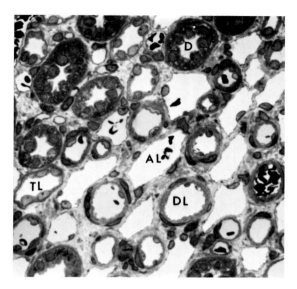

24–48 Light micrograph of a cross section through a
bundle of vasa recta (center) from the outer
medulla of a human kidney. Note the patterned array
with thick-walled descending limbs of the vasa recta
(DL) being surrounded by thin-walled ascending limbs
of the vasa recta **(AL)**. The straight part of the distal
tubule **(D)** and some thin limb sections **(TL)** can also
be identified. × 420.

trunks that exit via the renal hilus. The lymph is
then drained into nodes along the inferior vena
cava and aorta. The lymphatics that accompany
the interlobular vessels anastomose with a rich
supply of lymphatics in the renal capsule and
perirenal tissue. Medullary lymphatics have not
been clearly demonstrated in electron micrographs.

Innervation

Many autonomic nerve fibers that form the renal
plexus accompany the renal artery and its
branches to the kidney. Most of these fibers are
from the sympathetic division of the autonomic
nervous system. The fibers are derived from cell
bodies located mainly in the celiac and aortic
ganglia. The sympathetic fibers innervate renal
blood vessels to cause vasoconstriction. In addition, some authors believe that parasympathetic
fibers of the autonomic nervous system derived
from the vagus nerve also enter the kidney. Sensory fibers have been described as well. When
these sensory fibers are cut, renal pain is
blocked. Although numerous light microscopists

describe nerve endings along the wall of the renal tubules and within the renal corpuscle, electron microscopists have not recognized them and have identified nerve endings only along the renal vessels, in the juxtaglomerular apparatus, and in the renal interstitium. Nerves have not been identified penetrating the basement membrane of any tubule or within the renal corpuscle. Because the nerve fibers to the kidney are cut during renal transplantation, it is obvious that the kidney can function adequately without an extrinsic nerve supply.

Extrarenal Collecting System

Excretory Passages

Urine is conveyed from the kidney to the bladder where it is stored. When the bladder becomes appropriately distended, the micturition reflex causes emptying of the bladder, and the urine leaves via the urethra. Urine is excreted through the minor calyxes (Fig. 24–49), the major calyxes, the renal pelvis, the ureter (Fig. 24–50), the bladder, and the urethra. The walls of all but the last are similar in their basic structure, being

composed of an inner mucosal layer, a middle muscularis layer, and an external adventitial coat of connective tissue that binds the structure to the surrounding connective tissue. The upper portion of the bladder extends into the pelvic cavity; it therefore is covered by parietal peritoneum and hence has a serosa. The thickness of the three layers of the wall increases from the minor calyxes to the bladder.

Mucosa. While the urine is being conveyed and stored within the extrarenal collecting system, only small changes occur in its composition. A specialized lining layer called *transitional epithelium* along the lumen of the excretory passages and the bladder is responsible for this low permeability (Fig. 24–51). This intact epithelium seems to be a barrier to the rapid diffusion of salt and water. In addition, transitional epithelium gives a distensibility to the lining layer. The epithelium is generally said to be two to three cells thick in the minor calyxes, four to five cells thick in the ureter, and six or more cells thick in the empty bladder. The superficial cells of the transitional epithelium appear large

24–49 Light micrograph showing the wall of a calyx. The calyx is lined by transitional epithelium **(TE)**, a lamina propria **(LP)**, and muscularis **(M)**.

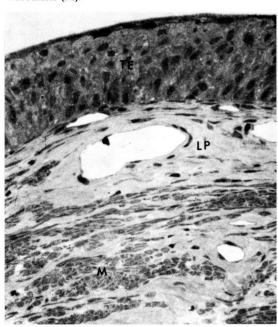

24–50 Light micrograph showing the wall of a dog ureter lined by transitional epithelium **(TE)**, lamina propria **(LP)**, muscularis **(M)**, and a layer of adventitia **(A)** containing vessels.

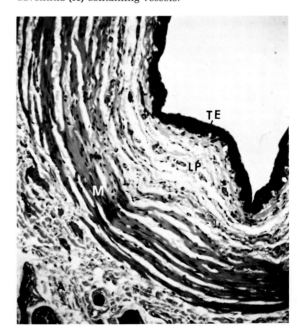

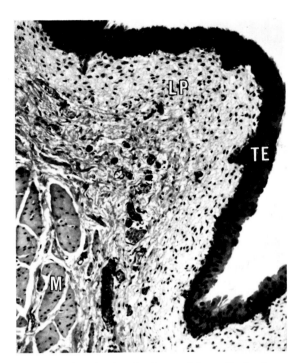

24–51 Light micrograph of part of the wall of a dog bladder, showing the transitional epithelium **(TE)**, the lamina propria **(LP)**, and part of the muscularis **(M)**. × 500.

and rounded and sometimes contain large polyploid nuclei. When the epithelium is stretched, such as in the filling bladder, it becomes much thinner and the surface cells are stretched into a squamous layer. The distensibility of the transitional epithelium results not only from a change in shape of the cells from rounded to flat but also from certain other anatomic features. The surface of the luminal cells is characterized by an irregular contour with small **V**-shaped indentations that penetrate into the cell (Figs. 24–52 and 24–53). The apical cytoplasm contains stacks of fusiform vesicles that are limited by a membrane of the same thickness as the apical plasma membrane (12 nm). It seems that the fusiform vesicles are formed from the surface membrane when the bladder is relaxing. This is demonstrated by placing a marker such as ferritin in the lumen of the bladder and observing its uptake into the fusiform vesicles (Porter and Bonneville, 1968). In addition, the epithelial cells beneath the surface appear to have numerous lateral interdigitations and projections that disappear during distension. Only a few small desmosomes are seen between the cells of the transitional epithelium.

Lamina Propria. The lamina propria is composed of a fairly dense layer of collagenous connective tissue that becomes somewhat looser in the lower region near the muscularis. There is no submucosa in the wall. When the excretory passages are empty, the mucosa is folded. When the organ is distended, the mucosa can be stretched flat; this folding allows for considerable increase in luminal diameter.

Muscularis. The muscular layer of the excretory passages usually consists of two layers of smooth muscle. Although the precise orientation of the muscle is complex, the inner layer appears to be oriented predominantly in a longitudinal fashion, whereas the outer layer is oriented predominantly in a circular fashion. In addition, the layers of smooth muscle differ from those of the gastrointestinal tract in that they are penetrated by connective tissue in such a manner that bundles of oriented smooth muscle are seen instead of a true layer.

The muscle layers are thinnest in the minor calyxes, but two layers of muscle are present (Fig. 24–49). The inner layer is attached to the base of the medulla and contains longitudinal fibers. The outer layer follows a more circumferential path with anterior and posterior loops that cross on the anterior and posterior sides of the calyx (Van den Bulcke et al., 1970). This layer extends higher up and forms a ring around the base of the medullary pyramid. The calyxes act as funnels whose walls contract in waves that move the fluid from the medullary pyramid into the renal pelvis.

The walls of the renal pelvis and the upper two-thirds of the ureter contain the same two layers of smooth muscle, which continue to be found in bundles; however, they are thicker than in the walls of the calyxes. In the lower third of the ureter, an additional outer longitudinal layer of smooth muscle is found. Periodic peristaltic waves proceed down the ureter, forcing urine into the bladder. No definite pacemaker initiating these waves has been found.

The ureters pierce the bladder wall obliquely, and the inner longitudinal layer of smooth muscle inserts into the lamina propria of the bladder. Because of the oblique course of the ureters

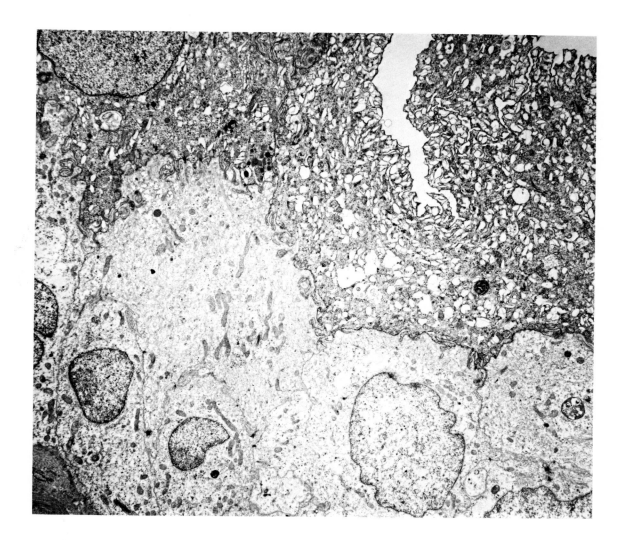

through the wall of the bladder, their walls are pressed together as the bladder distends. The likelihood of urine refluxing into the ureters is therefore decreased.

Bladder

The bladder is a reservoir for urine and varies in size and shape as it is filled (Fig. 24–51). Three layers of smooth muscle with complex orientation have been described in the thick wall of the bladder. The middle layer is the most prominent. Because of the tortuosity of the muscle, it is difficult to delineate clearly these various layers in a random histological section. In the region of the trigone, an internal sphincter is formed by

24–52 Electron micrograph showing the transitional epithelium of a rat bladder. The large cells lining the apical surface are characterized by an irregular contour to their apical plasma membrane and by numerous fusiform vesicles within their cytoplasm. × 31,500. (Courtesy of F. Remington.)

the orientation of smooth muscle around the opening of the urethra.

Blood Vessels. Blood vessels penetrate the walls of the excretory passages and enter the muscularis where they supply it with an abundant capillary network. A plexus is then formed within the lamina propria of the mucosa, and branches form a rich plexus of capillaries located

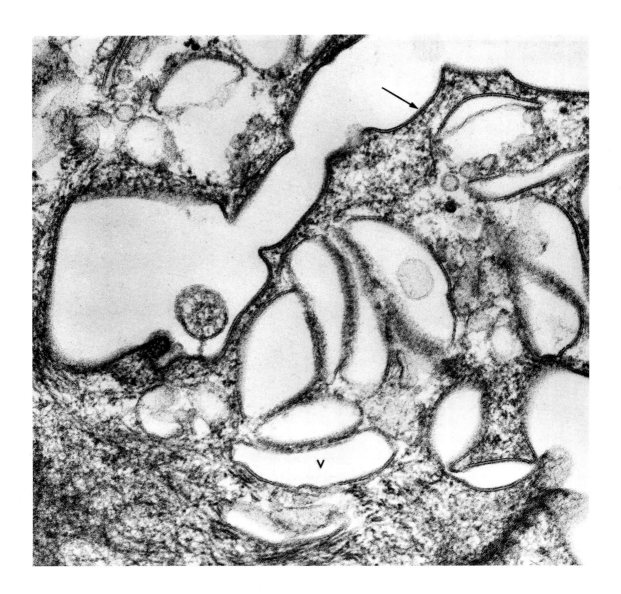

24–53 Electron micrograph of the surface cell membrane of a transitional epithelial cell, showing the 120-Å thick apical plasma membrane **(arrow)** and similar membranes surrounding fusiform vesicles **(V)** in the cytoplasm. × 6,600.

just beneath the epithelium. In the deeper layers of the walls of the pelvis and ureters, abundant lymph vessels are seen accompanying these blood vessels.

Nerves. The bladder is supplied by both sympathetic and parasympathetic divisions of the autonomic nervous system. The sympathetic fibers traverse the inferior hypogastric plexus and form a plexus in the adventitia of the bladder wall, the *plexus vesicalis*. These sympathetic fibers appear to play little role in micturition. The preganglionic fibers of the parasympathetic division that supply the bladder arise from the spinal cord in the second, third, and fourth sacral levels. The fibers traverse to the bladder via the pelvic nerve and the inferior hypogastric plexus where they intermingle with the sympathetic fibers and synapse with ganglion cells located within the adventitia and muscularis of the bladder wall. These fibers are important for micturition. Afferent sensory fibers from the bladder traverse the pelvic and hypogastric nerves.

Urethra

The urethra is a fibromuscular tube through which urine passes from the urinary bladder to the exterior. In the male (Fig. 24–54), the urethra is long (approximately 20 cm) and also serves for the passage of seminal fluid during ejaculation. In the female (Fig. 24–55), it is short (approximately 3 to 5 cm). Because the male and female urethra differ in structure, they will be considered separately.

Male Urethra. The male urethra can be divided into three segments. It begins at the neck of the bladder and extends through the prostate gland (prostatic portion), though the pelvic and urogenital diaphragm (membranous portion), and finally through the root and body of the penis to the tip of the glans penis (spongy, or anterior, part).

The *prostatic portion* of the urethra is approximately 3 to 4 cm in length. It extends through the prostate gland where multiple small prostatic ducts enter. On the posterior wall of the prostatic urethra, a conical elevation called the *veru montanum* (or *colliculus seminalis*) is located. A blind invagination called the *prostatic utricle* extends into the substance of the prostate at the summit of this region. The prostatic utricle is thought to represent a vestige of the fused caudal ends of the müllerian or paramesonephric duct, which in the female form the uterus and most of the vagina. The ejaculatory ducts enter the urethra on each side of the opening of the prostatic utricle. The urethra in this region is lined by transitional epithelium. The lamina propria is highly vascular. Two coats of smooth muscle bundles surround the mucosa; the bundles of the inner coat are oriented longitudinally and those of the outer coat are circular in orientation. The circular muscular bundles are a continuation of the thickened circular region at the bladder outlet, called the *internal sphincter* of the bladder.

The *membranous portion* of the male urethra runs from the apex of the prostate to the bulb of the corpus cavernosus penis, traversing the urogenital and pelvic diaphragms. It is therefore surrounded by striated muscle fibers that form the *external sphincter* of the bladder. The epithelium in this region is stratified or pseudostratified columnar.

The *spongy portion* (anterior) is approximately 15 cm long and extends through the bulb, body, and glans of the penis encased by the corpus cavernosum urethrae (spongiosum). The lumen of the urethra is dilated within the region of the bulb (intabulbar fossa) and in the glans (novicular fossa). The epithelium lining most of the urethra in this region is pseudostratified columnar (Fig. 24–54), with patches of stratified squamous epithelium. In the novicular fossa the epithelium becomes stratified squamous. The ducts of the bulbourethral glands enter the spongy seg-

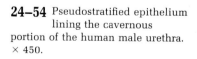
24–54 Pseudostratified epithelium lining the cavernous portion of the human male urethra. × 450.

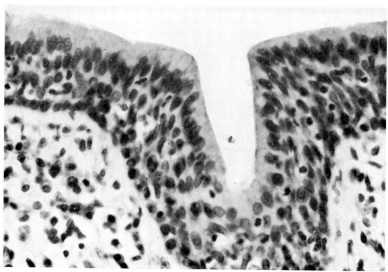

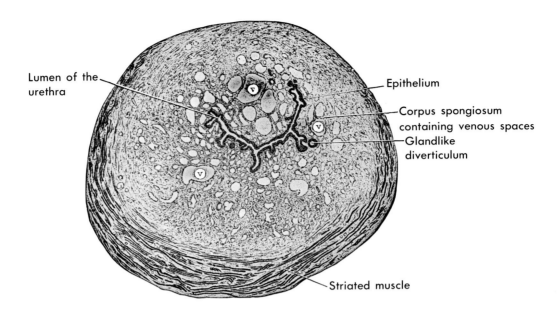

Lumen of the urethra

Epithelium

Corpus spongiosum containing venous spaces

Glandlike diverticulum

Striated muscle

24–55 Transverse section of the human female urethra. Picric acid–sublimate fixation. × 10. (From Von Ebner.)

ment of the urethra. Mucus-secreting glands (glands of Littre) also empty into the urethra throughout its length. However, they are most frequently found within this spongy portion.

Female Urethra. The female urethra is relatively short, approximately 3 to 5 cm long. The lumen is crescentic in outline, and most of it is lined with stratified squamous epithelium (Fig. 24–55). Pseudostratified columnar epithelium may also be found. Within the epithelium some nests of mucus glands may be found. The lamina propria consists of a wide zone of vascular connective tissue that contains many thin-walled veins. The muscularis of the female urethra is similar to that in the bladder neck. An inner longitudinal layer of smooth muscle bundles is surrounded by a thicker layer of smooth muscle with circular orientation. The outer circular fibers are continuous with those in the internal sphincter of the urethra. The outer circular layer is reinforced with striated muscle fibers of the constrictor muscle of the urethra.

References and Selected Bibliography

General

Bulger, R. E., Siegel, F. L., and Pendergrass, R. 1974. Scanning and transmission electron microscopy of the rat kidney. Am. J. Anat. 139:483

Kaissling, B., and Kriz, W. 1979. Structural Analysis of the Rabbit Kidney. Advances in Anatomy, Embryology, and Cell Biology, Vol. 56. Berlin: Springer-Verlag.

Porter, K. R., and Bonneville, M. A. 1968. Fine Structure of Cells and Tissues. Philadelphia: Lea and Febiger.

Rambourg, A., and Leblond, C. P. 1967. Electron microscopy observations on the carbohydrate-rich cell coat present at the surface of cells in the rat. J. Cell Biol. 32:27.

Rouiller, C. 1969. General anatomy and histology of the kidney. In C. Rouiller and A. F. Muller (eds.), The Kidney, Vol. 1. New York: Academic Press, Inc., p.61.

Zimmermann, K. W. 1911. Zur Morphologie der Epithelzellen der Saugetierniere. Arch. Mikrobiol. Anat. 78:199.

Kidney
Juxtaglomerular Apparatus:

Ausiello, D. A., Kreisberg, J. I., Roy, C., and Karnovsky, M. J. 1979. Contraction of cultured rat mesangial cells after stimulation with angiotensin II and arginine vasopressin. Kidney Int. 16:804A.

Barajas, L. 1970. The ultrastructure of the juxtaglomerular apparatus as disclosed by three-dimensional reconstructions from serial sections. J. Ultrastruct. Res. 33:116.

Barajas, L., and Latta, H. 1967. Structure of the juxtaglomerular apparatus. Circ. Res. 20,21 (Suppl. II):15.

Renal Corpuscle:

Blau, E. B., and Haas, J. E. 1973. Glomerular sialic acid and proteinuria in human renal disease. Lab. Invest. 28:477.

Brenner, B. M., Troy, J. L., and Daugharty, T. M. 1971. The dynamics of glomerular ultrafiltration in the rat. J. Clin. Invest. 50:1776.

Chang, R. L. S., Deen, W. N., Robertson, C. R., and Brenner, B. N. 1975. Perselectivity of the glomerular capillary wall: III. Restricted transport of polyanions. Kidney Int. 8:212.

Hollinshead, W. H. 1966. Renovascular anatomy. Postgrad. Med. 40:241.

Jorgensen, F. 1966. The Ultrastructure of the Normal Human Glomerulus. Copenhagen: Munksgaard.

Ryan, G. B., and Karnovsky, M. J. 1976. Distribution of endogenous albumin in the rat glomerulus: Role of hemodynamic factors in glomerular barrier function. Kidney Int. 9:36.

Seiler, M. W., Venkatachalam, M. A., and Cotran, R. S. 1975. Glomerular epithelium: Structural alterations induced by polycations. Science (Wash., D.C.) 189:390.

Venkatachalam, M. A., Cotran, R. S., and Karnovsky, M. J. 1970. An ultrastructural study of glomerular permeability in aminonucleoside nephrosis using catalase as a tracer protein. J. Exp. Med. 132:1168.

Tubules and Collecting Ducts:

Berger, S. J., and Sacktor, B. 1970. Isolation and biochemical characterization of brush borders from rabbit kidney. J. Cell Biol. 47:637.

Bulger, R. E. 1965. The shape of rat kidney tubular cells. Am. J. Anat. 116:237.

Bulger, R. E., and Trump, B. F. 1966. Fine structure of the rat renal papilla. Am. J. Anat. 118:685.

De Duve, C., and Baudhuin, P. 1966. Peroxisome (microbodies and related particles). Physiol. Rev. 46:323.

Harper, J. T., Puchtler, H., Meloan, S. N., and Terry, M. S. 1970. Light-microscopic demonstration of myoid fibrils in renal epithelial, mesangial and interstitial cells. J. Microscopy 91:71.

Myers, C. E., Bulger, R. E., Tisher, C. C., and Trump, B. F. 1966. Human renal ultrastructure. IV. Collecting duct of healthy individuals. Lab. Invest. 15:1921.

Osvaldo, L., and Latta, H. 1966. The thin limbs of the loop of Henle. J. Ultrastruct. Res. 15:144.

Pricam, C., Humbert, F., Perrelet, A., and Orci, L. 1974. A freeze-etch study of the tight junctions of the rat kidney tubules. Lab. Invest. 30:286.

Rhodin, J. 1958. Anatomy of kidney tubules. Int. Rev. Cytol. 7:485.

Schwartz, M. M., and Venkatachalam, M. A. 1974. Structural differences in thin limbs of Henle: Physiological implications. Kidney Int. 6:193.

Tisher, C. C., Bulger, R. E., and Trump, B. F. 1966. Human renal ultrastructure. I. Proximal tubule of healthy individuals. Lab Invest. 15:1357.

Tisher, C. C., Bulger, R. E., and Trump, B. F. 1968. Human renal ultrastructure. III. The distal tubule in healthy individuals. Lab. Invest. 18:655.

Ureter and Bladder

Hicks, R. M., and Ketterer, B. 1970. Isolation of the plasma membrane of the luminal surface of rat bladder epithelium, and the occurrence of a hexagonal lattice of subunits both in negatively stained whole mounts and in sectioned membranes. J. Cell Biol. 45:542.

Van den Bulcke, C., Keen, E. N., and Fine, H. 1970. Observations on smooth muscle disposition in the urinary tract. J. Urol. 103:783.

Development

Clark, S. L., Jr. 1957. Cellular differentiation in the kidneys of newborn mice studied with the electron microscope. J. Biophys. Biochem. Cytol. 3:349.

Du Bois, A. M. 1969. The embryonic kidney. *In* C. Rouiller and A. F. Muller (eds.), The Kidney, Vol. 1. New York: Academic Press, p. 1.

Pathology

Darmady, E. M., and Stranack, F. 1957. Microdissections of the nephron in disease. Br. Med. Bull. 13:21.

Muehrcke, R. C., Mandal, A. R., and Volini, F. I. 1970. IV. Renal interstitial cells: Prostaglandins and hypertension. A pathophysiological review of the renal medullary interstitial cells and their relationship to hypertension. Circ. Res. 26, 27:1-109.

Westura, E. E., Kannegiesser, H., O'Toole, J. D., and Lee, J. B. 1970. IV. Renal interstitial cells: Prostaglandins and hypertension. Antihypertensive effects of prostaglandin A₁ in essential hypertension. Circ. Res. 26, 27:1-131.

Physiology

Gottschalk, C. W., and Mylle, M 1959. Micropuncture study of the mammalian urinary concentrating mechanism: Evidence for the countercurrent hypotheses. Am. J. Physiol. 196:927.

Pitts, R. F. 1963. Physiology of the Kidney and Body Fluids. Chicago: Year Book Medical Publishers, Inc.

Richet, G., Hagege, J., and Gabe, M. 1970. Correlation between bicarbonate transfer and morphology of tubular cells distal to Henle's loop in the rat. Nephron 7:413.

Vasculature

Rennke, H. G., Cotran, R. S., and Venkatachalam, M. A. 1975 Role of molecular charge in glomerular permeability. Tracer studies with cationized ferritins. J. Cell Biol. 67:638.

Trueta, J., Barclay, A. E., Daniel, P., Franklin, K. J., and Prichard, M. M. L. 1947. Studies of the Renal Circulation. Oxford: Blackwell Scientific Publications, Ltd.

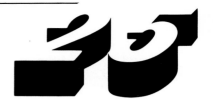

The Female Reproductive System

Richard J. Blandau

The female reproductive system (Fig. 25–1) is composed of an internal group of organs situated within the pelvis, consisting of the ovaries, the oviducts (also called uterine or fallopian tubes), the uterus, and the vagina. The external genitalia comprise the mons pubis, the labia minora, the labia majora, and the clitoris. The mammary glands, although not genital organs, are an important appendage to the reproductive system.

The ovaries are paired organs situated on either side of the uterus, each 2 to 5 cm long, 1.5 to 3 cm wide, and 0.8 to 1.5 cm thick. The size of the ovaries varies greatly from week to week during each menstrual cycle and during pregnancy; this variation is related to the number and stage of development of the growing follicles and corpora lutea. To study the ovaries intelligently, it is important to know at which stage of the menstrual cycle they were removed.

Each ovary is attached to the broad ligament by a double fold of peritoneum, the mesovarium (Figs. 25–1 and 25–2). The mesovarium is attached to the ovary only along one margin, the hilum. The suspensory ligament of the ovary (Fig. 25–1) is a fold of peritoneum that is directed upward over the iliac vessels and contains the ovarian vessels. The mesovarium and the suspensory ligaments often contain significant amounts of smooth muscle fibers whose rhythmic contractions, particularly at the time of ovulation, move the ovaries closer to the fimbriae of the oviducts.

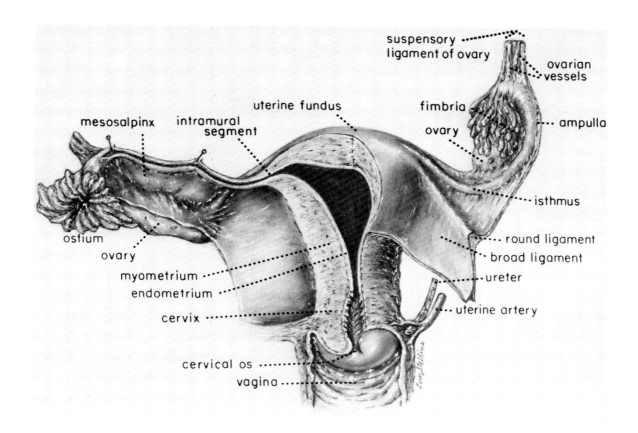

suspensory ligament of ovary

ovarian vessels

uterine fundus

fimbria

ovary

ampulla

mesosalpinx

intramural segment

isthmus

ostium

ovary

round ligament

broad ligament

myometrium

ureter

endometrium

uterine artery

cervix

cervical os

vagina

25–1 Reproductive organs of the human female.

Sexual Maturation (Puberty)

The female sexual organs normally remain in an immature state during approximately the first 10 years of life. In the succeeding 2 to 4 years there occurs a gradual enlargement of the reproductive organs, accompanied by growth of the breasts, changes in the contours of the body, and the appearance of axillary and pubic hair. This period of sexual development culminates in the appearance of the first menses (menarche) at an average age of 13.5 years. In a recent study of 30,000 menstrual cycles in women between 15 and 39 years of age, the average cycle length was 29 days with a standard deviation of 7.46 days. Mature reproductive life, characterized by recurring menstrual cycles, lasts until about age 45 to 50. Women then enter a period known as the menopause (also called the climacteric or "change of life") during which reproductive cycles become irregular, lengthen, and eventually cease. Thereafter, in the postmenopausal period, the reproductive organs are atrophic and functionless.

The Internal Organs

The Ovaries

The ovaries are remarkable organs that store from the time of birth all the eggs the human female will ever have. They also cyclically secrete hormones that are essential for the postnatal growth and development of the pelvis, the secondary sex organs, and the mammary glands.

Each ovary is covered by a continuous mesothelium composed of a single layer of cuboidal epithelium. Because of the tenuous attachment of this layer of cells to the underlying stroma, it is often accidentally removed in making the histological preparation. Each ovary consists of an outer cortex and a central medulla (Fig. 25–2). Embedded within the loose connective tissue of the medulla are nerves, lymph vessels, and many large blood vessels. In the adult ovaries, the arteries are often coiled and tortuous as they pass

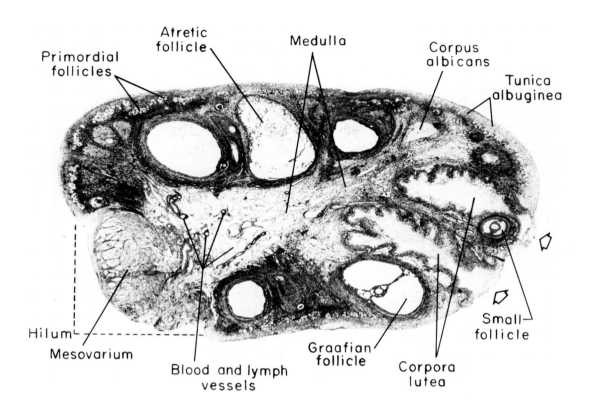

Primordial follicles · Atretic follicle · Medulla · Corpus albicans · Tunica albuginea · Hilum · Mesovarium · Blood and lymph vessels · Graafian follicle · Corpora lutea · Small follicle

25–2 Unretouched photomicrograph of a longitudinal section of an ovary of the cat. **Arrows** point to the site of the recent rupture of two ovarian follicles that are being transformed into corpora lutea. ×12.

toward the cortical zone. This arrangement allows them to adapt readily during the phases of rapid ovarian enlargement, ovulation, and corpus luteum formation. The medulla may also contain remnants of a closed ductular system, the rete ovarii. They are small and irregularly arranged ducts lined by a single layer of low cuboidal epithelium. Embryologically, they are homologous to the rete testes in the male gonads.

The stroma of the cortex is composed of closely packed spindle-shaped cells (Fig. 25–3) arranged in irregular whorls except near the periphery where the stroma forms a dense, fibrous, collagenous connective tissue layer, the tunica albuginea (Figs. 25–2 and 25–3). Elastic fibers are few or absent. A few smooth muscle cells have been described as scattered in the cortical stroma and in the walls of preovulatory follicles

in the ovaries of rats and monkeys. Contractions of the smooth muscles, particularly in the ovulatory follicles, may play a role in ovulation.

At the time of birth, in the human female 300,000 to 400,000 oocytes are embedded in the stroma of the cortex of both ovaries. Of them, only 420 to 480 may ovulate during the entire reproductive life of the individual and less than 5% of them may be fertilized. Less than one-half of the fertilized eggs will develop normally and go to term. During each menstrual cycle, 5 to 20 follicles may grow to a considerable size (Fig. 25–3). Only one of these follicles will ovulate; the rest will degenerate by the process of atresia. Atresia begins during the fetal period, is accentuated postnatally, and continues throughout the reproductive life span. More will be said about the various types of atresia later in this chapter.

Primordial or Unilaminar Follicles. The cortex of the ovary, particularly in the young woman, contains many individual primordial unilaminar follicles (Fig. 25–3), each consisting of a large oocyte enclosed in a single layer of cuboidal or columnar cells resting on a basement

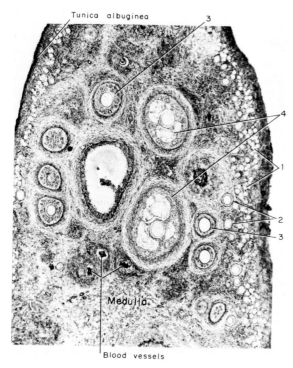

Tunica albuginea

3

4

1

2

3

Medulla

Blood vessels

25–3 Photomicrograph of a rabbit ovary showing (1) numerous primordial follicles with a single layer of flattened follicular cells, (2) unilaminar follicles with a single layer of cuboidal epithelium, (3) multilaminar follicles without antra, and (4) vesicular follicles with follicular antra. Note the increase in size of the egg as the follicle grows and the presence of the zona pellucida in 2, 3, and 4. ×50.

Growth of Follicles. Follicular growth is a continuous process. Follicles begin to grow under almost all physiological circumstances. Growth is not interrupted by ovulation, periods of anovulation, or pregnancy. Growth continues at all ages from infancy to the time of the menopause.

In the normal menstrual cycle a rise in follicle-stimulating hormone (FSH) affects follicular growth whereas the luteinizing hormone (LH) stimulates steroidogenesis. However, it is the interrelationship and the cooperative efforts among estradiol, FSH, and LH that regulate the growth and steroidogenesis of the ovarian follicles (Fig. 25–30). As the oocyte begins to grow, the flattened follicular cells become cuboidal (Fig. 25–5) and proliferate rapidly to form a stratified epithelium. These cells are called multilaminar primary follicles.

The multilaminar epithelium rests on a distinct basement membrane (membrana limitans externa) (Fig. 25–5), which stains brilliantly red with the periodic acid Schiff (PAS) technique. The basement membrane is exceptionally homogeneous and relatively highly polymerized, and it separates the stratum granulosum from the theca interna (Fig. 25–6). As the egg grows, a clear, refractile, highly polymerized membrane, the zona pellucida (mucoid oolemma) (Fig. 25–7), is interposed between the oocyte and the immediately adjacent follicular cells. The zona pellucida is a noncellular glycoprotein-mucopolysaccharide membrane that also stains a brilliant red with the PAS technique. The origin of the zona pellucida is uncertain; some investigators believe it is formed from secretions of the follicular cells that immediately surround the egg, whereas others suggest that peripheral Golgi bodies in the oocyte itself have some function in its formation. The zona pellucida usually appears first in the unilaminar follicle with but a single layer of cuboidal or columnar cells.

As the zona pellucida appears, the plasma membrane of the oocyte forms numerous microvilli (Fig. 25–7) that extend into the zonal membrane. At the same time, irregularly arranged and sinuous cytoplasmic projections from the follicular cells (Fig. 25–7) penetrate the zona and make contact with the plasma membrane of the egg. Thus, despite the presence of a rather thick zona pellucida (5 μm in the mature ovum), the egg and follicular cells maintain plasma membrane contact throughout the period of growth until the time of ovulation.

membrane. Because the oocyte is so large (25 to 30 μm), its circumference may be surrounded by several flattened follicular cells in sectioned material. The plasma membranes of the oocyte and the follicular cells at this stage are relatively smooth, closely apposed to one another, and at certain places connected by desmosomes. The oocyte (Fig. 25–4) has a large vesicular nucleus with finely dispersed chromatin and one or more large nucleoli. The nuclear envelope has well-developed pores. A well-developed Golgi apparatus with short tubular profiles may be located near the nucleus. The round mitochondria have typical cristae. The endoplasmic reticulum (ER) is represented by numerous small vesicles. The cytological characteristics of the oocytes easily distinguish them from the follicular cells or any of the other cells in the cortical stroma (Fig. 25–3).

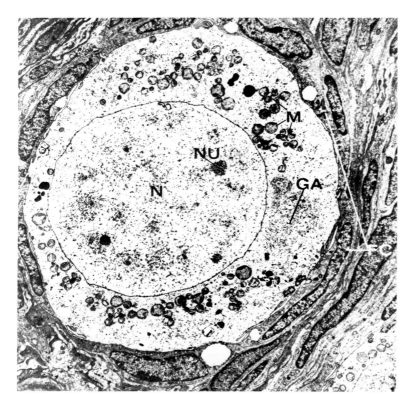

25–4 Electron micrograph of a primordial follicle of a rabbit. Notice the oocyte surrounded by flattened follicular epithelium (**FC**) and the absence of zona pellucida. The cytoplasm of the oocyte contains some characteristic round mitochondria (**M**), a few strands of endoplasmic reticulum, and numerous free ribosomes. **N**, nucleus; **NU**, nucleolus; **GA**, Golgi apparatus. (Courtesy of F. J. Silverblatt.) ×2,800.

25–5 A multilaminar growing follicle in a rabbit ovary showing a distinct basement membrane separating the follicular epithelium from the theca folliculi. ×260. ▽

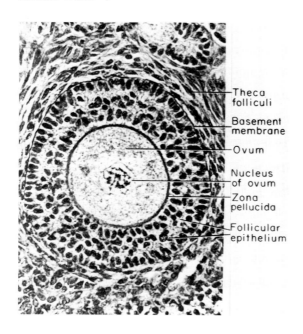

- Theca folliculi
- Basement membrane
- Ovum
- Nucleus of ovum
- Zona pellucida
- Follicular epithelium

The Theca Cone. As the follicle begins to grow and becomes multilaminar, it tends to sink deeper into the cortical stroma, while the surrounding stromal cells arrange themselves into a circumferential sheath to form the theca folliculi (Fig. 25–5). The growing follicle is then directed toward the ovarian surface by the formation of a wedge-shaped thecal cone (Fig. 25–8) whose details are not seen unless the follicle is sectioned in the proper plane. The directional movement of the thecal cone toward the surface displaces the numerous oocytes stored in the cortex (Fig. 25–8) laterally so that they are not unduly compressed by the rapidly growing and expanding follicles. The stromal cells constituting the theca folliculi differentiate into an inner glandular and vascularized layer, the theca interna (Fig. 25–6), and an outer layer of connective tissue cells, the theca externa. The boundary between the two thecal layers is indistinct, as is that between the theca externa and the surrounding stroma. The theca interna is composed of fibroblast-like cells that multiply to form several concentric layers of cells. In later stages of follicular growth these cells enlarge and differentiate into steroid-secreting cells. They appear either ovoid or spindle-

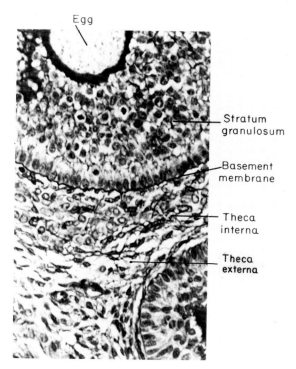

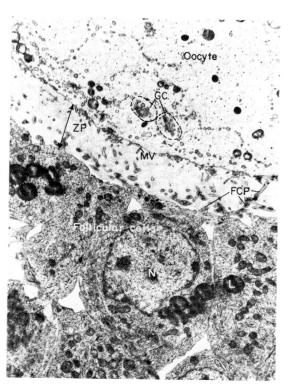

25–6 Section from a multilaminar follicle of a rabbit, showing the thickness of the basement membrane and the transformation of the theca interna into steroid-secreting cells. ×650.

25–7 Electron micrograph of a peripheral sector of a mouse oocyte, its zona pellucida, and the associated follicular cells. Notice the numerous microvilli from the oocyte and the sinuous processes from the follicle cells penetrating the zona pellucida. **ZP,** zona pellucida; **MV,** microvillus; **GC,** Golgi complex; **L,** lipid; **FCP,** follicle cell processes; **N,** nucleus. ×4,200. (Courtesy of D. L. Odor.)

shaped and have rounded nuclei. Lipid droplets are abundant and may be visualized if they are appropriately fixed and stained. When the follicle ovulates, the thecal gland cells persist for only a short time before undergoing degeneration, and they soon disappear completely. Numerous small blood vessels penetrate the theca externa to supply the complex vascular plexus of the theca interna. Blood vessels do not enter the follicular epithelium until after ovulation when the ovulated follicle is transformed into a corpus luteum (See Fig. 25–15).

Development of the Vesicular Follicle. When the follicular cells have proliferated into six to 12 layers, small lakes of follicular fluid appear among them, which stain positively with the PAS technique and are called the Call-Exner bodies (Fig. 25–9). They are thought to represent the precursors of follicular fluid. In some animals such as the rabbit, the Call-Exner bodies are numerous and much more obvious than those in the ovarian follicles of women. The accumulations of follicular fluid enlarge and coalesce to

form a fluid-filled cavity, the follicular antrum (Figs. 25–9, 25–10, and 25–11A). The liquor folliculi is a clear, viscid fluid rich in hyaluronic acid. In sectioned material it often has a granular appearance and stains a pale pink with the PAS technique. An ovarian follicle with a completely formed antrum is described as a secondary or vesicular follicle. By the time antrum formation begins, the oocyte has attained its full size (125–150 μm in human beings) and is encompassed by a fully developed zona pellucida. The follicle continues to enlarge until it reaches a diameter of 8 to 10 mm or more (Fig. 25–11A and B).

In most vesicular follicles the egg, surrounded by several layers of follicular cells, assumes an eccentric position and appears as a small hillock, the cumulus oophorus, which protrudes into the antrum (Fig. 25–11A).

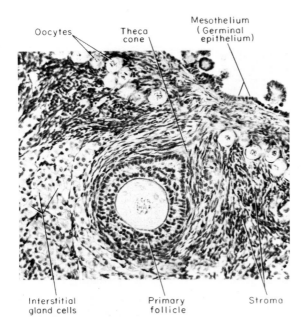

Oocytes   Theca cone   Mesothelium (Germinal epithelium)

Interstitial gland cells   Primary follicle   Stroma

25–8 The appearance of the theca cone in a growing follicle of a rabbit. Note how the primary oocytes are moved aside as the follicle expands toward the surface. × 175.

25–9 A multilaminar, vesicular follicle of a rabbit in which the Call-Exner vacuoles are prominent. Fusion of these vacuoles results in an enlarged antrum filled with follicular fluid. × 85.

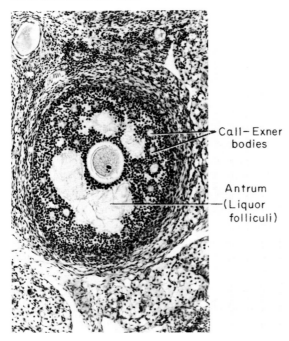

Call-Exner bodies

Antrum (Liquor folliculi)

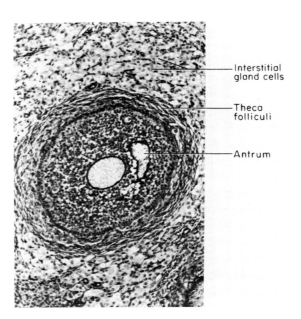

Interstitial gland cells

Theca folliculi

Antrum

25–10 The early formation of an antrum, the concentric arrangement of the cells of the stroma to form the theca folliculi and the arrangement and appearance of the interstitial gland cells of a rabbit ovary. × 75.

The zona pellucida is surrounded by a single continuous layer of follicular cells, the corona radiata (Fig. 25–9), which is anchored to the zona by cytoplasmic processes that penetrate it (Fig. 25–7). The follicular or granulosa cell layer that lines the inside of the follicle is called the stratum granulosa.

The Preovulatory Follicle. The discharge of a mature ovum at ovulation results from a series of complex cytological and growth changes within the egg itself and in the follicular and thecal cells surrounding it. Why only certain of the primordial follicles begin to grow and develop during any particular menstrual cycle is still a mystery.

In the human female, follicles require 12 to 14 days to reach maturity and attain the preovulatory stage. As the follicles reach their maximum size, they may occupy the full thickness of the ovarian cortex and bulge above the surface of the ovary (Fig. 25–11A).

The Follicle as an Endocrine Organ. The initial recruitment and growth of a primordial follicle begins either autonomously or under the trophic influence of unknown hormonal factors.

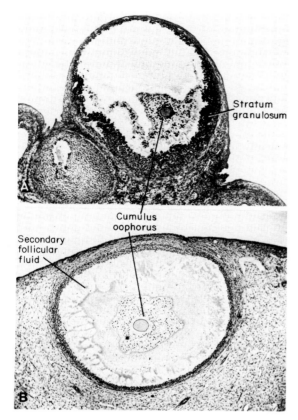

Stratum
granulosum

Cumulus
oophorus

Secondary
follicular
fluid

25–11 Photomicrograph of preovulatory follicles of
(A) rat and **(B)** rabbit. Notice the separation of
the cumulus oophorus from the stratum granulosum.
Notice also the secretion of the secondary follicular
fluid, especially in **B**.

After the follicle is selected, its continued
growth depends on the presence of FSH, a glycoprotein hormone produced by the adenohypophysis and delivered to the ovary by the blood
stream. Follicle-stimulating hormone acts directly and selectively on granulosa cells by
means of specific cell-surface receptors. Granulosa cells also contain receptors specific for estrogen and testosterone. Under the influence of
another adenohypophyseal glycoprotein, LH, the
theca interna cells produce androgens, principally androstenedione and testosterone. The thecal androgens are transported to the granulosa
cells where aromatizing enzymes catalyze their
conversion to estrogen. The aromatization process is induced by FSH. These estrogens, principally estradiol-17β are then transported into the
follicular antrum where they act to promote the
synthesis of their own receptors and to stimulate

the proliferation of the granulosa cells; hence,
the follicle grows. Ovarian estrogens are also released into the perifollicular capillary network
and from there into the general circulation. The
increasing plasma levels of estradiol-17β, late in
the follicular phase serve as a positive feedback
signal at the central nervous system–hypophyseal
axis to cause the preovulatory LH surge (Fig.
25–30). The rising concentration of intrafollicular
estrogen acts on the granulosa cells to induce LH
receptor formation, and, shortly before ovulation,
LH directs the granulosa cells to begin producing
progesterone. The increasing levels of LH act to
reduce the receptor sites available on the granulosa cells for FSH and estradiol-17β, thus reducing estrogen production and shifting to that of
progesterone. The granulosa and theca cells act
interdependently to produce ovarian estrogens.
The "two-cell hypothesis" appears to present the
most logical explanation that brings together recent information on the site of specific steroid
hormone production with that on the appearance
and importance of hormone receptors.

In addition to estrogen and progesterone biosynthesis, the granulosa cells produce a protein
hormone called folliculostatin, which acts as a
negative feedback inhibitor of FSH secretion.
Whereas considerable physiological evidence
supports claims for the existence of folliculostatin, its chemical identity remains unknown.

The complexity of ovarian follicular development and function has been summarized suc-
cinctly in a symposium sponsored by the National Institutes of Child Health and Human
Development and edited by Midgley and Sadler.

Maturation Division (Meiosis) of the Ovum.
Before an egg can be fertilized, it is essential that
its diploid number of chromosomes (46) be reduced to the haploid number (23). This process
begins before the egg is discharged from the follicle and involves the formation of the first polar
body (Fig. 25–12), an event that results in a very
unequal cytoplasmic division. In order to understand fully the various steps in this complex process, the reader is urged to review the process of
meiosis in Chap. 1.

In the human female, all oocytes complete the
earliest stages of meiosis during the fetal period,
so that postnatally the chromosomes are in the
diplotene, or "resting" stage of meiosis. They
will remain in this stage throughout the reproductive life or until the oocyte begins the period
of preovulatory growth, at which time the process of meiosis is resumed. In the formation of

922

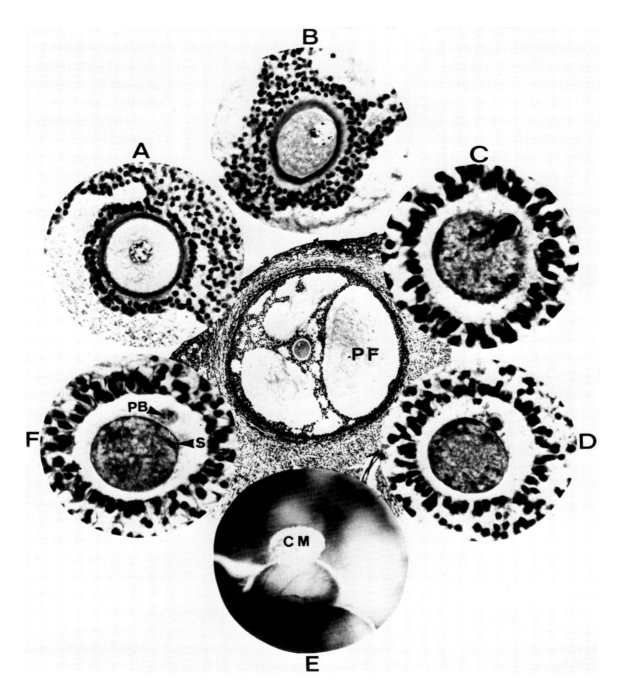

25–12 Stages in the formation of the first polar body in a preovulatory follicle **(PF)** of the rat.
A. The centrally located vesicular nucleus at the beginning of the preovulatory growth phase. **B.** The movement of the nucleus to the periphery of the egg. **C.** Formation of the first polar body. **D.** Abstriction of the polar body vesicle and compacted chromosomes remaining within the egg. **E.** An ovulated follicle from a 16-mm motion picture. **CM,** cumulus mass. **F.** Section of this cumulus mass, showing the first polar body **(PB)** and the second maturation spindle **(S),** with the remaining chromosomes arranged on the metaphase plate.

the first polar body, the vesicular nucleus or germinal vesicle moves to a position just beneath the oolemma, the plasma membrane of the egg (Fig. 25–12B); the chromatids, still attached at their chiasmata, condense and become visible at the microscopic level. The nuclear membrane disappears, and a spindle with fine spindle fibers is formed and assumes a position paratangential to the surface. The chromosomes are grouped on the metaphase plate of the spindle. The spindle then rotates 90° to the egg surface. A small bleb of clear cytoplasm is extruded from the egg and half of the chromosomes are discharged into it (Fig. 25–12C). The first polar body is quickly pinched off and comes to lie free within the perivitelline space (Fig. 25–12D). A second spindle forms immediately and the chromosomes remaining in the egg become arranged on the metaphase plate. This is the condition of the egg at the time of ovulation (Fig. 25–12E and F), and it has required approximately 8 to 10 h to attain this condition. The formation of the second polar body in the second meiotic division must await the transport of the ovulated egg into the ampulla of the oviduct and its penetration by a spermatozoon.

The size of the preovulatory follicle increases significantly during the 12 to 15 h before rupture, the period of preovulatory swelling. It involves (1) a rapid growth of the follicle itself; (2) the secretion of a thinner secondary follicular fluid (Fig. 25–11B) at an increased rate; and, late in this phase, (3) an increased inward folding of the stratum granulosum and theca (Fig. 25–11A; and also Fig. 25–15). Changes occur also in the cumulus oophorus preparatory to freeing the ovum from the stratum granulosum. The intercellular cement anchoring the cumulus cells to one another depolymerizes so that they separate (Fig. 25–11A and B). This separation appears to be related to the action of the LH.

In some animals the cumulus mass, with its enclosed egg, floats free within the antrum (Fig. 25–11B); in others, the strands of cumulus remain attached to the follicle wall until ovulation.

Ovulation. The mechanism of events leading to the rupture of the follicle and expulsion of the egg is still a mystery. The appearance of a bulging follicle above the surface of the ovary may give the impression that increasing intrafollicular pressure leads to its rupture. However, careful measurements of intrafollicular pressure just before ovulation reveal that there is no signifi-

cant increase in pressure even at the moment of rupture. Approximately 30 min before a follicle ruptures, the stratum granulosum, the theca folliculi, and tunica albuginea become thinned out progressively (Fig. 25–13A to C) in a restricted area on the surface of the follicle. This bulging area is called the stigma or macula pellucida. It has been suggested that proteinase, collagenase, or plasmins may depolymerize the collagen fibers in the region of the stigma, weakening the follicular wall. Although these theories are attractive, conclusive evidence as to the role of these substances in follicle rupture is not yet available.

Just before ovulation, a nipple-like cone bulges above the surface of the follicle. Its membranous covering appears similar to the basement membrane that separates the follicular cells from the theca. Within a few minutes this membrane ruptures (Fig. 25–13D), expelling the ovum enclosed in the cumulus oophorus. This event is called ovulation (Fig. 25–13E), and the ovulated egg can now be termed the gamete. Ovulation has been observed in various living anesthetized laboratory animals and recently in the human female, recorded cinematographically. In rats, rabbits, monkeys, and humans, a rather slow extrusion of the follicular contents was observed. The time between rupture of the stigma and discharge of the ovum averaged 72 sec. In many mammals, including primates, the viscous follicular fluid is not completely expressed from the antrum during ovulation. It may remain adherent to the site of the stigma (Fig. 25–13E) until it is swept from the ovarian surface by the cilia lining the fimbriated end of the oviduct.

Formation of the Corpus Luteum. The ovulated follicle is transformed rapidy into a new, highly vascularized, glandular structure, the corpus luteum or luteal gland. It is called the corpus luteum of ovulation if pregnancy does not follow. If pregnancy ensues, it is called the corpus luteum of pregnancy. In pregnancy, the corpus luteum grows much larger and lasts longer.

Even before ovulation the wall of the follicle tends to become folded or plicated (Fig. 25–14A). The plicae are retained (Fig. 25–14B) as the follicle is transformed into a corpus luteum and are a characteristic feature of the fully formed luteal body. The transformation of the ovulatory follicle into a corpus luteum involves, first, the depolymerization of the basement mem-

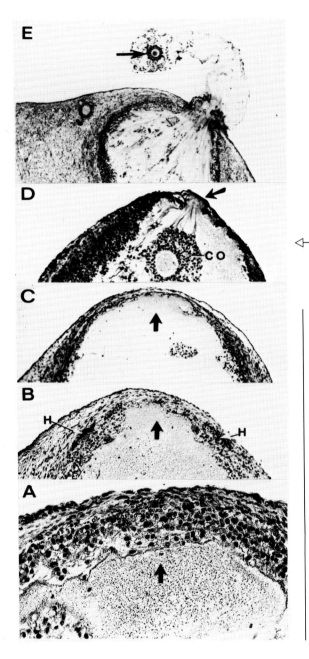

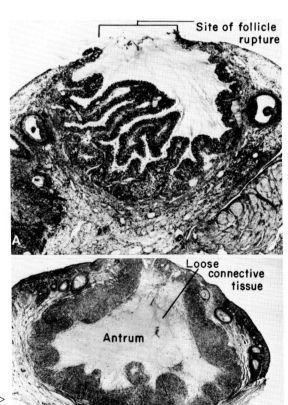

25–13 Stages in the formation of the stigma or macula pellucida in an ovulating follicle in a rabbit. **A.** Several hours before ovulation the stratum granulosum is still quite thick, as are the theca and tunica albuginea. **B.** One-half hour before ovulation hemostasis **(H)** appears in the region of the stigma. There is a significant thinning out of the follicular cells and underlying stroma. **C.** A few minutes before rupture the follicular cells in the region of the stigma have almost disappeared, as has the stromal tissue. **D.** The stigmal cap **(arrow)** lifts away and the free cumulus oophorus **(CO)** streams toward the opening. **E.** Ovulation is completed but the viscous antral fluid still adheres to the site of rupture. The **arrow** points to the egg enclosed by the corona cells, which are in close association with the zona pellucida and the surrounding cumulus oophorus.

25–14 Photomicrograph of two stages in the development of the corpus luteum of the cat. **A.** The recent site of rupture as well as the remarkable foldings of the stratum granulosum. **B.** Several days later the luteal cells appear glandular and the antrum is being invaded by a loose connective tissue.

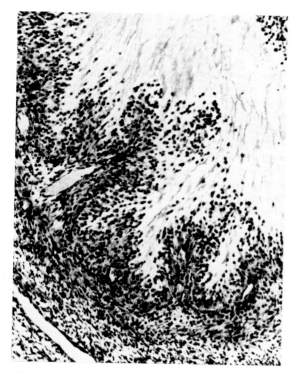

25–15 Section of the wall of a corpus luteum of a monkey 1 day after ovulation. The basement membrane has disappeared. Note that the connective tissue and blood vessels are invading the stratum granulosum. ×70.

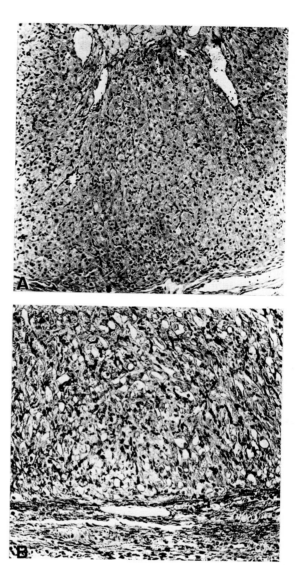

25–16 Corpus luteum at the peak of development (A) and early degeneration (B) in the monkey. A. A section through a corpus luteum 8 or 9 days after ovulation. B. Corpus luteum on first day of menstrual flow. Cells shrunken, extensive lipid vacuolation, nuclei pyknotic. ×75. (Courtesy of G. W. Corner.)

brane that originally separated the granulosa cell layers from the theca. This depolymerization allows the connective tissue cells and blood vessels to invade the stratum granulosum (Fig. 25–15). The granulosa cells of the ovulatory follicle that will become the luteal cells of the corpus luteum begin to undergo cytomorphosis even before ovulation. The large preovulatory follicle secretes both estrogen and progesterone. Mitoses are seldom seen in the glandular parenchymal cells of the developing corpus luteum but are noted in the rapidly developing endothelium of the blood vessels which invade it.

The luteal cells enlarge, become polyhedral, and are filled with lipid droplets (Fig. 25–16A). In ordinary histological preparations the cytoplasm of the luteal cells contains numerous empty vacuoles whose lipid contents are dissolved by the organic solvents used in processing the tissues. It is not known whether the several types of luteal cells that have been described are transitional stages in the differentiation of a single cell type or represent distinct cell species. An interesting feature of the developing corpus luteum is the rapid invasion of the stratum granulosum with connective tissue elements of the theca interna and sprouts of capillary endothelium. The connective tissue forms a delicate reticulum supporting the luteal cells. A com-

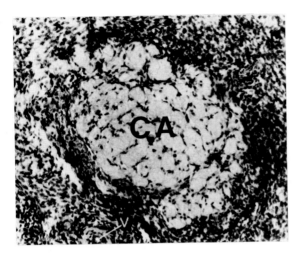

25–17 Corpus albicans **(CA)** in human ovary.

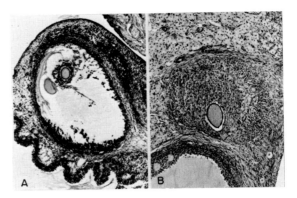

25–18 Follicular atresia. **A.** Cat. Large follicle; cells of stratum granulosum and egg degenerating. **B.** Rabbit. Antrum filled with glandular-appearing cells, egg degenerated but zona pellucida still intact. The theca interna contributes to the interstitial gland tissue.

plex rete network of capillaries forms rapidly throughout the gland. With time, larger blood vessels are formed. The formation of the vascular network in the developing corpus luteum is remarkably similar to that seen during the development of the vascular supply in any embryonic organ.

In electron micrographs of the corpus luteum, the luteal cells have mitochondria with tubular cristae and an abundant smooth ER so characteristic of steroid-secreting cells. The fully formed corpus luteum secretes both estrogens and progestins. If the egg is not fertilized, the corpus luteum lasts for about 14 days. With the egg's demise (Fig. 25–16B), the rate of secretion of estrogens and progestins drops and the corpus luteum begins to undergo involution. The luteal cells become filled with complex lipids and degenerate. With time, a hyaline intercellular material accumulates, and the former corpus luteum assumes the appearance of an irregular white hyaline scar, the corpus albicans (Fig. 25–17). The corpus albicans may persist for many months before it gradually disappears. If, on the other hand, the egg is fertilized and implants into the endometrium of the uterus, the corpus luteum persists. It enlarges to 2 to 3 cm to become the corpus luteum of pregnancy. During pregnancy, the corpus luteum remains functional for several months and then gradually declines as the placenta takes over the task of steroid hormone synthesis and secretion. Involution is accelerated after delivery, leading to the formation of a corpus albicans. A corpus albicans formed from a corpus luteum of pregnancy may last for years.

Atresia of Follicles. As mentioned earlier, atresia, or degeneration of eggs and follicles, at all stages of follicular development is a prominent feature in the life of the ovaries. Large numbers of oocytes degenerate and disappear during the fetal and early postnatal periods. It has been proposed that a primary cause of atresia during these early periods is the disruption or loss of the follicular cells encompassing each oocyte. This possibility suggests that if the life of the oocyte is to be maintained, the follicular cells must be in continuous and intimate contact with the plasma membrane of the egg. Among the groups of follicles that grow to a large size in each menstrual cycle, only one, as a rule, attains full maturity and ovulates. All the remaining large vesicular follicles and many of the smaller ones undergo atresia.

Atresia of a vesicular follicle may occur in many different ways (Fig. 25–18A and B) but always with the usual signs of cell degeneration, such as pyknosis and chromatolysis of the nuclei and shrinkage and dissolution of the cytoplasm. The ooplasm cytolyzes, often leaving only the remnant of the zona pellucida to mark the location of the ovum. Macrophage invasion of atretic follicles is a regular feature. The zona pellucida, composed of complex mucopolysaccharides, is

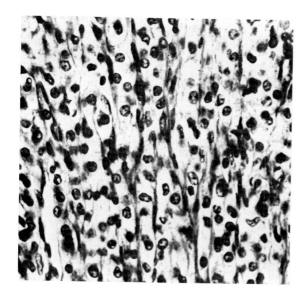

25–19 Mature interstitial gland tissue at 8.5 months of gestation in a woman. Notice the arrangement of the glandular cells and the nuclei of the capillary endothelium between the rows of cells. ×520. (Courtesy of H. W. Mossman.)

more highly polymerized, but eventually it, too, is broken down and engulfed by macrophages. Occasionally, the basement membrane separating the follicular cells from the theca interna increases in thickness, assumes a corrugated hyaline-like appearance, and is then called the glassy membrane. In some atretic follicles the cells of the theca interna enlarge, become epithelioid, and may be arrayed in a radial or cord-like fashion (Fig. 25–19). These cords of cells may be separated from one another by delicate connective tissue fibers and a capillary network. The cells are often filled with lipid droplets, giving them an appearance of an old corpus luteum.

The Interstitial Gland. The origin, development, and endocrine function of the interstitial gland or interstitial cells of the ovary have been the subject of much confusion and controversy. In many mammals, such as the rabbit (Figs. 25–8 and 25–9) and women (Fig. 25–19), clusters or cords of large, epithelioid cells with cytology and vascularity typical of endocrine glands are dispersed in the cortical stroma. These cells are referred to collectively as the interstitial gland or interstitial cells. Cytologically, they resemble luteal cells to a remarkable degree.

The interstitial gland is present periodically in the ovary of the human female from before birth until well after the menopause. The interstitial cells are thought to originate from the cells of the theca interna of degenerating large secondary follicles or degenerating vesicular follicles of all sizes. Thecal gland cells are formed from the theca interna cells of ripening follicles that are not destined to ovulate. They are present only in sexually mature individuals and only at or near the time of ovulation. The thecal gland is an important source of estrogens.

Differentiation of interstitial gland tissue is cyclic and is probably related to the rhythmic atresia of the various crops of vesicular follicles during the menstrual cycle or pregnancy. The role of the interstitial gland cells in normal ovarian physiology is yet to be completely defined. Studies on steroidogenesis in the ovarian stroma in women show that it principally synthesizes estrogens. In rabbits, on the other hand, interstitial cells are stimulated directly by gonadotrophins to synthesize and secrete 20α-OH-progesterone. Many researchers believe that the interstitial gland plays a significant role in providing estrogens for the growth and development of the secondary sex organs during the prepubertal period.

Other groups of epithelioid cells may be found in the region of the hilum of the ovary in the human and are called hilus cells. These cells are usually associated with vascular spaces and unmyelinated nerve fibers. They appear glandular; contain lipids, cholesterol esters, and lipochrome pigments; and are identified best during pregnancy and at the onset of the menopause. The common finding of Reineke crystalloids suggests a kinship to the interstitial cells of the testes. Tumors or hyperplasia of the hilus cells usually leads to masculinization. Although the evidence is tenuous, it is suggested that these cells secrete steroids related to androgens.

Vessels and Lymphatics. The ovaries have a rich blood supply from several sources. The principal arteries are the ovarian arteries, which arise from the aorta below the level of the renal vessels. They travel a relatively long course through the infundibulopelvic ligaments to reach the ovaries. The ovarian arteries anastomose with the uterine arteries, which are branches of the hypogastrics.

The veins accompany the arteries and often

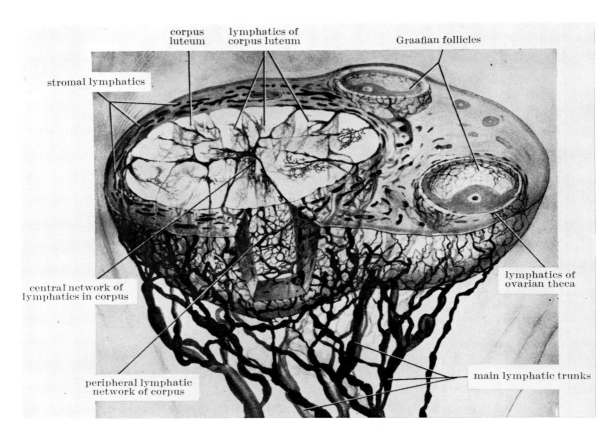

corpus luteum

lymphatics of corpus luteum

Graafian follicles

stromal lymphatics

central network of lymphatics in corpus

lymphatics of ovarian theca

peripheral lymphatic network of corpus

main lymphatic trunks

25–20 Diagram showing the arrangement of lymphatics within and around a corpus luteum, Graafian follicles, and stroma in the ovary of the ewe. (Courtesy of B. Morris.)

form a complex plexus of vessels in the hilum. Of principal interest are the cyclic change and continuous reorganization of the vascular pattern of the ovaries as crops of follicles and corpora lutea grow, perform their function, and degenerate. Thus, with each cycle, an extensive blood and lymphatic system develops to support the growth and cytodifferentiation of various cells.

The ovary has a lymphatic system (Fig. 25–20) whose ubiquity and complexity are seldom appreciated. Large numbers of lymphatic vessels are organized around the developing follicles and corpora lutea. The extrinsic lymphatic drainage follows a course to the aortic, preaortic, and paraaortic lymph nodes in the pelvis.

In developing follicles, the lymphatics are arranged in a basket-like network within the theca folliculi but, like the blood vessels, do not penetrate into the stratum granulosum. The corpora lutea, however, are heavily infiltrated by lymphatic vessels (Fig. 25–20). The lymphatic capillaries often have open intercellular junctions so that materials from the interstitial pores can readily enter the vessels. It has been shown in the ewe, for example, that coincident with the formation of the corpus luteum, lymph flow from the ovary increases significantly. It has been suggested that there may be an association between the synthesis and secretion of steroid hormones by the corpus luteum and an increase in capillary permeability.

Nerves. The nerves of the ovaries are derivatives of the ovarian plexus and uterine nerves. All vessels and nerves enter the ovary through the hilum. Most of the nerves are nonmyelinated and sympathetic and supply the muscular coats of arterioles. Some nonmyelinated fibers form plexuses around multilaminar follicles. Whether nerves are associated also with the generalized smooth muscle cells in the ovary is unknown. A few sensory nerve endings have been described in the ovarian stroma.

The Oviducts

The oviducts extend bilaterally from the uterus to the region of the ovary (Fig. 25–1). They provide the necessary environment for fertilization and segmentation of the egg until it attains the morula stage of development. The fertilized egg remains within the oviduct for approximately 3 days before it enters the uterus.

The oviducts in the sexually mature human female are 10 to 12 cm in length. They are suspended by a rather loose mesentery, the mesosalpinx (Fig. 25–1), a derivative of the broad ligament. In the human, each oviduct may be divided into several linear segments distinguishable by gross examination and by studying transverse sections taken at different levels throughout the tube. These segments consist of the interstitial segment, which pierces the uterine wall; the isthmus (Fig. 25–1), which constitutes approximately two-thirds of the oviduct; and the somewhat more dilated ampulla (Fig. 25–1), which extends from the isthmus to the infundibulum. The free margin of the funnel-shaped infundibulum is extensively folded and fluted, giving it a fimbriated or tentacle-like appearance (Fig. 25–1). These folds are called fimbriae. At the time of ovulation the fimbriated end of the infundibulum embraces the ovary, almost completely enclosing it and forming the ovarian bursa. At least 50% of the surface epithelial cells are ciliated. All of the cilia, irrespective of their location on the surface of the fimbriae and in the ampullae beat toward the uterus. The wall of the oviduct consists of a complex mucous membrane, several muscle layers, and, peripherally, a serosa.

The Mucosa. Throughout the length of the oviduct the mucous membrane extends into the lumen in a linear system of complex folds. These mucosal folds are so elaborately branched, especially in the ampulla, that normally there is only a potential lumen (Fig. 25–21). Approximately 50% of the cells lining the ampullary mucosa are ciliated and are arranged in irregular rows. The secretory cells appear in groups between the ciliated cells. They often bulge above the surface, the extent of the bulging depending on the time

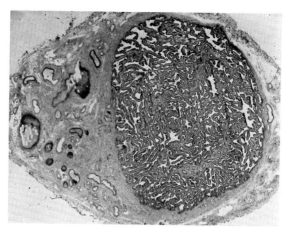

25–21 A cross section of a human ampulla removed surgically at midcycle. To avoid shrinkage the oviduct was frozen in liquid nitrogen and then sectioned and stained. Note the complexity of the mucosal folds that almost completely fill the lumen.

in the menstrual cycle (Fig. 25–22). The mucosal folds of the isthmus are much less complicated and have fewer ciliated cells (Fig. 25–23). As the isthmus approaches the uterus, the diameter of its lumen is greatly decreased.

25–22 Photomicrograph showing ciliated and glandular cells **(arrow)** of the surface epithelium of the ampulla of the oviduct of the monkey. (Courtesy of R. Brenner.)

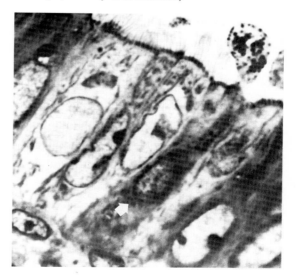

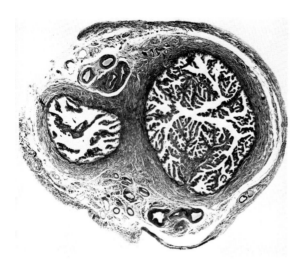

25–23 A cross section of a human isthmus removed surgically at midcycle, frozen in liquid nitrogen, and then sectioned and stained. Note that the mucosal folds are far less complicated than those of the ampulla.

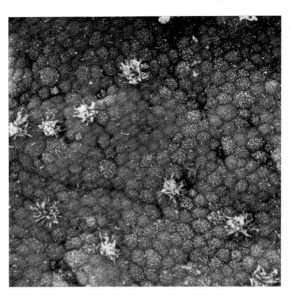

25–24 A scanning electron micrograph of the surface of the ampulla from a postmenopausal woman. Note that a few ciliated cells are present.

It has been frequently stated that at about the time of ovulation, steroid hormones, such as progesterone, accelerate the rate of ciliary beating. Recent studies in which the newer techniques of laser spectrometry were used have revealed that the rate of ciliary beat before and after ovulation remains extraordinarily constant (approximately 22 beats/sec) and that estrogen and progestogens do not affect the rate of beat.

Although there are rhythmic contractions of the ampullae in primates, they do not appear to affect the rate of movement of the ovulated cumulus egg mass within the ampullar lumen. Direct observations of egg transport through this segment in the living primate clearly show that the cilia play the primary role in transporting the eggs through the ampulla to the ampullo-isthmic junction, the normal site of fertilization.

The development of cilia in the oviduct is dependent on the presence of the ovary. In women born without ovaries, no ciliated cells develop and the mucosal folds are little more than broad ridges.

It has now been clearly established that ciliogenesis in the primate oviductal epithelium is an estrogen-driven phenomenon. That estrogens are important in ciliogenesis may be dramatically demonstrated in oviducts from postmenopausal patients. After the menopause, the epithe-

lium normally is of the low cuboidal type and there are few ciliated cells (Fig. 25–24). If postmenopausal patients have been on long-term estrogen therapy, one often sees a richly ciliated epithelium similar to those in women in the reproductive age at midcycle (Fig. 25–25).

Muscularis. The muscularis of the oviduct consists, in general, of an inner circular or spiral layer and an external layer of rather poorly defined longitudinal fibers. There is no distinct boundary between the two. A third, inner layer of longitudinal muscles has been described in the proximal isthmus in the oviducts of the human female. There is an obvious increase in the thickness of the circular muscle layers as the isthmus approaches the uterus. The thickness of the muscularis decreases significantly, particularly in the ampulla and infundibulum. As the muscularis thins, it is increasingly difficult to decipher the orientation and delineate the planes of smooth muscle layers in the ampulla, particularly as they approach and enter the fimbriae. The peritoneal coat of the oviduct is covered by a thin serosa.

Blood Vessels, Lymphatics, and Nerves. The arterial blood supply of the oviducts is derived from both the uterine and ovarian arteries. In hu-

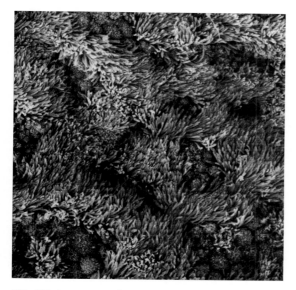

25–25 A scanning electron micrograph of the surface of the ampulla from a postmenopausal woman who had been on continuous estrogen therapy for more than 10 years. The richly ciliated surface is remarkably similar to that of a young woman during the active reproductive period.

mans the amount contributed by each varies among individuals. Borell and Fernström found that occasionally in women only one of the arteries supplied the entire oviduct and that the endocrine status of the woman determined the width of its adnexal branches. Anastomoses of the ovarian and uterine arteries are common. The venous drainage, although often showing significant variation, generally follows the arterial blood supply. The lymphatic supply is extensive and elaborately developed.

The nerve fibers of the oviducts originate in the sympathetic division of the autonomic nervous system and are conveyed in the hypogastric nerves to both the isthmus and ampulla. Other sympathetic preganglionic fibers synapse in the ovarian plexus and from there supply the fimbriae and part of the ampulla. The parasympathetic innervation of the oviduct is derived also from two sources. The interstitial portion of the isthmus is innervated by the pelvic nerve, and the distal portion of the oviduct is innervated via the vagus nerve through the ovarian plexus.

It is generally believed that cholinergic fibers supply the mucosa whereas the muscularis is under adrenergic control. The extent to which the various subdivisions of the oviduct are innervated and the function of the cholinergic and adrenergic fibers in oviductal physiology remains controversial.

Uterus

The human uterus is a hollow, pear-shaped organ with a thick muscular wall. It receives the oviducts and opens into the vagina through the cervical canal (Fig. 25–1). It lies in the pelvic cavity interposed between the bladder and rectum. Its size varies among nonpregnant women. The average dimensions are: length, 6.3 cm; breadth, 4.5 cm; and thickness, 2.5 cm. The expanded rostral portion is called the body or corpus uteri, and the caudal portion, a part of which protrudes into the upper vagina, is the cervix. The cervical canal passes from the uterine cavity through the cervix and opens into the vagina. The opening visible from within the vagina is called the external os (Fig. 25–1). The term fundus refers to the dome-shaped upper portion of the body of the uterus from which the oviducts extend. The body of the uterus is flattened anteroposteriorly, and the lumen appears as a transverse slit. The cavity of the uterus is confluent with the lumina of the oviducts.

The wall of the uterus is composed of an internal layer, the endometrium (glandular mucosa); a middle layer, the myometrium (muscularis); and an external layer, the perimetrium (serosa) (Fig. 25–1). It should be noted that the posterocaudal third of the uterus does not have a serosa, since this portion of the uterus lies below the peritoneal reflection. The connective tissue of the broad ligament at the lateral edges of the uterus is termed the parametrium.

Endometrium. In humans, beginning at puberty and continuing until the menopause, the uterine mucosa undergoes cyclic changes in structure and secretory activity. The terminal event in each cycle is a partial destruction and sloughing of a portion of the endometrium, accompanied by some extravasation of blood, an event termed menstruation. The endometrium is a complex mucous membrane (Fig. 25–26). Its height varies from 1 to 7 mm with the phases of the menstrual cycle and in early pregnancy (Fig. 25–27A, B, and C). It consists of a simple columnar epithelium and a wide lamina propria, the endometrial stroma. It is firmly attached to the myometrium without any intervening submu-

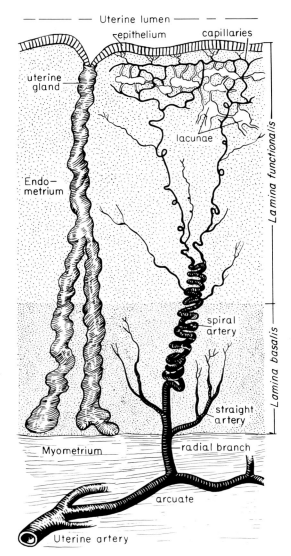

25–26 Diagrammatic representation of the glands and vasculature of the human endometrium.

epithelium of both the glands and surface epithelium. The stroma in which the uterine glands are embedded resembles mesenchymal tissue (Fig. 25–27C); the cells, stellate in appearance, are loosely arranged and often have oval nuclei.

The endometrium is usually divided into two layers or zones (Fig. 25–26), differing in their morphology and function: a lamina basalis or basal layer and a lamina functionalis or functional layer.

The basal layer is attached directly to the myometrium and occasionally may extend into small pockets in the muscularis. Dr. Carl Hartman once removed all the endometrial tissue from the uterus of a menstruating rhesus monkey with scalpel and scissors and then scrubbed away the remaining bits of tissue with cotton swabs. At the end of the next menstrual cycle, he was surprised to find a completely regenerated endometrium. This was a dramatic demonstration of the regenerative capacity of the endometrium even from the bits of tissue tucked into the small pockets of the myometrium (Fig. 25–27B and C).

There is considerable variation among women in the thickness of the basal layer of endometrium. Its stroma is much more cellular and fibrous than that of the functional zone. The basal layer undergoes few obvious microscopic changes during a menstrual cycle and serves principally as a source of tissue for the cyclic regeneration of the functional layer. The functional layer rises from the basal layer toward the lumen of the uterus and is the site of the principal cyclic changes in the endometrium, which prepare a bed for the fertilized ovum. The endometrial tissue, particularly in its functional zone, undergoes constant histological change, which is related directly to the secretion of the various hormones by the ovary.

The epithelial cells during the early follicular phase are tall columnar cells (Fig. 25–28) with numerous long, narrow microvilli extending from their surfaces. Their nuclei may be elongated or quite irregular in shape, their mitochondria are relatively small, and their Golgi complexes assume a supranuclear position. Many cells show cytoplasmic inclusions and granules of varying size and shape. At this stage in the cycle, glycogen is not discernible by electron microscopy. Dramatic changes in the cytology of cells (Fig. 25–29) are seen during the mid luteal phase, when the corpus luteum is actively secreting both estrogens and progestogens. The mi-

cosa. The stroma contains many simple tubular uterine glands (Fig. 25–27B) that open onto the surface of the mucosa, extend deep into the endometrial stroma, and end blindly near the muscularis. Occasionally, they are branched in the area adjacent to the myometrium. The epithelium lining the glands and that covering the surface appear identical. Occasionally, patches of ciliated cells may be seen either within the glands or on the surface epithelium facing the lumen. There is a basement membrane beneath the

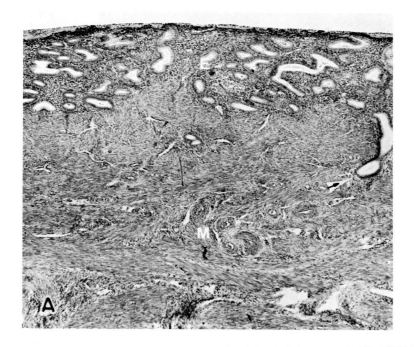

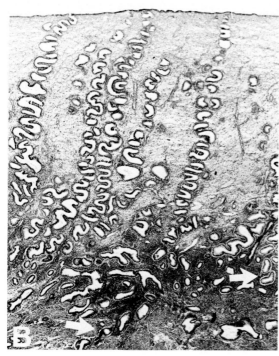

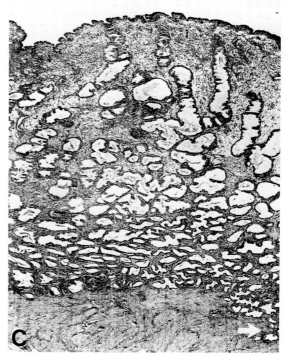

25–27 Photomicrographs of human endometria
during the menstrual cycle and pregnancy.
A. Shedding of the stratum functionalis has been
completed. Regeneration of the endometrium has just
begun. **E,** endometrium; **M,** myometrium. **B.** Early
secretory endometrium. **C.** Gestational endometrium,
fourteenth day of pregnancy. Notice the arrows
pointing out stratum basalis tissue in crypts of
myometrium.

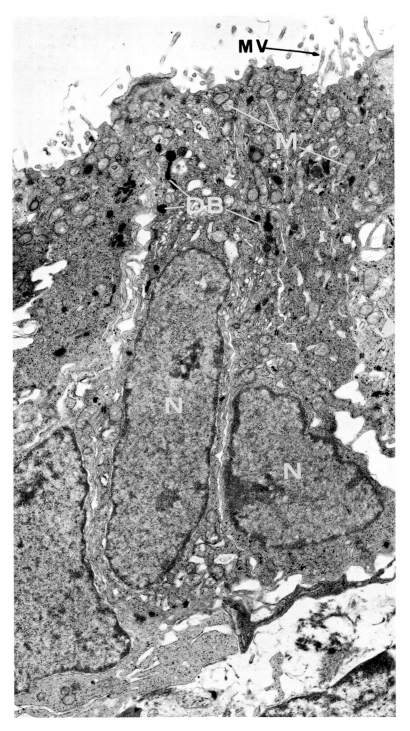

25–28 Electron micrograph of human epithelial endometrial cells during the early follicular phase. **N**, nucleus; **M**, mitochondria; **DB**, dense bodies; **MV**, microvilli. ×10,500. (Courtesy of E. R. Friedrich.)

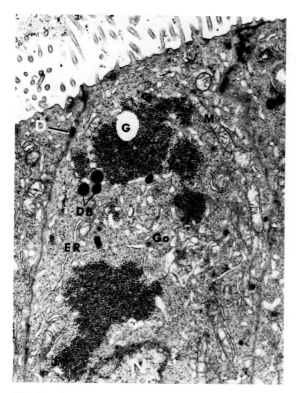

25–29 Electron micrograph of the apical portion of the midsecretory phase of human endometrium. Notice the large glycogen deposits **(G)**, the slightly dilated Golgi structure **(Go)**, and a few remaining dense bodies **(DB)**. **D**, desmosome; **ER**, endoplasmic reticulum; **M**, mitochondria. (Courtesy of E. R. Friedrich.)

tween the outer and middle third of the myometrium and from which radial branches extend inward to supply the endometrium. There may be 20 or more radial branches (sometimes called submucous vessels) from each arcuate artery. The spiral arteries (Fig. 25–26) are particularly characteristic of the endometrium. They pass through the basalis and extend into the functional zone. The proximal part of the vessel is an unchanging segment, whereas the distal end is subject to repeated degeneration and regeneration with each menstrual cycle. The typical development of the spiral arteries is dependent on a certain ratio of estrogens and progestins. Branches of the spiral vessels serve the tissues of the basalis as independent arteries or arterioles. The straight arteries (Fig. 25–26) are not subject to the actions of hormones.

As the spiral vessels traverse the functionalis, they divide into several terminal arterioles that frequently anastomose with one another. These arterioles, in turn, connect with a complex rete network of capillary units and lacunas (Fig. 25–26). The lacunas are very thin, dilated vessels that vary greatly in size. These structures are ordinarily not classified as part of the venous system but rather are terminal ectatic capillaries or connecting lacunas and are defined as part of the arterial vasculature. The venules and veins also form an irregular network with sinusoidal enlargements called collecting lacunas (Fig. 25–26). The endometrial veins flow into a venous plexus concentrated at the basalis-myometrial border.

Cyclic Changes in the Endometrium. The cyclic changes in the tissues of the endometrium are a direct response to the fluctuating concentrations of the various ovarian steroids (Fig. 25–30). The synthesis of the ovarian steroids and their rate of secretion are regulated by the cyclic secretions of neurohormones produced by a network of secretory neurons in the hypothalamus that are carried via the pituitary portal system to the adenohypophysis and effect the release of FSH and LH. All of these cyclic, secretory functions are modulated by a series of feedback mechanisms initiated by the ovarian steroids. Much information is now available about the elaborate enzymatic and cytochemical interrelationships of steroid hormone synthesis and metabolism involved in the control of the normal menstrual cycle (Yen and Jaffe, 1978).

tochondria are larger and are surrounded by narrow tubules of rough ER. Large aggregates of glycogen, as well as numerous polyribosomes, are present. During the later luteal phase, the apical portions of the cells are filled with glycogen. The apical cell membrane becomes distended and ruptures, releasing glycogen and other cytoplasmic components into the lumen. During the premenstrual or degenerative phase, the mitochondria are significantly smaller and lysosomes increase in number. Myelin figures or lipid droplets form within the remaining glycogen deposits.

A unique and very elaborate vascular system is developed in anticipation of an implanting embryo. The uterine artery gives off six to 10 arcuate arteries (Fig. 25–26), which extend be-

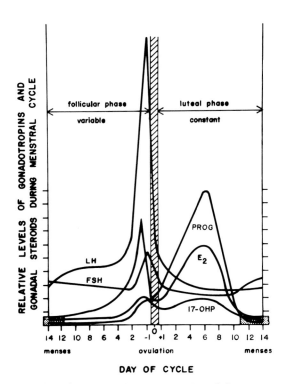

25–30 A diagrammatic representation of the secretions of the various pituitary and ovarian hormones during a single menstrual cycle in the human.

The endometrium passes through three successive phases that correspond to the functional activity of the ovary. The follicular phase, which varies in length, is concurrent with the growth of the follicles and estrogen secretion. The luteal phase, which is more constant in length, coincides with the functional length of the corpus luteum, and the menstrual phase lasts through the period of menstrual bleeding.

FOLLICULAR PHASE. During the follicular phase, the endometrium increases in thickness from 1 to 3 mm. The endometrial glands become longer and more numerous. Many mitoses may be seen throughout the epithelium and the stroma. The epithelial cells, particularly in the glands, become taller and accumulate a considerable store of glycogen basal to the nucleus. No doubt other presecretory substances accumulate as well. The surface epithelium is simple columnar. A few ciliated cells may be scattered here and there but may be more numerous around the openings of the glands. The glands are either straight-walled or slightly wavy. They secrete a thin mucoid layer. The stroma during this time is rich in mucoid substance.

In the follicular phase, the coiled arteries lengthen with the regrowth of the endometrium and extend through more than half its thickness. They are lightly coiled.

LUTEAL PHASE. Remarkable modifications of the endometrium ensue within a day or two after ovulation. The glands become irregularly coiled and the glandular epithelium begins to secrete. The lumen of each gland becomes filled with a mucoid fluid rich in nutrients, particularly glycogen. The glycogen moves from a subnuclear position to the apical surface and is discharged from the cells. The glands enlarge and often become sacculated, especially in the deeper third of the mucosa. The endometrium gradually becomes more edematous and may increase in thickness to 5 or 6 mm. This increase is primarily due to swelling of the tissues rather than to proliferation of cells. The mesenchymatous cells of the stroma share in this edematous condition. During the luteal phase, the coiled arteries lengthen and become more spiral. Near the end of the cycle, rather characteristic decidual changes are often seen in the stromal cells.

Decidual cells differentiate from stromal fibroblasts. When fully formed they appear as large "epithelial" cells usually with two or more nuclei, each with several nucleoli. They contain significant stores of glycogen and fat. The decidual cells probably have a nutritive function during the implantation process.

MENSTRUAL PHASE. Reduction in hormonal activity of the corpus luteum 4 to 5 days before menstruation has a profound effect on the endometrium. Changes in the hemodynamics of blood flow in the functionalis are of primary significance in understanding the process of menstruation. The endometrium becomes ischemic and stops secreting. The functionalis shrinks, owing to loss of ground substance and water. The stromal cells become closely packed and densely stained. The lumina of the glands are reduced or obliterated in the general collapse of the endometrium. There is an intermittent constriction of the spiral vessels, resulting in reduced arterial and venous blood flow and stasis in the capillaries. Approximately 2 days after the endometrium begins its decline, the epithelium becomes disrupted, and blood, uterine fluid, and desquamated bits of the mucosa are sloughed from the functionalis and discharged via the vagina. This period of bloody vaginal discharge, lasting roughly 5 days, is termed the menses. The menstrual process begins with extravasation of blood from capillaries or from arterioles into the stroma. These localized accumulations of blood "lakes" or hematomas cause further endometrial ischemia and pressure necrosis as they coalesce and then rupture onto the mucosal surface. Fragments of mucosa detach, leaving exposed stroma and naked vessels. The disintegrating functionalis becomes tattered and soaked with blood. Desquamation of tissue continues until the stratum functionalis is discarded.

Menstrual blood is both arterial and venous. Clotting is inhibited, and hemostasis is dependent on vasoconstriction. Arterial bleeding is intermittent and brief, coincident with the period of relaxation of the coiled arteries, whereas bleeding from veins is a light but protracted seepage. The coiled arteries are shed piecemeal and more slowly than the neighboring stroma and glands, so they often protrude from the denuded surface of the menstruating endometrium. Small tufts of clotted blood fill the lumina at the tips of the coiled vessels. The straight arteries serving the stratum basalis do not become constricted during menstruation; hence, the stratum basalis remains well supplied with blood while the functionalis is being sloughed.

The functionalis is usually lost entirely, leaving only the basalis with the exposed blind ends of the glands. Elsewhere the mucosal surface is denuded and raw. When hemorrhage stops and a new set of ovarian follicles begins to develop, remnants of healthy uterine epithelium, particularly from the mouths of the glands, proliferate rapidly and provide the denuded areas with an epithelial covering.

THE GRAVID CYCLE. It takes about 3 days for the fertilized ovum (zygote) to reach the uterus. The zygote undergoes rapid embryonic growth and by the fifth day develops into a blastocyst. By the early part of the second week of the luteal phase, it becomes embedded in the uterine mucosa (implantation, nidation). At this time, the peripheral cellular elements of the blastocyst (the chorion, consisting of the trophoblast and extraembryonic mesoderm) begin secreting a hormone known as human chorionic gonadotropin (hCG), which is a factor in maintaining the life and function of the corpus luteum beyond the usual limits of a menstrual cycle. The growth of the endometrium is not interrupted; there is no menstrual flow, and this circumstance is commonly denoted as the first missed period. A secretory or progestational endometrium becomes a gestational endometrium (Fig. 25–27C) by the fact of pregnancy. The endometrium undergoes further progestational development to become the decidua of early pregnancy. Placentation is discussed fully in Chap. 27.

Myometrium. The musculature of the uterus forms a thick tunic that is composed of three muscle layers somewhat blended because of complex interconnecting bundles, yet interspersed by considerable connective tissue. Well-defined muscle layers are not easily discernible over the body of the uterus. In general, the cells in the central portion of the muscularis are more circularly disposed, whereas those to either side tend to be directed obliquely or longitudinally. The middle region of the muscularis contains many large blood and lymphatic vessels (stratum vasculare). Over the cervix, the muscularis is layered in a relatively defined manner; there are an inner and outer longitudinal layer and a middle circular layer. Elastic fibers, although few and peripherally located in the uterus, are abundant in the outer wall of the cervix.

In the nonpregnant uterus the muscle cells are about 0.25 mm in length. During pregnancy, they increase in number and in size and may reach a length of 5 mm by the end of gestation, with a commensurate increase in cell thickness. New smooth muscle cells are added by differentiation from undifferentiated connective tissue cells and probably by division of preexisting smooth muscle cells. Because many of these muscle cells remain after childbirth, the uterus does not revert to its virginal size. Other changes accompanying the distension of the pregnant uterus are an increase in elastic tissue peripheral to the myometrium and a striking growth of the blood vessels; during the last 20 weeks of gestation the uterus ceases to increase in weight and the myometrium becomes progressively thinner.

Perimetrium. The pelvic peritoneum surrounding the uterine tubes and most of the uterus constitutes their serosa. It extends from the sides of the uterus, forming the broad ligaments through which blood and lymph vessels and nerves reach the uterus on each side. The larger vessels are exceptionally tortuous.

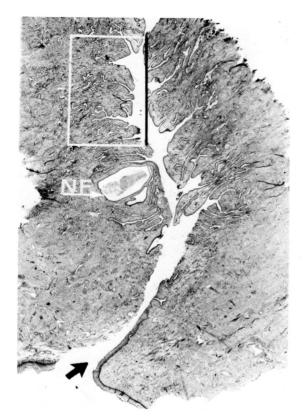

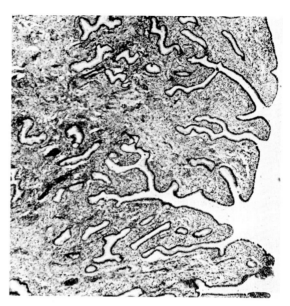

Embedded in the perimetrium are the sympathetic ganglia and plexuses. The sympathetic supply to the uterus is derived from the hypogastric plexus, and the parasympathetic supply is by the way of rami from the second, third, and often the fourth sacral nerves. Large nerve trunks enter the uterus at the cervix and extend to all parts of the body and fundus. The musculature and blood vessels are abundantly supplied, and some fibers ramify in the endometrium, forming a network around the glands. Nothing is known about the significance of these fibers or what happens to them during the cyclic sloughing and regeneration of the superficial layer of the endometrium. No ganglia have been found within the wall of the uterus.

The Cervix. The cervix uteri (Fig. 25–31) encloses the cervical canal, which is approximately 3 cm long and slightly distended in the middle

portion. The mucosal lining of the cervix, the endocervix, is continuous with that of the body of the uterus (Fig. 25–1) but differs sharply in both its epithelium and underlying stroma. The mucous membrane, 3 to 5 mm thick, forms very complex deep furrows or compound clefts called the plicae palmatae (Fig. 25–32). These folds run in longitudinal, transverse, and oblique directions and form a very irregular arrangement that may penetrate the entire thickness of the mucosa. This arrangement of folds is often misinterpreted as being a system of branching tubular glands of the compound racemose variety. The basic pattern, then, of the epithelium of the cervical canal is a complex system of clefts with accessory folds and tunnel-like projections. The lining epithelium of the plicae palmatae consists of a single layer of tall mucus-secreting cells. Some of the epithelial cells are ciliated, with the cilia beating toward the vagina. There is no hard evidence that the ciliated cells play any significant role either in sperm transport through the cervix or in the flow of mucus from the surface of the secretory cells. The height of the cells and the position of their nuclei vary with the time of the cycle and their secretory activity. During the follicular and luteal phases, the epithelial cells synthesize mucus and other substances and

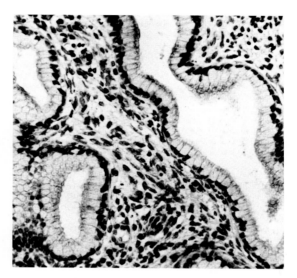

25–34 Epithelium of human cervical glands. Cells laden with mucus. Notice the basal position of the nuclei. H&E stain. ×240. (Courtesy of E. R. Friedrich.)

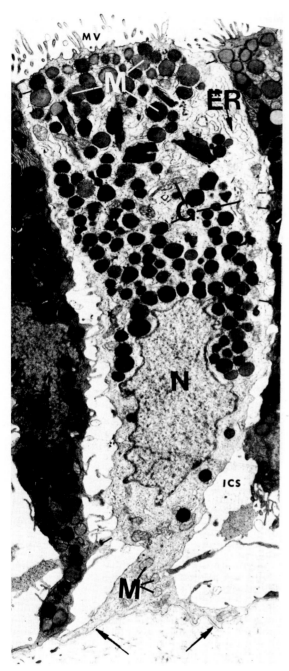

25–33 Electron micrograph of human endocervical epithelial cells. **Arrows,** basement membrane; **N,** nucleus; **G,** Golgi complexes; **ER,** granular endoplasmic reticulum; **M** (white), mucous granules; **MV,** microvilli; **M** (black), mitochondria; **ICS,** intercellular pores. ×7,800. (Courtesy of E. R. Friedrich.)

package them in membrane-bounded vacuoles (Fig. 25–33). The cells laden with these materials stain poorly, and their nuclei are pushed to the base of the cells (Fig. 25–34). During active secretion, the nuclei rise to the center of the cells (Fig. 25–35) as the secreted mucus distends the lumina of the glands. The cervical mucus has its origin in this single layer of columnar secretory cells that line the intricate system of crypts. The biophysical properties of the cervical mucus are largely determined by the action of estrogens and progestogens on the secretory cells and are responsible for the complex rheological properties of the mucus, attributes that vary dramatically at different times in the menstrual cycle. Cervical mucus is a concentrated solution of glycoprotein rich in carbohydrates. It is a colloid with rheological characteristics of viscoelasticity, which implies that it possesses both solid and fluid-like properties. In humans, at about the time of ovulation the cervical mucus is a voluminous hydrophilic gel. It is composed of a high-viscosity component (gel phase) and a low-viscosity component that consists of a variety of electrolytes and organic compounds such as glucose, amino acids, and soluble proteins. It consists of approximately 99.5% water, which is bound within the complex of mucins. When the molecular arrangement of the glycoproteins in mid cycle cervical mucus is determined by laser light-

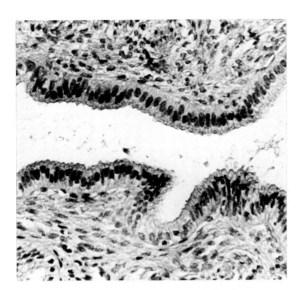

25–35 Epithelium of human cervical glands in active secretion. Notice the change in the position of the nuclei and the secretory materials within the lumen. H&E stain. ×240. (Courtesy of E. R. Friedrich.)

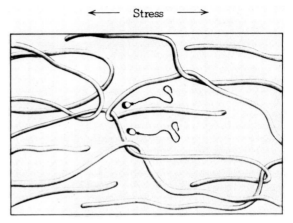

25–36 The hypothetical arrangement of the mucin macromolecules in stretched human cervical mucus at midcycle. Active flagellation of the spermatozoa realign the macromolecules in a linear direction.

scattering spectroscopy (Lee et al., 1977), it can be shown that the mucus is composed of an ensemble of entangled randomly coiled macromolecules. As spermatozoa penetrate the mucus they reorient the entangled macromolecules in a linear arrangement (Fig. 25–36). The reorientation is effected by the mechanical forces generated by the active flagellations of the spermatozoa (Fig. 25–37). It is well known that spermatozoa can penetrate mid cycle cervical mucus much more readily than the mucus secreted during the luteal phase of the cycle. In fact, luteal cervical mucus acts as a barrier to sperm transport into the uterus. The luteal mucus is composed also of an ensemble of macromolecules, but they are much more tightly packed because the mucus contains less water. Thus the cyclic changes in the macrorheological properties of mucus appear to be due simply to changes in the degree of hydration of the entangled molecular network.

The mucosa of the cervix does not take part in the menstrual changes, so it is not sloughed. After the menopause, the mucosa shrinks, the glandular epithelium becomes gradually flattened, and the secretory activity is arrested. The subepithelial tissue of the human cervix is composed predominantly of a dense connective tissue. Smooth muscle makes up approximately 15% of the tissue, and the distal portion of the cervix (partio vaginalis) contains no smooth muscle. The connective tissue and smooth muscle are arranged in a very complex pattern.

Vagina

The vagina is a thick-walled fibromuscular tube that forms the lowermost segment of the reproductive tract and connects the uterus with the outside of the body. The wall consists of a mucosa, a muscularis, and a heavy covering of connective tissue. The lumen of the vagina is flattened anteroposteriorly. The mucosa is thrown into numerous transverse folds or rugae (Fig. 25–1).

The mucous membrane consists of a stratified squamous epithelium many cell layers thick, resting on a papillated lamina propria (Fig. 25–38). Cells in the outer layers are greatly flattened and may contain keratohyaline granules, but they are not strictly cornified. At midcycle they all contain an abundance of glycogen. Some of the superficial layer of the vaginal epithelium may be shed at or near the time of menstruation (Fig. 25–39) and is called, in parallel with the uterine mucosa, the functionalis.

In the lamina propria subjacent to the vaginal epithelium, there is a wide band of rather dense fibrous connective tissue that is succeeded peripherally by a layer of loose connective tissue with many blood vessels. Beyond this layer lies

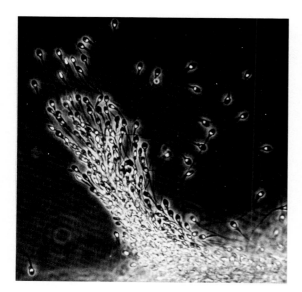

25–37 Human spermatozoa penetrating human midcycle cervical mucus. Note the unidirectional movement of almost all of the spermatozoa.

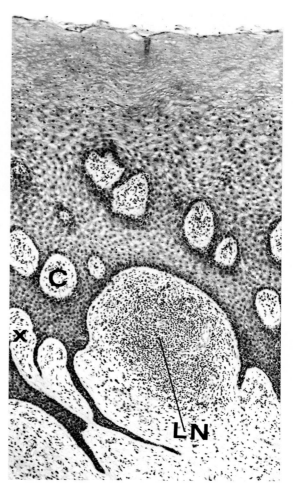

25–38 Photomicrograph of an oblique section through the vaginal wall of a monkey obtained a few hours after ovulation. Notice the lymph nodule (**LN**) in the submucosa. **C** is a cross section of a connective tissue core. Imagine the deep papilla at **X** cut in cross section.

the muscle coat. Elastic fibers are plentiful beneath the epithelium and sparse elsewhere in the fibromuscular wall. Diffuse lymphoid tissue and solitary nodules (Fig. 25–38) are present occasionally in the mucous membrane. Lymphocytes, along with granulocytes, invade the epithelium in large numbers in each menstrual cycle. The great increase, particularly of granulocytes, before, during, and after menstruation is apparent also in vaginal smears.

The muscularis of the vagina is composed of an inner and an outer layer. In the outer portion there are bundles of longitudinal smooth muscle cells that are continuous with corresponding cells in the myometrium. Where the two muscle layers meet, the inner circular cells are interwoven with the outer longitudinal ones. Striated muscle cells form a sphincter around the introitus of the vagina.

The vagina has an external coat composed of a firm inner layer well supplied with elastic fibers and an outer layer of loosely arranged connective tissue, which blends with that of surrounding organs.

Blood and lymphatic vessels are abundant in the wall of the vagina. The veins in the rugae are particularly numerous and large, and during sexual excitement they simulate erectile tissue. The

vaginal wall receives mylinated and unmyelinated nerve fibers. The latter form a ganglionated plexus in the external fibrous coat and supply the muscularis and blood vessels. The myelinated fibers terminate in special sensory organs in the mucosa.

The surface cells of the vaginal epithelium undergo continuous desquamation and constitute the bulk of the cells seen in a vaginal smear. In subhuman primates and many lower forms, the free cells in the vagina vary in number, type, and form in a regular and predictable manner,

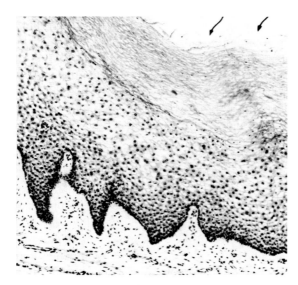

25–39 Photomicrograph of the vaginal mucosa in the fornix near the cervix of a monkey. Notice that the papillae are not as extensive. There is some peeling off of the superficial layers **(arrows)** of stratified squamous epithelium. H&E stain. ×300.

correlating with events in the reproductive cycle. In women the vaginal epithelium varies little with the cycle, and smears are mainly useful for determining whether the vaginal mucosa is atrophic or under effective estrogen stimulation.

The glycogen stores in the superficial cells of the vaginal epithelium are fermented to lactic acid by certain acid-forming bacteria, which thus influence the pH of the vaginal fluid. The glycogen accumulation correlates with the amount of estrogen stimulation, being greatest at the time of ovulation. With diminished estrogen titer, as after ovulation, less glycogen is formed and less is broken down so the pH of the vaginal fluid shifts toward alkalinity; this shift favors the development of infectious organisms such as staphylococci, *Escherichia coli*, trichomonas, and *Monilia albicans*. The ability of estrogen to reduce the vaginal pH and increase the thickness of the epithelial wall accounts for its effectiveness in the treatment of various vaginal infections that are especially common in children and postmenopausal women.

External Sex Organs (External Genitalia)

The external sex organs consist of the labia majora and minora, clitoris, and vestibular glands. The labia majora are homologous with the scro-

tum of the male. They are composed of skin and a thin layer of smooth muscle. In adulthood, the outer surface is covered with coarse pubic (genital) hair, with numerous sebaceous and sweat glands. The labia minora are devoid of hair, are covered by a stratified squamous epithelium, and enclose a highly papillated vascular core of loose connective tissue. Sebaceous glands, not connected with hair follicles, occur on both sides. Enhanced pigmentation is due to melanin.

The clitoris is an erectile body and is the homolog of the corpora cavernosa of the penis. It is mainly composed of two small cavernous bodies and a poorly developed glans clitoridis. The clitoris is covered with a thin layer of stratified squamous epithelium overlying a vascular stroma with high papillae. It contains many such specialized sensory nerve terminations as Meissner's corpuscles, Pacinian corpuscles, and Krause's end bulbs.

The vestibule is the space at the vaginal portal flanked by the labia. The epithelium differs from that of the vagina in possessing glands. The lesser vestibular glands secrete mucus and are situated mainly about the clitoris and urethral outlet. There is in addition a pair of large vestibular glands (glands of Bartholin), which are located in the lateral walls of the vestibule. They correspond to the bulbourethral glands of the male and are similar in structure; they are the tubuloacinar type and are lined with columnar cells that produce a whitish, mucoid, lubricating fluid.

The hymen consists of fine-fibered vascular connective tissue covered on both sides with a mucous membrane similar to that of the vagina.

References and Selected Bibliography

General

Blandau, R. J. 1955. Biology of eggs and implantation. In W. C. Young (ed.), Sex and Internal Secretions, 3rd ed., Vol. 2. Baltimore: The Williams and Wilkins Co., p. 797.

Yen, S. S. C., and Jaffe, R. B. 1978. Reproductive Endocrinology, Physiology, Pathophysiology and Clinical Management. Philadelphia: W. B. Saunders.

Development

Witschi, E. 1948. Migration of the germ cells of human embryos from the yolk sac to the primitive gonadal folds. Carnegie Inst. Contrib. Embryol. 32:67.

Ovary

Baker, T. G., and Franchi, L. L. 1967. The fine structure of oogonia and oocytes in human ovaries. J. Cell Sci. 2:213.

Bassett, D. L. 1943. The changes in the vascular pattern of the ovary of the albino rat during the estrous cycle. Am. J. Anat. 73:251.

Blandau, R. J. 1955. Ovulation in the living albino rat. Fertil. Steril. 6:391.

Block, E. 1951. Quantitative morphological investigations of the follicular system in women. Acta Endocrinol. (Copenh.) 8:33.

Corner, G. W., Jr. 1956. The histological dating of the human corpus luteum of menstruation. Am. J. Anat. 98:377.

Crisp, T. M., Dessouky, D. A., and Denys, F. R. 1970. The fine structure of the human corpus luteum of early pregnancy and during the progestational phase of the menstrual cycle. Am. J. Anat. 127:37.

Hertig, A. T. 1968. The primary human oocyte: Some observations on the fine structure of Balbiani's vitelline body and the origin of the annulate lamellae. Am J. Anat. 122:107.

Hertig, A. T., and Adams, E. C. 1967. Studies on the human oocyte and its follicle. I. Ultrastructural and histochemical observations on the primordial follicle stage. J. Cell Biol. 34:647.

Morris, B., and Sass, M. B. 1966. The formation of lymph in the ovary. Proc. R. Soc. (Lond.) Ser. B 164:577.

Mossman, M. H., Koering, M. J., and Ferry, D., Jr. 1964. Cyclic changes of interstitial gland tissue of the human ovary. Am. J. Anat. 115:235.

Odor, D. L. 1955. The temporal relationship of the first maturation division of rat ova to the onset of heat. Am. J. Anat. 97:461.

Ryan, K. J., Petro, Z., and Kaiser, J. 1968. Steroid formation by isolated and recombined ovarian granulosa and thecal cells. J. Clin. Endocrinol. Metab. 28:355.

Ryan, K. J., and Short, R. V. 1965. Formation of estradiol by granulosa and theca cells of the equine ovarian follicle. Endocrinology 76:108.

Strassman, E. O. 1941. The theca cone and its tropism toward the ovarian surface, a typical feature of growing human mammalian follicles. Am. J. Obstet. Gynecol. 41:363.

Oviduct

Brenner, R. M. 1969. Renewal of oviduct cilia during the menstrual cycle. Acta Radiologica 40:561.

Brenner, R. M., Resko, J. A., and West, N. B. 1974. Cyclic changes in oviductal morphological and residual cytoplasmic estradiol binding capacity induced by sequential estradiol-progesterone treatment of spayed Rhesus monkeys. Endocrinology 95:1094.

Hafez, E. S. E., and Blandau, R. J. 1969. The Mammalian Oviduct, Comparative Biology and Methodology. Chicago: The University of Chicago Press.

Uterus, Vagina, and Adnexa

Bartelmez, G. W. 1933. Histological studies on the menstruating mucous membrane of the human uterus. Carnegie Inst. Contrib. Embryol. 24:141.

Borell, U., and Fernstrom, I. 1953. The adnexal branches of the uterine artery. Acta Radiologica 40:561.

Danforth, D. N. 1947. The fibrous nature of the human cervix, and its relation to the isthmic segment in gravid and nongravid uteri. Am. J. Obstet. Gynecol. 53:541.

Fluhman, C. F. 1958. The glandular structures of the cervix uteri. Surg. Gynecol. Obstet. 106:515.

Hartman, C. G. 1944. Regeneration of the monkey uterus after surgical removal of the endometrium and accidental endometriosis. West. J. Surg. Obstet. Gynecol. 52:87.

Jacobson, H. N., and Nieves, O. 1961. Intrinsic nerve fibers of the primate endometrium. Exp. Neurol. 4:180.

Lee, W. I., Verdugo, P., Blandau, R. J., and Gaddum-Rosse, P. 1977. Molecular arrangement of cervical mucus: A reevaluation based on laser light-scattering spectroscopy. Gynecol. Invest. 8:254.

Markee, J. E. 1940. Menstruation in intraocular endometrial transplants in the Rhesus monkey. Carnegie Inst. Contrib. Embryol. 28:220.

Markee, J. E. 1950. The morphological and endocrine basis for menstrual bleeding. Prog. Gynecol. 2:63.

Papanicolaou, G. N. 1933. The sexual cycle in the human female as revealed by vaginal smears. Am. J. Anat. 52:519.

Pribor, H. C. 1951. Innervation of the uterus. Anat. Rec. 109:339.

Schmidt-Matthiesen, H. 1963. The Normal Human Endometrium. New York: McGraw-Hill Book Company.

Vickery, B. H., and Bennett, J. P. 1968. The cervix and its secretion in mammals. Physiol. Rev. 48:135.

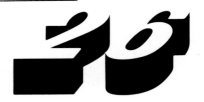

The Mammary Gland

Dorothy R. Pitelka

The mammary gland *(mamma)* is a compound tubuloalveolar gland of cutaneous origin. It is unique to the class Mammalia, and its function in infant nutrition is vital to most mammalian species. It is of extraordinary biological interest, inasmuch as its complex secretory product contains proteins, fats, and a sugar, all of which are organ-specific. Moreover, its major phases of development, function, and regression occur repeatedly in the adult female in response to a complex sequence of both internal (hormonal) and external (suckling) stimuli.

Mammae develop in pairs along embryonic *milk lines* running bilaterally from the axilla to the groin. A single pectoral pair is the rule for humans, but adventitious nipples or glands may appear elsewhere along the milk line. Each mamma consists of (1) the glandular epithelium, which is suspended in (2) subcutaneous connective tissue stroma within a more or less abundant bed of (3) adipose tissue, and (4) a *nipple*, or *teat*, where the gland's collecting ducts open to the skin surface. The epithelium is organized as a branching duct system terminating, when fully developed, in secretory *ductules* and *alveoli*. Contractile *myoepithelial cells* arranged in varying patterns surround the ductal and alveolar epithelium, within a continuous basement membrane that encloses the whole epithelial system.

General Morphology and Histology of the Adult Gland

The Nipple and Areola

Ten to 20 independent excretory ducts (*lactiferous ducts, galactophores*), each leading from one of the lobes of the gland, open at the tip of the human nipple (Fig. 26–1). Packed among them are large sebaceous glands that often empty into the lactiferous ducts rather than at the surface. Keratinizing stratified squamous epithelium, continuous with that of the skin, lines the outer parts of the lactiferous ducts, and horny cell debris usually plugs their openings. Among the epithelial cells of the outer parts of the lactiferous and sebaceous ducts, as well as the skin of the nipple and the surrounding *areola*, are variable numbers of dendritic melanocytes, giving these areas a darker pigmentation than the neighboring skin. Scattered over the areola are sebaceous glands, some sweat glands, and the clustered openings of *Montgomery glands*. Once thought to be modified sebaceous glands, Montgomery glands recently have been characterized as mammary glands comparable in development to those opening on the nipple. The epidermis at the tip of the nipple is fissured and pitted externally; basally it interdigitates deeply with long dermal papillae (Fig. 26–1). The sides of the relaxed nipple are marked by circular wrinkles. Hair is absent from nipples and areola.

The dense collagenous connective tissue of the nipple and areola (Figs. 26–2 and 26–4) con-

26–1 Galactophore opening at the tip of a human nipple. It is lined by keratinizing stratified squamous epithelium continuous with the nipple epidermis **(Ep)**; the latter is deeply ridged externally and invaded basally by long dermal papillae **(DP)**. The apparent bifurcation of the galactophore is probably the effect of oblique sectioning of a gently folded wall. At right are several sebaceous gland acini **(SG)**. Hematoxylin and eosin. × 40. (Histological preparation courtesy of J. J. Elias.)

26–2 Connective tissue in the cross-sectioned nipple of a pregnant mouse. The basal cells of the nipple epidermis **(Ep)** appear at the top, and the tip of a fold in the galactophore **(G)** is just visible at the bottom. Elastic fibers **(El)** are numerous, oriented circularly near the epidermis and mainly longitudinally (seen in cross section as dense dots) elsewhere. Several smooth muscle bundles **(SM)** are cut in cross section. Epon embedment, Mallory's azure II-methylene blue. × 540.

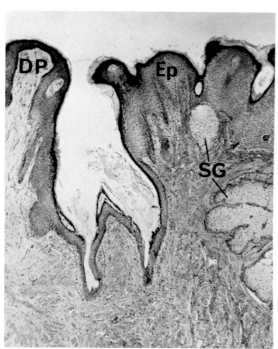

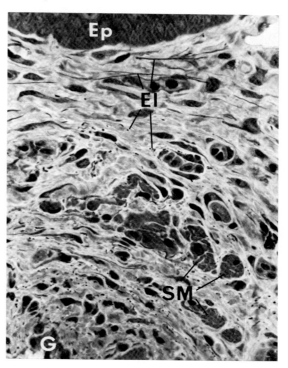

tains bundles of elastic fibers that fan out to attach to the overlying epidermis, particularly of the tip of the nipple. Abundant smooth muscle bundles, both radial and circular in arrangement, also attach to the overlying skin. Their contraction effects a wrinkling of the areola and erection of the nipple in response to cold, touch, or psychic stimuli.

Nipples and teats of other mammals are similar in basic structure (Fig. 26–3); erection of the nipple in many species aids the suckling young in grasping it. In ruminants, the complex of smooth muscles and elastic connective tissue may be responsible for sphincter-like closure of the teat canal, but such sphincters have not been demonstrated in the human nipple.

Duct System

From their openings at the tip of the human nipple (Fig. 26–1), the galactophores descend a short distance and then may branch into smaller lactiferous ducts, which radiate under the areola and expand as variably swollen ampullae, or *lactiferous sinuses* (Fig. 26–4), with folded walls. These sinuses in turn give rise to the branching smaller ducts leading ultimately in postpubertal females into the *lobules*, which are clusters of secretory alveoli.

The stratified squamous epithelium near the opening of the lactiferous duct shows a gradual transition to two approximately cuboidal layers in the lactiferous sinus. Through the remainder

26–3 Nipple and adjacent tissues from a lactating mouse. The single galactophore **(G)**, cut obliquely within the nipple, leads down into an expanded ampulla **(A)** below. Deep folds in the surface of the nipple allow for erection and elongation during suckling. The spongy material at the left is lobuloalveolar tissue. Scanning electron micrograph; glutaraldehyde fixation, Freon critical-point drying. × 40. (Courtesy of M. K. Nemanic.)

26–4 Lactiferous sinus under the areola of a woman in the eighth month of pregnancy. The wall of the sinus is wrinkled and folded. Around the deeply stained epithelium of the sinus is a layer of relatively cellular connective tissue. In the more peripheral, densely fibrous connective tissue are empty blood vessels and, at the left, some of the smooth muscle bundles **(SM)** that run under the skin of the areola. Hematoxylin and eosin. × 40. (Histological preparation courtesy of J. J. Elias).

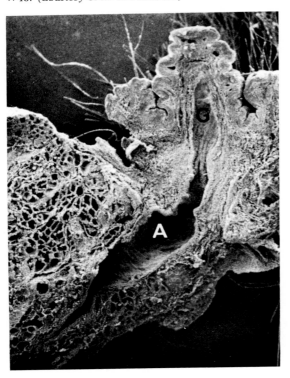

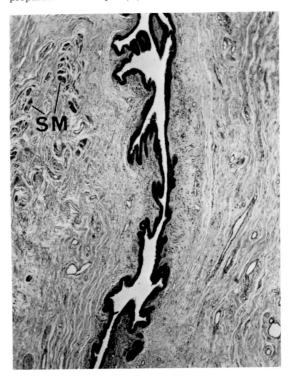

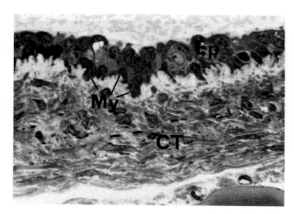

26–5 Major duct from an adult virgin mouse; the lumen is at the top, connective tissue sheath **(CT)** below. Beneath the superficial epithelial layer **(Ep)** are myoepithelial cells **(My)**, with smaller, more distorted, darkly stained nuclei; the basal surface of the myoepithelial layer is characteristically serrated. Epon embedment, Paragon stain. × 680.

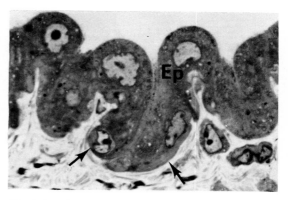

26–6 Distal duct from a lactating mouse. The lumen is at the top; connective tissue is at bottom. The folded wall consists of a discontinuous myoepithelial layer **(arrows)** and epithelial cells **(Ep)** that are much larger than those in major ducts. Epithelial nuclei are not noticeably different from those in Fig. 26–5, but the more abundant cytoplasm contains scattered, clear vesicles suggesting modest secretory activity. Epon embedment, Mallory's azure II-methylene blue. × 1,250.

of the duct system, the superficial epithelial cells are cuboidal to columnar. They have scant cytoplasm and a central, oval nucleus containing one or more nucleoli and scattered or marginal heterochromatin (Fig. 26–5). The basal layer consists of myoepithelial cells, smaller than the luminal cells and often more deeply stained, and with smaller and more contorted nuclei. They form a virtually continuous circumferential stratum in major duct branches. The cells are spindle-shaped, oriented with the long axis of the duct, and frequently longitudinally ridged, giving the duct a characteristically serrated peripheral contour in cross or oblique section (Fig. 26–5).

As the duct system extends distally and its branches become smaller, the investment of myoepithelial cells becomes discontinuous and the cells begin to assume a stellate form, with long processes extending from a central perinuclear zone to form an open basket around the duct wall. The epithelial cells of distal ducts during pregnancy and lactation often enlarge and become slightly to fully secretory (Fig. 26–6); even in major ducts, occasional patches of secretory cells may appear.

Alveoli

The secretory unit of the mammary gland is the lobule. It consists of a cluster of alveoli around the single small duct that drains it and from which it originated (Fig. 26–7). Alveoli develop during pregnancy (or to a lesser and variable degree during postovulatory phases of the menstrual or estrous cycle) as blunt tubular or spherical outgrowths from the side or end of the duct. Their arrangement in lobular units is clearest when the gland is not fully developed (Figs. 26–7 and 26–8).

The alveolar wall is a single layer of epithelial cells, embraced by a loose network of myoepithelial cells with their long, slender processes. Until specific hormonal stimulation at some stage of pregnancy induces secretory differentiation, the epithelial cells resemble those of ducts. Upon stimulation, cytoplasmic volume increases and evidence of secretion becomes visible histologically in the form of vesicles in the cytoplasm and fat droplets in cells and lumen (Fig. 26–9). The extent of lobular differentiation at any given stage before or during pregnancy may vary widely within a single gland (Fig. 26–8 and 26–9) as well as among individuals and species.

If nursing takes place, full secretory development is reached some days after parturition. In a lactating gland, alveoli are distorted by close packing and by the partial fusion of neighbors (Figs. 26–10 and 26–11); thus alveoli may drain into other alveoli within the lobule. Further-

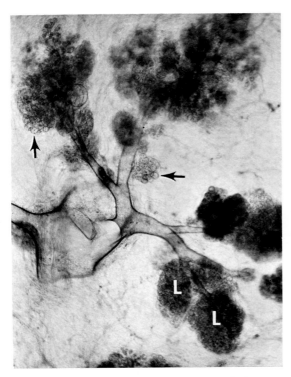

26–7 Persisting lobules in the resting gland of a 25-year-old woman who had had one child. A single terminal branch from a small duct enters each lobule **(L)**. Bubble-like alveoli **(arrows)** can be distinguished at the edges of some lobules. 2-mm section in methylsalicylate, hematoxylin. × 20. (Courtesy of H. M. Jensen and S. R. Wellings.)

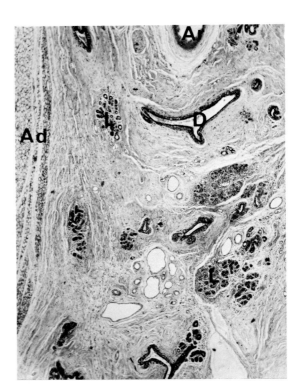

26–8 Relatively undifferentiated area of a human breast at 8 months of gestation. At the left is part of a lobe of adipose tissue **(Ad)**; the edge of a cross-sectioned artery **(Ar)** is at the top right. Below it is a branching duct **(D)**. Elsewhere are sections of smaller ducts and developing lobules **(L)**. Thin-walled veins, lymph vessels, and arterioles are scattered throughout the abundant fibrous connective tissue. Immediately adjacent to ducts and within lobules, the connective tissue is more cellular, and the many nuclei at this low magnification create a densely stippled effect. Hematoxylin and eosin. × 35. (Histological preparation courtesy of J. J. Elias.)

more, cells of the terminal branches of the intralobular duct typically are fully secretory, so that these ductules are identifiable as drainage pathways only if one can follow their course for some distance (Fig. 26–10). The lactating lobule in histological section therefore has a spongy appearance, as of many irregular, intercommunicating chambers. Adjacent lobules in lactation may also be close-packed, their limits indicated in section only by the connective tissue septa that bound them. When lactation ceases, lobules decrease greatly in size and many of them regress partially or completely, leaving a resting gland that again is predominantly ductal.

Stroma

Connective tissue of the mamma is basically of two types: (1) variously dense, fibrous connective tissue enclosing the ducts and lobules and supporting the breast in its subcutaneous position; and (2) loose, cellular connective tissue surrounding the ductules and alveoli within each lobule.

The dense collagenous tissue of the nipple and the interlobar and interlobular septa in the adult gland contains occasional elastic fiber bundles (becoming more abundant with age) and relatively few fibroblasts (Figs. 26–2, 26–4, and 26–8). In addition to the glandular parenchyma, it encloses blood and lymph vessels, nerves, and occasional macrophages and mast cells. Peripherally, the septa merge with fibrous fascia that suspend the human breast from the sternum and pectoral muscle fascia and that connect via

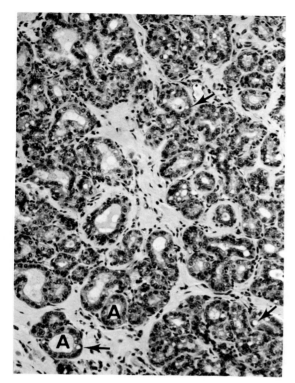

26–9 Another area of the same prelactating human gland as Fig. 26–8. Lobules here are well developed, and some of the alveoli **(A)** (or ductules—the two are not distinguishable) are enlarged. Secreted material, including spherical residues of extracted fat droplets, fills the lumina, and some cells contain clear fat vacuoles **(arrows)**. Hematoxylin and eosin. × 135. (Histological preparation courtesy of J. J. Elias.)

mammary ligaments with the overlying dermis. Within the supporting septa, each major lactiferous duct is surrounded by a sheath of concentrically layered fibroblasts, collagenous fiber bundles, and frequent elastic fibers (Figs. 26–2, 26–5, and 26–12). At the internal limit of the fibrous sheath, the basement membrane is a narrow, cell-free zone that contains the basal lamina of the epithelium and many collagenous fibers (Fig. 26–12). The sheath diminishes in thickness, density, and elastic fiber content as the duct divides into successively smaller branches.

Within lobules, frequent fibroblasts and abundant capillaries are enclosed in a loose collagenous network. At certain times associated with stages of menstrual or lactational cycles, lymphocytes, plasma cells, or macrophages may be present in large numbers.

Lobules of adipose tissue are also enclosed in the supporting stroma in most species, forming a special mammary fat pad. In rodents, the septa are relatively thin, and fat lobules interdigitate abundantly with lobules of glandular tissue; in bovine and human mammae, connective tissue is more abundant and separates most fat-cell tracts from epithelial lobules.

The amount of mammary connective tissue increases as ducts and blood vessels extend during pregnancy, but within lobules it appears to become attenuated as expanding alveoli, which fill all available space, displace the stromal elements. Adipose cells may be progressively depleted of their fat stores in late pregnancy and lactation. They generally do not disappear even if fully depleted (Fig. 26–15) and can accumulate fat again after lactation ends.

Circulation and Innervation

The mamma is a skin gland, and its blood vessels and nerves are those of the skin where the gland is located. The human breast is supplied by the intercostal, lateral thoracic, and internal mammary (a branch of the subclavian) blood vessels. The developing duct system, growing from the nipple within the connective tissue septa of the subcutaneous mammary fat pad, adopts the existing vascular system of the stroma, with the result that the mammary ducts and the blood vessels have different branching patterns. Duct epithelium is separated from its blood supply by the thickness of its fibrous sheath, whereas growing end buds and secretory alveoli are more closely invested by capillary plexuses (Fig. 26–11).

Lymph flow from the lactating gland is high. Lymphatic capillaries are not present within the lobules, but fine lymphatic vessels surround them. Large lymphatics are frequent in the connective tissue septa; in the human, they lead mainly to the axillary lymph nodes.

Innervation of the mamma includes somatic sensory and sympathetic motor fibers. In the human breast, nonencapsulated, single or branching sensory end organs are numerous around the galactophores and in the dermis at the tip of the nipple; smaller numbers are associated with Montgomery galactophores on the areola. Such receptors in experimental animals are known during suckling to trigger the neuroendocrine reflex discharge of hormones responsible for milk ejection and for maintaining lactation. Histological evidence for sensory endings elsewhere in the gland is equivocal. However, receptors sen-

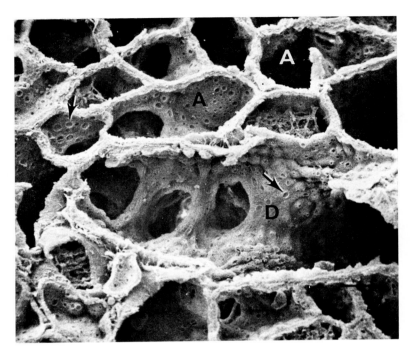

26-10 Mammary gland of a lactating mouse. In this scanning electron micrograph, close-packed alveoli **(A)** washed almost free of milk surround a small secreting ductule **(D)** with several openings. Secreting epithelium is distinguished by the flat craters **(arrows)** left by fat globules extracted during processing. Glutaraldehyde fixation, Freon critical-point drying. × 220. (From Nemanic, M. K., and Pitelka, D. R., 1971, J. Cell Biol. 48:410.)

sitive to intramammary pressure do exist; afferent discharges in mammary nerves of rabbits have been recorded after ductal fluid pressure has been experimentally increased.

The smooth muscles of the teat or nipple and areola are liberally innervated by sympathetic fibers, as are arteries and arterioles throughout the gland. In the various species investigated, the rate of mammary blood flow is under nervous as well as hormonal control and is very labile. It increases sharply at parturition and remains remarkably stable from day to day during lactation under normal conditions but is readily diminished by stress. The consensus of recent investigators is that mammary myoepithelial and epithelial elements are not innervated.

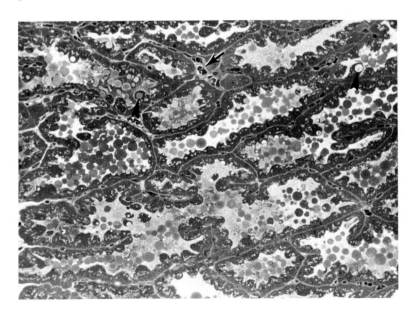

26-11 Mammary gland of a lactating mouse comparable to that in Fig. 26-10. Alveolar lumina contain spherical fat globules and finer particulate material. Within the cells are clusters of tiny, clear Golgi vesicles and some larger, round fat globules **(arrowheads)**. The small blood vessels (for example, see **arrow** at top) and abundant capillaries between alveoli are identifiable by the presence of darkly stained erythrocytes. Epon embedment, Mallory's azure II-methylene blue. × 200.

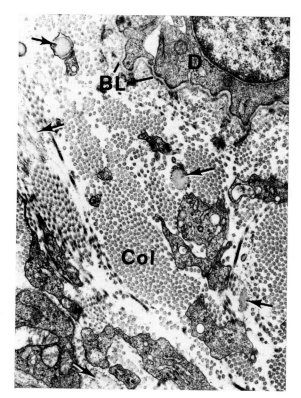

26–12 Connective tissue adjacent to a major lactiferous duct **(D)** of a midpregnant mouse. Most of the field is filled with large bundles of collagenous fibrils **(Col)**; dispersed among them are several elastic fibers **(arrows)** and numerous fibroblast cell processes of various sizes. Close to the duct, the collagenous fibrils are more loosely and irregularly arrayed. Some of them appear to make contact with the basal lamina **(BL)**. Electron micrograph. × 13,400.

The Cytology of Secretion

To appreciate the special properties of the mammary gland's organization and ultrastructure, some familiarity with the nature of milk is necessary. The whole biological function of the gland is to provide, only at the proper time, a fluid that will meet all of the nutritional needs of the newborn young. The composition of milk is basically similar in all mammals; hence, it is not surprising that the internal structure of the gland differs very little among them.

Milk

Milk is a watery solution, or suspension, of proteins, lipids, carbohydrates, vitamins, salts, im-munoglobulins, and many other substances in small quantities. The predominant proteins, lipids, and carbohydrates are synthesized by the mammary epithelium and are unique to it; other components are synthesized there or are selectively transferred from the blood. The three major specific proteins are: the abundant, nutritionally important caseins; α-lactalbumin, nutritional and also essential for lactose synthesis; and (at least in ruminants) β-lactoglobulin, the significance of which, apart from nutrition, is unknown. Caseins are released from secreting cells mainly as micellar particles; the other two proteins are released in solution. The major milk fats are neutral triglycerides. They are characterized by a higher proportion of short- and medium-chain and unsaturated fatty acids and a higher degree of molecular asymmetry than are found in other body fats; this composition causes the fats to remain liquid and mobile at body temperature. They are secreted as droplets surrounded by a coat that prevents coalescence. The disaccharide lactose, composed of glucose and galactose, is the major carbohydrate of most milks; it is released in solution. Certain classes of immunoglobulins are present in milk in varying amounts and in proportions differing from those in blood plasma. The intestinal epithelium in the newborn of many species—but not the human—can transfer some of these antibodies intact to the circulation. Unabsorbed immunoglobulins, especially IgA, serve an antimicrobial protective function in the infant's gut.

Milk is isosmolar with blood plasma. Because lactose is so abundant in milk as to be its major osmole, the transfer of osmotically active components from blood must be selectively controlled. Levels of sodium, potassium, and chloride differ in the two fluids, and they seem in milks of different species to be inversely related to lactose content. Calcium and phosphates, of great nutritional importance, are present in solution but are secreted in much larger quantities insolubly complexed with casein micelles. One or more iron-binding proteins are present in most milks, but the iron content is variable.

Alveolar Cells and the Formation of Milk

Surface Characters. Like other active transporting epithelia, lactating mammary epithelium consists of a sheet of firmly joined, strongly asymmetric cells (Figs. 26–13, 26–14, and 26–18). Apical cell surfaces, facing the central

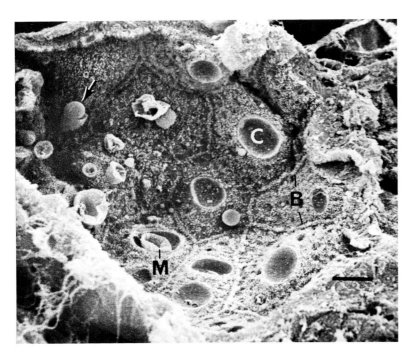

26–13 Luminal surface of an alveolus. The polygonal cell surfaces are thickly dotted with microvilli, and distinct rows of close-set microvilli mark the cell borders **(B)**. Large, flat, empty craters **(C)** are left by extraction of large superficial fat droplets; in some instances the collapsed membrane envelope **(M)** remains, and in one case **(arrow)**, a preserved fat globule still lies partly within the ruptured membrane. Scanning electron micrograph; glutaraldehyde fixation, Freon critical-point drying. × 1,250. (From Nemanic, M. K., and Pitelka, D. R. 1971. J. Cell Biol. 48:410.)

lumen where milk is deposited, bear irregularly distributed microvilli, which tend to be longer and more numerous along cell borders than elsewhere. These borders are joined to one another laterally in a continuous mosaic. Below this zone of tight contact, contiguous lateral cell surfaces show varying contours: for part of their course, they are closely parallel and gently undulating; elsewhere they extend long, contorted cytoplasmic processes into intercellular spaces, or the spaces may be closed and the processes compressed into interdigitating folds. The basal cell membrane is thrown intermittently into series of extensions and infoldings (Figs. 26–14, 26–15, and 26–18). Evidence of pinocytosis at this surface is seen in the form of vesicles of various sizes in the subjacent cytoplasm and occasional membrane invaginations suggesting vesicle formation.

Inserted between the bases of epithelial cells are myoepithelial cell bodies or their slender processes (Figs. 26–14, 26–18, and 26–19); the latter can be seen indenting the basal surface of nearly every secretory cell. Myoepithelial membranes are studded with clusters of tiny, open plasmalemmal vesicles, similar to those characteristic of smooth muscle cells. Externally, a distinct, continuous basal lamina is present.

The structure that maintains continuous close contact of luminal cell borders is a tight-junction belt, or occluding zone (Figs. 26–14, 26–16, and 26–18), encircling every cell (see Chap. 3). Desmosomes are abundant in major ducts at all times and in alveoli during development, but there are few or none in lactating cells. Hence, the tight junctions here are essential to provide mechanical adhesion as well as to limit transepithelial permeability. As in other transporting epithelia, the occluding zone provides a permeability barrier by restricting diffusion of substances across the epithelium through intercellular spaces.

Gap junctions, thought to be the sites of direct transfer of ions and small molecules between

26–14 Typical mammary alveolar cells from a mouse at full lactation; electron micrograph. Note the irregularly distributed microvilli on the luminal surface and the membrane convolutions at the basal surface. Very dense, round bodies in the lumen and secretory vacuoles are casein micelles. **C,** capillary; **ER,** rough endoplasmic reticulum; **F,** fat globule; **G,** Golgi complex; **L,** lumen; **M,** mitochondrion; **My,** myoepithelial cell process; **N,** nucleus; **TJ,** tight junction. × 13,000.

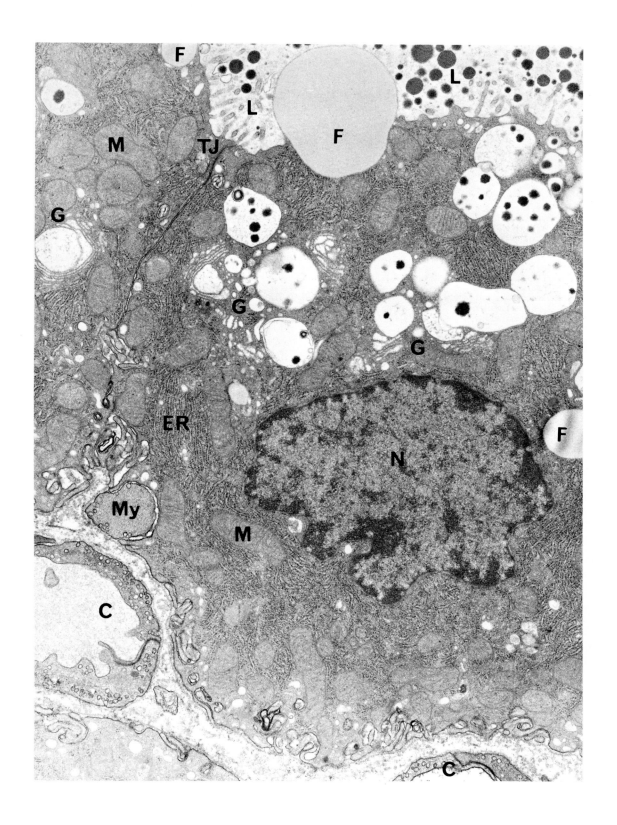

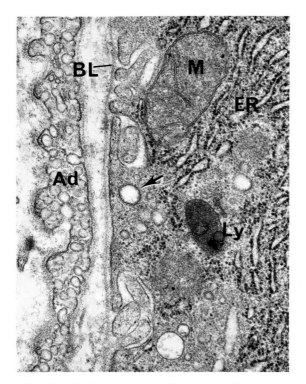

cells in contact, are present rather frequently in or near the occluding zone and erratically elsewhere in mammary epithelium. They link epithelial and myoepithelial cells in all combinations.

Cytoplasmic Structure and Function. The general architecture of the secreting mammary cell is that of any protein-synthesizing exocrine cell. It is dominated by flattened cisternae of rough endoplasmic reticulum (ER) filling most of the cytoplasm and by many Golgi complexes lateral and apical to the nucleus (Figs. 26–14 and 26–18). The Golgi region (Fig. 26–17) contains abundant microvesicles in addition to flattened proximal and inflated distal cisternae. Secretory vesicles are common between the Golgi region and the apical cell surface. Near the cell base are small, membrane-limited bodies with a dense matrix that presumably are lysosomes (Fig. 26–15). Activity of several lysosomal enzymes has been demonstrated biochemically and cytochemically in lactating cells. More complex ly-

26–15 A depleted adipose cell process **(Ad)**, with △ contorted surface and abundant plasmalemmal vesicles crowding the visible cytoplasm, lies next to the base of an alveolar epithelial cell in a lactating mouse. A distinct basal lamina **(BL)** extends smoothly over the membrane convolutions of the alveolar cell; a less distinct lamina coats the fat-cell surface. Assorted vesicles are present in the alveolar cell; one **(arrow)** bears on its cytoplasmic surface a coat of short bristles often seen on pinocytic vesicles. **M,** mitochondrion; **ER,** cisternae of rough ER containing fine particulate material; **Ly,** probable lysosome. Electron micrograph. × 31,000.

26–16 Freeze-fracture replica of the occluding ▽ junction in lactating mouse mammary gland. Electron micrograph. Between the particle-studded lateral cell membrane, extending across the top of the picture, and the microvilli protruding into the lumen at the bottom is the network of gently undulating ridges and grooves. Meshes in the network are spindle-shaped next to the lumen and rounded abluminally. The number of ridges in any one transect of the band averages six to eight in lactating cells. At **Cy,** the fracture plane has left the membrane and passed through a projecting lip of cytoplasm. × 48,700. (From Pitelka, D. R., Hamamoto, S. T., Duafala, J. G., and Nemanic, M. K. 1973. J. Cell Biol. 56:797.)

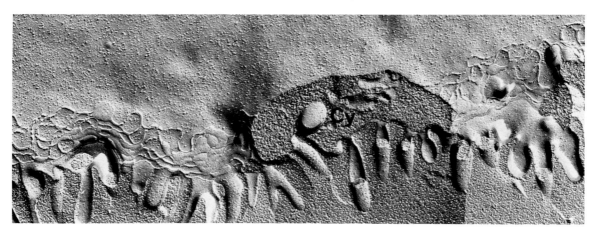

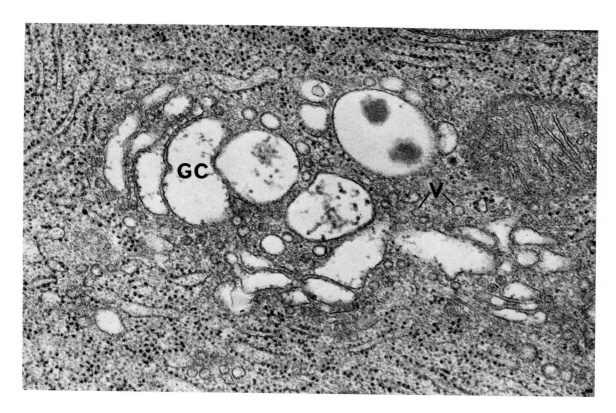

sosomal derivatives, apparently autophagic, are occasionally seen. Rod-shaped mitochondria are distributed through the cytoplasm (Fig. 26–14). Fat globules of various sizes are present in the cytoplasm of most cells. In the dense cytoplasmic matrix are scattered microtubules, most frequent in the Golgi region, and filaments in small bundles or forming a mat of variable thickness beneath surface membranes. Smooth-membraned vesicles other than those of the Golgi complex are present chiefly near cell surfaces; there is no conspicuous smooth ER.

Caseins, α-lactalbumin, and other proteins synthesized on the ribosomes of the rough ER pass into the lumina of its cisternae, which become filled with fine particulate material of moderate electron density (Figs. 26–15 and 26–17). This material is transferred to the Golgi complex probably by migration of microvesicles. Dispersed particles appear in the proximal, flat Golgi cisternae and accumulate in inflated distal sacs. Condensation of most casein protein into dense micelles occurs here or during migration of the secretory vacuole to the cell surface. The micelles have a highly characteristic granular substructure; a typical inflated vesicle encloses several of them (Fig. 26–14). The noncasein

whey proteins, including α-lactalbumin, remain dissolved in the fluid that fills the vesicle. Secretory vesicles reaching the apical plasmalemma fuse with it and release their contents to the lumen in a conventional exocytic process. A full discussion of exocrine secretion is presented in Chap. 21.

Milk fats contain, in various proportions, dietary fatty acids (mainly long-chain) from the blood as well as fatty acids (C4–C16) synthesized in mammary cells. Triglyceride synthesis occurs in the regions of the cell occupied by ER, where bound and free ribosomes are abundant. Fat droplets appear in the cytoplasm, without any enclosing membrane. Increase in size occurs by accretion or fusion as the globule moves to the cell surface, where it is extruded into the lumen (Fig. 26–14). The plasmalemma is carried out with it and pinches off behind it, enclosing it in a mem-

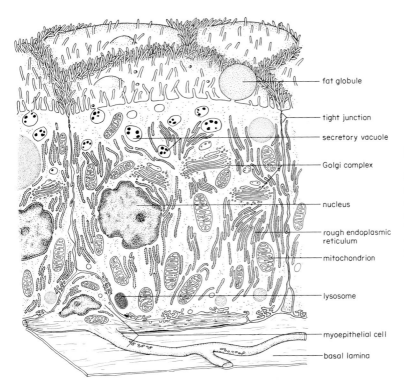

fat globule

tight junction

secretory vacuole

Golgi complex

nucleus

rough endoplasmic
reticulum

mitochondrion

lysosome

myoepithelial cell

basal lamina

26–18 Schematic drawing of alveolar cells in a lactating mammary gland. Microvilli, concentrated along the cell borders, are shown in three-dimensional view on the apical surfaces. At the base of the cells, the basal lamina is indicated extending forward, with a branching myoepithelial cell process lying on it. Organelles are not drawn to scale.

brane envelope. In some instances, secretory vacuoles collect around the globule and may contribute their membranes to it directly during the pinching off. Fragments of cytoplasm are sometimes included within the envelope. Fat secretion thus contributes to the milk not only lipids and fat-soluble vitamins but membrane phospholipids, cholesterol, glycoproteins, and enzymes, plus cytoplasmic constituents in small amounts.

Lactose synthesis requires two proteins. One of them is a common galactosyl transferase in the Golgi membranes of many cell types; its usual function is to transfer galactose from UDP galactose to N-acetylglucosamine in the formation of glycoproteins. In the presence of the second protein, α-lactalbumin, the specificity of the galactosyl transferase activity changes so that glucose in low concentrations can serve as the galactose acceptor. Because cytoplasmic membranes are impermeable to disaccharides, lactose draws water osmotically into the distal Golgi sacs and young secretory vacuoles, and they swell. Consequently, most of the volume of the secretory vacuole is occupied by fluid, in which the lactose, whey proteins, and other substances are dissolved.

The discharge of bits of cytoplasm with milk fat droplets is a form of apocrine secretion. Although histological evidence of more extensive sloughing in healthy glands is scant, large fragments of organelle-filled cytoplasm and a few viable epithelial cells are typically present in normal milk; their numbers may be increased by mechanical milking. In addition, macrophages and lymphocytes are abundant, particularly in the first days of nursing. Together with immunoglobulins, they protect against invading organisms in the maternal ducts and in the infant's gut.

Of the serum immunoglobulins, IgG is most abundant in the milk of species whose young can acquire passive immunity by absorbing it. Human infants obtain IgG by placental transfer before birth, and IgA is the major immunoglobulin in human milk. The selective uptake of particular immunoglobulins from among those in the circulating blood or those released by locally concentrated plasma cells probably is attributable to binding by specific receptors on the basolateral membranes of secretory cells, followed by transcellular transport in endocytic vesicles. Secretory IgA is released into the milk (and other external secretions) as a dimer to which a component has been added during transit by the epithelial cells, the complex being more resistant than serum IgA to proteolysis and pH changes.

Membrane flux in the lactating cell is extensive and differs significantly from that in most secreting cells. Membrane is added as usual to the apical surface by exocytosis of secretory vesicles; in mammary cells, membrane is also extruded from the apical surface as fat globule envelopes. Whereas disassembly or recycling of excess surface membrane is necessary in other cells, totally new membrane constitutents must continually be synthesized by mammary cells to replace all of the membrane secreted with milk fat. Biochemical evidence that apical surface membrane originates from the ER–Golgi system is particularly good in the case of mammary cells, where it has been drawn from comparisons of purified fat globule membrane with internal cytomembrane fractions (Keenan et al., 1978).

The Cytology of Milk Excretion

Milk secretion by lobuloalveolar tissue of the lactating mammary gland is slow but continuous. Suckling is intermittent, occurring only once a day in some species. In the intervals, milk accumulates, gradually inflating the alveolar lumina and seeping into the available ducts. The nursing infant, by its own action, can remove only that part of the milk lying in the ducts or sinuses near the nipple. The bulk of the milk in the ductal and alveolar lumina must be moved out into the larger ducts during nursing by contraction of myoepithelial cells. Milk excretion thus requires the myoepithelial network to eject milk from the blind terminal chambers of the gland and the ducts to contain it and channel it to the nipple.

Myoepithelium

Myoepithelial cells are distinguished by their basal position (they never abut on the lumen), their abundant plasmalemmal vesicles, and their content of tracts of actin microfilaments 5 to 7nm in diameter (Fig. 26–19). These tracts occupy the long cell processes of the alveolar myoepithelium (Figs. 26–14 and 26–18) and most of the basal cytoplasm, including the ridges, of ductal myoepithelium (Fig. 26–21). Irregularly distributed in islands within or around the filament tracts are cisternae of rough or smooth ER, small

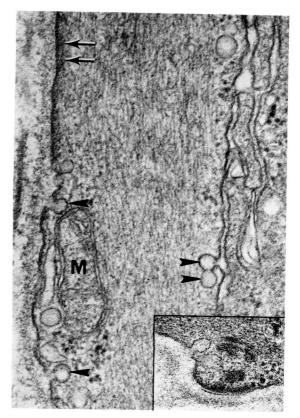

26–19 Myoepithelial cell process lying next to an alveolar cell on the right. Electron micrograph. At both edges of the myoepithelial process are plasmalemmal vesicles **(arrowheads)**, most of them clearly open to the surface. Ribosomes and a mitochondrion **(M)** lie in islands in a cytoplasm otherwise occupied by parallel filaments. Under the cell membrane at upper left is a dense plaque **(arrows)**; the space between the cell membrane and the basal lamina over this area is filled with filamentous material. × 60,000. **Inset.** A well-developed hemidesmosome at the surface of a differentiating myoepithelial cell from a 3-week-old mouse (same duct seen in Fig. 26–23). A typical hemidesmosome consists of a thin, dense plate outside the plasma membrane, filamentous material between it and the basal lamina, a dense plaque on the cytoplasmic side of the membrane, and two or three dense nodes associated with cytoplasmic filament tracts. Electron micrograph. × 62,000.

mitochondria, and ribosomes. Some filaments appear to insert in dense plaques under the cell membrane, and at these sites there often are hemidesmosomes (inset, Fig. 26–19) or simpler fibrillar connections to the basal lamina (Fig.

26–19). Nodes of a density similar to the plaques are scattered within the larger filament bundles.

Myoepithelial contraction occurs in response to the hormone oxytocin in the milk-ejection reflex. Sensory stimuli from receptors in the nipple, or stimuli of sight and sound associated by conditioning with nursing, are conveyed to the hypothalamus, triggering the neurohypophysis to release oxytocin into the blood. Myoepithelial contraction can be induced experimentally by oxytocin applied topically or injected, by mechanical or electrical stimuli, and by a variety of physiological and pharmacological agents known to induce contraction of smooth muscle. Contraction of myoepithelial cell processes embracing the alveoli and secretory ductules compresses their lumina, expressing the milk into the ducts. The contraction is accompanied or rapidly followed by a marked change in epithelial cell shape, from cuboidal or even squamous in engorged alevoli to pseudocolumnar, with the apical surface bulging far into the alveolar lumen (Fig. 26–20). The effects of contraction on duct shape are less clear. Milk inevitably drains from major ducts during tissue dissection; hence ducts in histological samples are usually empty and their walls folded. Ducts in milk-filled glands of living mice shorten and widen after oxytocin application. This increase in cross-sectional area could decrease resistance to milk flow, so that milk forced out of alveoli can continue down the ductal tree. Any significant increase in total ductal volume probably results from flattening of folds in the walls.

In the human and some other mammals without large gland cisterns, oxytocin release occurs in waves, evoking repeated myoepithelial response over a protracted suckling period

Ducts

The epithelial lining of major ducts consists of cells of unremarkable structure, showing little change during pregnancy and lactation. Both cells and nuclei often have convoluted surfaces; interdigitating processes between neighboring cells are abundant (Fig. 26–21). Apical surfaces bear microvilli that often are shorter than those of secretory cells. Prominent junctional complexes (Fig. 26–22), consisting of occluding junctions, intermediate junctions, and desmosomes, link epithelial cells at their apical borders; desmosomes and gap junctions are variably frequent elsewhere.

Cytoplasmic organelles—mitochondria, Golgi complexes, and rough ER—are sparse. Only filaments of various diameters appear more frequently than in secretory cells. The structure of

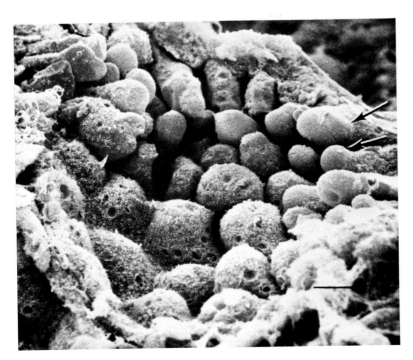

26–20 Luminal surface of a contracted alveolus in a lactating mouse mammary gland. Scanning electron micrograph. Most of the cells bulge deeply into the lumen. Apical membranes are covered with microvilli and fat craters except where large subsurface fat droplets occupy the apical bulge; here the membranes become smooth **(arrows)**. Compare the cell shapes here and in the more inflated alveoli in Figs. 26–10 and 26–13. Glutaraldehyde fixation, Freon critical-point drying. ×1,250. (From Pitelka, D. R., Hamamoto, S. T.,.Duafala, J. G., and Nemanic, M. K. 1973. J. Cell Biol. 56:797.)

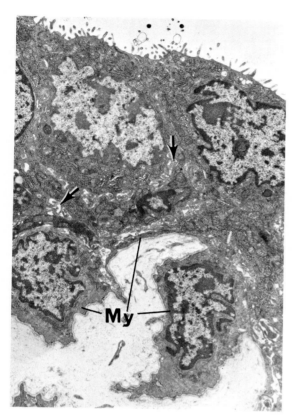

26–21 Major lactiferous duct from a lactating mouse. As compared with secretory alveolar cells, ductal epithelial cells have a small cytoplasmic volume. They bear typical microvilli on their apical surfaces and many irregular processes extending from their lateral and basal surfaces **(arrows)** and interdigitating with those of adjacent epithelial and myoepithelial cells. In the myoepithelial cell **(My)** layer, cell bodies occupy angular basal protrusions and in addition have peripheral ridges and valleys, with the result that the duct profile in cross section appears serrated at both low and high magnification. Nuclei of both epithelial and myoepithelial cells have irregular contours. Electron micrograph. × 7,300.

the major ducts is thus consistent with their function as conduits and storage spaces, mechanical integrity and flexibility being the most important requirements. There is no evidence that the mammary ducts are capable of selective reabsorption of any constituent of the secreted fluid, as are those of some other exocrine glands.

In the lactating gland, gradations in a number of characteristics associated with secretion appear between the typical major duct cells at one extreme and the fully developed ductular and alveolar cells at the other. As the ducts approach their intralobular endings, increasing prominence of the synthetic and secretory organelles, a decrease in frequency of desmosomes, progressive development of the basal membrane convolutions in epithelial cells, increasing discontinuity of the myoepithelial layer, and thinning of the connective tissue sheath are evident.

Mammary Development and Its Hormonal Control

Morphogenesis and Cyclic Differentiation

The human embryonic milk line is a low ectodermal ridge extending from forelimb to hindlimb in the 9-mm embryo. It regresses caudally but thickens in the thorax to form a solid epithelial bud by the end of the second month. Relatively little development occurs in the next month. A 13-week anlage examined with the electron microscope by Salazar and Tobon consisted of a solid mass of undifferentiated epithelial cells, beginning to form small branches in the upper dermal mesenchyme. The cells ultrastructurally resembled those of the neighboring epidermis. During the second trimester of gestation, continued proliferation and branching produce the 10 to 20 major duct rudiments, which bifurcate and develop lumina. Luminal epithelial cells are cuboidal to columnar and well polarized, with apical microvilli and junctional complexes; some of the basal cells are undifferentiated and some are distinct myoepithelial cells. The dermal mesenchyme surrounds the growing buds with more or less concentrically oriented cellular and fibrous layers. During the next 3 months, ducts elongate and branch, reaching the subcutaneous connective tissue. The nipple is first apparent as an external prominence at about 20 weeks. In the last trimester, its superficial cells are sloughed and the deeper cells form the keratinized, stratified, squamous lining of the galactophores.

The sequence of prenatal development is similar in other mammals. Mammary anlagen differentiate in embryos of both sexes. In the human and some other species, similarity in kind and rate of development continues after birth until the approach of puberty. In the male mouse and rat, the stalk between the growing rudiment and the epidermis ruptures at about the time fetal androgens begin to appear; the gland rudiment per-

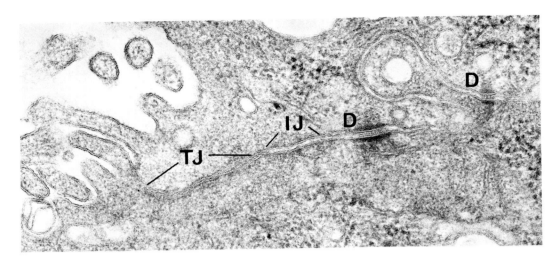

26–22 Junctional complex linking cells in a major mammary duct from a lactating mouse. Electron micrograph. The outer leaflets of the cell membranes are fused at several points in the tight junction **(TJ)**. Next to this are a poorly developed adhering, or intermediate, junction **(IJ)**, a distinct desmosome **(D)**, and, farther along the interdigitating membranes, a smaller desmosome. A meshwork of filaments occupies the cytoplasm adjacent to the junctional zone in the cell at the bottom. × 64,000.

sists and develops further, but the nipple is lacking. Castration in either sex or growth of rudiments in organ culture without hormones, results in female-type development (Kratochwil).

A brief burst of ductal proliferation occurs in glands of both sexes in the human and some other species at birth, accompanied by secretion of a fluid called witch's milk. Hormonal stimulation is presumably the cause, but whether of fetal or maternal origin is unknown.

Mammary growth from birth to the approach of puberty usually parallels body growth. The histology and ultrastructure of the established ducts are essentially as in the adult gland, with a luminal epithelial lining surrounded by a myoepithelial layer. At growing tips or new branching points, cell proliferation may create multilayered thickenings. In the wake of active growth, cells gradually become aligned in two layers and the basal ones differentiate as myoepithelial cells (Fig. 26–23).

At some time before the appearance of other external signs of puberty in females, growth in all tissues of the mammary gland accelerates, and the duct system proliferates to a variable ex-

tent through the connective tissue septa of the mammary fat pad. With the onset of ovarian cycles, further ductal growth may occur during the first several preovulatory phases. Postovulatory phases are characterized by varying degrees of ductular or alveolar development; in the human and some other mammals with relatively long luteal phases, the general pattern of lobule development may be laid down in the postpubertal nulliparous female. Further proliferation may occur in succeeding cycles, but this is followed by corresponding regression, and the ducts remain well spaced within the stroma. Cyclic ultrastructural changes have been described in ductule cells in the adult human gland, modest secretory differentiation appearing during the luteal phase. Individual variation is great, however.

During pregnancy, ductal elongation and branching resume, and lobuloalveolar development fills the stroma between ducts. Epithelial cell proliferation continues through pregnancy and into lactation. When first formed, alveolar cells resemble those of small ducts. The various signs of preparation for lactation—growth in cytoplasmic volume; quantitative increase in cytoplasmic RNA, rough ER, Golgi membranes, and mitochondria; rise in synthetic enzyme levels; and accumulation of secretory products in cells and lumina—occur at different relative times in the gestation span in different species. By the end of pregnancy, there is usually a considerable but not maximal development of the morphological secretory apparatus (Fig. 26–24), the enzyme complement characteristic of lactation is present, and lumina are engorged with fat and protein. Milk available to the nursling during the first day

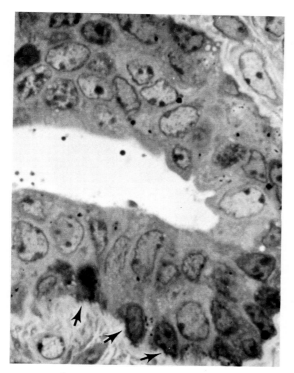

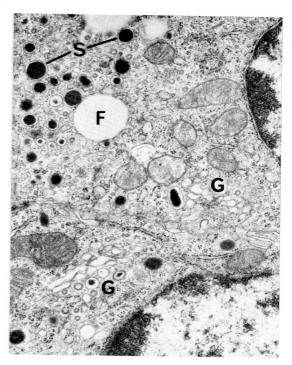

26–23 Major duct in the gland of a 3-week-old mouse. The epithelium in the upper half of this cross section adjoins a branching site and appears multilayered. The epithelium in the lower half is predominantly double-layered, the basal layer of cells showing the smaller nuclei, increased density, and serrated external surface characteristic of ductal myoepithelium **(arrows)**. Epon embedment, Mallory's azure II-methylene blue. × 1,450.

26–24 Supranuclear cytoplasm in two alveolar cells from a midpregnant mouse. Ribosomes are abundant, rough ER is sparse. Fat droplets **(F)** are present, and secretory vesicles **(S)** are numerous but small, each containing a single dense protein granule and little fluid. Golgi complexes **(G)** are evident, but their cisternae are not conspicuously inflated. Electron micrograph. × 19,400.

or so is mainly that accumulated before birth. It is called colostrum and has a high antibody content. Its composition is more similar to blood plasma than is that of typical milk, probably owing to leakiness of occluding junctions in the prelactating epithelium. Soon after parturition, the rates of all secretory activities rise rapidly, the permeability of the junctions drops, and typical milk appropriate for the needs of the young is secreted.

Regression and Involution

Lactation can be terminated and regression induced at any time by the cessation of nursing, but under natural conditions the size and secretory activity of the gland decline slowly as the growing young resort increasingly to other foods.

The histology and ultrastructure of regression have been most extensively examined in laboratory animals—usually mice—after abrupt premature removal of the young. In these cases, secretion continues for a day or more and the glands become greatly distended with milk. There follows a period in which several processes appear to participate. Rupture of some cells and alveolar walls releases cytoplasm into the lumen and luminal contents into the interstitial spaces. How much of this is the mechanical result of handling glands already under the tension of abnormal engorgement is unknown. Autophagic and perhaps heterophagic activity becomes intense in the mammary epithelium. The concentrations of several lysosomal enzymes increase after the young are removed, and these levels persist while other enzymatic activities decline. Large cytoplasmic vacuoles appear.

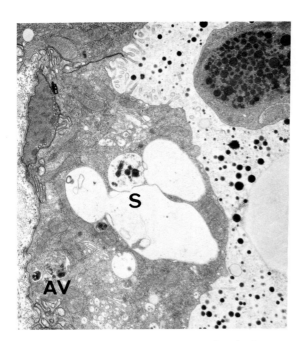

26–25 Alveolar cells in a mouse gland 24 h after removal of the young. The mother had nursed the pups for 3 weeks, approximately a normal span. There has been little regression of ER or Golgi complex, but grossly swollen and fused secretory vesicles are present **(S)**, and some possible autophagic vacuoles have appeared **(AV)**. In the lumen is a cellular structure that may represent sloughed cytoplasm, containing a vacuole packed with casein-like granules. Electron micrograph. × 5,800.

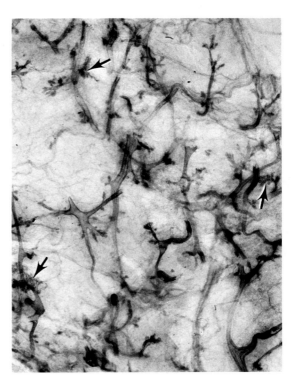

26–26 Breast of a 52-year-old woman showing persistence of ducts but involution of almost all alveoli; only tiny, shrunken lobular structures remain **(arrows).** A 2-mm section in methylsalicylate; hematoxylin. × 5.6 (Courtesy of H. M. Jensen and S. R. Wellings.)

Many of these vacuoles enclose aggregates of protein particles, some perhaps taken up from the lumen, and the contents lose the characteristic structure of casein micelles (Fig. 26–25). Cytoplasmic organelles soon are seen in stages of degradation within vacuoles. Finally, degenerating cells and debris apparently are removed by macrophages or other phagocytic cells. As a result of these processes, whether abrupt and drastic in premature regression or more gradual during normal weaning, some secretory cells revert to a resting stage whereas most are destroyed. Myoepithelial cells and the basal lamina generally persist, condensing around the remaining epithelium.

Senile involution of the human breast typically begins well before menopause with gradual reduction of lobular tissue, especially peripherally. Ultimately, with advancing age, almost all the finer ducts and alveoli disappear (Fig. 26–26) and the connective tissue becomes thickened and hyaline. Local abnormal configurations of ductal or alveolar tissue may be frequent in breasts of postmenopausal women or of old females of other species.

Hormones

Hormonal control of mammary growth and activity is known to be of paramount importance. The kinds and sequences of hormones involved have been extensively studied in experimental animals by administration of hormones to intact animals, by extirpation of endocrine organs and replacement of specific hormones, or by hormonal induction of differentiation in organ culture. Because of species differences, variations in experimental technique, and the synergistic and antagonistic hormonal and metabolic actions that may come into play in a normal animal, the picture that emerges is neither clear nor complete. Certain effects are generally recognized.

Ovarian steroid hormones stimulate mammary growth at puberty and during pregnancy. Estrogens are considered to promote ductal growth, and estrogens plus progesterone to promote lobuloalveolar development. Essential to these effects are the hypophyseal protein hormones prolactin and growth hormone. The placenta secretes estrogens, progesterone, and prolactinlike hormones; they can replace or augment the effects of ovarian steroids and hypophyseal prolactin during pregnancy. Adrenal corticoids, insulin, and thyroid and parathyroid hormones are also involved in mammary maintenance and growth, directly or in synergism with the other essential hormones.

Appropriately scheduled increases in the quantity of glandular tissue are thus ensured by the actions of hormones that also regulate ovarian and uterine cycles. Apart from growth itself, intracellular differentiation during pregnancy and the activation of lactogenesis at parturition also are dependent on hormone combinations and sequences. The onset of active lactation is partly due to an abrupt fall in progesterone level at the end of pregnancy. Progesterone has been shown to block the production of α-lactalbumin and to inhibit a stimulatory effect of estrogen on circulating prolactin levels. Estrogen, prolactin, and corticosteroid levels in the circulation increase in late pregnancy; injection of glucocorticoid or prolactin or both can initiate lactation in pregnant animals.

Hormonal requirements for maintaining milk secretion also vary considerably among species. Prolactin is probably universally necessary, and adrenal corticoids usually are, whereas the ovarian steroids are not required and may even be inhibiting. The continuing availability of the requisite hormones is governed by neuroendocrine mechanisms. Sensory stimuli of suckling lead to release of several hormones from the anterior pituitary (as well as of oxytocin from the posterior pituitary), the most important being prolactin and ACTH. A complex of releasing and inhibiting factors in the hypothalamus mediates these responses.

Breast Cancer

Pathological states affecting the human mammary gland include microbial infections; endocrine malfunctions causing abnormal lactation; congenital anomalies in size, shape, or number of glands; and many kinds of abnormal growth. The last range from chronic mild proliferation and sloughing of ductal epithelium, occurring in many premenopausal breasts, through a variety of benign, localized tumors to cancer. In both incidence and mortality, breast cancer is the major cancer in women; the lifetime probability of developing it is about 7% for a woman born in the United States.

Tumor development can affect both the epithelial and the connective tissues of the breast. The transformation to malignancy (defined as progressive growth with invasion of surrounding tissues or metastasis to other sites) may involve either tissue. Pure connective tissue cancers (sarcomas) are rare, however; most breast cancers—and more than 85% of all human cancers—are of predominantly epithelial origin (carcinomas). They vary widely in growth rate and in the extent to which cell and tissue differentiation are lost (anaplasia). Many malignant breast tumors are believed to originate with proliferation of duct lining cells. These cells are contained for variable periods within the duct, gradually filling its lumen. Subsequent growth may involve the extension of ductlike tubules or solid cords of epithelium through the surrounding connective tissues, or rows or sheets of cells without glandular organization may infiltrate among stromal elements. The growth may ultimately reach and invade the pectoral muscles or the skin of the breast.

Metastases in the lungs, brain, bone, or other sites are the most common direct causes of death. Clumps of cells dislodged from the tumor are carried by the lymph and blood circulation until they lodge in a small vessel and grow in the new site (Fig. 26–27).

Possible factors in human breast carcinogenesis are suggested by epidemiological studies. Genetics or environment or both appear to be significant: breast cancer incidence is much higher in North America and Northern Europe than in most of Asia and Africa. It is higher among whites than among blacks in the United States, but Japanese populations in this country have higher incidences than in Japan. Close blood relatives of breast cancer patients have a higher probability of developing the disease than unrelated controls; this is not attributable to milk transmission of an infective agent, as the great decline in breast feeding over the past 50 years has not been accompanied by a significant decline in the incidence of breast cancer. Other epidemiological evidence implicates diet: national rates of mortality from breast cancer appear to be positively correlated with obesity and with con-

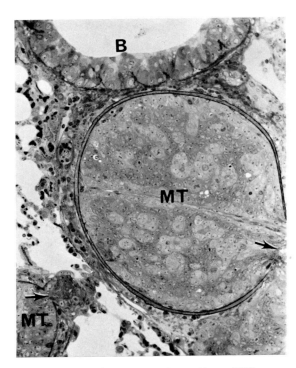

26–27 Metastatic mammary tumor tissue **(MT)** within two arterioles in a mouse lung; part of a bronchiole **(B)** is seen at the top and partially collapsed pulmonary alveoli at the left and bottom. The arteriolar tunica media, with its darkly stained elastic lamellae, is stretched by the tumor mass, and both arterioles have ruptured **(arrows)**, permitting the tumor to expand into the pulmonary tissues. Epon, Mallory's azure II-methylene blue. × 190.

sumption of fat, animal protein, and refined sugar. Reproductive physiology probably plays a role. The most complete current statistics indicate that the age of a woman at her first childbirth is related to her breast cancer risk. For a woman bearing her first child at the age 30, the risk is about the same as that for a nulliparous woman and about twice as high as that for a woman bearing her first child before the age of 20.

Hormone therapy for breast cancer has been developed empirically and on the basis of data from experimental animals. Some human tumors are unresponsive to any hormonal manipulation; others respond to the addition of hormones or to their deletion by endocrinectomy. Demonstration of specific hormone receptors in cells of the tumor may be useful in predicting hormone re-

sponse. Other treatments for breast cancer include drugs and irradiation; immunological methods are also being explored. Reduction of mortality rests primarily on diagnosis and treatment of a tumor before it has spread beyond the breast. Improvement in histological or biochemical techniques for identifying premalignant lesions is therefore a continuing research goal.

References and General Bibliography

General

Cowie, A. T. 1974. Overview of the mammary gland. J. Invest. Dermatol. 63:2.

Dabelow, A. 1957. Die Milchdrüse. In Handbuch der mikroskopischen Anatomie des Menschen, Vol. III/3. Berlin: Springer-Verlag OHG, p. 277.

Fanger, H., and Ree, H. J. 1974. Cyclic changes of human mammary gland epithelium in relation to the menstrual cycle. An ultrastructural study. Cancer 34:574.

Hems, G. 1978. The contributions of diet and childbearing to breast-cancer rates. Br. J. Cancer 37:974.

Wellings, S. R. 1980. Development of human breast cancer. Adv. Cancer Res. 31:287.

Lactation

Ahmed, A. 1978. Atlas of the Ultrastructure of Human Breast Diseases. Edinburgh: Churchill Livingston.

Bauman, D. E., and Davis, C. L. 1974. Biosynthesis of milk fat. In B. L. Larson and V. R. Smith (eds.), Lactation, Vol. II. New York: Academic Press, Inc., p. 31.

Brennan, M. J. 1978. Lactation and the breast cancer process. In B. L. Larson (ed.), Lactation, Vol. IV. New York: Academic Press, p. 313.

Ceriani, R. L., Taylor-Papadimitriou, J., Peterson, J. A., and Brown, P. 1979. Characterization of cells cultured from early lactation milks. In Vitro 15:356.

Cowie, A. T., Forsyth, I. A., and Hart, I. C. 1980. Hormonal Control of Lactation. Berlin: Springer-Verlag.

Head, J. R., and Beer, A. E. 1978. The immunologic role of viable leukocytic cells in mammary exosecretions. In B. L. Larson (ed.), Lactation, Vol. IV. New York: Academic Press, Inc., p. 337.

Helminen, H. J., and Ericsson, J. L. E. 1971. Effects of enforced milk stasis on mammary gland epithelium, with special reference to changes in lysosomes and lysosomal enzymes. Exp. Cell Res. 68:411.

Hollmann, K. H. 1974. Cytology and fine structure of the mammary gland. In B. L. Larson and V. R. Smith (eds.), Lactation, Vol. I. New York: Academic Press, Inc., p.3.

Jenness, R. 1974. Biosynthesis and composition of milk. J. Invest. Dermatol. 63:109.

Jones, E. A. 1978. Lactose biosynthesis. In B. L. Larson (ed.), Lactation Vol. IV. New York: Academic Press, Inc., p. 371.

Keenan, T. W., Franke, W. W., Mather, I. H., and Morré, D. J. 1978. Endomembrane composition and function in milk formation. *In* B. L. Larson (ed.), Lactation, Vol. IV. New York: Academic Press, Inc., p. 105.

Kraehenbuhl, J. P., Racine, L., and Galardy, R. E. 1975. Localization of secretory IgA, secretory component, and α chain in the mammary gland of lactating rabbits by immunoelectron microscopy. Ann. N.Y. Acad. Sci. 254:190.

Lascelles, A. K., and Lee, C. S. 1978. Involution of the mammary gland. *In* B. L. Larson (ed.), Lactation, Vol. IV. New York: Academic Press, Inc., p. 115.

Linzell, J. L. 1955. Some observations on the contractile tissue of the mammary glands, J. Physiol. (Lond.) 130:257.

Linzell, J. L. 1974. Mammary blood flow and methods of identifying and measuring precursors of milk. *In* B. L. Larson and V. R. Smith (eds.), Lactation, Vol. I. New York: Academic Press, Inc., p. 143.

Mayer, G., and Klein, M. 1961. Histology and cytology of the mammary gland. *In* S. K. Kon and A. T. Cowie (eds.), Milk: The Mammary Gland and Its Secretion, Vol. I. New York: Academic Press, Inc., p. 47.

Montagna, W., and MacPherson, E. E. 1974. Some neglected aspects of the anatomy of human breasts. J. Invest. Dermatol. 63:10.

Peaker, M. 1978. Ion and water transport in the mammary gland. *In* B. L. Larson (ed.), Lactation, Vol IV. New York: Academic Press, Inc., p. 437.

Pitelka, D. R., Hamamoto, S. T., Duafala, J. G., and Nemanic, M. K. 1973. Cell contacts in the mouse mammary gland. I. Normal gland in postnatal development and the secretory cycle. J. Cell Biol. 56:797.

Raynaud, A. 1961. Morphogenesis of the mammary gland. *In* S. K. Kon and A. T. Cowie (eds.), Milk: The Mammary Gland and Its Secretions, Vol. I. New York: Academic Press, Inc., p. 3.

Saacke, R. G., and Heald, C. W. 1974. Cytological aspects of milk formation and secretion. *In* B. L. Larson and V. R. Smith (eds.), Lactation, Vol. II. New York: Academic Press, Inc., p. 147.

Salazar, H., and Tobon, H. 1974. Morphologic changes of the mammary gland during development, pregnancy and lactation. *In* J. B. Josimovich, M. Reynolds, and E. Cobo (eds.), Lactogenic Hormones, Fetal Nutrition, and Lactation, New York: John Wiley & Sons, Inc., p. 221.

Sasaki, M., Eigel, W. N., and Keenan, T. W. 1978. Lactose and major milk proteins are present in secretory vesicle-rich fractions from lactating mammary gland. Proc. Natl. Acad. Sci. U.S.A. 75:5020.

Tindal, J. S. 1978. Neuroendocrine control of lactation. *In* B. L. Larson (ed), Lactation, Vol IV. New York: Academic Press, Inc. p. 67.

Tobon, H., and Salazar, H. 1975. Ultrastructure of the human mammary gland. II. Postpartum lactogenesis. J. Clin. Endocrinol. Metab. 40:834.

Tucker, H. A. 1974. General endocrinological control of lactation. *In* B. L. Larson and V. R. Smith (eds.), Lactation, Vol. I. New York: Academic Press, Inc., p. 277.

Vorherr, H. 1978. Human lactation and breast feeding. *In* B. L. Larson (ed.), Lactation, Vol. IV. New York: Academic Press, Inc., p. 182.

Woessner, J. R., Jr. 1969. The physiology of the uterus and mammary gland. *In* J. T. Dingle and H. B. Fell (eds.), Lysosomes in Biology and Pathology, Vol. I. Amsterdam: North-Holland Publishing Co., p. 299.

The Human Placenta

Helen A. Padykula

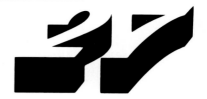

The human placenta is a transient organ that mediates physiological exchange between the mother and the developing embryo fetus. It is genetically programmed for an existence of 9 months. It is important to realize that the placenta has both fetal and maternal parts and is therefore composed of cells of two different genotypes. This is a biological situation with important immunological implications, since the placental–fetal complex may be viewed as a natural allograft resistant to rejection. The following general definition, derived from Mossman's (1937) monograph, is a useful one to remember: The placenta consists of "an apposition or fusion of the fetal membranes with the uterine mucosa for the purpose of carrying out physiological exchange." To understand placental structure, it is thus essential to know the structure of the extraembryonic membranes and also of the uterine endometrium.

The placental association places the fetal blood stream in close proximity with the maternal blood stream, but normally these two bloodstreams do not mix. They are separated by tissue layers called the *placental barrier*. Oxygen and nutrients are transferred across the placenta from the maternal blood to the fetal blood; carbon dioxide and various metabolic waste products are transported in the reverse direction. A vast transport surface is created that functions temporarily as a fetal lung, intestine, kidney, and liver. As a complex endocrine organ the placenta assumes aspects of ovarian, anterior pituitary, and quite likely hypothalamic function. This remarkable role reflects considerable functional autonomy in the endocrine regulation of pregnancy.

The placenta varies considerably in its morphology among the orders of mammals. This diversity makes it unique when compared with organs, such as the lung, kidney, or liver, that are relatively similar among different mammals. Placental diversity has phylogenetic significance related to the evolutionary modifications that occurred in the vertebrate extraembryonic membranes as they were modified for intrauterine development. In this chapter the discussion is limited to the human placenta. However, it should be emphasized that thorough understanding of the placenta of primates is derived only through a knowledge of comparative placentation (Mossman, 1937; Amoroso, 1952; Steven, 1975) and, going even further back phylogenetically, through a knowledge of the development of birds and reptiles. The reader is advised to review the structure and function of the extraembryonic membranes of the chick and pig as well as the histophysiology of the primate uterus (see stan-

dard texts of embryology and Chap. 25). The most complete collection of human placental specimens ever gathered together may be studied in the monograph by Boyd and Hamilton (1970), which is a rich source of information on placental morphology.

Fertilization and Early Development

The ovulated human *ovum* is a large cell (diameter 100–150 μm) that contains little stored nutrient. It is surrounded by a thick glycoprotein coat, the *zona pellucida* (Fig. 27–1), and ovarian corona radiata cells. Fertilization occurs in the

27–1 A living human secondary oocyte cultured in pyruvate Krebs-Ringer medium. Under in vitro conditions, human oocytes obtained from ovarian follicles proceed with meiosis, form the first polar body **(PB)**, and mature to the metaphase II stage. The cumulus cells have been removed; the zona pellucida **(ZP)** is present. Scale marker, 20 μm. (From Kennedy, J. F., and Donahue, R. P. 1969. Science 164:1292.)

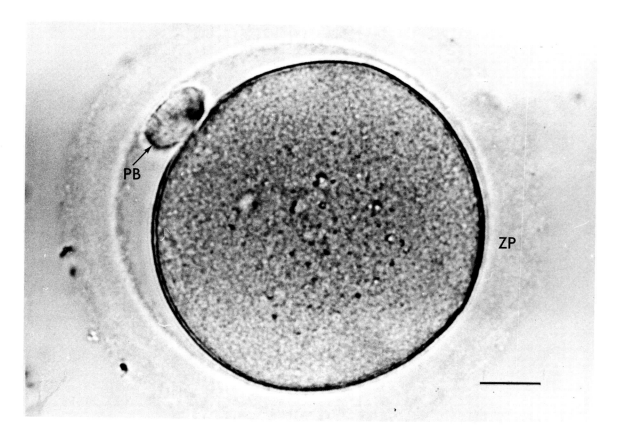

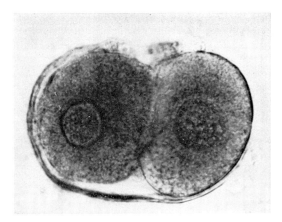

27-2 Two-cell stage of the human zygote, probably 1.5 to 2.5 days old, obtained from the fallopian tube. The zona pellucida still surrounds the blastomeres. × 400 (Courtesy of A. T. Hertig and J. Rock.)

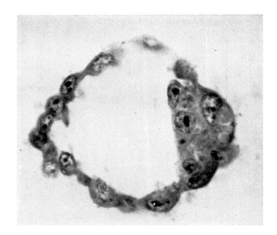

27-4 Normal human free blastocyst approximately 4.5 days old obtained from the uterine cavity. Observe the layer of primitive trophoblastic cells surrounding the blastocyst cavity, and the inner cell mass located at one pole (to the right). The zona pellucida has almost completely disappeared. × 600. (Courtesy of A. T. Hertig and J. Rock.)

ampulla of the fallopian tube. As the newly formed zygote passes through the fallopian tube, it undergoes holoblastic cleavage (Fig. 27–2) and forms a solid mass of cells called the *morula* (Fig. 27–3). Between 84 and 96 h after ovulation, the morula enters the uterus, fluid begins to accumulate among the cells, a central cavity ap-

27-3 Phase contrast micrograph of a seven-cell human morula, obtained approximately 72 h after ovulation as determined by urine LH levels and histology of the corpus luteum. Polar bodies **(arrow)** and 7 blastomeres are located within a cavity surrounded by the zona pellucida. × 360. (From Pereda, J. and H. B. Croxatto 1978 Biol. Reprod. 18:481)

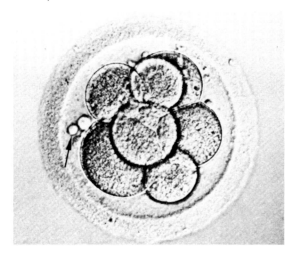

pears, and the *free blastocyst* is formed (Fig. 27–4). The blastocyst exists free in the uterine secretions for approximately 3 days, since the youngest attached human blastocyst is estimated to be 7.5 days of age (Fig. 27–6).

The human blastocyst is nearly spherical (Fig. 27–4). At this early stage, the principal precursor of the fetal placenta, the *trophoblast,* is evident as a thin cellular layer surrounding the blastocyst. The embryo-forming cells are localized in the *inner cell mass* at one pole of the inner surface of the trophoblast. The trophoblast is the outer component of the *chorion,* the outermost extraembryonic membrane. At implantation the zona pellucida is shed, and the trophoblast at the embryonic pole of the blastocyst begins to implant in the highly glandular progestational uterus on approximately day 21 to 22 of the menstrual cycle. Human differentiation has been achieved in vitro from the fertilization of preovulatory oocytes to the blastocyst stage (Steptoe et al., 1971). Return of such early stages to the human uterine cavity has resulted in the birth of "test tube babies" (Edwards, 1980).

Implantation

The human blastocyst usually implants on the upper posterior wall of the body of the uterus near the midsagittal plane. As the trophoblastic cells come into contact with the uterine epithe-

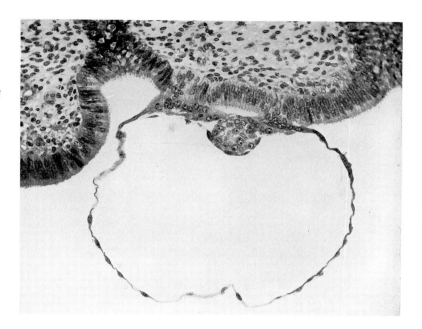

27–5 An 8- to 9-day blastocyst of a rhesus monkey attached to the endometrium. Syncytial trophoblast is conspicuous at the embryonic pole and is penetrating the uterine epithelium. The embryo-forming cells (future germ disc) form a discrete mass separated from the cavity of the blastocyst by primitive endoderm. ×200. (Courtesy of C. H. Heuser and G. L. Streeter.)

lium they proliferate and soon form an attachment to the uterine wall. As we trace placental differentiation, it will become evident that the trophoblast will form the regulatory component of the placental barrier.

The blastocyst of the rhesus monkey begins to implant on the ninth day after fertilization (Fig. 27–5). The trophoblastic cells proliferate rapidly in a coronal area at the embryonic pole, and several points of attachment to the uterine epithelium are established. In the rhesus monkey the trophoblast forms desmosomal association with the uterine epithelium. This intimate ultrastructural association suggests that the uterine epithelium does not recognize the genetic "foreignness" of the trophoblast.

The youngest known human blastocyst is shown in Fig. 27–6.[1] The local surface epithelium has disappeared, and the trophoblast is in contact with endometrial connective tissue. The trophoblast, which is in the form of a thick plate, has differentiated into the *syncytiotrophoblast*, a multinucleated cytoplasmic mass or syncytium that arises by the fusion of separate cells of the underlying *cytotrophoblast*. Intact

superficial maternal capillaries are in close association with the syncytial trophoblast of this early implant.

The human embryonic complex penetrates farther into the highly vascular endometrial connective tissue and becomes enclosed by it (interstitial implantation). By the eleventh day the interstitial position is achieved and the uterine epithelium covers over the site (Figs. 27–7 to 27–9). A view of the endometrial surface at the implantation site of a normal 11-day human embryo is shown in Fig. 27–7. The embryonic complex resides in a slightly raised, glistening translucent area, about 1 mm in diameter, surrounded by a bright red area that reflects a modification of blood vessels in the adjacent stroma. Microscopic examination of sections of this 11-day implant reveals that rapid growth and differentiation of the trophoblast has occurred around the entire circumference (Fig. 27–9). The trophoblast now has differentiated into two types: an inner layer of cytotrophoblast composed of individual cells and a broad outer layer of syncytial trophoblast. The syncytium now possesses spaces called lacunae that contain maternal blood, which communicate with each other and with maternal sinusoids and veins; these vascular connections allow the initiation of the maternal circulation. The presence of the placental protein hormone *human chorionic gonadotropin* (hCG) in the maternal circulation at this time provides evidence of a functional ma-

---

[1]Our knowledge of early human development is derived primarily from the important studies of A. T. Hertig and J. Rock. For a comprehensive bibliography of their work, see the paper by Hertig, Rock, and Adams published in 1956. See also O'Rahilly's (1973) survey of the Carnegie collection of human embryos of the first 3 weeks of development.

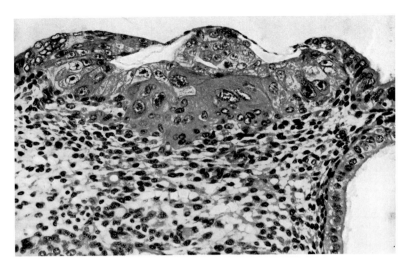

27–6 A 7-day human implantation site in the edematous 22-day secretory endometrium. The trophoblast is in direct contact with the uterine stroma and has proliferated to form a thick solid plate of syncytiotrophoblast and cytotrophoblast. The inner cell mass is now a bilaminar germ disc. The blastocyst cavity is collasped. The uterine luminal epithelium has not yet covered over the site of penetration. × 300. (Courtesy of A. T. Hertig and J. Rock.)

ternal vascular connection. This first rise in circulating hCG "rescues" the corpus luteum by stimulating ovarian progesterone secretion, which maintains pregnancy during the first 10 weeks. Later, hCG promotes placental synthesis of progesterone. The presence of hCG in the maternal blood and urine provides a convenient basis for early recognition of pregnancy.

Two extraembryonic membranes not involved in the formation of the human placenta—the am-

27–8 Section through an 11-day human implantation site in the 25-day secretory endometrium. The invading blastocyst is situated in the stroma just below the endometrial surface. The whole expanse of the endometrium is evident with its dilated, coiled glands. See Fig. 27–9 for enlargement of the implantation site. × 20 (Courtesy of A. T. Hertig and J. Rock.)

27–7 Surface view of the human endometrium and implantation site on the eleventh day of development. Sections through this specimen are shown in Figs. 27–8 and 27–9. × 8 (Courtesy of A. T. Hertig and J. Rock.)

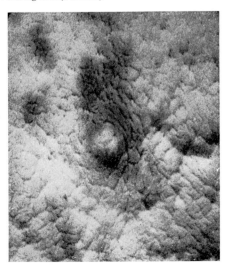

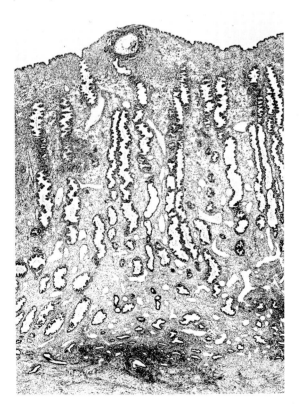

27–9 Section through an 11-day human implantation site in the 25-day secretory endometrium. Within the syncytial trophoblast **(k)** is an intercommunicating network of lacunar spaces that contain some maternal blood **(c).** The bilaminar embryonic germ disc is apparent in the center of the implant, with the amniotic cavity above and the yolk sac cavity below. Above the embryo and to the right is an enlarged uterine gland **(d).** Coiled arteries **(a)** occur near the implant. **b,** edematous stroma; **e,** exocoelom; **f,** endoderm forming part of the yolk sac; **g,** ectodermal embryonic shield; **h,** amniotic cavity enclosed by amnion that is delaminating in situ; **i,** repairing endometrial epithelium; **j,** cytotrophoblast. ×100. (Courtesy of A. T. Hertig and J. Rock.)

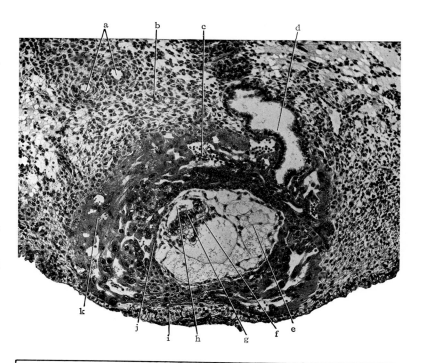

27–10 Diagrams illustrating placental differentiation during the early weeks of pregnancy. **A,** 3 weeks; **B,** 5 weeks; **C,** 8 weeks. (From Corliss, G. E. 1976. Patten's Human Embryology. New York: McGraw-Hill, Inc.)

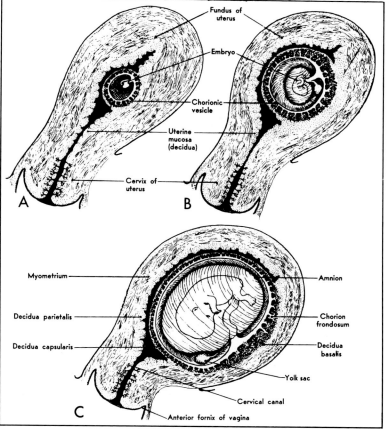

nion and the yolk sac—are also being differentiated (Fig. 27–10). The *amnion* is a domelike membrane that encloses a fluid-filled cavity over the embryonic disc. The bilaminar embryonic disc consists of a thick plate of ectoderm and a thin ventral layer of endoderm. The *yolk sac* is attached to the ventral surface of the embryonic disc; its cavity is lined dorsally by the primitive endoderm and elsewhere by a layer of flattened cells. The confluent spaces in the extraembryonic mesenchyme surrounding the yolk sac represent the exocoelom. Although the yolk sac is involved in placentation in subprimate mammals, it never establishes contact with the chorion in primates (Fig. 27–18). The human yolk sac is the initial site of fetal blood cell formation (see Chap. 12).

Establishment of the Placental Villi and Circulation

The third week of pregnancy (days 14 to 21) is a period of intense trophoblastic growth as the placenta expands to broaden its contact with the maternal circulation. By the fifteenth day the maternal circulation becomes fully functional, when lacunae in the placental syncytium become confluent and connect with open-ended uterine coiled arteries and veins.

Rapid proliferation of the cytotrophoblast pro-

vides a fundamental cellular mechanism for expansion of the fetal placenta. Cords of trophoblast, called *primary chorionic villi*, begin to extend outward from the surface of the chorion. After the fifteenth day, mesenchyme appears in the base of the primary villi and extends progressively toward their growing distal ends (Fig. 27–11). This process gradually converts the primary chorionic villi into *secondary villi*. Each secondary villus contains a core of mesenchyme surrounded by a continuous sheath of cytotrophoblast that is covered by a mantle of syncytial trophoblast. Maternal blood now flows through large intercommunicating spaces that collec-

27–11 Section through a 16-day human implantation site. Compare with Fig. 27–10A. Observe the embryonic shield with the amniotic cavity **(i)** above it and the yolk sac cavity **(c)** below it. The dark chorion encloses the large exocoelom **(j)** and is connected to the embryo by the mesodermal allantoic body stalk **(b)**. Secondary villi containing cores of mesoderm and angioblasts are differentiating **(d)**. Peripheral to them is a lamina composed largely of cytotrophoblast, constituting cell columns **(f)** and the developing trophoblastic shell **(e)**. Surrounding the latter is the decidua. Below, separating the implant from the uterine cavity, is a broad zone of decidua capsularis **(g). a,** decidua basalis; **k,** intervillous space; **h,** dilated maternal venous sinus. × 30. (Courtesy of A. T. Hertig and J. Rock.)

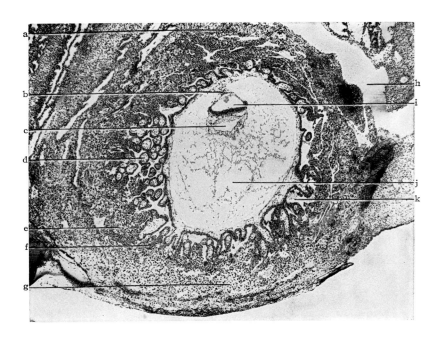

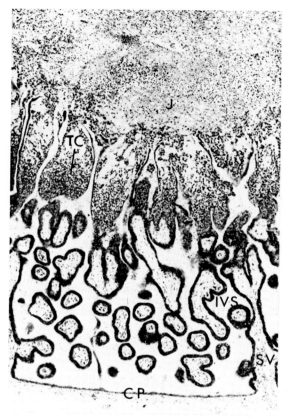

27–12 Normal rhesus monkey placenta, 29 days gestation. The relationship of the early placental villi to the chorionic plate (CP) and fetal–maternal junction (J) is shown. The stem villus (SV) originates from the chorionic plate and is anchored at this stage by the trophoblastic cell columns (TC) to the fetal–maternal junction. IVS, intervillous space. × 50. (From Wislocki, G. B., and Streeter, G. L. 1938. Contrib. Embryol., 160:3.)

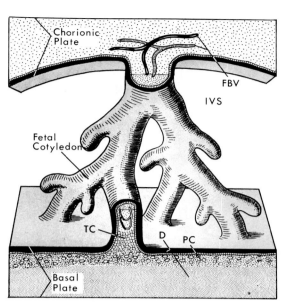

27–13 Diagrammatic representation of the relationship of the fetal cotyledon (stem villus) to the chorionic plate and to the basal plate (or trophoblastic shell). FBV, Fetal blood vessel; IVS, intervillous space; TC, trophoblastic cell columns; PC, peripheral cytotrophoblast; D, decidua. (From Boyd, J. D., and Hamilton, W. J. 1970. The Human Placenta. Cambridge, England: W. Heffer and Sons, Ltd.)

tively are called the *intervillous space* (Figs. 27–12 and 27–13). The syncytial trophoblast lines the intervillous space and is bathed directly by circulating maternal blood throughout pregnancy.

The distal tips of the secondary villi develop into solid columns (cytotrophoblastic cell columns) that unite peripherally to form the *trophoblastic shell* (Figs. 27–12 to 27–14). The cell columns represent the first stage in the formation of the *anchoring villi* (see later stage in Fig. 27–33A). The trophoblastic shell encloses the entire implant and is the frontier of embryonic tissue. It is composed principally of cellular tro-

phoblast but also contains irregular strands of syncytial trophoblast. The arrangement of the cytotrophoblast in the columns and shell provides a mechanism for lengthening the villi and for circumferential expansion of the fetal placenta. Trophoblastic cells come into close association with maternal *decidual cells* (altered stromal cells) (Figs. 27–33 to 27–35). This intimate intermingling of cells with different genotypes is of considerable interest immunologically and has been designated the "deciduotrophoblastic complex" (Tekelioglu-Uysal et al., 1975). Later in pregnancy, the cytotrophoblast proliferates in localized areas on some villi, creating the *cytotrophoblastic islands* (Fig. 27–31).

Embryonic blood vessels appear in the cores of the villi and form the *tertiary* placental villi. The primordium of the umbilical cord also makes its appearance through the formation of the *body stalk* (Fig. 27–14), which is the homolog of the allantoic stalk in other groups of mammals. The mesodermal primordium connects the caudal part of the embryo with the chorion (tro-

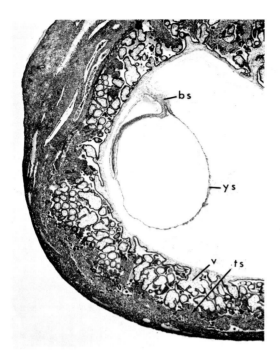

27–14 Section through the 18- to 19-day human placental site. The curved embryonic disc has differentiated to the stage of Hensen's node and the primitive groove. The yolk sac **(ys)** contains blood islands. From the hindgut the body stalk **(bs)**, which is partly penetrated by an endodermal diverticulum, connects with the chorionic mesoderm. Secondary placental villi **(v)** are evident; their distal ends are solid masses of cytotrophoblast that fuse peripherally to form the trophoblastic shell **(ts)**. × 15. (Courtesy of A. T. Hertig and J. Rock.)

phoblast) to form a *chorioallantoic placenta*. By subsequent differentiation and elongation, the body stalk forms the *umbilical cord* and *umbilical vessels*. The early embryonic placental vasculature thus becomes connected through the umbilical vessels with the embryonic heart; toward the end of the third week, fetal blood begins to circulate in the capillaries of the villi. The placental villi are now supplied by both maternal and fetal blood, and physiological exchange is greatly facilitated.

The allantoic stalk of most mammals contains an endodermal diverticulum of the hindgut, which in association with the allantoic mesoderm forms the allantoic sac. In humans and monkeys the endodermal diverticulum of the hindgut remains rudimentary and microscopic (Fig. 27–14).

Placental Villi

Gross Relationships

The structural and functional unit of the human fetal placenta is the *stem villus* with its branches that become increasingly abundant as pregnancy proceeds. It places the fetal blood stream into close association with the maternal blood stream. The villous structure creates a tremendous absorptive surface to facilitate transport. Each stem villus with its branches has a separate fetal blood supply; this unit has been called the *fetal cotyledon*. The size, shape, and distribution of the fetal cotyledons change during pregnancy (Fig. 27–10).

The stem villus or fetal cotyledon originates at the *chorionic plate* (see Figs. 27–14A and 27–36, here and color insert). During pregnancy each stem villus subdivides longitudinally at its distal end to create villi of a second and third order. These villi, in turn, form still smaller branches. The placental stem villus has been likened to a tree or shrub rooted in the chorionic plate, with branches extending into the intervillous space filled with maternal blood (Figs. 27–15 and 27–36, here and color insert). Some large trunks of villi terminate in the trophoblastic shell (later called *basal plate*) and are called *anchoring villi* (Figs. 27–12, 27–13, and 27–33A). The anchoring villi possess contractility comparable to that of a smooth muscle. Such activity would alter the distance between the chorionic plate and trophoblastic shell and thus affect placental blood flow.

The fetal cotyledon brings its separate fetal blood supply into close topographic association with the open maternal coiled artery (Figs. 27–16B and 27–36). In the human placenta only abour half the fetal cotyledons are aligned with coiled arteries (Freese, 1974). The cotyledons directly aligned with a spiral artery may have a barrel-like configuration that encloses a central cavity devoid of villi (Fig. 27–16A and B). The possible significance of a hollow cotyledonary form will be pursued below in the discussion on placental circulation.

The morphology of the villi is difficult to interpret at the microscopic level because only pieces of the branches are seen in sections (Fig. 27–17). The total surface area for transport is expanded by an increase in the number of terminal villi. Scanning electron microscopy provides a promising new approach for analyzing the progressive differentiation of the villous tree (Fig. 27–18).

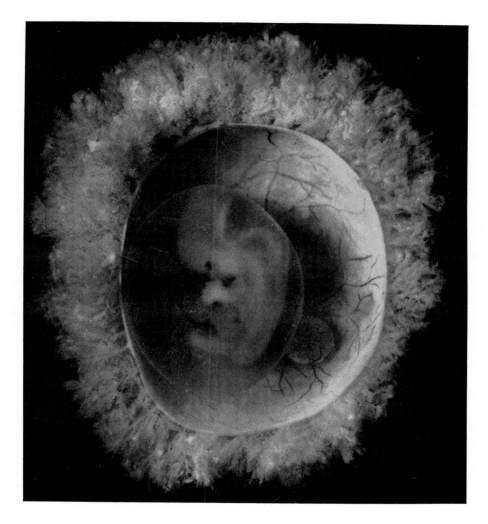

In the early placenta the villi occur all over the surface of the chorion (Fig. 27–15). Basally, in association with the thick and well-vascularized endometrium, the villi grow more elaborately. They constitute the *chorion frondosum* and eventually give rise collectively to the gross discoidal form of the definitive placenta (Fig. 27–19). The endometrial connective tissue in this region is called the *decidua basalis*. Over the outer chorionic wall, which bulges toward the uterine cavity, the villi are much shorter and there, by the third month of gestation, the villi and the associated *decidus capsularis* dwindle, leaving the *chorion laeve*. As the fetus enlarges and its membranes expand, the chorion laeve eventually fuses with the *decidua vera* of the opposite uterine wall, thereby obliterating the uterine cavity. Figure 27–10 illustrates some of these gross relationships.

27–15 Normal human gestation sac at 40 days, separated from the uterus. The chorion laeve was removed to reveal the relationships of the embryo with the extraembryonic membranes. The embryo is most immediately enclosed by the amnion. The chorionic membrane encloses the exocoelom into which the small yolk sac extends. The placental villi project outward from the chorionic plate: at this early stage the villi are diffusely distributed over the entire chorionic surface. Compare with Fig. 27–10B. × 3.5. (Carnegie Institution of Washington.)

Cellular Organization

The villus of the early placenta has a loose mesenchymal vascular core covered by two layers of trophoblast (see Figs. 27–20 and 27–21; see also Figs. 27–22 and 27–23, here and color insert). The basal layer consists of one category of cyto-

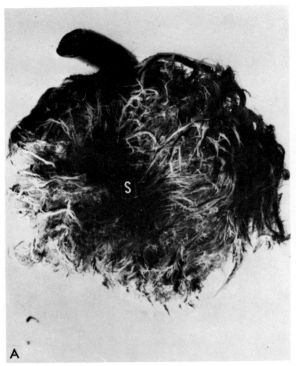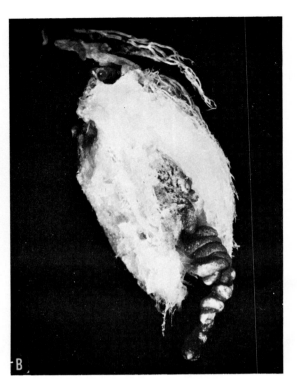

Figure 27–16

trophoblastic cells (*Langhans' cells*) that have large euchromatic nuclei and a lightly basophilic cytoplasm. The Langhans' cells are stem cells for the overlying *syncytial trophoblast* with its small heterochromatic nuclei and strong cytoplasmic basophilia. The Langhans' cells multiply, transform, and fuse with the syncytium to effect its progressive expansion (Fig. 27–21). These stem cells decrease in number after the fifth month of pregnancy; at term, relatively few remain. They store glycogen only during the first 4 to 6 weeks of gestation. Because the cytotrophoblastic cells of the villi differ in several ways from those in the trophoblastic shell, it is recommended that the terms *Langhans' cytotrophoblast* and *peripheral cytotrophoblast* be used to distinguish them.

The undifferentiated state of the Langhans' cells is evident in their ultrastructure (Fig. 27–24). Free ribosomes are common in the cytoplasm, whereas rough endoplasmic reticulum (ER) is relatively sparse. The mitochondria are larger than those of the syncytium. The Langhans' cells are associated with each other and with the syncytium by desmosomes and tight junctions; their basal surfaces rest on the basal lamina. Transitional cells occur with ultrastructural characteristics intermediate between those

27–16 Isolated human fetal cotyledons. **A.** The fetal vasculature was injected with a plastic material. The elaborate branching of the stem villus is evident. The dark central area **(S)** represents the intracotyledonary space (or central cavity). **B.** A highly coiled maternal uteroplacental (spiral) artery is aligned with the entrance to the intracotyledonary space. The fetal villi appear as a white mass here. (From Freese, U. E. 1974. *In* L. Longo and H. Bartels [eds.], Respiratory Gas Exchange and Blood Flow in Placenta. Washington, D. C.: Department of Health, Education and Welfare Publication [NIH] 73–361.)

27–17 Human placental villi at 10 weeks **(A)** and at term **(B)**. Both photomicrographs were taken at the same magnification. Note that as gestation proceeds, the branches of the villous tree become progressively finer and more numerous. Also, the placental barrier becomes thinner and fetal capillaries come in close apposition to the trophoblastic cover. Compare with Fig. 27–18. H&E. × 100.

27–18 Scanning electron micrographs of human placental villi. **A.** 10 to 14 weeks' gestation. From the thick stem villus, more slender branches are originating. **B.** Term placenta. Note the profusion of slender villi. (From King, B. F., and Menton, D. N. 1975. Am. J. Obstet. Gynecol. 122:8248.)

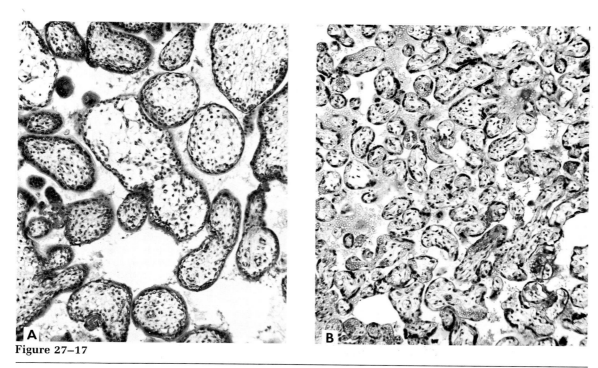

Figure 27–17

Figure 27–18

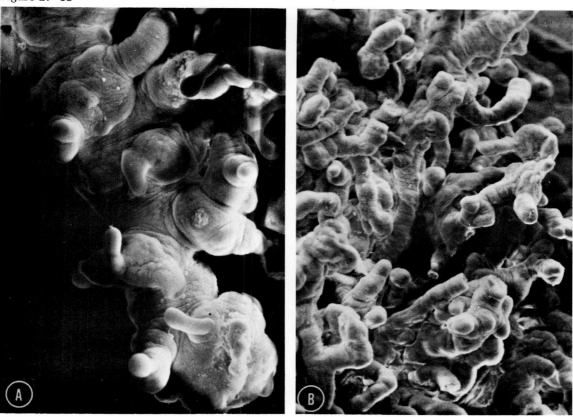

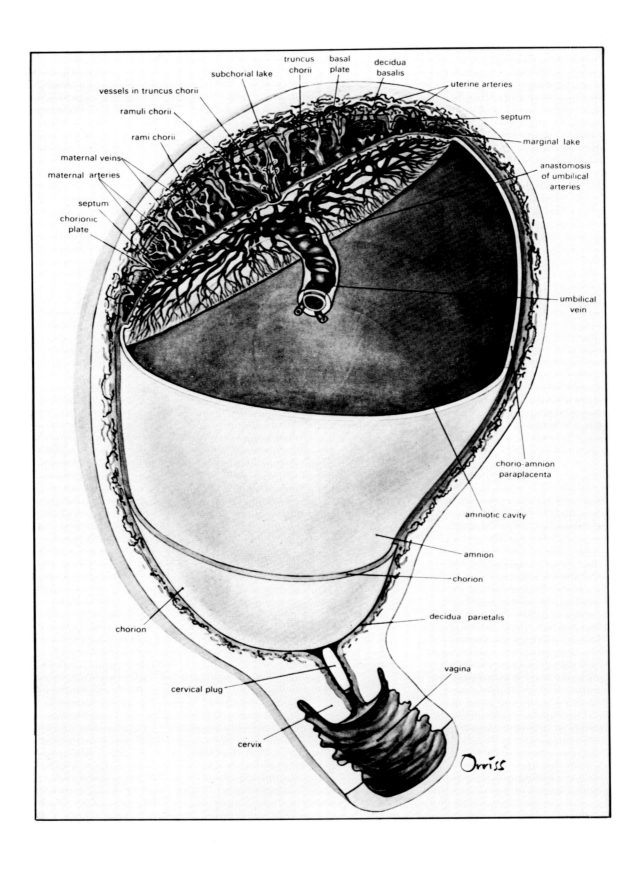

27–19 Schematic representation of a full-term human placenta in situ. A portion of the chorion and amnion, as well as the fetus, has been removed. The branching pattern of the two fetal umbilical arteries and the umbilical veins along the fetal surface of the discoidal placenta is shown. The highly specialized feto-maternal tissue and vascular interactions of the definitive discoidal placenta are illustrated. Note particularly the chorionic plate and the fetal placental villi (rami chorii) with their anchorage in the basal plate. Note the rich uterine arterial and venous supplies to the decidua basalis. The extent of the chorionic and amniotic sacs is shown. (From Boyd, J. D., and Hamilton, W. J. 1970. The Human Placenta. Cambridge, England: W. Heffer and Sons, Ltd.)

$\Longleftarrow$

of Langhans' cells and syncytium, and evidence of cell fusion between these transitional cells and the syncytium has been obtained. Remnants of fusion are represented in the syncytial cytoplasm by fragments of cell membranes, desmosomes, and even intercellular spaces.

The placental syncytium is a remarkable structural differentiation (Figs. 27–20 to 27–25). By position and prevalence, it is the chief regulator of transport as well as the site of synthesis of both the steroid and protein placental hormones (see below). The synctiotrophoblast is a continuous layer of multinucleated cytoplasm that forms a complete covering over multitudinous villi. A significant structural–functional feature is the apparent absence of intercellular

space in this absorptive surface. All substances entering or leaving the fetal blood must therefore pass through the syncytium. This layer is thick early in gestation and becomes progressively thinner as gestation advances (Fig. 27–25). Regional differences in the thickness of the syncytium exist in the maturing placenta. As the Langhans' layer becomes discontinuous, the syncytium comes increasingly in contact with the basal lamina.

The free surface of the syncytium interacts directly with the maternal blood and is modified into a profusion of highly pleomorphic microvilli (Fig. 27–24). In addition, the syncytial surface is extended by larger projections in the form of ridges that are studded with microvilli. The irregular form of the microvilli suggests tremendous mobility. Some microvilli are pseudopods and contain cytoplasmic organelles; others are clublike. Like the conspicuous microvillous borders of the small intestine and proximal tubule of the kidney, this placental border is rich in alkaline phosphatase activity. Between the microvilli are small coated pits that may be involved in macromolecular uptake. Relatively large tabs of syncytium, such as that illustrated in Fig. 27–23 (see here and color insert), often project into the intervillous space. In normal pregnancy, such nucleated syncytial masses are released into the intervillous space and enter the maternal venous system. They get as far as the maternal pulmonary capillaries but apparently do not enter the systemic arterial system. Later in preg-

27–20 Cross section of a young human placental villus, showing an axial mesenchymal core surrounded by the two-layered trophoblastic epithelium composed of an inner cellular layer of Langhans' cells (cytotrophoblast) and an outer layer of syncytium (syncytial trophoblast). Vacuoles of various sizes occur in the syncytium. × 550. (Courtesy of W. J. Hamilton and R. J. Gladstone.)

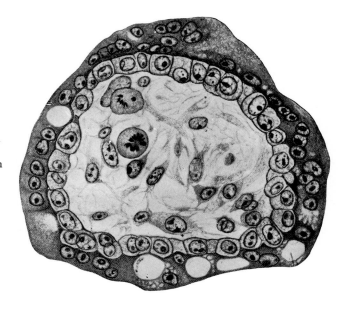

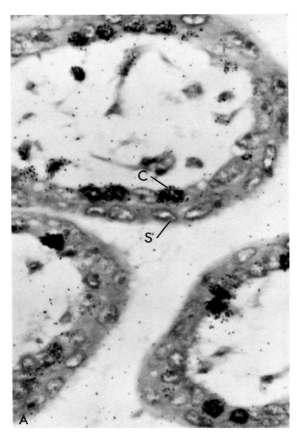 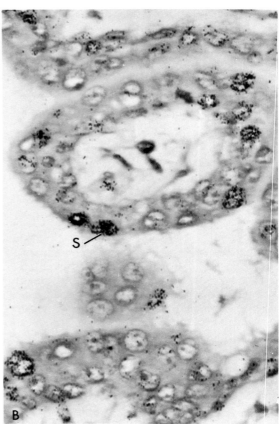

27–21 Radioautographs showing the incorporation of tritiated thymidine into the placental villi of the rhesus monkey. **A.** One hour after intravenous injection of [³H]thymidine, only the nuclei of the cytotrophoblastic **(C)** or Langhans' cells are labeled. **B.** However, 48 h after such an injection, a high percentage of syncytiotrophoblastic **(S)** nuclei carry the label. × 600. (Courtesy of A. R. Midgley and G. B. Pierce.)

nancy, even whole villi are released into the maternal circulation (Ramsey, 1973). The significance of this surprising phenomenon is unknown.

A conspicuous feature of the nuclei of the syncytiotrophoblast is their tendency to clump close together (Figs. 27–23, here and color insert, and 27–38). They are usually located in the basal cytoplasm and are larger in earlier stages of gestation than later. Cytoplasmic vacuolation is common during the first 3 months (Fig. 27–23). The superficial cytoplasm, especially in the early syncytium, is distinctly acidophilic; in this re-

gion tubules as well as smooth-surfaced vesicles of various sizes are concentrated. In contrast, the basal and perinuclear cytoplasm is intensely basophilic (Fig. 27–23), reflecting a high concentration of both free polysomes and rough ER (Fig. 27–24). The elaborate system of rough ER indicates that this trophoblastic region is involved in the synthesis of proteins for export, such as the placental protein hormones hCG, human chorionic somatomammotropin (hCS), and perhaps human chorionic thyrotropin (hCT) (see below). Golgi complexes are distributed at intervals in the syncytium. Slender filamentous mitochondria that have both lamellar and tubular cristae occur throughout the cytoplasm. Glycogen is stored in the syncytiotrophoblast only during the first 2 months.

Both endocytosis and exocytosis are well developed in the syncytiotrophoblast and may be, for example, related to the transport of maternal antibodies to the fetal blood and to the secretion of hCG and hCS into the maternal blood. This two-way intrasyncytial traffic offers chal-

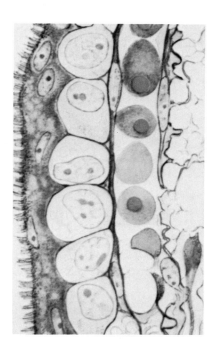

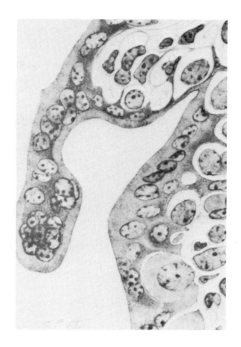

27–22 Drawing illustrating the structure of the human placental villus at 3 months of gestation. × 1,520. (Courtesy of G. B. Wislocki and H. S. Bennett.) This is a black-and-white rendition of a color plate. See color section.

27–23 Drawing of a section of human placental villus at 13 weeks. × 1,140. (Courtesy of E. W. Dempsey and G. B. Wislocki.) This is a black-and-white rendition of a color plate. See color section.

lenge to analysts. Ultrastructural evidence suggests that the syncytium possesses endocytic mechanisms for macromolecular uptake. Various populations of cytoplasmic granules limited by smooth membranes form a conspicuous feature of the syncytium. Current evidence indicates that the lysosomal system is represented primarily in the form of multivesicular bodies (Fig. 27–26A and B).

A significant cytochemical feature of the syncytium is the presence of numerous birefringent sudanophilic droplets throughout gestation. These cholesterol-rich lipid droplets have cytochemical properties similar to those of steroid-producing cells of the gonads and adrenal cortex. The mitochondria of the syncytium have both tubular and lamellar cristae, another feature associated with steroid-producing cells. Various evidence now indicates that the syncytium secretes the placental steroids, estrogen and progesterone.

The stroma of the villi is initially a loose mesenchyme that becomes more densely collagenous with advancing gestation. Two types of cells oc-

cur in this fetal connective tissue, fibroblasts and a unique cell type called the *Hofbauer cell*. The fibroblasts have the usual ultrastructural features of fibroblasts in other organs where they are known to elaborate the precursors of the macromolecules of the extracellular matrix. The Hofbauer cells are large, elliptical, and vacuolated and have eccentrically placed nuclei. They are most numerous in the early placenta (Fig. 27–27) where they occur within distinct fluid-filled stromal channels (Fig. 27–28). Ultrastructural and cytochemical evidence suggests that they are similar to macrophages (Fig. 27–29). Although the specific function of the Hofbauer cells is unknown, they may participate in the removal and remodeling of the extracellular stromal material that would necessarily occur in relation to the lengthening, branching, and vascularization of the villi.

Branches of the umbilical arteries and vein course through the stroma of the stem villi and their branches (Fig. 27–36, see here and color insert). The terminal (free) villi possess an anasto-

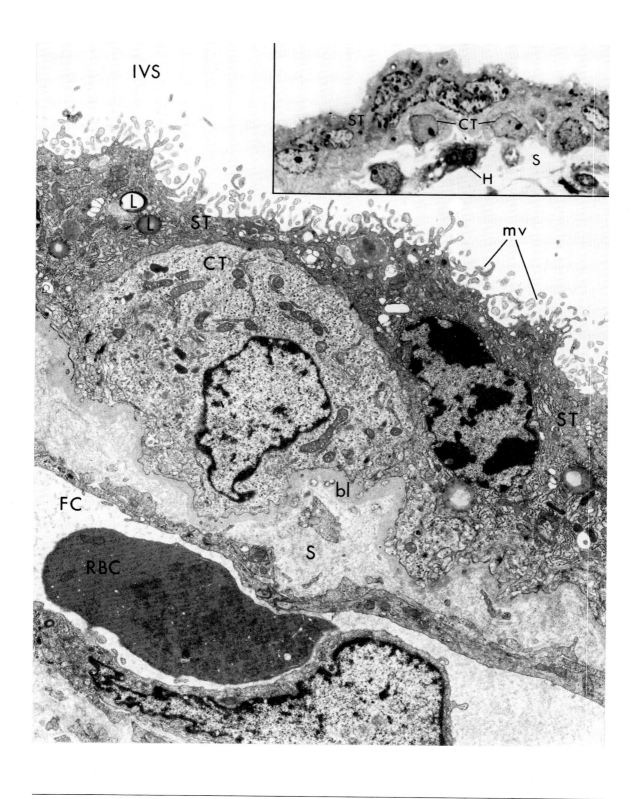

27–24 Normal human placental barrier at 24 weeks of pregnancy. Photomicrograph (× 1,240) at upper right: The multinucleate syncytial trophoblast **(ST)** overlies the cytotrophoblastic Langhans' cells **(CT).** The syncytial nuclei are more heterochromatic than the Langhans' nuclei. **H,** Hofbauer cell; **S,** fetal stroma. Electron micrograph (× 8,800): Besides differences in nuclear structure, note the contrasting ultrastructure of the cytoplasm of the syncytial **(ST)** and Langhans' trophoblast **(CT).** The Langhans' cells, as stem cells of the syncytium, are relatively undifferentiated whereas the highly differentiated syncytium has an abundance of cytoplasmic membranes, pleomorphic microvilli **(mv),** lipid droplets **(L),** and membrane-limited granules. The trophoblastic basal lamina **(bl)** is thick. **S,** fetal stroma; **FC,** fetal capillary; **RBC,** fetal red blood cell with mitochondria and ribosomes; **IVS,** intervillous space. (From Cardasis, Padykula, and Driscoll.)

mosing network of *sinusoidal capillaries* that may exceed 50 μm in diameter (Fig. 27–38). These wide vessels allow an unusually small decrease in the blood pressure from the umbilical arteries to the umbilical vein.

Junction of Maternal and Fetal Tissues

The outermost frontier of the trophoblast is called the *trophoblastic shell* or early *basal plate* (Figs. 27–30 to 27–32). It is attached firmly to modified gestational endometrium called *decidua*. Conspicuous large maternal *decidual cells* (20–30 μm in diameter) appear in great number and intermingle with the fetal cytotrophoblastic cells of the shell (Figs. 27–33 to 27–35). This immunological confrontation between cells of different genotypes is tolerated, whereas at other maternal sites an allograft would be rejected. Antigenic stimuli are present in the form of fetal antigens inherited from the

27–25 Diagram of the human placental barrier near term. The maternal blood **(MB)** is separated from the fetal blood **(FB)** by the syncytiotrophoblast **(S),** occasional Langhans' cells **(L),** basal lamina **(bl)** of the trophoblast, fetal connective tissue **(CT),** basal lamina **(bl)** of the fetal capillary, and the fetal endothelium **(E).** (Courtesy of A. C. Enders. 1965. Obstet. Gynecol. 25:378.)

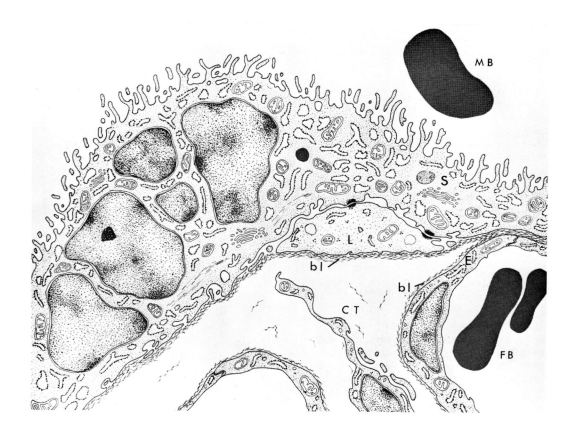

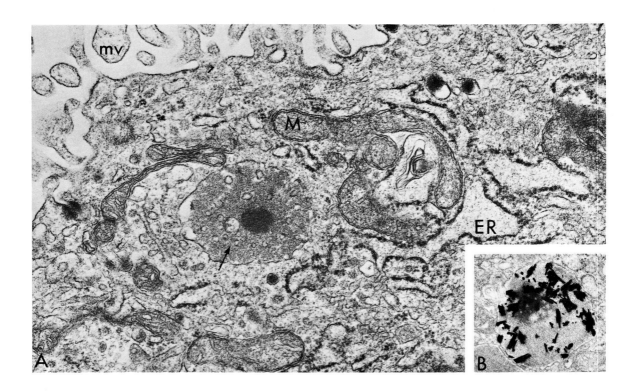

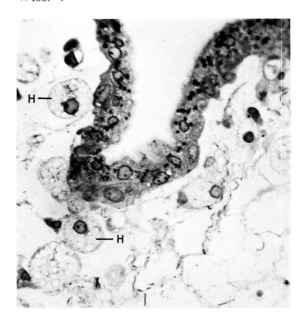

27–26 Multivesicular bodies in the human
△   syncytiotrophoblast. **A.** A multivesicular body
(arrow) contains a dark nucleoid. Note also the
abundant rough endoplasmic reticulum **(ER)**,
mitochondria **(M)** with lamellar and tubular cristae,
and microvilli **(mv).** × 30,000. **B.** Acid phosphatase
activity in the multivesicular bodies. (Part A from
Martin, B. J., and Spicer, S. S. 1973. Anat. Rec.
175:15; part B from Hoffman, L. H., and Di Pietro,
D. L. 1972. Am. J. Obstet. Gynecol. 114:1087.)

27–27 Human placental villus at 10 weeks. The two-
layered trophoblast rests on a rather loose
mesenchymal stroma. The highly vacuolated Hofbauer
cells **(H)** are located within stromal compartments that
occur within a fibroblastic meshwork. See Figs. 27–28
and 27–29. Plastic section, 2 μm, toluidine blue.
× 450. ▽

father that are not present in the mother. Much
remains to be learned about the mechanisms underlying this immunological tolerance as well as
about the strong cohesive forces that unite these
maternal and fetal tissues. At birth this region of
attachment becomes the region of separation.

Decidual and cytotrophoblastic cells can be
distinguished from each other at the light-microscopic level, particularly by the stronger cytoplasmic basophilia of the cytotrophoblastic cells
(Fig. 27–33A and B). Also, it is useful to remember that the decidual cells are derivatives of the
uterine connective tissue, whereas the trophoblastic cells are epithelial derivatives held together by desmosomes.

From the time of implantation a peculiar acidophilic extracellular material called *fibrinoid*

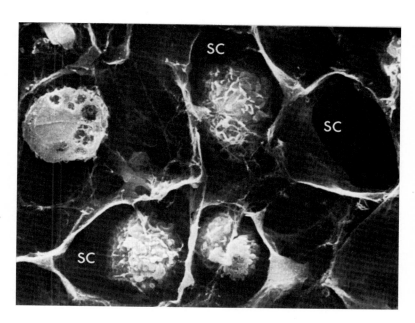

27–28 Hofbauer cells in stromal channels **(SC)** of human placental villi at 12 weeks of pregnancy. The highly pleomorphic surfaces of the Hofbauer cells are evident. At the upper left, the cleavage plane passed through the cell interior. ×1,500. (From Castellucci, M., Zaccheo, D., and Pescetto, G. 1980. Cell Tissue Res. 210:235.)

accumulates around the fetal cytotrophoblasts (Figs. 27–33B and 27–35); the term fibrinoid describes a group of substances related to fibrin. Comparable cells occur in cytrotrophoblastic islands on the villi (Fig. 27–31) and as cell columns (Figs. 27–12 and 27–13).

The appearance of numerous *decidual cells* in the uterine stroma is an early sign of pregnancy.

27–29 Hofbauer cell in the stroma of human placenta villus at 24 weeks of pregnancy. Hofbauer cells have ultrastructural features resembling those of tissue macrophages. The mobile cell surface has broad cytoplasmic extensions. Various vacuoles and dense granules **(arrows)** occur in the cytoplasm. **CF,** collagen fibers; **ECM,** extracellular matrix. ×9,500. ▽

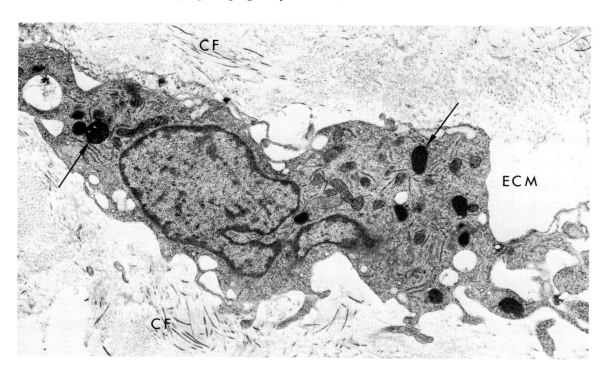

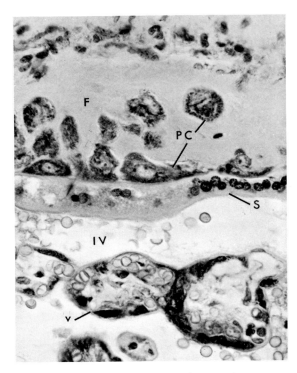

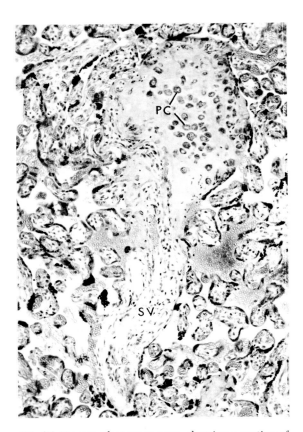

27–30 Human placenta at term, showing the composition of the basal plate. The upper part of the photomicrograph shows the basal plate, whereas the lower part contains placental villi **(v)** and the intervillous space **(IV)**. In the basal plate, the peripheral or basal cytotrophoblastic cells **(PC)** possess conspicuous cytoplasmic basophilia, a major cytochemical feature of this cell type. Note also that these epithelial cells are embedded in fibrinoid **(F)**. Maternal blood is evident in the intervillous space, and the fetal sinusoids are packed with erythrocytes. Note that syncytium **(S)** clothes the fetal aspect of the basal plate. Eosin-methylene blue. × 450.

27–31 Human placenta at term, showing a portion of a large branch of a stem villus **(SV)** with an associated island of cytotrophoblast **(PC)**. The large stem villus is surrounded by numerous sections through the finely branched villous tree. The trophoblastic cells of the island stain darkly because of their high cytoplasmic content of ribonucleoprotein. Eosin–methylene blue. × 100.

These large cells occur not only in the decidua basalis but also in the decidua capsularis and parietalis. The precise origin of the human decidual cells is unknown. It is generally assumed that they arise from precursor periarteriolar cells ("predecidual cells") produced by a wave of mitosis just before implantation. Although the specific function of decidual cells remains unknown, their close proximity to the fetal cytotrophoblastic cells suggests that the process of decidualization may be a component of a local immunological regulation or placental attachment, or both.

The ultrastructural features of decidual cells resemble those of protein-secreting cells, espe-

cially the fibroblasts (Fig. 27–34). The nuclei are euchromatic with large nucleoli. The moderately basophilic cytoplasm contains free polysomes and diffusely distributed rough ER and Golgi membranes. The decidual cells are separated from each other by extracellular matrix. The ground substance of the extra cellular matrix surrounding the decidual cells is strongly metachromatic. Also, collagen fibrils as well as various connective tissue cells occur in the matrix surrounding the decidual cells. A likely function for decidual cells may be to produce and maintain a special gestational extracellular matrix. An unusual feature of this cell type is the presence of a thick, PAS-positive cell coat that covers all or portions of the surface. In early pregnancy this

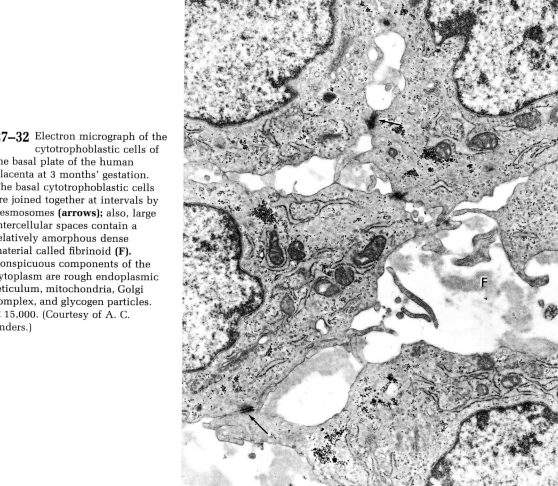

27–32 Electron micrograph of the cytotrophoblastic cells of the basal plate of the human placenta at 3 months' gestation. The basal cytotrophoblastic cells are joined together at intervals by desmosomes **(arrows)**; also, large intercellular spaces contain a relatively amorphous dense material called fibrinoid **(F)**. Conspicuous components of the cytoplasm are rough endoplasmic reticulum, mitochondria, Golgi complex, and glycogen particles. × 15,000. (Courtesy of A. C. Enders.)

cell coat is interrupted intermittently by ultramicroscopic cytoplasmic processes (1–1.5 μm long) that extend into the extracellular matrix. The surface processes are structurally heterogenous. A curious structural feature is the occurrence of gap junctions between the surface projections of a single decidual cell. A role in prolactin secretion has been indicated for the decidua in several investigations.

The peripheral cytotrophoblastic cells differ considerably in location, ultrastructure, and presumably function from the Langhans' cytotrophoblastic cells of the villus. The peripheral cytotrophoblastic cells possess abundant rough ER and Golgi membranes (Fig. 27–35), features indicating secretory protein synthesis. The secretory function of these cells is unknown, although they may synthesize the fibrinoid matrix in which they are embedded. The nature of the immunological relationship of the trophoblast first with the uterine epithelium and then with decidual cells is of considerable theoretical and practical importance. After maternal circulation is established, the maternal blood cells in the intervillous space are washed against the fetal syncytium. Early embryonic tissue is antigenic and the uterus is immunologically competent, yet gestation proceeds to term without rejection by the mother. In the feto-maternal confrontation at the placental attachment site, modified cell

988

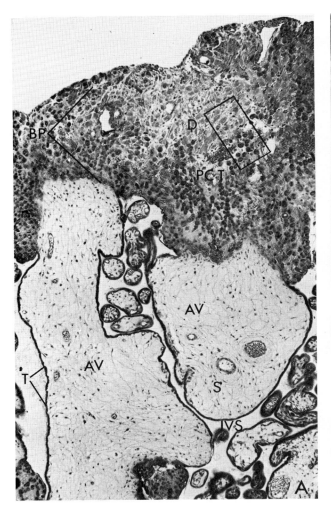

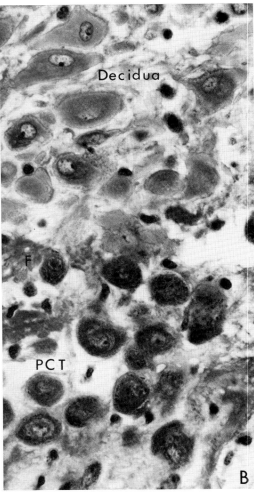

27–33 Fetal–maternal junction, normal human placenta, 24 weeks of pregnancy. **A.** Anchoring villi **(AV)** are continuous with the basal plate **(BP)**, which is composed of fetal peripheral cytotrophoblast **(PCT)** and maternal decidua **(D). IVS,** intervillous space; **S,** fetal stroma; **T,** trophoblastic cover of the villi. The region of the fetal–maternal junction inside the **box** is enlarged in part B.

B. Peripheral cytotrophoblastic cells (lower half) have rounded contours and a distinctly basophilic cytoplasm. Decidual cells vary more in shape (upper half) and have lightly basophilic cytoplasm. **F,** fibrinoid. See Figs. 27–34 and 27–35 for ultrastructural features. Eosin-methylene blue. Part A, × 69; part B, × 530. (From Cardasis, Padykula, and Driscoll.)

coats and extracellular matrixes may be components of the immunological barrier. In addition, maternal antibodies may act locally as "blocking antibodies" that mask fetal antigens.

The separated uterine surface of the delivered placenta shows elevated convex subdivisions of *maternal cotyledons* (lobes) that are demarcated by grooves. *Placental septa,* which project into the intervillous space, occur at these intercoty-

⟶

27–34 Decidual cells from the human placental basal plate at 24 weeks of pregnancy. Note the irregular cell surface in association with clumps of adherent cell coat **(CC)** material. Unusually slender mitochondria **(arrows),** cisternal rough endoplasmic reticulum **(RER),** and Golgi **(G)** membranes are widely distributed throughout the cytoplasm. The cytoplasmic matrix is densely packed with microfilaments. **ECM,** extracellular matrix. × 8,500.

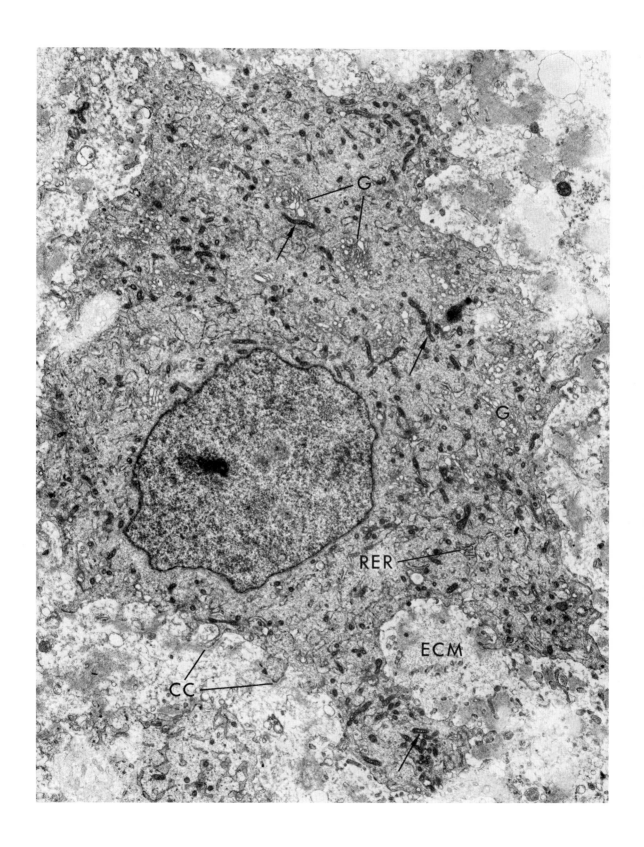

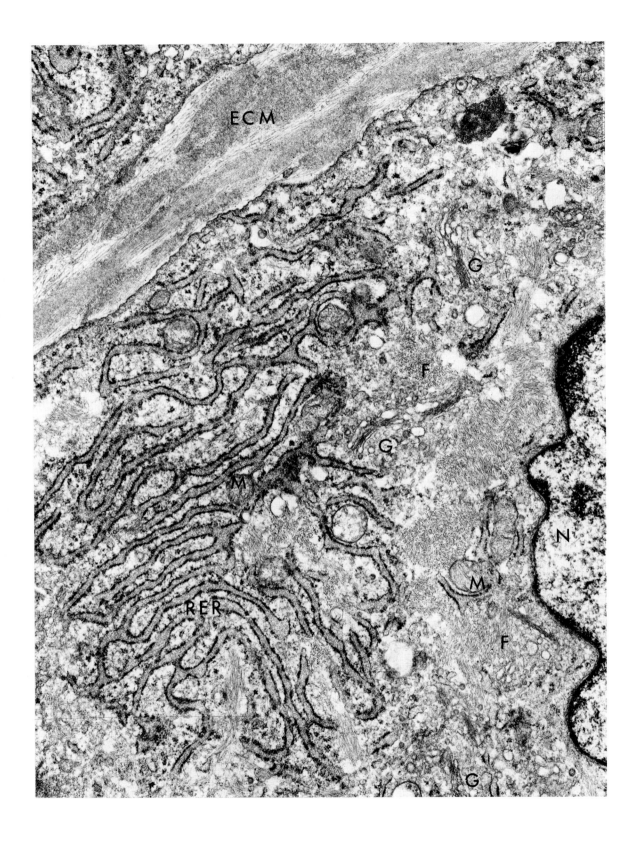

27–35 Peripheral cytotrophoblastic cell, basal plate, 24 weeks of pregnancy. Principal cytoplasmic characteristics of these fetal placental cells are the abundance of oriented cisternae of rough endoplasmic reticulum **(RER)** and the closely packed filaments **(F)** in the cytoplasmic matrix. A distinctive filamentous extracellular matrix **(ECM)** separates trophoblastic cells. **G,** Golgi complex; **M,** mitochondria; **N,** nucleus. × 18,250.

ledonary grooves of the basal plate. Investigators disagree about whether the origin of these septa is maternal, fetal, or dual.

Placental Circulation

The gross anatomy of the placenta reflects strongly the vascular arrangement. A pattern of blood flow through the *definitive discoidal placenta* was illustrated by Harris and Ramsey (1966) (Fig. 27–36; see here and color insert). The two *umbilical arteries* are continuous with the fetal internal iliac arteries and carry blood rich in carbon dioxide from the fetus to the placenta. In the chorionic plate they divide into numerous placental arteries that spread fanwise; from these radial trunks, vertical branches are given off that ramify into the stem villi (fetal cotyledons) and their numerous branches. The configuration of the fetal cotyledon has been depicted as treelike (Fig. 27–36) or barrel-shaped (Fig. 27–16). The branching form of the villus is followed by the blood vessels (Fig. 27–37). The fetal umbilical arteries branch and rebranch to break up finally into the *sinusoidal capillary bed* of the smallest villi (Fig. 27–38). Newly formed capillaries invade the syncytial buds on the growing tips of the villi and thus the volume of the capillary bed increases steadily during pregnancy. Each fetal cotyledon with its ramifications is autonomous. To keep pace with the fetal growth, fetal cotyledons increase in weight and length instead of spreading the area of placental attachment.

The circulation of maternal blood commences during the second week; the fetal circulation is established by the end of the third week. The vascularity becomes increasingly rich on both maternal and fetal sides. Early in pregnancy, the fetal capillaries lie in a central position in the villus, but as pregnancy advances, these thin-walled, anastomosing, endothelial tubes with

their large lumina come to lie just beneath the surface of the trophoblast (Fig. 27–38). Venous blood is returned from the terminal villi through a system of veins that accompany the arteries. They lead eventually to the single *umbilical vein* that carries oxygenated blood back to the fetus where it connects with the ductus venosus.

The fetal circulation through the placenta is maintained by a pressure head; it has been demonstrated in the fetal lamb that at term the pressure gradient between the umbilical arteries and umbilical vein is approximately 65 mm Hg. The placental capillary pressure is much above that of other capillary beds and also exceeds the pressure in the maternal intervillous space. The umbilical arteries, as well as the sinusoidal capillaries, have large lumina, and this feature keeps the local blood pressure high.

Maternal blood enters the intervillous space through open-ended *uteroplacental arteries* (endometrial coiled arteries) that penetrate the basal plate. At the point of entry the arteries have terminal dilations. These dilations are the remarkably modified coiled arteries of the nonpregnant endometrium that have been rebuilt from invading cytotrophoblasts. The tunica media is largely replaced by trophoblast. The trophoblast does not, however, invade the uteroplacental veins.

There is often one maternal arterial entry opening at the center of a fetal cotyledon (Fig. 27–16B). Where such alignment occurs, there is an intracotyledonary villus-free space that would offer low resistance to the pulsatile flow of maternal arterial blood (Fig. 27–16A). Where such alignment is absent, the fetal cotyledon lacks a central cavity (Freese, 1974).

The maternal blood from the uteroplacental artery spurts into the intervillous space in fountain-like jets. It has been assumed that the force of this pulsatile jet stream sweeps aside the free terminal villi, especially near the point of arterial entry (Fig. 27–36). According to another interpretation, the jet stream may be directed into a central, villus-free cavity of the fetal cotyledon. Because the maternal arterial blood pressure is considerably greater than that in the intervillous space, the arterial stream is driven toward the chorionic plate; then as the pressure of the stream decreases, lateral dispersion occurs. Lateral dispersion has been visualized in living pregnant rhesus monkeys by x-ray cinematography. The blood then falls back in a fountain-like spray to bathe the surface of the syncytiotrophoblast, and exchanges between the two

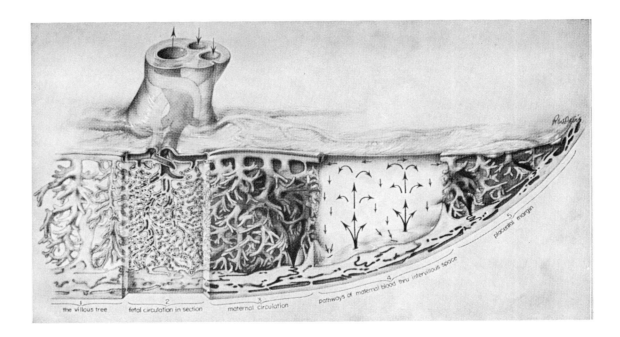

the villous tree   fetal circulation in section   maternal circulation   pathways of maternal blood thru intervillous space   placenta margin

27–36 Structural organization and blood circulation in the human placenta. This is a black-and-white rendition of a color plate. See color section.

bloodstreams occur. Finally it drops back into venous openings that are distributed along the basal plate. The venous pressure is lower than that of the intervillous space; thus differences in the blood pressure of the arteries, intervillous space, and veins control the maternal circulation in the placenta. The maternal and fetal blood streams move in more or less opposite directions, but investigators tend to agree that countercurrent flow does not occur, at least in the primate placenta. Further functional interpretation must, however, await agreement on the three-dimensional form of the human stem villus and its branches.

The Human Placental Barrier

Early in implantation the hemochorial nature of the human placental barrier is established, as maternal blood circulates through the lacunae lined by syncytium (Fig. 27–9). While the villi form and expand, the thickness of the barrier decreases progressively as the Langhans' cells disappear, the syncytium flattens into a thin layer, and the sinusoidal capillaries assume a position closer to the trophoblastic basement membrane. The barrier is thus composed entirely of fetal tissue (Fig. 27–25). The branches of the stem villi become progressively smaller and more numerous, and thus the area of the transport surface increases. The placental barrier at term varies in its thickness; it can be as thin as 2 μm but in some areas as thick as 60 μm. Evidence is gathering that regional differences exist along the barrier.

Small molecules are most likely transferred via the microvilli along the free syncytial surface in accordance with their concentration gradients at rates related to lipid solubility and ionization. Macromolecular substances are presumably taken up via pinocytosis since coated pits and vesicles are numerous. Membrane-limited granules occur in the syncytium and might represent secretory (exocytosis) or absorptive (endocytosis) processes. The ultrastructure of the syncytium resembles that of thyroid follicular cells, which are also involved in the two-way traffic of secretory and absorptive functions.

The basal surface of the syncytial trophoblast borders on either Langhans' cells or the epithelial basal lamina directly; the latter relationship becomes more common as gestation proceeds (Fig. 27–25). At term the basal cytoplasm is modified to form narrow infoldings as well as footlike processes. This structural amplification may be

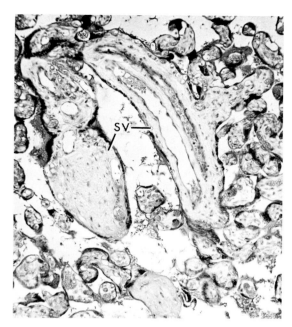

27–37 Branches of the stem villi in the human placenta at term. In the branches of the stem villus **(SV)** at the right, a fetal artery and vein course through its core. In addition, a branch point is evident in this stem villus. Eosin-methylene blue. × 100.

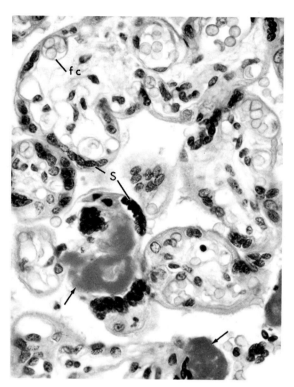

27–38 Human placental villi at term. Fetal sinusoidal capillaries **(fc)** are now closely apposed to the syncytiotrophoblast **(S)**. The stroma is denser than in early gestation. Hyalinization of the villi is evident **(arrows)**. In certain areas the nuclei of the syncytium are crowded together and form dense clusters. Eosin-methylene blue. × 450.

related to transport from the fetal toward the maternal blood. The epithelial basal lamina rests on a thin layer of connective tissue, and occasionally the processes of fibroblasts intervene between the epithelium and the capillary. In some regions the connective tissue layer may be obliterated and the two basal laminae become closely apposed or fused.

Thus at the ultrastructural level, the three-layered hemochorial placental barrier becomes further subdivided into five ultrastructural components: syncytium, trophoblastic basal lamina, connective tissue layer, endothelial basal lamina, and endothelium. There is considerable regulation of the substances transferred between the two bloodstreams. It is generally agreed that such regulation is exerted principally by the syncytial trophoblast.

Functions of the Placenta

The transport activities of the placenta are complex because numerous materials required for the synthesis of fetal tissues must be transferred and the waste products of fetal metabolism re-

moved. In general, small molecules cross more readily than larger ones. The building blocks for proteins, phospholipids, and polysaccharides are transferred from the maternal blood to support the synthesis of the macromolecules in the fetus. A well-known exception to this is the transfer of antibodies across the human placenta; prenatal transmission of passive immunity depends on the placental capacity to transport intact protein molecules. Considerable attention centers now on the teratogenic effects of alcohol which, like other molecules with molecular weights of 600 to 1,000, crosses the placental barrier freely. Fetal alcohol syndrome has been associated with chronic maternal alcoholism.

Although it is generally believed that gases pass by simple diffusion, evidence indicates that the arrangement of the microcirculation is a major factor in placental gas exchange. In the human placenta the free-flowing maternal blood cascades over the villous branches of the fetal cotyledon, an arrangement that presents a strong challenge to physiological interpretation of transport activities. Glucose transport into placental cells occurs by facilitated diffusion. The regulation of glucose across the placental barrier is illustrated in the example of the diabetic mother. Her high blood glucose results in some increase in fetal blood sugar, but the fetal level is always considerably less than the maternal level. Amino acids are normally more concentrated in fetal blood than in maternal blood. This situation reflects specific active transport mechanisms in the placenta, most likely located in the syncytium.

The placenta is a multiorgan that performs the functions usually associated with the lungs, kidneys, anterior pituitary, ovaries, liver, and intestinal mucosa of the adult organism. Its metabolic activities are both anabolic and catabolic. It synthesizes amino acids, glucose, fatty acids, cholesterol, triglycerides, and steroids. It performs conversions of substrate; for example, androgens are converted to estrogens, and glucose to fructose.

The placenta is a multipotential endocrine gland that can perform some of the functions of the ovary, anterior pituitary, and most likely also the hypothalamus. In some species, including humans, the ovaries can be removed quite early in pregnancy without affecting its course; the placental steroids maintain an appropriate gestational environment. Human placental steroidogenesis starts after the seventh week of pregnancy. Placental enzymes synthesize progesterone from acetate or cholesterol, but the placenta lacks two enzymes needed for estrogen synthesis; however, these enzymes are present in the fetal adrenal gland and possibly the fetal liver. Estrogen is therefore synthesized by the integrated endocrine activity of the *feto-placental unit*. The concept of the feto-placental unit was introduced in 1962 by Diczfalusy who defined it as follows: "the fetus and placenta form a functional unit to carry out biosynthetic reactions together, which the placenta per se or the fetus per se is incapable of completing."

Three peptide placental hormones mimic certain functions of the adult pituitary, hCG, hCS, and hCT. Human chorionic gonadotropin is a glycoprotein hormone with inherent FSH and LH activities; although its full role remains to be defined, hCG stimulates initial production of estrogen and progesterone by the corpus luteum of early pregnancy. Human chorionic somatomammotropin [hCS] (also known as human placental lactogen [hPL]) is a single polypeptide chain that is remarkably similar to human growth hormone (hGH) of the pituitary in molecular weight and in the number and sequence of amino acids. Both hGH and hCS have growth-promoting, lactogenic, metabolic effects, which has led to the suggestion that hCS is the growth hormone of pregnancy.

Immunocytochemical procedures have shown that hCG and hCS are localized almost exclusively in the syncytiotrophoblast of the placenta. Thus it is likely that the syncytium is the site of synthesis of both of these protein hormones. A hypothalamic function by placental cells has been identified recently. Placental LH–RH (luteinizing hormone–releasing factor) is present in the Langhans' trophoblastic cells (Fig. 27–39C and D). This peptide hormone may regulate the secretion of hCG by the adjacent syncytium. This regulation, in turn, may influence placental steroidogenesis, which also occurs in the syncytium.

These multilevel endocrine mechanisms endow the fetus with a unique capacity for autonomous control of the gestational milieu. The extraordinary autonomy of the placenta has been well expressed by Ginsburg: "The placenta is a unique organ—an allograft resistant to immunological destruction and functioning to a large extent autonomously, independent of homeostatic regulatory mechanisms in the mother."[2]

Biologists have considered the placenta as a factor in the forces that initiate birth. It has been suggested that the placenta undergoes age changes as gestation proceeds. The principal morphological age changes in the human placenta are the accumulation of fibrin and fibrinoid and the hyalinization of the syncytium. (Fig. 27–38). However, whether these changes limit placental function is not at all certain. There is some evidence of waning physiological activity near term, but on the whole it has been difficult to pinpoint the functional changes as being related to senescence. As fetal organs differentiate and acquire their characteristic functions, the placenta may relinquish some of its activities. However, interrelationships between placental differentiation and fetal differentiation are in-

---

[2]Ginsburg, J. 1971. Annu. Rev. Pharmacol. 11:387.

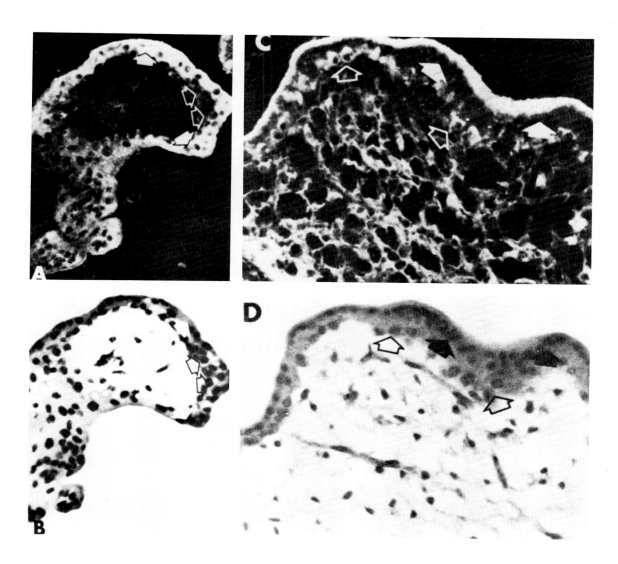

completely defined. The concept of the feto-placental unit, which rests primarily, so far, on evidence related to steroid metabolism, is an important step in this direction. The life span of the human placenta is normally less than 266 days. Thus the placenta provides an interesting model for studying differentiation, since kaleidoscopic changes in morphology, function, and chemical composition occur in a relatively short time.

Comparative Placentation

The human placenta may be described as *hemochorial, villous, discoidal,* and *deciduate.* To understand the meaning of this classification, it

27–39 Immunocytochemical localization of human chorionic gonadotropin (hCG) and luteinizing hormone–releasing factor(LH–RF) in normal human placental villi (first trimester). **Arrows** serve as reference points for cell identification. Comparison of **A** and **B** indicates that a high concentration of fluorescent anti-hCG occurs in the syncytiotrophoblast **(white arrow)** but not in the Langhans' cytotrophoblast. Conversely, comparison of **C** and **D** demonstrates that fluorescent anti-LRF is localized in the Langhans' cytotrophoblast but not in the syncytial trophoblast. Anti-LRF occurs also at the free surface of the syncytial trophoblast. Parts A and C, immunofluorescence preparations; parts B and D, H&E. × 430. (From Khodr, G. S., and Siler-Khodr, T. 1978. Fertil. Steril. 29:523.)

is necessary to appreciate comparative placentation, a topic beyond the scope of this chapter. Detailed information on comparative placentation can be found in the works of Grosser (1927), Mossman (1937), and Amoroso (1952), Wislocki and Padykula (1961), Enders (1965) and Steven (1975). Briefly, however, the yolk sac and allantois fuse with the chorion in different mammals to form various placental relationships. In human beings, only a chorioallantoic placenta is formed.

The chorioallantoic placentas of mammals are classified according to gross form or on the basis of the ultrastructure of the placental barrier. The gross form is related to the distribution of villi (or lamellae) over the surface of the chorion. The early human placenta starts out with the villi quite uniformly distributed over the outer surface of the chorion; this gross arrangement is described as a *diffuse placenta* (Fig. 27–10). It differentiates into a definitive form that is discoidal in shape; that is, the villi are arranged in the form of a disc (Fig. 27–19). Other gross forms are cotyledonary (ruminants) or zonary (carnivores).

The histological classification introduced by Grosser is based on the light microscopic structure of the placental barrier. Grosser's classification is derived from the number of maternal tissue layers that intervene between the maternal and fetal circulations (Fig. 27–40) and thus has functional implications. When the chorion is apposed to an intact endometrium, this relationship is described as *epitheliochorial* (for example, pig, horse). In the *syndesmochorial* placenta (ruminants), the uterine epithelium is destroyed, leaving the connective tissue stroma exposed to the trophoblast. In the *endotheliochorial* placenta (for example, carnivores) most of the connective tissue surrounding the maternal capillaries is destroyed, thus placing the trophoblast in close association with the maternal endothelium. In the *hemochorial* placenta (for example, bats, higher primates, some insectivores, and rodents), the maternal blood comes into direct contact with the chorionic villi or lamellae through the destruction of the maternal capillary endothelium. In this type of placenta the remaining endometrium becomes transformed into decidua. At birth there may be considerable bleeding (in humans and monkey) as the *deciduate* placenta is shed. Although Grosser's scheme is generally

27–40 Chorioallantoic barriers of sow, sheep, cat, and humans near full term. This reinterpretation of Grosser's classification indicates that the differences in the widths of the various types of placental barriers may not be as great as is generally believed. The fetal capillaries **(fc)** and maternal capillaries **(mc)** are heavily outlined. In the human placenta, the maternal capillaries have been eroded, and the maternal blood circulates through the intervillous space. In the epitheliochorial placenta of the sow and in the syndesmochorial placenta of the sheep, the fetal capillaries penetrate deeply into the trophoblast, and the maternal capillaries push into the overlying tissue. These morphological modifications decrease significantly the distance between the two bloodstreams. Furthermore, the placental barriers of the sheep and cat are practically identical with respect to the number of layers separating the two blood streams. (Prepared by G. B. Wislocki in consultation with E. C. Amoroso.)

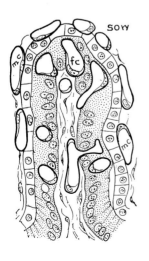
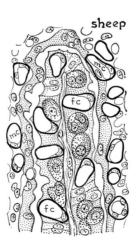
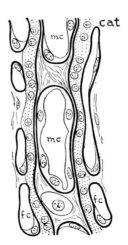
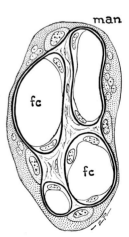

Umbilical Cord

The human umbilical cord is a translucent, glistening, white "rope" of tissue of fetal allantoic origin. It extends from the umbilicus to the placenta and reaches a length of 35 to 50 cm at term. It consists of two *umbilical arteries* and one *umbilical vein* embedded in an abundant mucous connective tissue (Fig. 27–41; see here and color insert). It is covered by an epithelium that is initially single-layered and becomes stratified late in gestation. In transverse sections, the arteries usually appear constricted, whereas the vein is generally open. The umbilical cord and its blood vessels usually exhibit torsion; there is an average of 11 spiral turns, with the number being proportional to the length of the cord. From the umbilicus to the placenta, the caliber of the blood vessels increases, but the vein normally remains larger than the arteries.

Mucous connective tissue is highly characteristic of the umbilical cord. In this specialized stroma, the ground substance is unusually abundant. This slippery, gelatinous material, rich in proteoglycan, is also called *Wharton's jelly*. It fills the large intercellular spaces that are located among the interlacing bundles of collagenous fibers. The intense metachromasia of Wharton's jelly indicates the presence of sulfated proteoglycan (Fig. 27–41). Collagen fibers are plentiful, but elastic fibers are scarce except in the umbilical vessels. The cells of this connective tissue are a primitive form of fibroblast, which are stellate in shape in collapsed cord and elongate in distended cord. They resemble fibroblasts ultrastructurally but have usually thick bundles of microfilaments (Parry, 1970). In routine preparations, the outlines of these cells are difficult to recognize, and only their nuclei are evident. Like many other embryonic cells, they have a rich store of glycogen. Fetal autonomic nerve fibers occur in the cord.

The *umbilical arteries* are peculiar in their structure. Their relatively thick muscular walls are heavily impregnated with metachromatic ground substance. Unlike muscular arteries elsewhere, they do not have an elastica interna. In-

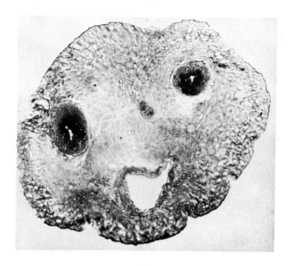

A

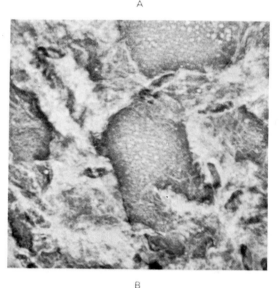

B

27–41 Human umbilical cord at full term stained with toluidine blue. × 500. (Courtesy of E. H. Leduc and G. F. Odland.) This is a black-and-white rendition of a color plate. See color section.

stead, their walls contain a diffuse network of elastic fibers that is especially dense beneath the intima. The arteries have a thick muscular coat, but there is lack of agreement about the arrangement and number of layers of smooth muscle fibers. There is no elastica externa, and the tunica adventitia is replaced by mucous connective tissue.

The wall of the *umbilical vein* is quite muscular, being composed of intermingled longitudinal, oblique, and circular smooth muscle fibers. Elastic fibers are limited to an elastica interna, which is a primary feature used to distinguish the vein from the arteries. The smooth muscle cells of both umbilical arteries and vein are rich in glycogen.

The human umbilical cord is a derivative of the body stalk (Fig. 27–19), which is the homolog of the allantoic mesoderm. The endodermal component of the allantois extends the entire length of the cord as a slender epithelial tube. At birth, however, it is represented by only a strand of epithelial cells in the vicinity of the umbilicus. In addition, the stalk of the yolk sac, surrounded by an extension of the body cavity, occurs in the umbilical cord in early development. This stalk contains the endodermal vitelline duct and the vitelline vessels enclosed in a slender strand of mesoderm. The loop of intestine from which the yolk stalk originates may also extend into the cord; ordinarily it is retracted into the abdomen by the time of birth; if it is not, umbilical hernia results. Usually the stalk of the yolk sac and its vitelline vessels, together with the coelom of the cord, have been obliterated some time before birth.

References and Selected Bibliography

Amoroso, E. C. 1952. Placentation. *In* A. S. Parkes (ed.), Marshall's Physiology of Reproduction, Vol. 2. London: Longmans, Green & Co., Ltd., chap. 15.

Atkinson, L. E., Hotchkiss, J., Fritz, G. R., Surve, A. H., Neill, J. D., and Knobil, E. 1975. Circulating levels of steroids and chorionic gonadotropin during pregnancy in the rhesus monkey, with special attention to the rescue of the corpus luteum in early pregnancy. Biol. Reprod. 12:335.

Beaconsfield, P., and Villee, C. (eds.). 1979. Placenta—A Neglected Experimental Animal. New York: Pergamon Press.

Boyd, J. D., and Hamilton, W. J. 1970. The Human Placenta. Cambridge, England: W. Heffer & Sons, Ltd.

Castellucci, M., Zaccheo, D., and Pescetto, G. 1980. A three-dimensional study of the normal human placental villous core. Cell Tissue Res. 210:235.

Chatterjee, M., and Munro, H. N. 1977. Structure and biosynthesis of human placental peptide hormones. Vitamins and Hormones 35:149.

Crawford, J. M. 1962. Vascular anatomy of the human placenta. Am J. Obstet. Gynecol. 84:1543.

Dreskin, R. B., Spicer, S. S., and Greene, W. B. 1970. Ultrastructural localization of chorionic gonadotropin in human term placenta. J. Histochem. Cytochem. 18:862.

Edwards, R. G. (ed.). 1980. Conception in the Human Female. New York: Academic Press.

Enders, A. C. 1965. A comparative study of the fine structure of the trophoblast in several hemochorial placentas. Am. J. Anat. 116:29.

Enders, A. C. 1965. Formation of the syncytium from cytotrophoblast in the human placenta. Obstet. Gynecol. 25:378.

Enders, A. C., 1968. Fine structure of anchoring villi of the human placenta. Am. J. Anat. 122:419.

Enders, A. C., and King, B. F. 1970. The cytology of Hofbauer cells. Anat. Rec. 167:231.

Enders, A. C., and Schlafke, S. J. 1969. Cytological aspects of trophoblast–uterine interaction in early implantation. Am. J. Anat. 125:1.

Finn, C. A. 1971. The biology of decidual cells. Adv. Reprod. Physiol. 5:1.

Freese, U. E. 1974. Vascular relations of placental exchange areas in primates and man. *In* L. Longo and H. Bartels (eds.), Respiratory Gas Exchange and Blood Flow in Placenta. Washington, D.C.: Department of Health, Education, and Welfare Publication (NIH) 73–361.

Grosser, O. 1927. Frauenentwicklung, Einhautbildung und Plazentation der Menschen und der Saügetiere. Munich: Bergmann.

Harris, J. W. S., and Ramsey, E. M. 1966. The morphology of human uteroplacental vasculature. Contrib. Embryol. 38:45.

Heinrich, D., Metz, J., Raviola, E., and Forssmann, W. G. 1976. Ultrastructure of perfusion-fixed fetal capillaries in the human placenta. Cell Tissue Res. 172:157.

Hertig, A. T., Rock, J., and Adams, E. C. 1956. A description of 34 human ova within the first 17 days of development. Am. J. Anat. 98:435.

Kaufmann, P., Stark, J., and Stegner, H. E. 1977. The villous stroma of the human placenta. Cell Tissue Res. 177:105.

Khodr, G. S., and Siler-Khodr, T. 1978. Localization of luteinizing hormone-releasing factor in the human placenta. Fertil. Steril. 29:523.

Martin, B. J., and Spicer, S. S. 1973. Multivesicular bodies and related structures of the syncytiotrophoblast of human term placenta. Anat. Rec. 175:15.

Martin, C. B., Jr., and Ramsey, E. M. 1970. Gross anatomy of the placenta of rhesus monkeys. Obstet. Gynecol. 36:167.

McWilliams, D., and Boime, I. 1980. Cytological localization of placental lactogen messenger RNA in syncytiotrophoblast layers of human placenta. Endocrinology 107:761.

Midgley, A. R., Jr., Pierce, G. B., Jr., Deneau, G. A., and Gosling, J. R. G. 1963. Morphogenesis of syncytiotrophoblast in vivo: An autoradiographic demonstration. Science (Wash., D.C.) 141:349.

Mossman, H. W. 1937. Comparative morphogenesis of the foetal membranes and accessory uterine structures. Carnegie Inst. Contrib. Embryol. 26:129.

O'Rahilly, R. 1973. Developmental stages in human

embryos, Part A. Embryos of the first three weeks (stages 1–9). Washington, D.C.: Carnegie Institute Publication 631.

Parry, E. W. 1970. Some electron microscope observations on the mesenchymal structures of full term umbilical cord. J. Anat. 107:505.

Ramsey, E. M. 1973. Placental vasculature and circulation. In R. O. Greep (ed.), Handbook of Physiology, Vol. 3, Part 2, Sec. 7. Washington, D.C.: American Physiological Society, chap. 47.

Steptoe, P. C., Edwards, R. G., and Purdy, J. M. 1971. Human blastocysts grown in culture. Nature (Lond.) 229:132.

Steven, D. H. (ed.). 1975. Comparative Placentation, Essays in Structure and Function. New York: Academic Press.

Tekelioglu-Uysal, M., Edwards, R. G., and Kismisci, H. 1975. Ultrastructural relationships between decidua, trophoblast, and lymphocytes at the beginning of human pregnancy. J. Reprod. Fertil. 42:431.

Wilkin, P. 1965. Organogenesis of the human placenta. In R. L. DeHaan and H. Ursprung (eds.), Organogenesis. New York: Holt, Rinehart and Winston, Inc., chap. 30.

Wislocki, G. B., and Bennett, H. S. 1943. Histology and cytology of the human and monkey placenta, with special reference to the trophoblast. Am. J. Anat. 73:335.

Wislocki, G. B., and Padykula, H. A. 1961. Histochemistry and electron microscopy of the placenta. In W. C. Young (ed.), Sex and Internal Secretions, 3rd ed., vol. 2. Baltimore: The Williams & Wilkins Company, chap.15.

Wislocki, G. B., and Streeter, G. L. 1938. On the placentation of the macaque (Macaca mulatta), from the time of implantation until the formation of the definitive placenta. Contrib. Embryol. 160:3.

Wynn, R. M. 1973. Fine structure of the placenta. In R. O. Greep (ed.), Handbook of Physiology, Vol. 2, Part 2, Sec. 7. Washington, D.C.: American Physiological Society, chap. 42.

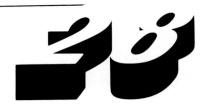

The Male Reproductive System

Martin Dym

Differentiation of the Male Reproductive System

Sexual characteristics of adults are a result of a series of developmental events that occur mainly in the prenatal period (Fig. 28–1). The genes guiding gonadal sex differentiation into the male are most probably located in the Y chromosome. Immunological studies suggest that the H-Y antigen is the regulatory factor for the sexual differentiation of the male gonad. After the male gonads have differentiated, testicular hormones regulate the subsequent steps of sexual differentiation. Sertoli cells produce anti-müllerian hormone, which leads to a regression of the Müllerian (paramesonephric) duct. Androgen secretion from Leydig cells induces male differentiation in the mesonephric duct, the accessory sex glands, external genitalia, and the neuroendocrine system.

Thus differentiation into a male is determined by the action of testis-determining genes. When the testis-determining genes are inactive, the undifferentiated gonad develops into an ovary and the individual is female. The female genital tract, external genitalia, and neuroendocrine system, moreover, differentiate without any known hormonal control or other factors. Similarly, the mesonephric duct in the female regresses because of lack of testosterone to maintain it (Fig. 28–1).

General Features

The male reproductive system (Fig. 28–2) consists of the primary sex organs, the two testes, and a set of accessory sexual structures. The testes function both as an exocrine gland that produces the male germ cells and an endocrine gland that produces the male sex hormone, testosterone. This hormone is responsible for germ-cell production, growth, and function of the accessory male sex organs, and the development of other attributes of masculinity, such as beard, deep voice, and strong musculature. The accessory sexual organs include: (1) the copulatory organ, the penis; (2) a complicated set of tubules leading from the testes to the penis; and (3) an associated group of glands, called the male accessory glands, that contribute fluid secretions to the semen upon ejaculation. In the adult human male, each testis is an ovoid organ weighing approximately 12 g. Its average dimensions are 4.5 cm in length, 2.5 cm in breadth, and 3 cm in the anteroposterior diameter. The testes are suspended in the scrotum and are invested anteriorly and laterally by a serous cavity, the tunica vaginalis, derived from the peritoneum (Fig. 28–3).

Immediately deep to the tunica vaginalis, the testis is covered with a thick fibrous capsule, the tunica albuginea. The inner aspect of the tunica

28–1 The proposed regulatory mechanisms in prenatal sexual differentiation as presented in the text. The indifferent stages are in the middle ovals. Female structures differentiate upwards **(thick arrows)** and male structures downward **(thick arrows).** Regulatory factors and their source and target are indicated by **thin arrows.** Regression is indicated by **dashed arrows. F,** gene for ovarian differentiation; **M,** structural gene for testicular differentiation; **O,** gene for further ovarian development; **R,** regulatory gene for testicular differentiation. (Courtesy of L. J. Pelliniemi and M. Dym, 1980, In D. Tulchinsky and K. J. Ryan [eds.], Maternal–Fetal Endocrinology. Philadelphia: W. B. Saunders.)

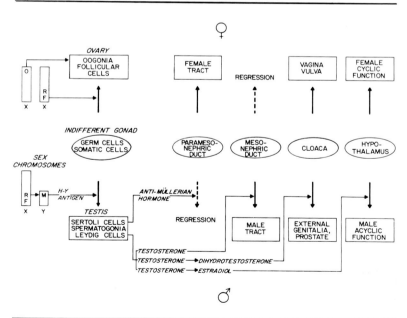

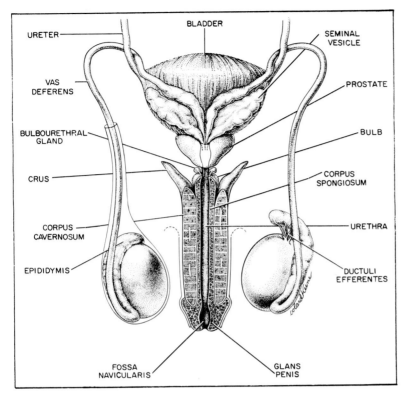

28–2 Posterior view of the human male reproductive system.

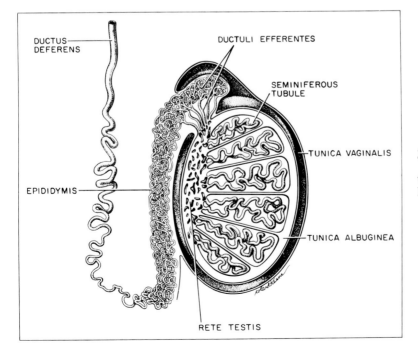

28–3 Diagram demonstrating the seminiferous tubules and the excurrent duct system of the human testis.

albuginea, the tunica vasculosa, consists of loose connective tissue and contains the large blood vessels of the testis. At the posterior margin of the testis, the tunica albuginea thickens and is projected into the interior of the gland as the mediastinum testis. Ducts, blood vessels, lymphatics, and nerves enter or leave the testis through the mediastinum.

From the mediastinum, delicate septa of connective tissue pass into the interior of the organ, subdividing it into about 250 lobules. Each testicular lobule contains one to four sperm-producing, convoluted seminiferous tubules. The connective tissue spaces occupying the intervals between the seminiferous tubules are filled with blood vessels, lymphatics, nerves, macrophages, monocytes, mast cells, fibrocytes, lymphocytes, and Leydig cells—the endocrine cells responsible for testosterone production.

The seminiferous tubules form coiled loops that empty at both ends into the rete testis, a series of epithelium-lined channels within the mediastinum. Spermatozoa and testicular fluid produced within the tubules pass into the ductuli

28–4 Photomicrograph of a human testis and its excurrent duct system. × 1.35 (Courtesy of A. F. Holstein.)

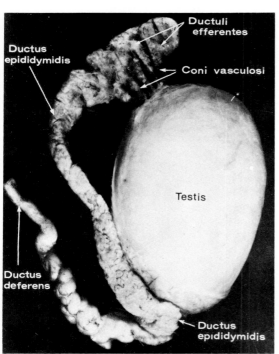

efferentes and epididymis via the rete testis (Fig. 28–4). Anastomoses and branching of the seminiferous tubules are common in man.

Occasionally the tubules may terminate blindly at one end. Uncoiled, each seminiferous tubule can measure up to 80 cm in length and 150 to 250 μm in width. In man, the combined length of the tubules in one testis is approximately 255 m.

Vascular and Nervous Connections to the Testis

It is a distinctive feature of mammals that the testicular artery becomes highly convoluted as it approaches the testis and is surrounded by the venous pampiniform plexus, a thermoregulatory device for precooling arterial blood. Some branches of the testicular artery enter the testis through the mediastinum, whereas others pass over the periphery of the testis in the tunica vasculosa. Arterioles enter the septula from both the mediastinum and the periphery. Branches leave the septula and form capillary plexuses around the convoluted seminiferous tubules. Veins accompany the arteries. Lymphatic vessels are numerous in the tunica albuginea and extend along the tubules. The testes have both a vasomotor and a sensory innervation. Nerves from the spermatic plexus form a net in the deeper part of the tunica albuginea and from there reach the walls of the tubules and the Leydig cells. The blood vessels and nerves do not penetrate into the seminiferous epithelium.

Boundary Layers of the Seminiferous Tubules

The seminiferous tubules of common laboratory rodents are bounded by a constant number of clearly defined cellular and acellular layers (Fig. 28–5). Adjacent to the seminiferous epithelium is its basal lamina. Outside the basal lamina is a clear zone containing collagen fibrils of varying orientation. Peripheral to this zone is a layer of flattened cells, the myoid cells, followed by a layer containing lymphatic vessels. Collectively, the structures surrounding the epithelium may be referred to as the tunica propria or the limiting membrane. In monkeys and humans, the seminiferous tubules are ensheathed by a basal lamina adjacent to which are collagen elastic fibrils and multiple layers (three to five) of flattened myoid cells (Fig. 28–6). The myoid cells

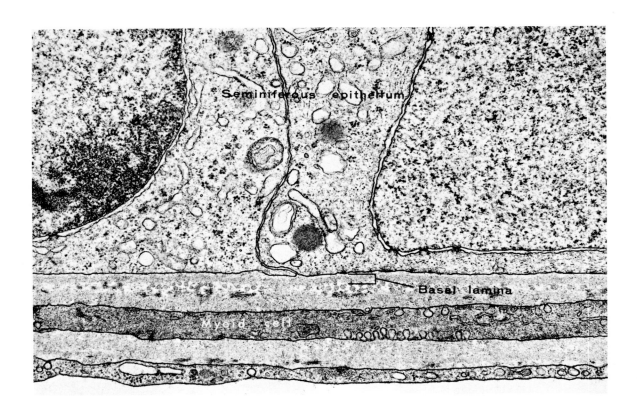

28–5 Electron micrograph of the rat tunica propria.
Deep to the basal lamina, collagen fibrils are
seen in transverse section. The myoid cells
(peritubular contractile cells) are characterized by
densely packed filaments and pinocytotic vesicles.
Note the endothelium of a lymphatic sinusoid
adjacent to the external glycoprotein coat of the myoid
cell. × 27,270. (From Dym, M., and Fawcett, D. W.
1970. Biol. Reprod. 3:308.)

(peritubular contractile cells) contain many fine
cytoplasmic filaments believed to be actin and
therefore contractile. These filaments can combine with heavy meromyosin.

Individual seminiferous tubules contract rhyth-
mically in vitro, and it is likely that the myoid
cells are responsible for these movements. In addition to maintaining the integrity of the seminiferous epithelium, the myoid cells may assist
in the propulsive movements of sperm and testicular fluid from the seminiferous tubules to the
rete testis. In many instances of male infertility
the boundary layers of the tubules become
greatly thickened.

Seminiferous Epithelium

The seminiferous tubules are lined by a highly
complex and specialized stratified epithelium,
termed the seminiferous or germinal epithelium.
In the adult, this epithelium is composed of two
populations of cells: (1) a nonproliferating population of supporting cells, the Sertoli cells; and
(2) a proliferative population of germ cells that
migrates continuously from the periphery of the
tubule to the luminal free surface. The germinal
elements consist of successive generations of
cells arranged in well-defined concentric layers
within the epithelium. These cells include, from
the periphery to the lumen of the tubule, spermatogonia, spermatocytes, and immature and
mature spermatids (Figs. 28–7 and 28–8).

Spermatogenesis

Spermatogenesis refers to the process whereby
the spermatogonial stem cells at the base of the
seminiferous tubules divide and differentiate to
give rise ultimately to spermatozoa at the luminal free surface.

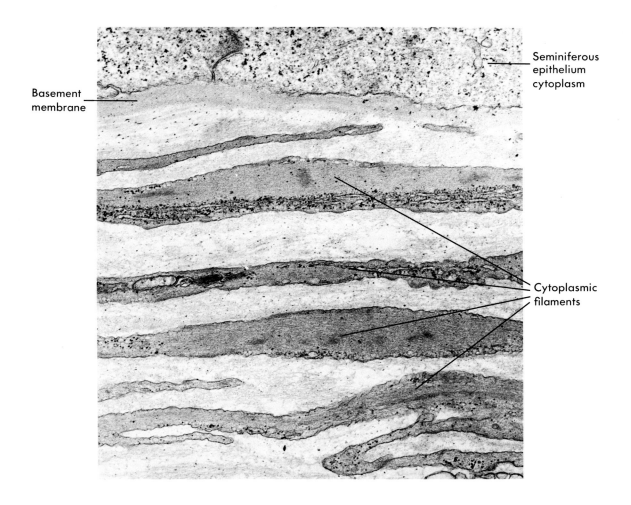

Basement
membrane

Seminiferous
epithelium
cytoplasm

Cytoplasmic
filaments

Spermatogonia and Stem-Cell Renewal

On the basis of nuclear staining, three types of spermatogonia have been described in man: (1) dark type A(Ad) spermatogonia; (2) pale type A (Ap) spermatogonia; (3) type B spermatogonia (Figs. 28–7 and 28–8). Generally, the spermatogonia are approximately 12 μm in diameter and border the limiting membrane of the seminiferous tubules. Their nuclei are round or slightly ovoid, approximately 6 to 7 μm in diameter, with nucleoli usually attached to the nuclear envelope. The Ad spermatogonium has a dark nucleus containing a deeply stained, finely granulated chromatin, whereas the Ap cell possesses a pale nucleus showing a finely granulated but pale-stained chromatin. Frequently, a large pale-staining nuclear vacuole is found within the type A dark cell. Type B spermatogonia are character-

28–6 Electron micrograph of the myoid cells surrounding a human seminiferous tubule. × 20,000. (Courtesy of M. H. Ross.)

ized by spherical nuclei containing large clumps of chromatin adjacent to the nuclear envelope and a centrally located nucleolus. The cytoplasm of the spermatogonia stains lightly, has a faint granular texture, and may possess a crystal of Lubarsch, approximately 1.0 × 7.0 μm. This inclusion is composed of closely packed parallel arrays of dense filaments interspersed with dense granules.

In rodents, four successive generations of undifferentiated type A spermatogonia have been described: A_1, A_2, A_3, A_4. The type A_1 cells divide by mitosis to give rise to type A_2; the type A_2 in turn yield type A_3, which finally produce type A_4

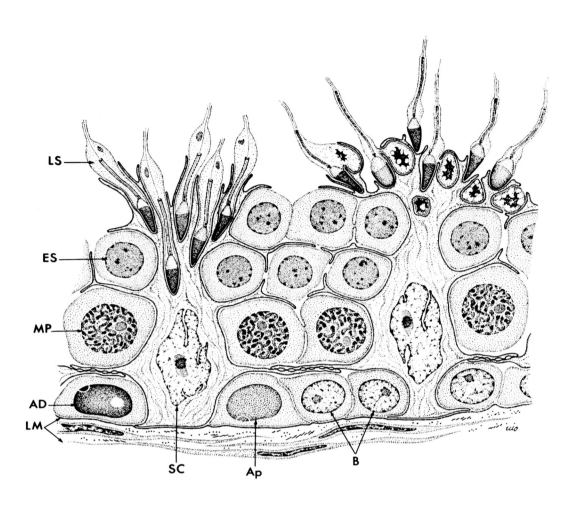

LS —
ES —
MP —
AD —
LM —

SC   Ap   B

28–7 A drawing of the seminiferous epithelium showing the relationship of the Sertoli cells and germ cells. Middle pachytene spermatocytes **(MP)**; early spermatids **(ES)**; late spermatids **(LS)**; type A dark spermatogonium **(AD)**; type A pale spermatogonium **(Ap)**; limiting membrane **(LM)**; Sertoli cell **(SC)**; B spermatogonia **(B).** (Courtesy of Y. Clermont.)

For spermatogenesis to continue indefinitely, without exhausting the supply of spermatogonia, some type A spermatogonia must serve as stem cells and give rise to other type A stem cells. The identity of the stem cells in the seminiferous tubules has still not been fully clarified. Some investigators believe that the undifferentiated type

spermatogonia. Type A$_4$ spermatogonia divide and give rise to intermediate (In) spermatogonia, which in turn yield type B cells. The latter spermatogonia (In, B) are the differentiated elements, committed to the production of spermatocytes. In addition, another group of spermatogonia is present in the seminiferous epithelium. These cells either rarely divide or have a very long cell-cycle time. They have been referred to as "reserve" stem cells (Ao).

28–8 A schematic drawing of the six stages (cell associations) of the cycle of the seminiferous epithelium in man. Sertoli cell, **Ser;** dark and pale type A spermatogonia, **Ad** and **Ap;** type B spermatogonia, **B;** preleptotene spermatocyte, **Pl;** leptotene spermatocyte, **L;** zygotene spermatocyte, **Z;** pachytene spermatocyte, **P;** primary spermatocyte in division, **Im;** secondary spermatocyte, **II;** spermatids in various steps of differentiation, **Sa, Sb, Sc, Sd;** residual bodies, **RB.** (From Clermont, Y. 1963. Am. J. Anat. 112:35.)

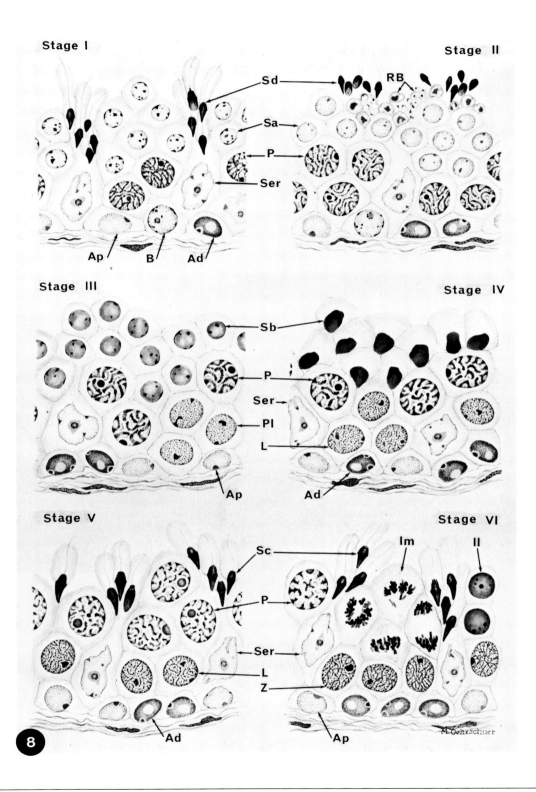

Stage I

Stage II

Sd
RB
Sa
P
Ser
Ap   B   Ad

Stage III

Stage IV

Sb
P
Ser
Pl
L
Ap
Ad

Stage V

Stage VI

Sc
Im   II
P
Ser
L
Z
Ad   Ap

M. Oehzschner

8

A_4 spermatogonia serve as stem cells; others believe that the long-cycling population of cells, the type Ao, are in fact the stem cells (As).

In man and monkeys, 3 h after a single injection of ^{3}H-thymidine, the type Ad spermatogonia remain unlabeled, thus indicating that they are not actively undergoing mitosis. The Ad may be the "reserve" stem cells or the long-cycling spermatogonia population in the primates and perhaps sporadically give rise to type Ap spermatogonia in order to maintain their numbers at normal levels. The type Ap spermatogonia divide by mitosis to give rise to type B cells.

Spermatocytes and Meiosis

Meiosis is a type of nuclear division restricted to gametes, that is, spermatocytes and oocytes, wherein the number of chromosomes characteristic of somatic cells, the diploid number (2n), is halved to the haploid number (1n). For this reason meiosis is termed a reduction division. The haploid nuclei of the gametes unite and the diploid number of chromosomes is restored in the process of fertilization. The fertilized ovum and all its descendents except the gametes divide by mitotic division, and the diploid number is therefore maintained in somatic cells. Meiosis has the second major function of providing genetic variation by the exchange of segments of homologous chromosomes and the random selection of one of the two homologs during the reduction division.

Meiosis involves two successive nuclear divisions with one division of chromosomes (Chap. 1). Preleptotene spermatocytes produced as a result of the mitotic divisions of the type B spermatogonia closely resemble the parent type B cells, although their nuclei are somewhat smaller. They are located at the periphery of the tubule and are frequently in direct contact with the basal lamina of the epithelium (Fig. 28–8). Soon after their formation the preleptotene spermatocytes duplicate their DNA in preparation for the first meiotic division, which reduces the number of chromosomes to the haploid condition. After the incorporation of nucleotides and other substances for DNA synthesis, the preleptotene spermatocytes migrate away from the basal lamina. The lengthy prophase of this division involves extensive rearrangement of the chromatin as the cells progress through leptotene, zygotene, pachytene, and diplotene stages.

In the leptotene stage the chromosomes are evident as thin and delicate filaments. This stage is followed by zygotene, where pairing of homologous chromosomes occurs (synapsis). As the cells enter pachytene, the chromosomes become shorter and thicker and each one splits into two chromatids, attached by a centromere. There is a marked increase in nuclear and cellular volume as the cells progress through the pachytene stage. It is also at this stage that an exchange of genetic material occurs between pairs of homologous chromosomes.

During synapsis, as the homologous chromosomes pair, unusual tripartite structures become visible in the nuclues (Fig. 28–9). They are composed of two parallel bands separated by a clearer interval in which a thin dense line is found. These structures are called synaptonemal complexes and are typically found in zygotene and pachytene spermatocytes. The synaptonemal complexes appear to be sites of attachment of the two homologous chromosomes. Each pair of homologous chromosomes is attached at both ends to the nuclear envelope. The homologous paired chromosomes, called a bivalent, therefore consist of four chromatids. The pachytene stage is very long, occupying about 16 days in humans; these cells are therefore visible in most cross sections of seminiferous tubules.

After the pachytene stage, the two chromosomes of each bivalent separate sufficiently to become visible (diplotene stage), but at certain points along their length they remain attached. These attachment sites are termed chiasmata. The final stage of prophase of the first meiotic division is called diakinesis. During diakinesis the chromosomes of each bivalent pair move farther apart, thicken even more, and stain very deeply.

At the end of prophase, after the dissolution of the nuclear envelope, the two bivalents (four chromatids) align themselves at the equatorial plate in metaphase I. During anaphase I the daughter chromatids of each homolog, united by their centromeres, move to opposite poles. In contrast to mitosis, the centromeres of the first meiotic division do not divide. Anaphase I and telophase I quickly follow and two new cells, namely, the secondary spermatocytes, are formed, each containing the haploid number of chromosomes.

Secondary spermatocytes (8 to 9 μm) are much smaller than primary spermatocytes and, in addition to size differences, may be identified in sections by their spherical nuclei containing pale granular chromatin. Since they have a relatively short duration (8 h), they are infrequently found

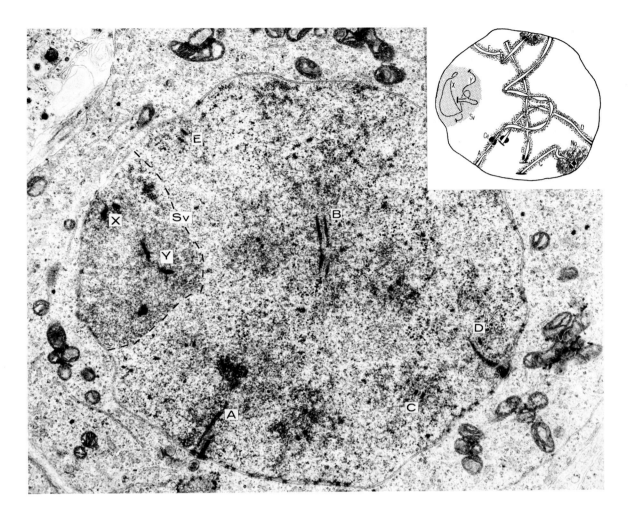

in sections of seminiferous tubules. The secondary spermatocytes quickly enter the prophase of the second maturation division without duplicating their DNA. During metaphase II, the chromosomes line up on the equatorial plane; whereas in anaphase II, the centromeres divide and each chromatid moves to the opposite pole in a manner identical to that seen in mitosis. After telophase II, the young spermatids are formed, each containing the haploid number of chromosomes.

Spermatids and Spermiogenesis

Spermiogenesis refers specifically to the differentiation of the newly formed spermatids to mature spermatids just before their release into the tubule lumen. The major features of this extraordinarily complex process involve elaboration of the acrosome from the Golgi apparatus, conden-

29–9 An electron micrograph of a rat pachytene spermatocyte. Portions of five synaptonemal complexes (**A, B, C, D,** and **E**) can be seen. Inside the sex vesicle (**Sv**), portions of the X and Y chromosomes are seen. (Courtesy of A. Hugenholtz.) **Inset.** Five synaptonemal complexes (**A, B, C, D,** and **E**) shown in the electron micrograph are depicted in this drawing, based on serial sectioning of the entire nucleus. Each complex represents a set of paired chromosomes, has a centromere (**Ce**), and is attached with both ends to the nuclear envelope. A is the longest pair of chromosomes and C and E are nucleolar-bearing (**No**) chromosomes. The sex vesicle (**Sv**) contains the cores of the X and Y chromosomes. (Courtesy of P. B. Moens.)

sation and elongation of the nucleus, formation of a motile flagellum, and extensive shedding of cytoplasm. The factors responsible for these dramatic nuclear and cytoplasmic changes are still poorly understood.

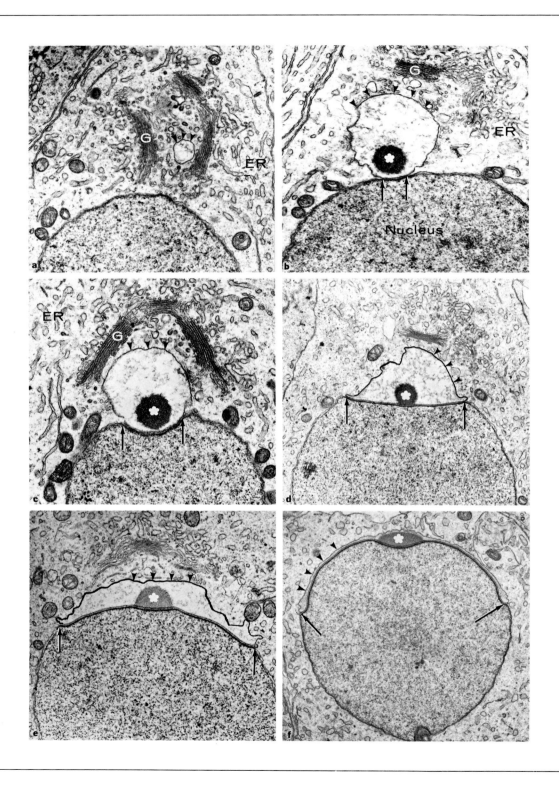

28–10 Electron micrographs of successive steps in the development of the acrosome in monkey spermatids. During early spermiogenesis **(a)** a small forming acrosomic vesicle **(arrowheads)** is visible in the juxtanuclear Golgi **(G)** region. The acrosomic granule **(white asterisk)** soon forms within the vesicle and both migrate to the nuclear envelope **(b)**. Gradually the acrosomic vesicle **(arrowheads)** spreads to cap more than one-half of the nuclear surface **(c, d, e, and f)**. Arrows in b–f mark boundaries of cover of nuclear membrane by the acrosome. The acrosomic granule appears to redistribute and form the acrosomal contents **(f)**. Note the well-developed smooth endoplasmic reticulum **(ER)** and its intimate association with the Golgi complex. Parts a, b, and c, × 11,000; d, e, and f, × 8,700; d and e were slightly retouched. (From M. Pladellorens and M. Dym.)

It is convenient for descriptive purposes to subdivide spermiogenesis into four successive phases: Golgi, cap, acrosome, and maturation (Figs. 28–10 to 28–12).

Golgi Phase. The newly formed spermatids closely resemble the secondary spermatocytes from which they are derived although their nuclei are somewhat smaller (5 to 6 μm). The cytoplasm is pale-stained and contains a juxtanuclear Golgi complex. Perinuclear mitochondria, a pair of centrioles, free ribosomes, smooth endoplasmic reticulum, and a few lipid droplets characterize the cytoplasm. An irregularly shaped basophilic mass, the chromatoid body, is also visible. An early sign of spermatid differentiation is the appearance of periodic acid Schiff–positive granules in the region of the Golgi apparatus (Fig. 28–10). These proacrosomic granules, rich in glycoprotein, soon coalesce within a membrane-bounded acrosomic vesicle, containing a single large granule, the acrosomic granule, that becomes closely applied to the nuclear envelope. The acrosomic granule appears to be surrounded by the less dense acrosomic vesicle. The vesicle and granule continue to enlarge through further contributions from the surrounding Golgi substance. There are numerous communications between the extensive smooth endoplasmic reticulum and the Golgi complex. The position of the acrosomic region on the nucleus identifies the anterior pole of the spermatid. During this phase of spermatid development, in many species, the mitochondria suddenly migrate toward the periphery of the cytoplasm to lie very close to the plasma membrane. In 1-μm sections of epon-embedded seminiferous tubules examined with the light microscope, the spermatid plasma membrane appears thickened and somewhat irregular as a result of the close association of the mitochondria.

While the acrosomic granule and vesicle are being elaborated, the two cylindrical centrioles, situated at right angles to each other, move from a position near the nucleus to the periphery of the cell opposite the forming acrosome (Fig. 28–12). Formation of the characteristic axoneme of the sperm tail (nine peripheral doublets plus a central pair of microtubules) is initiated by the distal centriole, which is now oriented perpendicular to the cell surface. The centrioles migrate back to the nucleus along the long axis of the cell without interrupting the formation of the microtubular core of the tail. The proximal centriole attaches itself to the caudal pole of the nucleus (implantation fossa) while the distal centriole continues to induce the production of the flagellum.

Cap Phase. During this phase a head, or acrosomic cap, develops from the acrosomic vesicle and granule and spreads eventually to overlie the entire anterior half of the nucleus (Figs. 28–10 and 28–12). The acrosomal cap, derived through reshaping of the membrane of the acrosomal vesicle, consists of an outer and inner acrosomal membrane enclosing the acrosomal contents. Between the nuclear envelope and the inner acrosomal membrane, a granular-filamentous material forms. Furthermore, in the region of the acrosome, the nuclear envelope loses its nuclear pores and appears denser, possibly because of chromatin condensation on its inner aspect. The chromatoid body migrates to the region of the centrioles and appears to surround the origin of the flagellum near the distal centriole.

Acrosome Phase. The main characteristics of this phase are the orientation of the anterior pole of the spermatid nucleus (acrosomic region) toward the base of seminiferous tubules and the elongation and condensation of the nucleus itself (Fig. 28–11). The spermatid cytoplasm is displaced toward the luminal region of the seminiferous tubules. In this manner the acrosomal region of the nucleus closely approximates the plasma membrane and the cell becomes somewhat elongated. The nucleus begin to progressively flatten and elongate while the chromatin

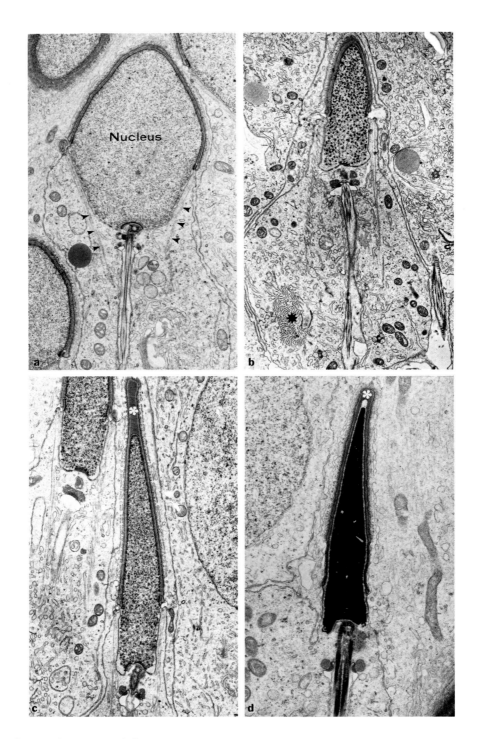

28–11 Nuclear condensation and elongation are demonstrated in these electron micrographs. The arrowheads in **a** point to the manchette. Note the unusual pattern of endoplasmic reticulum **(black asterisk)** in **b.** The **white asterisks** demonstrate the apical segment of the acrosome. Parts a, b, c, and d approximately × 8,000. (From M. Pladellorens and M. Dym.)

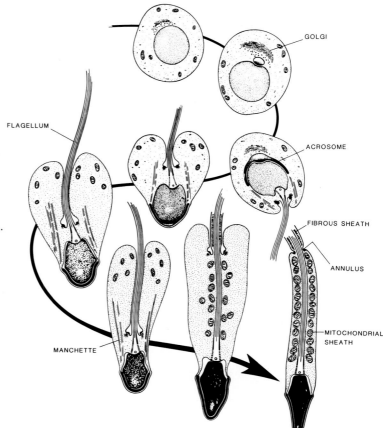

28–12 A schematic drawing of spermiogenesis in the human.

granules enlarge and become uniform in size and evenly dispersed, except for some clear spaces. These vacuoles mostly disappear, and in the final stages the nuclei assume a homogeneous appearance, stain very deeply, and are devoid of visible substructure (Fig. 28–11).

The Golgi complex detaches itself from the anterior pole of the nucleus and migrates freely in the cytoplasm when the acrosome ceases growing. About the same time, cytoplasmic microtubules are assembled and form a cylindrical sheath that attaches itself to the caudal pole of the nucleus close to the posterior margin of the acrosome cap. This sheath is called the manchette, or caudal tube, the function of which remains unknown (Figs. 28–11 and 28–12).

In the region of the implantation fossa there are modifications in the centriolar apparatus that result in the formation of the neck region or connecting piece of the spermatozoa (Fig. 28–13). As the tail differentiates further, nine longitudinally

oriented coarse fibers form along the flagellum adjacent to the microtubules. These nine columns of dense fibers are firmly united to nine segmented columns in the connecting piece of the neck (Fig. 28–13).

The annulus, a ringlike structure near the centrioles, migrates down the flagellum. The mitochondria, which up to now were dispersed in the spermatid cytoplasm, line up along the coarse fibers of the flagellum from the neck region to the annulus (Fig. 28–14). This portion of the tail is called the midpiece. As the mitochondrial migration ends, the caudal tube disappears. Distal to the midpiece a fibrous sheath develops to surround the nine longitudinally oriented coarse fibers (Fig. 28–15). The plasma membrane of the spermatid follows closely the contours of the developing flagellum.

Maturation Phase. The main features of this phase are the pinching off and phagocytosis of

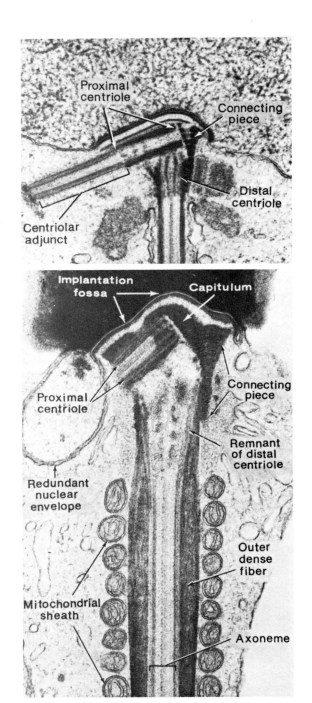

28-13 These electron micrographs demonstrate the neck region of the developing spermatids. The segmented connecting piece appears to be continuous with the outer dense fibers. During further development, the centriolar adjunct and the distal centriole disappear. A, × 14,560; B, × 20,800. (From Bloom, W., and Fawcett, D. W. 1975. A Textbook of Histology, 10th ed. Philadelphia: W. B. Saunders Co.)

the residual spermatid cytoplasm by the Sertoli cells. Finally, the Sertoli cells engineer the release of the late spermatids into the tubule lumen. In some species there may be further condensation of the nucleus and shape alterations in the acrosome during this final phase of spermiogenesis.

The Spermatozoon

The mature human spermatozoon is approximately 60 μm long and may be subdivided into two major parts, the head and the tail. The principal components of the head are the acrosome and the nucleus. Segments of the tail, in order of their proximity to the head, are designated the neck, the middle piece, the principal piece, and the end piece (Figs. 28–16; 28–17, see here and color insert; and 28–18).

The head, which consists mostly of nucleus and acrosome, has a flattened pyriform shape and is 4.5 μm long, 3.0 μm wide, and 1 μm deep. The condensed nucleus is a compact mass of chromatin that appears very dense and homogeneous in electron micrographs. The acrosome overlies the anterior two-thirds of the nucleus like a cap and contains glycoprotein and numerous lysosomal enzymes that are important in fertilization. In some species the acrosome projects well beyond the anterior tip of the nucleus and has a volume many times that of the nucleus. In the human, however, the acrosome is relatively small and closely follows the nuclear contours.

The neck region consists of a pair of centrioles and nine segmented columns (connecting piece) that appear to merge with the nine outer dense fibers of the rest of the tail. The middle piece, a segment about 5 to 7 μm long and a little over 1 μm thick, extends from the neck to the annulus. It contains the proximal portion of the characteristic 9 + 2 flagellum, the nine coarse fibers, and the circumferentially oriented mitochondria. The mitochondria adhere tightly to the coarse fibers and are packed very close to each other in a helical arrangement.

The principal piece, extending from the annulus nearly to the end of the tail, forms the main portion of the flagellum and is about 45 μm in length. The axoneme and the nine longitudinally oriented dense fibers are enclosed in a sheath of circumferential fibers that extend the length of the principal piece. These fibers are semicircular in shape and end on opposite sides in two longitudinal columns, which are really thickenings of the sheath. The circumferential fi-

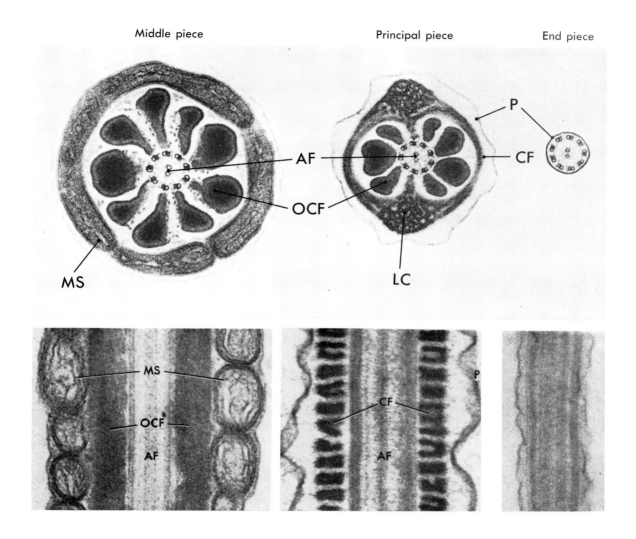

Middle piece   Principal piece   End piece

bers branch and anastomose. The end piece is
simply the terminal segment (5 μm) of the flagellum, in which the central microtubular complex
is bare.

Intercellular Bridges

It is well established that large clusters of similar
types of germ cells differentiate simultaneously
within the seminiferous tubules. This very precise synchronous development may be partially
attributed to the fact that germ cells in the same
step of differentiation are connected to one another by intercellular bridges; that is, cytokinesis
is incomplete. These bridges are enduring structures that persist until the late spermatids are released into the tubule lumen as free spermatozoa
(Fig. 28–19).

28–14 Transverse and longitudinal sections through
the middle piece, principal piece, and end
piece of guinea pig spermatozoa. The internal core of
the middle piece consists of a central pair of
microtubules, the axoneme **(AF)**, surrounded by nine
peripheral pairs of microtubules and nine outer course
fibers **(OCF)**. **MS,** mitochondrial sheath. In the
principal piece the circumferential fibers **(CF)** of the
sheath are continuous with the apposed longitudinal
columns **(LC)**. **P,** plasmalemma. All similar
magnifications. (Courtesy of D. W. Fawcett.)

In rodents, clusters of 16 or more type A_1
spermatogonia may be interconnected by cytoplasmic bridges. These cells divide a total of
eight times during spermatogenesis, and if the
progeny of all divisions remain joined, upward
of 4,000 spermatids might be found intercon-

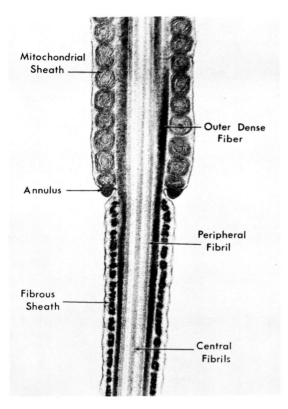

28–15 An electron micrograph demonstrating the annulus at the junction of the middle and principal pieces of the spermatozoon. × 33,000. (Courtesy of D. W. Fawcett.)

nected. These theoretical maximum numbers are in fact never achieved, because numerous germ cells degenerate during normal spermatogenesis. In the human, the clusters of synchronously developing germ cells are much smaller; therefore, far fewer germ cells are joined by cytoplasmic bridges.

The cytoplasmic bridges appear to form during mitosis as a result of incomplete cytokinesis. They are usually 2 to 3 μm in width and are locally reinforced or stiffened by a layer of dense material on the inner or cytoplasmic surface (Fig. 28–20). Bridges are usually not evident in routine histological sections of paraffin-embedded material, but they may be seen with the light microscope in 1-μm plastic sections of material fixed and embedded for electron microscopy (Fig. 28–21). In the thinner plastic sections there is less superimposition of structure and one can utilize more effectively the resolving power of the light microscope and obtain images of surprising clarity.

The occurence of bridges among spermatogonia may have implications for stem-cell renewal in the testis. It is possible that once incomplete cytokinesis of the type A stem spermatogonia has been initiated, then all linked daughter cells are equally commited to progressive differentiation; this means that when two completely separate type A spermatogonia result from a type A mitotic division, the cells probably remain as stem cells.

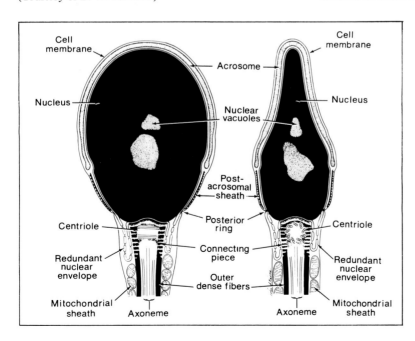

28–16 Drawings of the head and neck regions of human spermatozoa. The **left** drawing depicts the oval outline seen in a frontal view; the **right** drawing is of a section perpendicular to the left one and depicts the pyriform shape of the spermatozoon. (From Pedersen, H., and Fawcett, D. W. 1976. In E. S. E. Hafez (ed.), Human Semen and Fertility Regulation in the Male. St. Louis: Mosby.)

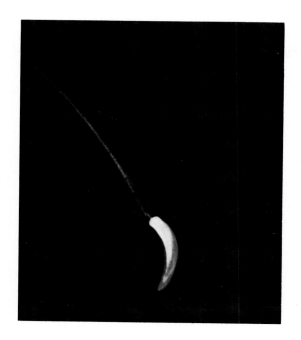

28–17 Hamster sperm stained by fluorescence microscopy for acrosome, nucleus, and tail. This is a black-and-white rendition of a portion of a color plate. See color section.

Cycle of the Seminiferous Epithelium

Examination of the seminiferous epithelium in all mammals, including humans, reveals that the germ cells are not arranged at random but are organized into well-defined cellular associations. For instance, in a particular region of the seminiferous tubules, late spermatids at a given step in spermiogenesis occur only in specific combination with early spermatids, spermatocytes, and spermatogonia at respective steps of their development (Fig. 28–22). These groupings of cells succeed one another in any given area of the seminiferous tubules and the sequence repeats itself indefinitely. Each recognized cell grouping represents a stage in the cyclic process; the series of successive stages occuring between two appearances of the same cellular association, in a given area of the seminiferous tubule, is defined as the cycle of the seminiferous epithelium. The

28–18 A schematic drawing of the mammalian spermatozoon, as revealed by electron microscopy, showing transverse sections at different locations along its length. (Slightly modified from Bloom, W., and Fawcett, D. W. 1975. A Textbook of Histology, 10th ed. Philadelphia: W. B. Saunders Co.)

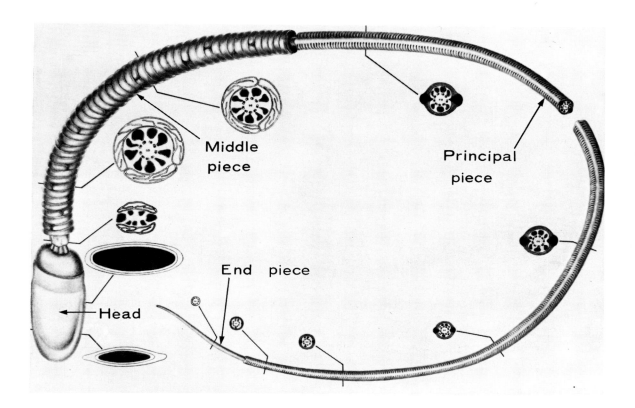

Middle piece

Principal piece

End piece

Head

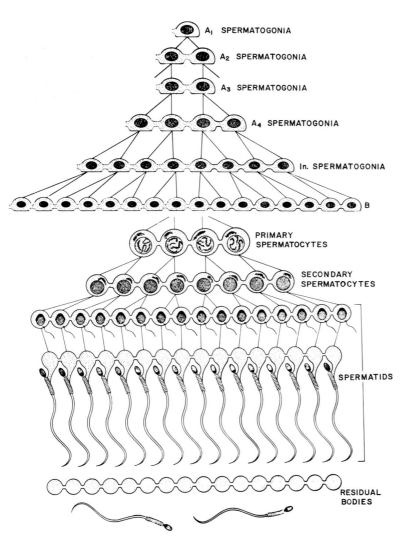

28–19 A model depicting intercellular bridges connecting the germ cells. Individual spermatozoa are separated just prior to their release into the tubule lumen. For the sake of simplicity, the cells are shown in linear array. (From Dym, M., and Fawcett, D. W. 1971. Biol. Reprod. 4:195.)

number of such stages in a cycle is constant for any given species; the rat has 14 (Fig. 28–23), the guinea pig and monkey 12, and man 6 (Fig. 28–24); the stages are designated by Roman numerals (see page 1023).

If it were possible to continuously examine in the living animal a portion of a seminiferous tubule, all 14 stages (in the rat) would occur in succession in that particular region, and the series (cycle) would repeat itself time after time. During one cycle, a type A₁ spermatogonium in stage VIII would evolve to a preleptotene spermatocyte in the same stage; the preleptotene cell would differentiate to a pachytene cell; the pachytene would become a step 8 spermatid, and the step 8 spermatid, a step 15 spermatid. Thus, it is obvious that there are four to five successive

generations of germ cells within the seminiferous epithelium and that the development of any single generation occurs concomitantly with the development of the earlier and later generations. The cells in each generation are all at precisely the same step of development.

Wave of the Seminiferous Epithelium

In all mammals examined, except humans and possibly baboons, a given cellular association occupies a relatively long length or segment of the seminiferous tubules. Each such segment corresponds to a stage of the cycle of the seminiferous epithelium and is numbered accordingly. The segments are disposed along the tubule in consecutive order to form what is termed, somewhat

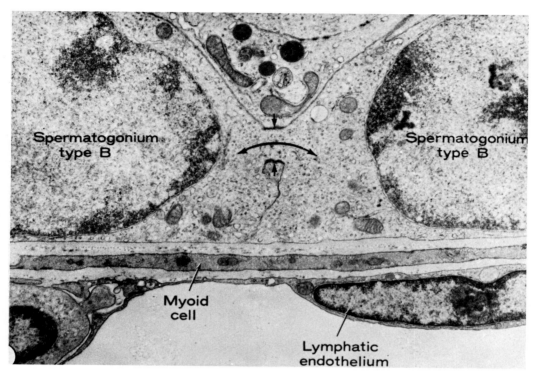

28–20 Electron micrograph of
△ two type B spermatogonia
connected by an intercellular
bridge. **Arrowheads** indicate the
width of the cytoplasmic bridge
connecting the two spermatogonia;
the **double-headed curve arrow**
lies in the center of the bridge and
indicates the continuity. × 11,000.
(From Dym, M., and Fawcett,
D. W. 1971. Biol. Reprod. 4:195.)

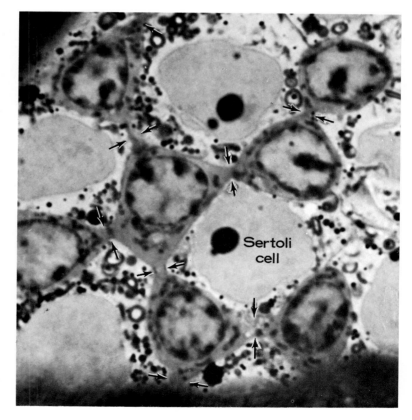

28–21 Light micrograph
▷ depicting at least eight
type B spermatogonia in the rat
connected by intercellular bridges
(arrows). × 1,200. (From Dym, M.,
and Fawcett, D. W. 1971. Biol.
Reprod. 4:195.)

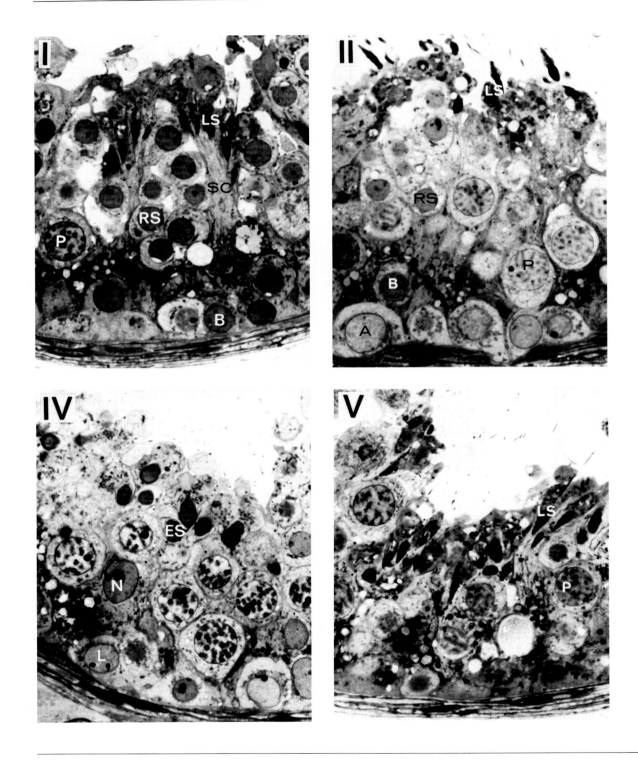

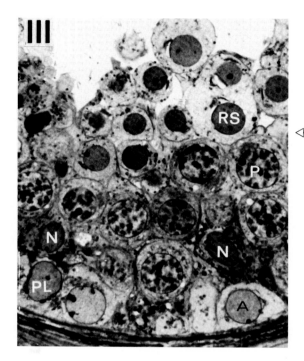

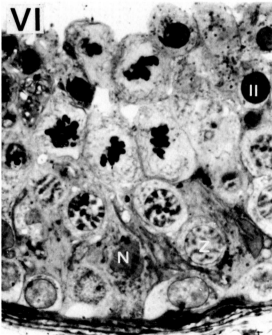

28–22 Light micrographs of the six stages of the cycle of the seminiferous epithelium in man. **A,** type A spermatogonia; **B,** type B spermatogonia; **PL,** preleptotene spermatocytes; **L,** leptotene spermatocytes; **Z,** zygotene spermatocytes; **P,** pachytene spermatocytes; **II,** secondary spermatocytes; **RS,** round spermatids; **ES,** elongating spermatids; **LS,** late spermatids; **SC,** Sertoli cell cytoplasm; **N,** Sertoli cell nuclei. Epon sections, I μm. × 500. (Courtesy of A. F. Holstein.)

inaccurately, the wave of the seminiferous epithelium. Each wave consists of the complete series of segments representing the recognized cellular associations for that species (Fig. 28–25). The segments are disposed distally along the seminiferous tubule in descending order and form a continuous succession of waves. Rats, for example, have an average of 12 waves per tubule. The descending order in the sequence of segments applies to both limbs of the tubular arches, reading distally from the rete testis. The continuous successions of waves in each limb meet distally near the midpoint of the arch. At this point, designated the site of reversal, the order of sequence of segments reverses. The reversal is owing to the shift in the direction of progression from distal to proximal along the tubule. At points where the seminiferous tubules branch, the continuity of the descending order is not broken.

In distinguishing between waves and cycles of the seminiferous epithelium, it is important to bear in mind that the cycle refers to changes taking place over a period of time in a given area of the seminiferous tubule, whereas the wave refers to the distribution of different cellular associations along the length of the tubule.

The average length of each tubular segment correlates roughly with the relative duration of the corresponding cellular association or stage of the cycle. In rats, the several segments in a wave vary in average length from 0.4 to 3.2 mm, and the stages they represent vary from 6 to 63 h. However, there is no strict proportionality between segmental length and duration of the stages of the cycle. For example, in rats, segment VI has a length equal to about 2% of the wave, whereas the duration of stage VI is 9.2% of the cycle. The length of segments and waves varies considerably but the duration of the stages and of the cycle is constant.

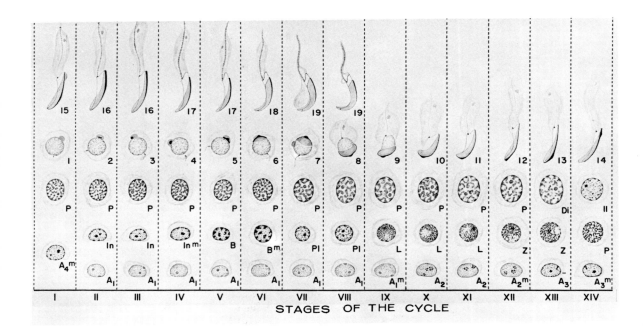

STAGES OF THE CYCLE

28–23 The cellular composition of the 14 stages of
the cycle of the seminiferous epithelium in
the rat. Each column numbered with a Roman
numeral shows the cell types present in one of the
cellular associations found in cross sections of
seminiferous tubules. The cellular associations or
stages of the cycle succeed one another in time in any
given area of the seminiferous epithelium in the rat.
Following cellular association XIV, cellular
association I reappears, so that the sequence starts
over again. The stages of the cycle were identified by
means of 14 of the 19 steps of spermiogenesis
(numbers 1 to 19). These steps were defined by the
changes observed in the nucleus and in the acrosomic
structure (acrosome and head cap seen applied to the
surface of the nucleus) in sections stained with the
PA-Schiff-hematoxylin technique. Letters: A_1, A_2, A_3,
and A_4 represent four generations of type A
spermatogonia; **In,** intermediate spermatogonia; **B,**
type spermatogonia; the subscript m next to a
spermatogonium indicates occurrence of mitosis; **Pl,**
preleptotene spermatocyte; **L,** leptotene spermatocyte;
Z, zygotene spermatocyte; **P,** pachytene spermatocyte;
II, secondary spermatocyte. (From Dym, M., and
Clermont, Y. 1970. Am. J. Anat. 128:265.)

Seminiferous Tubule Differences Between Human and Subhuman Species

In subhuman primates and in lower species a
particular cell association occupies an extensive
area along the length of a seminiferous tubule

(up to 10 mm); therefore, any tubule cross section examined with the light microscope will
usually reveal the same cellular association
throughout (Fig. 28–26). In human seminiferous
tubules, each cellular association occupies a very
small area along the length of a seminiferous tubule. Indeed, each patchlike cellular grouping
does not even extend around the circumference
of the tubule; cross sections of human seminiferous tubules thus frequently reveal two to four
cellular associations (Figs. 28–26 and 28–27).
Humans, furthermore, do not exhibit a wave of
the seminiferous epithelium. However, the fundamental pattern of the cycle of the seminiferous
epithelium is as characteristic of humans as of
other mammalian species.

Duration of Spermatogenesis

Preleptotene spermatocytes are the most advanced germ cells in the human testis to incorporate tritiated thymidine in preparation for the
DNA synthesis of the first meiotic division. One
hour after a single injection of ³H-thymidine, the
preleptotene spermatocytes in stage III of the cycle were labeled (Fig. 28–24). As the cells pro-
gressed through leptotene, zygotene, and pachytene stages, the pachytene spermatocytes in the
same stage of the cycle demonstrated the label 16
days later. As expected, after a further 16 days,
round spermatids in stage III were labeled; and

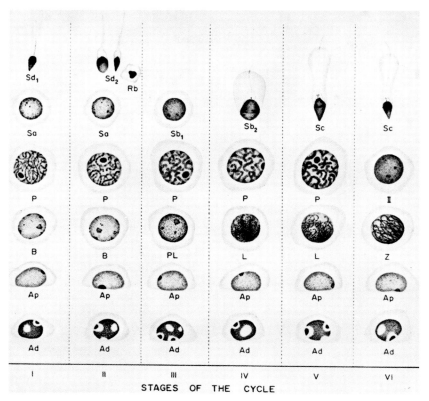

28–24 The six stages or cellular associations in
△ humans. See Fig. 28–8 for a description of
lettering. (Courtesy of Y. Clermont.)

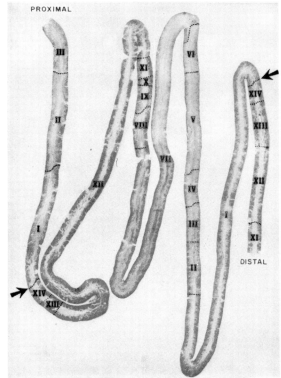

28–25 An isolated seminiferous tubule of rat testis,
▷ showing a wave of the seminiferous
epithelium. Fourteen segments representing the 14
stages of the cycle of the seminiferous epithelium are
arranged in continuous numerical and distally
descending order to form a so-called wave. The limits
of the wave are indicated by **arrows.** Note the
difference in lengths of the several segments and the
variability in length of segments of a given type
(compare segments I, II, and XII). (From Perey, B.,
Clermont, Y., and Leblond, C. P. 1961. Am. J. Anat.
108:55, Fig. 7.)

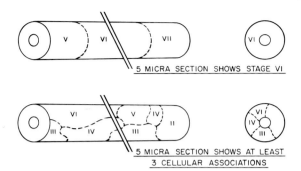

5 MICRA SECTION SHOWS STAGE VI

5 MICRA SECTION SHOWS AT LEAST 3 CELLULAR ASSOCIATIONS

28–26 Diagrammatic representation of the major difference in the organization of the seminiferous epithelium between humans (**lower**) and most subhuman species (**upper**). In humans the cell associations occupy small patchlike areas along the length of the tubule. In the subhuman species each cell association occupies a more extensive area along the length of the tubule.

finally, 16 days later, mature spermatids retained the label, just prior to their release into the tubule lumen. From these studies it was determined that the duration of the cycle in humans occupied an interval of 16 days and that the time

28–27 Photomicrograph showing in a single cross section of a seminiferous tubule four different and well demarcated stages of the cycle of the seminiferous epithelium × 40. (From Clermont, Y. 1963. Am. J. Anat. 112:50.)

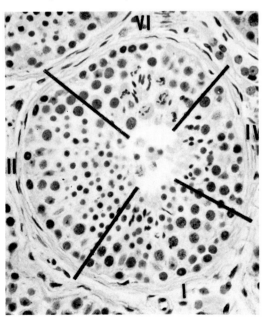

taken for spermatogonia to evolve into spermatozoa is about 64 days. The duration of the cycle and the duration of spermatogenesis are constant and species-specific. Furthermore, they cannot be altered by hormone withdrawal or by other deleterious actions on the testis. Either the germ cells differentiate at their normal speed or they degenerate and die.

Structure and Function of Sertoli Cells

The Sertoli cells are nondividing tall columnar elements that extend from the base of the seminiferous epithelium to the tubule lumen (Fig. 28–28). This elaborate cell type consists of a narrow portion resting on the basal lamina, an intermediate portion that provides lateral processes around which the spermatocytes and spermatids are arranged, and apical projections that enclose the late spermatids, just before their release into the tubule lumen. The basal portion of the cell is voluminous and is characterized by an irregularly shaped nucleus and abundant profiles of smooth endoplasmic reticulum (Fig. 28–29). Lipid droplets, thin filaments, glycogen granules, numerous spherical and elongated mitochondria exhibiting transverse cristae of orthodox lamellar configuration, and a very large well-developed Golgi complex are also evident. Isolated patches of rough endoplasmic reticulum are present and occasionally several such cisternae can be found arranged circularly around a single lipid droplet. Other characteristics of the basal cytoplasm are membrane-limited bodies of various sizes, shapes, and densities, and, in humans only, inclusion bodies of Charcot-Böttcher (Fig. 28–30). The latter are irregularly shaped filamentous structures about 20 μm long and 1 μm wide. The intermediate and apical portions of the columnar Sertoli cells contain rod-shaped mitochondria and logitudinally oriented microtubules and filaments. The Sertoli cell nucleus is large and is characterized by a homogeneous nucleoplasm and a distinctive tripartite nucleolus (Fig. 28–31). A sheath of fine cytoplasmic filaments completely surrounds the Sertoli cell nucleus and separates it from other organelles. Near the base of the seminiferous epithelium, adjacent Sertoli cells are joined by tight junctions. These cells are frequently found overlying the spermatogonial population and early spermatocytes and are characterized by subsurface filaments, hexagonally packed, and cisternae of endoplasmic reticulum subjacent to the filaments (Fig. 28–32). The Sertoli cell cytoplasm immediately adjacent

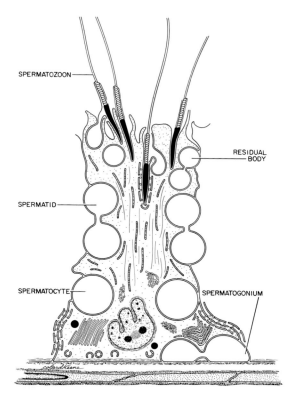

SPERMATOZOON

RESIDUAL BODY

SPERMATID

SPERMATOCYTE

SPERMATOGONIUM

28–28 Diagram illustrating the fine structure of the Sertoli cell and the cellular tight junctions separating adjacent Sertoli cells. The occluding junctions between Sertoli cells subdivide the seminiferous epithelium into two compartments: a *basal compartment* containing the spermatogonia, preleptotene and leptotene spermatocytes, and an *adluminal compartment* containing the more advanced spermatocytes and spermatids. (After Dym, M., and Fawcett, D. W. 1970. Biol. Reprod. 3:308.)

to acrosomic and maturation-phase spermatids contains filaments and a flattened cistern of endoplasmic reticulum, resembling one-half of a typical Sertoli–Sertoli junctional complex (Fig. 28–28).

Because the germ cells develop in the microenvironment provided by the Sertoli cells, it is possible that the full control of germ-cell differentiation is mediated by the Sertoli cell. The various functions that may be ascribed to the Sertoli cell are listed below.

Support and Nutrition of Germ Cells. On the basis of shape and strategic position within the seminiferous epithelium, it has been suggested that the Sertoli cell provides nutrients for the avascular germinal epithelium. Although it is likely that the Sertoli cell transports nutrient material from the capillaries to the germ cells, no direct evidence exists for this function.

Release of Late Spermatids into the Tubule Lumen. It has been suggested that the Sertoli cells engineer the release of late spermatids into the tubule lumen. They may also be involved in the movement of germ cells from the basal lamina to the tubule lumen. Recent work has shown that the Sertoli cell filaments contain actin and are therefore probably contractile.

Steroidogenic Function. An early step in the synthesis of testosterone is the side-chain cleavage of cholesterol to form the C_{21} steroid pregnenolone (Fig. 28–33). In vitro studies on cultured Sertoli cells have demonstrated that the enzymes required for this cleavage are not present in Sertoli cells. Therefore, it may be concluded that de novo synthesis of testosterone does not occur in the Sertoli cells. On the other hand, under certain experimental conditions, the Sertoli cell is able to convert C_{21} steroids such as pregnenolone and progesterone to testosterone, but this role may not be significant in normal spermatogenesis.

Phagocytosis. It is well known that during the normal process of spermatogenesis, numerous germ cells degenerate at specific stages of the cycle of the seminiferous epithelium. In addition, as late spermatids are released into the tubule lumen, the residual cytoplasm is shed and retained within the seminiferous epithelium. The Sertoli cells effectively phagocytize these vast numbers of degenerating entities, but the mechanism by which this is accomplished remains obscure.

Secretory Function. If the ductuli efferentes are ligated in experimental animals, the testis soon swells and becomes turgid. This increase in weight and size of the organ is attributed to a continuous production of fluid by the Sertoli cells plus a lack of a normal egress route. In addition to fluid secretion, the Sertoli cells elaborate a specific protein referred to as androgen-binding protein (ABP). This protein is found within the lumen of the seminiferous tubules and proximal portion of the excurrent duct system of the testis. More recently, ABP has been found in the circulation; however, the mechanism of secretion by the Sertoli cells remains to be clarified. Secretion of ABP appears to be under dual control of follicle-stimulating hormone

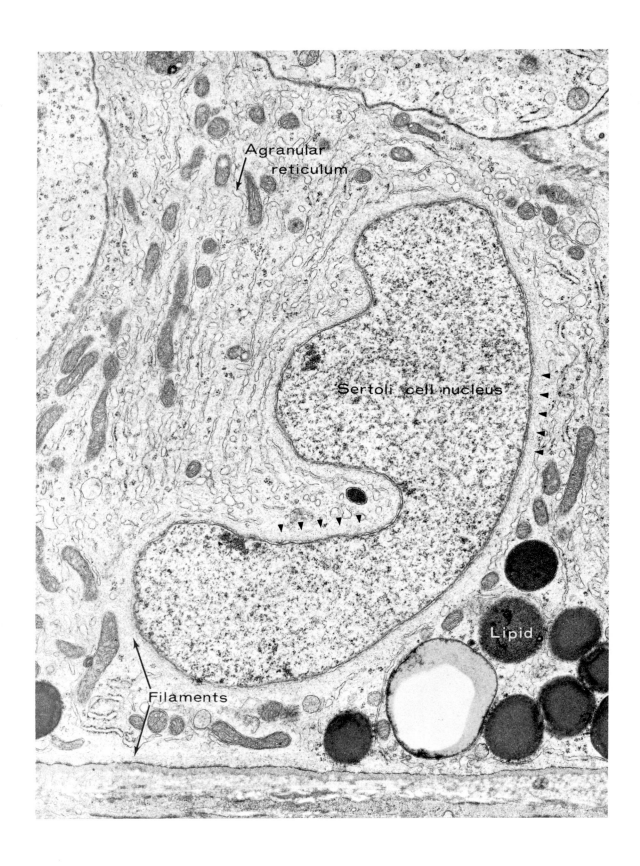

28–29 Electron micrograph of the basal portion of a monkey Sertoli cell. Note the filamentous zone surrounding the nucleus (**arrowheads**) and the abundant agranular reticulum. × 8,190. (From Dym, M. 1973. Anat. Rec. 175:639.)

(FSH) and testosterone. The role and importance of ABP are still under investigation, but it may serve as a means of concentrating testosterone within the seminiferous epithelium, thereby providing the high local concentrations necessary for spermatogenesis and sperm maturation in the epididymis.

Recent work has demonstrated that calmodulin, a Ca^{++}-dependent regulatory protein, is found in Sertoli cells. Calmodulin appears to play a pivotal role in mediating Ca^{++} functions in eukaryotic cells. Plasminogen activator is also found in large concentrations within Sertoli cells. It has been speculated that this protein may serve to unzipper the Sertoli–Sertoli tight junctions, permitting migration of spermatocytes from basal to adluminal compartments (see below). The Sertoli cells produce inhibin, a protein that may be involved in the selective feedback inhibition of FSH production in the pituitary gland.

Cell-to-Cell Communication. Gap junctions are located between adjacent Sertoli cells. A central pore in the junctional complex extends between the connected cells and permits ions and small molecules to pass from cell to cell. In this manner one Sertoli cell may communicate with its neighbor. This arrangement may partially explain the synchrony in the wave that is observed among adjacent segments of the seminiferous tubules.

Role of the Sertoli Cell in the Blood–Testis Barrier. Tight junctions between adjacent Sertoli cells delimit two compartments within the seminiferous epithelium (Fig. 28–28): (1) a *basal compartment* between the junctional complexes and the basal lamina containing the spermatogonia, preleptotene and leptotene spermatocytes, and (2) an *adluminal compartment* between the junctions and the tubule lumen containing the more mature spermatocytes and spermatids. Circulating plasma proteins are excluded from the lumen of the seminiferous tubules and it is likely that the Sertoli–Sertoli junctional complexes are the morphological site of the barrier (Figs. 28–34 and 28–35).

The subdivision of the seminiferous epithelium into two compartments may be important for a number of reasons. The germ cells in the basal compartment synthesize DNA and, as such, they have direct access to blood-borne substances associated with this process. On the other hand, soon after the spermatocytes are formed, they migrate from the basal compartment to the specialized environment of the adluminal compartment. The tight junctions may permit the accumulation of high concentrations of ABP within the epithelium. Finally, haploid germ cells contain antigens that are "foreign" to the body. The barrier may serve to isolate these proteins from the general circulation, thereby preventing an immune response. The full biological significance of the blood–testis barrier remains to be elucidated. Certain amino acids and ions are found in very high concentrations in the lumina of the seminiferous tubules, whereas cholesterol is excluded. These latter observations cannot be explained simply by the presence of junctions between Sertoli cells.

Interstitial Tissue, Lymphatics, and Leydig Cells

The seminiferous tubules are bound together by the interstitial tissue, which consists of loose connective tissue septa with lymphatic vessels, capillaries, arterioles, venules, fibrocytes, macrophages, mast cells, lymphocytes, and Leydig cells (Fig. 28–36). In rodents the lymphatic capillaries have an unusually large lumen and lie among the tubules (Fig. 28–37). Leydig cells appear to be directly exposed to the lymph. In primates lymphatics are more typical, discrete vessels (Fig. 28–38). The interstitial lymphatics drain into those of the rete testis, which in turn form the two or three large vessels of the spermatic cord.

The clusters of Leydig cells are located in the angular spaces among the seminiferous tubules and are frequently associated with blood vessels. These cells have a spherical or irregularly polyhedral shape and are about 20 μm in diameter. Occasionally fusiform or elongated cells are found. The nuclei are usually rounded and the cell surface is characterized by numerous small microvilli. The most prominent cytoplasmic organelle is the abundant smooth endoplasmic reticulum (Fig. 28–39). This feature is characteristic of steroid-secreting cells. Mitochondria, patches of rough endoplasmic reticulum, a large Golgi complex, centrioles, and lipid droplets are

1028

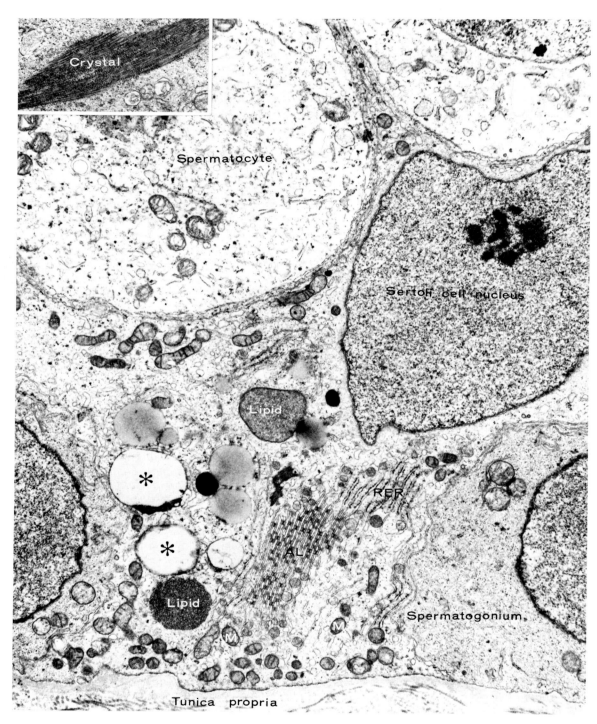

28–30 Electron micrograph showing the basal portion of a human Sertoli cell and several germ cells. Note the mitochondria (**M**), annulate lamellae (**AL**), rough endoplasmic reticulum (**RER**), and lipid droplets. The content of several lipid droplets (**asterisks**) has been extracted during processing of the tissue. A crystalloid of Charcot-Böttcher is seen in the **inset.** × 8,000; inset, × 15,000. (Courtesy of H. E. Chemes.)

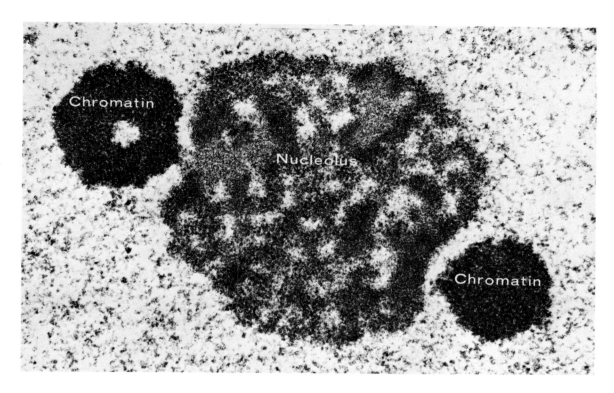

also located within the acidophilic cytoplasm. Lipochrome pigment granules are abundant, especially in older men, and are seen as heterogeneous conglomerations of dense granules.

In humans, conspicuous cytoplasmic crystals of Reinke are characteristic features (Fig. 28–39). Their occurrence is inconstant among individuals and among the cells of a given individual. The crystals vary widely in size and form but are often rectilinear and may be 20 μm long and 3 μm thick. The angles may be sharp or rounded. The crystals are composed of macromolecules

28–31 The tripartite nucleolar complex of Sertoli cells is depicted in this electron micrograph. The nucleolus proper is surrounded by two satellite bodies of perinucleolar chromatin. × 48,000.

28–32 Electron micrograph of a Sertoli–Sertoli intercellular junction. Tight junctions **(arrowheads)** and 90-Å "narrow" junctions **(arrows)** are apparent. Subsurface cisternae of endoplasmic reticulum **(asterisks)** are separated from the cell surface by bundles of filaments that are hexagonally arranged. × 63,000. (From Dym, M., and Fawcett, D. W. 1970. Biol. Reprod. 3:308.)

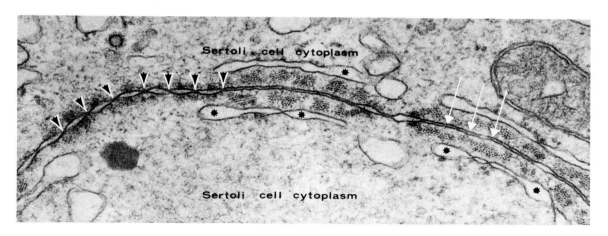

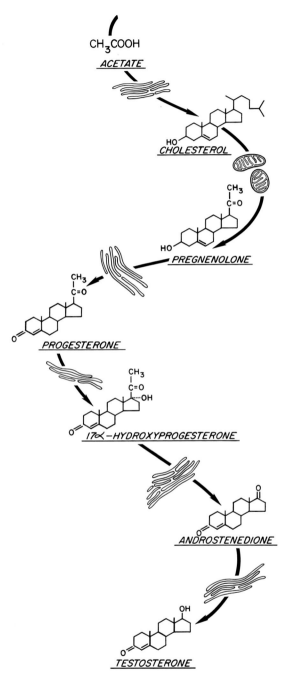

28–33 A schematic representation of the steps in the conversion of acetate to testosterone. All the enzymes are present in the microsomal fraction except for the cholesterol side-chain cleaving enzymes, which are found in the mitochondria.

about 50 Å in diameter, which, being evenly spaced at about 190 Å, present a highly ordered pattern of internal structure.

By the use of histochemical techniques, the Leydig cells have been shown to contain cholesterol, ascorbic acid, lipases, esterases, leucylamino peptidase, succinic dehydrogenase, cytochrome oxidase, and 3-B-ol dehydrogenase. Recent work has shown that the Leydig cells secrete glycoprotein for export. The Leydig cells produce testosterone from the precursor cholesterol. Most of the enzymes necessary for this conversion are located within the smooth endoplasmic reticulum, although the cholesterol side-chain cleavage enzymes are located in the mitochondria.

Hormonal Control of Spermatogenesis

In addition to producing spermatozoa, the testis secretes into the bloodstream an androgenic steroid hormone, testosterone, which is essential for puberal development, spermatogenesis, and structural and functional maintenance of the male accessory organs. In fact, testosterone probably acts on most tissues and organs in the body. The Leydig cells are responsible for secreting testosterone (Fig. 28–40).

The characteristic structure and endocrine function of the interstitial cells are sustained and controlled by the hypophyseal gonadotrophic hormone LH (luteineizing hormone), also known as ICSH or interstitial cell–stimulating hormone. In the absence of LH, the interstitial cells undergo severe atrophy and cease producing testosterone. The completely atrophic Leydig cell is spindle-shaped, the amount of cytoplasm is greatly reduced, and the nucleus is smaller and its chromatin is denser and more compact. The lipid droplets also disappear.

Very high concentrations of testosterone adjacent to the seminiferous tubules are required to maintain spermatogenesis in the adult; however, lower peripheral levels will maintain secondary sex characteristics and male libido. Lowered circulating levels of testosterone will result in an increased release of LH from the pituitary and an increased production of testosterone by the Leydig cell.

The role of LH in the male, therefore, is clear. It stimulates the Leydig cells to produce testosterone, which is required for spermatogenesis. Testosterone alone can maintain spermatogenesis, male libido, and the accessory glands follow-

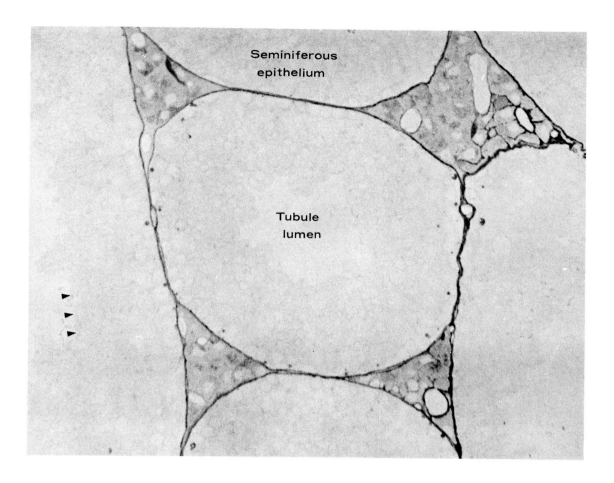

28-34 Light micrograph of several seminiferous tubules showing the distribution of vascularly injected horseradish peroxidase. The black reaction product is present in the interstitial tissue and surrounds the seminiferous tubules. No peroxidase is found inside the lumen of the seminiferous tubules. × 180. (From Dym, M. 1973. Anat. Rec. 175:639.)

ing hypophysectomy in adult humans and experimental animals. This appears to indicate that FSH is not required for male reproductive function in the adult. However, many biochemical data have accumulated indicating that the Sertoli cell is the primary target for FSH in the testis. When FSH is administered to immature rat testes, there is (1) a binding of FSH to receptors present on the plasma membrane of the Sertoli cell; (2) a stimulation of the membrane-bound adenylate cyclase and a concomitant increase in the intracellular accumulation of cyclic AMP; and (3) an activation of cyclic AMP-dependent protein kinases and an eventual increase of protein synthesis. Other work has demonstrated that the Sertoli cells respond to FSH by increasing the secretion of ABP. Autoradiographic studies with labeled FSH demonstrated that this hormone is localized to the Sertoli cells. Thus, it is obvious that there are many important actions of FSH on the seminiferous tubules at the biochem-

ical level; however, it has proved difficult to assign a definitive requirement for this hormone in the biological process of spermatogenesis. On the other hand, in the immature testis, abundant evidence exists to indicate that FSH is required for spermatogenesis.

Factors Influencing Testicular Function

Heat. The germinal cells in the seminiferous tubules are particularly susceptible to injury by temperatures above that of the scrotum, which in

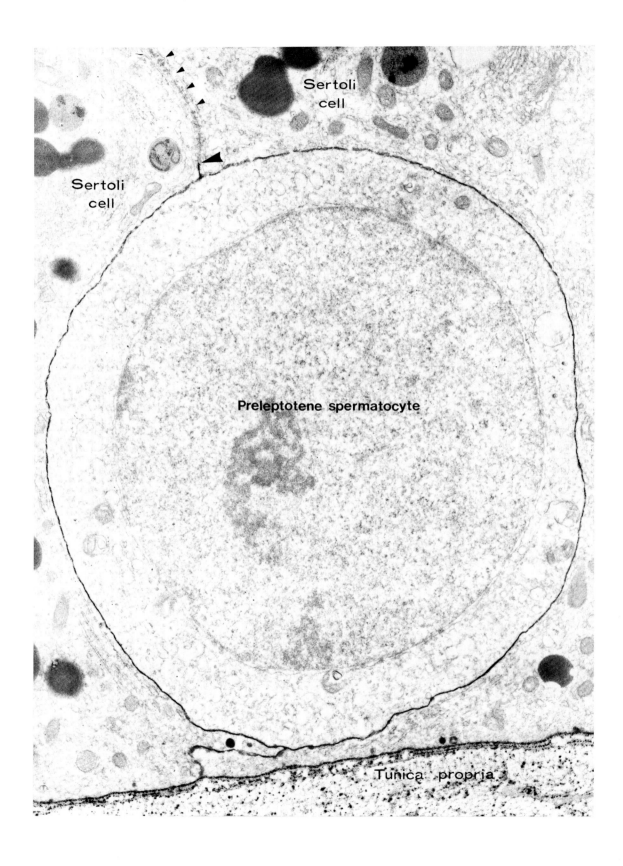

Sertoli
cell

Sertoli
cell

Preleptotene spermatocyte

Tunica propria

28–35 An electron micrograph of a monkey preleptotene spermatocyte surrounded by lanathanum nitrate. The lanathanum was perfused into the monkey's testis with the fixative. The junctional complexes between Sertoli cells **(arrowheads)** above the spermatocyte prevent the electron-opaque tracer from penetrating deeper into the seminiferous epithelium. × 11,000.
(From Dym, M. 1973. Anat. Rec. 175:639.)

28–36 A scanning electron micrograph of a portion ▽ of a rat's testis showing a number of seminiferous tubules in transverse section. The interstitial tissue is seen among the tubules. × 33.
(Courtesy of A. K. Christensen.)

men is 1.5 to 2.5°C lower than that of the abdominal cavity. The vascular connections of the testis are so arranged, as discussed above, that the arterial blood is cooled by yielding heat to the surrounding pampiniform venous plexus. When the testes of mature male animals are surgically retracted into the abdomen, the seminiferous epithelium degenerates. The Sertoli cells are not reduced in number nor does this procedure cause an early impairment of the androgenic function of the Leydig cells, as shown by the fact that the accessory sexual organs are maintained at normal adult size for at least 6 to 8 months, after

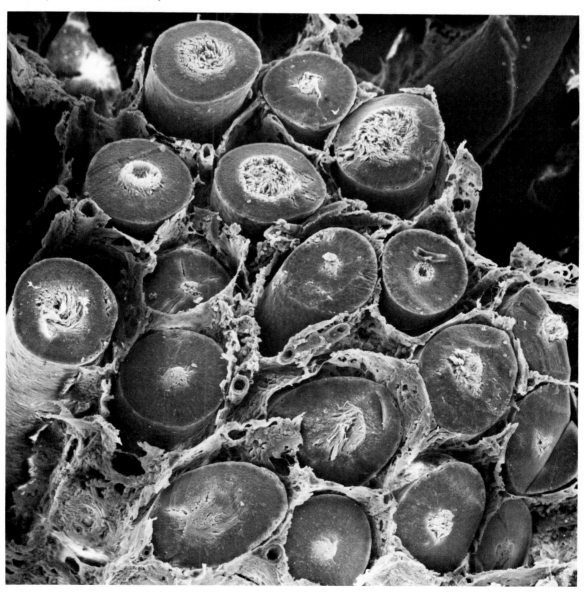

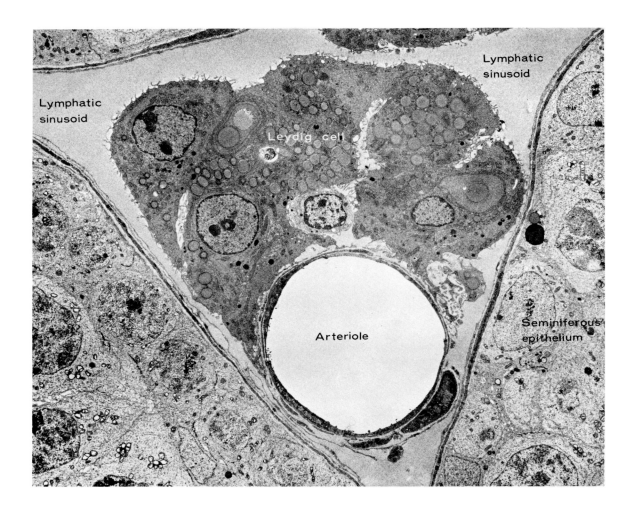

Lymphatic sinusoid

Lymphatic sinusoid

Leydig cell

Arteriole

Seminiferous epithelium

28–37 An electron micrograph of an interstitial region in the rat's testis. The close association of the Leydig cells to the blood vessels is seen. The Leydig cells appear to be directly exposed to lymph in the lymphatic sinusoids. Note the microvilli at the surface of the Leydig cells. × 3,000. (Courtesy of R. Vitale.)

which they may gradually become smaller. In addition to tubular injury at body temperatures, fevers are well known to induce temporary infertility. Frequent immersions in hot baths or wearing close-fitting, tight trousers may also result in fewer sperm in the ejaculate.

Cryptorchidism. Ten percent of newborn males have testes that are not fully descended into the scrotum. This condition is referred to as cryptorchidism. Most of these testes descend spontaneously; however, if this does not occur, surgical intervention is usually carried out before 5 years of age. Beyond the age of 5 there is evidence that irreversible changes occur. A prolonged residence of the testis within the abdomen results in progressive degeneration of germ cells. If the testis is not in the scrotum at puberty, spermatogenesis is likely never to occur. Beyond the age of 30, fibrosis takes place, which frequently impairs Leydig cell function. At this age the abdominal testis may also develop neoplastic changes and must therefore be removed.

Irradiation. Dividing populations of cells are very sensitive to radiation. Graded doses of ionizing radiation, administered directly to human testes, evoke correspondingly graded biological

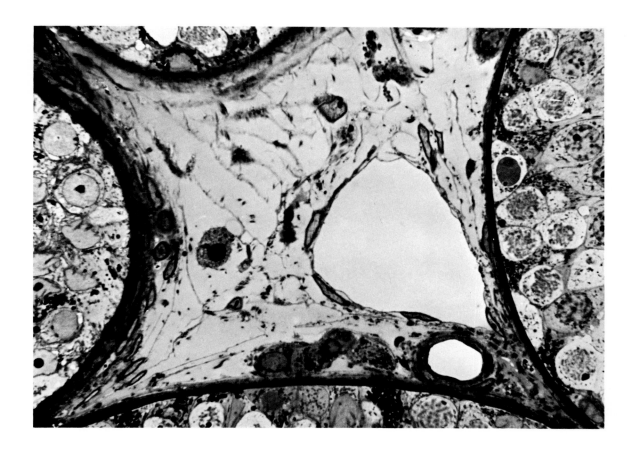

28–38 A light micrograph of the interstitial region of a monkey's testis. A small capillary is located below a larger lymphatic vessel. A few Leydig cells are noted adjacent to the seminiferous tubule below. × 450.

responses that lead eventually to a denuding of the germinal epithelium and a reduction in sperm count. In general, the lower the dosage, the less dramatic is the cell loss and the more rapid the recovery. However, even a few rads will destroy a significant number of the spermatogonial population.

Age. After the age of 55, spermatogenesis decreases very gradually, although the Sertoli cells and Leydig cells appear unaltered. There is also an increase in the number of abnormal, nonviable sperm in the ejaculate. However, men in their 80s and 90s still have adequate spermatogenesis with sperm counts within the normal range and they can father children.

Vasectomy. After ligation of the vas deferens (vasectomy) the seminiferous tubules continue to produce spermatozoa. The fate of these sperm in vasectomized men remains an enigma. In some species after vasectomy, spermatozoa are resorbed in the male reproductive tract or stored in

cysts and distended portions of the epididymis. In the human and monkey, epididymal macrophages appear to be involved in the sperm resorption. Because spermatozoa possess antigens that are foreign to the body, this resorption may lead the immune system to produce circulating antisperm antibodies. These immunoglobulins can immobilize and destroy the sperm on contact. The antibodies do not penetrate the seminiferous tubules because of the effective blood–testis permeability barrier. However, evidence is accumulating that these high-molecular-weight proteins may enter the lumen of the rete testis and epididymis and possibly affect the fertilizing capacity of spermatozoa in these regions. This may partially explain why men who have

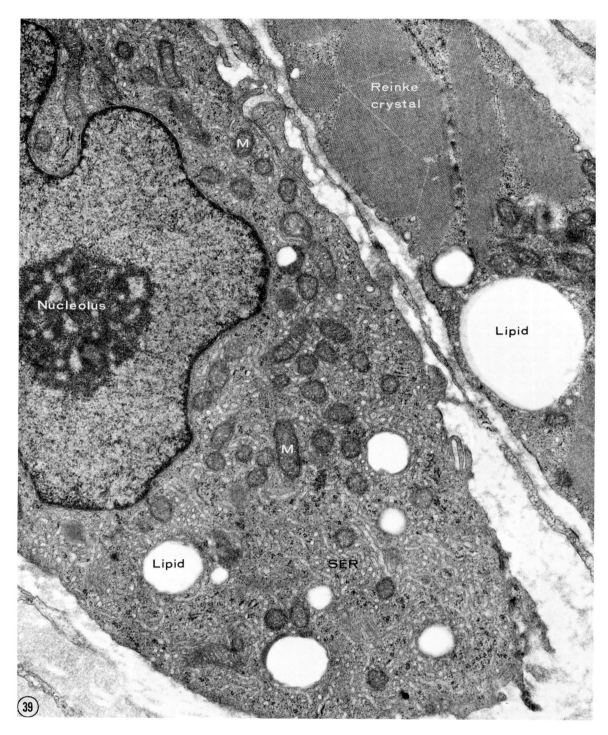

28–39 An electron micrograph of human Leydig cells. The cytoplasm is characterized by smooth endoplasmic reticulum **(SER)**; lipid droplets, partially extracted; and numerous mitochondria **(M)**. A Reinke crystal is also noted. × 17,640. (Courtesy of A. K. Christensen.)

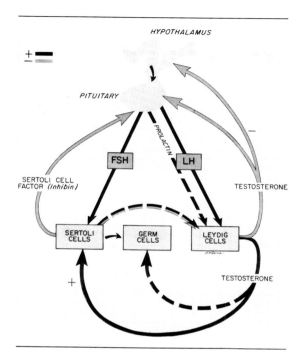

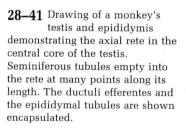

28–40 Diagrammatic representation of the hormonal control of male reproductive function.

reanastomoses of the vas deferens after vasectomy may possess normal numbers of sperm in their ejaculate but their sperm appear incapable of fertilizing the egg. It has recently been shown that long-term vasectomy may result in irreversible changes within the germinal epithelium.

Excurrent Duct System of the Testis

Tubuli Recti and Rete Testis

The convoluted seminiferous tubules within a given testis lobule are arranged mainly in the form of loops (Fig. 28–41), each end of which joins the rete testis (Fig. 28–42, see here and color insert). As the seminiferous tubules approach the rete there is a gradual depletion of the germinal elements until the tubules are lined only by Sertoli cells. This portion of the tubule without germ cells is very short and ends in an abrupt transition to the simple cuboidal epithelium characteristic of the tubuli recti. The tubuli recti, or straight tubules, are confluent with the rete testis. The rete testis consists of a series of channels or interconnected chambers lined by simple cuboidal or low columnar epithelium within a bed of highly vascular loose connective tissue. The luminal surface of the epithelial cells

28–41 Drawing of a monkey's testis and epididymis demonstrating the axial rete in the central core of the testis. Seminiferous tubules empty into the rete at many points along its length. The ductuli efferentes and the epididymal tubules are shown encapsulated.

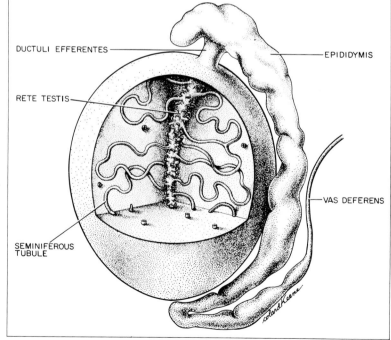

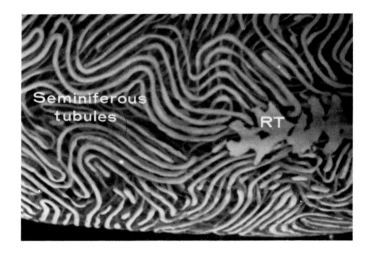

28–42 Microphil injection of the microvasculature and seminiferous tubules. This is a black-and-white rendition of a color plate. See color section.

is covered with short microvilli and a single long flagellum (Fig. 28–43). In most mammalian species the rete occupies an axial position in the testis extending from the ductuli efferentes at the upper pole of the testis to the lower pole (Fig. 28–41). The seminiferous tubules release their contents into the axial rete at many points along its entire length. In men, the rete testis is present in the posterior portion of the testis within the mediastinum; in rats, mice, and hamsters, the rete is located in a superficial position immediately deep to the tunica albuginea (Fig. 28–42; see here and color insert).

Ductuli Efferentes

In men 10 to 15 ductules, the ductuli efferentes (Fig. 28–44, see here and color insert), emerge from the mediastinum and connect the rete testis with the ductus epididymidis. Each ductulus efferens is coiled into a cone-shaped mass in the head of the epididymis. The epithelium consists of alternating patches of tall and low columnar cells. Two cell types are present, the ciliated and the nonciliated cell (Fig. 28–45). Both contain abundant supranuclear granules and most of the common cellular organelles. The cilia beat in the direction of the epididymis and may assist in the movement of sperm. The nonciliated cells are absorptive in function and bear numerous microvilli on their free surface. In addition to acting as a conduit for sperm, the ductuli efferentes absorb most of the fluid produced within the seminiferous tubules.

The epithelium of the ductuli is surrounded by a layer of circular, smooth muscle several cells thick. It is significant that from the ductuli efferentes to the urethra the sperm duct has a muscular coat. After spermatozoa have been carried to the ductuli efferentes by the flow of luminal fluid, their further transport is assured by muscular action. The muscle layer thickens toward the ductus epididymidis. Among the muscle cells there are elastic fibers that, like those of the ductus epididymidis and ductus deferens, first appear at puberty.

Ductus Epididymis

The ductus epididymis in mammals is a highly tortuous tube 4 to 5 m in length. The coils of this duct, together with the entwining vascular connective tissue, smooth muscle, and surrounding tunic, form the epididymis. The epithelium is pseudostratified columnar and rests on a basal lamina and a thin lamina propria encircled by the smooth muscle, with the fibers oriented circularly. The muscle layer is very thin over most of the length of the tube, but it thickens markedly and longitudinal fibers appear near the ductus deferens. Outside the muscle layer, loose connective tissue is molded about the duct and constitutes the interstitium of the epididymis. Blood vessels, lymphatic vessels, and nerves occur in the fibrous stroma. The nerves form a thick myenteric plexus with autonomic ganglia in addition to perivascular nets. The plexus is more highly developed in the vas deferens and seminal vesicles.

For descriptive purposes the epididymis may be subdivided into three portions: head, body, and tail (Fig. 28–46). The segment of the head

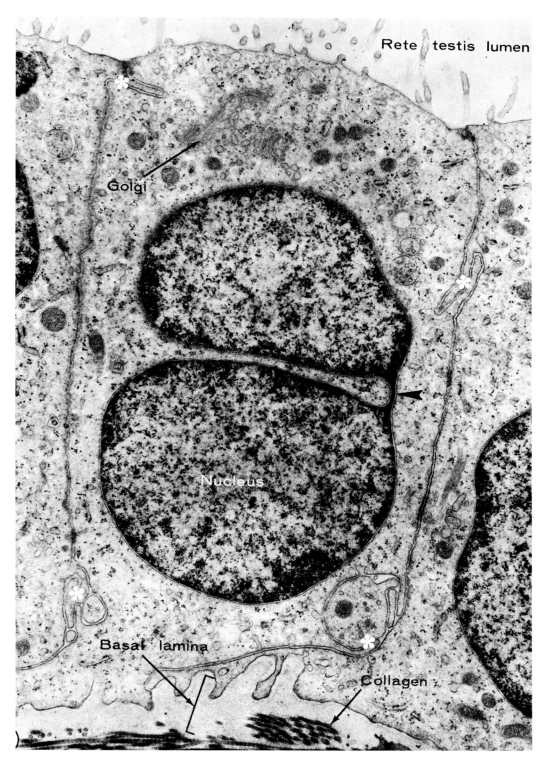

28–43 Electron micrograph of the monkey's rete testis epithelium. **Arrowhead,** chromatin bridge between two nuclear lobes; **asterisk,** lateral interdigitation with contiguous cells. × 7,500.

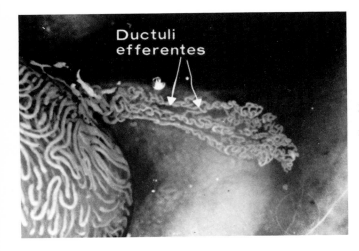

28–44 Microphil injection of the rete testes and ductuli efferentes. This is a black-and-white rendition of a color plate. See color section.

28–45 Light micrograph of a transverse section through a ductus efferens in a monkey. Both the ciliated and nonciliated cells are densely packed with granules. × 650. (Courtesy of A. S. Ramos, Jr.)

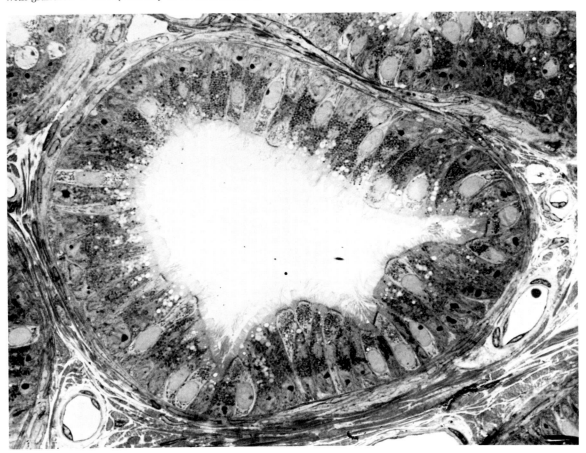

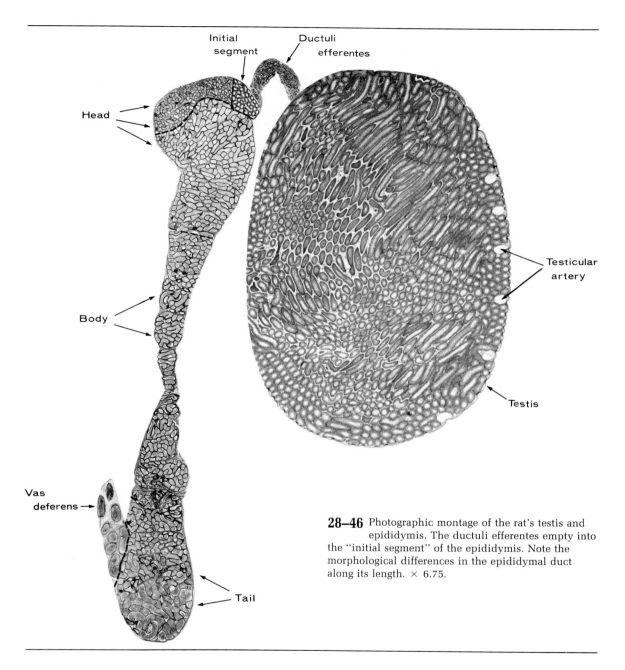

28–46 Photographic montage of the rat's testis and epididymis. The ductuli efferentes empty into the "initial segment" of the epididymis. Note the morphological differences in the epididymal duct along its length. × 6.75.

into which the ductuli efferentes empty is called the initial segment. Spermatozoa leaving the testis exhibit weak, random, circular motion and are incapable of fertilizing ova. On the other hand, sperm taken from the tail of the epididymis have a strong unidirectional motility and are able to fertilize ova. Thus, it is clear that the sperm require the epididymal environment to become mature; furthermore, this maturation is androgen-dependent. The mechanism by which the epididymis induces the functional maturation of spermatozoa is now under intensive investigation. It is known that the epithelium secretes glycerylphosphorylcholine, carnitine, sialic acid, glycoproteins, and possibly steroids into the tubule lumen.

It is not surprising that various segments of the epididymis exhibit different morphological

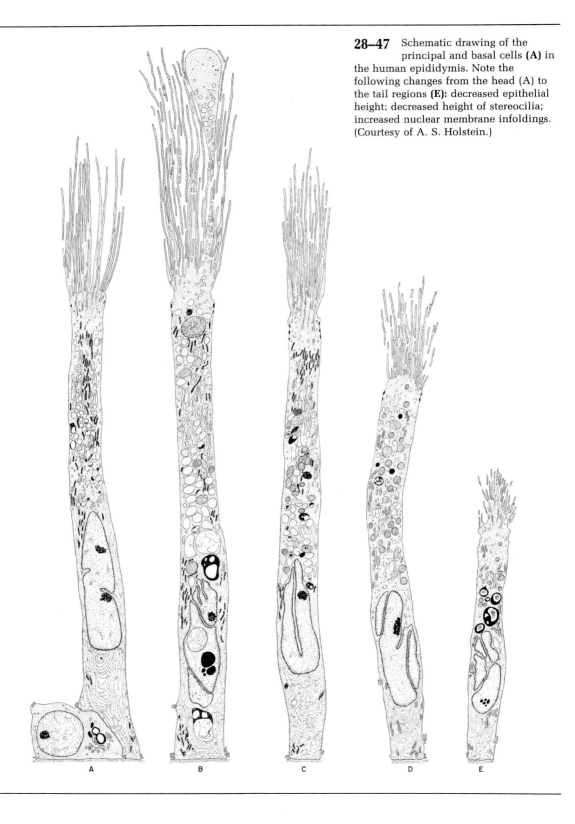

28–47 Schematic drawing of the principal and basal cells **(A)** in the human epididymis. Note the following changes from the head (A) to the tail regions **(E)**: decreased epithelial height; decreased height of stereocilia; increased nuclear membrane infoldings. (Courtesy of A. S. Holstein.)

A B C D E

characteristics, since the respective regions perform various functions. For example, the head region absorbs fluid and particulate matter readily; the tail acts as a sperm reservoir and can contract forcefully upon appropriate nervous stimulation.

The epididymal duct is lined by tall columnar cells resting on a well-defined basal lamina (Fig. 28–47). The luminal free surface of the epithelium bears long nonmotile microvilli (stereocilia), the height of which decreases from 80 μm in the head region to 40 μm in the tail. The principal cell is the most abundant and is characterized by an impressively large supranuclear Golgi complex and abundant profiles of rough endoplasmic reticulum in the basal cytoplasm. The apical cytoplasm contains numerous micropinocytotic vesicles, multivesicular bodies and lysosomes, lipid droplets, coated vesicles, and mitochondria. The nucleus in the head region is cigar-shaped with the long axis parallel to the long axis of the cell. Nuclear membrane infoldings are present in the distal part of the head and in the body and reach a maximum in the tail region where most nuclei have very bizarre shapes.

Small round cells containing spherical nuclei are found at the base of the epididymal epithelium insinuated among the principal cells. These basal cells contain few organelles and appear lightly stained in electron micrographs. The function of the basal cells remains obscure. Intraepithelial lymphocytes are located at all levels in the epithelium. In rodents and monkeys they represent about 2% of the total cell population.

Ductus Deferens

The ductus deferens is a thick-walled tube that is continuous with the tail of the epididymis and extends to the prostatic urethra. Near the prostate the lumen widens and appears as a spindle-shaped enlargement, the ampulla. At the distal end of the ampulla the duct is joined by the duct of the seminal vesicles. From this point it continues to the urethra as the ejaculatory duct (Fig. 28–2). The wall of the ductus deferens is composed of three well-defined layers, the mucosa, muscularis, and adventitia.

The mucosa protrudes into the lumen in several low longitudinal folds (Fig. 28–48). The epithelium is similar in structure to, but not as tall as, that in the epididymis. Some of the columnar cells are exceedingly rich in mitochondria. Stereocilia are present on the free surface of the cells, and frequently they are matted together and form

cones. The stereocilia tend to disappear toward the ampulla. A thin basal lamina is present. The lamina propria is very dense, largely because of a heavy infiltration of elastic fibers. The vas deferens is surrounded by a three-layered smooth muscle coat 1 to 1.5 mm thick. The fibers of the inner and outer layers are arranged longitudinally and those of the middle layer circularly. The adventitia is composed of a fibrous covering of the muscle layer and loose connective tissue, which blends with that of contiguous structures.

Ampulla of the Vas Deferens

The longitudinal folds in the mucosa of the ductus deferens extend into the ampulla, where they increase in height and become branched. The ampulla has a wide lumen and its muscular coat is thinner, with less distinct layers, than elsewhere in the ductus deferens. The longitudinal muscle layers separate into long strands that terminate toward the ejaculatory duct. The epithelium of the ampulla is pseudostratified columnar similar to the rest of the vas. Glandular diverticula showing evidence of secretion extend deep into the surrounding muscle layer.

Ejaculatory Duct

The portion of each ductus deferens that extends from the ampulla to the urethra is reduced in width and receives the duct of the seminal vesicle. The conjoined duct is known as the ejaculatory duct. These ducts, 1 cm in length, penetrate the prostate gland and open into the prostatic urethra on a thickened portion of the urethral mucosa known as the colliculus seminalis, or verumontanum. The mucous membrane, cast into numerous thin folds, forms glandular diverticula that are similar to, but less elaborate than, those in the ampulla. The epithelium is pseudostratified or simple columnar.

Male Accessory Sex Organs

Seminal Vesicles

The seminal vesicles arise as outgrowths from the vas deferens distal to the ampulla. They develop into elongated, hollow organs 5 to 10 cm long, whose walls are packed with small, saclike evaginations. The proximal extremity of each vesicle joins the vas deferens to form the ejaculatory duct (Fig. 28–2). Each vesicle is honeycombed by thin primary folds of mucosae that

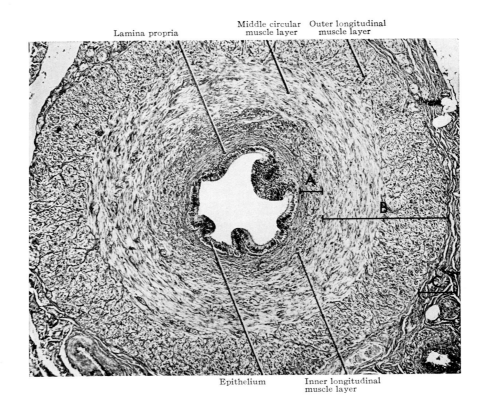

Lamina propria   Middle circular   Outer longitudinal
                        muscle layer   muscle layer

Epithelium   Inner longitudinal
                        muscle layer

28–48 Photomicrograph of a transverse section of the human ductus deferens. **A,** mucosa; **B,** muscularis; **C,** adventitia. × 50.

extend deep into the lumen. These folds branch and anastomose into secondary and tertiary folds that join to form numerous irregular chambers, all of which communicate with the large central lumen. This arrangement increases the surface area of the secretory epithelium. The folds are covered with a pseudostratified epithelium consisting of tall columnar, nonciliated cells that reach the luminal surface, and basal cells identical with those seen elsewhere in the excurrent duct (Fig. 28–49). The secretory cells have a single ovoid nucleus and contain numerous granules, clumps of lipochrome pigment, and some lipid droplets.

The lamina propria contains many elastic fibers. A layer of smooth muscle consisting of inner circular and outer longitudinal fibers and an external sheet of loose connective tissue complete the wall of the seminal vesicle.

Fine-structural observations on the epithelium of the seminal vesicles reveal characteristics usually identified with active secretion of protein. The cytoplasm is packed with rough endoplasmic reticulum. The apical cytoplasm exhibits large vacuoles containing dense secretory granules.

The abundant secretion formed in the seminal vesicles is a viscid material with a whitish yellow color. This gland produces a substantial portion of the whole ejaculate and contains many reducing substances. Prostaglandins were first discovered in sheep seminal vesicles and these glands are frequently used to study the mechanism of prostaglandin secretion. The most important free sugar produced is fructose, and an analysis of this compound in semen may be used to evaluate the secretory activity of the gland. The height of the cells and their functional activity are dependent on the action of testosterone. After castration, the seminal vesicles shrink and cease forming fluid, and the epithelium is reduced to low cuboidal.

Prostate

The prostate, like the seminal vesicles, is a major secretory contributor to the seminal plasma. It is a compact musculoglandular organ, 20 g in weight, in contact with the inferior surface of the

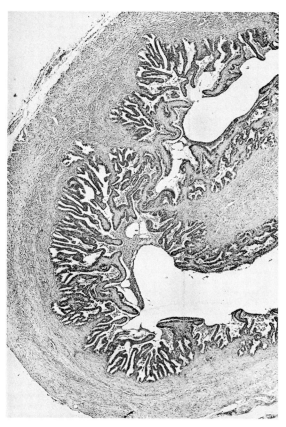

28—49 Longitudinal section of a diverticulum of a human seminal vesicle. ×27.

bladder (Fig. 28–2). The prostate surrounds the first portion of the urethra as it leaves the bladder and consists of three groups of glands arranged somewhat concentrically around the urethra (Fig. 28–50). The smallest are the periurethral mucosal glands. This area of the prostate is involved in producing nodular hyperplasia but is not related to the main function of the prostate or to the origin of cancer. The periurethral glands are separated from the true prostate by a mass of smooth muscle tissue. Previous descriptions subdivided the true prostate into (1) submucosal glands and (2) main prostatic glands (Fig. 28–50). Cancer of the prostate originates in the true prostate, mainly from the "peripheral zone." The prostate consists of 30 to 50 tubuloalveolar glands opening directly into the prostatic urethra through 15 to 30 ducts. The ducts of the mucosal glands open at various points into the urethra, whereas those of the true prostate open onto the posterolateral urethral sinus near the verumon-

tanum. In each lobe the glands are embedded in a markedly fibromuscular stroma, which aids in the ejaculatory discharge of the prostatic fluid.

The glandular epithelium in the prostate is normally simple columnar or pseudostratified (Fig. 28–51). Basal cells resting on the basal lamina are insinuated among the columnar cells. Near the urethra the lining of the epithelium changes to the transitional type characteristic of the bladder and prostatic urethra. Histochemically, the prostatic epithelium is remarkable for the abundance of acid phosphatase.

The prostatic secretion is a colorless fluid, pH 6.5, rich in proteolytic enzymes. The most potent one is fibrinolysin, which plays a role in the liquefaction of semen. Zinc, citric acid, and acid phosphatase also occur in high concentrations in prostatic fluid. The last two products provide a reliable and sensitive test for assessing prostatic function.

As seen by electron microscopy, the prostatic epithelial cells possess luminal microvilli and an abundance of rough endoplasmic reticulum, except in the region of the Golgi complex (Fig. 28–52). Numerous vacuoles containing secretory granules are a common feature of the apical cytoplasm. Castration changes are marked by a reduction in height of the epithelial cells and a loss of the secretory products. These and other cellular changes are reversed by the administration of testosterone.

In the prostatic alveoli, especially of older men, there are concretions of various forms, 0.2 to 2 mm in diameter; in sections they may exhibit concentric layers and show double refraction with polarized light (Fig. 28–53). These structures are believed to be condensations of secretory material and are probably deposited around fragments of cells. The larger concretions sometimes obstruct the prostatic ducts and cause distension of the gland. Octahedral crystals also occur in the prostatic secretion.

The prostate is surrounded by a fibroelastic capsule with some smooth muscle fibers on its inner aspect. These muscle fibers connect with others that penetrate between the prostatic lobules. In many rodents one pair of the lobes of the prostate, the coagulating gland, is differentiated to supply a secretion that coagulates the seminal fluid in the vagina, forming a plug.

The utriculus masculinus is a small pouch on the dorsal wall of the urethra that opens on the verumontanum between the orifices of the two ejaculatory ducts. This a remnant of the müllerian duct.

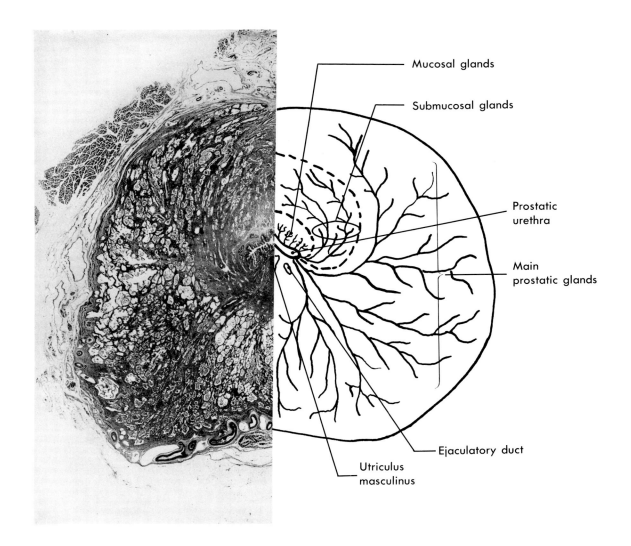

28–50 Normal human prostate in transverse section at left. × 4. (From Franks, L. M. 1954. Ann. R. Coll. Surg. Eng. 14:92.) Diagram of the glandular composition added at right.

Bulbourethral Glands

The two bulbourethral glands or Cowper's glands, are pea-sized structures situated one on each side of the urethral bulb and connected with the penile urethra by fairly long ducts (Fig. 28–2). They are compound tubuloalveolar glands; the end pieces may be rounded sacs or simple tubes (Fig. 28–54). The cells of the simple epithelium vary greatly in height and appearance. In the resting state, they are columnar with granular cytoplasm and have a spherical nucleus. At the peak of secretion, the cells appear to be filled with mucus and have their nuclei flattened against the basal lamina. The glands are divided into small lobules by septa composed of connective tissue and skeletal muscle. The excretory ducts are lined with simple columnar epithelium, except near the urethral orifice where it becomes pseudostratified columnar. The coating of the ducts is made of fibrous tissue and a thin layer of smooth muscle. The secretory product is a clear, viscous, mucus-like substance composed of galactose, galactosamine, galacturonic acid, sialic acid, and a methylpentose. It is poured into the urethra under erotic stimulation and probably acts as a lubricant.

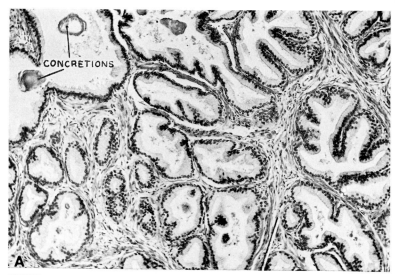

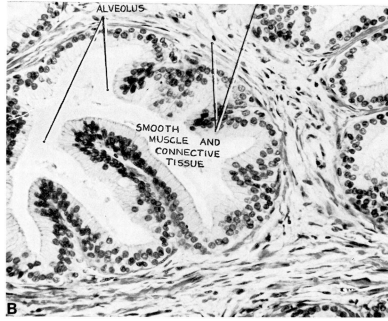

28–51 Human prostate. **A.** Note fibromuscular stroma. **B.** Note simple columnar epithelium, few basal cells, secretion in lumen. A, × 90; B, × 275.

Penis

The penis is an elongate organ consisting principally of the urethra and three parallel cavernous bodies (Figs. 28–2 and 28–55). The paired corpora cavernosa penis are placed dorsally, and beneath them in the midline is the single corpus cavernosum urethrae (spongiosum) that originates as an expanded portion, the bulbous urethrae, and terminates as the glans penis, a structure at the end of the penis having the appearance of a blunted cone. The urethra lies in the center of the spongiosum. A dense, fibroelastic connective tissue layer, the tunica albuginea, binds the three cavernous bodies together and also provides an attachment to the skin over the shaft of the penis. The deepest fibers of this tunic are organized as a capsule around each cavernous body. Those surrounding the corpora cavernosa penis fuse in the midline to form a septum

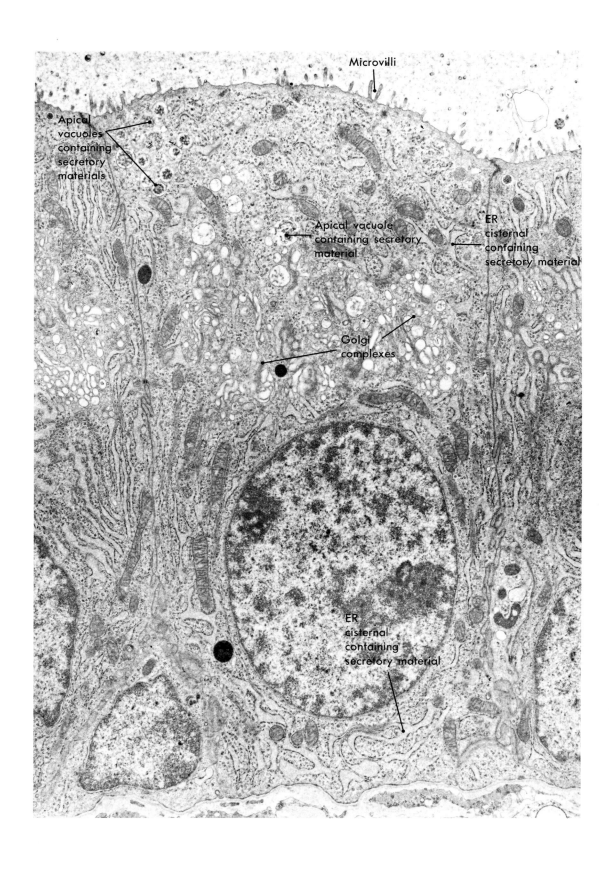

Microvilli

Apical
vacuoles
containing
secretory
materials

Apical vacuole
containing secretory
material

ER
cisternal
containing
secretory material

Golgi
complexes

ER
cisternal
containing
secretory material

28–52 Columnar cells of the epithelium of ventral prostate of a 28-day-old rat. These cells possess enlarged Golgi complexes, dilated cisternae of rough endoplasmic reticulum, and vacuoles containing dense secretory material. × 12,000. (Courtesy of C. J. Flickinger.)

in the penis that becomes incomplete distally. The albuginea enclosing the spongiosum is thinner and contains circularly arranged smooth muscle fibers and more elastic fibers than that of the paired cavernous bodies.

The cavernous bodies are composed of true erectile tissue that increases in size by filling with blood and changing from a flaccid to a rigid state, therby producing an erection of the penis. These bodies are honeycombed by a complex network of venous spaces separated by trabeculae. The trabeculae are lined with typical vascular endothelium and have connective tissue and smooth muscle in the wall. Blood enters these spaces from two sources: from capillaries in the walls of the trabeculae that drain into the spaces, but more importantly for the purpose of erection, from the terminal branches of arteries that course through the walls of the trabeculae and empty

28–53 Section of the human prostate, showing concretions. × 90.

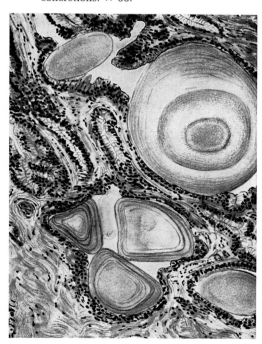

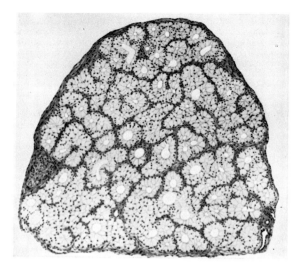

28–54 Section through part of a lobule of the bulbourethral gland. (Stieve.) × 90.

directly into the spaces. These vessels are the helicine arteries, so called because they are coiled and twisted in the flaccid penis. They have heavy muscular walls, with subendothelial thickenings of the longitudinal muscle fibers that partly occlude the lumen. The veins draining the cavernous bodies have such thick walls that they resemble arteries; they contain abundant col-

28–55 Cross section of the penis of a 23-year-old man. The septum between corpora cavernosa penis is incomplete. Section is that from distal one-third of the organ. (Stieve.) × 2.5.

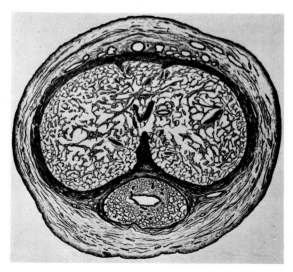

umns of inner logitudinal muscle fibers that make the lumen crescentic or star-shaped. The erectile tissue of the glans penis consists only of convolutions of large veins, and it does not reach the same state of rigidity as the shaft of the erect penis.

Recent studies of the vascular events associated with the process of erection and detumescence of the penis have clarified our understanding of these important processes (Fig. 28–56). The presence of arteriovenous (AV) anastomoses between the deep artery of the penis and the peripheral venous return has been reaffirmed. Hemodynamic experimental work in humans has shown that blood flow into the cavernous spaces of 20 to 50 ml per min will produce erection

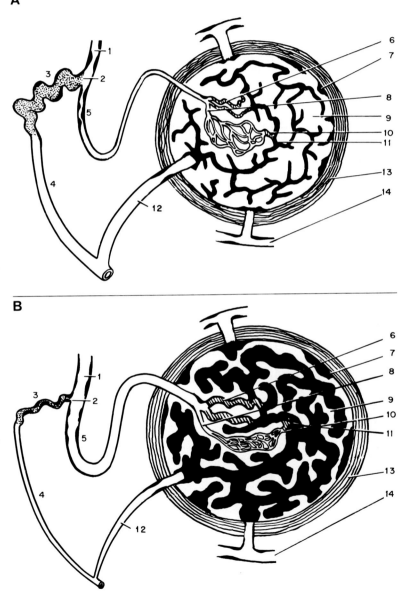

28–56 Vascular relationships of the human penis. **A.** In the flaccid state, blood flows toward the corpora cavernosa in the deep artery of the penis (1). This vessel possesses intimal cushions that tend to regulate blood flow. Almost all the blood passes directly into (2) an arteriovenous anastomosis (3), which is usually dilated in this state and connects with efferent veins (4). Minimal amounts of blood pass to the corpora cavernosa. At a point inside the corpora this artery (5) divides into two branches, the helicine artery (6) that empties almost immediately into the blood spaces of the erectile tissue (7, 11) and the nutritive artery (8) of the trabeculae (9), which, after breaking up into a capillary network re-forms into a small vein (10) and empties into the cavernous space (11). Cavernous spaces are drained by veins that have internal cushions (12, 14). These veins pierce the tunica albuginea (13) and constitute the efferent venous return. **B.** During erection, blood flow in the deep artery of the penis (1) increases. The opening (2) of the arteriovenous anastomosis (3) is reduced by active vasoconstriction resulting in a slight dilated artery (5) passing through the tunica albuginea (13) into the cavernous body. The helicine arteries (6) dilate the cavernous spaces (7) and fill with blood while the nutritive vessel (8) and its venous junction (10) with the cavernous space (11) become compressed. Blood flow leaving the cavernous body (12, 14) is not reduced despite the internal structure of these emergent veins. (Adapted and modified from Conti, G. 1952. Acta Anat. 5:217.)

without the necessity of postulating a venous-closing mechanism. Because parasympathetic activity on the AV complex is required to increase blood flow to the cavernous spaces, it is suggested that concomitant sympathetic activity produces contraction of arterioles supplying the rest of the penis. This combined autonomic interplay ensures a rigid intromittent organ through which sperm can be discharged into the vaginal vault. Relaxation of such autonomic activity after sexual excitement reduces blood flow to the cavernous spaces and shunts most of the blood to the peripheral venous vessels, thereby returning the penis to its flaccid condition.

The skin of the penis is thin, elastic, fat-free, and somewhat more deeply pigmented than that covering the body. Coarse pubic hairs are present at the root of the organ; elsewhere over its shaft there are only lanugo hairs. At the forward end of the penis, the skin is attached to the corona of the glans and forms a circular fold, the prepuce (foreskin) that overlies the glans. The inner surface of the prepuce differs from the skin elsewhere on the penis by having a thinner epidermis and being free of sebaceous and sweat glands. Over the body of the penis there is a subcutaneous layer of smooth muscle fibers that is continuous with the tunica dartos of the scrotum. On the corona glandis, sebaceous glands occur in the absence of hair follicles.

The penis is abundantly supplied with spinal, sympathetic, and parasympathetic nerve fibers. The sensory fibers of the medullated spinal nerves (dorsal nerves of the penis) terminate in many types of sensory endings; as tactile corpuscles in the papillae of the dermis, as end bulbs of Krause and Pacinian corpuscles in the superficial connective tissue, and as genital corpuscles found in or near the cavernous bodies. Free sensory endings also occur. The sympathetic and parasympathetic nerves are a continuation of the prostatic plexus and supply the numerous smooth muscles of the trabeculae and the cavernous blood vessels. The glans is peculiar in that it has no receptors for light, touch, warmth, or cold; however, cylindrical end bulbs of Krause are present.

Semen

This secretion consists of spermatozoa suspended in a complex fluid derived from the testis, epididymis, vas, and accessory sex glands that empties into the excurrent duct system. The ejaculate is about 3 ml in volume and contains approximately 200 to 300 million spermatozoa. In humans, three main glandular systems contribute successively to the ejaculate. The first portion comes from the prostate gland and is a thin, milky emulsion that is slightly acid. In addition, the acid phosphatases are mainly derived from the prostate. The second portion comprises the secretions from the testes, ductus epididymidis, and ductus deferens and therefore contains the highest concentration of spermatozoa. The third portion possesses the highest concentration of fructose, a substance specific for the seminal vesicles and a prime energy source for motile sperm. Prostaglandins, a family of biologically active lipids found in high concentrations in human seminal plasma, are derived from the seminal vesicles. Their biological properties as regulators of smooth muscle activity may influence sperm transit in the male and female and the implantation process.

The average transit time of human spermatozoa from their release into the lumen of the seminiferous tubules through the ductular system to their appearance in the ejaculate is 12 days (with a range of 1 to 21 days).

References and Selected Bibliography

General Literature

Brandes, D. 1974. Male Accessory Sex Organs. Structure and Function in Mammals. New York: Academic Press.

Gorland, M. 1975. Normal and Abnormal Growth of the Prostate. Springfield, Ill.: Charles C. Thomas.

Hamilton, D. W., and Greep, R. O. (eds.). 1975. Handbook of Physiology; Endocrinology, vol. 5, sec. 7, Male Reproductive System. Washington, D.C.: American Physiological Society.

Johnson, A. D., Gomes, W. R., and Vandemark, N. L. (eds.). 1970. The Testis: vol. 1, Development, Anatomy, and Physiology; vol. 2, Biochemistry; vol. 3, Influencing Factors. New York: Academic Press.

Mann, T. 1964. Biochemistry of Semen and of the Male Reproductive Tract. London: Methuen and Co.

Steinberger, E. 1971. Hormonal control of mammalian spermatogenesis. Physiol. Rev. 51:1.

Specific References

Bartke, A., Harris, M. E., and Voglmayr, J. K. 1975. Regulation of testosterone and dihydrotestosterone levels in rete testis fluid. Evidence for androgen biosynthesis in seminiferous tubules in vivo. In F. S. French, V. Hansson, E. M. Ritzén, and S. N. Nayfeh (eds.), Hormonal Regulation of Spermatogenesis. New York: Plenum Press.

Christensen, A. K. 1975. Leydig cells. In D. W. Hamilton and R. O. Greep (eds.), Handbook of Physiology; Endocrinology, vol. 5, sec. 7, Male Reproductive

System. Washington, D.C.: American Physiological Society.

Christensen, A. K., and Fawcett, D. W. 1966. The fine structure of testicular interstitial cells in mice. Am. J. Anat. 118:551.

Clermont, Y. 1963. The cycle of the seminiferous epithelium in man. Am. J. Anat. 112:35.

Clermont, Y. 1966. Renewal of spermatogonia in man. Am. J. Anat. 118:509.

Clermont, Y. 1969. Two classes of spermatogonial stem cells in the monkey (Cercopithecus aethiops). Am. J. Anat. 126:57.

Clermont, Y. 1972. Kinetics of spermatogenesis in mammals: Seminiferous epithelium cycle and spermatogonial renewal. Physiol. Rev. 52:198.

Clermont, Y., and Bustos-Obregon, E. 1968. Re-examination of spermatogonial renewal in the rat by means of seminiferous tubules mounted "in toto." Am. J. Anat. 122:237.

Clermont, Y., and Harvey, S. C. 1967. Effects of hormones on spermatogenesis in the rat. In Endocrinology of the Testis, Ciba Foundation Colloquia on Endocrinology 16:173.

Clermont, Y., and Leblond, C. P. 1955. Spermiogenesis of man, monkey, ram and other mammals as shown by the "periodic acid–Schiff" technique. Am. J. Anat. 96:229.

Conti, G. 1952. L'érection du pénis humain et ses bases morphologico-vasculaires. Acta Anat. (Basel) 14:217.

DeKretser, D. M., Catt, K J., and Paulsen, C. A. 1971. Studies on the in vitro testicular binding of iodinated luteinizing hormone in rats. Endocrinology 88:332.

Dorr, L. D., and Brody, M. J. 1967. Hemodynamic mechanisms of erection in the canine penis. Am. J. Physiol. 213:1526.

Dym, M. 1973. The fine structure of the monkey (Macaca) Sertoli cell and its role in maintaining the blood–testis barrier. Anat. Rec. 175:639.

Dym, M. 1974. The fine structure of monkey Sertoli cells in the transitional zone at the junction of the seminiferous tubules with the tubuli recti. Am. J. Anat. 140:1.

Dym, M. 1976. The mammalian rete testis—A morphological examination. Anat. Rec. 186:493.

Dym, M., and Clermont, Y. 1970. Role of spermatogonia in the repair of the seminiferous epithelium following x-irradiation of the rat testis. Am. J. Anat. 128:265.

Dym, M., and Fawcett, D. W. 1970. The blood–testis barrier in the rat and the physiological compartmentation of the seminiferous epithelium. Biol. Reprod. 3:308.

Dym, M. and Fawcett, D. W. 1971. Further observations on the numbers of spermatogonia, spermatocytes, and spermatids connected by intracellular bridges in the mammalian testis. Biol. Reprod. 4:195.

Fawcett, D. W. 1975. The mammalian spermatozoon. Dev. Biol. 44:395.

Fawcett, D. W. 1975. Ultrastructure and function of the Sertoli cell. In D. W. Hamilton and R. O. Greep (eds.), Handbook of Physiology; Endocrinology, vol. 5, sec. 7, Male Reproductive System. Washington, D.C.: American Physiological Society.

Fawcett, D. W., and Burgos, M. H. 1960. Studies on the fine structure of the mammalian testis. II.The human interstitial tissue. Am. J. Anat. 107:245.

Fawcett, D. W., Heidger, P. M., and Leak, L. V. 1969. Lymph vascular system of the interstitial tissue of the testis as revealed by electron microscopy. J. Reprod. Fertil. 19:109.

Fawcett, D. W., and Hollenberg, R. D. 1963. Changes in the acrosome of guinea pig spermatozoa during passage through the epididymis. Z. Zellforsch. 60:276.

Fawcett, D. W., and Phillips, D. M. 1969. Observations on the release of spermatozoa and on changes in the head during passages through the epididymis. J. Reprod. Fertil. (Suppl.) 6:405.

Flickinger, C. J. 1971. Ultrastructural observations on the postnatal development of the rat prostate. Z. Zellforsch. 113:157.

French, F. S., and Ritzén, E. M. 1973. Androgen binding protein in efferent duct fluid of rat testis. J. Reprod. Fertil. 32:479.

Hamilton, D. W. 1971. Steroid function in the mammalian epididymis. J. Reprod. Fertil. (Suppl.) 13:89.

Hamilton, D. W. 1975. Structure and function of the epithelium lining the ductuli efferentes, ductus epididymis, and ductus deferens in the rat. In D. W. Hamilton and R. O. Greep (eds.), Handbook of Physiology; Endocrinology, vol. 5, sec. 7, Male Reproductive System. Washington, D.C.: American Physiological Society.

Heller, C. G., and Clermont, Y. 1964. Kinetics of the germinal epithelium in man. Recent Prog. Horm. Res. 20:545.

Heller, C. G., Lalli, M. F., and Rowley, M. J. 1968. Factors affecting the testicular function in man. In Pharmacology of Reproduction, vol. 2. New York: Pergamon Press.

Holstein, A. F. 1969. Morphologische Studien am Nebenhoden des Menschen. In W. von Bargmann and W. Doerr (eds.), Zwanglose Abhandlungen aus dem Gebiet der normalen und pathologischen Anatomie. Stuttgart: G. Thieme.

Huckins, C. 1971. The spermatogonial stem cell population in adult rats. I. Their morphology, proliferation and maturation. Anat. Rec. 169:533.

Kormano, M., and Suoranta, H. 1971. Microvascular organization of the adult human testis. Anat. Rec. 170:31.

Lam, D. M. K., Furrer, R., and Bruce, W. R. 1970. The separation, physical characterization and differentiation kinetics of spermatogonial cells of the mouse. Proc. Natl. Acad. Sci. U.S.A. 65:192.

Leblond, C. P., and Clermont, Y. 1952. Spermiogenesis of rat, mouse, hamster, and guinea pig as revealed by the periodic acid–fuchsin sulfurous acid technique. Am. J. Anat. 90:167.

Mason, K. E., and Shaver, S. L. 1952. Some functions of the caput epididymis. Ann. N.Y. Acad. Sci. 55:585.

McNeal, J. E. 1972. The prostate and prostatic urethra: A morphological synthesis. J. Urol. 107:1008.

Means, A. R., Fakunding, J. L., Huckins, C., Tindall, D. J., and Vitale, R. 1976. Follicle stimulating hormone, the Sertoli cells and spermatogenesis. Recent Prog. Horm. Res.

Moens, P. B. 1973. Mechanisms of chromosome synapsis at meiotic prophase. Int. Rev. Cytol. 35:117.

Newman, H. F., Northrup, J. D., and Devlin, J. 1964. Mechanism of human penile erection. Invest. Urol. 1:350.

Nicander, L. 1958. Studies on the regional histology and cytochemistry of the ductus epididymis in stallions, rams and bulls. Acta Morphol Neerl. Scand. 1:337.

Orgebin-Crist, M. C. 1969. Studies on the function of the epididymis. Biol. Reprod. (Suppl.) 1:155.

Perey, B., Clermont, Y., and Leblond, C. P. 1961. The wave of the seminiferous epithelium in the rat. Am. J. Anat. 108:47.

Roosen-Runge, E. C. 1962. The process of spermatogenesis in mammals. Biol. Rev. 37:343.

Rowley, M. J., Berlin, J. D., and Heller, C. G. 1971. The ultrastructure of four types of human spermatogonia. Z. Zellforsch. 112:139.

Rowley, M. J., Teshima, F., and Heller, C. G. 1970. Duration of transit of spermatozoa through the human male ductular system. Fertil. Steril. 21:390.

Setchell, B. P., and Waites, G. M. H. 1975. The blood–testis barrier. In D. W. Hamilton and R. O. Greep (eds.), Handbook of Physiology; Endocrinology, vol. 5, sec. 7, Male Reproductive System. Washington, D.C.: American Physiological Society.

Sohval, A. R., Suzuki, Y., Gabrilove, J. L., and Churg, J. 1971. Ultrastructure of crystalloids in spermatogonia and Sertoli cells of normal human testis. J. Ultrastruct. Res. 34:83.

Stieve, H. 1930. Mannliche Genitalorgane. In W. von Möllendorff (ed.), Handbuch mikroskopischen Anatomie des Menschen, Vol. 7, Part 2. Berlin: Springer-Verlag OHG.

Zamboni, L., Zemjanis, R., and Stefanini, M. 1971. The fine structure of monkey and human spermatozoa. Anat. Rec. 169:129.

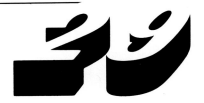

The Hypophysis

Nicholas S. Halmi

Introductory Remarks on Endocrine Tissues

The *endocrine glands* are also known as *ductless glands or glands of internal secretion.* Their parenchymal cells manufacture specific products, termed *hormones,* which they usually secrete into the blood stream. Hormones act as chemical regulators of the functions of specific tissues elsewhere in the body or of the somatic cells in general. The specific structure affected is called the *target organ* of the hormone concerned. The endocrine glands constitute one of the great coordinating mechanisms of the body; the other is the nervous system. The two systems are intimately linked in their functions. The focus of neuroendocrine integration is the adenohypophysis, which regulates a number of target glands (thyroid, adrenal cortex, gonads) and is in turn controlled by "release" and "inhibitory" factors (hypophyseotropic hormones) produced in hypothalamic neurons and conveyed to the adenohypophysis through blood vessels. Also, hormones from the hypophysis may be secreted toward the brain and modulate its functions. Furthermore, according to Pearse, many peptide-producing endocrine cells, APUD cells, are actually derived from neuroectoderm and share histochemical characteristics (amine precursor uptake and decarboxylation) with neural elements. APUD cells are scattered in the epithelium of organs such as the intestine and are believed to have a controlling influence on nearby cells by secreting their products into their immediate environment (paracrine secretion). Finally, some nerve cells in the central nervous system have been found to elaborate peptide hormones akin to or identical with those synthesized in endocrine cells (e.g., ACTH, αMSH, prolactin, and insulin). These peptides may act as neurotransmitters. Both the nervous and the endocrine systems participate in the maintenance of a steady physiological state and are therefore described as having a *homeostatic* or *homeokinetic* role.

The glands universally recognized as endocrine glands are the hypophysis, thyroid, parathyroids, adrenals, gonads, and islets of the pancreas. The placenta, when present, also elaborates hormones. Some other organs (e.g., intestine and kidney) have endocrine functions in addition to their dominant activity. The number of hormones produced by the endocrine glands ranges from one (parathyroid) to 10 or more (hypophysis).

Because endocrine glands have no ducts, their cells secrete into vascular channels. Most endocrine glands are primarily composed of parenchyma and blood vessels, with relatively little stroma. The parenchymal cells are usually polyhedral epithelial cells, arranged with at least one surface abutting upon the wall of a blood or lymph vessel. Their cytoplasm generally contains either clear vacuoles filled with lipid material or granules that are denser than the cytoplasm and have specific affinities for certain dyes. Cells that produce steroid hormones (for example, those of the adrenal cortex) contain lipid droplets; those whose products are peptide or protein hormones (such as the cells of the anterior pituitary lobe) have secretion granules in their cytoplasm. The abundance of these droplets or granules correlates better with the amounts of hormones stored than with their secretion rate.

The endocrine glands have an exceptionally rich blood supply; the thyroid and adrenals are among the most vascular tissues in the body. This feature reflects their intense metabolic activity and the fact that the blood stream both supplies the materials from which hormones are synthesized and carries away the released hormones.

Hypophysis (Pituitary Gland)

Gross Structure and Subdivisions

The hypophysis lies at the base of the brain, to which it is linked by a stalk, the *infundibular* or *pituitary stalk*. In human beings, the stalk is long and slants forward from the brain to the hypophysis. The hypophysis is flattened on the superior surface and is distinctly elongated in the transverse plane. Average measurements of the gland are 1.3 cm (transverse) × 1 cm (sagittal) × 0.5 cm (vertical). It weighs less than 1 g in adults, being somewhat heavier in women than in men. The hypophysis undergoes some enlargement during pregnancy and may weigh up to 1.5 g in multiparae. It rests in a depression in the sphenoid bone, the *sella turcica*. The dura mater of the brain extends across this bony depression as a diaphragm, the *diaphragma sellae*, and is reflected over the surface of the hypophysis to form a fibrous connective tissue capsule that is fused with the periosteum lining the sella.

The hypophysis consists of a glandular portion, the *adenohypophysis,* and a neural portion, the *neurohypophysis* (Table 29–1). The part of the adenohypophysis that forms the bulk of the bulbous main part of the gland is the *pars distalis* or *anterior lobe*. Behind it lies the considerably smaller contribution of the neurohypophysis to the body of the pituitary gland, the *pars nervosa* or *infundibular process*. Between them there is, in most animals and in the fetus but not in the postnatal human gland, a thin cellular partition derived from the adenohypophysis. This partition is the *pars intermedia* or *intermediate lobe*. The core of the infundibular stalk is formed by a neurohypophyseal structure, the *infundibular stem*.This stem connects the infundibular process to a portion of the neurohypophysis called the *median eminence*, which is attached to the hypothalamus of the brain. In humans, the median eminence is poorly developed. A sleeve-like and usually incomplete cranial extension of the adenohypophysis, the *pars tuber-*

Table 29–1 Divisions of the Hypophysis

Major division	Subdivisions
Adenohypophysis	Pars tuberalis
	Pars intermedia–intermediate lobe
	Pars distalis–anterior lobe
Neurohypophysis	Pars nervosa or infundibular process–posterior lobe

	Infundibulum
	  Infundibular stem
	  Median eminence (of tuber cinereum)

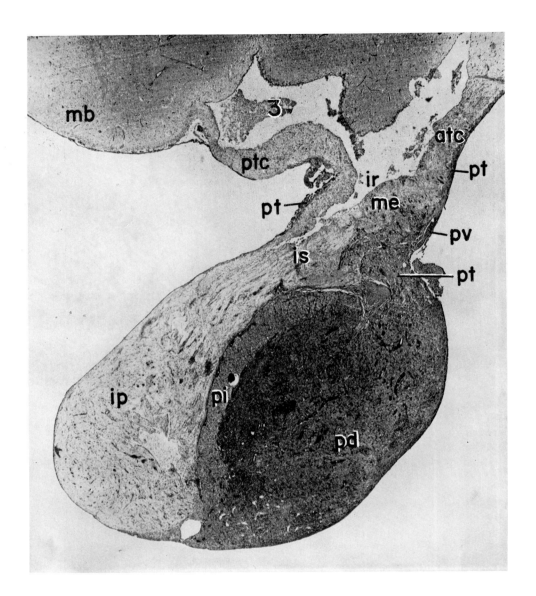

29–1 Midsagittal section through a rabbit hypophysis that is in connection with the hypothalamus. This shows the pars distalis **(pd)**, the pars intermedia **(pi)**, the infundibular process or pars nervosa **(ip)**, the infundibular stem **(is)**, the pars tuberalis **(pt)**, a portal vessel **(pv)**, the median eminence **(me)**, anterior and posterior portions of the tuber cinereum **(atc** and **ptc)**, the third ventricle **(3)** with its infundibular recess **(ir)**, and the mammillary body **(mb)**. Azan stain.

alis, invests the infundibular stem and furnishes the outer layers of the pituitary stalk. These relationships are shown in Fig. 29–1.

Histogenesis of the Hypophysis

The adenohypophysis and the neurohypophysis have different embryological origins. The former arises as an evagination (Rathke's pouch) of the lining of the future oral cavity, whereas the nervous component develops as a downgrowth (infundibulum) from the floor of the diencephalon (Fig. 29–2A).

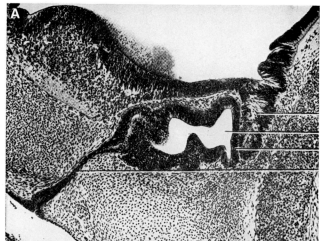

Infundibulum

Rathke's pouch

Pars intermedia

Cellular
attachment

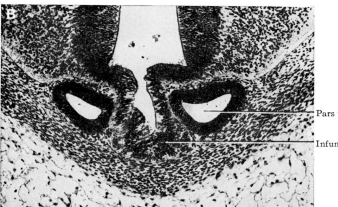

Pars tuberalis

Infundibulum

29–2 Development of the human hypophysis. **A.** A 17-mm embryo. Midsagittal section through the bulbous end of Rathke's pouch and the adjacent infundibulum. The cellular strand marks the point of origin of the epithelial component of the hypophysis. **B.** Median section through the hypophysis of a midterm fetus. Pars tuberalis points to lateral extensions of Rathke's pouch, which later become obliterated. The pars tuberalis is formed by the walls of these recesses. (Courtesy of B. Romeis.)

The two anlagen are closely situated and soon establish contact. The stem of tissue connecting the nervous lobe to the brain is retained in the adult as the core of the pituitary stalk. The attachement of Rathke's pouch to the roof of the oral cavity is lost early in embryonic life, but rudiments are sometimes found as a cellular strand in the sphenoid bone and as a nest of glandular tissue, known as the *pharyngeal pituitary,* at the site of origin in the nasopharynx. The pharyngeal pituitary may produce functional pituitary tumors. At least one hormone (growth hormone) has been identified in its cells.

Figure 29–2 illustrates well what happens as the development of Rathke's pouch proceeds. It aligns itself early against the rostral surface of the infundibulum and develops into three separate glandular portions: (1) the rostral wall of the pouch, which thickens very markedly to form the pars distalis; (2) the caudal wall, which becomes a very thin layer of cells that fuses with the neural outgrowth and is known as the pars intermedia; and (3) the bilateral thickenings of the wall on the dorsolateral aspects of Rathke's pouch, which form two hornlike extensions that pass around the infundibular stem, one on each side, creating a collar of tissue, the pars tuberalis.

In birds, Rathke's pouch is of neuroectodermal origin; there is no conclusive evidence for this origin in mammals.

Blood Supply of the Hypophysis

The hypophysis derives its blood supply from two sets of arteries: inferior hypophyseal arteries that arise from the internal carotids and supply

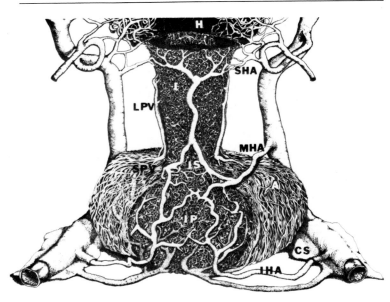

29–3 Drawing of the vasculature of the rhesus monkey pituitary (posterior view) based on vascular casts. **I,** infundibulum; **IS,** infundibular stem, lower end; **IP,** infundibular process; **H,** hypothalamus; **CS,** cavernous sinus; **A,** adenohypophysis; **SHA, MHA, IHA—** superior, middle, and inferior hypophyseal arteries; **LPV, SPV—**long and short portal vessels. The main source of blood to the anterior lobe is the SHA; the MHA and IHA supply primarily the infundibular process. Veins draining the infundibular process also have tributaries from the adenohypophysis and are **Y**-shaped. These features do not show up from behind. Whereas blood flow in the LPV is mainly toward the adenohypophysis, that in the SPV is believed to be to or from the adenohypophysis, depending on prevailing pressure conditions. The capillary network of the neurohypophysis (IP, IS, I) anastomoses with that of the hypothalamus, thus providing a pathway from the hypophysis to the brain. (From Bergland, R. M., and Page, R. B. 1978. Endocrinology 102:1325.)

mainly the pars nervosa, and several superior hypophyseal arteries emanating from the internal carotids and from the posterior communicating artery of the circle of Willis. The superior arteries feed a capillary plexus in the pars tuberalis that gives off capillary loops that penetrate the median eminence and infundibular stem. This plexus is drained by long portal vessels that pass down the pars tuberalis and supply the capillaries in the pars distalis. The portal vessels are so called because, like the portal vein of the liver, they are interposed between two sets of capillaries, one in the pars tuberalis and infundibular stem, and another in the pars distalis. In addition, a set of short inferior hypophyseal arteries feeds the outer layer of the pars distalis. Bergland and Page (1979) have proposed an unorthodox concept regarding the vascular drainage of the hypophysis. They believe that only a small portion of the blood in the pars distalis drains directly into the cavernous sinus and that there is ample opportunity for blood to be shunted from the pars distalis to the pars nervosa, via short portal vessels and **Y**-shaped veins that drain both the anterior and the posterior lobes. The capillary bed of the neurohypophysis, in turn, is envisaged as being subject to regulatory influences that induce its blood to flow mainly into the cavernous sinus or mainly toward the hypothalamus (Fig. 29–3).

The hypophyseal "portal circulation" is a remarkably constant feature throughout the vertebrate groups. The portal vessels provide the morphological basis for the regulation of the anterior lobe by the hypothalamus. Hypothalamic nerve fibers end around the capillary loops in the infundibular stem, and substances that have traveled along them (neurohormones and hypophyseotropic factors) are released there into the blood stream. The blood, thus enriched, is carried to the pars distalis by the portal vessels, and the neurohormones can then influence the cells of this part of the adenohypophysis. The hypophyseal portal circulation provides the vascular part of what is called the *neurovascular link* between the hypothalamus and the pituitary (see section on Hypothalamic Regulation). Connections between the blood supplies of the neurohypophysis and the hypothalamus, on the other hand, provide an anatomical basis for possible humoral influences of the anterior lobe on the brain.

Nerve Supply of the Hypophysis

Nerve fibers originating from hypothalamic cells are an integral part of the neurohypophysis and are discussed in that context. Nerve fibers of the infundibular stalk do not appear to extend into the pars distalis, but in some mammals nerve fibers leave the pars nervosa to terminate around cells of the pars intermedia. Although some post-ganglionic sympathetic and possibly also para-sympathetic nerve fibers can be found in the adenohypophysis, there is no evidence that their function is anything other than vasomotor.

Adenohypophysis

Despite its small size, the adenohypophysis elaborates numerous hormones: growth hormone (GH, or somatotropin, STH); prolactin; thyrotropin (TSH); the gonadotropins, follicle-stimulating hormone (FSH) and luteinizing hormone (LH); and a glycoprotein prohormone molecule that is cleaved into adrenocorticotropin (ACTH); the lipotropins (LPH); peptides with morphine-like activity, the endorphins; and the melanocyte-stimulating hormones (MSH).

Microscopic Structure

Pars Tuberalis. The pars tuberalis forms a collar of cells 25 to 60 μm thick around the neural stalk. It is thickest anterior to the stalk and frequently incomplete on the posterior aspect. The cells are arranged in short cords or globular clusters and occasionally as small folli-

cles. Nests of squamous cells are often found in or around the pars tuberalis. The pars tuberalis contains some functional cells, among which gonadotropic cells predominate.

Pars Intermedia. In most species this portion of the adenohypophysis is quite distinct. It is lacking in some mammals (for example, whales) and in birds. In such animals, a dural septum separates the pars distalis from the pars nervosa. In human beings, the pars intermedia is rudimentary and is composed of chromophobic and basophilic cells. These cells often surround colloid-filled cysts and merge imperceptibly with those of the pars distalis. Sometimes a remnant of Rathke's cleft persists; in such cases the pars intermedia cells are those posterior to the lumen. The cells lining follicles may be ciliated. A unique feature of the human gland is the invasion of the pars nervosa by basophilic cells sim-

29–4 Portions of the human pars nervosa.
A. Basophilic cells of the anterior lobe (top) invading the pars nervosa. Masson's trichrome.
B. Salivary-type glands **(t)** surrounded by lymphocytes in the pars nervosa. Note a blood vessel **(v)** and a large intermediate lobe cyst **(ic).** Gomori's trichrome.

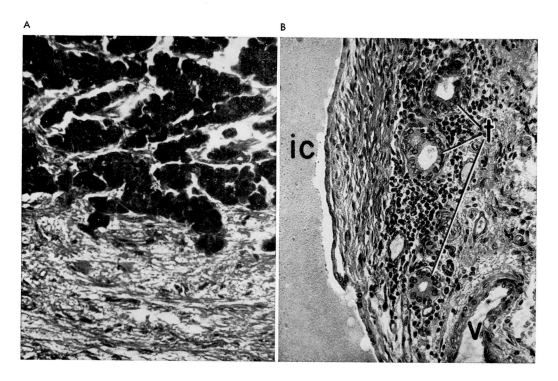

ilar to those in the pars distalis (Fig. 29–4A). Such displaced cells may be quite numerous or altogether absent. Tubular (salivary type) glands surrounded by loose lymphatic tissue (Fig. 29–4B) can often be seen in the pars nervosa next to the pars intermedia.

Pars Distalis. The pars distalis forms about 75% of the hypophysis. The cells in the pars distalis are arranged mainly in cords between which are large-bore capillaries. Some cells appear to be in clusters and others in twisted cords; still others form small, well-defined follicles whose lumina may contain colloid. There is rather little connective tissue in any part of the hypophysis. In the pars distalis, there are two symmetrical, posterolateral foci of fibrous connective tissue; elsewhere, only fine reticular fibers are entwined around the parenchymal cells and the capillaries (Fig. 29–5).

The classic nomenclature distinguishes three main types of cells in the pars distalis: *acidophils*, *basophils*, and *chromophobes*. These types were said to constitute about 40, 10, and

29–5 Portion of a human pars distalis. Note reticular fibers dividing cell nests; see also acidophils **(a)**, basophils **(b)**, and γ cells **(γ)**. PAS–hematoxylin–orange G.

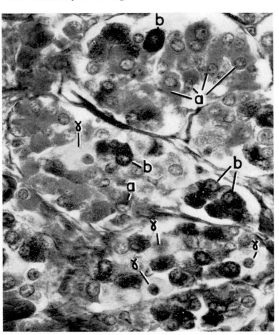

50 % of the anterior lobe cells, respectively, but more recent observations by both light and electron microscopy have shown that chromophobes are much less numerous and largely supportive elements (follicular cells) forming a network within the parenchyma. "Basophil cells" is a misnomer, because these cells are actually characterized by blue staining of their granules with the aniline blue component of triacid stains such as Mallory's. A better term for them is "mucoid," which is based on the fact that their granules stain reddish with periodic acid Schiff (PAS) because of their glycoprotein content. The old nomenclature of pars distalis cells became obsolete when Romeis (1940) realized that with sophisticated staining techniques both the acidophil and the basophil category could be broken down into additional cell types, which he designated by Greek letters. Subsequent recognition of further subdivisions among Romeis's cell types necessitated the addition of subscript numerals and, because several other new nomenclatures were concurrently developed, terminological chaos ensued. Fortunately, the advent of immunocytochemistry has made it possible to classify adenohypophyseal cell types on the basis of the one or more hormones they contain, and a detailed discussion of nomenclatures based on empirical histological techniques is no longer necessary. The only cell type delineated by Romeis that is difficult to characterize immunocytochemically is the γ cell, a large, faintly PAS-positive cell that may be functionally heterogeneous (partly thyrotropic, partly gonadotropic) (Fig. 29–5).

Among the *acidophils* of the human hypophysis, small cells that are generally rounded and most numerous in the posterolateral parts of the pars distalis predominate. They are usually packed with highly refractile granules that stain immunocytochemically for GH (STH) (Fig. 29–6A). These cells are therefore best designated as *somatotrops* or *growth hormone cells*. Acidophils of another type, quite variable in shape and apparently wedged between adjacent cells, are revealed by immunocytochemistry as the source of prolactin (Fig. 29–6B). The prolactin cells are called *lactotrops* or *mammotrops*. When they enlarge in response to elevated levels of estrogen, as in pregnancy, they become stainable with carmoisine or erythrosin, dyes that stain normal prolactin cells erratically at best. These hypertrophic-hyperplastic prolactin cells were first described as "pregnancy cells" in 1909 (Fig. 29–6C).

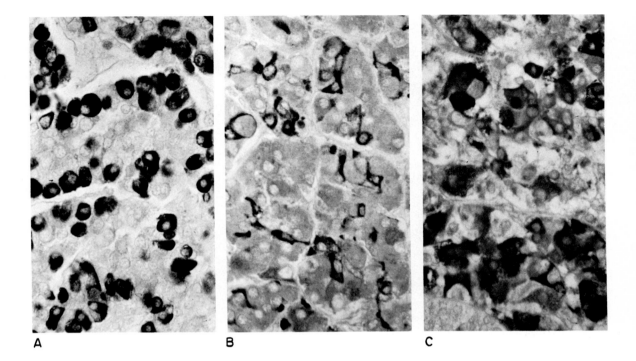

A   B   C

The commonest *basophil* cells are usually round or ovoid, and contain many granules that are intensely PAS-positive. This cell type predominates among the cells that invade the pars nervosa. Immunocytochemically, these cells react with anti-ACTH and also anti-LPH, evidently because they contain these petides in the free form or as part of the common precursor molecule, or both. In humans LPH is not further broken down as it is in some animal species. The best name for the predominant basophil of the human pars distalis is therefore *adrenocorticolipotrop*, or *ACTH/LPH cell*. Adrenocorticolipotrop cells occur most commonly in anteromedian portions of the pars distalis. Almost entirely confined to this part of the lobe are rather large, angular cells that stain intensely blue with aldehyde thionin but only faintly with PAS (Fig. 29–7). Immunocytochemistry has shown that these cells stain for TSH, and hence can be called *thyrotrops*. The third category of basophil cells is composed of small cells that are most common in the posterolateral part of the anterior lobe. They contain rather coarse granules that stain with aldehyde thionin and less well with PAS. These granules are very vulnerable to postmortem changes. Immunocytochemistry has revealed both FSH and LH in the great majority of

29–6 Human anterior hypophyseal lobes immunocytochemically stained by the unlabeled antibody peroxidase-antiperoxidase **(PAP)** complex method. **A.** Growth hormone cells in a normal hypophysis. **B.** Prolactin cells in the same hypophysis. **C.** Hypertrophic, hyperplastic prolactin cells from the hypophysis of a lactating woman. A and B, × 400; C, × 250. (Rearranged from Halmi, N. S., Parsons, J. A., Erlandsen, S. L., and Duello, T. 1975. Cell Tissue Res. 158:497.)

these cells, which are therefore best designated as *gonadotrops* or *FSH/LH cells* (Fig. 29–8).

True *chromophobes* (other than follicular cells) are much less numerous than counts based on conventionally stained material indicate, if they indeed exist. Most of the apparently chromophobic cells certainly have a few specific granules. It is commonly believed that the cells of the pars distalis show cyclic secretory activity, that is, that they first accumulate and then release their specific granules. "Chromophobes" may therefore be transitionally degranulated cells. Because large shifts in the distribution of granulated cells may occur and mitoses are infrequent in the anterior lobe, the apparent chromophobes are the probable reservoir from which more fully granulated cells of different types originate.

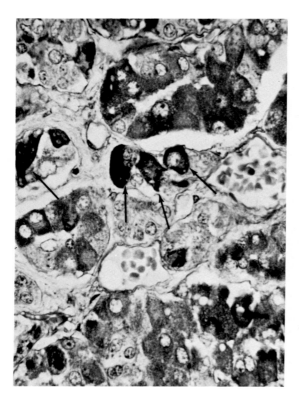

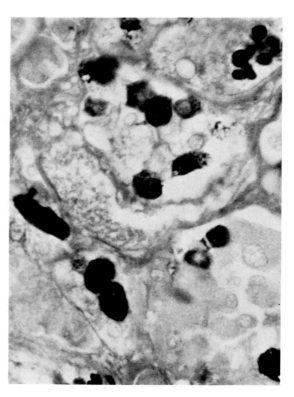

29–7 Anteromedian portion of a human pars distalis stained with aldehyde thionin–PAS–orange G. The ACTH/LPH cells, stained with PAS, are those with variable gray granulation. The angular or irregularly shaped TSH cells, stained with aldehyde thionin, appear dark **(arrows).**

29–8 Gonadotropic cells of human adenohypophysis immunocytochemically stained with antibody against LH. Unlabeled antibody–PAP complex method. Staining of red blood cells is a result of their peroxidase activity and not an immunocytochemical reaction.

Ultrastructure of the Adenohypophyseal Cells

Among the *acidophils,* the *somatotrops* have granules that are densely packed and average 370 nm in diameter. The rough endoplasmic reticulum is moderately well developed. The *prolactin cells* in the resting state have small granules (average, less than 200 nm in diameter). The enlarged prolactin cells in pregnancy and lactation are characterized by relatively sparse granules that may be quite large (over 600 nm in maximal diameter). The rough endoplasmic reticulum is exceptionally well developed in these cells. In tumors arising from prolactin cells, the granules are variable, and their mode of extrusion from the cell is unusual: they leave parts of the cell not adjacent to capillaries ("misplaced exocytosis").

Among the *basophils,* the *ACTH/LPH cells*

are round or ovoid, with granules at random throughout the cytoplasm. Granule size overlaps so much with that of GH cells that distinction on this basis is tenuous. The two cell types can be readily distinguished, however, by electron-microscopic immunocytochemistry. Often, ACTH/LPH cells contain large lipids droplets. A feature unique to them is the presence in the cytoplasm of a small number of fibers about 60 to 80 Å in diameter. These fibers can become much more numerous in pathological states (see Crooke cells below.) Immunostaining reveals a single set of granules reactive for ACTH, βLPH, and βMSH (because antibodies against βMSH crossreact with its parent molecule, βLPH (Figs. 29–9 and 29–10)). The *TSH cells* have the smallest secretory granules of all hypophyseal cells (150 nm or less across) (Fig. 29–9). The *gonadotrops* have granules intermediate in size between those of TSH and GH cells. Their electron density is quite

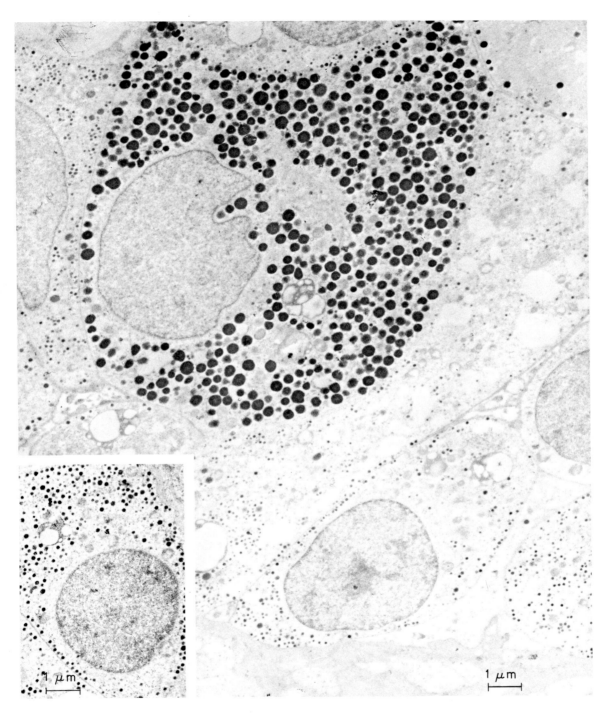

29–9 Electron micrograph of ACTH/LPH cell (upper part of field) whose granules were immunocytochemically stained with antibody against [17-39]ACTH. Unlabeled antibody–PAP complex method. The adjacent cells with considerably smaller, unstained granules are TSH cells. The **inset** (lower left) shows the granules of TSH cells immunocytochemically stained with antibody against the hormone-specific β chain of TSH. (The glycoprotein hormones of the pituitary, TSH, FSH and LH, share a virtually identical α chain.) (Courtesy of Gwen V. Childs.)

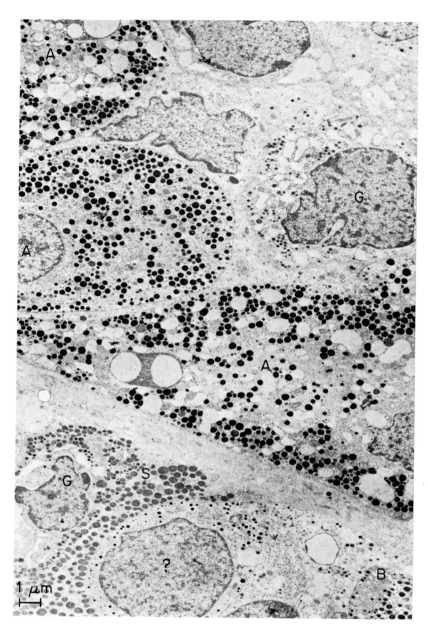

29–10 Electron micrograph of ACTH/LPH cells immunocytochemically stained with antibody against βMSH **(A).** Unlabeled antibody–PAP complex method. Also shown are an unstained growth hormone cell **(S)** and gonadotrops **(G).** (Courtesy of Gwen V. Childs.)

variable. These cells often contain lipid droplets and lysosomes (Fig. 29–11). The γ *cells* are characterized by few secretion granules and an abundance of smooth endoplasmic reticular sacs. They resemble the hypertrophic-hyperplastic TSH cells in the pituitaries of hypothyroid rats ("thyroidectomy cells").

The *follicular cells* are stellate or elongated, and their apexes may join together to line small spaces filled with homogeneous colloid, into which they extend microvilli.

Histochemistry of the Adenohypophysis
The basophil cells of the adenohypophysis, including the γ cells, can be best defined as the cells whose secretory granules give a positive PAS reaction after digestion with amylase; that

is, they contain glycoproteins. These granules, which usually appear coarse, must correspond to aggregates of those seen with the electron microscope. The cells that produce the glycoprotein hormones TSH and the gonadotropins are only weakly PAS-positive in humans. In human beings, the cells with the most markedly PAS-reactive granules produce the simple peptides ACTH and βLPH. This is not surprising, however, since both are derived from a common glycoprotein precursor. The colloid droplets seen in some hypophyseal cells are intensely PAS-positive and sudanophilic, and they may contain a lipid pigment. Intercellular colloid also stains with PAS. Basophilia due to rough endoplasmic reticulum is found in the cytoplasm of anterior lobe cells. It is most prominent in active lactotrops.

Histophysiology of the Adenohypophysis

Because the adenohypophysis is known to produce a number of hormones and contains several cell types, many efforts have been made to identify the cellular source of individual hormones. Even before the immunocytochemical studies, whose success has permitted the functional classification of human adenohypophyseal cell types, much light was shed on the function of pituitary cell classes by (1) bioassays of different parts of large hypophyses in which cell types are unevenly distributed, and (2) correlation of cytological and functional changes in various physiological, pathological, and experimental conditions. Because target-organ hormones act back on the cells that produce the tropic hormones, experimental changes in the levels of target-gland hormones have been especially useful in eliciting characteristic responses in the hypophysis. Experimentally induced or spontaneously arising tumors of individual cell types often produce an excess of the hormone normally elaborated by these cells and have thus furnished important information on the cellular sources of different hormones.

Growth Hormone (Somatotropin). Growth hormone is a simple protein that enhances body growth after birth. Its absence results in *pituitary dwarfism*; its oversecretion in childhood leads to *gigantism* and during adult life to *acromegaly* (enlargement of hands, feet, mandible, and viscera). In addition to the immunocytochemical staining of the most numerous form of acidophils

for GH (Fig. 29–6A), the origin of GH from these cells is affirmed by tumors (adenomas) arising from them that are found in gigantism or acromegaly.

Prolactin. Prolactin is a simple protein that promotes mammary development and lactation. It also participates in the maintenance of corpora lutea in rodents, whose prolactin has therefore been called *luteotropin (LTH)*. In the pituitary of a number of species (for example, rabbit and cat), staining with azocarmine and orange G reveals two types of acidophils, carmine cells and orange cells. The former are consistently prominent when prolactin secretion is enhanced (Fig. 29–12, see here and color insert). As indicated, the human "resting" prolactin cell does not stain well differentially, except by immunocytochemistry (Fig. 29–6B), but the hypertrophic, hyperplastic, and hyperactive prolactin cell in pregnancy and lactation (Fig. 29–6C) does. Human pituitary tumors composed of prolactin cells are fairly common. They cause elevated levels of plasma prolactin and cessation of menses (amenorrhea) with or without milk flow (galactorrhea).

Thyrotropin (Thyroid-Stimulating Hormone). This glycoprotein hormone stimulates many functions of the thyroid. In human beings with primary thyroid failure, hypersecretion of TSH is accompanied by the appearance of large, lightly granulated basophils containing colloid droplets. These basophils are derived from TSH cells. Conversely, in Graves' disease, a condition characterized by hypersecretion of thyroid hormones in response to a nonpituitary thyroid stimulator, the negative feedback effect of these hormones on the TSH cells of the pituitary causes such basophils to regress. Adenomas of TSH cells are rare: most of them occur in people with longstanding hypothyroidism, but some cause hyperthyroidism by hypersecreting TSH and thereby overstimulating a responsive thyroid.

Gonadotropins: Follicle-Stimulating Hormone and Luteinizing Hormone. Follicle-stimulating hormone, a glycoprotein, stimulates the growth of ovarian follicles past the primordial stage and activates the spermatogenic epithelium of the testis. Luteinizing hormone, also a glycoprotein, is necessary for ovulation and the secretion of estrogen by the follicle; it also stimulates the Leydig cells of the testis to secrete androgen. In human beings, the most convincing proof for the

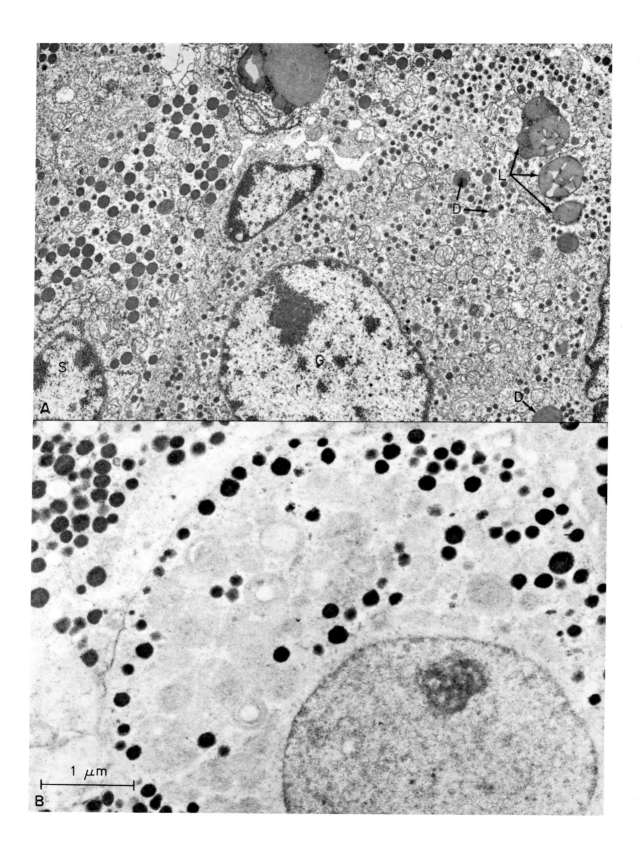

29–11 **A.** Conventional electron micrograph of a gonadotrop **(G)** from a normal human hypophysis. Note relatively small granules of variable size and electron density, several lipid droplets **(L),** and dense bodies **(D).** Portions of a GH cell **(S)** show the larger size of its secretion granules. **B.** Secretion granules of a gonadotrop immunocytochemically stained with antibody against the β chain of FSH. Unlabeled antibody–PAP complex method. The unevenness of the outline of the granules is due to the ring-shaped PAP complex molecules deposited on them. (Part A courtesy of S. S. Schochet, Jr.; part B courtesy of Gwen V. Childs.)

identity of gonadotrops (FSH/LH cells) is immunocytochemical (Fig. 29–8). These cells regress during pregnancy, when placental estrogen exerts a negative feedback effect on them, and they are usually small and few in childhood, when gonadotropin secretion is at a low level. However, they do not show the expected hypertrophy and hyperplasia after the menopause, when secretion of gonadotropins is elevated. This is in contrast to the marked enlargement and multiplication of gonadotrops in castrated rats.

Adrenocorticotropin (Adrenocorticotropic Hormone) and Related Peptides. Adrenocorticotropin is a polypeptide containing 39 amino acids. It stimulates the adrenal cortex to secrete glucocorticoids such as cortisol. In human beings ACTH has been immunocytochemically localized in anterior and posterior lobe basophil cells with anti-[1-39]ACTH or antiserum against the biologically inactive C-terminal sequence of the molecule ([17-39]ACTH) (Fig. 29–9). The latter has the advantage of circumventing immunoreactivity due to MSH or LPH, which share a number of amino acids with the N-terminal portion of ACTH, and the disadvantage of not necessarily demonstrating biologically active ACTH. Spontaneous hypersecretion of ACTH, which leads to adrenal cortical hyperplasia and hypercortisolism (Cushing's disease), is often associated with relatively small "basophilic" tumors of the hypophysis. If a patient with Cushing's disease is bilaterally adrenalectomized, his pituitary sometimes develops relatively large tumors. These tumors were believed to be chromophobic, but electron microscopy has shown that they are composed of ACTH/LPH cells. Such tumors secrete large amounts of both ACTH and βLPH. Furthermore, Cushing's disease or administration of glucocorticoids leads to a pathognomonic alteration of the ACTH/LPH cells. Their granules are in part or totally replaced by PAS-negative material that is homogeneous under the light microscope (Crooke's hyalin change, Fig. 29–13) and revealed by the electron microscope as being due to an accumulation of the fibrils characteristic of ACTH/LPH cells. Crooke's change is seldom seen in posterior lobe basophils. Its functional significance is obscure, but it undoubtedly reflects the effects of the negative feedback of excess glucocorticoids on the cells that secrete ACTH.

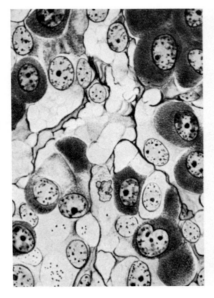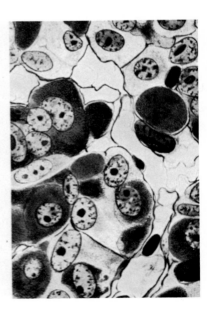

29–12 Anterior lobe of the cat hypophysis. This is a black-and-white rendition of a color plate. See color section.

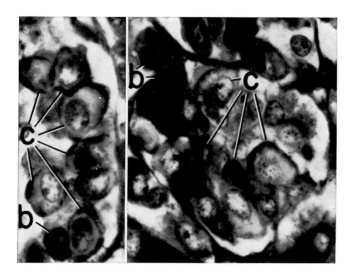

29–13 Pars distalis from a patient who was treated with large doses of cortisone before his death. Note contrast between fully granulated ACTH/LPH cells **(b)** and cells showing Crooke's hyaline change **(c)**. The annular distribution of the hyaline material is particularly obvious in the cell near the left lower corner. PAS–hematoxylin–orange G.

In the ACTH/LPH cells of the adult human pars distalis, the precursor molecule is cleaved to ACTH as well as βLPH and its smaller derivative γLPH. No function of LPH is known. In the pars intermedia of animals, LPH is further metabolized to βMSH and β-endorphin. Melanocyte-stimulating hormone causes dispersal of melanin in the melanophores of amphibians, but it has no established physiological function in mammals. Large doses of injected MSH can cause hyperpigmentation in humans. β-Endorphin is a potent opoid, i.e., it acts like morphine. Adrenocorticotropin itself is cleaved in the pars intermedia to αMSH. Such a breakdown occurs only in a small fraction of pars distalis ACTH/LPH cells and of the ACTH/LPH cells that invade the pars nervosa.

Hypothalamic Regulation of the Adenohypophysis

Many of the functions of the adenohypophysis depend on its connections with the hypothalamus. Furthermore, some of the negative feedback effects of target-gland hormones on the respective tropic hormones are mediated by way of the hypothalamus. In rats, hypophyses transplanted under the kidney capsule show total or substantial loss of gonadotropic, thyrotropic, and adrenocorticotropic function. The basophils in such grafts are decreased in number and size or are absent. When such transplants are placed back under the median eminence and reestablish normal vascular connections, their structural and functional integrity returns. More or less selective interference with the secretion of various hypophyseal hormones can be achieved by appropriately placed hypothalamic lesions. These functional changes are accompanied by corresponding morphological alterations of the adenohypophysis. It is likely that circumscribed hypothalamic regions produce specific substances that govern the release (and also the production) of different hypophyseal principles. These factors must reach the adenohypophysis via the portal vessels. The thyrotropin-releasing hormone (TRH) has been chemically identified as pyroglutaminyl-histidylprolineamide and synthesized, as have the decapeptide that releases gonadotropins (GnRH, LHRH), a 14-amino-acid inhibitor of GH secretion (somatostatin), and a 41-amino acid stimulator of adrenocorticotropin secretion (CRF). Prolactin secretion seems to be tonically inhibited rather than stimulated by the hypothalamus, although TRH releases prolactin as well as TSH. Transplanted pituitaries of rats are eventually transformed so as to consist largely of acidophils of the prolactin-producing type. In such animals, corpora lutea are maintained much beyond the normal physiological limit. Even tissue cultures of pituitary cells secrete prolactin and respond to estrogen, which is also a stimulus to prolactin production in vivo. The intermediate lobe also seems to be restrained by the hypothalamus. Section of the hypophyseal stalk or transplantation of the adenohypophysis in amphibians leads to hyperplasia of the isolated pars intermedia and to blackening of the skin due to enhanced production of MSH. The regulation of βLPH secretion in human beings is different: βLPH and ACTH are generally released in parallel, both being under predominantly stimulating hypothalamic influences.

Neurohypophysis

The neurohypophysis secretes two hormones into the systemic circulation: *vasopressin (antidiuretic hormone (ADH))* and *oxytocin*. In addition, it is in this part of the pituitary that the "release" and inhibitory hypophyseotropic factors regulating functions of the adenohypophysis are discharged into the portal vascular system that feeds the pars distalis.

Structure

The neurohypophysis is a complex of structures that include the axon terminations of secretory nerve cells of the hypothalamus. The neurosecretory cells are distinct from other neurons in that their axons do not terminate on other nerve cells or on other effector cells but store the secretory product and release it into the blood stream. Neurosecretory cells that conform to this definition have been found in many species from arthropods up. Although these cells resemble the neurosecretory cells of mammals even ultrastructurally, having granules that measure 100 to 300 nm across, their functions can be quite dissimilar among species.

Developing from the floor of the diencephalon behind the optic chiasma, the *infundibulum* (median eminence and infundibular stem) and the *pars nervosa* at first contain the continuation of the cavity of the third ventricle (infundibular recess). This cavity is usually obliterated during development, except for remnants lined by ependymal cells. After this obliteration, the hilar or central portion of the pars nervosa is formed by a densely packed bundle of about 50,000 nonmyelinated fibers known as the *hypothalamohypophyseal tract* (Fig. 29–14).

The origins of the nerve fibers of the hypothalamohypophyseal tract have been precisely determined by experiments in animals in which the hypophyseal stalk was sectioned. The resultant interruption of the nerve fibers in the infundibular stem is followed by chromatolysis and retrograde degeneration of their nerve cell bodies in the supraoptic and paraventricular nuclei of the hypothalamus and in more scattered nerve

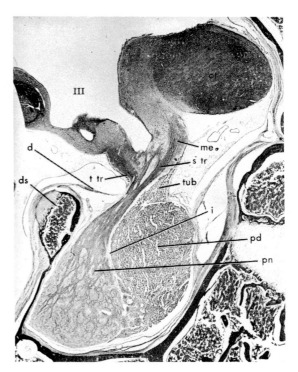

29–14 The primate neurohypophysis. Sagittal section of the neurohypophysis of a cynomolgus monkey, in situ in meninges and sella turcica. Protargol silver stain shows rostral and caudal contributions to the hypothalamohypophyseal tract, which sweeps from the infundibulum into the pars nervosa; **III,** third ventricle; **me,** median eminence; **tub,** pars tuberalis; **i,** pars intermedia; **pd,** pars distalis; **pn,** pars nervosa; **s tr,** supraopticohypophyseal tract; **t tr,** tuberohypophyseal tract; **d,** diaphragma sellae; **ds,** dorsum sellae. × 12. Bodian stain.

cells caudally in the tuber cinereum. Nerve fibers arising from cell bodies in the infundibular and tuberal regions *(tuberohypophyseal tract)* terminate mainly in the median eminence, whereas nerve fibers originating in the supraoptic and paraventricular nuclei *(supraopticohypophyseal tract)* end mostly in the pars nervosa. In human beings, however, the median eminence is not prominently developed and does not have the characteristic neurohypophyseal structure seen in other vertebrates, including lower primates. The nerve endings of the human tuberohypophyseal tract and of some of the fibers of the supraopticohypophyseal tract can be found around the capillary loops in the infundibular stem.

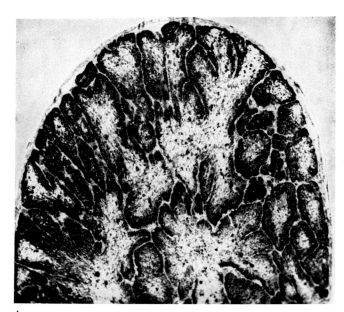

A

29–15 Opossum neural lobe. **A.** Low-power view. The lobules are outlined by the dense staining of the palisade zone surrounding the pale hilum of each lobule. Note deeply stained Herring bodies in the hilum of each lobule. Chrome alum–hematoxylin. × 70. **B.** Schematic representation of the histological organization of a neural lobe lobule. Nerve fibers of the hypophyseal tract **(f)**, pituicyte cell bodies **(pit)**, and three Herring bodies **(HB)** are shown in the hilum of the lobule (lower right). Surrounding this region, the palisade zone **(p)** is seen to be formed by rodlike nerve fiber terminals containing the stained neurosecretory substance. Although light micrographs have suggested that the nerve fiber terminals are coated with neurosecretory substance, electron micrographs indicate that the granules that probably represent neurosecretory substance are confined within the plasma membrane of the axon terminals. The central core of the cylindrical axon terminals often contains a cluster of neurofilaments that may represent the axon terminal as seen in silver impregnations at the light-microscopy level. Interspersed among axon terminals are pituicyte fibers that extend to the vascular-collagenous septal layer **(s).** Axon **(ax).** Bodian stain.

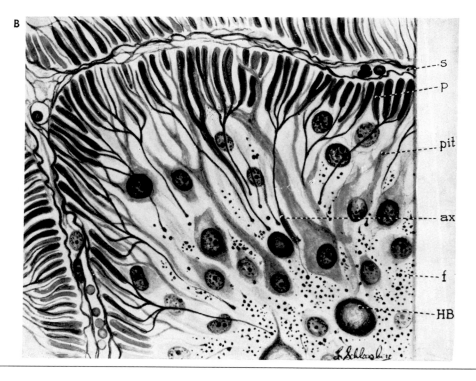

B

The hypothalamohypophyseal tract branches as it enters the hilum of the pars nervosa, and the branches are dispersed to form the core of the irregular lobules of which the pars nervosa is composed. An analysis of the structure of the pars nervosa of a primitive mammal, the opossum, has revealed the fundamental plan of the neurohypophyseal lobule (Fig. 29–15). In the "typical" lobule, the central core of nerve fibers extends to the margin of the lobule as parallel arrays of blindly ending nerve fiber terminals, the *palisade zone*. The lobule is surrounded by a *septal zone* of loose collagenous tissue containing a rich network of capillary vessels, which in some fashion receive the secretory products contained in the nerve terminals. Among the nerve fibers are dispersed the dominant intrinsic cells of the neurohypophysis, the neuroglia-like *pituicytes,* whose short processes often extend out to the septal zone between the nerve terminals. They have been described in detail by Romeis (1940), who emphasized the occurrence of a variety of pituicytes and a variety of inclusions within them. In most mammals, including human beings, the lobular pattern is greatly distorted, but careful inspection may reveal "typical" lobules as well as lobules so modified as to appear "inverted," with a central rather than peripheral septal or vascular zone.

In about 5% of human hypophyses, aggregates of large, round cells with coarse PAS-positive granules can be seen in the neurohypophysis. The origin and significance of these so-called choristomas are not known.

A histological key to the role of the neurohypophysis was supplied by the finding of Bargmann (1966) that the abundant gelatinous material in the pars nervosa could be selectively stained and shown to be present not only in the pars nervosa but also in the nerve fibers of the hypothalamohypophyseal system. In some mammals the stainable material is also readily demonstrable in nerve cell bodies in the hypothalamus. By means of certain stains (chrome alum hematoxylin, aldehyde fuchsin, or aldehyde thionin after permanganate oxidation), this *neurosecretory substance* (Figs. 29–13 and 29–14) is stained a brilliant blue or purple. Thickenings or outpocketings of the axons in the hypothalamo-hypophyseal tract, the so-called *Herring bodies* (Fig. 29–16), have similar staining characteristics. A physiological role of the neurosecretory substance is documented by its drastic depletion in response to osmotic stimuli that cause massive release of ADH (Fig. 29–17). The ADH content of neurohypophyses whose neurosecretory substance content is thus reduced is quite low. Immunocytochemical evidence for the relationship of the neurosecretory substance and the neurohypophyseal hormones is discussed below.

Fine Structure

Electron-microscopic observations have revealed that electron-dense membrane-bounded granules of the order of 100 to 300 nm in axons and axon terminals of the neurohypophysis disappear in

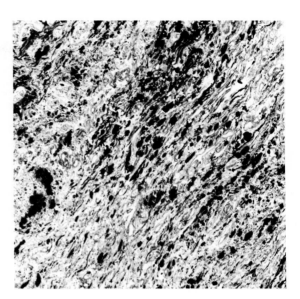

29–16 Neurosecretion-laden fibers of the human infundibular stem are shown in contact with or near Herring bodies (dark, irregular blobs). Aldehyde thionin after permanganate oxidation. × 160.

response to the same stimuli that cause depletion of the neurosecretory substance and of posterior lobe hormones. Electron-microscopic studies of the secretory process in the neurohypophysis have shown that neurosecretory granules are found only within the cytoplasm of nerve cells, and especially in the nerve fiber terminals (Fig. 29–18), where they can be stained immunocytochemically for hormones (for example, ADH; Fig. 29–19) and their associated carrier peptides, the neurophysins. Other fibers contain smaller granules (50–80 nm) reminiscent of membrane-bounded granules found in adrenal medulla (catecholamine granules) (Fig. 33–16) and in adrenergic nerve endings. In addition to neurosecretory granules, smaller vesicles (30 nm) have been observed in the nerve fiber terminals in the pars nervosa. They resemble synaptic vesicles. The specific granules of the posterior pituitary have been isolated in relatively pure form by centrifugal sedimentation in a fraction containing most of the hormone of the gland. Some evidence was obtained that ADH and oxytocin are stored in different granules.

In light-microscopic preparations stained with silver, the Herring bodies are revealed as greatly expanded axon portions, containing a more densely stained core. In electron-microscopic preparations (Fig. 29–18), the core appears as a

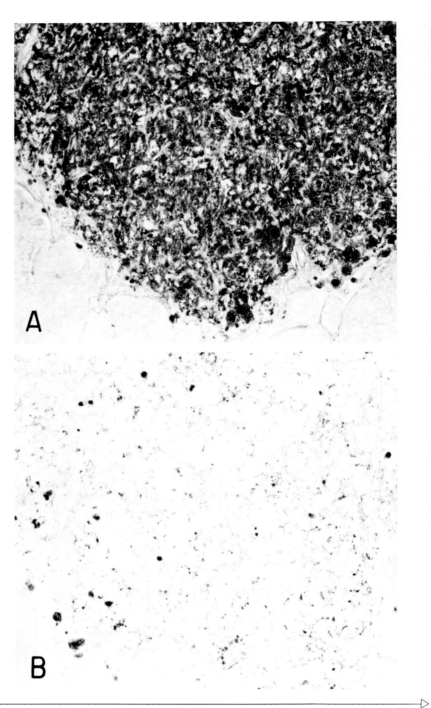

29–17 **A.** Normal pars nervosa of a rat. It is loaded with neurosecretory substance. **B.** Pars nervosa of a rat that had received a 2.5% sodium chloride solution instead of drinking water for 4 days. Note almost complete disappearance of the neurosecretory substance. Aldehyde fuchsin after permanganate oxidation. × 160.

29–18 Diagram illustrating, at the electron-microscopic level, the principal features of organization of the zone of hormone transfer in the opossum. Capillary lumen **(c)** lined by endothelium with abundant vesicles indicating active pinocytosis, and numerous "pores"; septal zones **(s)**, composed of collagen space, bounded by basement membranes **(b)**, and separating palisade axon terminals **(t)** from endothelium. Septal zone contains fibroblasts **(f)** and mast cells (tip of mast cell shown at **m**). Isolated depleted palisade terminals **(x)** occur in the normal animal, unassociated with an increase of synaptic

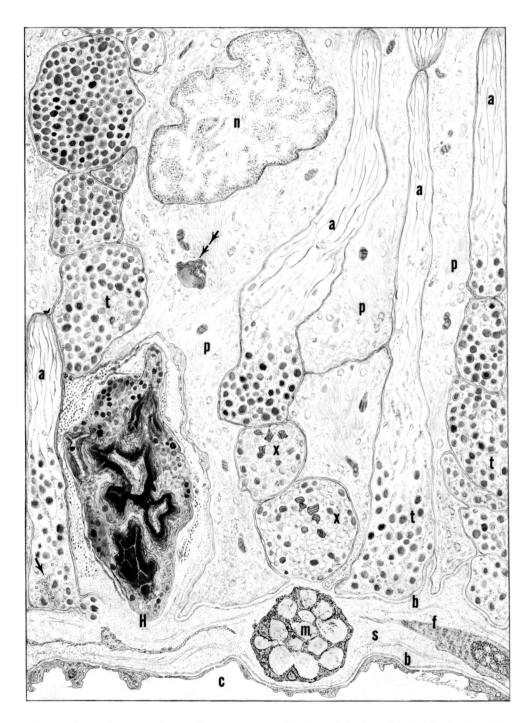

microvesicles. Such vesicles **(arrow)** typically occupy the tips of palisade terminals near the septal zone. Axons and palisade axon terminals are interspersed with pituicytes and their processes **(p),** which may extend down to the septal zone. Pituicytes occasionally contain dense inclusions **(double arrow).**

Nucleus of pituicyte **(n).** Herring bodies **(H)** are axon terminals apparently formed by development of a central cavity, which becomes surrounded by densely packed membranous lamellae. Approximately × 8,000. Bodian stain. Drawn by Eleanor Bodian: provided by courtesy of David Bodian.

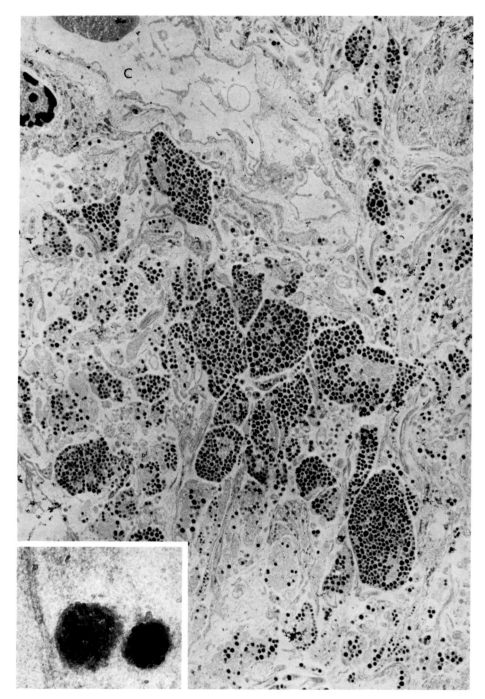

29–19 Electron micrograph of the posterior pituitary of a guinea pig, immunocytochemically stained for ADH (with the unlabeled antibody–PAP complex method). ADH is confined to the neurosecretory granules in axons and nerve terminal. The **inset** shows that the round PAP complex molecules corresponding to the sites of ADH storage are strictly limited to the neurosecretion granules. × 8,400; inset, × 110,000. (From Silverman, A. J., and Zimmerman, E. A. 1975. Cell Tissue Res. 159:291.)

densely osmiophilic mass of tightly packed concentric membranes, or it may contain a number of smaller laminated bodies. The peripheral axoplasm contains numerous neurosecretory granules that are usually more electron-opaque than those seen in the palisade-zone terminals. It is more difficult to deplete granules of Herring bodies by osmotic stimulation than to deplete those in the palisade zone.

Histochemistry

The localization of the active principles of the neurohypophysis by chemically specific methods rests on the finding that both ADH and oxytocin are octapeptides that contain cystine, as do the carrier peptides (neurophysins) to which they are linked. Histochemical techniques for the disulfide groups of cystine have been successfully applied to the demonstration of neurosecretory substance. The selectivity of chrome alum hematoxylin and of other staining methods for the neurosecretory substance also appears to be based on these disulfide groups.

Histophysiology

Of the two hormones of the neurohypophysis, *vasopressin* was named for its pharmacological effect of raising blood pressure. The term *antidiuretic hormone* is preferable because it refers to a physiological function of the hormone: it makes the distal convoluted tubules and collecting ducts of the kidney permeable to water and thereby enables the solute pool in the renal medulla to cause water absorption from these ducts. In the absence of ADH, a large volume (sometimes 20 liters per day or more) of dilute urine is voided (diabetes insipidus). *Oxytocin* is named after the effect that relatively large doses of this hormone have on the parturient uterus: by enhancing contractions, the hormone "speeds up birth." Whether this is a normal physiological function of the hormone is questionable. However, oxytocin is known to play a role in the evacuation of the lactating breast. It squeezes milk from mammary alveoli by causing contraction of the myoepithelial cells surrounding them.

Antidiuretic hormone and oxytocin are manufactured in the perikarya of the supraoptic and paraventricular nuclei and travel with the axoplasmic flow along the axons arising from these nuclei, to be discharged at or near the nerve endings in the posterior lobe. Section of the pituitary stalk or removal of the posterior lobe alone does not cause permanent diabetes insipidus: the median eminence in experimental animals subjected to these procedures is readily transformed into a miniature infundibular process. Antidiuretic hormone and oxytocin are extractable from the hypothalamus, not only the neurohypophysis, although in small amounts. The classic observations of Fisher, Ingram, and Ranson (1938), who produced diabetes insipidus by placing lesions in the hypothalamus of cats, are easily explained: by severing the hypothalamohypophyseal tract before it reaches the neurohypophysis, such lesions prevent the normal flow of hormones to their site of delivery into the blood and even cause retrograde degeneration of the nerve cells in the supraoptic and paraventricular nuclei. There is evidence that the supraoptic nucleus contains about equal amounts of ADH and oxytocin, and the paraventricular nucleus more oxytocin than ADH, but less than there is in the supraoptic nucleus. Antidiuretic hormone and oxytocin are apparently produced in separate cells, since, as shown in Fig. 29–20, different cells stain immunocytochemically with antibodies against ADH or oxytocin. The same cells can be demonstrated with antibodies against ADH-associated and oxytocin-associated neurophysin, respectively. Antidiuretic hormone and oxytocin are synthesized as larger molecules encompassing both the hormones and their associated neurophysins. These precursor molecules are cleaved into neurophysin and hormone as they travel toward the nerve terminals with the axoplasmic flow. In the neurosecretory cell processes, ADH and oxytocin are linked to their respective neurophysins by noncovalent bonds and in a 1:1 molar ratio. In several species, two neurophysins (I and II) have been found, and in some a third (neurophysin III). In the rat, neurophysin I is associated with ADH and neurophysin II (and III) with oxytocin. The convection of the neurophysin–hormone complexes to the neurohypophyseal axon terminals seems to occur with the aid of neurotubules. Hormone content and the density per area of neurosecretory granules correlate well if measured along the hypothalamohypophyseal tract, or during dehydration experiments (Fig. 29–17).

An instructive experiment of nature is a strain of rats (Brattleboro strain) that have hereditary diabetes insipidus. In these animals, the cells that would ordinarily produce ADH and neurophysin I are immunocytochemically negative for both, whereas those that manufacture oxytocin

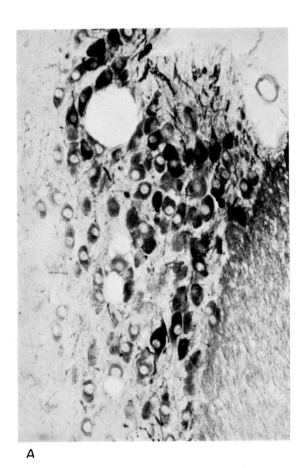

A

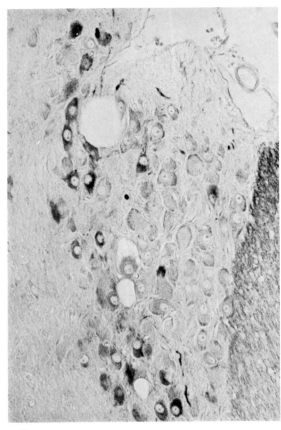

B

29–20 Supraoptic nucleus of a rat, stained immunocytochemically for ADH **(A)** and oxytocin **(B)**. Note the dissimilar distribution of the perikarya containing these hormones. (Courtesy of E. A. Zimmerman.)

and neurophysin II are immunocytochemically and functionally normal.

Release of ADH and oxytocin (which can occur independently) takes place when the neurosecretory granules are extruded by exocytosis at the nerve terminals. The contents enter the perivascular spaces and there quickly lose their electron density. Only in exceptional circumstances does stainable neurosecretory material appear in the blood vessels. When oxytocin or ADH is discharged, the appropriate neurophysin is also released into the circulation. The most descriptive nomenclature applied to human neurophysins is based on the stimuli that cause their

secretion: the neurophysin linked to oxytocin is, like the hormone itself, released in response to estrogen and hence is called estrogen-stimulated neurophysin; that attached to ADH is secreted, along with ADH itself, after the administration of nicotine, and therefore is called nicotine-stimulated neurophysin. The role of the small synaptic-like vesicles in the nerve endings of the hypothalamohypophyseal tract is not clear. Some investigators believe that they are remnants of the membranes of neurosecretion granules; others believe that they produce acetylcholine, which is involved in hormone discharge. The release of hormones occurs in response to impulses that travel along the axons of neurosecretory cells. What role, if any, the pituicytes play in the discharge of neurohypophyseal hormones is obscure.

The physiological stimuli for ADH secretion are an increase in plasma osmolality and a decrease of blood volume in certain pressure-sensitive portions of the vascular system. The perikarya of the supraoptic and paraventricular nuclei themselves may be osmoreceptors, since they are in unusually intimate contact with capillaries. The question arises why secretion of neurohypophyseal hormones cannot occur into such hypothalamic capillaries themselves. It may be pertinent that the hypothalamus has and the neurohypophysis lacks a blood–brain barrier. The hypothalamus does not whereas the neurohypophysis does stain with vital dyes injected into animals. It is conceivable that the blood–brain barrier permits the passage of the constituent amino acids of the peptide hormones but prevents the entry of these hormones into blood after their synthesis, whereas the passage of hormones is not impeded in the neurohypophysis. Discharge of ADH also occurs in response to stressful stimuli or upon electrical excitation of the hypothalamus. Oxytocin is released after stimulation of the nipple, as by suckling, or after vaginal distension. These stimuli are conveyed to the hypothalamus along neural pathways.

The hypophyseotropic release and inhibitory factors through which the hypothalamus exerts control over the adenohypophysis are elaborated in the perikarya of scattered hypothalamic neurons and then travel to the capillaries of the median eminence and the infundibular stem along the axons of the tuberohypophyseal tract, much as described for the hormones released into the systemic circulation in the infundibular process. Some of the fibers of the supraopticohypophyseal tract also end along capillary loops in the median eminence and stalk. Fibers from both tracts occasionally end along the processes of specialized ependymal cells in the median eminence called tanycytes. The tanycytes have their cell bodies near the third ventricle, and they span the entire width of the median eminence, with their processes terminating near the capillaries of the superior portal plexus. Some investigators believe that the tanycytes transport neurosecretions from nerve fibers (and possibly the cerebrospinal fluid) to the portal vascular system. Several workers have found them immunoreactive for neurophysin. The nerve cells and fibers containing gonadotropin-releasing hormone (GnRH, LHRH) have been identified immunocytochemically, as have those carrying the inhibitor of GH release, somatostatin, TRH, and CRF. It has been suggested that ADH or neurophysin released into the portal circulation from nerve terminals of the paraventriculohypophyseal tract may be involved in regulating the secretion of ACTH and possibly of other pars distalis hormones. Nerve fibers containing neuropeptides (hypophyseotropic factors, the opioid peptides Met- and Leu-enkephalin) have been found terminating in the pars nervosa. Their functional significance is unknown.

References and Selected Bibliography

General

Bergland, R. M., and Page, R. B. 1979. Pituitary–brain vascular relations: A new paradigm. Science (Wash., D.C.) 204:18.

Daniel, P. M. 1966. The anatomy of the hypothalamus and pituitary gland. *In* L. Martini and W. F. Ganong (eds.), Neuroendocrinology, vol. 1. New York: Academic Press, p. 15.

Fawcett, D. W., Long, J. A., and Jones, A. L. 1969. The ultrastructure of endocrine glands. Recent Prog. Horm. Res. 25:315.

Ganong, W. F., and Martini, L. (eds.). 1978. Frontiers in Neuroendocrinology, vol. 5. New York: Raven Press.

Pearse, A. G. E., and Takor-Takor, T. 1976. Neuroendocrine embryology and the APUD concept. Clin. Endocrinol. (Suppl.) 5:229s.

Reichlin, S., Baldessarini, R. J., and Martin, J. B. (eds.). 1978. The Hypothalamus. New York: Raven Press.

Romeis, B. 1940. Hypophyse. *In* W. von Möllendorff (ed.), Handbuch der mikroskopischen Anatomie des Menschen, vol. 6, part 3. Berlin: Springer-Verlag OHG.

Adenohypophysis

Baker, B. L. 1974. Functional cytology of the hypophysial pars distalis and pars intermedia. *In* R. O. Greep and E. B. Astwood (eds.), Handbook of Physiology, sec. 7, vol. 4, part 1. Washington, D.C.: American Physiological Society, p. 45.

Celio, M. R., Pasi, A., Bürgisser, E., Buetti, G., Höllt, V., and Gramsch, G. H. 1980. Pro-opiocortin fragments in normal adult pituitary. Distribution and ultrastructural characterization of immunoreactive cells. Acta Endocrinol. (Copenh.) 95:27.

Duello, T. M., and Halmi, N. S. 1979. Ultrastructural-immunocytochemical localization of growth hormone and prolactin in human pituitaries. J. Clin. Endocrinol. 49:189.

Ezrin, C., and Murray, S. 1963. The cell of the adenohypophysis in pregnancy, thyroid disease, and adrenal cortical disorders. *In* J. Benoit and C. da Lage (eds.), Cytologie de l'Adénohypophyse. Paris: Editions du C. N. R. S. (No. 128), p. 183.

Halmi, N. S. 1974. The current status of pituitary cytophysiology. N. Z. Med. J. 80:551.

Halmi, N. S., Parsons, J. A., Erlandsen, S. L., and Duello, T. 1975. Prolactin and growth hormone cells in the human hypophysis: A study with immunoenzyme histochemistry. Cell Tissue Res. 158:497.

Herlant, M., and Pasteels, J. L. 1967. Histophysiology of human anterior pituitary. Meth. Achievm. Exp. Pathol. 3:250.

Moriarty, G. C. 1973. Adenohypophysis: Ultrastructural cytochemistry. A review. J. Histochem. Cytochem. 21:855.

Nakane, P. 1970. Classifications of anterior pituitary cell types with immunoenzyme histochemistry. J. Histochem. Cytochem. 18:9.

Pelletier, G., Robert, F., and Hardy, J. 1978. Identification of human pituitary cell types by immunoelectron microscopy. J. Clin. Endocrinol. 46:534.

Phifer, R. F., Midgley, A. R., Jr., and Spicer, S. S. 1973. Immunohistologic and histologic evidence that follicle-stimulating hormone and luteinizing hormone are present in the same cell type of the human pars distalis. J. Clin. Endocrinol. 36:125.

Phifer, R. F., Orth D. N., and Spicer, S. S. 1974. Specific demonstration of the human hypophyseal adrenocortico-melanotropic (ACTH/MSH) cell. J. Clin. Endocrinol. 39:684.

Phifer, R. F., and Spicer, S. S. 1973. Immunohistochemical and histologic demonstration of thyrotropic cells of the human adenohypophysis. J. Clin. Endocrinol. 36:1210.

Phifer, R. F., Spicer, S. S., and Orth, D. N. 1970. Specific demonstration of human hypophysial cells which produce adrenocorticotropic hormone. J. Clin. Endocrinol. 31:347.

Purves, H. D. 1966. Cytology of the adenohypophysis. In G. W. Harris and T. Donovan (eds.), The Pituitary Gland, vol. 1. Berkeley: University of California Press, p. 147.

Tixier-Vidal, A., and Farquhar, M. G. (eds.). 1975. The Anterior Pituitary. New York: Academic Press, Inc.

Neurohypophysis

Baker, B. L., Dermody, W. C., and Reed, J. R. 1975. Distribution of gonadotropin-releasing hormone in the rat brain as observed with immunocytochemistry. Endocrinology 97:125.

Bargmann, W. 1966. Neurosecretion. Int. Rev. Cytol. 19:183.

Bindler, E., La Bella, F. S., and Sanwal, M. 1967. Isolated nerve endings (neurosecretosomes) from the posterior pituitary. Partial separation of vasopressin and oxytocin and the isolation of microvesicles. J. Cell Biol. 34:185.

Dierickx, K., and Vandesande, F. 1977. Immunocytochemical localization of the vasopressinergic and oxytocinergic neurons in the human hypothalamus. Cell Tissue Res. 184:15.

Dierickx, K., and Vandesande, F. 1979. Immunocytochemical demonstration of separate vasopressin-neurophysin and oxytocin-neurophysin neurons in the human hypothalamus. Cell Tissue Res. 196:203.

Fisher, C. V., Ingram, W. R., and Ranson, S. W. 1938. Diabetes Insipidus and the Neurohumoral Control of Water Balance: A Contribution to the Structure and Function of the Hypothalamicohypophysial System. Ann Arbor, Mich.: J. W. Edwards, Publisher, Inc.

Gainer, H., Sarne, Y., and Brownstein, M. J. 1977. Biosynthesis and axonal transport of rat neurohypophysial proteins and peptides. J. Cell Biol. 73:366.

Morris, J. F., Nordmann, J. J., and Dyball, R. E. 1978. Structure-function correlation in mammalian neurosecretion. Int. Rev. Exp. Pathol. 18:1.

Sachs, H., Fawcett, P., Takabatake, Y., and Portanova, R. 1969. Biosynthesis and release of vasopressin and neurophysin. Recent Prog. Horm. Res. 25:447.

Scharrer, B. 1969. Neurohumors and neurohormones: Definitions and terminology. J. Neurovisc. Rel. (Suppl.) 9:1.

Silverman, A. J., and Zimmerman, E. A. 1975. Ultrastructural immunocytochemical localization of neurophysin and vasopressin in the median eminence and posterior pituitary of the guinea pig. Cell Tissue Res. 159:291.

Sloper, J. C. 1966. The experimental and cytopathological investigation of neurosecretion in the hypothalamus and pituitary. In G. W. Harris and B. T. Donovan (eds.), The Pituitary Gland, vol. 3. Berkeley: University of California Press, p. 130.

Zimmerman, E. A., Defendini, R., Sokol, H. W., and Robinson, A. G. 1975. The distribution of neurophysin-secreting pathways in the mammalian brain. Ann. N. Y. Acad. Sci. 248:92.

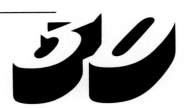

The Pineal Gland

W. B. Quay

Functional Relationships

The pineal gland (pineal body or epiphysis cerebri) of humans and other mammals is now usually considered to be endocrine in its functional activity. However, in its origin and evolution within vertebrate animals it has had other functional relationships. In lower forms pineal photoreceptive capacity is the major activity suggested on the basis of both microscopic structure and neurophysiology.

The mammalian pineal gland is a distinctive component of the neuroendocrine system. Within the pineal gland, neural and hormonal inputs interact to regulate the synthetic and secretory activities of the pineal's unique parenchymal cells, the pinealocytes. These cells are believed to synthesize and secrete hormones of two chemical families: indoleamines such as melatonin, and peptides resembling those of the hypothalamohypophyseal system.

Investigations with laboratory mammals show that the major endocrine role of the pineal gland, as it is currently understood, is mediation or modulation of the timing of some biological rhythms. This modulation relates to changes in the timing of the phases of the 24-h (circadian) and seasonal or annual (circannual) rhythms in response to environmental cues, such as the daily start and ending of light. The pineal gland's rich sympathetic innervation and physiological interrelationships with stress and arousal have suggested that its endocrine activity probably is tied to these factors as well. Furthermore, there is experimental evidence for pineal actions on aspects of brain chemistry and excitability under certain conditions. The clearest demonstration of pineal function has been made with the seasonal regression of reproductive organs in several photoperiodic species. In the golden hamster, the best studied of these species, the reproductive regression that is prompted by darkness or short-day photoperiods depends on the presence of the pineal gland. It remains to be shown which human physiological rhythms or mechanisms are under a pineal influence. Nevertheless, in humans as in other species, marked 24-h and seasonal rhythms occur in blood levels of the pineal hormone melatonin.

Evolutionary Relationships

The pineal complex is a characteristic of vertebrates (subphylum Vertebrata). One or more components of this organ complex occur in representatives of all Classes, from cyclostomes to birds and mammals. Photoreceptors and acces-

30–1 Sagittal section of a human pineal organ and adjacent structures of the dorsal junction of diencephalon **(left)** and mesencephalon **(right).** Loyes iron–hematoxylin technique for myelin. × 8. (Courtesy of P. I. Yakovlev.)

sory components of diminutive eyelike structures dominate the pineal complex of "lower" vertebrates. A more or less solid parenchymatous and presumably nonsensory pineal gland has evolved within several different groups of "higher" vertebrates (turtles, snakes, birds, and mammals). It is generally thought that the remaining endocrine portion of the pineal complex in humans and other mammals has lost its direct photosensory capability. However, some recent evidence suggests that this supposition may not be entirely true, particularly in young mammals. Presumably lost also during the pineal gland's evolution are direct neural interconnections with the brain. However, this interpretation also has been challenged by several recent studies, especially in terms of photic information reaching the pineal gland by way of nerve fibers from the brain as well as from the cervical sympathetics.

Comparative electron microscopic studies have provided strong circumstantial evidence that at least many of the glandular pinealocytes of humans and other vertebrates evolved from pineal photoreceptor cells. From this and other available information, one conclusion is inescapable: the pineal gland is unique among vertebrate endocrine organs in the remarkable magnitude and diversity of its evolutionary remodeling.

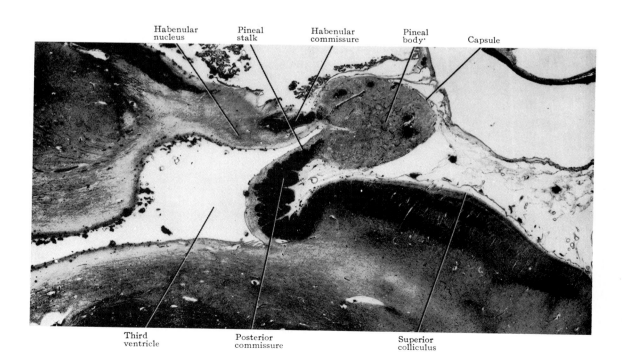

Habenular nucleus   Pineal stalk   Habenular commissure   Pineal body·   Capsule

Third ventricle   Posterior commissure   Superior colliculus

Development and Histogenesis

The human pineal gland develops early during the second month of embryonic life. Although it is a single median structure in the adult (Fig. 30–1), in the embryo it often has two parts, an anterior and solid part originating from the region of the habenular commissure, and a posterior and hollow part originating from a saccular evagination of the diencephalic roof between the habenular and posterior commissures. Cellular proliferation is earlier and greater in the anterior part. With light microscopy it is difficult to distinguish human pinealocytes from glia-like cells until about the 150th day. Neuroepithelial proliferations forming pineal parenchyma consist at first of cords and follicles of cells, which become invested with embryonic connective tissue. Pineal neuroepithelial cells give rise to parenchymal cells or pinealocytes and to neuroglial cells (Fig. 30–2). Later in development most signs of parenchymal cords and follicles are lost, as the lobules composed chiefly of pinealocytes, increase in size and distinctness. Stromal tissue forms septa and trabeculae between the lobules and is continuous with a thin connective tissue capsule. Capsular and septal tissues are mostly derived from embryonic meningeal mesenchyme, but with cellular contributions from neural crest and vascular systems (Fig. 30–2).

The mammalian pineal gland grows from infancy to adulthood mainly by an increase in the size of the pinealocytes and, secondarily and more variably, by an increase in glial and stromal cells and their products. Extreme examples of such increases are called gliosis and fibrosis, respectively. In the human pineal gland, these processes are seen most clearly in the variable, but usually increasing, width with age of the interlobular septa (Fig. 30–3). Maximum pineal weight (150–160 mg) occurs in the fifth decade, with a larger and heavier gland in females from the fourth decade onward. Pineal weight usually falls in the sixth decade. This decrease does not, however, represent a selective atrophy of the pineal gland, since pineal weight is essentially constant relative to either hypophyseal or brain weight.

Neither notable increase in numbers of pinealocytes nor pineal regeneration has been demonstrated in any adult mammal, excluding the abnormal cellular capacities in pineal tumors and some heterotopic transplants. Thus pineal growth and regenerative abilities resemble those of the central nervous system, from which its parenchyma is derived.

Anatomy and Histology

Adult human pineal glands are 5 to 8 mm long and 3 to 5 mm wide. Their thin connective tissue capsule is externally continuous with meningeal (pial and arachnoid) tissues and is basally interrupted by the pineal stalk (Fig. 30–1). At its base the stalk region contains the pineal recess, an extension of the third ventricle lined by ependymal cells (Fig. 30–4). The pineal stalk also contains nerve fibers from the adjacent habenular and posterior commissural regions of the brain, lying at the junction of the diencephalic roof anteriorly and the tectum of the midbrain posteriorly. The bundles of nerve fibers running through the stalk have usually been considered to be merely aberrant commissural loops, pulled out developmentally with the basal pineal tissue in which they are embedded. Although they are usually

30–2 Developmental origins of cells found in mammalian pineal glands. Relative thicknesses of **arrows** for cellular descents are intended to suggest relative numbers of cells in the different lines. **Dashed arrows** signify cell types and origins that are variable in relation to pineal region, species, age, or pathological processes.

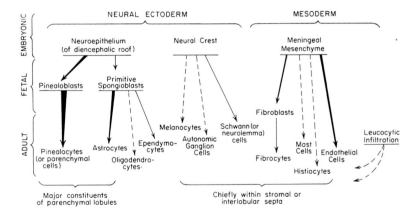

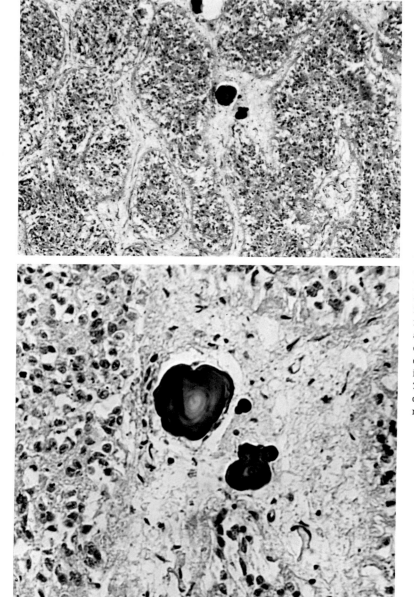

30–3 Low-power **(above)** and intermediate-power **(below)** views of the same human pineal tissue section stained with acid alum hematoxylin and eosin. At these magnifications the usually distinct lobulation and often present concretions in the stroma are features useful in tissue identification. At higher magnification the characteristic and unique features of the nuclei of pinealocytes are the most consistently present aids for identifying pineal tissue. (From a 78-year-old woman; death due to cardiovascular disease and myocarditis.)

thought to lack either synaptic relationships or functional importance within the pineal gland, recent neurophysiological observations have re-opened the question of their true relationships and possible significance.

Other recent studies suggest also that human pineal innervation may be more complex than is generally appreciated. They have provided evi-dence for neural connections between pineal and the habenular and posterior commissural regions and findings of nerve cell bodies or ganglion cells at three sites, rostral, distal and intrapineal. Even so, the dominant view continues to be that pineal innervation is exclusively autonomic and that the endocrine functioning of the pinealo-cytes depends on their sympathetic innervation.

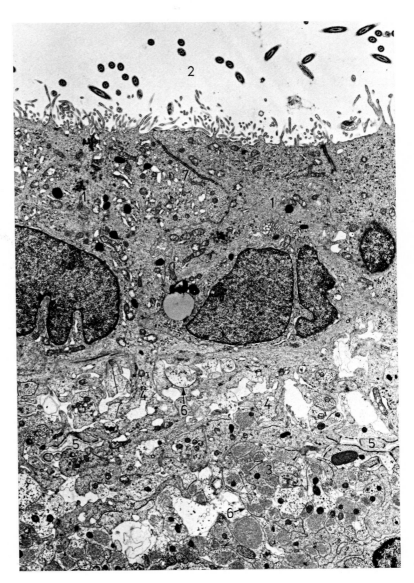

30–4 Ependymal cells (1) covering the proximal or ventricular surface of the pineal gland (squirrel monkey) where it faces on the pineal recess (2), an extension of the third ventricle. Ependymal cilia and microvilli are seen in the recess. Below the ependymal cells, filamentous glial processes (3) intermingle with processes of the ependymal cells (4). Nearby are extravascular spaces (5) lined by basal lamina and in continuity with the perivascular space. Tight junctions (6) occur between glial cell processes, and a junctional complex (7) joins the ependymal cells to each other. × 6,800. (Courtesy of H. Wartenberg and Springer-Verlag.)

Pineal sympathetic fibers are in two morphological configurations: (1) small fascicles penetrating the capsular surface in many places along with small blood vessels, and (2) a *nervus conarii* entering the posterior and distal pole of the organ. This nerve is formed by the fusion in the midline of bilateral component trunks that ascend intracranially along the tentorium cerebelli on each side. These trunks originate on each side from the superior cervical sympathetic ganglion. Nevertheless, it is probable that some of the contributing postganglionic nerve cell bodies lie more peripherally and intracranially.

Pineal blood is supplied by small arteriolar branches from offshoots of the two posterior choroid arteries. Each of these arteries in turn stems from the posterior cerebral artery on the same side. Shortly after penetrating the capsule, pineal arterioles lead into a capillary or sinusoidal network, which extends throughout the interior of the organ. Ultrastructural fenestration of the capillary endothelium is reported in some species. In the human fetus tight junctions between the endothelial cells indicate the presence of a blood–brain barrier. In some species of experimental mammals, such a barrier within the pineal gland appears to be deficient or lacking. Perivascular spaces and variably defined channels or canaliculi occur along and outside of the capillary walls. These canaliculi and the cells of the small blood vessels are regulated by the biogenic amines released nearby by the pinealocytes and sympathetic nerve terminals, respectively. Sympathetic nerve processes and cytoplasmic terminations of pinealocyte process often lie in or close to the perivascular spaces and their intercellular extensions (Fig. 30–5). The extent and degree to which these components are invested by a basal lamina, connective tissue, and glial cell cytoplasm vary among species of mammals. Vascular drainage of the pineal is provided by venules that course beneath the capsule before passing through to the adjacent meningeal tissue. They drain eventually into larger veins or dural

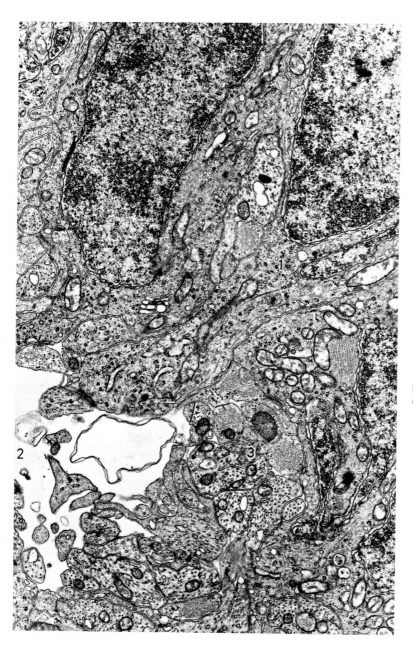

30–5 Structural interrelationships of cell processes and sympathetic nerve fibers in the vicinity of an intercellular space in the pineal gland (squirrel monkey). A short cytoplasmic process from a pinealocyte (1) courses toward the space (2); nerve (3), glial, and pinealocyte processes are intermingled. × 15,000. (Courtesy of H. Wartenberg and Springer-Verlag.)

venous sinuses in the vicinity. In humans they drain primarily into the great cerebral vein (of Galen).

Small striated muscle fibers are sometimes found within the pineal gland. Electron microscopy has revealed that these fibers in pineal tissue are more common than previously thought. However, we still do not know whether they have a function here, or merely represent some evolutionary remnant of pineal or parietal eye musculature in a reptilian ancestor.

The anatomical position of the pineal gland is critical to intracranial venous drainage. It lies close to the union of outflow from the deep cerebral veins with the median and deep dural venous sinuses. Pineal tumors often impede or divert this outflow by compressing it against the splenium of the corpus callosum.

Human pineal tissue by light microscopy and the usual histological staining procedures shows few features useful in tissue identification. The two most obvious features are lobulation and concretions (Fig. 30–3). They are useful when present, but their occurrence is variable, even in adults and older individuals. Most dependable of the criteria for histological identification are size and structure of the pinealocytes' nuclei. They are large, deeply creased, polymorphic, and contain one to several large nucleoli.

Pinealocytes

Pinealocytes, or pineal parenchymal cells, constitute the majority of the cells seen within lobules (Fig. 30–6). They are often seen to be connected to each other by gap junctions, desmosomes, and intermediate types of junctions. The gap junctions are especially interesting. They are seen between pinealocytes in all developmental stages, and they suggest electrotonic coupling of the pinealocytes to one another as well as interflow of small molecules. Like neurons, pinealocytes usually have two or more cytoplasmic extentions or processes, numerous cytoplasmic cisterns, microtubules, vesicles of several kinds, organelles for active oxidative metabolism and protein synthesis, and at least parts of structures usually associated with synaptic contacts in central nervous or retinal tissues (Fig. 30–7). The cytoplasmic extensions of the pinealocytes sometimes include shorter and thinner types that terminate within the group of adjacent cells and longer, thicker types that terminate within or close to the perivascular space or intercellular channels or canaliculi. Within the swol-

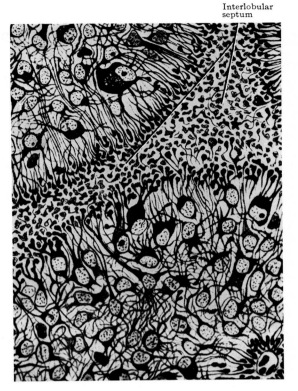

Interlobular septum

30–6 A classic and semidiagrammatic interpretation of the organization of pinealocytes within a small region of the adult pineal gland, based on metallic impregnations and light microscopy. Parts of two parenchymatous lobules are shown. In each, polymorphic pinealocytes have club-shaped processes, which often terminate in the vicinity of small blood vessels in the interlobular tissue. (After Del Rio-Hortega.)

len, clublike endings of the latter processes are vesicles and grumose or dense bodies that some authors believe to contain presecretory materials (Fig. 30–7). However, the local concentrations and numbers of these vesicles and bodies are generally not great, and they do not indicate that the pinealocyte has much capacity for storing any known presecretory product. Pinealocyte mitochondria are notable for their relatively great number or concentration in the perikaryon, their polymorphism, and frequently large size (up to 4 μm long in the rat). Various mitochondrial inclusions have been described, particularly in pinealocytes of adult or old individuals; they include concentrically lamellated bodies, clusters of osmiophilic granules within the mitochon-

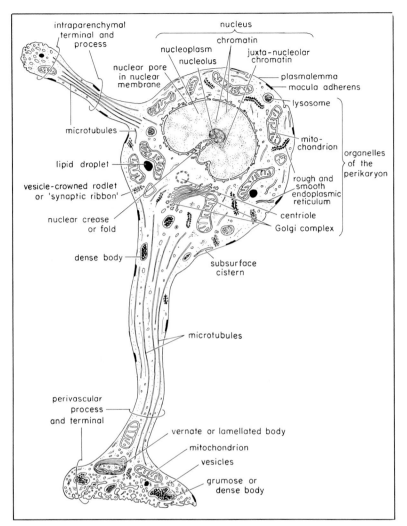

30–7 Composite diagram of a typical mammalian pinealocyte. In order to include all of the usually encountered organelles and inclusions in their characteristic locations, some liberties have been taken in the relative sizes of some of them and of representations of intracellular membrane systems.

drial matrix, dense intracristal layers, and dense-core microcylinders 270 to 330 Å wide.

Many of the organelles and inclusions of the pinealocytes follow 24-h cycles of change. Interest in this subject started with the discovery of high-amplitude 24-h rhythms in pineal serotonin (5-HT, 5-hydroxytryptamine), and subsequently in the enzyme activities contributing to the synthesis of melatonin. The chemical and ultrastructural elements contributing to melatonin synthesis and secretion lie within the pinealocytes. In the pinealocytes, cytoplasmic vesicles, microtubules, glycogen granules, synaptic ribbons, and synaptic ribbon fields similarly show marked 24-h cycles. Many of these elements have their daily peak, or *acrophase*, during the night or

dark phase of the daily cycle. This is as true for higher primates as for lower mammals. Interestingly, the phase relationships of these rhythms are not reversed in diurnal as compared with nocturnal species.

One of the most enigmatic of these cyclic organelles of the pinealocyte is the synaptic ribbon ("vesicle-crowned rodlet," "vesicle-crowned lamellae"). This structure was demonstrated first in retinal photoreceptor cells and has been found subsequently in many other sensory cells, as, for example, those of the inner ear. In these sensory cells the synaptic ribbons are part of the presynaptic complex, in which they appear to be engaged in transferring neurotransmitter from synaptic vesicles to the cell membrane. This concept falls apart, however, when we come to the mammalian pinealocyte. On the "postsynaptic" side of the pinealocyte's "synaptic" ribbon there may be another pinealocyte, an astrocytic glial cell, extracellular space, or cerebrospinal fluid, depending partly on species and pineal region. It has been suggested that "synaptic" ribbons in mammalian pinealocytes may be involved more diffusely in the transport and release of chemical mediators than is true for their antecedents in pineal photoreceptor cells.

It remains uncertain whether in humans and other mammals the pinealocytes belong to one or more cell types or subtypes. Variation in the cytoplasmic density of these cells in electron micrographs has led to the descriptive distinction of "light" and "dark" pinealocytes. More recently it has been suggested that one subtype manufactures material in the Golgi apparatus and secretes it from granular vesicles, whereas another secretes material that forms within the granular endoplasmic reticulum. More information is needed to rule out the possibility that what is observed pertains only to differences in phase or level of activity within a single cell type. It also remains to be determined, as with immunocytochemical methods, whether specific mRNAs and peptides characterize pinealocytes or particular subtypes.

Histochemistry and Histophysiology

Pineal products that may be hormonal in function are of two biochemical types, indoleamines, and peptides or proteins. Melatonin (5-methoxy-N-acetyltryptamine) is the best known and most studied of the pineal's indoleamine products. Its effects on reproductive and nervous tissues vary depending on circumstances such as dosage, time of administration, and species. Although melatonin can cause rapid blanching of some amphibian skin, a property useful in bioassays, it has little if any physiological effect on mammalian pigment cells. The tissue site with the greatest biochemical capacity for synthesizing melatonin is the pineal gland, despite the fact that this capacity and melatonin itself occur in other places as well, including the retina, Harderian gland, and gastrointestinal mucosa. The pineal gland is required for normal levels of melatonin in the blood, since these levels are diminished in pinealectomized animals. Plasma melatonin concentrations in humans and other studied species vary with time of day and with season or time of year. The half-life of melatonin in blood has been estimated to be from 1 to about 20 min.

The control and mediation of control of the synthesis and release of melatonin by the pineal gland have been defined experimentally in laboratory mammals. An apparently innate 24-h rhythmicity in pineal biosynthetic and metabolic activities in the early postnatal animal comes under sympathetic control when the organ acquires sympathetic innervation. This sympathetic control occurs through the agency of norepinephrine and cyclic AMP (adenosine 3′,5′-monophosphate). Cellular localizations and daily changes in norepinephrine and serotonin, a precursor of melatonin, have been described in studies using the method of Falck and Hillarp, in which catecholamines such as norepinephrine are converted to a green fluorescent product, and tryptamines such as serotonin form a yellow fluorescent product. By this and other procedures, pineal synthesis of serotonin and related compounds is seen to be localized to the pinealocytes, whereas norepinephrine originates from sympathetic nerve fibers and terminals.

Much less is known about all aspects of the peptides or proteins in pineal glands. Many of the peptides found in the hypothalamohypophyseal system have been found, or claimed to occur, within the pineal gland as well. In the pineal gland, however, their concentrations are much lower, and their anatomical origins and exact chemical identities are still questioned. The site in the pineal of arginine vasopressin (AVP), oxytocin, and related amounts of their respective neurophysins, has been suggested to be within neurosecretory fibers originating at least partly from the magnocellular hypothalamic nuclei. Identifications and localizations claimed for other pineal peptides are disputed. These peptides include arginine vasotocin (AVT), LH-RH, TRH, somatostatin, alpha-MSH, angiotensin II, and substance P. It is likely that there are pineal-specific peptides that may be important as hormones, but their chemical identification is still in progress.

It has been known for many decades that human and cattle pineal glands often contain calcareous concretions, known also as corpora arenacea, psammoma bodies, acervuli, and brain sand (Fig. 30–3). Recently they have been found in some other species of mammals, and sometimes with different cellular relationships and chemical compositions. Those in human and cattle pineal glands appear to be glial or stromal in origin and localization. They do not differ structurally or chemically from such deposits in a wide variety of other tissues and regions. Their primary microcrystalline structure is that of hydroxyapatite. Their occurrence in human pineal glands is not associated with decrease in pineal enzymic or metabolic activities. Thus, the presence of such concretions in a particular pineal gland is not a reliable indicator of reduced or impaired pinealocyte function. The prevalence of human pineal corpora arenacea increases with age, and for many years these concretions have been useful to the radiologist in providing an intracranial and normally nearly medial intracranial "landmark" in radiographs. A recent study in Scotland used skull radiographs and CT scans of 1,000 consecutive patients to study calcification in the pineal region. Pineal calcification was seen in films from 61% and in CT scans from 83% of patients over 30 years old. By either technique of visualization, prevalence of pineal calcification was 10% greater in males.

Various other structural, histological, and cytological features of the human pineal gland change or increase during either youth or older age, but these changes are subject to wide individual variation, even in the eight or ninth decades of life. Fibrosis and gliosis increase throughout life, but in the pineal gland no consistent or typical pattern is evident in these changes. Sexual differences have been claimed, as for example, greater variability in fibrosis and a different pattern and greater amount of gliosis in men than women.

In conclusion, recent ultrastructural and biochemical studies are in accord with the belief that pineal functional activity follows postnatal differentiation and continues into adult and older ages in humans and most other mammals.

References and Selected Bibliography

General

Axelrod, J. 1974. The pineal gland: A neurochemical transducer. *Science* (Wash., D.C.) 184:1341.

Kappers, J. A., and Pévet, P. (eds.). 1979. The Pineal Gland of Vertebrates Including Man. *Prog. Brain Res.* 52.

Pévet, P., Buijs, R. M., Dogterom, J., Vivien-Roels, B., Holder, F. C., Guerné, J. M., Reinharz, A., Swaab, D. F., Ebels, I., and Neaçsu, C. 1981. Peptides in the mammalian pineal gland. *In* C. D. Matthews and R. F. Seamark (eds.), Pineal Function. Amsterdam: Elsevier/North Holland Biomedical Press, p. 173.

Quay, W. B. 1974. Pineal Chemistry in Cellular and Physiological Mechanisms. Springfield, Ill.: Charles C. Thomas Publ.

Reiter, R. J. 1980. The pineal and its hormones in the control of reproduction in mammals. *Endocrine Rev.* 1:109.

Reiter, R. J. (ed.). 1981. The Pineal Gland. Boca Raton, Fla.: CRC Press.

Tapp, E., and Huxley, M. 1972. The histological appearance of the human pineal gland from puberty to old age. *J. Pathol.* 108:137.

Vollrath, L. 1980. The Pineal Organ. *Handbuch der mikroskopischen Anatomie des Menschen* 6 (7). Berlin: Springer-Verlag.

Wartenberg, H. 1968. The mammalian pineal organ: Electron microscopic studies on the fine structure of pinealocytes, glial cells and on the perivascular compartment. *Z. Zellforsch.* 86:74.

Wetterberg, L. 1978. Melatonin in humans. Physiological and clinical studies. *J. Neural Transmission* (Suppl.) 13:289.

Specific

Cardinali, D. P. 1981. Melatonin. A mammalian pineal hormone. *Endocrine Rev.* 2:327.

Ebels, I., and Benson, B. 1978. A survey of the evidence that unidentified pineal substances affect the reproductive system in mammals. *Prog. Reprod. Biol.* 4:51.

Hewing, M. 1980. Cerebrospinal fluid–contacting area in the pineal recess of the vole (*Microtus agrestis*), guinea pig (*Cavia cobaya*), and rhesus monkey (*Macaca mulatta*). *Cell Tissue Res.* 209:473.

Hewing, M. 1981. Topographical relationships of synaptic ribbons in the pineal system of the vole (*Microtus agrestis*). *Anat. Embryol.* 162:313.

Hülsemann, M. 1971. Development of the innervation in the human pineal organ. Light and electron microscopic investigations. *Z. Zellforsch.* 115:396.

Ito, T., and Matsushima, S. 1968. Electron microscopic observations on the mouse pineal, with particular emphasis on its secretory nature. *Arch. Histol. Jpn.* 30:1.

Kachi, T. 1979. Demonstration of circadian rhythm in granular vesicle number in pinealocytes of mice and the effect of light: Semiquantitative electron microscopic study. *J. Anat.* 129:603.

Karasek, M. 1981. Some functional aspects of the ultrastructure of rat pinealocytes. *Endocrinol. Exp.* 15:17.

Krstić, R. 1976. Ultracytochemistry of the synaptic ribbons in the rat pineal organ. *Cell Tissue Res.* 166:135.

Lew, G. M., Payer, A., and Quay, W. B. 1982. The pinealocyte nucleolus: Ultrastructural and stereological analysis of twenty-four-hour changes. *Cell Tissue Res.* 224:195.

Macpherson, P., and Matheson, M. S. 1979. Comparision of calcification of pineal, habenular commissure and choroid plexus on plain films and computed tomography. *Neuroradiology* 18:67.

Matsushima, S., and Ito, T. 1972. Diurnal changes in sympathetic nerve endings in the mouse pineal: Semiquantitative electron microscopic observations. *J. Neural Transmission* 33:275.

Møller, M. 1976. The ultrastructure of the human fetal pineal gland. II. Innervation and cell junctions. *Cell Tissue Res.* 169:7.

Møller, M. 1978. Presence of a pineal nerve (nervus pinealis) in the human fetus; a light and electron microscopical study of the innervation of the pineal gland. *Brain Res.* 154:1.

Mullen, P. E., Leone, R. M., Hooper, J., Smith, I., Silman, R. E., Finnie, M., Carter, S., and Linsell, C. 1979. Pineal 5-methoxy tryptophol in man. *Psychoneuroendocrinology* 2:117.

Perlow, M. J., Reppert, S. M., Tamarkin, L., Wyatt, R. J., and Klein, D. C. 1980. Photic regulation of the melatonin rhythm: Monkey and man are not the same. *Brain Res.* 182:211.

Pévet, P. 1977. On the presence of different populations of pinealocytes in the mammalian pineal gland. *J. Neural Transmission* 40:289.

Quay, W. B. 1970. Physiological significance of the pineal during adaptation to shifts in photoperiod. *Physiol. Behav.* 5:353.

Quay, W. B. 1974. Pineal canaliculi: Demonstration, twenty-four-hour rhythmicity and experimental modification. *Am. J. Anat.* 139:81.

Rix, E., Hackenthal, E., Hilgenfeldt, U., and Taugner, R. 1981. Neuropeptides in the pineal gland? A critical immunocytochemical study. *Histochemistry* 72:33.

Smith, J. A., Mee, T. J. X., Padwick, D. J., and Spokes, E. G. 1981. Human post-mortem pineal enzyme activity. *Clin. Endocrinol.* 14:75.

Tetsuo, M., Polinsky, R. J., Markey, S. P., and Kopin, I. J. 1981. Urinary 6-hydroxymelatonin excretion in patients with orthostatic hypotension. *J. Clin. Endocrinol. Metab.* 53:607.

Theron, J. J., Biagio, R., and Meyer, A. C. 1981. Circadian changes in microtubules, synaptic ribbons and synaptic ribbon fields in the pinealocytes of the baboon *(Papio ursinus)*. *Cell Tissue Res.* 217:405.

Ueck, M., and Wake, K. 1977. The pinealocyte—A paraneuron? A review. *Arch. Histol. Jpn.* (Suppl.) 40:261.

Vaughan, G. M., McDonald, S. D., Jordan, R. M., Allen, J. P., Bell, R., and Stevens, E. A. 1979. Melatonin, pituitary function and stress in humans. *Psychoneuroendocrinology* 4:351.

Vaughan, G. M., Pelham, R. W., Pang, S. F., Loughlin, L. L., Wilson, K. M., Sandock, K. L., Vaughan, M. K., Koslow, S. H., and Reiter, R. J. 1976. Nocturnal elevation of plasma melatonin and urinary 5-hydroxyindoleacetic acid in young men: Attempts at modification by brief changes in environmental lighting and sleep and by autonomic drugs. J. Clin. Endocrinol. Metab. 42:752.

Vollrath, L. 1973. Synaptic ribbons of a mammalian pineal gland. Circadian changes. *Z. Zellforsch.* 145:171.

Vollrath, L., and Howe, C. 1976. Light and drug induced changes of epiphysial synaptic ribbons. *Cell Tissue Res.* 165:383.

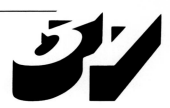

The Thyroid Gland

Lois W. Tice

Although the thyroid is classified as an endocrine gland, its cells perform both exocrine and endocrine secretory functions as they manufacture and release thyroid hormone. Recognition of their dual function provides a key to understanding thyroid histology. In the exocrine phase of secretion, thyroid follicular cells synthesize and secrete thyroglobulin, a large glycoprotein (MW 660,000). Thyroglobulin is stored extracellularly in the interior of the thyroid follicles where it is partially iodinated. In the endocrine phase of secretion, stored thyroglobulin is taken up by the follicular cells and broken down to active thyroid hormones. These hormones are then released into the blood and lymph. The active hormones are iodinated amino acids, L-thyroxine (tetraiodo-L-thyronine) and 3,5,3′-triodo-L-thyronine. They function to stimulate metabolism, particularly oxidative metabolism, and have important effects on maturation (brain development and amphibian metamorphosis, for example). In addition, the thyroid in mammals contains C cells (parafollicular cells or light cells). These cells produce another hormone, calcitonin or thyrocalcitonin, which acts to lower blood calcium.

Origin and Development

The parenchyma of the thyroid gland is of entodermal origin and arises by a median downgrowth of the base of the tongue. The developing gland is connected to its point of origin by the thyroglossal duct, which usually becomes obli-

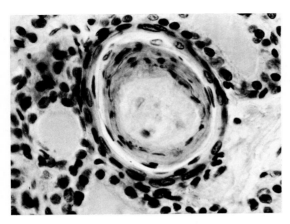

31–1 Ultimobranchial tubule in a normal rat thyroid. This micrograph is of the oval cross section of a closed tube lined by stratified squamous epithelium. The lumen contains desquamated cells with pycnotic nuclei, and debris. (Courtesy of C. P. Leblond.)

terated during later development but which may give rise to persisting structures such as the pyramidal lobe, thyroglossal cysts, or thyroid tissue within the tongue (lingual thryoid). The thyroid may include branchial pouch derivatives such as parathyroid glands and C cells. However, transplantation experiments have shown that C cells originate in the neural crest and migrate into the ultimobranchial body during development. Remnants of the ultimobranchial body also produce ultimobranchial tubules (Fig. 31–1) or follicles lined by stratified squamous epithelium. Other unusual types of follicles containing, for example, ciliated cells have been observed in some species. In nonmammals the ultimobranchial body may remain a separate organ.

The proliferating mass of embryonic thyroid cells breaks up into small cords and sheets of cells. Only late in development do recognizable thyroid follicles with follicular lumina appear. The appearance of follicles with stored colloid seems to coincide with the onset of mature function and iodination of thyroglobulin. With the appearance of follicular lumina containing extracellular stored colloid, the cells around the colloid become arranged into a single continuous layer surrounded by basement membrane. The cell layers together with the colloid that they enclose are called *follicles*; they constitute the basic functioning unit of the adult thyroid gland. They are variable in shape, and they range in humans from 50 to 900 μm in diameter.

Gross Structure

In human beings the thyroid gland normally weighs from 15 to 30 g. It consists of two lateral lobes connected by an isthmus, which lies close to the second and third tracheal rings. It is located near the shield-shaped thyroid cartilage of the larynx, from which it takes its name. The thyroid is surrounded by a fibrous capsule from which connective tissue septa may extend into the interior of the gland, separating it into lobules. The follicles are separated by a loose connective tissue, the stroma, containing blood vessels, nerve fibers, and lymphatics. Its rich blood supply is via the superior and inferior thyroid arteries. Smaller arteries within the gland may have intimal thickenings or endothelial cushions. These arteries break up into an extensive capillary network that comes into close contact with the basement membranes of the follicles. A network of lymphatic vessels is also found between the follicles. These vessels drain into larger vessels beneath the capsule and ultimately into cervical or retrosternal lymph nodes.

Small nerve bundles enter the thyroid together with the larger blood vessels. They consist primarily of postganglionic sympathetic fibers that originate in the middle and superior cervical ganglia, although cholinergic fibers are also contributed by the recurrent laryngeal branch of the vagus. Many of these fibers synapse on blood vessels and are therefore probably vasomotor in function. In some species (mouse and human) nerve fibers are also found terminating in close contact with the follicles themselves. The physiological function of these fibers is not known in normal animals. In animals in which pituitary function has been suppressed, sympathetic stimulation can mimic the effects of TSH, thyroid-stimulating hormone.

Light Microscopy

With the light microscope, the thyroid follicle is the dominant feature of the gland. This follicle consists of a cuboidal (in humans) epithelium that forms a continuous cell layer around the central mass of colloid (Fig. 31–2A). The colloid is amphoteric, staining with both acidic and basic dyes. Because it contains thyroglobulin, a glycoprotein, it is PAS-positive. The relative height of the epithelial cell layer and the relative size of the mass of colloid depend on the activity of the follicle as well as the species studied.

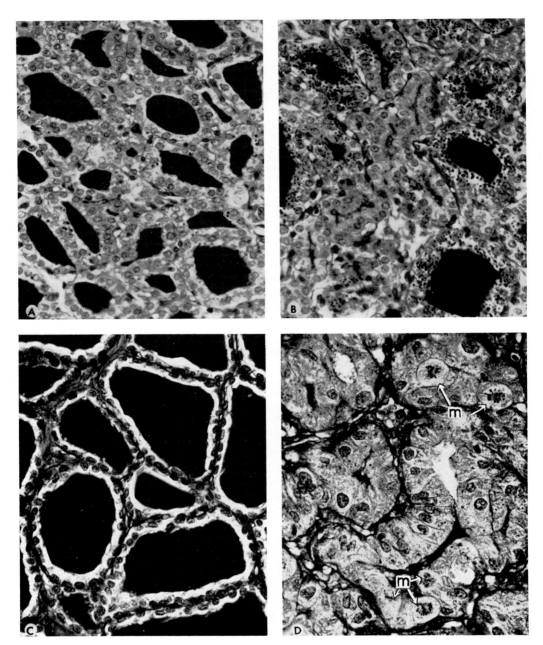

31–2 Rat thyroid in normal and experimental states.
A. Normal thyroid. Note "cuboidal" follicular cells and a few intracellular colloid droplets. **B.** Thyroid 3.5 h after intravenous injection of 250 mU of thyrotropin. Many follicles contain only traces of colloid. Intracellular colloid droplets are abundant in the follicular cells of follicles that have larger amounts of colloid in their lumina. **C.** Thyroid several weeks after hypophysectomy. Note distention of lumina by colloid, which shows some shrinkage in the periphery. The follicular cells are flat. **D.** Thyroid of a rat that was fed an iodine-deficient diet for several weeks and then injected for 10 days with the thiocarbamide propylthiouracil. The collapsed lumina contain little colloid. The follicular cells are tall columnar; several mitoses **(m)** can be seen. The capillaries are engorged. All sections stained with PAS-hematoxylin. (Parts A and B from Wollman, S. H. 1964. J. Cell Biol. 21:191.)

When the gland is inactive, the mass of colloid is large and the cells around it flattened (Fig. 31–2C). In hyperactive states the cells are tall and may be in mitosis, and the mass of colloid is relatively small (Fig. 31–2D). In normal animals an intermediate situation is seen, and considerable variation in activity exists from follicle to follicle, with a corresponding variation in histological appearance.

Two kinds of epithelial cells are present in the follicles—typical follicular epithelial cells and parafollicular or C cells (Fig. 31–3). The follicular cells, unlike the parafollicular cells, show a definite polarity in the arrangement of their organelles. The nucleus at the base of the cell varies in shape depending on the height of the follicular epithelium. It is relatively flat in flattened follicular cells and round or ovoid in columnar cells. In flattened epithelia the Golgi apparatus may be displaced to one side of the nucleus, whereas in cuboidal or columnar epithelial cells it lies above it. Mitochondria are found throughout the cytoplasm, which varies in its basophilia

depending on the state of activity of the cells. Colloid droplets may be present, particularly after TSH stimulation. Rarely, degenerating cells with pyknotic nuclei (colloid cells of Langendorff) are observed.

Parafollicular cells (often called C cells because of their calcitonin secretion) are relatively uncommon and may occur singly or in groups. They have no obvious polarity and never contain colloid droplets. They are larger than follicular cells and their cytoplasm appears pale with many staining methods; hence, their other name of light or clear cells. They may stain intensely with silver impregnation techniques, probably because of their catecholamine content.

Ultrastructure

With the electron microscope, the follicular colloid is homogeneous or faintly reticular with a moderate electron density. It is bounded by the follicular cells, which have microvilli at their apical border (Figs. 31–4, 31–5, and 31–8A). The microvilli tend to vary in height depending on the functional activity of the cell (Fig. 31–5). Between the microvilli, bristle-coated pits are sometimes observed. The tight junction at the apical end of the lateral plasma membrane forms a continuous seal between adjacent follicular cells. This seal probably functions to prevent leakage of the antigenically active thyroglobulin from the lumen of the follicle. Desmosomes, gap junctions, and interdigitations of the lateral plasma membranes of adjacent cells are also present. The basal plasma membrane has many infoldings.

The nucleus of the follicular cells varies in height depending on the height of the cell. In active cells the nucleolus may be prominent. Long filamentous mitochondria are randomly distributed. Ribosomes and polysomes are scattered through the cytoplasm.

Many ultrastructural features of thyroid follicular cells are typical of cells that produce protein for export. Cisternae of rough-surfaced endoplasmic reticulum (RER), usually distended, are found throughout the cytoplasm and are largely responsible for its basophilia. The well-organized Golgi apparatus lies between the nucleus and the apical end of the cell or may be displaced laterally. The apical cytoplasm contains many small vesicles, some of which are bristle-coated. Other vesicles have a moderately electron-dense homogeneous content and have been

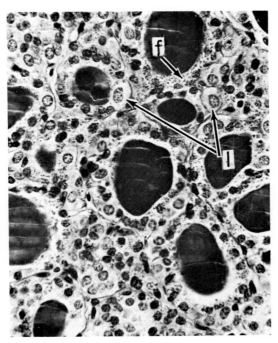

31–3 Normal rat thyroid. Note differences between follicular cells proper **(f)**, which contain numerous colloid droplets, and the larger C cells (light cells) **(I)**, which do not. PAS-hematoxylin stain. (Courtesy of C. P. Leblond.)

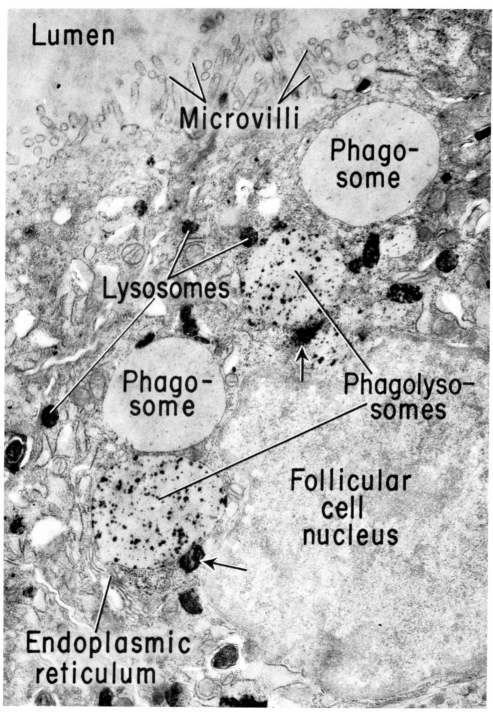

31–4 Electron micrograph of the apical portion of a follicular cell stained for acid phosphatase. Note the presence of the enzyme in the darkly stained lysosomes, some of which are closely attached to the much larger colloid droplets (phagosomes) **(arrows).**

The two large droplets with irregular black speckling are phagolysosomes, whose colloid has become intermingled with lysosomal contents, as demonstrated by the irregular staining for acid phosphatase. × 20,000. (From Wollman, S. H. 1965. J. Cell Biol. 25:593.)

shown to empty their contents into the follicular lumen. The apical vesicles are probably the means by which thyroglobulin is transported from the Golgi apparatus to the follicular lumen.

Other organelles appear to function in the retrieval of thyroglobulin from the follicular lumen, its subsequent digestion, and the ensuing endocrine secretion of thyroid hormone. In occasional cells pseudopods are seen, which are projections of the apical plasma membrane into the follicular lumen (Fig. 31–8B). These pseudopods sequester bits of colloid, and their membranes fuse to form intracellular colloid droplets or phagosomes, which then sink into the apical cytoplasm of the follicular cells. The colloid droplets (Figs. 31–4 and 31–5B) are relatively large cytoplasmic bodies, with a homogeneous, moderately electron-dense content bounded by a membrane. *Lysosomes* appear to fuse with the colloid droplets to form larger phagolysosomes during colloid digestion (Fig. 31–4). Coated vesicles formed from coated pits also participate in protein uptake by thyroid cells, but their quantitative importance in colloid resorption has not been evaluated and may be quite small.

The follicular cells lie on a homogeneous basement membrane with a delicate network of collagen fibers beneath it. The abundant capillary network, often with fenestrated endothelial cells, comes in close contact with the basement membrane and its associated fibrils.

Although parafollicular, or C, cells (Fig. 31–6) may occur in groups outside the thyroid follicles, others are enclosed within the basement membrane of the follicles. In this location they are never in contact with the follicular colloid, although the cytoplasm of the intervening follicular cells may be very attenuated. They vary widely in shape and may have cell processes that seem to extend toward nearby capillaries. They have large, pale nuclei and abundant narrow cisternae of RER, which sometimes form whorls or spirals. Nearby is their extensive Golgi apparatus.

The predominant ultrastructural feature of parafollicular cells is their small secretory granules 1,000 to 1,800 Å in diameter (Fig. 31–6A). In well-fixed cells they have a finely granular content separated from the membrane by a clear space. The granules appear to be formed by budding off of lamellae of the Golgi apparatus, and transitional forms between the Golgi apparatus and secretory granules may be seen in many cells. Their long mitochondria are randomly distributed.

Histochemistry and Histophysiology

Many cytochemical and autoradiographic studies have been directed to the question of where in thyroid cells various events occur in the synthesis of thyroglobulin and its breakdown into an active thyroid hormone. As we have noted earlier, it is convenient to separate the two phases of secretion, the exocrine phase in which thyroglobulin is secreted apically into the colloid, and the endocrine phase in which resorbed colloid is broken down into active thyroid hormone and secreted into the blood. However, it must be emphasized that in the living thyroid cell, both phases of secretion take place simultaneously.

Thyroglobulin Synthesis and Secretion

Iodide and amino acids are actively transported into the follicular cells via the basal plasma membrane. Autoradiographic studies have shown that thyroglobulin protein precursors are synthesized in the RER (Fig. 31–7), and some of the carbohydrate residues (mannose) are added. Further carbohydrate residues (galactose and fucose—the terminal carbohydrate residue of one carbohydrate side chain) are added in the Golgi apparatus, and the uniodinated molecule is assembled. The uniodinated thyroglobulin is then transported via apical vesicles to the follicular lumen where it is added to the colloid mass (Fig. 31–8).

Concurrently, a peroxidase, thyroperoxidase, is synthesized by the follicular cells and is transported to the follicular lumen via the same route (RER, Golgi apparatus, and apical vesicles) and is also released into the follicular lumen (Fig. 31–5). This enzyme, like other peroxidases, can iodinate proteins, and thyroperoxidase is responsible for iodinating thyroglobulin. Iodination apparently occurs only in the follicular lumen (Fig. 31–9) despite the probable coexistence of the two proteins within the same organelles in the follicular cells. The reason for the absence of intracellular iodination is not known. (This situation is reminiscent of the fetal thyroid, where iodination of thyroglobulin seems to begin concomitantly with the appearance of follicular lumina.) The process of iodination has been intensively studied. It appears to involve the oxidation of iodide to a higher valence state, but the details of its mechanism are still in doubt. Iodotyrosyl groups couple within the thyroglobulin molecule to produce peptide-linked hormone (iodothyronyl) groups. This is the storage form of thyroid hormone.

Secretion of Thyroid Hormone

The second phase of thyroid secretion involves the reuptake of thyroglobulin by the follicular cells and its breakdown to active hormone. The production of pseudopods and colloid droplets has been described above. This process may require the participation of microtubules and microfilaments, because it is inhibited by colchicine and cytochalasin B. Subsequently, lysosomes fuse with colloid droplets to form phagolysosomes, large bodies that contain cytochemically demonstrable acid-phosphatase and esterase, classic marker enzymes for lysosomes (Fig. 31–4). It is presumed that the lysosomes, which also contain a protease active at acid pH, contribute their enzymes to the colloid droplet and that the acid proteases are responsible for the breakdown of thyroglobulin. Iodotyrosine precursors, which make up most of the iodine in thyroglobulin, are enzymatically deiodinated, releasing their iodine to be reused by the cells. The details of the process by which the active hormones are subsequently released from the cell are not well understood, but it is assumed that they diffuse from the base of the follicular cell

31–5 Rat thyroids incubated in a medium for demonstration of peroxidase activity. **A.** Three weeks after hypophysectomy. The flattened follicular cells **(FC)** are at the top of the figure. Beneath them are the basement membrane **(B)** and narrow processes of connective tissue cells. A blood vessel **(BV)** with an endothelial cell nucleus is at the bottom of the figure. The follicular cells have peroxidase activity in the nuclear envelope **(ne)** and in a few flattened cisternae of RER **(R).** The small Golgi apparatus **(g)** is relatively inactive. No peroxidase activity is present at the cell apexes. **B.** This rat was hypophysectomized for 3 weeks and then given TSH for 2 days before autopsy.

The follicular lumen **(L)** is at upper right, the basement membrane **(B)** at lower left. The nuclear envelope of the follicular cell has intense peroxidase activity. Cisternae of RER **(RER)**, now somewhat expanded, have greatly increased in number. These cisternae, and some vesicles and lamellae of the expanded Golgi appartus **(g)**, are peroxidase-positive. A few peroxidase-positive apical vesicles are present near the cell apex. Some peroxidase activity is also present in the follicular lumen **(*).** Note the colloid droplets **(C)** and lysosomes **(L).** Part A, × 15,950; part B, × 16,250.

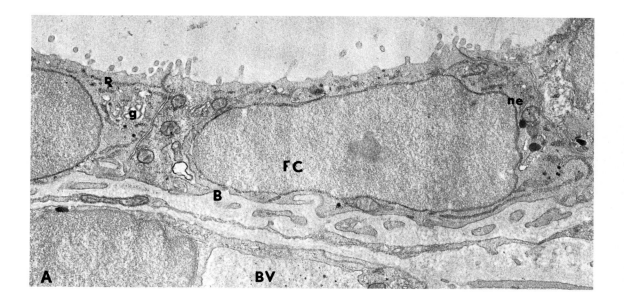

into the blood and lymph. The active hormones are the iodinated amino acids L-thyroxine (tetraiodo-L-thyroxine) and L-thyronine (3,5,3′-triiodo-L-thyronine).

C Cells

As befits their neural crest origin, C cells have much of the biochemical machinery of the sympathetic neuron or the adrenal medulla. Fluorescence microscopy and autoradiographic studies have shown that they take up catecholamines or their amino acid precursors, decarboxylate the precursors to catecholamines, and store them together with their protein hormone calcitonin in a reserpine-sensitive granule. They thereby seem to be part of the APUD system, defined in Chap. 29. Cytochemically, they also contain monamine oxidase, an enzyme capable of oxidizing cytoplasmic catecholamines. When experimental animals are injected with calcium, the cells rapidly degranulate (Fig. 31–6B), and concomitantly blood calcitonin levels increase. Degranulation, together with loss of catecholamine-induced fluoresence, can also be produced more slowly in animals fed diets high in vitamin D_2. The pri-

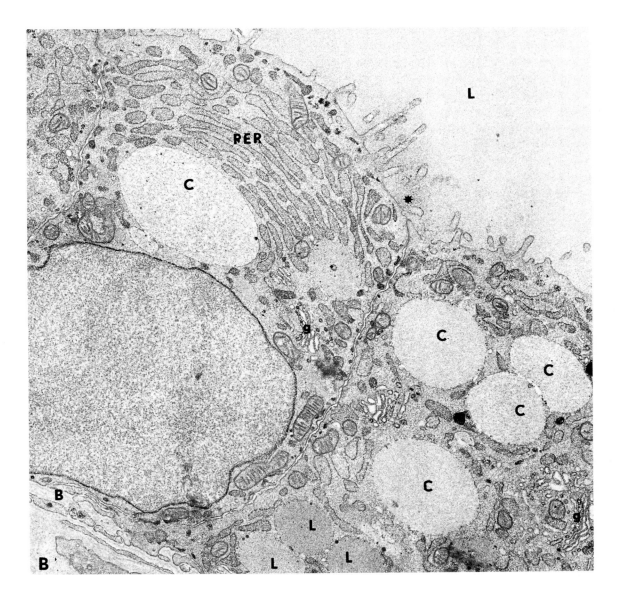

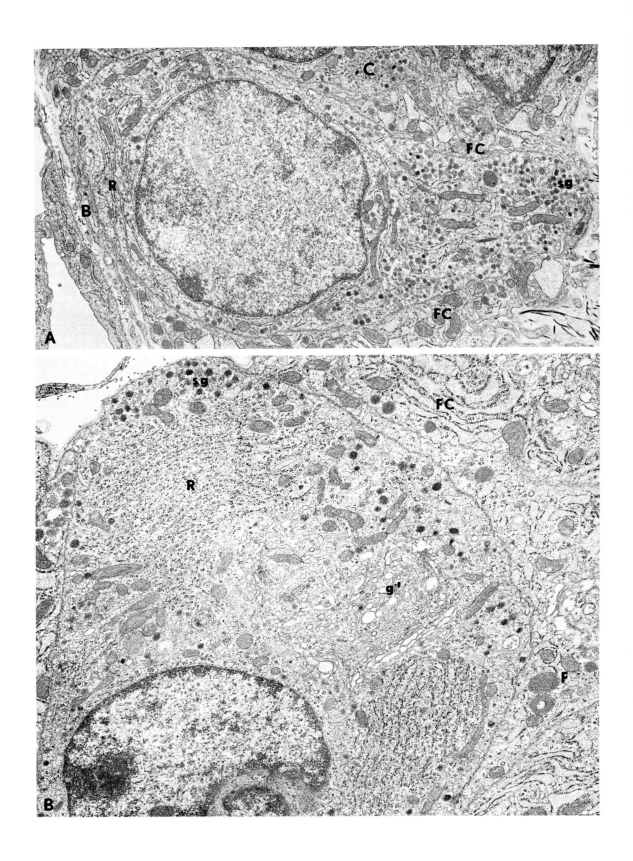

31–6 **A.** Parafollicular cell from normal mouse thyroid. This cell lies within the basement membrane **(B)** of the follicle and is flanked by another C cell **(C)** and by follicular cells **(FC).** The somewhat elongated cell contains long mitochondria, narrow RER cisternae **(R)**, and many small, moderately electron-dense secretory granules **(sg).** The Golgi apparatus is not included in the section. **B.** Mouse C cell 4 h after the start of hourly calcium injections. Note the surrounding follicular cells **(FC).** Only a few secretory granules **(sg)** are observed, and they tend to be peripherally placed. Cisternae of RER **(R)** are abundant, and the prominent Golgi apparatus **(g)** has an unusually large number of associated vesicles. Part A, × 10,000; part B, × 12,800.

31–7 Autoradiographs of thyroids from rats killed at various intervals after the injection of [³H]-labeled leucine. The dark grains indicate the locations of proteins (largely thyroglobulin) synthesized from the labeled leucine. **A.** At 30 min, the grains overlie the cytoplasm of the follicular cells. They are located throughout the cell but are scarce at the apical edge in contact with the colloid. No grains are over the colloid. **B.** At 4 h, the grains predominate in the apical end of the cells. **C.** At 36 h, the grains are distributed uniformly over the colloid. All three sections are counterstained with PAS-hematoxylin. (Courtesy of N. J. Nadler, K. Harrison, and C. P. Leblond.)

mary effect of calcitonin is to inhibit the resorption of bone calcium salts, which results in a fall in blood calcium levels.

Regulation of Thyroid Activity

The pituitary hormone TSH is the most important regulator of thyroid activity, although, as noted earlier, sympathetic activity may also mimic TSH effects under circumstances in which TSH secretion is minimal or absent. The pituitary–thyroid axis appears to form a feedback loop, for elevated blood levels of thyroid hormone act to suppress TSH secretion. In part, this appears to be a direct pituitary effect; and in part, pituitary function is affected when hypothalamic production of a thyroid-releasing hormone (TRH) is suppressed.

Because of this feedback loop, the thyroid gland may appear hyperactive when blood levels of circulating thyroid hormone are normal or low. Iodine deficiency, or administration of drugs that interfere with production of thyroid hormone, leads to increased TSH production, which in turn results in a hyperactive gland. Conversely, administration of thyroxine can suppress TSH secretion with the consequence that the thyroid gland comes to resemble the gland seen after hypophysectomy.

The mode of action of TSH appears, at least in part, to be via a specific TSH receptor. When TSH combines with the receptor, adenyl cyclase is activated and intracellular levels of cyclic

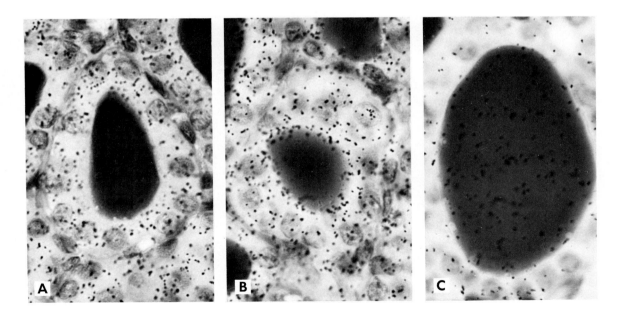

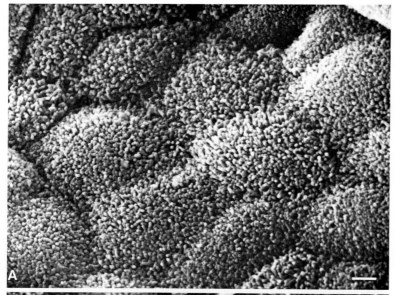

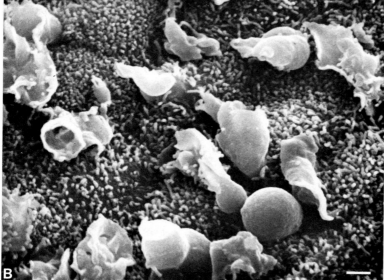

31–8 Scanning electron micrographs of the apical surfaces of thyroid follicular cells. The glands were fixed and subjected to critical point drying. **A.** Microvilli cover the apical surface of unstimulated thyroid follicles from a hypophysectomized rat for 24 h. Each cell appears to be slightly elevated in its center. The depressed regions mark the boundary between adjacent cells. **B.** Thyrotropin **(TSH)** elicits these large apical pseudopods in many follicles within 5 to 20 min in hypophysectomized animals. Pseudopods evidently form as broad flat lamellae that curl up and overlap, engulfing droplets of colloid; the pseudopods then assume a globular form, retract into the cell, and disappear from the apical surface. Under these conditions, new pseudopods are continually initated for approximately 1 h and cells of a given follicle tend to respond synchronously. Responding cells generally display a single pseudopod, and individual pseudopods usually engulf multiple droplets of varied sizes. Part A, × 499; part B, × 4,914. (Micrographs courtesy of B. K. Wetzel.)

AMP increase. Cyclic AMP or dibutyryl cyclic AMP can mimic TSH stimulation.

The morphological effects of TSH are best studied in hypophysectomized or thyroxine-suppressed animals. All follicles and cells do not respond at the same rate to the hormone, possibly because of local variations in blood flow. Within a short but variable time (usually a few minutes but depending on the species studied) after TSH administration, pseudopods are observed, fol-

lowed by the appearance of intracellular colloid droplets (Fig. 31–2B). Lysosomes migrate apically from their former position at the base of the cell. Lysosome migration and pseudopod formation do not appear to be interdependent, since migration of lysosomes can still be observed when pseudopod formation has been inhibited. Exocytotic release of apical vesicles is also observed after TSH administration. Thyroid blood flow increases. Later there are signs of increased

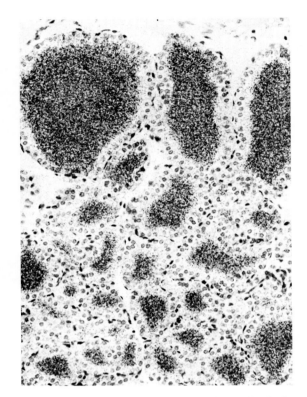

31–9 Autoradiograph of the thyroid of a rat that had received ^{125}I-labeled iodide in its drinking water long enough to have its body iodine stores labeled to the same specific radioactivity (that is, the same number of counts per minute per unit mass of iodine). In this condition of so-called radioisotopic equilibrium, the distribution of radioactivity reflects that of nonradioactive iodine faithfully. Note that essentially all the blackening of the emulsion due to the radioactive iodine is over the colloid in the lumina rather than in the follicular epithelium. × 240. (From Wollman, S. H. 1967. Endocrinology 81:1074.)

synthetic activity by the follicular cells. Synthesis of both thyroglobulin and thyroperoxidase (Fig. 31–5) appears to be TSH-stimulated. Eventually, if stimulation is prolonged, increased cell division and hyperplasia of the gland occur (Fig. 31–2D).

References and Selected Bibliography

Andros, G., and Wollman, S. H. 1967. Autoradiographic localization of radioiodide in the thyroid gland of the mouse. Am. J. Physiol. 213:198.

Brown-Grant, K. 1966. Regulation of TSH secretion. In G. W. Harris and B. T. Donovan (eds.), The Pituitary Gland, vol. 2. Berkeley: University of California Press, p. 235.

Dumont, E. 1971. The action of thyrotropin on thyroid metabolism. Vitam. Horm. 29:289.

Ekholm, R., and Ericson, L. E. 1968. The ultrastructure of the parafollicular cells of the rat. J. Ultrastruct. Res. 23:378.

Heimann, P. 1966. Ultrastructure of human thyroid: A study of normal thyroid, untreated and treated diffuse toxic goiter. Acta Endocrinol. (Suppl.) (Copenh.) 53:110.

Loewenstein, J. E., and Wollman, S. H. 1967. Distribution of ^{125}I and ^{127}L in the rat thyroid gland during equilibrium labeling as determined by autoradiography. Endocrinology 81:1074.

Nadler, N. J., Sarkar, S. K., and Leblond, C. P. 1962. Origin of intracellular colloid droplets in the rat thyroid. Endocrinology 71:120.

Pitt-Rivers, R., and Trotter, W. R. (eds.). 1964. The Thyroid. London: Butterworth & Co., Ltd.

Seljelid, R., Reith, A., and Nakken, K. F. 1970. The early phase of endocytosis in the rat thyroid follicle cell. Lab. Invest. 23:595.

Strum, J. M., and Karnovsky, M. J. 1970. Cytochemical localization of endogenous peroxidase in thyroid follicular cells. J. Cell Biol. 44:655.

Taylor, S. (ed.). 1968. Calcitonin: Proceedings of the Symposium on Thyro Calcitonin and the C Cells. London: Heinemann Educational Books, Ltd.

Wetzel, B. K., Spicer, S. S., and Wollman, S. H. 1965. Changes in fine structure and acid phosphatase localization in rat thyroid cells following thyrotropin administration. J. Cell Biol. 25:593.

Whur, P., Herscovics, A., and Leblond, C. P. 1969. Radioautographic visualization of the incorporation of galactose-^{3}H and mannose-^{3}H by rat thyroids in vitro in relation to the stages of thyroglobulin synthesis. J. Cell Biol. 43:289.

Wollman, S. H., Spicer, S. S., and Burstone, M. S. 1964. Localization of esterase and acid phosphatase in granules and colloid droplets in rat thyroid epithelium. J. Cell Biol. 21:191.

Wollman, S. H., and Wodinsky, I. 1955. Localization of protein-bound I^{131} in the thyroid gland of the mouse. Endocrinology 56:9.

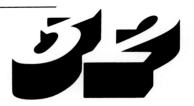

The Parathyroid Glands

John T. Potts, Jr.

Anatomy and Embryology of the Parathyroid Glands

The biological function of the parathyroids is to raise blood calcium concentrations by multiple actions on several organ systems, the bone, kidney, and gut. The glands, so named because of their anatomic proximity to the thyroid, are paired structures, usually four in number. Each gland in adults has an average weight of 100 to 140 mg and measures approximately 6 × 4 × 2 mm. The upper or superior pair of parathyroids, supplied by the inferior thyroid artery or, rarely, the superior thyroid artery, is located on the posterior capsule of the thyroid at the dorsal or dorsomedial aspect of the lateral lobe or within the substance of the thyroid; the lower or inferior pair, supplied by the inferior thyroid artery, has a more variable location near the lower pole of the thyroid, usually associated with remnants of the thymus. Occasionally variation is noted in the number and location of the glands; this issue is of clinical importance to surgeons exploring the neck to find and remove enlarged, hyperfunctioning glands that develop in the disease hyperparathyroidism. Accessory glands result from division of one or more of the four glands during embryogenesis. There are almost always four glands; additional glands are reported in 2% to 6% of individuals, although some estimates suggest an even higher incidence of accessory glands.

The variation in location of the glands is best understood in terms of the embryogenesis of the parathyroids. The glands arise from the third and fourth branchial pouches. The superior glands (referred to as parathyroid IV) arise from the fourth branchial pouches; the gland analage is closely associated with the ultimobranchial body (the structure within which the parafollicular cells concerned with biosynthesis of calcitonin are found in later phases of embryogenesis). As the ultimobranchial body becomes incorporated into the posterior lateral portion of the thyroid, parathyroid IV becomes closely associated with the thyroid at this site. The inferior glands of the adult human (parathyroid III) arise from the third branchial pouch and hence are originally more cephalad than parathyroid IV. The eventual inferior and more variable anatomic location of parathyroid III relates to its extensive migration caudally, closely associated with the thymus, as the two embryonic bodies migrate toward the thorax. Parathyroid III usually separates from the thymus and ceases migration in the lower neck at the level of the lower pole of the thyroid. The location in the adult of either of the glands representing parathyroid III (inferior glands) within thymic remnants at the thoracic inlet or even within the mediastinum seems explained by a failure to arrest the caudad migration during embryogenesis.

Parathyroids are first recognized in amphibians and higher orders; fishes lack definable parathyroid glands. In the orders studied, the glands arise from the branchial pouches as in humans; anatomic and histological similarities of the parathyroids are noted throughout the vertebrates. Some mammals, such as the rat, have only two glands, but most mammalian species have four.

That the parathyroids appeared in the animal kingdom as a discrete gland during the evolutionary period of the first life on land has been interpreted as an adaptation needed to ensure an adequate supply of calcium. Calcium is abundant in seawater; the concentration of calcium in the sea exceeds that in the blood and extracellular fluid of fishes and other vertebrates. Calcium is not plentiful in the food chain on land; hence, teleologically, it is reasoned that the parathyroids evolved to help ensure an adequate assimilation of calcium. It is unknown, at present, however, if glandular tissue or hormonal substances analogous to the parathyroids and parathyroid hormone are present in fishes or even in life forms appearing earlier in evolutionary history.

Microscopic Structure of the Parathyroid Glands

The parathyroid glands are encapsulated and well vascularized with a rich capillary network supplied by arterioles derived from branches of the inferior thyroid artery. They are drained by multiple venules into various portions of the anatomic venous plexus formed by the anastamosis of the superior, middle, and inferior thyroid veins. The vessels enter and leave the gland through trabeculae that traverse the gland from the fibrous capsule. It is possible, by using carefully placed catheters, to sample blood from each of the thyroid veins. Assay of hormone content in each sample is useful in identifying which of the parathyroid glands is overactive in patients with hyperparathyroidism. Although the glands are innervated, neural control of parathyroid function may not be physiologically important, because parathyroid transplants function normally.

The glands continue to grow in size and weight from birth through adolescence; maximum weight is attained at about age 20 and remains constant thereafter. Numerous qualitative changes in the parathyroids occur throughout life. In children, the glands show a uniformity of appearance; the principal cell type, the *chief cell,* predominates and few other nonvascular cellular elements are present. Connective tissue increases in the glands of the young adult. The parenchyma become arranged in visible cords and nests, separated by the collagenous bands, and the glands thus exhibit a more lobulated appearance than in infancy (Fig. 32–1). With advancing age the number of fat cells increases; these cells may occupy 60 to 70% of the volume of the gland in the elderly adult (Fig. 32–1). Hence, although weight remains constant, the functional mass of chief cells decreases with age. In a person 70 years old, a uniform appearance of the glands, composed entirely of chief cells and devoid of fat cells, would be abnormal and indicate functional overactivity.

Two principal types of cells are identified by characteristic light-microscopic and ultrastructural analyses, the chief cell and the oxyphil cell (Figs. 32–2 and 33–3). A third cell type, a transitional cell, is recognized by some histologists (Fig. 32–3). Chief cells are believed to be responsible for hormone production. The chief cell is typically 4–8 μm in diameter with a clear cytoplasm and a small and centrally located nucleus.

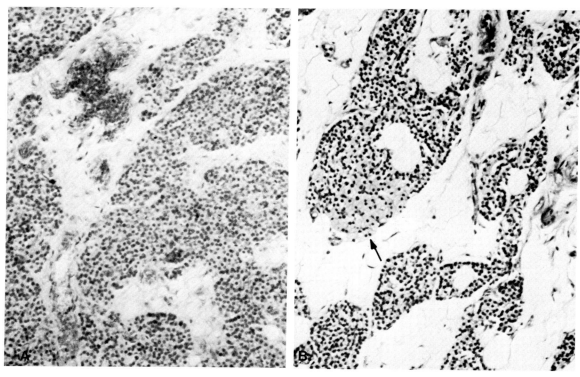

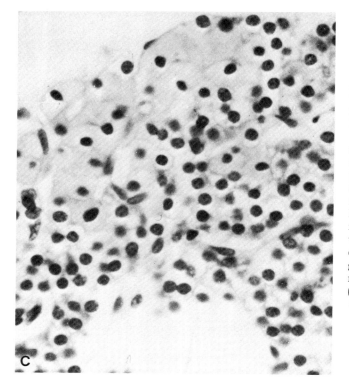

32–1 **A.** Photomicrograph of a normal human parathyroid gland from a 20-year-old man. Stroma largely free of fat is present between uniform sheets and cords of cells. × 25. (Courtesy Edith Robbins.) **B.** Photomicrograph of normal parathyroid gland from a 60-year-old man. Stromal fat occupies more than 50% of the gland. Note near center of picture **(arrow)** an area of larger cells with more abundant cytoplasm and smaller nuclei than the predominant chief cells; the large cells termed oxyphil cells (see part 6). × 35. (Courtesy of Edith Robbins.) **C.** Higher magnification of a region of a parathyroid gland containing a small nodule of oxyphil cells (upper left) adjacent to chief cells; the larger size, more abundant cytoplasm, and smaller nuclei of the oxyphil cell are apparent. With hematoxylin and eosin stain and color reproduction, the oxyphil cells are eosinophilic with granular cytoplasm, prominent cytoplasmic borders, and dark small nuclei. The granules are presumably the abundant mitochondria characteristic of the oxyphil cell (see electron micrograph, Fig. 32–3). × 150. (Courtesy of Edith Robbins.)

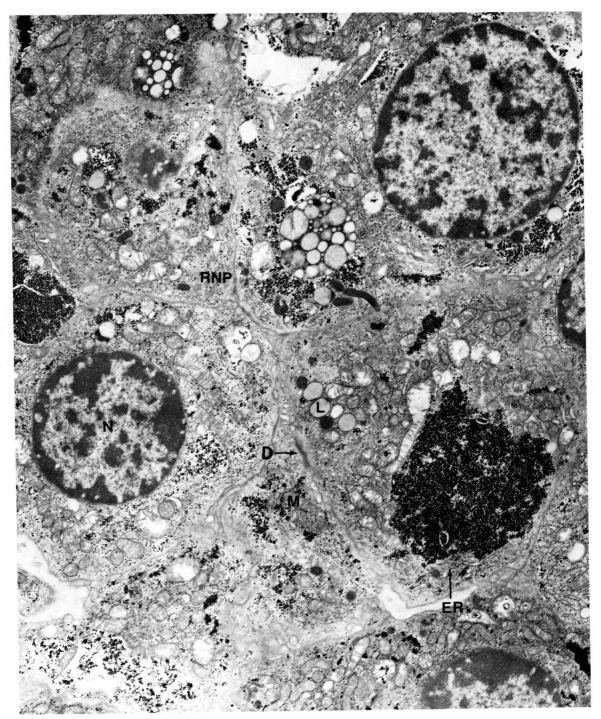

32–2 Group of chief cells from a normal human parathyroid gland. Note the variation in abundance of glycogen and number of mitochondria. **G**, glycogen; **L**, lipid; **D**, desmosome; **M**, mitochrondria; **N**, nucleus; **RNP**, ribonucleoprotein; **ER**, endoplasmic reticulum. See Figs. 32–6 to 32–8 for details of cytoplasmic elements (endoplasmic reticulum, Golgi apparatus, and secretion granules) associated with active secretion. (Courtesy of R. J. Weymouth and H. R. Seibel.)

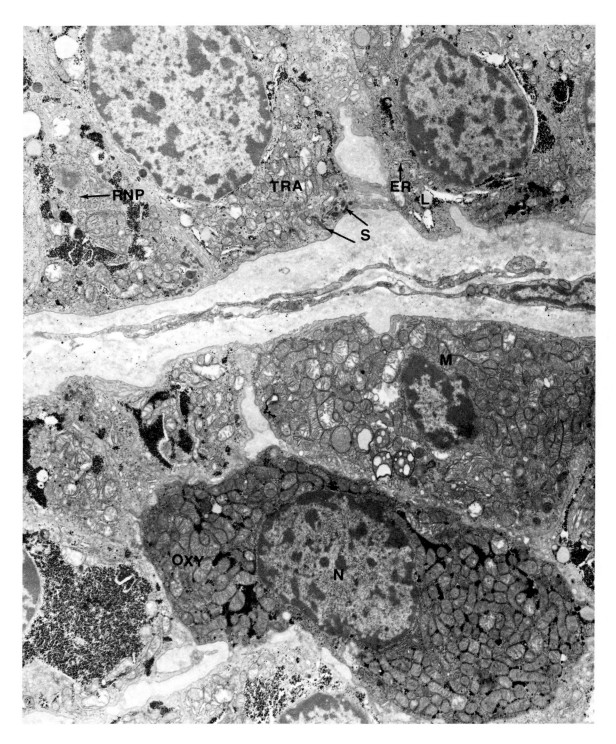

32–3 Oxyphil cell in a normal human parathyroid gland shown in comparison with chief cells and a transitional cell. Note the range in density of mitochondria and the presence of glycogen in granules. **OXY,** oxyphil cell; **C,** chief cell; **TRA,** transitional cell; **S,** secretory material. Other abbreviations as in Fig. 32–2. (Courtesy of R. J. Weymouth and M. N. Sheridan.)

Many chief cells are detected in a phase apparently inactive in hormone production; endoplasmic reticulum and Golgi apparatus are not prominent and membrane-bounded granules are rare or absent. In these cells, glycogen, lipid, and lipofuscin bodies are abundant (Fig. 32–2). In cells with this appearance there are also more lysosomes, rich in acid-phosphatase, seen near the Golgi apparatus and elsewhere. Certain chief cells are detected in phases believed to be associated with active hormone production or secretion. In these cells large numbers of mature secretory granules are seen near the cell periphery; at times the limiting membranes of the secretory granules fuse with the cell membrane. Often these cells have a prominent endoplasmic reticulum with numerous associated ribosomes (RER) which are detected as basophilic bodies by light microscopy. The Golgi apparatus is often enlarged, with numerous parallel arrays of enlarged membrane spaces filled with vesicles and membrane-limited granules. Cells that appear morphologically to be in a state of relative secretory inactivity outnumber cells with prominent endoplasmic reticulum and Golgi apparatus by 3 to 1 or more in the normal human gland (Fig. 32–2), accounting for the relatively clear cytoplasm of most chief cells.

The oxyphil cell, 6 to 10 μm in diameter, is larger than the chief cell and contains a granular cytoplasm that avidly binds eosin. Its nucleus is usually smaller and more heterochromatic than the nucleus of the chief cell; the cells contain an abundance of mitochondria (Fig. 32–3) that account for the granular, eosinophilic character of the cytoplasm. Endoplasmic reticulum and Golgi apparatus are scanty in the oxyphil cells of normal glands, and secretory granules are usually absent. The transitional cell (Fig. 32–3) has a variable quantity of mitochondria and glycogen; the cells are less granular in appearance than the oxyphil cell.

Chief cells are the exclusive parenchymal cell recognized in the gland of infants and children before puberty. The oxyphil cell, first recognized at puberty, increases in number with increasing age; oxyphil cells are detected adjacent to chief cells or occasionally in clusters arranged as nests or follicles distributed within various sites within the gland (Fig. 32–1). Although some morphologists have believed that oxyphil cells do not produce parathyroid hormone (PTH), certain evidence contradicts this view. Microscopic examination of the abnormal parathyroid tissue removed from patients with hyperparathyroid-

ism reveals, in rare cases, only oxyphil cells. Because excessive hormone production ceases when the gland containing only these cells is removed, oxyphil cells in such abnormal states must secrete the hormone.

There are not yet correlations between the morphological characteristics of the individual types of parathyroid cells and the biological functions such as hormone production, storage, and release. Such techniques as immunocytolocalization and radioautography (discussed below under Endocrine Function) are just beginning to be applied to the study of cell function; hence, firm conclusions about morphological and functional correlations cannot yet be made. A plausible hypothesis, based on the accumulated morphological and physiological data, is that there is one principal parenchymal cell, seen usually in an appearance that leads to its classification as a chief cell, but occasionally seen in a different cellular configuration leading to classification as an oxyphil or transitional cell.

Endocrine Function

Physiology of the Parathyroid Glands

Physiologists and cell biologists have become increasingly aware of the multiple regulatory and metabolic roles played by calcium ion in extracellular fluid and within cells. Maintenance of extracellular fluid calcium concentration is essential for life. In terrestrial existence calcium may often be limited in the diet; under such circumstances, the conservation of calcium concentration in blood requires efficient uptake of available dietary calcium from the intestine, energy-requiring transport of calcium to extracellular fluid from the large compartment of calcium present in an insoluble form in bone, and reduction of calcium losses by lowering urinary calcium clearance. These considerations seem to explain the coincident appearance of the parathyroids with evolution of life on land.

The physiological function of PTH is to maintain extracellular fluid calcium concentration. The hormone raises blood calcium by its actions on bone and kidney directly and, indirectly, by action on the intestine. In the intestine it affects the synthesis of 1α, 25-dihydroxyvitamin D_3 [1α, 25-$(OH)_2D_3$], which acts to increase serum calcium. In turn PTH production is closely regulated by serum calcium concentration. This feedback system involving the parathyroids is one of the most important homeostatic mechanisms for the close regulation of extracellular fluid calcium concentration. Any tendency toward hypocalcemia, as might be induced by calcium-deficient diets, is counteracted by an increased rate of secretion of PTH. This increased secretion, in turn, acts to (1) increase the rate of dissolution of bone mineral, thereby providing an increased flow of calcium from bone into extracellular fluid; (2) reduce the renal clearance of calcium, returning more of the calcium filtered at the glomerulus into extracellular fluid; and (3) increase the efficiency of calcium absorption in the intestine. Rapid changes in blood calcium are due to effects of the hormone on bone and, to a lesser extent, on renal calcium clearance. The action of the hormone on bone would preserve calcium concentration in blood at the cost of bone destruction and release of bone mineral. Maintenance of calcium balance or the total body content of calcium, on the other hand, is due to the effects of the hormone, via control of $1\alpha,25$-$(OH)_2D_3$ levels, on the efficiency of intestinal calcium absorption.

Blood calcium concentration controls the secretion of PTH. Hormone secretion increases steeply to a maximum value of fivefold above basal rates whenever calcium concentration falls below normal. When calcium concentration returns to normal, PTH secretion is rapidly reduced. This regulation of PTH by the controlled variable, calcium, accomplishes a homeostasis of calcium; that is, it maintains calcium concentration within narrow limits by rapidly correcting any tendency of the level to rise or fall. Factors such as epinephrine may also increase hormone secretion, but the physiological significance of noncalcium secretagogs is not yet established.

Parathyroid hormone also has important effects on the metabolism of inorganic phosphate. The hormone causes obligatory release of phosphate with calcium from bone whenever the hormone mediates an increase in the dissolution of bone matrix and mineral. The action of PTH on the kidney is opposite in direction to its action on calcium; the hormone increases the renal clearance of phosphate. The latter effect of PTH on phosphate metabolism is biologically predominant over actions on bone; in animals, experimental parathyroidectomy leads to an increase in blood phosphate associated with a marked reduction in urinary phosphate concentration. The overall physiological significance or homeostatic role of the effects of PTH on phosphate metabolism is less certain than for calcium. Phosphate ion itself, unlike calcium ion,

has no direct effect on PTH secretion; hence, unless accompanied by corresponding changes in calcium levels, wide swings in blood or extracellular fluid phosphate would not be countered by any change in the rate of hormone secretion or, therefore, the biological effect of the hormone. It has been reasoned that the action of the hormone on phosphate metabolism is best understood as a secondary rather than homeostatic action, and its role on phosphate metabolism arises because of the abundance of phosphate in the terrestrial food chain. Because phosphate deficiency, in health, is an unlikely environmental challenge, it seems beneficial to eliminate in the urine the additional phosphate mobilized from bone while conserving renal calcium when both mineral ions are liberated by the action of PTH on bone in response to calcium deficiency. A high blood phosphate level, per se, tends to lower calcium concentration by multiple actions related in part to the finite solubility product of the mineral ions. Hence, the calcium-elevating action of the hormone when required by dietary calcium deficiency is more effective if skeletal phosphate, mobilized along with calcium, is excreted via the kidney and the calcium retained.

The mode of action of PTH at the biochemical level involves effects of the hormone on adenylate cyclase in the cells of the target tissue. Stimulation of enzyme activity during specific hormone–target cell membrane interaction leads to an increase in intracellular cyclic adenosine monophosphate (cyclic AMP). It seems likely that this rapid rise in intracellular cyclic AMP is the initial biochemical step in all the physiological effects of PTH. There are as yet few data concerning the cellular mechanism whereby an increased intracellular concentration of cyclic AMP leads to changes in calcium and phosphate ion translocation. In a number of tissues responsive to hormones through a cyclic AMP mechanism there is evidence for stimulation of protein kinases causing, in turn, phosphorylation of critical proteins that initiate the hormonal effect.

Biosynthesis of Parathyroid Hormone

Biochemistry. The biosynthesis of PTH, as with other polypeptides and proteins destined for secretion from cells, involves the synthesis of several molecular forms larger than the polypeptide of 84 amino acids eventually secreted from the cell. These larger molecules are the precursor of the hormone. In the smaller, intermediate precursor, proparathyroid hormone (proPTH), a six-

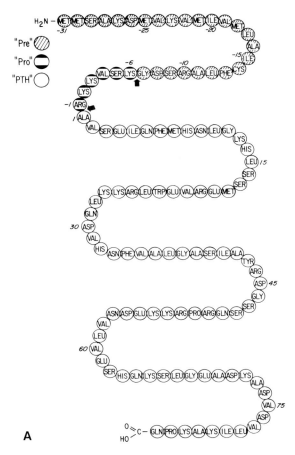

32-4 A. The amino acid sequence of pre-proPTH.
Residues in **hatched circles** constitute the NH$_2$-terminal leader sequence, the hydrophobic region that brings about attachment to the membrane of the endoplasmic reticulum. **Shaded** residues are specific to the prohormone. Residues in **open circles** denote PTH, the principal secreted form of the hormone. The **arrows** indicate the peptide bonds cleaved during removal of the leader sequence and the specific peptide of the hormone (part B). **B.** Schema depicting the proposed intracellular pathway of the biosynthesis of PTH. In the nucleus, PTH-specific messenger ribonucleic acid (mRNA) is transcribed from parathyroid genomic deoxyribonucleic acid (DNA). In the cytoplasm, the mRNA, with additional polyadenine added to one end (3') of the mRNA (AAAA 3'), directs the synthesis of pre-proPTH on ribosomes that attach to the membrane of the endoplasmic reticulum. The mRNA is read from the 5' to the 3' end. Pre-proparathyroid hormone, the initial product of synthesis on the ribosomes, is converted into proPTH by removal of (1) the NH$_2$-terminal methionyl residues (by methionyl aminopeptidase) and (2) the NH$_2$-terminal sequence (-29 through -7) of 23 amino acids during or within seconds after synthesis (by a second enzyme, called a "clipase"). The conversion of pre-proPTH probably occurs during transport of the polypeptide into the cisterna of the rough endoplasmic reticulum. By 15 to 20 min after synthesis, proPTH reaches the Golgi region and is converted to PTH by (3) removal of the NH$_2$-terminal hexapeptide (through action of a tryptic-like enzyme and carboxypeptidase B-like enzyme). Parathyroid hormone is stored in the secretory granule until released into the circulation in response to a fall in the blood concentration of calcium. The estimated time needed for each of these events is given below the schema. Fragments as well as intact PTH (1–84) may be released from the gland; in peripheral sites, a fragment, 1–33, and related fragments are cleaved from the intact PTH (see text for details).

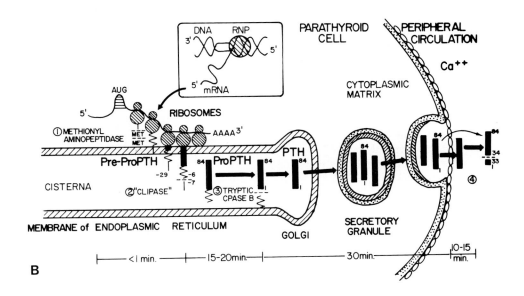

amino-acid peptide present at the amino terminus of the hormone, is cleaved off, liberating PTH itself (Fig. 32–4A). Analyses of the biosynthesis of PTH employing translation of messenger RNA for PTH in heterologous cell-free systems led to the identification of a still larger molecular-weight precursor termed pre-proparathyroid hormone (pre-proPTH). The larger precursor, consisting of 115 amino acids, contains the complete sequence of proPTH plus an additional 25 amino acids added to the amino terminus of proPTH; the prehormone is rapidly converted to the prohormone (Fig. 32–4A).

In all, there are four proteolytic processing events between initial synthesis of PTH and its final disappearance from blood or tissue fluids after interacting with receptors in target organs. The first three cleavages occur intracellularly; the fourth cleavage occurs after the hormone is secreted into the circulation. The intracellular cleavages have been studied by adding radioactive amino acids to slices of parathyroid tissue (pulse-labeling) and then extracting the tissue at intervals of seconds to minutes after synthesis of hormone that incorporates the radioactive amino acids has begun. The conversion of pre-proPTH to proPTH was found to occur within seconds of synthesis; in the second cleavage, occurring after a delay of 15 to 20 min, proPTH, the intermediate biosynthetic precursor, is converted to PTH. Two other cleavages not involving conversion of precursor to product occur with PTH; these additional cleavages reflect the complexity of the sequential modification of polypeptide hormones central to the role of a particular protein in endocrine homeostasis and metabolism. Evidence, still largely indirect, indicates that during hypercalcemia and limited secretion of PTH, there is extensive intracellular degradation of the polypeptide, a process that limits the amount of hormone available for secretion. With hypocalcemia there appears to be a sudden reduction of intracellular degradation, which rapidly increases quantities of hormone available to meet increased secretory demands. Certain evidence relating to the heterogeneity of circulating PTH suggests that fragments resulting from this cleavage may in some circumstances be secreted into peripheral blood.

The chief cells detected with increased numbers of lysosomes may, through the process of lysosomal fusion with secretory granules, be involved in hormone destruction. When this phenomenon is considered along with evidence of varying phases of synthetic activity versus inactivity of chief cells (discussed above), it seems that intracellular signals, not yet understood, dictate alternating phases of increased hormone production and hormone destruction by the parathyroid cells.

A most intriguing posttranslational cleavage is an extracellular proteolytic modification of PTH that results from efficient and selective uptake of circulating hormone by cells in liver, kidney, and perhaps other sites, followed by cleavage of the polypeptide. The Kupffer cells of liver rapidly degrade the hormone by one or more enzymes apparently located on the cell surface; the enzymes convert the hormone to an amino-terminal fragment (approximately one-third of the molecule) and a larger fragment consisting of the middle and carboxyl regions. The significance of this cleavage in peripheral tissues is not known. Systematic studies, employing chemical synthesis of fragments and analogs of PTH followed by assays of biological activity of these synthetic peptides in a variety of appropriate test systems, have established that the amino-terminal one-third of the molecule contains all the structure needed for expression of all known actions of the hormone. Because studies of the site where the hormone is cleaved by Kupffer cell enzymes have indicated that the minimum active fragment might be released intact, the peripheral metabolism of the hormone may represent a final activation step occurring outside the parathyroid cell. Alternatively, the peripheral metabolism may represent an important route of destruction and metabolic clearance of the hormone that controls the rate of expression of its biological activity.

Ultrastructure. Studies in vitro of PTH biosynthesis and analogous studies in vitro with other hormones and secretory proteins have provided strong evidence as to the probable sequence of biosynthetic events for secretory proteins, as well as the role of various cellular organelles in this process. It is generally appreciated, however, that information is still limited about details of the early phases of biosynthesis and the specific function of cellular elements in hormone processing. Current theories concerning the possible function of precursors in cellular biosynthesis of proteins destined for secretion indicate that prehormones with their hydrophobic leader sequences may serve a critical cellular role as short-lived intermediates that direct the

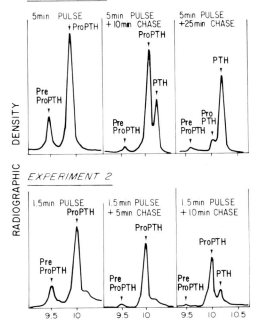

EXPERIMENT 1

EXPERIMENT 2

DISTANCE FROM ORIGIN (cm)

32–5 Electrophoretic patterns obtained from polyacrylamide gels of labeled proteins with radioactivity intensity of each band recorded by densitometric tracing of exposed x-ray film in extracts of parathyroid gland slices incubated for the times indicated. The pulse incubations were done with [^{35}S]methionine. Results in the lower panel (Experiment 2) show that there is no detectable PTH until 11.5 min after initiating pulse–chase analysis; upper panel results indicate that PTH is not the predominant form of radioactive protein until 30 min.

transport of hormone from the site of synthesis in the cytosol on the polyribosomes of the endoplasmic reticulum, across the endoplasmic reticular membrane into the interior of the cisternae—the inferior, extracytosolic space within the reticular channels (Fig. 32–4A and B). The theory predicts that after such transmembrane transport, the secretory proteins are protected and directed through the cisternal space to the site of hormone packaging in granules in the Golgi complex. Subsequently, the secretory granules are translocated to the cell membrane for release by granule rupture to the cell exterior and entry into the circulation (Fig. 32–4B). Recently, histological studies were undertaken to examine

directly the cellular sites involved in hormone synthesis, modification, and secretion. Serial studies with tissue slices were performed by autoradiography after pulse-labeling of PTH precursors by incorporation of radioactive amino acids. The locations of radioactivity detected by autoradiographs in various portions of the cytoplasm of the cells were studied as a function of time after initial incubation. The studies were combined with extraction of other aliquots of the same tissue incubates to determine with gel analytical systems the rates of formation of pre-proPTH and proPTH, as well as the rate of the interconversion of the precursor forms to PTH (Fig. 32–5). Such studies afford the opportunity to test the Palade hypothesis that synthesis of all secreted proteins, including hormones generally and PTH specifically, begins on the endoplasmic reticulum. The newly synthesized hormone, such as PTH, is subsequently transported through the cells to the Golgi apparatus and finally incorporated into secretory granules. At the completion of a cycle of synthesis and packaging, these granules should be found in mature form at the periphery of the cell under the cell membrane. This hypothesis was confirmed. At the end of 5 min of pulse-labeling, which results in the incorporation of radioactivity into newly synthesized hormonal protein, all of the radioactive counts are detected in the region of the endoplasmic reticulum (Fig. 32–6). At this time, only prehormone and prohormone are detected on analytical gels (Fig. 32–5). (There is less prehormone than prohormone because the former is so rapidly converted to the latter.) At 10 min after completion of the pulse labeling, counts are first detected in abundance in the region of the Golgi apparatus (Fig. 32–7A and B). At this time, PTH is first detected, as well as proPTH on analytical gels; pre-proPTH is no longer detected (Fig. 32–5). At 55 min after the pulse, most of the counts are present in mature secretory granules, many of which are found just underneath the cell membrane (Fig. 32–8). After 25 min the analytical gels show principally PTH. Thus, excellent temporal correlation was found in these studies between the cellular location predicted by the Palade formulation of hormonal precursors and the rates of interconversion of prehormone to prohormone to hormone as analyzed by electrophoresis of labeled hormone extracted from the tissues at the same time periods that ultrastructural autoradiography was performed. Studies of this type provide the first opportunity

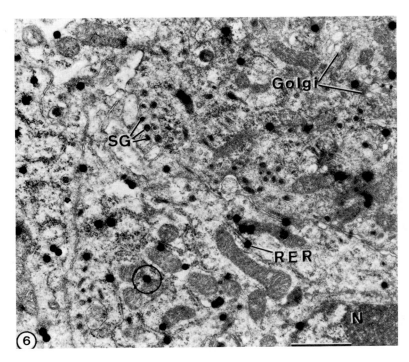

32–6 Autoradiograph of parathyroid cells at the end of a 5-min pulse of [³H]leucine. The three main intracellular membrane compartments of the parathyroid cell are identified: rough endoplasmic reticulum **(RER)**, Golgi apparatus, and secretory granules **(SG)**. At this time, many autoradiographic grains **(black dots)** relate to RER cisternae. Around one developed grain, the probability circle, used for quantitative evaluation of the labeling, has been drawn. **N**, nucleus. Bar, 1 μm; × 21,800.

to make careful functional correlations between hormonal production and the function of cell organelles in initial synthesis and sequential transformation of biosynthetic precursors. Figure 32–4B summarizes these overall concepts concerning the synthesis of PTH. Pre-proparathyroid hormone made initially on the ribosomes in the rough endoplasmic reticulum is converted within seconds of synthesis, perhaps even before the parathyroid polypeptide chain is completed, to proPTH. The additional hydrophobic sequence in the prehormone apparently serves an important intracellular function in securing attachment of the ribosomes to the endoplasmic reticulum, facilitating the transfer of the hormone from the cytosol where it is synthesized to the protected extracytosolic space within the endoplasmic reticulum so that directed transport and packaging can be accomplished. The prehormone is then discharged down the cisternal space of the endoplasmic reticulum and reaches the Golgi apparatus at about 15 to 20 min. At this point, conversion of the prohormone by proteolytic enzymes results in the initial appearance of PTH; hormone thereafter is found in progressively more mature membrane-limited granules. After 55 min have elapsed from initial pulsing,

when counts are abundant in mature, membrane-limited granules, other studies have established that the first appearance of radioactive amino acids is detected in hormone secreted from all parathyroid tissue slices. This correlative temporal evidence linking the time of appearance of radioactive counts in membrane-limited granules with hormone secreted into the medium around the cells, plus immunocytolocalization studies with antisera to the hormone that have shown specific antibody staining of the membrane-limited granules, have provided the needed verification that these granules indeed contain hormone and are involved in the secretory process.

Pathophysiology of the Parathyroid Glands

A failure of normal production or secretion of PTH results in a state of calcium deficiency called hypoparathyroidism. Such disorders are very rare in clinical medicine. Patients have a low blood calcium (hypocalcemia) and a high blood phosphate (hyperphosphatemia). Multiple symptoms are attributable to the hypocalcemia, including spasms of skeletal and bronchial musculature and convulsions. The nature of the

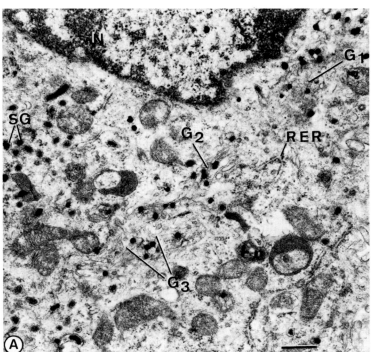

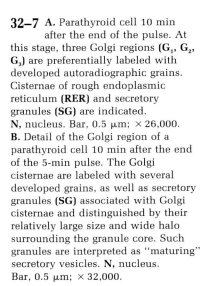

32–7 A. Parathyroid cell 10 min after the end of the pulse. At this stage, three Golgi regions **(G₁, G₂, G₃)** are preferentially labeled with developed autoradiographic grains. Cisternae of rough endoplasmic reticulum **(RER)** and secretory granules **(SG)** are indicated. **N,** nucleus. Bar, 0.5 μm; × 26,000. **B.** Detail of the Golgi region of a parathyroid cell 10 min after the end of the 5-min pulse. The Golgi cisternae are labeled with several developed grains, as well as secretory granules **(SG)** associated with Golgi cisternae and distinguished by their relatively large size and wide halo surrounding the granule core. Such granules are interpreted as "maturing" secretory vesicles. **N,** nucleus. Bar, 0.5 μm; × 32,000.

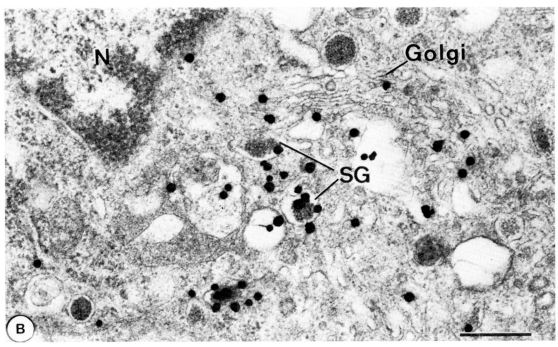

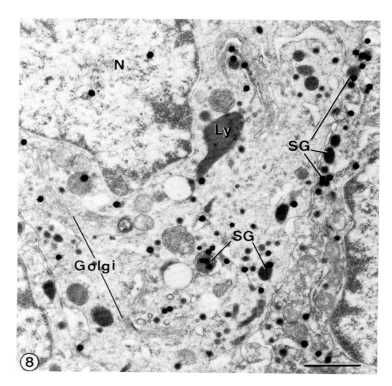

32–8 Parathyroid cell 55 min after the end of the 5-min pulse. This time point is characterized by the presence of numerous labeled secretory granules **(SG)**, several of them marginated at the cell periphery. A moderate degree of Golgi labeling is still present. **N,** nucleus; **ly,** lysosome. Bar, 1 μm; × 21,000.

cellular defects in hormone synthesis and processing, which presumably explain the hypoparathyroid state, are not understood.

The more important clinical issue, owing to a substantial frequency of occurrence (one new case per 1,000 people per year), is hyperparathyroidism. Hyperparathyroidism refers to a clinical state in which there is continued excessive production of PTH; hormone production is no longer responsive to the control by calcium levels in blood that normally regulate secretion and production according to need. As a result of continued overproduction of hormone, patients develop hypercalcemia, hypophosphatemia, and a number of deleterious consequences that result from abnormalities in mineral ion concentration such as excessive bone destruction and calcium deposits in the urinary tract (kidney stones). The pathological defect in the parathyroid gland may be either an adenoma, which is a benign tumor involving a single parathyroid gland, or hyperplasia, involving all glands. Chief cells predominate in such diseased glands; fat cells and stromal elements are greatly reduced. Adenomas are much more common than hyperplasia. A sin-

gle adenoma is the cause of approximately 80% of clinically recognized cases of primary hyperparathyroidism; hyperplasia accounts for 15%.

Histopathologists note that one occasionally useful histological criterion in defining an adenoma is that the masses of chief cells, devoid of fat cells, that constitute the functioning core of the adenoma are surrounded by a capsule of normal tissue with a normal distribution of fat cells and connective tissue. In hyperplasia, on the other hand, the entire cut surface of the gland reveals replacement by chief cells.

A third pathophysiological defect in the parathyroid glands that is encountered in hyperparathyroidism is parathyroid carcinoma (accounting for less than 4% of cases). Parathyroid carcinoma is usually of low-grade malignancy and recurrence is rare after the tumor is removed. Occasionally, however, especially if the capsule of the gland is ruptured during surgical excision, there may be local seeding of metastases in the lymph nodes of the neck or, rarely, hematogenous spread of the tumor.

The histological criteria associated with carcinoma of the parathyroid include detectable mitotic figures (rarely seen in normal glands, adenomas, or hyperplastic glands) and an increase in fibrous tissue within the stroma of the glands. Such criteria alone, without evidence of blood vessel invasion, are diagnostic for parathyroid carcinoma.

References and Selected Bibliography

Cohn, D. V., MacGregor, R. R., Chu, L. L. H., Kimmel, J. R., and Hamilton, J. W. 1972. Calcemic fraction-A: Biosynthetic peptide precursor of parathyroid hormone. Proc. Natl. Acad. Sci. U.S.A. 69:1521.

Greep, R. O. 1948. Parathyroid glands. *In* U. S. Von Euler and H. Heller (eds.), Comparative Endocrinology, vol. 1. New York: Academic Press.

Habener, J. F., and Potts, J. T., Jr. 1974. Chemistry, biosynthesis, secretion, and metabolism of parathyroid hormone. *In* R. O. Greep and E. B. Astwood (eds.), Handbook of Physiology, sec. 7, vol. 4. Baltimore: Williams and Wilkins Co., p. 313.

Habener, J. F., and Potts, J. T., Jr. 1978. Biosynthesis of parathyroid hormone. N. Engl. J. Med. 299:580 and 635.

Habener, J. F., Amherdt, M., Ravazzola, M., and Orci, L. 1979. Parathyroid hormone biosynthesis: Correlation of conversion of biosynthetic precursors with intracellular protein migration as determined by electron microscope autoradiography. J. Cell Biol. 80:715.

Krebich, G., Czako-Graham, M., Grebenau, R. C., and Sabatini, D. S. 1980. Functional and structural characteristics of endoplasmic reticulum proteins associated with ribosome binding sites. Ann. N. Y. Acad. Sci. 343:17.

Palade, G. E. 1975. Intracellular aspects of the process of protein synthesis. Science (Wash., D.C.) 189:347.

Potts, J. T., Jr., Kronenberg, H. M., Habener, J. F., and Rich, A. 1980. Biosynthesis of parathyroid hormone. Ann. N.Y. Acad. Sci. 343:38.

Roth, S. I. 1971. Anatomy of the parathyroid glands. *In* L. J. DeGroot, G. F. Cahill, Jr., L. Martini, D. H. Nelson, W. D. Odell, J. T. Potts, Jr., E. Steinberger, and A. I. Winegrad (eds.), Endocrinology, vol 2. New York: Grune and Stratton, p. 587.

Roth, S. I. 1971. Recent advances in parathyroid gland pathology. Am. J. Med. 50:612.

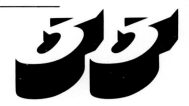

The Adrenal Gland

John A. Long

The adrenal glands constitute one of the major homeostatic organs of the mammalian body. They are composed of two separate endocrine organs that differ in embryological origin, type of secretion, and function. In mammals, the two organs are arranged as an outer cortex and an inner medulla surrounded by a common capsule (Fig. 33–1). In the other vertebrate classes, the two tissues may be completely unassociated or intermingled to a greater or lesser degree. In these cases, the homolog of the mammalian medulla is called *chromaffin tissue*, whereas the tissue corresponding to the cortex of mammals is called *interrenal tissue*.

The cortex, whose secretory rate is controlled by hormones produced in the adenohypophysis and the kidney, produces steroid hormones that affect carbohydrate and protein metabolism, resistance to physiological stresses, and electrolyte distribution. The medulla, under nervous control, secretes catecholamines that affect heart rate and smooth muscle function in blood vessels and the viscera; various aspects of carbohydrate and lipid metabolism are also influenced by catecholamines.

It is convenient to describe the two components of the gland separately; it should be kept in mind, however, that there appears to be a phylogenetic trend toward the more intimate structural relationship between the two glandular tissues as seen in mammals. In addition, an interesting functional relationship has been described, which will be discussed below.

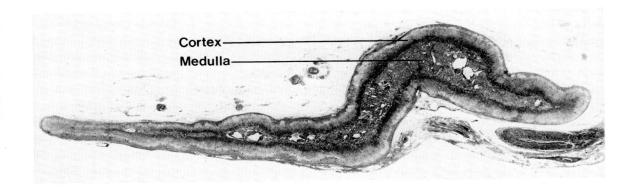

Cortex

Medulla

Gross Anatomy

The adrenal glands (called *suprarenal glands* in human beings because of their upright posture) lie retroperitoneally near the anterior poles of the kidneys and embedded in the perirenal adipose tissue. The right and left glands have somewhat different shapes in human beings, the left gland being somewhat broader. The combined weight of the adrenals from human adults dying immediately of accidental causes is about 8 g. It should be remembered that both weight and size of the glands vary considerably with age and physiological condition of the organism. In gross section, the cortex, which constitutes the largest part of the gland, appears yellow because of the presence of lipids. The medulla, which represents approximately 10% of the weight of the adrenal gland is reddish or brown.

Blood Supply

Three main groups of arteries supply the human adrenal gland: (1) superior suprarenal arteries, which arise as branches of the inferior phrenic artery and are the major blood supply, (2) middle suprarenals arising from the aorta, and (3) inferior suprarenals, which arise from the renal artery (Fig. 33–2). The adrenal arteries form a plexus in the capsule from which three types of intraglandular vessels arise: (1) Arteriae capsulae supply the connective tissue capsule of the organ. (2) Arteriae corticis arise from the capsular plexus by repeated branching and then descend into the cortex to break up into the capillary bed supplying the cortical parenchyma. These capillaries anastomose in the inner cortex and empty into the medullary vascular bed via relatively few small channels. (3) Arteriae medullae pene-

33–1 Section of a human adrenal gland. The cortex is of uniform thickness and surrounds the medulla, which is more variable in thickness. × 4.

trate the cortex via connective tissue trabeculae and directly supply the medullary tissue (Fig. 33–3).

Thus, the medulla has two blood supplies—one via the cortical capillaries and the other directly from the medullary arteries. Several orders of venules ultimately join to form the large central vein, which in human beings has conspicuous bundles of longitudinally oriented smooth muscle in the intraglandular portions of its wall. The adrenal vein exits at the hilum of the gland and on the left side empties into the left renal

33–2 Diagram of the major arterial supply and venous drainage of the human adrenal gland.

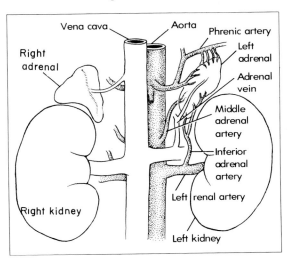

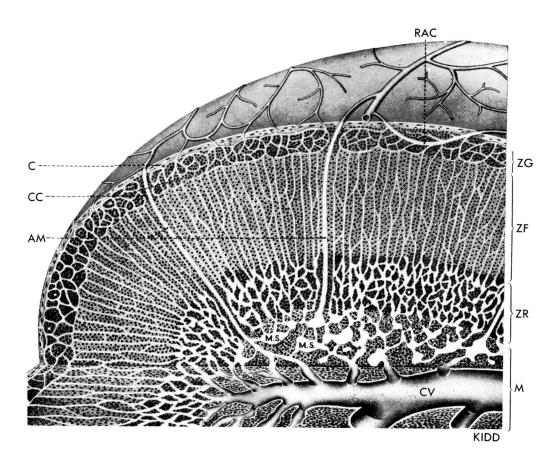

33–3 Stereogram of a mammalian adrenal gland
    showing the medulla **(M)** with its central vein
(CV), and the cortex with its three zones, the zona
glomerulosa **(ZG)**, zona fasciculata **(ZF)**, and zona
reticularis **(ZR)** enclosed by the capsule **(C)**. Two
arteriae medullae **(AM)** and an arteria corticis **(RAC)**
are shown. (Reproduced by permission from Harrison,
R. G. 1959. A Textbook of Human Embryology, 1st ed.
Oxford: Blackwell Scientific Publications, Ltd.)

vein; the right adrenal vein joins the vena cava
directly.

Lymphatics

The lymphatic drainage is not well delineated,
but it appears that the capsule possesses a set of
lymphatics that pass out along the adrenal arteries; the central vein has a separate set that follows this vein to the exterior of the gland. No
small lymphatic vessels have been detected
within the parenchyma of the adrenal gland.

Innervation

The main innervation of the adrenal gland is
composed of preganglionic sympathetic fibers
arising from T_8 to T_{11} and passing to the gland
via the greater and lesser splanchnic nerves.
These fibers penetrate to the medulla and synapse with the chromaffin cells, which are thus
homologous with sympathetic ganglion cells.
There is no parasympathetic innervation of medullary parenchymal cells. Recent ultrastructural
studies have revealed efferent nerve endings
(possibly adrenergic) on a small proportion of
the endocrine parenchymal cells of the adrenal
cortex in several species including humans. Similar nerve endings are seen in the thyroid gland
and the endocrine pancreas. There is some evidence that these nerves are involved in the compensatory hypertrophy that occurs when one
adrenal is removed from a rat (Dallman et al.,
1977). There is no evidence that these nerves
have a role in the short-term secretory response.
If there were any effect, it would have to spread

from to cell to cell via gap junctions because very few of the adrenocortical cells are innervated.

Histology of the Adrenal Cortex

In all mammals except montremes, the adrenal cortex can be divided into three concentric zones, which were named zona glomerulosa, zona fasciculata, and zona reticularis by Arnold in 1866 (Fig. 33–4). These structural subdivisions of the cortex have functional implications that will be mentioned below. In humans, the zona glomerulosa accounts for approximately 15% of the total cortical volume, the zona fasciculata about 78%, and the zona reticularis about 7%. The gland is surrounded by a capsule composed of fibroblasts and collagenous and elastic fibers, as well as a few smooth muscle fibers in some species. Connective tissue trabeculae penetrate the cortex, carrying nerves and blood vessels to the medulla. Reticular fibers, which are continuous with the fibers of the capsule, form a meshwork around the parenchymal cells of the cortex and medulla.

Lying immediately beneath the capsule, the cells of the zona glomerulosa are ovoid to columnar in shape and are arranged in spherical masses or arcades. These cells are relatively small (12–15 μm in diameter), contain a single spherical nucleus, and possess a small amount of homogeneously staining cytoplasm in which a few small lipid droplets are suspended. In the adrenal of humans, the zona glomerulosa may be absent in restricted areas of the cortex; in these regions, cells of the zona fasciculata are found immediately beneath the capsule.

The zona fasciculata is composed of long, radially arranged cords that are generally one or two cells thick and are separated from adjacent cords by capillary vessels that form the blood supply of the cortex. The cells are larger than those of the other zones (approximately 20 μm in diameter) and are packed with numerous large lipid droplets in the living state. After treatment with the organic solvents necessary to prepare routine histological sections, lipids are extracted and leave spaces that give the cytoplasm a reticulated appearance and a poor affinity for the usual histological stains. These cells have sometimes been called spongiocytes or clear cells because of this artifact of specimen preparation.

The innermost zone of the adrenal cortex, the zona reticularis, is characterized by the disruption of the regular, parallel alignment of the

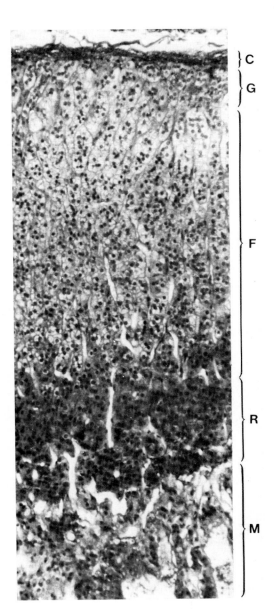

33–4 Cross section of a human adrenal gland, showing division of the cortex into three concentric zones. **C,** capsule; **G,** zona glomerulosa; **F,** zona fasciculata; **R,** zona reticularis; **M,** medulla. × 100.

cords of the zona fasciculata and the formation of an anastomosing network of cellular cords interspersed by capillaries. The component cells are smaller than those of the zona fasciculata and contain relatively few small lipid inclusions. Hence, the cytoplasm is compact and readily stained. Cells of this zone are notable for large accumulations of lipofuscin pigment, which is visible with the light microscope as golden-brown deposits.

Ultrastructure of the Adrenal Cortex

The ultrastructure of adrenocortical cells is similar in many ways to that of other steroid-secreting cells, including the corpus luteum of the ovary and interstitial cells of the testis. These similarities include a large amount of smooth endoplasmic reticulum (ER), numerous lipid inclusions, and the frequent occurrence of mitochondria with tubular or vesicular cristae. Despite these general similarities, cells of each of the zones of the adrenal cortex are sufficiently different to warrant separate description. Each cell of the zona glomerulosa has a spherical nucleus. The cytoplasm is full of smooth ER (Fig. 33–5), which forms a tubular, anastomosing network. A few profiles of rough ER are seen; most of the ribosomes are free in the cytoplasm, many being arranged in spirals and rosettes. Stacks of smooth

membrane-bounded cisternae associated with numerous small vesicles constitute the Golgi complex, usually seen close to the nucleus. A pair of centrioles is present. The mitochondria are usually elongated and the cristae are broad and flat.

Cells of the zona fasciculata differ from those of the zona glomerulosa in several respects. Most prominent is the large number of lipid droplets, which may be so numerous as to almost fill the cell (Fig. 33–6). Mitochondria are distinctive in this zone, usually being more rounded than those of the zona glomerulosa. Their cristae are short and tubular. The rough ER is well developed. It is common to find several cisternae aligned parallel to one another forming structures that may be seen, in appropriate light-microscopic preparations, as basophilic bodies. The plasma membrane is thrown into short, irregular microvilli over parts of the cell surface, whereas in other regions the membranes of adjacent cells are parallel and separated by a space of approximately 20 nm. In restricted regions, the membranes of adjacent cells are much closer together and form "gap junctions."

The ultrastructure of the zona reticularis differs slightly from that of the zona fasciculata. In the reticularis, mitochondria tend to be more elongate, and fewer lipid droplets are present (Fig. 33–7). Many membrane-limited inclusions

33–5 Electron micrograph of a cell of the zona glomerulosa of the human adrenal cortex. N, nucleus; M, mitochondrion; SER, smooth-surfaced endoplasmic reticulum; L, lipid droplet; LF, lipofuscin; G, Golgi complex. × 22,500.

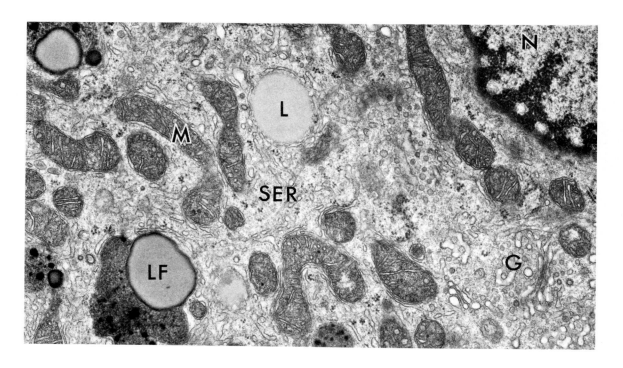

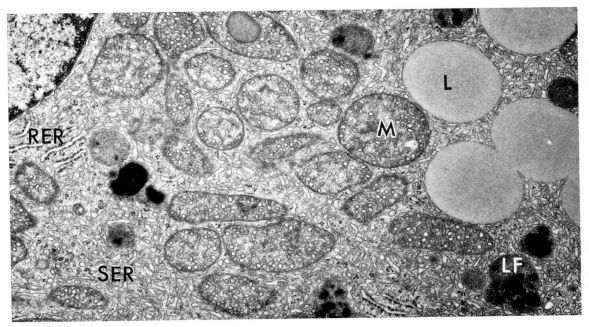

33–6 Electron micrograph of a cell of the zona
△ fasciculata from the human adrenal cortex. **M,**
mitochondrion; **RER,** rough-surfaced endoplasmic
reticulum; **SER,** smooth-surfaced endoplasmic
reticulum; **L,** lipid droplet; **LF,** lipofuscin pigment.
× 19,250.

33–7 Electron micrograph of a cell from the zona
reticularis of the human adrenal cortex.
SER, smooth-surfaced endoplasmic reticulum;
M, mitochondrion; **LF,** lipofuscin pigment.
× 32,500. ▽

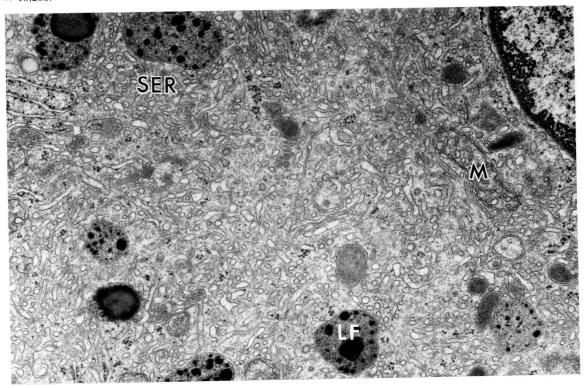

with heterogeneous contents are present. These structures correspond to the lipofuscin pigment granules seen by light microscopy. They seem to be accumulations of waste materials, some of which are probably oxidized, polymerized products of hydrolysis of unsaturated lipids. Acid phosphatase, a typical lysosomal enzyme, has been detected in lipofuscin granules. These granules increase in number with age; hence, their alternative names "wear and tear pigment" and "aging pigment."

Certain ultrastructural changes in adrenocortical cells can be observed when the rate of synthesis of adrenocortical steroids is caused to decrease or increase (for example, when the animal is hypophysectomized or injected with adreno-

33–8 Some of the cytological changes in typical lipid-containing adrenocortical cells **(A)** when their activity is stimulated or inhibited. **Left:** With stimulation, adrenocortical cells, their nuclei, and the nucleoli enlarge. With acute **(B)** or prolonged **(D)** stimulation, there may be a loss of lipid stores; with more moderate but chronic **(C)** stimulation, the lipid droplets become small and lose detectable cholesterol stores but retain a high titer of unsaturated fatty acids. **Right:** With removal of stimulus, adrenocortical cells, their nuclei, and their nucleoli shrink **(E to G)**. The lipid droplets apparently coalesce and gradually disappear. Initially there may be an increase in cholesterol concentration. Gradually both the fatty acids and the cholesterol stores decline. Both the severely stimulated and long-term inactive cells lack lipid stores; they are distinguishable only by size. (From Deane, H. W. 1962. *In* Handbuch der Experimentellen Pharmakologie, vol. 14. Berlin: Springer-Verlag OHG, p. 1, by permission from Springer-Verlag.)

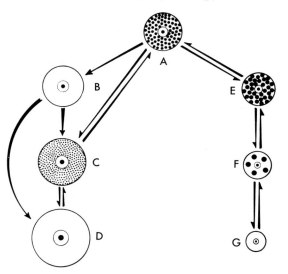

corticotropic hormone). When adrenocortical cells are stimulated, their cytoplasmic volume enlarges and the quantity of smooth ER increases. The fate of the lipid droplets depends on the degree of stimulation (Fig. 33–8). It is now appreciated that the minute-to-minute precursor of adrenal steroids is cholesterol derived from circulating plasma low-density lipoproteins (LDL) (Brown et al., 1979). These lipoproteins are taken up by adrenal cells via specific receptors in the plasma membrane. After internalization, LDL is hydrolyzed by lysosomal enzymes, freeing cholesterol esters that are subsequently broken down to free cholesterol and free fatty acids. This cholesterol is then used as a precursor for steroid synthesis when the cell is in the steady state. Upon acute stimulation by adrenocorticotropic hormone (ACTH), cholesterol esters stored in lipid droplets are hydrolyzed, yielding additional free cholesterol to satisfy the increased demand for precursor.

If stimulation by ACTH persists, new LDL receptors are added to the plasma membrane permitting an increased rate of uptake of lipoprotein. With prolonged stimulation, lipid droplets become smaller and may finally disappear altogether. When stimulation is withdrawn, as in hypophysectomy, there is atrophy of the cells of the zonae fasciculata and reticularis and a decrease in the quantity of smooth ER. Lipid droplets at first enlarge and coalesce, reflecting decreased utilization for hormone production. Eventually lipid droplets disappear altogether. Close study of adrenocortical cells has not revealed visible evidence for the mechanisms of intracellular transport and release of secretory products. Present evidence indicates that steroid hormones are not stored in large quantity in adrenocortical cells and that they are released continuously as individual molecules, not discontinuously in packets as is the case in many protein-secreting cells. A few workers have suggested that steroids are stored in granules and released by exocytosis. The evidence for this hypothesis is rather poor.

Capillary Endothelium

The endothelium of the capillary vessels of the cortex is of the fenestrated or visceral type (Fig. 33–9). The cell is quite thin except near the nucleus, where thickenings occur to accommodate the nucleus and most of the other cytoplasmic organelles such as Golgi material and mitochondria. Individual profiles of granular reticulum are sometimes found in the thin cytoplasmic exten-

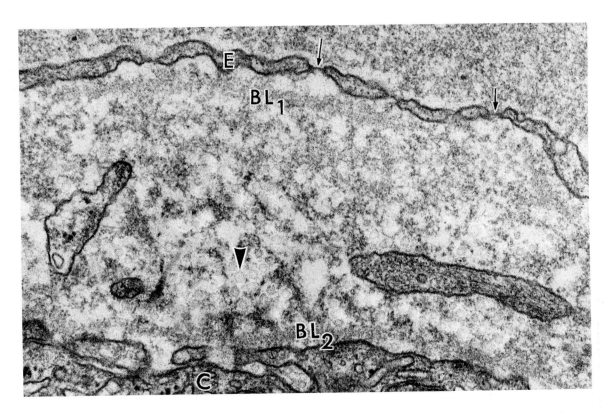

33–9 Electron micrograph of capillary endothelium in the human adrenal cortex. Endothelial cell **(E)** with fenestrae at **arrows;** basal lamina beneath endothelium labeled **BL₁**. Cross sections of reticular fibers are faintly seen at the end of the **arrowhead.** Basal lamina adjacent to cortical parenchymal cell **(C)** labeled **BL₂.** × 66,000.

sions. At intervals, the wall becomes so thin that it appears to be a single layer that lacks the structure of a unit membrane. These regions are termed fenestrae. A continuous basal lamina is present beneath the endothelium. A space that may be occupied by fibroblasts and macrophages is present between the endothelium and the endocrine parenchyma. There is no evidence that the endothelial cells of adrenal capillaries are avidly phagocytic. Therefore, these cells do not belong to the mononuclear phagocyte system (reticuloendothelial system) as is so commonly, but erroneously, stated in older works. Collagen fibrils with the characteristic 64-nm repeat lie subendothelially. They correspond to the elements demonstrated by silver-impregnation methods and are termed reticular fibers by light microscopists. A basal lamina is present on the surfaces of parenchymal cells that abut on the subendothelial space.

Histophysiology of the Adrenal Cortex

A wide variety of steroid hormones is secreted by the adrenal cortex. These hormones can be derived from cholesterol stored in the lipid inclusions as fatty acyl esters of cholesterol.

However, in human beings, the most important source of substrate for adrenocorticoid biosynthesis is cholesterol derived from LDL taken up from the blood plasma.

Although almost 100 different steroids have been extracted from adrenal glands of humans and experimental animals, only a few are normally released from the gland and are hormonally active. In human beings, the most important adrenal steroid is cortisol, an example of a class of hormones called glucocorticoids because of their pronounced effects on carbohydrate metabolism. Another member of this class is corticosterone, which is secreted in small amounts by the human adrenal gland but is the principal glucocorticoid secreted by the rat. Aldosterone is the most potent mineralocorticoid, so called because of the effects of this class of corticosteroid

1124

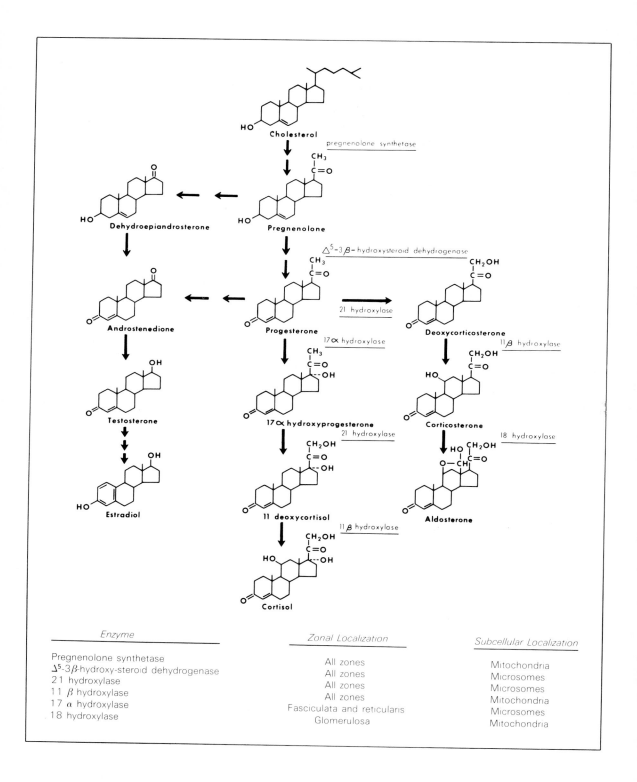

33–10 Diagram showing the pathways taken in the biosynthesis of the principal corticosteroids.

The zonal distribution and subcellular distribution of the most important enzymes are given in the table.

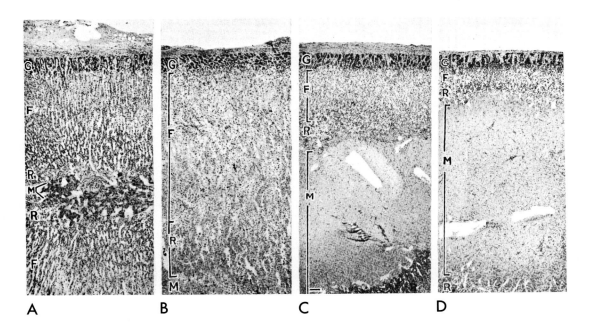

A   B   C   D

on electrolyte balance. A weak androgen (dehydroepidandrosterone and its sulfate) is secreted in large quantities by the human adrenal. The secretion of estrogens has not been unequivocally demonstrated and it is probable that the estrogens found in postmenopausal or oophorectomized women originate from the aromatization of precursors, such as dehydroepiandrosterone (DHA), in the liver and in adipose tissue.

The morphological zonation of the adrenal cortex is paralleled by an important functional zonation: cells of a given zone are specialized for the synthesis and release of certain classes of steroid hormones. Thus, aldosterone is secreted by cells of the zona glomerulosa, whereas cortisol and DHA are formed by cells of the zonae fasciculata and reticularis. There are some indications that the zona reticularis may be more active in androgen secretion than the zona fasciculata.

Steroid hormones are formed from cholesterol by removal of a six-carbon fragment of the side chain followed by a dehydrogenation at carbon-3 and a series of hydroxylations at specific sites. A simplified scheme showing the biosynthesis of the principal adrenal steroids is given in Fig. 33–10, together with the subcellular localization of the enzymes involved. Note that a precursor may move from one compartment to another (for example, mitochondria to microsome) several times before the final product is formed. How this is accomplished in a controlled fashion is not understood.

33–11 Sections of rhesus monkey adrenal glands.
A. Normal adrenal cortex. **B.** After treatment with ACTH. Note the increase in width of zonae fasciculata **(F)** and reticularis **(R)**. **C.** After treatment with cortisone. The inner zones are reduced in width. **D.** Hypophysectomized for 90 days. Extensive atrophy of inner zones. Note that the width of the zona glomerulosa **(G)** is the same in each instance. **M,** medulla. × 36. (By permission from Knobil et al. 1954. Acta Endocrinol. (Copenh.), 17:229.)

Control of Secretion

The adenohypophysis is essential for maintaining the structure and function of the adrenal cortex. If the pituitary gland is removed from an animal, a striking decline in the weight of the adrenal gland ensues and is paralleled by a decline in secretion of most of the adrenal hormones. Histologically, the inner zones of the cortex are atrophied whereas the zona glomerulosa is well maintained (Fig. 33–11). The hormone secreted by the adenohypophysis that maintains the adrenal cortex is ACTH. Adrenocorticotropic hormone is a polypeptide composed of 39 amino acids whose sequence is known for a number of species, including humans. The main effects of ACTH are to stimulate steroid synthesis and release, to promote growth of the adrenal cortex, to increase blood flow through the adrenal, and to cause ascorbic acid depletion in a few species, most notably the rat.

If ACTH is given to a hypophysectomized animal, it will prevent the decline in weight and secretory activity of the adrenal cortex that would ordinarily ensue. If ACTH is given to an animal with an intact pituitary gland, this hormone will cause a hypertrophy of the inner zones of the adrenal cortex and an elevation of the circulating levels of many of the adrenal corticoids. Adrenocorticotropic hormone will not cause a hypertrophy of the zona glomerulosa, nor will it increase the secretory rate of aldosterone except when given in large doses and then only transiently. It has been concluded that the inner zones of the adrenal cortex, the zona fasciculata and the zona reticularis, are regulated by ACTH and that the zona glomerulosa is controlled by a different mechanism. This evidence also indicates that aldosterone is formed only by cells of the zona glomerulosa, and careful microchemical investigations have shown that the enzymes necessary for the final steps in aldosterone biosynthesis are found only in these cells. The zona glomerulosa is found to hypertrophy if the animal is maintained on a sodium-deficient diet, but if a potent mineralocortoid such as aldosterone or deoxycorticosterone is given over a long period, the zona glomerulosa will atrophy and the other zones will remain normal.

If experimental animals or human beings are given large quantities of a glucocorticoid such as cortisol over a long period of time, subsequent histological examination of the adrenal glands will reveal a pronounced atrophy of the zona fasciculata and zona reticularis. For many years it was thought that the high levels of glucocorticoids directly suppressed the synthesis and release of ACTH by the adenohypophysis, which led, in turn, to atrophy. It is now known that an additional link in the feedback loop is present: the hypothalamus. Certain neurons in this region of the brain (specifically, the arcuate nucleus) are believed to produce a substance called corticotropin-releasing factor (CRF). Corticotropin-releasing factor was the first hypothalamic factor postulated to regulate anterior pituitary secretory rate. Recently, a 41 residue peptide has been isolated from sheep hypothalami and the amino acid sequence determined. This peptide elicits a dose-related increase in plasma ACTH concentration (Rivier et al., 1982). The rate of secretion of CRF is inversely related to the circulating levels of glucocorticoids to which neurons in the arcuate nucleus are exposed. The axons of these hypothalamic neurons end on portal blood vessels in the median eminence, which transport CRF to the adenohypophysis. Here, CRF stimulates the synthesis and release of ACTH. Figure 33–12 diagrams the feedback loop.

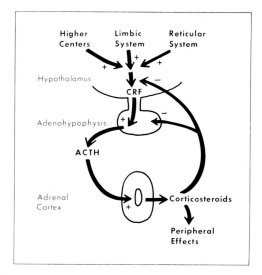

33–12 Diagram illustrating current concepts of the neuroendocrine control of the adrenal cortex.

The effects of glucocorticoids are numerous and widespread. Most cells possess cytoplasmic receptors for glucocorticoids that bind the steroid. The complex then migrates into the nucleus where it interacts with chromatin and, in some way, modifies the transcription of DNA into messenger RNAs. These RNAs then code for specific proteins that elicit the observed hormonal effects. In general, glucocorticoids are catabolic in the periphery (muscle, lymphoid tissue, skin, and adipose tissue) and anabolic in the liver.

Glucocorticoids cause inhibition of protein synthesis in fibroblasts and other cells, but protein catabolism continues normally or is increased. This mechanism provides amino acids that can enter the gluconeogenesis pathway in the liver. These hormones decrease uptake of glucose by such peripheral cells as muscle and skin and are necessary for lipolysis to occur under the influence of catecholamines or glucagon. Glucocorticoids enhance uptake of amino acids by the liver and appear to induce the formation of certain key enzymes for gluconeogenesis in this organ. The net result is increased glucose concentration in the blood (hyperglycemia), increased urinary nitrogen excretion, and fat loss.

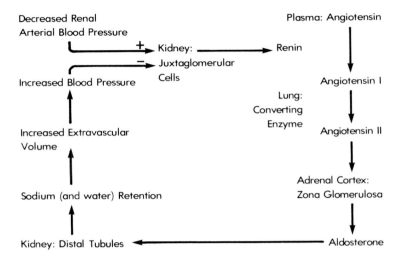

33–13 Diagram illustrating one of the mechanisms controlling secretion of aldosterone by the zona glomerulosa.

Glucocorticoids also depress the inflammatory response, and wounds heal poorly when high levels of these hormones are present. In order for the organism to cope with stresses such as burning, cold, or starvation, glucocorticoid hormones are necessary. Finally, glucocorticoids such as cortisol have a feedback influence on the hypothalamic neurons that produce CRF, as well as a direct inhibitory effect on corticotrophs of the anterior pituitary gland.

Aldosterone, the principal secretory product of cells of the zona glomerulosa, is a potent mineralocorticoid first identified in 1953. Aldosterone promotes the resorption of sodium ions in the distal tubule of the nephron, increases potassium excretion by the kidney, and causes a lowering of the sodium concentration in sweat, saliva, and intestinal secretions.

The rate of aldosterone secretion is regulated by the renin–angiotensin system, ACTH, and the plasma concentrations of potassium and sodium. The primary control system is the renin–angiotensin mechanism, which is a complex feedback loop involving the kidney (Fig. 33–13). The signal sensed by the juxtaglomerular apparatus is not certain. It may be a decrease in the degree of stretch of the juxtaglomerular cells themselves or it may be a decrease in the sodium load at the macula densa. In either case, this signal causes renin to be released from the juxtaglomerular cells. Renin is an enzyme that catalyzes the conversion of angiotensinogen, a circulating α_2-globulin, to angiotensin I. Angiotensin I is then converted to angiotensin II, which acts on the zona glomerulosa of the adrenal to stimulate the secretion of aldosterone. Aldosterone acts on the distal tubules of the nephron to promote sodium retention, leading to an increase in intravascular fluid volume and consequent increase in blood pressure. As a result, the receptor cells of the juxtaglomerular apparatus are stretched and the feedback loop is closed.

Adrenal Medulla

The adrenal medulla is composed of an endocrine parenchyma (chromaffin cells) supported by connective tissue elements and profusely supplied with nerves and blood vessels (Fig. 33–14). Ganglion cells are present but are usually difficult to find in routine sections. Chromaffin cells have been defined by Coupland (1965) as cells, derived from neuroectoderm and innervated by preganglionic sympathetic fibers, that synthesize and release catecholamines (epinephrine and norepinephrine). These cells show a brown coloration when exposed to an aqueous solution of potassium dichromate. This "chromaffin reaction" is thought to result from the oxidation and polymerization of catecholamines contained within granules in the cells. Catecholamines also form yellow-green fluorescent compounds after reacting with formaldehyde. This technique has been of great value in recent years for mapping the distribution of catecholamines in organs such as the adrenal medulla and the nervous system. Adrenal medullary cells also form a part of the widespread APUD system of cells. This system is more fully discussed in Chapter 29.

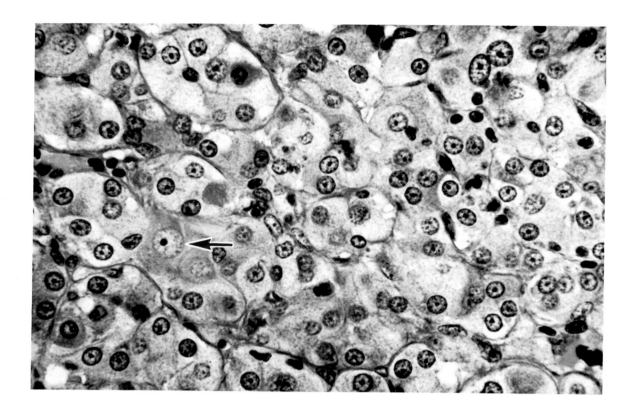

33–14 Photomicrograph of a section of the human adrenal medulla. A ganglion cell is indicated by the **arrow.** × 600.

Chromaffin cells are arranged as epithelioid cords in close association with vascular spaces. The cells are round, polyhedral, or in some species, columnar. In most species, the application of histochemical methods permits the identification of two types of cells, one of which contains norepinephrine and the other epinephrine. When viewed with the electron microscope, the most prominent feature of these cells is the abundance of membrane-bounded electron-dense granules, 150 to 350 nm in diameter, which are the sites of storage of catecholamines (Fig. 33–15). These granules also contain high concentrations of ATP, specific proteins called chromogranins, as well as soluble dopamine β-hydroxylase. After special preparative methods, it is possible to demonstrate with the electron microscope that two populations of cells exist. Some of the cells, which are thought to store norepinephrine, have granules of very high electron density, whereas most of the cells have granules

of lesser electron density and correspond to epinephrine-storing cells (Fig. 33–16).

Typical elongate mitochondria and rough ER are present in both cell types. A Golgi apparatus is situated close to the nucleus, and within the cisternae of this organelle a dense material may be seen. It is believed that the chromaffin granules are formed in the Golgi complex in a manner similar to that described for zymogen granules in pancreatic acinar cells. A few microvilli may be present at the cell surface, and a single cilium is probably present on each cell. Maculae adherantes occur as junctional complexes between parenchymal cells. Each chromaffin cell is innervated by a cholinergic preganglionic sympathetic nerve, the stimulation of which initiates the release of stored catecholamine (Fig. 33–17).

Morphological events accompanying the release of catecholamines are the subject of controversy. Some workers have reported that chromaffin granules retain their integrity and that catecholamine diffuses out of, or is actively transported out of, the granules and the cell. Others have reported that the granule membrane fuses with the plasmalemma and that the entire content of the granule is emptied into the extra-

33–15 Electron micrograph of an epinephrine-storing cell from the rat adrenal medulla. **C,** chromaffin granules; **M,** mitochondrion; **G,** Golgi complex. × 11,200.

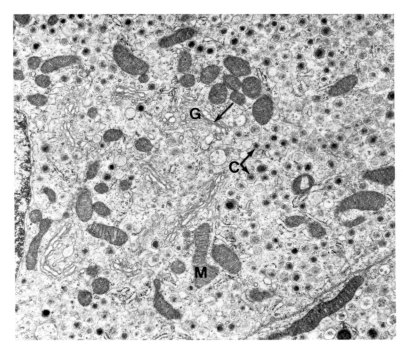

33–16 Electron micrograph to compare the chromaffin granules in a norepinephrine-storing cell (upper left, **NE**) and an epinephrine-storing cell (lower right, **E**) in the cat adrenal medulla. × 33,600.

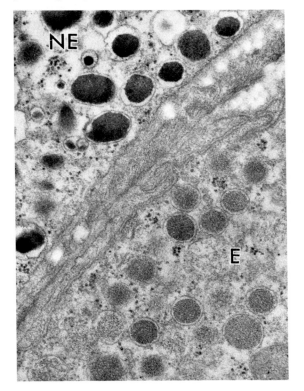

33–17 Electron micrograph showing cholinergic preganglionic fiber **(S)** ending on a chromaffin cell **(C)** in the rat adrenal medulla. × 34,700.

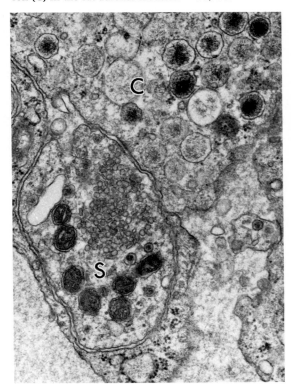

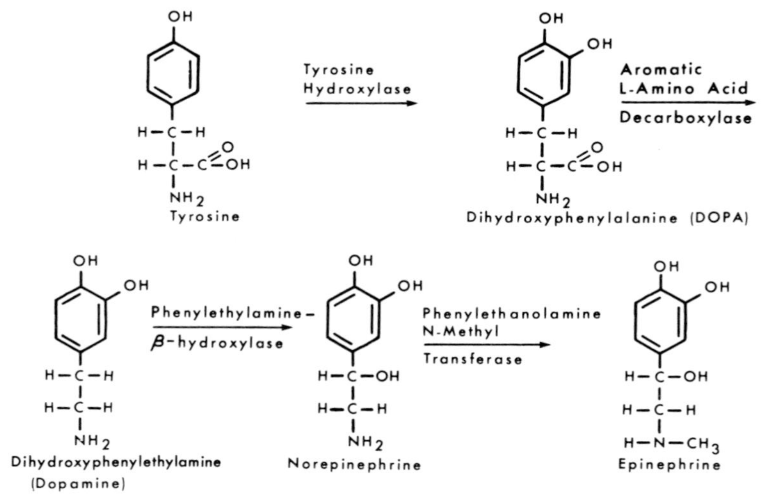

33–18 Biosynthetic pathway of catecholamines in the adrenal medulla.

cellular space and eventually enters the circulation (quantal release). Physiological evidence is consistent with the mechanism of quantal release.

As previously noted, the adrenal medulla receives a dual blood supply, one from the arteriae medullae and the other from capillary vessels that are continuous with the capillaries of the cortex. It has been reported that norepinephrine-storing cells are usually more closely associated with vessels arising from arteriae medullae, whereas epinephrine-storing cells are supplied with blood that has previously perfused the cortex and thereby contains a higher concentration of corticosteroids. There is evidence that phenylethanolamine-N-methyl transferase, the enzyme that transfers a methyl group from S-adenosyl methionine to norepinephrine, yielding epinephrine, is induced in the presence of glucocorticoids (Fig. 33–18).

In a hypophysectomized animal that does not secrete ACTH and thus does not secrete normal levels of glucocorticoids, the amount of epinephrine that can be isolated from the adrenal medulla declines, with a concomitant slight rise in the concentration of norepinephrine. In rat and rabbit fetuses, the accumulation of epinephrine in the adrenal medulla coincides with the initiation of adrenocortical function. If the fetus is deprived of its hypophysis by decapitation in utero, the rise in epinephrine content is not seen, but the levels of norepinephrine are above normal. Injection of ACTH or cortisol into the de-

capitated fetuses restores the normal ratio of epinephrine to norepinephrine. Comparative histological and endocrinological studies provide additional evidence for this interesting interaction between cortex and medulla. In the shark, where interrenal and chromaffin tissues are separate, norepinephrine is the main catecholamine, whereas in mammals where the cortex (interrenal tissue) surrounds the medulla (chromaffin tissue) the principal catecholamine is epinephrine.

The effects of the hormones of the adrenal medulla are widespread and will be considered only briefly here. Epinephrine causes the breakdown of glycogen to glucose (glycogenolysis) in the liver and skeletal muscle, with a consequent rise in blood glucose levels. Free fatty acids are mobilized from adipose tissue under the influence of catecholamines. Epinephrine causes an elevation of blood pressure, an acceleration of the heartbeat, cutaneous vasoconstriction, and dilation of coronary and skeletal muscle vessels, but vasoconstriction in other organs such as the intestinal tract. Under the influence of catecholamines, the threshold of the reticular-activating system of the brain is lowered and the subject becomes more alert. It can be seen that all these effects have an obvious adaptive value when the organism is confronted with an emergency situation.

Secretion of adrenal medullary hormones is under sympathetic nervous control. During sleep or narcosis, little or no secretion can be detected;

while the organism is carrying on normal activities, low quantities of catecholamines can be detected in the circulation. When the animal is exposed to pain, cold, anoxia, hypoglycemia, emotional excitement, or other stress, the secretion of catecholamines rises sharply and the homeostatic mechanisms mentioned above are brought into play.

Development

In 4- to 5-week-old human fetuses, mesothelial cells in the region of the dorsal mesentery and near the cranial pole of the mesonephros begin to proliferate and penetrate into the subjacent, highly vascular mesenchyme. Continued growth of these primordia results in bilateral organs that protrude into the coelomic cavity and become encapsulated. The gland becomes differentiated into two regions: an outer zone composed of small, compact cells, which will form the definitive cortex of the adult; and an inner zone of larger, eosinophilic cells, which is called the fetal zone (Fig. 33–19). The fetal zone constitutes approximately 80% of the cortex at term, but it undergoes rapid degeneration after birth; the definitive cortex enlarges and eventually becomes differentiated into the familiar three zones of the adult gland.

Chromaffin cells from the neural crest begin to migrate into the adrenal anlage at 6 to 7 weeks of fetal life and subsequently aggregate in the center of the gland to form the adrenal medulla.

Cells of the fetal cortex have the ultrastructural appearance of other steroid-secreting cells (Fig. 33–20). The smooth ER is elaborately developed, lipid droplets are abundant, and the Golgi complex is prominent. The mitochondria in cells of the fetal zone resemble those of the adult zona fasciculata. The fetal adrenal gland is under the control of ACTH secreted by the pituitary gland of the fetus. Anencephalic fetuses possess very small adrenal glands, and the fetal zone is lacking. The physiological role of the fetal zone of human adrenals in intrauterine life is slowly becoming clearer, but progress is hampered by the fact that only a few other species of primates have a comparable fetal zone.

The human fetal adrenal gland is a steroidogenic organ that is part of a "fetal–placental" unit. The fetal adrenal is incapable of carrying out certain steroidogenic reactions; in particular, the Δ-hydroxysteroid dehydrogenase system

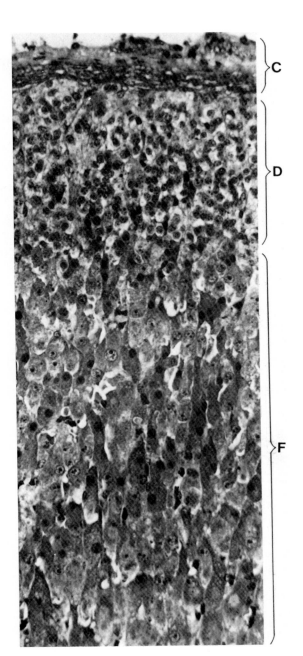

33–19 Section of a human fetal adrenal at 18 weeks of gestation, showing the division into fetal and definitive cortex. × 300.

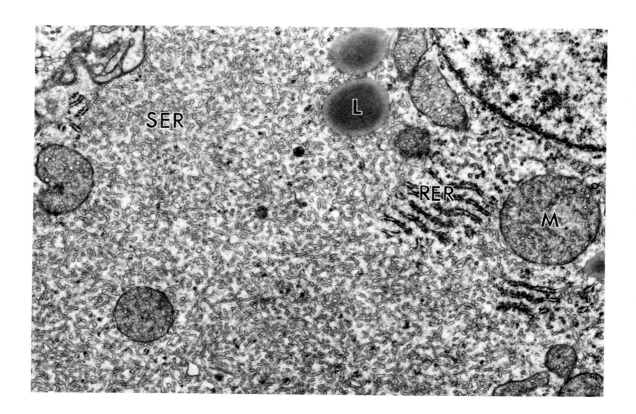

33–20. Electron micrograph of a cell of the human fetal adrenal cortex at 14 weeks of gestation. **SER,** smooth-surfaced endoplasmic reticulum; **RER,** rough-surfaced endoplasmic reticulum; **M,** mitochondrion; **L,** lipid inclusion. × 13,000. (Courtesy of N. S. McNutt and A. L. Jones.)

has very low activity in the gland. This enzyme is present in high quantity in the placenta. The products of this enzymatic reaction are transferred to the fetus where the adrenal gland carries out a series of hydroxylations that result in the production of cortisol, corticosterone, deoxycorticosterone, and aldosterone. A 17-21 hydroxylase is present that converts C_{21} steroids to C_{19} products, particularly DHA. This enzyme is not found in the placenta. A sulfokinase is present in the adrenal gland that converts DHA to DHA sulfate, the principal precursor of estrogens synthesized by the placenta.

Although much as been learned about the role of the fetal adrenal in steroidogenesis, the full biological significance of this activity during pregnancy remains to be elucidated.

References and Selected Bibliography

General

Blaschko, H., Sayers, G., and Smith, A. D. (eds.). 1975. Handbook of Physiology, sec. 7, Endocrinology, vol. 6, Adrenal Gland, Washington, D.C.: American Physiological Society.

Christy, N. P. (ed.). 1971. The Human Adrenal Cortex. New York: Harper & Row, Publishers, Inc.

Coupland, R. E. 1965. The Natural History of the Chromaffin Cell. London: Longmans, Green and Co., Ltd.

Deane, H. W. 1962. The anatomy, chemistry and physiology of adrenocortical tissue. In Handbuch der Experimentellen Pharmakologie, vol. 14 Berlin: Springer-Verlag OHG, p. 1.

Eisenstein, A. B. (ed.). 1967. The Adrenal Cortex. Boston: Little, Brown and Co.

Jones, I., Chester, and Henderson, I. W. (eds.). 1978. General Comparative and Clinical Endocrinology of the Adrenal Cortex, vol. 2. New York: Academic Press.

Symington, T. 1969. Functional Pathology of the Human Adrenal Gland. Baltimore: The Williams & Wilkins Company.

Specific

Baxter, J. D., and Rousseau, G. G. 1979. Glucocorticoid hormone action: An overview. In J. D. Baxter and G.

G. Rousseau, eds., Glucocorticoid Hormone Action. Monographs on Endocrinology, vol. 12. p. 1.

Black, V. H., Robbins, E., McNamara, N., and Huima, T. 1979. A correlated thin-section and freeze-fracture analysis of guinea-pig adrenocortical cells. Am. J. Anat. 156:453.

Brown, M. S., Kovanen, P. T., and Goldstein, J. L. 1979. Receptor-mediated uptake of lipoprotein-cholesterol and its utilization for steroid synthesis in the adrenal cortex. Recent Prog. Horm. Res. 35:215.

Dallman, M. F., Engeland, W. C., and McBride, M. H. 1977. The neural regulation of compensatory adrenal growth. Ann N.Y. Acad. Sci. 297:373.

Gill, G. N. 1976. ACTH regulation of the adrenal cortex. Pharmacol. Ther. B 2:313.

Griffiths, K. and Cameron, E. H. D. 1970. Steroid biosynthetic pathways in the human adrenal. Adv. Steroid Biochem. Pharmacol. 2:223.

Johannisson, E. 1968. The foetal adrenal cortex in the human. Its ultrastructure at different stages of development and in different functional states. Acta Endocrinol. (Suppl.) (Copenh.) 130.

Lanman, J. T. 1953. The fetal zone of the adrenal gland. Medicine 32:389.

Long, J. A. 1975. Zonation of the mammalian adrenal cortex. In H. Blaschko, G. Sayers, and A. D. Smith (eds.), Handbook of Physiology, Sec. 7, Endocrinology, vol. 6, Adrenal Gland. Washington, D.C.: American Physiological Society, p. 13.

Long, J. A., and Jones, A. L. 1967. Observation on the fine structure of the adrenal cortex of man. Lab. Invest. 17:355.

Migally, N. 1979. The innervation of the mouse adrenal cortex. Anat. Rec. 194:105.

Pohorecky, L. A., and Wurtman, R. J. 1971. Adrenocortical control of epinephrine synthesis. Pharmacol. Rev. 23:1.

Pollard, H. B., Pazoles, C. J., Creutz, C. E., and Zinder, O. 1979. The chromaffin granule and possible mechanisms of exocytosis. Int. Rev. Cytol. 58:159.

Rivier, C., Brownstein, M., Spiess, J., Rivier, J., and Vale, W. 1982. In vivo corticotropin-releasing factor-induced secretion of adrenocorticotropin, β-endorphin, and corticosterone. Endocrinology 110:272.

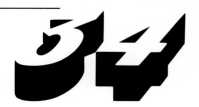

The Eye

Toichiro Kuwabara

The human eye is an approximate sphere, 2.5 cm in diameter. It forms an image of the environment on its photoreceptor layer, the retina, and transmits the information from that image to the optic nerve and thence to the brain. Human eyes have a wide range of motility. They can scan the visual field or track a moving object while maintaining precise coordination with one another. The histological architecture of the eye serves these optical, photoreceptive, and motility requirements.

The eye is often compared with a camera. The rigid box of the camera is analogous to the corneoscleral coat; the black lining of the camera is the uvea of the eye; and the photosensitive film of the camera is the retina of the eye. The mechanism for focusing differs, however, in that the lens of the camera moves back and forth, whereas the lens of the eye changes its accommodation by varying its convexity in situ. The diaphragm of the camera is analogous to the iris of the eye; both control the amount of entering light and the depth of field. With extremes of pupillary size at 2 and 7 mm, the f stop of the eye varies from 12.0 to 3.5.

The eyeball is positioned within the bony orbital socket, which contains the adipose tissue, extraocular muscle, blood vessels, and nerve fibers. Eyelids protect the anterior opening of the orbit.

Parts of Eye and Adnexa

The eye and adnexa lend themselves to the following divisions:

Protective Tissue

These tissues consist of *lids, conjunctiva,* and the surface of the *cornea* (Fig. 34–1). To them must be added *lacrimal glands* in the orbit and adnexal sebaceous glands of the lids. The orbital adipose tissue serves as a shock absorber.

Tissue Giving Form and Relative Rigidity to the Eye

This tissue is chiefly the corneoscleral coat, which together with the intraocular pressure maintains the relatively constant size and shape of the eye.

Nutritional and Light-Excluding Tissue

This layer lies just internal to the sclera and is called the *uvea.* Its major anatomic divisions are *choroid, ciliary body,* and *iris.* The uvea is heavily pigmented and vascularized.

Photoreceptive and Neural Tissues

These tissues are located in a membrane called the *retina,* lining much of the interior of the eye and connected with the brain by way of the *optic nerve* (Figs. 34–2 and 34–3).

Optical or Refractive Tissues

These tissues consist of the smooth anterior surface of the cornea (where most of the stationary refraction occurs), the *lens* (where the variable

34–1 Lids and eye. Noteworthy are the conspicuous folds of the upper lid, with the eyelashes coming from the anterior portion of the lid margin; the puncta **(arrows)** for drainage of tears; the white sclera covered by transparent conjunctiva; the iris with its characteristic radial structure; and the central black pupil. The cornea, being transparent, is not visible, but the central light spot reflected from the surface of the cornea indicates its smooth and convex surface.

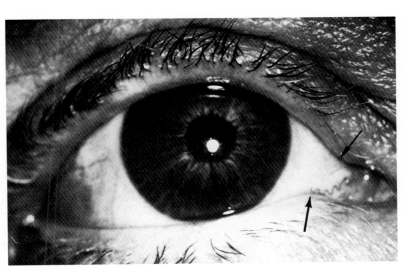

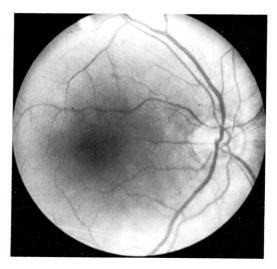

34–2 Ophthalmoscopic view of the interior of the eye. The nerve head, measuring about 1.5 mm in diameter, is the light, circular structure to the right of center. The blood vessels emerge from the center of this nerve. The smaller and lighter vessels are the arteries; the larger and darker vessels are the veins. The central, relatively dark area corresponds to the macula.

34–3 Schematic drawing of lids and eye. The interior of the eye has been exposed by removal of a calotte (section of a sphere) from the nasal side of the globe, as indicated in the **inset**.

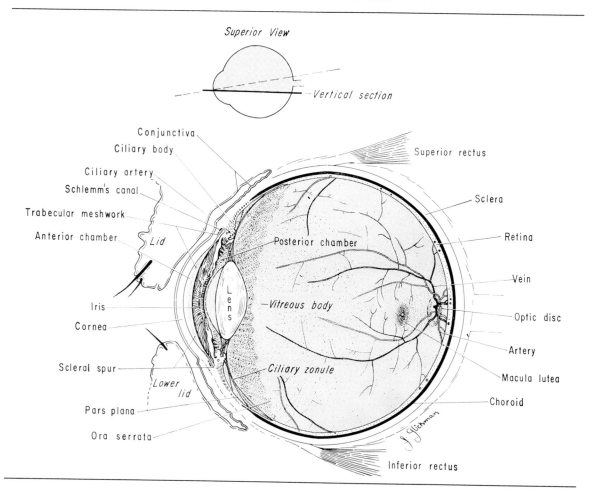

Superior View

Vertical section

Conjunctiva
Ciliary body
Ciliary artery
Schlemm's canal
Trabecular meshwork
Anterior chamber
Lid
Iris
Cornea
Scleral spur
Lower lid
Pars plana
Ora serrata

Superior rectus
Sclera
Retina
Posterior chamber
Vein
Lens
Vitreous body
Optic disc
Artery
Ciliary zonule
Macula lutea
Choroid
Inferior rectus

refraction occurs), and clear ocular media, consisting of *aqueous humor* in front of the lens and *vitreous humor* behind the lens (Fig. 34–3). Blood vessels are absent in these tissues.

Intraocular Fluid

Most of the fluid turnover in the eye occurs by way of the aqueous humor. This fluid is believed to be secreted by the *ciliary epithelium* into the *posterior chamber*, a pyramidal space bounded anteriorly by the iris, posteriorly by the lens and *zonular fibers*, and laterally by the ciliary body. The aqueous humor drains out of the eye at the periphery of the *anterior chamber* through the *trabecular meshwork* and *Schlemm's canal*.

Ocular Motor System

Each eye is provided with three sets of *extraocular muscles* that arise from the apex of the orbit (Fig. 34–4). The lateral and medial recti move the eye in the horizontal plane; the superior and inferior recti move the eye chiefly in the vertical plane but have a small torsional component; and the superior and inferior obliques have both a torsional component (increasing as the eye is turned outward) and a vertical component (increasing as the eye is turned inward). The two eyes are coordinated to move in remarkable symmetry.

The lids are provided with two sets of muscles. The *levator palpebrae* arise at the apex of

the orbit and open the eyes. The *orbicularis oculi* is a sphincter-like muscle within the skin of the lid and closes the eyes.

Development

The anlagen of the eyes are recognizable early in the embryo as a pair of lateral outpouchings of the diencephalon. As each pouch approaches the surface ectoderm, it invaginates to form an *optic cup*. The inner layer of this cup is destined to form the retina, nonpigmented ciliary epithelium, and posterior iris epithelium; the outer layer is destined to form the retinal pigment epithelium, pigmented ciliary epithelium, and anterior iris epithelium (Fig. 34–5).

The surface ectoderm overlying the optic cup thickens, invaginates, and eventually becomes the lens. The embryonic tissue surrounding the optic cup and lying in front of the lens then differentiates to form the outer structures of the eye.

By reason of this unique outpouching and subsequent invagination, the inner surfaces of the retina, ciliary body, and iris come to represent the basal surface of the tissue, whereas the intraocular contents (the vitreous space and anterior and posterior chambers) represent a modi-

34–5 Horizontal section of the eye and adjacent structures of a 7-week human embryo. **MR**, medial rectus; **LR**, lateral rectus; **ON**, optic nerve; **S**, sclera; **R**, retina; **V**, vitreous; **L**, lens; **C**, cornea. Note the hairpin folding of the neuroepithelium at the margin **(arrow)**.

34–4 Origins and insertions of the ocular muscles. (Reprinted with permission of Charles C. Thomas, Publisher.)

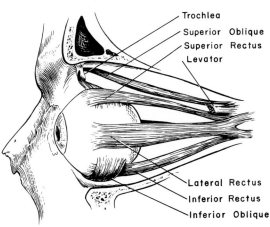

- Trochlea
- Superior Oblique
- Superior Rectus
- Levator
- Lateral Rectus
- Inferior Rectus
- Inferior Oblique

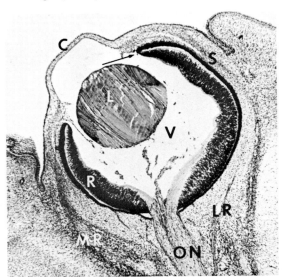

fied tissue space. During the embryonic period these spaces contain a rich vascular plexus, the *hyaloid system*, which disappears almost entirely before birth.

The invagination of the surface ectoderm has a similarly unique development so that the outer surface of the lens consists of the basement membrane.

By the third month of gestation the eye has already attained its definitive shape and structure. Differentiation of the neural elements of the retina occurs at a relatively late stage of gestation.

Lids

The upper and lower lids both protect and lubricate the anterior portions of the eyeballs. The skin surface is covered by stratified squamous epithelium like that of the rest of the face but the connective tissue stroma is more delicate and contains little fat. The superficial dermis also contains lymph vessels, sweat glands, and seba-

ceous glands (Fig. 34–6). Superficial muscle fibers, constituting the *orbicularis oculi*, are innervated by the VIIth nerve and serve to close the lids. The orbicularis muscle consists of bundles of fine striated muscle fibers. The transverse tube system is well developed in this muscle fiber. A small group of bundles of the similar striated muscle at the lid margin is called Riolan's muscle.

The deep stroma of the upper and lower lids contains a plaque of compact connective tissue containing large sebaceous glands that open onto

34–6 Vertical section of lids, globe, and orbit of a human adult. The upper lid has been somewhat displaced forward but otherwise shows an approximately normal relationship or structure. **UL**, upper lid; **LL**, lower lid; **C**, cornea; **AC**, anterior chamber; **I**, iris; **L**, lens (artifactually fragmented); **CB**, cillary body; **R**, retina (artifactually separated from choroid); **V**, vitreous body; **ON**, optic nerve; **Lev**, levator muscle; **MM**, Müller's muscle; **SR**, superior rectus; **CN**, ciliary nerve; **OF**, orbital fat. × 4.

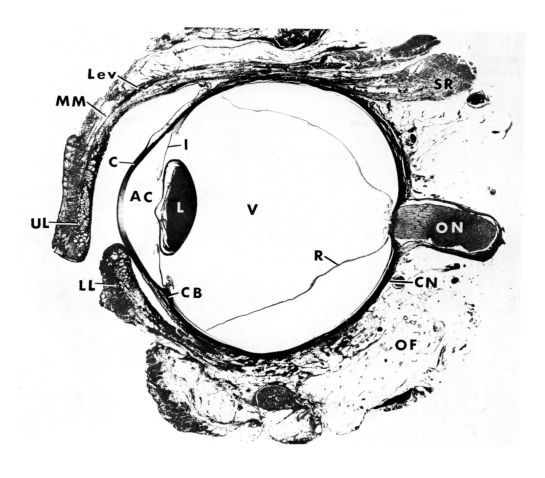

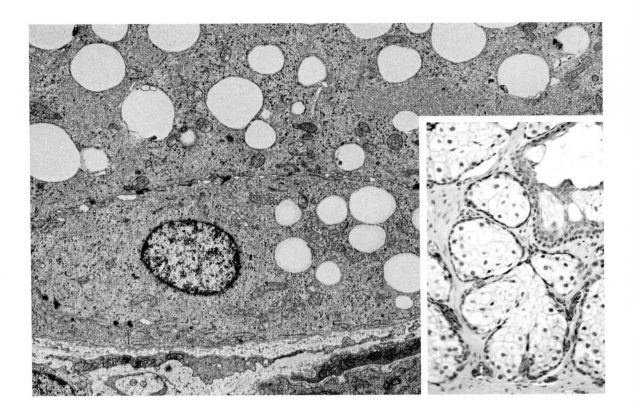

the lid margins. These plaques, called the *tarsal plates*, consist of compact collagen fibers and abundant elastica. The sebaceous structures within the plates are called *Meibomian glands* (Fig. 34–7); they secrete an oily material that seals the lid margins when the eyes are closed and prevents tears from overflowing when the eyes are open. Also, the lipid forms a thin film over the tear to prevent its evaporation. The glands consist of numerous alveoli that are connected to straight opening ducts and are arranged in a plane parallel to one another. Their orifices are situated slightly posterior to the row of the eyelashes. The gland cells at the margin of the alveoli are stratified epithelium, but the cells deposit abundant lipid droplets toward the center. Cells in the alveoli contain few microorganelles.

The levator palpebrae muscle that raises the upper lid inserts into the connective tissue in the subdermal zone and in the superior margin of the tarsus. Clusters of smooth muscle, *Müller's lid muscle*, intermingle with the striated muscle fibers at the anterior end of the levator muscle (Fig. 34–8). Similar smooth muscle cells are also present in the lower eyelids.

The lid margins mark the transition between

34–7 Meibomian gland. Electron micrograph shows a few cells in the basal portion of the acinus. Cells are joined to each other by desmosomes. Numerous lipid droplets are present. H & E stain. × 100; inset, × 7,000.

skin and mucous membrane. The stratified squamous ectoderm of the former becomes the mucous epithelium of the latter. The most noteworthy structures of these lid margins, however, are the *eyelashes*, which emerge from the anterior edge of the lid margin, and the 15 to 20 orifices of the Meibomian glands that open into the intermarginal space. The most medial portions of the upper and lower lid margins contain the orifices and canals that conduct the tears into the lacrimal sac and thence into the nose. These canals, called the *upper and lower canaliculi*, are lined by a stratified epithelium somewhat thicker than that of the conjunctiva.

The posterior surfaces of the lids are covered by a mucous membrane, the *palpebral conjunctiva*. The transitional zones where the palpebral conjunctiva is reflected onto the eye to become bulbar conjunctiva form cul-de-sacs or *fornices*.

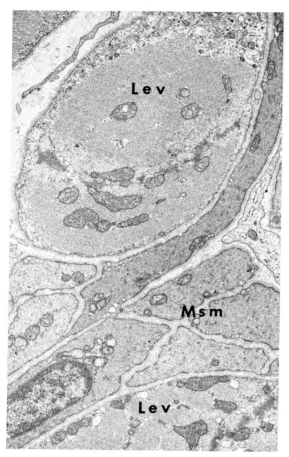

34—8 Anterior end of the levator muscle. Striated muscle fibers **(Lev)** are intermingled with Müller's smooth muscle cells **(Msm).** × 12,400.

Conjunctiva

Except for the cornea with which it is continuous, the conjunctiva provides the mucous membrane cover for the eye *(bulbar conjunctiva)* and posterior portion of the lids *(palpebral conjunctiva).*

Bulbar Conjunctiva

The epithelium of the bulbar conjunctiva is four to five cells thick, but the thickness increases to as many as 10 cells at the junction with the cornea. The epithelium of the conjunctiva is continuous with that of the cornea; the zone of transition is known as the *limbus.* The mucus-forming cells, *goblet cells,* are distributed in the epithelium and are especially abundant in the nasal angle of the bulbar conjuctiva. The folded conjunctiva is modified to form the *caruncle,* a skin tissue that contains hairs and sweat glands.

The epithelial cells are polygonal in shape and are loosely packed with a relatively small number of desmosomes (Fig. 34–9). Cell membranes are sparsely interdigitated and form intercellular spaces. The surface cells are held tightly with zonulae occludens. The cytoplasm consists of finely filamentous matrix and a moderate number of microorganelles. The goblet cells contain abundant mucin granules, rough endoplasmic reticulum, and Golgi apparatus.

Palpebral Conjunctiva

The palpebral conjunctiva has an epithelium only two to three cells thick and a variable abundance of subepithelial lymphatic tissue. The epithelial cells form large intercellular spaces in which wandering cells are commonly present. Intercellular spaces especially surround the tall epithelial cells in the fornix. Goblet cells are numerous in the palpebral conjunctiva (Fig. 34–10).

The subepithelial connective tissue consists of loose collagen fibers, occasional elastica, and abundant blood vessels, lymphatic vessels, and nerve fibers. The connective tissue has a great capacity for reversible swelling and congestion.

Cornea

The clear window comprising the most anterior portion of the eye is the *cornea.* In the adult it is about 11 mm in diameter and slightly more than 0.5 mm thick. Having a greater curvature than the sclera, the cornea has the gross appearance of a watch crystal (Figs. 34–1 and 34–3).

It is important, although possibly disappointing, to note that the cornea shows meager histological basis for its transparency. Except for the mucopolysaccharide stains, the corneal stroma is much like that of the sclera with no clear-cut demarcation at the limbus corresponding to the sharp optical difference that exists between cornea and sclera. The basis for transparency is physiological rather than anatomic: the optical homogeneity is maintained by a continual pumping out of the interstitial fluid across the semipermeable surface membranes so that the cornea is kept in a deturgescent state.

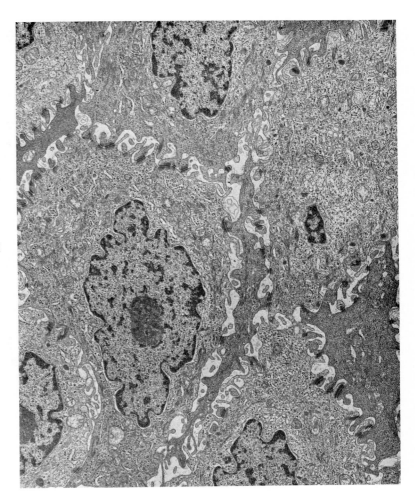

34–9 Bulbar conjunctiva. Polygonal epithelial cells are loosely packed. Cells are joined by a small number of desmosomes. Large intercellular spaces are present. × 13,300.

The histological composition of the cornea is notably uniform (Fig. 34–11). The constituent layers listed in an anterior-to-posterior direction are *epithelium*, *Bowman's membrane*, *stroma*, *Descemet's membrane*, and *endothelium* (or, as it is called by some authors, "mesenchymal epithelium"). The cornea is innervated, but totally avascular.

Epithelium

The epithelium, accounting for about one-tenth of the total corneal thickness, is five cells thick, with a uniquely smooth anterior surface (Fig. 34–12). The columnar basal layers have a robust basement membrane, as delineated by the PAS stain. Except for stratification, the epithelial cells show no differentiation toward either mucus formation or other specialization. However, the cells contain a large amount of glycogen. Mitoses are rarely seen in conventional sections but are readily found in flat whole mounts of the cornea.

By electron microscopy the epithelium is seen to consist of closely packed cells having a fine fibrillary cytoplasm with relatively few microorganelles (Fig. 34–13). The mitochondria are small and sparse. Only a small amount of rough endoplasmic reticulum and Golgi apparatus are present. The matrix contains a large number of glycogen particles, a moderate number of free ribosomes, and abundant keratofilaments. The cell boundaries show interlacing undulations and an abundance of desmosomes. The basal epithelial cells have numerous hemidesmosomes.

The superficial cells are nucleated and loosely attached to the underlying epithelial cells. The surface cell membrane has a structure of a fine vermiform ridge (Fig. 34–14). This structure may

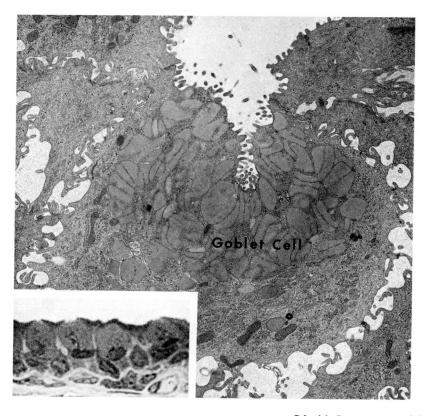

34–10 Palpebral conjunctiva. The goblet cell contains numerous mucin granules in the apical cytoplasm. Rough endoplasmic reticulum and Golgi apparatus are abundant in the rest of the cytoplasm. Intercellular spaces are extremely large. × 8,400. **Inset** shows light-microscopic view of the palpebral conjunctiva. × 400.

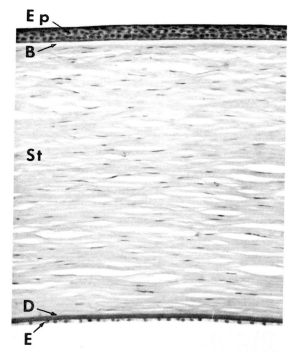

34–11 Cross section of the cornea. **Ep**, epithelium; **B**, Bowman's membrane; **St**, stroma; **D**, Descemet's membrane; **E**, endothelium. H & E stain. × 155. ◁

34–12 Anterior portion of the cornea. The ▽ epithelium shows columnar basal cells, polygonal wing cells, and flat superficial cells. **B**, acellular Bowman's membrane; **St**, stroma. × 380.

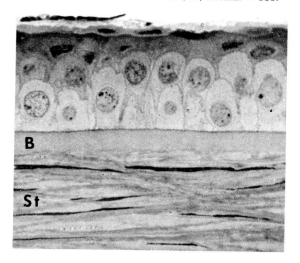

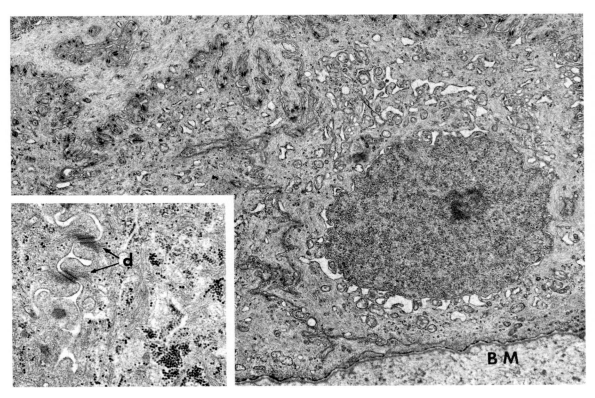

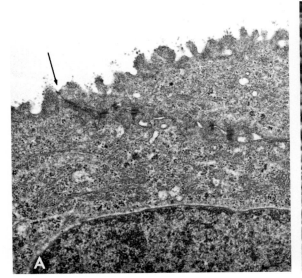

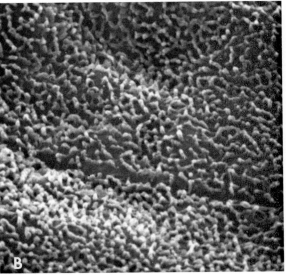

34–13 Basal cells of the corneal epithelium. The
△   lateral cell membranes are markedly
interdigitated and joined to each other by numerous
desmosomes. The basal surface is flat. **BM,** Bowman's
membrane. × 12,000. **Inset** shows details of the
cytoplasm: abundant keratofibrils; glycogen particles;
d, desmosome; membranous microorganelles are
sparse. × 30,400.

34–14 A. Superficial epithelial cell of the cornea.
▽   The most superficial cell is nucleated. Cells
are attached to each other by gap junctions **(arrow)**
and desmosomes. The cytoplasm contains rich
glycogen. The surface cells have fine ridges. × 20,000
B. Scanning electron-microscopic view of the corneal
surface. The surface is covered with vermiform ridges
except at the cell border. × 10,000.

aid in maintaining the moisture of the epithelial surface.

The corneal epithelium is richly innervated. The nerves enter the cornea at the limbus and lose the myelin sheath after passing through Bowman's membrane. The unmyelinated fibers reach the layer of the wing cell and end without forming any specific ending apparatus.

Bowman's Membrane

Named in honor of a nineteenth-century ophthalmologist and anatomist, Bowman's membrane is not a distinct membrane in the usual sense but is an acellular layer measuring approximately 30 μm in thickness. This layer stains negatively for mucopolysaccharide, but its other physical properties are similar to those of the rest of the corneal stroma (Figs. 34–12 and 34–15). It lies immediately beneath the epithelium throughout the entire extent of the cornea and terminates abruptly at the limbus. It is most highly developed in the human eye. Bowman's membrane maintains the optical smoothness of the anterior corneal layers. It consists of randomly arranged short collagen fibers and fine fibrils. The fibrils seemingly originate from the basement membrane of the basal epithelium (Fig. 34–15). The fine structure suggests that this layer is a newly formed connective tissue rather than a hyalinized stromal tissue.

Stroma

The *stroma* constitutes the bulk of the cornea and accounts for its characteristic shape and resistance. It consists of laminae of collagen fibers parallel to the surface, with *keratocytes* sandwiched between them (Figs. 34–11 and 34–16). When examined with the polarizing microscope, the corneal laminae, expecially in the posterior half, show a birefringence that differs from that of most collagenous structures in being unusually regular. Except for occasional wandering cells and inconspicuous nerves in its most anterior layers, the stroma shows no specialized elements. Specifically, no blood vessels, lymphatics, or other formed structures are present in the

34–15 **Left,** Bowman's membrane consists of fine fibrils and short collagen fibers. × 5,000. **Right,** higher magnification shows their randomly intermingled arrangement. × 30,000.

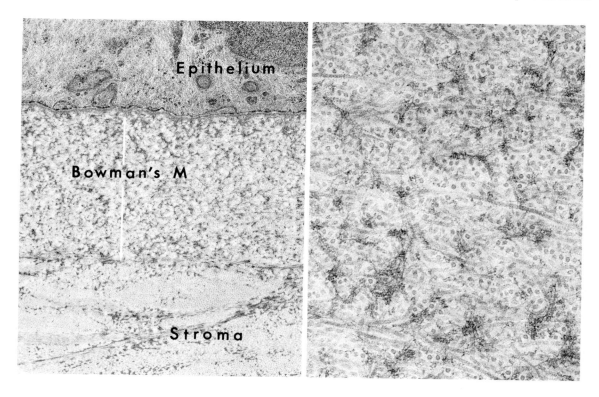

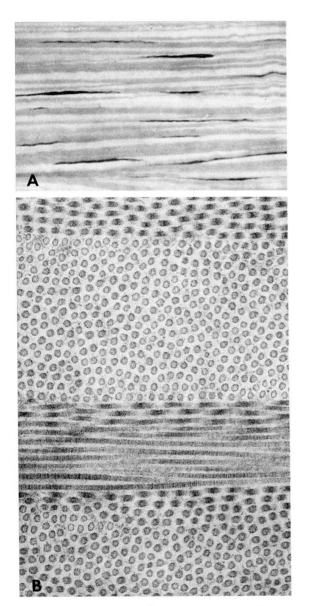

34–16 Lamellar arrangement of the corneal collagen fibers. **A.** Light micrograph of the central portion of the corneal stroma. Keratocytes distribute between lamellae. × 388. **B.** Collagen fibers are uniform in size (about 300 Å in diameter) and regularly spaced. Fibers are arranged parallel to the surface of the cornea. × 58,200.

normal cornea. The stroma stains, however, in a characteristically metachromatic fashion with toluidine blue and other thiazine dyes. The metachromatic substances, which have been identified chemically, are chondroitin sulfate and keratosulfate; they probably aid the reversible swelling properties (and transparency) of the cornea. These sulfated polysaccharides are not present in the sclera.

Collagen fibers are small (about 30 nm in diameter) and uniform in size. The 70-nm banding is present but not conspicuous by ordinary electron-microscopic staining. Abundant fine fibrils are present among the collagen fibers. Also, elastic fibrils measuring about 10 nm in diameter, often form bundles surrounding small elastin fibers among the collagen fibers. Collagen fibers form lamellae, approximately 2 μm in thickness, which are arranged parallel to the epithelial surface (Fig. 34–16). The lamellae in the anterior portion of the stroma are somewhat smaller and not so regular as they are in the central and posterior portion.

The keratocyte (stroma cell) is an extremely flat cell that projects stellate processes over a wide area. The cytoplasm consists of an electron-dense matrix in which moderate numbers of membranous microorganelles are present (Fig. 34–17). The amount of rough endoplasmic reticulum increases markedly in various pathological conditions. Small patches of basal lamina substances are present around the keratocytes, and the cells appear to attach to the collagen lamellae with occasional hemidesmosomes. However, the keratocyte easily changes its shape and location in pathological conditions.

Numerous macrophages and leucocytes are regularly present between the lamellae of collagen fibers. The phagocytic activity within the stroma is mostly carried out by these wandering cells.

Descemet's Membrane

Descemet's membrane, named for a Parisian ophthalmologist, botanist, and general physician of the eighteenth century, is an acellular layer about 10 μm thick, situated just posterior to the corneal stroma (Figs. 34–11 and 34–18). It stains lightly with eosin, lightly although definitely with elastic tissue dyes, but heavily with the PAS stain (like the lens capsule and certain other basement membranes). It does not stain metachromatically. When incised or ruptured, Desce-

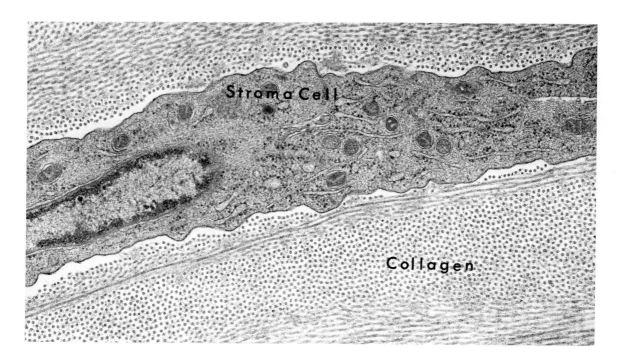

34–17 A portion of a stroma cell between collagenous laminae. The paranuclear cytoplasm contains rich mitochondria and rough endoplasmic reticulum. × 18,000.

met's membrane coils inward like a watch spring. At the periphery of the cornea it is frequently thickened by a bundle of circular fibers, forming *Schwalbe's line*.

The anterior border of Descemet's membrane is smooth and firmly attached to the deep corneal stroma. Its posterior surface is also smooth and attached to the endothelium, but wartlike excrescences develop regularly with age toward the periphery of the cornea.

Because of its coiling tendency, Descemet's membrane can take up slack with the reversible swelling of the cornea. Like the elastic lamina of blood vessels, it distributes tension evenly and prevents gross deformation of the tissue.

Descemet's membrane, which appears structureless by light microscopy, also shows little structure by electron microscopy. It is the thick basement membrane of the endothelial cell and is divided into two ill-defined layers (Fig. 34–18). The posterior half is made up chiefly of a uniform fine basal lamina substance, whereas the anterior half consists of aggregating fibril substances that are arranged somewhat regularly. The anterior portion of Descemet's membrane is considered to be an old form and it is absent in the embryonal and infantile corneas. The thickness of Descemet's membrane increases with age. Thick collagen fibers with a periodicity of 100 nm are often found in Descemet's membrane of senescent corneas. These fibers, thought to be a unique form of collagen, are common in the ocular connective tissue. Descemet's membrane becomes uneven toward the periphery, permitting processes of endothelial cells to insinuate into fine clefts in it. A deposit of lipid in the anterior half of Descemet's membrane is common in corneas of adults (arcus lipoides).

Endothelium

The endothelium, covering the posterior surface of the cornea, is a single layer of flat cells that appear as a regular mosaic of hexagonal cells in flat preparations (Fig. 34–19). Despite its thinness, the endothelium is an essential structure for maintaining normal deturgescence and transparency of the cornea. Mitoses are rarely seen, although the endothelium has the capacity for vigorous proliferation in pathological states.

At the periphery of the cornea, approximately 1 mm central to the termination of Descemet's

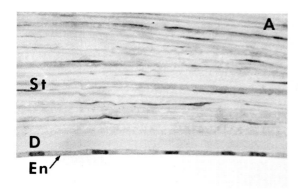

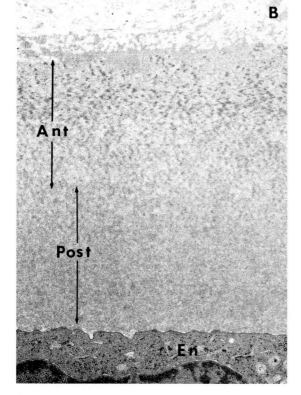

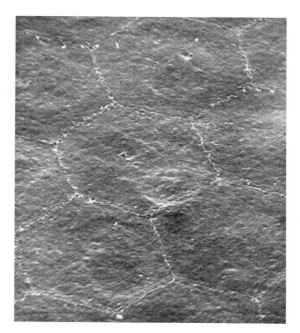

34–19 Scanning electron-microscopic view of the surface of the corneal endothelium. Hexagonal-shaped endothelial cells have a flat surface. × 4,850.

34–18 A. Posterior portion of the cornea. **St,** stroma; **D,** Descemet's membrane; **En,** endothelium. × 380. B. Two layers of Descemet's membrane. **Ant,** anterior; and **Post,** posterior portions; **En,** endothelium. × 15,800.

membrane, the normally thin endothelium becomes even more tenuous and then extends over the pores of the *trabecular meshwork.*

The endothelium consists of overlapping cells with marked interdigitations. However, desmosomes are seldom present. Cells are joined at the apical portion with zonulae occludens, but junctions are often small. In contrast to the epithelium, the endothelial cells are rich in mitochondria, vesicles, and Golgi complexes. Keratofibrils are absent in the cytoplasm. Metabolically, the endothelium appears to be the more active tissue (Fig. 34–20). Disruption of the endothelium causes sudden and severe edema of the corneal stroma.

Limbus

An imaginary line connecting the peripheral terminations of Bowman's and Descemet's membranes is the boundary of the cornea with the sclera. The region of this line is called the limbus; it corresponds to the abrupt optical change from the transparent cornea to the opaque *sclera.* Aside from the terminations of Bowman's and Descemet's membranes, it contains the sites of transition of conjunctival epithelium into corneal epithelium, the peripheral boundary of metachromatic staining of the corneal stroma, and the important trabecular meshwork in the angle of the anterior chamber.

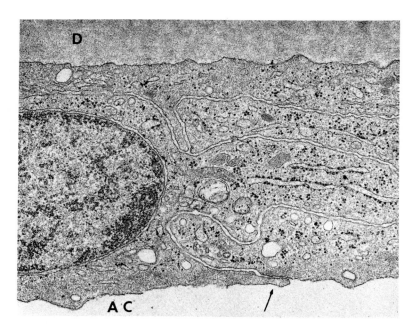

34–20 Endothelial cells have well-interdigitated lateral cell membranes. Apicolateral junction is not always conspicuous (**arrow**). The cytoplasm contains rich microorganelles. **D,** Descemet's membrane; **AC,** anterior chamber. × 28,600.

The corneal epithelium becomes seven to eight cells thick at the limbus and it gradually transforms into the conjunctival epithelium with the formation of intercellular spaces and basal infoldings. The subepithelial connective tissue, which contains abundant blood vessels, begins immediately peripheral to Bowman's membrane. The lamellar arrangement of the corneal collagen fibers becomes irregular, and individual collagen becomes larger as the fibers merge into the sclera. Numerous blood vessels and myelinated nerve fibers are present in the limbal sclera.

Trabecular Meshwork and Schlemm's Canal

Just peripheral to the end of Descemet's membrane is the *trabeculum,* or *trabecular meshwork,* that marks the site for drainage of aqueous humor (Fig. 34–21). The trabecular strands, which appear continuous with Descemet's membranes and endothelium, enclose spaces, called the *spaces of Fontana,* that communicate with the anterior chamber (Fig. 34–22). The central or axial border of the trabeculum coincides with Schwalbe's line and the peripheral border coincides with a prominent ridge, the *scleral spur,* from which the ciliary muscle arises.

Electron microscopy shows the trabecular strand to consist of central cores of elastica-rich collagenous connective tissue ensheathed by irregular amounts of basal lamina substances, and a lining of endothelial-like cells (Fig. 34–23). The covering of the trabecular strand is not always complete, and the connective tissue is often exposed to the meshwork spaces. Also, the trabecular endothelial cells form cellular bridges without forming prominent strands. The cell contains usual microorganelles and large vacuoles. Unlike other endothelium, cellular junctions and basal lamina layers beneath the cell are not striking. The trabeculae become less conspicuous toward the sclera and may disappear altogether, leaving a meshwork of connective tissue intermingled with numerous trabecular cells.

Anterior and lateral to the trabecular meshwork are one or more endothelial-lined channels coursing circumferentially about the cornea. These channels are collectively called *Schlemm's canal* (Fig. 34–22). They collect the aqueous humor that has filtered through the spaces of Fontana and that then passes out of the eye and into the episcleral vessels. The obstruction of drainage in these structures at the angle of the anterior chamber causes a pathological rise in the intraocular pressure and the eye disease *glaucoma.*

The endothelial cells of Schlemm's canal are uninterrupted and have prominent junctions. The cytoplasm consists of filamentous matrix

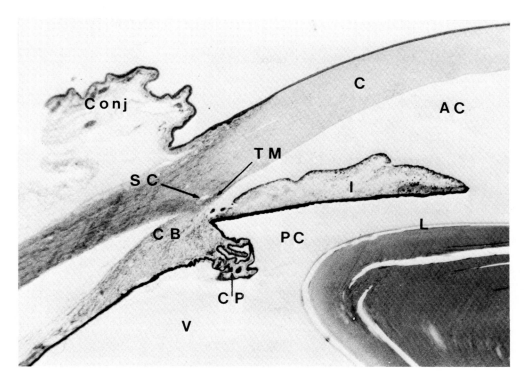

containing a small number of microorganelles. The cells that line the anterior chamber side of the canal have an appearance similar to that of the trabecular endothelium and have large vacuoles measuring 0.5 μm in diameter. The number of the vacuoles is variable. The cells covering the scleral side of the canal are thin and have spe-

34–21 Portion of the anterior segment of the eye. **C,** cornea; **Conj,** conjunctiva; **SC,** Schlemm's canal; **TM,** trabecular meshwork; **AC,** anterior chamber; **PC,** posterior chamber; **CP,** ciliary process; **CB,** ciliary body (artifactually separated from the sclera); **L,** lens; **V,** vitreous.

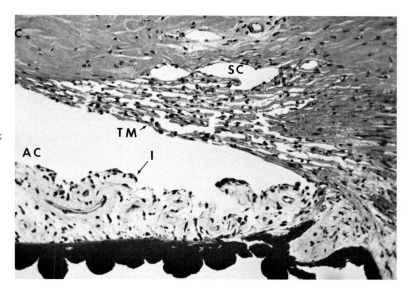

34–22 Angle of the eye. **C,** cornea; **SC,** Schlemm's canal; **TM,** trabecular meshwork; **AC,** anterior chamber; **I,** iris. × 180.

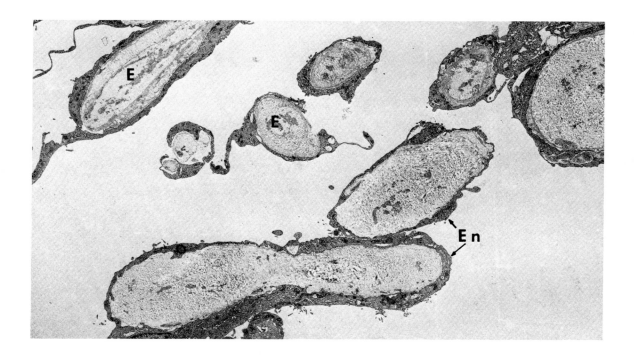

34–23 Trabecular meshwork. The trabecular connective tissue contains elastica **(E)**; **En,** endothelium-like covering cell. × 1,800.

cific structures. It is a moot question whether or not these vacuoles open directly into Schlemm's canal for passage of fluid and particles.

Anterior and Posterior Chambers

The *anterior chamber* is the area bounded by the cornea anteriorly and by the iris and lens posteriorly (Fig. 34–21). It has a depth of approximately 3 mm at its center, a volume of 0.2 ml, and a fluid turnover rate of 2 mm³ per min. The *aqueous humor,* which fills the anterior chamber, is a water-clear fluid containing most of the soluble constituents of the blood with an extremely small concentration of proteins (0.02% in contrast to 7% in the blood).

The *posterior chamber* is the pyramidal area bounded by the iris anteriorly, the lens and zonules posteriorly, and the ciliary body laterally (Fig. 34–21). The aqueous humor that fills the posterior chamber is believed to be secreted by the ciliary epithelium and circulates through the pupil into the anterior chamber. The pupillary

margin of the iris rests on the lens and thereby provides a ball valve that allows fluid to pass from posterior to anterior chamber but not in the reverse direction.

The posterior chamber is lined by the basement membrane of epithelial cells of the iris, lens, and ciliary body, and contains a large amount of filamentous material. In particular, the *zonules,* the posterior boundary of the chamber, form substantial bundles, although they are grossly inconspicuous. Because no apical cell surface bounds the space, the structure of the posterior chamber is not the same as the lumens of other cavity organs.

Sclera

The *sclera* is that portion of the outer tunic of the eye extending posteriorly to constitute about four-fifths of the eye's capsule (Fig. 34–3). With an average thickness of 0.5 mm, it varies from a maximal thickness at the posterior pole to a minimal thickness beneath the extraocular muscles. Like the corneal stroma with which it is continuous, the sclera consists chiefly of compact fibrous tissue and finely branched fibroblast-like cells. In contrast to the cornea, however, the collagenous laminae are less regularly arranged (seen especially well with crossed polaroids); there is more elastic tissue; blood vessels are present (especially at the limbus); the acidic mucopolysaccharides are absent; and there is no tendency to imbibe water.

The sclera shows several regional modifications. Abutting the limbus, the sclera contains a fairly rich plexus of blood vessels in anastomotic connection with Schlemm's canal and with the anterior ciliary vessels. The four rectus muscles insert in the superficial layers of the sclera at 5 to 8 mm from the limbus, and the two oblique muscles insert farther posteriorly. However, the most noteworthy modification is at the site of exit of the optic nerve. Here, the sclera is reduced to a fenestrated membrane, the *lamina cribrosa*, through which the nerves pass like filaments through a sieve. This "hole" has a diameter of a little more than 1 mm and is situated about 3 mm nasal to the posterior pole of the eye. It represents a weak spot in the sclera's resistance, and its fibers become bowed outward with abnormal elevations of the intraocular pressure (glaucoma).

Together with the corneal stroma, the sclera maintains the size and form of the eye. That this is of the utmost optical importance is evident from the observation that increasing the axial length of the eye by only 1 mm would cause a person to be severely incapacitated by nearsightedness *(myopia)*, whereas decreasing the length by only 1 mm from the norm would cause him to have a refractive deviation *(far-sightedness, hyperopia)* of the same magnitude in the opposite direction.

Uvea

The uvea is the pigmented and predominantly vascular coat of the eye. It consists of the *iris*, the *ciliary body*, and the *choroid*.

Iris

The *iris*, the most anterior portion of the uvea, extends from the angle of the anterior chamber to the pupillary margin (Figs. 34–3 and 34–21). It thus has the form of a disc with a hole in its center. Because of its reaction to light, it is properly considered the diaphragm of the eye.

The iris consists of a spongy *stroma* facing the anterior chamber, constituting the bulk of the iris, and a pigmented *epithelial layer* facing the posterior chamber and resting on the lens at the pupillary margin (Fig. 34–24). In addition, the iris contains a substantial *sphincter muscle* near its pupillary margin and a tenuous *dilator muscle* lying just anterior to the epithelium.

The tissue spaces of the iris stroma are continuous with the anterior chamber. There is no endothelium or epithelium at the anterior surface. No junctional apparatus is present between the cells at the anterior margin (Fig. 34–25). Collagen fibers often protrude into the anterior chamber through the wide intercellular spaces. Aside from the fibroblasts, the stroma contains pigmented cells of two distinctive shapes. One type, the melanophore, has elongated processes and melanin pigment granules in uniform sizes. Melanophores are most heavily concentrated along the anterior border layers of the iris. The number

34–24 Contrasting irises of **(A)** lightly pigmented (blonde) and **(B)** heavily pigmented (Negro) eyes. The former has a spongy stroma whereas the latter has a relatively compact stroma in which the pigment is concentrated anteriorly. The abundant blood vessels with their characteristically thick walls are seen especially well in the pigmented iris. The sphincter muscle forms a delicate lamina of smooth muscle fibers near the pupillary edge (to the left of center). Both irises contain a heavily pigmented epithelium lining their posterior surfaces.

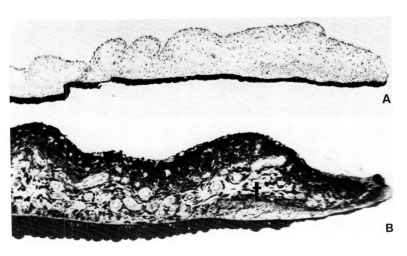

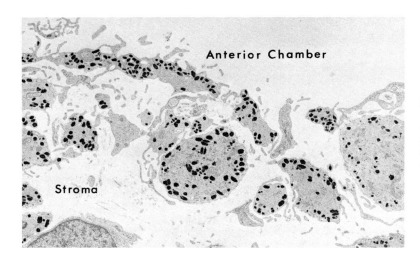

Anterior Chamber

Stroma

34–25 Anterior surface of the iris. There is no specific cell at the anterior surface. Tissue space of the spongy stroma is continuous to the anterior chamber. × 4,100.

of melanophores varies with the individual's complexion (Fig. 34–24). In dark-skinned people with brown eyes the pigment cells are abundant; in light-skinned people with blue eyes the stromal pigment may be absent altogether. *Clump cells* constitute the second type of pigmented cell in the stroma. They are round and more heavily pigmented and are more numerous toward the sphincter regions. These cells are phagocytes and become numerous in pathological conditions.

The blood vessels of the iris are noteworthy for having a thick, although not compact, layer around them. This layer forms a fibrous acellular "wall" that is unique for vessels of the iris. The blood vessel itself consists of a thin endothelial cytoplasm surrounded by a thin basement membrane and thin processes of the pericyte.

The *sphincter muscle,* which differentiated from the epithelial cells in the embryo, comprises a compact bundle of smooth muscle fibers arranged circularly near the pupillary margin. Muscle fibers are completely separated from the epithelial layer. The fine structure of the sphincter muscle cell is not different from that of other smooth muscles. It receives innervation for contraction from the parasympathetic ganglion in the orbit by way of the long ciliary nerves within the eye.

The *dilator muscle* is formed within the basal portion of the anterior epithelial cell layer (Fig. 34–26). There is no separated cellular layer of the dilator muscle. The apical half of the cell of the dilator muscle has all the characteristics of

the epithelial cell, but the basal half is markedly infolded and the cytoplasm contains smooth muscle elements. The muscle portion of the cell is ramified and covered with basal lamina. Numerous nerve fibers and their endings are present in the muscle tissue. Schwann's cells are often closely situated at the dilator muscle. Although the layer of the dilator muscle takes PAS staining because of its basement membrane, it is so indistinct that it can scarcely be identified by light microscopy. These dilator muscle fibers are arranged radially to the pupil, and they run the length of the iris except for the pupillary zone. They receive innervation for positive contraction from the sympathetic nervous system.

The dilator and sphincter muscles function reciprocally and provide an excellent example of the opposite action of the two components of the autonomic nervous system.

The pigment epithelium on the posterior surface of the iris, having developed from the anterior rim of the optic cup of the neuroepithelium, is a double layer of cells that are attached to each other apically. The basal surface of the posterior cell is markedly infolded and is covered with the basement membrane, which loosely attaches to that of the lens capsule. The anterior layer of cells has the muscular elements in its basal portion (dilator muscle). Cells of both layers are heavily pigmented, whether the eye is that of a light- or dark-skinned person (Fig. 34–26). The details of the cells are masked by the pigment, but both cells are relatively rich in microorganelles and glycogen particles. There are numer-

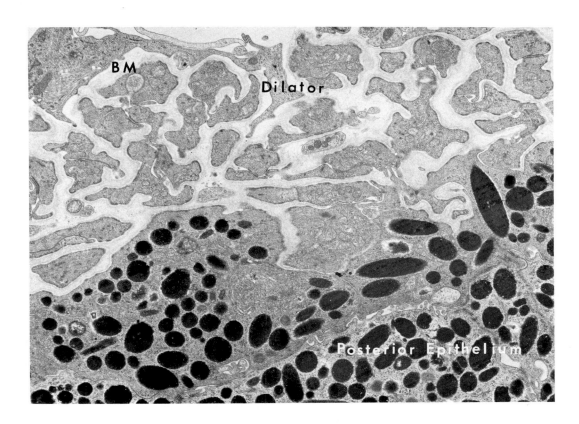

BM

Dilator

Posterior Epithelium

ous intercellular spaces between apexes of the epithelial cells. At the pupillary margin, the cells extend more centrally than does the stroma; hence, the pupillary border of the iris normally has a collarette of pigment epithelial cells. The cells of the two layers are continuous in a hairpin fashion at the pupillary margin.

Ciliary Body

The *ciliary body*, extending from the root of the iris anteriorly to the beginning of the retina at the ora serrata posteriorly, is the intermediate portion of the uvea (Fig. 34–21).

The anterior portion of the ciliary body is arranged in approximately 70 sagittally oriented folds or processes (pars plicata). In the opened eye these folds form regular ridges that radiate posteriorly (Fig. 34–27). These folds or processes contain a highly vascular stroma and are believed to be the main sites for the formation of the aqueous humor.

The posterior portion of the ciliary body is flat; accordingly, it is called *pars plana*. If the

34–26 Dilator muscle is developed within the basal infolds of the anterior epithelial cell. Apical portion of the dilator muscle cell is heavily pigmented. **BM,** basement membrane of the dilator muscle. × 18,000.

whole eye is cut coronally at its equator, the pars plana may be seen to join abruptly with the retina in a characteristically scalloped manner; this anatomic landmark is called the *ora serrata*.

Ciliary Muscle

In cross section the ciliary body has a roughly triangular shape, occupied chiefly with a smooth muscular mass, the *ciliary muscle*, which controls the focal power of the lens. The muscle is subdivided into a circular band situated at the inner anterior part of the triangle and a radial-meridional portion that extends from the scleral insertion just behind the trabecular meshwork to the posterior and inner portions of the ciliary body. The circular fibers, called *Müller's mus-*

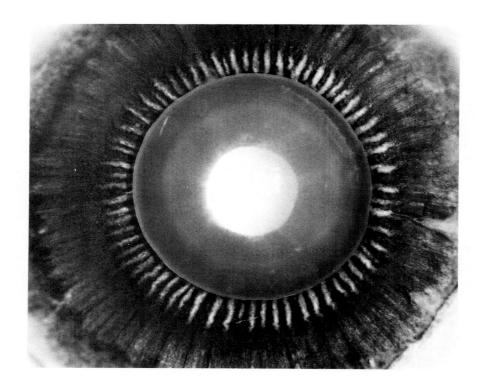

34–27 View of the lens and ciliary body from the back of the eye. The most central, white disc corresponds to the pupil: the lozenge-shaped structure is the lens; the radiating ridges constitute the processes of the ciliary body (pars plicata). Peripheral to the white ridges is the flat portion of the ciliary body (pars plana ending most peripherally in the ora serrata).

cle, relax the tension on the lens and cause the lens to accommodate for near vision; they are innervated by the parasympathetic system through the ciliary ganglion. The radial and meridional fibers (sometimes called *Brücke's muscle*) have no clearly proved function; some evidence suggests that they are innervated by the sympathetic system and cause the lens to focus for distant vision.

The ciliary muscle is divided into small compartments with a thick basement membrane. The general structure is identical to that of other smooth muscles, but the nerve element is more abundant (Fig. 34–28).

The anterior portion of the ciliary body contains a circular artery that provides the main blood supply to the iris and ciliary body. It is in turn connected with the anterior ciliary arteries and the long posterior ciliary arteries.

Ciliary Epithelium

The inner lining of the ciliary body comprises two layers of cuboidal cells of neuroectodermal origin and is derived from the marginal zone of the optic cup in the embryo. The inner layer with basement membrane abutting the vitreous is nonpigmented, whereas the outer layer with basement membrane abutting the stroma is pigmented (Figs. 34–29 and 34–30).

Cells of the two epithelial layers are joined to each other by their apical ends with a well-developed junctional complex. Small intercellular spaces are formed between the two cells (Fig. 34–30). The apical junctional complex transmits the movement of the ciliary muscle to the inner layer cell and also serves as the blood–aqueous barrier. The basal portion of the inner nonpigmented epithelial cells, which faces the posterior chamber, is markedly infolded. The cytoplasm of this zone contains numerous mitochondria. The apical portion of the cytoplasm is rich in rough endoplasmic reticulum and Golgi apparatus. Also, the cells have an active phagocytotic activity. The *zonule* fibers appear to be produced by the nonpigmented ciliary epithelium. They are especially abundant at the valley of the ciliary processes (Fig. 34–31).

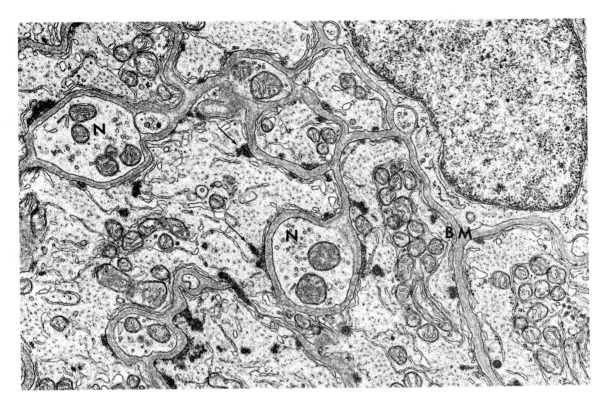

The pigmented cells in the outer layer also have well-developed basal infoldings. Several nerve fibers are present in the connective tissue between the infoldings. The cytoplasm contains rough endoplasmic reticulum among numerous melanin granules. Lateral cell membranes are closely apposed, but desmosomes are infrequent.

The structure of the nonpigmented epithelium of the pars plana is somewhat different from that of the pars plicata. Cells are tall and often their basal ends extend into the vitreous. In addition, large intercellular spaces are formed laterally. The cytoplasm contains numerous large mitochondria but only a moderate number of membranous microorganelles. The zonule fibers are mainly inserted to the basal surface of these cells.

Choroid

The *choroid* is the portion of the uvea that extends posteriorly from the region of the ora serrata. It lies immediately beneath the sclera and comprises a heavily vascularized and variably pigmented layer of choroid proper, a hyaline membrane called *Bruch's membrane*, and a pigment epithelial layer (Figs. 34–3 and 34–32).

34–28 Ciliary muscle. Smooth muscle cells are divided by thick basement membranes **(BM)**. Cells have rich mitochondria. Marginal patches are apparent **(arrow)**. Muscle is richly innervated. **N,** nerve endings. × 25,000.

34–29 Ciliary epithelium. The epithelium consists of two layers of cuboidal cells: the nonpigmented inner layer and the pigmented outer layer. **Arrows** indicate positions of the basement membranes. × 380.

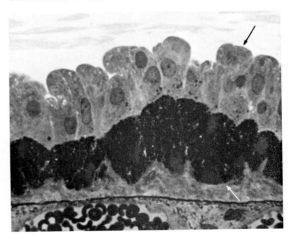

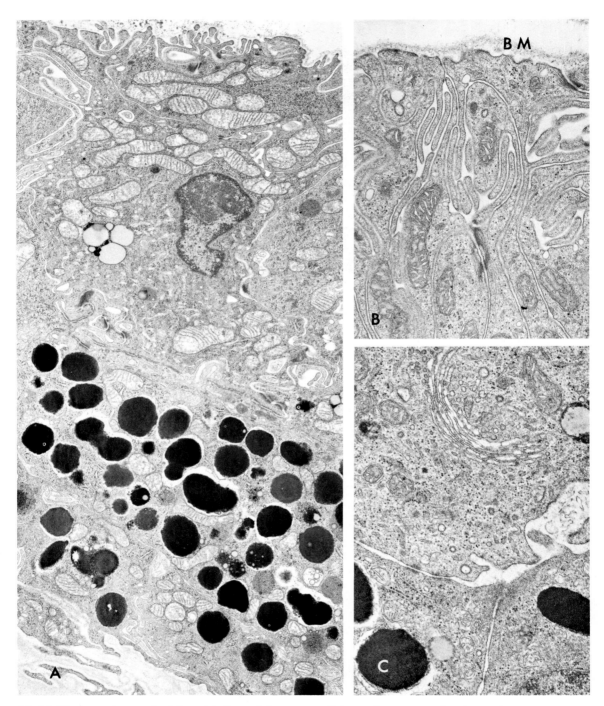

34–30 Electron micrograph of the epithelium of the ciliary body. Two-cell-layer epithelium has basement membranes **(BM)** on both surfaces. **A.** Outer layer cells contain abundant melanin pigment. Inner layer is rich in mitochondria. Base of the inner layer cell forms the posterior chamber surface. **B.** Inner layer adjacent to posterior chamber showing abundant infolding of the cell wall. **C.** Intercellular space is formed between the apical ends of the two cell layers.

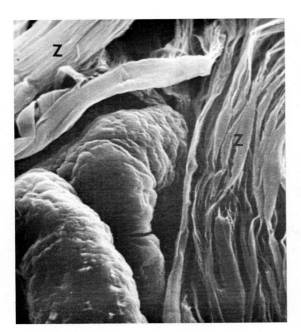

34–31 Scanning electron-microscopic view of the ciliary process and the zonule **(Z)**. × 2,900.

34–32 Left, choroid and the pigment epithelium. **PE,** pigment epithelium; **BM,** Bruch's membrane; **CC,** choriocapillaris; **V,** vein; **A,** artery. × 400. **Right,** electron micrograph shows that the choriocapillaris is fenestrated. **E,** elastica. × 28,000.

The choroid proper contains relatively large vessels, mostly veins, in its outer portions and a single layer of small sinuses called the *choriocapillaris* just beneath Bruch's membrane in its inner portions. The endothelial cell that lines the retinal side of the choriocapillaris is extremely thin and fenestrated (Fig. 34–32). The fenestrae have membranous diaphragms. The cytoplasm of the scleral side of the capillary is thick. Pericytes are present only in the scleral side of the choriocapillaris. This structure indicates an active fluid transport from the choriocapillaris to the pigment epithelium.

The blood drains out of the choroid by the four *vortex veins*, one in each posterior quadrant, and, to a lesser extent, by way of the ciliary body into the anterior ciliary vessels. The arterial supply to the choroid comes in part from the short ciliary arteries entering around the optic nerve and in part from anterior ciliary arteries entering the eye from the extraocular muscles. In addition, the choroid contains two large ciliary arteries and two long ciliary nerves passing to the ciliary body in the horizontal meridian.

The stroma of the choroid contains pigment cells, the *melanophores*, that vary in abundance according to the complexion of the individual (Fig. 34–32). These cells are also the sites of the common melanotic tumors of the eye. Less common in the choroid are mast cells, seen best with

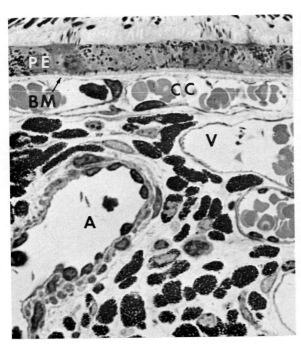

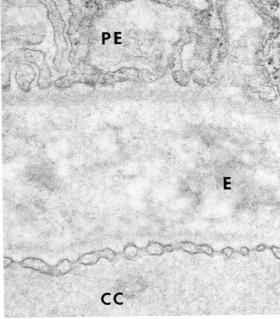

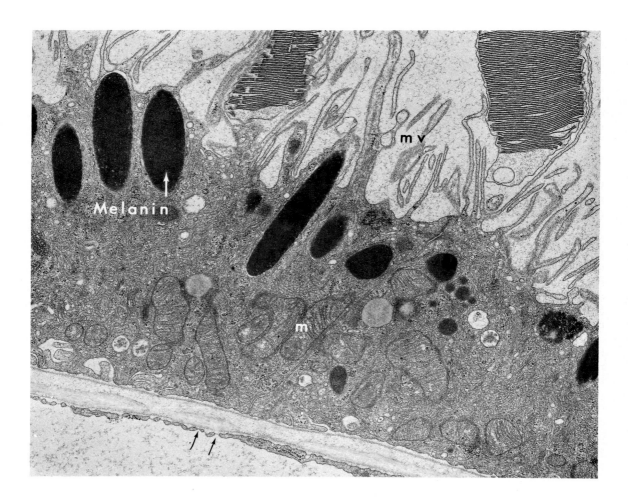

34–33 Electron micrograph of the junction between choroid and retina. In the lower left corner is a vessel of the choriocapillaris adjacent to Bruch's membrane. The endothelium of the choriocapillaris is fenestrated **(arrows)**. Occupying the center portion of the photograph is the pigment epithelium. The photoreceptor outer segments are interdigitating with microvilli of the pigment epithelium. **m**, mitochondria.

metachromatic stains, and, rarely, isolated ganglion cells.

Bruch's membrane is a thin lamina that interdigitates with the choriocapillaris on its outer surface and constitutes the basement membrane of the pigment epithelium on its inner surface. The basement membrane of the choriocapillaris forms the partial outer limit. The membrane consists of sparse collagen fibers and the centrally located elastic tissue (Fig. 34–32). Flat sections show that the elastica has a stellate configuration and forms a sievelike lamina at the center of the membrane. Bruch's membrane contains deposits of lipid and calcium in old age.

Pigment Epithelium

The pigment epithelium is a single layer of cuboidal cells situated just internal to Bruch's membrane. This layer is absent at the nerve head and it transforms into the pigmented layer of the ciliary epithelium at the ora serrata.

The pigment epithelium is of a neuroepithelial origin and is developed from the outer layer of the optic cup. This layer has a close anatomic and functional relationship with the retina and is often called *retinal pigment epithelium* (Fig. 34–33).

The *subretinal space*, containing a fluid rich in mucopolysaccharides, is formed between the pigment epithelium and the retina. This space corresponds to the embryonal neurovesicular space. The apical surface of the cell has a multitude of microvilli that extend forward to interdigitate with the rods and cones. Thus the rods and cones are not anatomically bound to the outer coats of the eye, and most histological sections show artifactual separation of the retina from the choroid. Separation of the retina is also a common clinical abnormality.

The pigment epithelial cell contains smooth endoplasmic reticulum that occupies the major part of the cytoplasm, numerous Golgi complexes in the perikaryon, rough endoplasmic reticulum in the apical zone, and abundant mitochondria in the basal portion. The cell contains a heavy concentration of melanin granules in the apical portion. These granules are round or oval, several times larger than the granules of melanocytes. Large spindle-shaped melanin granules are present in large microvilli (Fig. 34–33). Primary and secondary lysosomes are abundantly present in the cytoplasm, and the high activity of lysosomal enzymes has been demonstrated. Also, regularly contained with the epithelial cells are inclusion bodies with a laminated structure similar to that seen in photoreceptor outer segments (Fig. 34–34). The myelin bodies are the phagocytized tips of the outer segment of the photoreceptor element and are called *lamellar phagosomes*. Lamellar phagosomes and their degrading products in various appearances are abundant in the cytoplasm. These substances disappear from the cytoplasm within a short period of time, but certain remnants seem to change into lipofuscin granules. The number of lipofuscin granules increases with age whereas the number of melanin granules decreases in these cells (Fig. 34–34). Microperoxisomes, which contain catalases for digesting lipidic substances, are rich in this cell.

The pigment epithelium apparently secretes mucopolysaccharides. Pits and vacuoles are abundant in the apical cytoplasm together with rough endoplasmic reticulum and the Golgi apparatus. Incorporation of radioactive sulfate has been demonstrated experimentally.

Large oil droplets are present in the pigment epithelial cell of many animals (e.g., rabbits, birds, and frogs). Certain animals (e.g., opossum and fish) have reflectile substances within the cytoplasm. Also, *myeloid bodies*, regularly packed smooth endoplasmic reticulum are found in the pigment epithelial cells of lower animals.

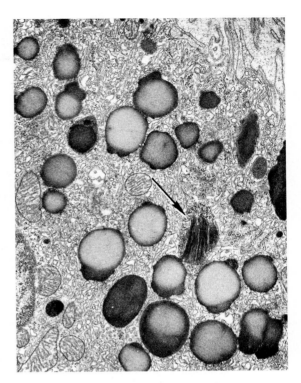

34–34 Pigment epithelial cell of an old person. Melanin granules are sparse whereas lipofuscin particles are abundant. **Arrow** indicates lamellar phagosome. × 14,500.

Lens

The lens is a transparent structure situated behind the iris and in front of the vitreous; it is held in place by the *zonular fibers*. In the adult human eye it measures approximately 10 mm in diameter and 5 mm in thickness. The anterior surface of the lens has an approximately spherical convexity, whereas the posterior surface has a paraboloid convexity (Figs. 34–3 and 34–21).

Changes in refraction of the lens occur by the interplay between its inherent tendency to become more spherical and the tension on the zonules, which flatten it.

One of the intriguing features of the lens is its isolation, not only from a blood supply but from interchange of cells with the rest of the body. The lens epithelium is derived from surface ectoderm and is enclosed in a permanent capsule early in gestation. This capsule is impermeable to cells and permits no ingress of macrophages or egress of the len's own cells; the lens carries

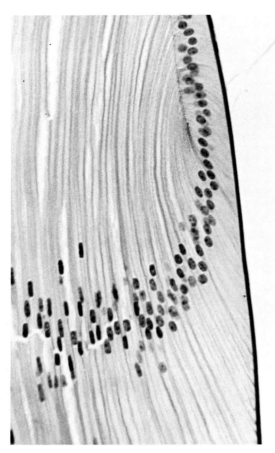

34–35 Equator of the lens of a child. The lens epithelial cells are differentiating into recognizable lens fibers. The nuclei are found at considerable depth in the cortex of the young lens. The capsule is heavily stained with PAS. × 150.

on its metabolism throughout life in a sort of tissue culture. Moreover, it permits an isolation of antigenic proteins that are foreign to the rest of the body.

Another intriguing feature is the remarkable transparency of the lens despite its densely proteinaceous nature. With age some of this transparency is lost; opacification of the lens sufficient to disturb vision is called *cataract.*

The outer surface of the lens is bounded by a *capsule,* the basement membrane of the lens cells, which has the same physical and tinctorial properties as Descemet's membrane (Fig. 34–35). The anterior portion of the capsule averages approximately 10 μm in thickness (disregarding

minor regional variations) whereas the posterior portion is less than half this thick.

Beneath the anterior capsule is a layer of cuboidal anterior lens cells that are remarkable for their uniformity and mode of differentiation. Although these cells are called *lens epithelium,* their structure is different from the conventional covering epithelium. The cell faces inwardly and its apical end attaches to the lens fibers; the outside is covered with the thick basement membrane (Fig. 34–35). The cytoplasm of the anterior lens cell contains a fine granular substance, a characteristic lens protein, and sparse microorganelles. The paucity of mitochondria accords with the relative insignificance of respiratory metabolism in the lens substance. The cells have conspicuous interdigitations, especially toward the equator. Cell membranes form junctional complexes with the lens fiber cells at the apical ends.

The anterior lens cell, which undergoes mitotic division at the paracentral zone, becomes the lens fiber cell at the equator. The elongating cells at the equator insinuate beneath the lens epithelium layer anteriorly and beneath the posterior capsule posteriorly. Because each nucleus retains its central location within the cell, the elongation of the cells causes a shifting of the nuclear distribution. Thus the *bow* configuration of the nuclei at the equator is formed (Figs. 34–35 and 34–36). The elongated cells eventually lose their nuclei and basal attachment. These differentiated cells are called *lens fibers.* The lens grows throughout life by continual addition of these fibers. (As in the growth of a tree trunk, the youngest fibers are just beneath the capsule.)

The *lens substance* consists of concentrically arranged lens fibers that have undergone varying degrees of condensation. The individual fiber structure is most evident in the superficial layers of the lens substance, called the *cortex.* Toward the center or *nucleus of the lens,* the fibers become progressively more homogeneous and less readily distinguishable as fibers histologically. The adult lens substance represents one of the most dense concentrations of protein in any tissue of the body. It stains strongly with eosin and other acid dyes. Because of its density, the adult lens substance is poorly infiltrated by ordinary embedding media; hence, except with embryonic or fetal specimens, sections of the lens are rarely obtained without disturbing artifacts.

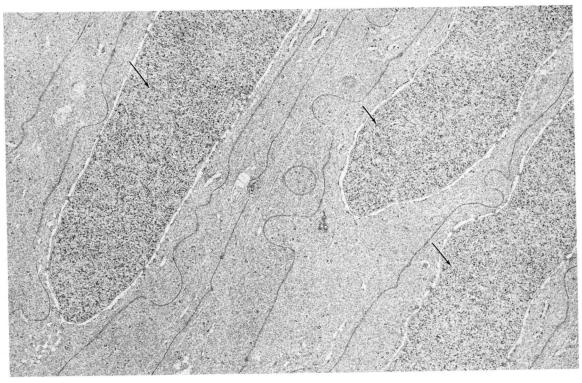

34–36 Bow zone of the lens. Lens cells have nuclei in this area **(arrows)**. Cell membranes are markedly interdigitated. Microtubules are seen frequently. Other microorganelles are sparse.

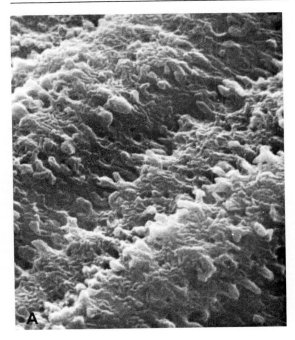

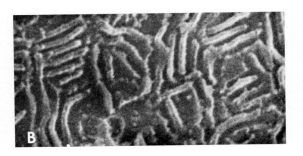

34–37 Electron-microscopic views of lens cells in the cortex. The cell has numerous knob and socket junctions. Also, the cell membrane is finely reticulated. **A,** × 3,000; **B,** × 20,000.

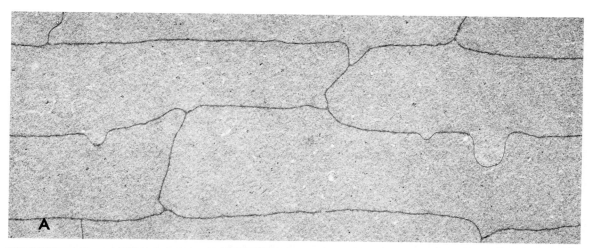

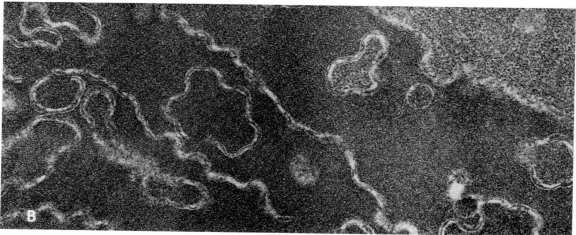

34–38 A. Cross section of lens fibers or cells in the superficial posterior cortex. The cytoplasm consists of fine granular substance. Except for scanty ribosomes, no microorganelles are seen. Cell membranes interdigitate. **B.** Cross section of the center of the lens. Cell membranes are attenuated. The cytoplasm is extremely compact and homogeneous.

The lens fibers have varying shapes according to their position. Cells in the bow zone have irregular large protrusions that interdigitate with those of adjacent cells. The protrusions become the regularly spaced knob and socket interlocking in the cortex (Fig. 34–37). Also, the cell surface of lens fibers in the cortex and deeper zones has fine ridges in a waffle-like pattern (Fig. 34–37).

Sections of the lens fiber show that the cells are closely packed without appreciable inter-spaces and that cell membranes form several junctions. Gap junctions are abundant, especially at the knob interlockings. Several desmosomes are also present. Except for occasional microorganelles in the cells at the bow zone, the lens cells contain only a uniform sprinkling or granules (Fig. 34–38). Cortical cells contain microtubules that run longitudinally in the marginal zone of the fiber cytoplasm. Toward the center of the lens, the cytoplasm becomes extremely homogeneous and dense. No microorganelles are present in these cells (Fig. 34–38).

Zonules

The *zonules* are hairlike filaments that connect the ciliary body with the lens. They insert, on the one hand, into the inner surface of the ciliary body, mainly at the pars plana and, on the other

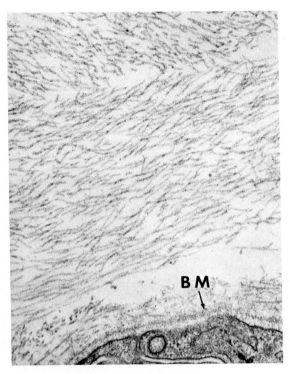

34–39 Vitreous at the ora serrata. Dense fibrils are present in this area. **BM,** basement membrane of the nonpigmented epithelium at the pars plana. × 34,900.

Vitreous

The large space between the lens, retina, and the pars plana of the ciliary body contains a viscid transparent fluid called the *vitreous*. Because of its embryological characteristics, the ocular cavity is basically different in structure from other body cavities: the space is lined by basement membranes of the cells forming the outer wall. Therefore, the vitreous is actually an extremely thin connective tissue, but not a cavity content in an ordinary histological sense.

The intraocular cavity of developing eyes of mammals is rich in blood vessels *(hyaloid vessels)*, which disappear when differentiation has been completed. The thin connective tissue including the basement membranes of the hyaloid blood vessels is called the *primary vitreous*.

The vitreous tissue is made up of minute amounts of fibrils and hydrophilic polysaccharides (especially hyaluronic acid) that stain faintly with the PAS stain. It is most dense anteriorly in the region of the ciliary body and behind the lens (Fig. 34–39). The vitreous shrinks considerably with most fixatives, however, so that one does not ordinarily find the normal distribution of vitreous in microscopic preparations.

The anterior border of the vitreous comprises an especially dense packing of the fibrils, thereby constituting the layer known as the *hyaloid membrane*. Also, a condensed layer of the vitreous fibrils is commonly present at the retinal inner limiting membrane. A few cells are present in the vitreous. They are affixed to the outermost portions of the vitreous or between the vitreous and the retina. It has been suggested that these cells are concerned with the formation and regeneration of the vitreous. The vitreous cell is small and its cytoplasm consists of fine filamentous matrix and a moderate number of microorganelles. A considerable number of macrophages is also present in the vitreous, especially in the anterior portion. These cells have numerous processes and the cytoplasm contains abundant vacuoles and inclusion bodies.

Electron microscopy of the vitreous is complicated by artifacts because of high water content (99.9%). However, specimens having survived the process of fixation, drying, and staining, show thin fibrils that have a periodicity of 12 nm. The fibrils are apparently of a collagenous nature and they attach to the basement membrane of the ciliary epithelium and the retina (Fig. 34–39).

hand, into the lens capsule just in front of and just behind the lens equator. They can be seen during life to be the suspensory filaments by which the lens is held in place and through which tension is varied on the lens by contraction of the ciliary muscle. The zonules form the posterior boundary of the posterior chamber and the anterior demarcation of the vitreous space.

The zonules stain poorly with acid dyes but well with the PAS reagent and slightly positive in elastic staining. By electron microscopy the zonules are seen to be dense aggregates of fibrils similar to those constituting the vitreous structure (Fig. 34–39). Fine fibrils measure about 7 to 8 nm in diameter and often show a tubular appearance. In addition, they show bandings at 12-nm intervals. Although the zonules are grossly and histologically inconspicuous, they are abundant (Fig. 34–31). Scanning electron microscopy reveals the substantial bundles connecting the ciliary epithelium and the lens, and their insertions to the lens are diffusely distributed.

Retina

Perhaps the most remarkable tissue of the eye, if not of the body, is the *retina*. In this membrane, which is no more than 0.5 mm thick, a light stimulus is received, converted into a neural impulse, integrated to some extent locally, and transmitted to the optic nerve for relay to the brain. All this is accomplished with an extraor-

dinary degree of adaptability to varying light intensities, discrimination of images, and color perception.

Because of its development, the retina is inverted from what one might expect. The inner surface of the retina is covered with the basement membrane and the outer surface is made up of the photoreceptor elements (Fig. 34–40). Therefore, light travels through the whole thickness of the retina before reaching the photoreceptors. The photoreceptor cells and the pigment epithelium of the choroid form the *subretinal space*, which corresponds to the embryonal neurovascular space. The sheetlike retina attaches to the optic nerve head posteriorly and to the ciliary epithelium anteriorly. The rest of the retina has no cytological attachment to the underlying tissue.

The retina consists of three main categories of neurons: photoreceptor, bipolar, and ganglion cells. These neurons form three clearly defined layers (Figs. 34–40 and 34–41). The photoreceptor cells are often called the *neuroepithelial portion* of the retina. They are analogous to the sensory receptors of the skin or to the first neurons in the efferent arc of other sensory systems. The bipolar cells are analogous to the cells in the dorsal ganglia; the ganglion cells of the retina are

34–40 Cross section of the retina. **ILM,** inner limiting membrane; **NFL,** nerve fiber layer; **GCL,** ganglion cell layer; **IPL,** inner plexiform layer; **INL,** inner nuclear layer; **OPL,** outer plexiform layer; **ONL,** outer nuclear layer; **OLM,** outer limiting membrane; **R & C,** rods and cones. **PE,** pigment epithelium; rods and cones are divided into **IS,** inner segment, and **OS,** outer segment. × 250.

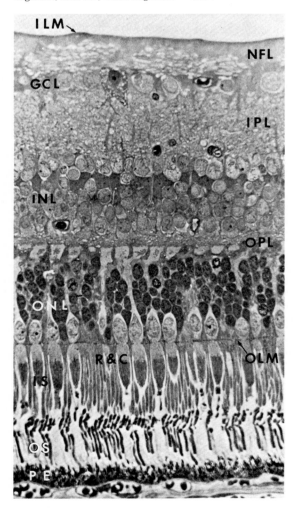

34–41 The major neuronal and glial organization of the retina and pigment epithelium. The Müller cell is shown unrealistically large to emphasize its distribution throughout the whole thickness of the retina.

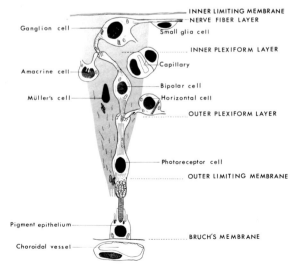

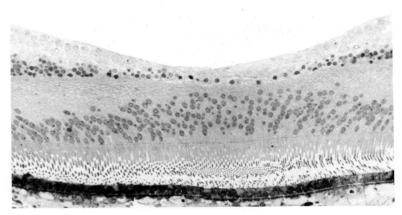

34–42 Cross section through macula. The macula consists of a central fossa in which all the layers, except that of the rods and cones, are displaced to the side. × 80.

analogous to the relay in the spinal cord and brainstem. The optic nerves, the counterparts of the lemnisci in the brainstem, conduct their impulses to the lateral geniculate bodies and thalami. The same number of neuronal relays are thus operative in the retina as in other sensory pathways.

Anterior to the outer nuclear layer is the outer plexiform layer, where synaptic connections occur between the axons of the rod and cone cells and the dendrites of the next order of cells. The layer between the bipolar cell and ganglion cell is the inner plexiform layer and consists of synaptic contacts between these cells.

Macula

The overall architecture of the retina is modified particularly in two areas. One of them is at the posterior pole of the eye where the retina forms the *macula* or *fovea* (Fig. 34–42). This area is about 1.5 mm in diameter at the posterior pole and constitutes the zone of greatest visual acuity. It is the zone of optimal image formation. (The name *macula lutea* refers to the yellow coloration of the retina in this region, which can be seen in the gross specimen but is not visible by ordinary histological examination.) At the macula the photoreceptors are modified into long, thin elements called *macula cones*. Morphologically, they resemble rods more closely than cones. The overlying retinal layers are greatly reduced at the center of the macula so that the inner surface of the retina forms a pitlike depression called the *foveola*. The nerve fibers from the regions of the retina that are lateral to the macula arch about it: the ganglion cells, inner plexiform

layer, and bipolar cells are displaced away from it; and the inner plexiform layer has a radiating pattern that has been called *Henle's fiber layer*. However, the most distinctive feature of the macula is the abundance of ganglion cells around the foveola.

The thinning of the retina at the macula serves the intensity of visual acuity by reducing to a minimum the overlying tissue through which light must pass before reaching the photoreceptors.

Müller's Cell and Limiting Membranes

Certain neuroepithelial cells of the embryonal optic cup keep their basal attachment during development. These cells extend fine cytoplasmic processes and become the retinal glial cell, *Müller's cell*. The basement membrane of these cells is the main part of the *inner limiting membrane* (Fig. 34–43). This membrane forms the inner boundary of the retina and stands out conspicuously with the PAS reagent. Flat preparations of the inner limiting membrane show a gyrate design impressed on it by the arborization of Müller's fibers.

The apical junctions of Müller's cells with photoreceptor cells form a sievelike structure at the outer limit of the outer nuclear layer. This structure is called the *outer limiting membrane* (Fig. 34–44). Fine microvilli of Müller's cells extend beyond the outer limiting membrane into the subretinal space.

Müller's cells have their nuclei in the bipolar cell layer, whereas the cytoplasm is distributed throughout the whole thickness of the retina. The cytoplasm of Müller's cells is most plentiful

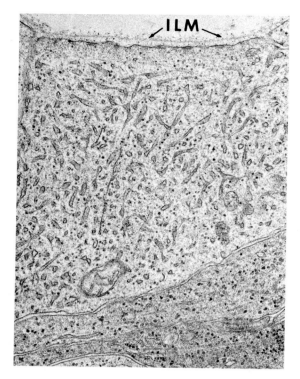

in the basal (inner) and apical (outer) layers. The cytoplasm, consisting of rich smooth endoplasmic reticulum, contains abundant glycogen particles (Fig. 34–43). Also, the cell has considerable glycolytic dehydrogenase activity. This cell serves for the structural as well as nutritional support system of the retina and is similar to the astrocyte of the central nervous system.

Other Glial Cells

A few spindle-shaped glial cells are present in the ganglion and nerve fiber layers. They usually surround bundles of nerve fibers and occasionally the blood vessels. At the posterior pole, these cells become the main glial element of the retina. The inner limiting membrane in the disc area is mainly made of the basement membrane of these glial cells. The cytoplasm of these cells contains fine neurofibrils and a small number of microorganelles. The number of glial cells in other layers of the retina is extremely small.

34–43 The inner (basal) portion of Müller's cells.
△   The cytoplasm is rich in smooth endoplasmic reticulum and glycogen particles. **ILM,** inner limiting membrane. × 26,200.

34–44 Outer limiting membrane **(arrow)** is a chain of apical junctions of Müller's cells. Microvilli of Müller's cells **(mv)** extend beyond the limiting membrane. × 20,000. ▽

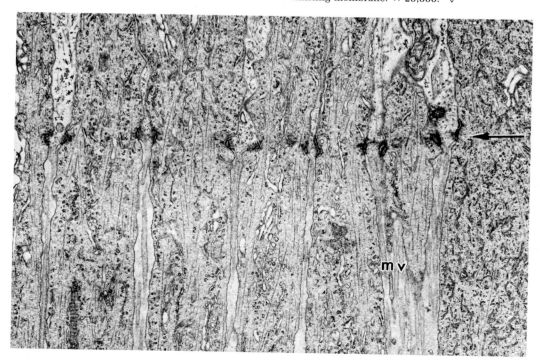

Photoreceptors

The *photoreceptors* are the *rods* and *cones* situated on the outer surface of the retina. The photoreceptor cells have their nuclei in the *outer nuclear layer* and extend their axon processes toward the *outer plexiform layer*. The photoreceptor elements protrude beyond the outer limiting membrane and are divided into two portions: *inner segment* and *outer segment*. The *outer segment* fingerlike body stains well with eosin and other acid dyes (Figs. 34–45 and 34–46). The outer segment contains the photoreceptive substance (*rhodopsin*, or visual purple, in the rods and *iodopsin* in the cones) and is responsible for the absorption of light that triggers off the visual stimulus. As their name implies, the rods have long, thin inner segments, whereas

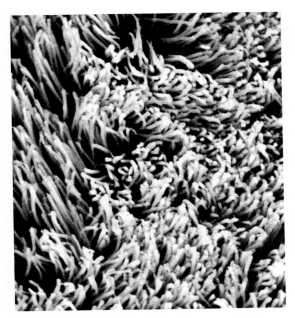

34–45 Scanning electron-microscopic view of the photoreceptor outer segments.

34–46 Photoreceptor elements of the retina. Inner segments of rods and cones contain packs of mitochondria. Outer segments **(OS)** consist of lamellar membranes. Pigment epithelium **(PE)** touches lightly at the tips of the outer segments. × 12,000.

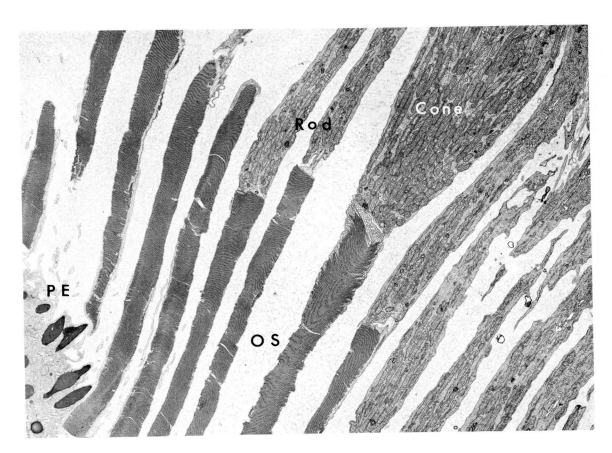

The inner half of the inner segment is called *myoid*, which contains abundant Golgi complexes, smooth endoplasmic reticulum, and microtubules. Glycogen particles are rich in this area. A specialized endoplasmic reticulum with abundant glycogen particles is developed in retinas of birds and frogs. The outer half of the inner segment is the *ellipsoid* in which a concentration of mitochondria is present (Fig. 34–46). Among mitochondria are wavy filamentous fibrils and scanty microtubules. The outer segment is connected with the inner segment by a ciliary connection having nine pairs of microtubules (Fig. 34–47). The central two pairs of the kinocilium are missing.

The *lamellar plates* of the outer segment are sacculated discs measuring about 1 μm in diameter. A stack of these discs is enveloped by the plasma membrane. The disc is formed by two apposing membranes measuring approximately 5 to 6 nm in thickness, and the marginal zone shows a loop configuration in cross sections (Fig. 34–48). These membranes of the rod outer segments are not continuous with the plasma membrane. On the other hand, membranes of the plates of the cone outer segment often connect with the outer plasma membrane (Fig. 34–49). This difference is most striking in the frog retina.

Lamellated rod membranes are formed at the ciliary connection zone and move centrifugally to be cast off at their outermost tips. They are then phagocytized by the pigment epithelium. In each monkey rod, there are approximately 1,300 plates, each with a life expectance of about 10 days (Young, 1967).

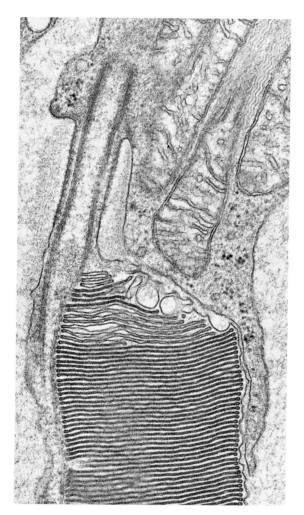

34–47 Electron micrograph through the junctions of the outer and inner segments of the rod. The upper portion of the photograph shows the inner segment containing a dense concentration of mitochondria, whereas the lower portion shows the outer segment, or photoreceptive end organ, containing laminated plates. The two portions are connected by modified cilia. × 32,200.

Outer Nuclear Layer

The perikaryon cell bodies of the rods and cones constitute the *outer nuclear layer* (Fig. 34–40). The cone nuclei are placed in the outermost portion of this layer. Rod and cone cell bodies are separated from each other by ramifications of the radial glia of the retina, Müller's cells.

The outermost limit of this layer is the *outer limiting membrane*, a zone of junctional complex between the photoreceptor cells and apical ends of Müller's cells.

The axonal (inner) and dendritic (outer) portions of the cytoplasm of photoreceptor cells contain regularly arranged microtubules. The scanty perikaryon cytoplasm also contains microtubules.

the cones have a broad base (Fig. 34–40 and 34–46). The rods have more photoabsorptive pigment, which, along with their cumulative neural connections, gives them greater sensitivity for low levels of illumination, that is, night vision. The cones, having less summation in the retina, permit greater resolution of images and therefore better visual acuity in daylight. The cones are also responsible for color perception.

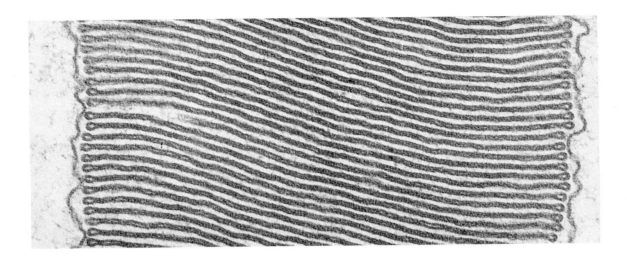

34–48 Higher magnification of the rod outer segment. Saccular discs are separated from each other. × 55,000.

34–49 Cone outer segment. Many membranes of the saccular discs constitute the outer wall of the photoreceptor. Inner side of the disc may communicate with the outside of the cell **(arrows).** × 50,000.

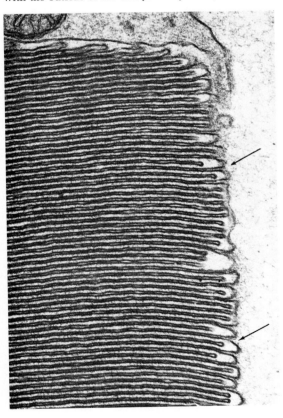

Outer Plexiform Layer

Axonal ends of the photoreceptor cells, dendritic processes of the bipolar cells, and processes of the horizontal cells constitute the *outer plexiform layer*. The cone synapses form a row at the center of the layer, and the rod synapses are situated at slightly outer zone. The inner half of this plexiform layer is composed of fine processes of bipolar and horizontal cells (Fig. 34–40). The cone cell forms a large *synaptic pedicle* in which more than 20 synaptic junctions are present (Fig. 34–50). The rod cell forms a small synaptic *spherule* that contains a few synaptic junctions. The synaptic junctions consist of invaginating processes of horizontal cells into the pedicle or spherule, and superficially located bipolar cell dendrites. The synaptic ends of the photoreceptors contain a few mitochondria and numerous *synaptic vesicles*, which particularly cluster around *synaptic bars*. The *synaptic bar*, a nonmembranous electron-dense body is usually situated between the invaginating horizontal cell processes.

The inner half of the outer plexiform layer consists of interwoven fine processes. Horizontal cell processes have well-developed gap junction–like attachments with other processes. Small blood capillaries are present in this layer.

Bipolar Layer

The middle lamina of cells is called the *bipolar cell* layer because it is chiefly made of bipolar neurons that relay impulses from the rod and cone cells inward to the next layer of cells. It

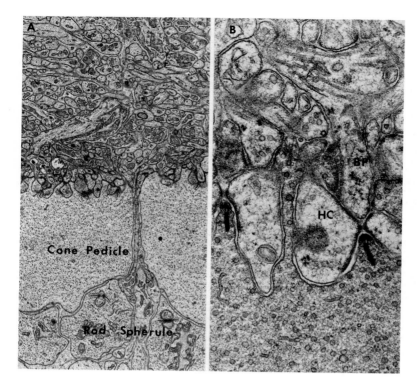

34–50 Outer plexiform layer.
    A. Pedicles of cones and spherules of rods constitute the outer half of the layer. The inner portion of the layer is occupied by processes of bipolar and horizontal cells. Synaptic junctions are seen in the terminal ends of the cones and rods. × 6,300. **B.** Higher magnification of a synaptic end of the cone pedicle. The synapse consists of large horizontal cell processes **(HC)** and the dendritic end of the bipolar cell **(BP).** The cone pedicle contains numerous vesicles and synaptic bars. × 37,000.

also contains the nuclei of Müller's cells, *horizontal cells,* and *amacrine cells* (Fig. 34–40). This layer effects some integration of the rods and cones and, in the case of the rods, a summation of impulses.

The outermost zone of the bipolar layer contains the horizontal cell, which sends fine processes to each synaptic junction (Fig. 34–51). The cytoplasm is electron lucent, contains mitochondria and Golgi apparatus, and has a high activity of lactic acid dehydrogenase. The tip portions of the processes contain fine vesicles. The bipolar cells have a relatively small soma cytoplasm but project a large axonal cytoplasm inwardly. By silver impregnation methods, several kinds of bipolar cells have been demonstrated. The amacrine cell, a monopolar cell, forms a layer in the innermost zone and is easeily distinguishable from other cells by its light staining and a lobulated nucleus. The cytoplasm contains an abundance of various microorganelles. The amacrine cell has a large cytoplasm that ramifies in the inner plexiform layer. Other nuclei in this layer belong to Müller's glial cells, which have a chromatin-rich almond-shaped nucleus. The perikaryon cytoplasm is usually electron-dense

34–51 Flat section through the outer zone of the bipolar cell layer stained for lactic acid dehydrogenase. Horizontal cells show their stretching processes. × 380.

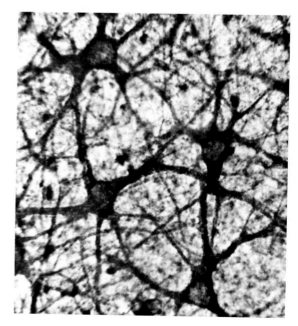

and contains lamellarly arranged rough endoplasmic reticulum. Processes of this cell are chief reservoirs for glycogen and for many enzymes concerned with energy metabolism.

Inner Plexiform Layer

Anterior to the bipolar cell layer is the *inner plexiform layer* for the synapses of the bipolar layer and the next order of cells. Three cell components contribute to synapes in this layer: the bipolar axons, ganglion cell dendrites, and amacrine cell processes. The bipolar cell axon has numerous synaptic junctions that are characterized by numerous vesicles clustering around

34–52 Synapses in the inner plexiform layer. The axonal end of the bipolar cell **(BP)** contains synaptic bars and clustering vesicles. Other cell components are ganglion cell **(G)** and amacrine cells **(A)**. The amacrine cell terminal contains clusters of vesicles. × 48,500.

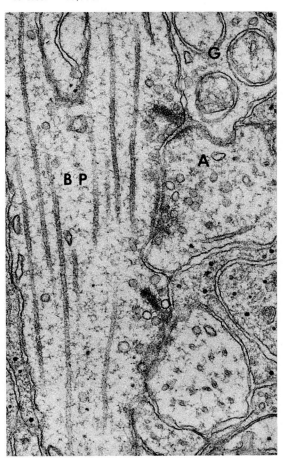

synaptic bars (Fig. 34–52). Attaching to this location are dendrites of the ganglion cells, which contain few large mitochondria, and amacrine cell processes which contain clusters of vesicles. In the complexity of interwoven processes of the neural and Müller cells, countless synaptic junctions are distributed throughout the layer. Relatively large Müller cell components often divide the tissue into insignificant groups. The inner plexiform layer contains blood vessels.

Ganglion Cell Layer

The ganglion cell layer is the most anterior lamina of cells. The ganglion cell layer may be eight to 10 cells thick at the posterior pole of the eye (at the macula), but it becomes reduced anteriorly to single scattered cells. Ganglion cells in the posterior retina are small, but those in the periphery are extremely large. A few glial cells are scattered among ganglion cells.

The ganglion cell has a relative abundance of cytoplasm containing rough endoplasmic reticulum organized in masses called *Nissl bodies*. Other prominent microorganelles are mitochondria, Golgi apparatus, and lysosomes. The nucleus contains prominent nucleoli (Fig. 34–53). Its dendrites connect with the bipolar cells in the outer plexiform layer and its axons form the nerve fiber layer and optic nerve. Both the axon and dendrite contain abundant microtubules.

Nerve Fiber Layer

The *nerve fiber layer* arises from the ganglion cells and leaves the eye by way of the optic nerve. The layer is, of course, thickest as it approaches the optic nerve. Along with the nerve fibers, this layer also contains large blood vessels, miscellaneous glia, and a plexus of Müller's fibers that compartmentalize the nerve fibers and fan out toward the innermost surface of the retina.

The axons form bundles of various sizes. Large bundles in the posterior portion of the retina are often surrounded by glial cells in addition to the Müller cell. Small bundles in the peripheral retina are enveloped by Müller cell cytoplasm. Axons are greatly variable in size from 0.2 to 3.0 μm in diameter. They are not myelinated or separated by glial cells. Axons contain regularly spaced microtubules and a few mitochondria. Scant smooth endoplasmic reticulum is present immediately inside the cell membrane.

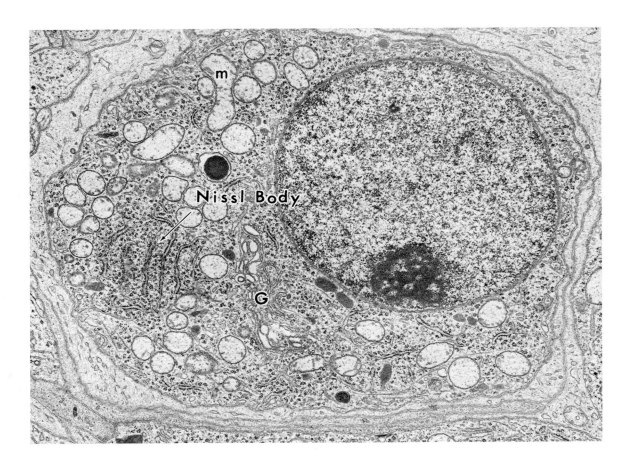

34–53 Ganglion cell in the macula area. The cell contains marked Nissl bodies. The nucleus is located at one edge of the cell and contains a prominent nucleolus. **G,** Golgi apparatus; **m,** mitochondria. × 20,000.

The inner limiting membrane (basement membrane) of this zone is formed mainly by astrocyte-like glial cells and is considerably thinner than the rest of the retina. Nerve fibers in this area are not myelinated.

Nerve Head

The second modification of retinal architecture occurs at the *nerve head*, or *papilla*. This is an area about 1 mm in diameter where the nerve fibers leave the eye to form the optic nerve (Figs. 34–2 and 34–56). The retina is absent in this region, and the visual field shows a corresponding "blind spot." The center of the nerve head is situated about 3 mm nasal to the center of the macula. Only cross sections of the eye cut near the horizontal meridian will show both macula and optic nerve. Cross sections through the center of the nerve head show a central depression, the *physiological cup*, through which the *central vessels* pass.

Retinal Vessels

The retinal arteries and veins traverse the nerve head but branch immediately after they are within the eye. The larger vessels course horizontally in the nerve fiber and ganglion cell layers but develop elaborate branching and capillary plexuses in all the inner layers of the retina.

The retinal vascular tree may be studied as whole mounts through injection of some material or may be digested with the rest of the retina by trypsin (Fig. 34–54). The latter technique permits subsequent staining of the vessels by ordinary dyes. The capillaries are then seen to contain an unusually thick basement membrane and two types of cell, one the endothelium lining

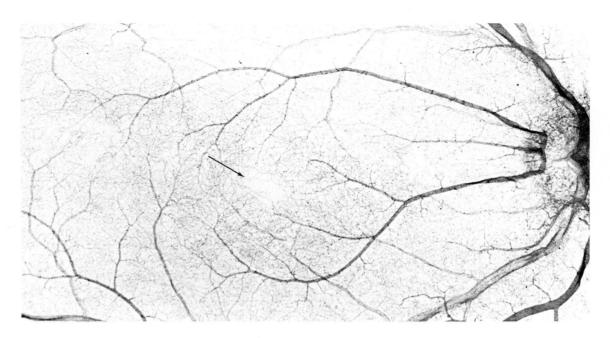

34–54 Flat preparation of the retinal vessels. Fine capillaries form a uniform meshwork. **Arrow** indicates the avascular zone of the fovea. × 60.

34–55 Capillary wall is made of two types of cell. Endothelial nuclei are ellipsoidal in shape and mural cells **(arrows)** have dark round nuclei. × 450.

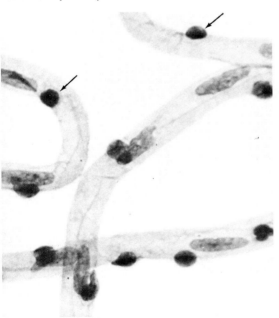

the capillary lumina and the other enclosed within the basement membrane; hence the name *mural cell* or intramural pericyte (Fig. 34–55). Cells of the latter type are believed to control the flow through the capillaries.

The endothelial lining is thick and uninterrupted. The cytoplasm of the mural cell contains abundant mitochondria, rough endoplasmic reticulum, Golgi apparatus, and glycogen particles. The cell matrix is filamentous and numerous dense bodies, which are common in smooth muscle cells, are regularly present.

The outer plexiform layer and outer nuclear layers of the retina are vessel-free zones that can derive sufficient nutrition from the choroid to survive when the retinal arteries are obstructed. The fovea is also a capillary-free zone that derives its nutrition from the choriocapillaris.

Optic Nerve

Axons of ganglion cells of the retina converge at the posterior pole and leave the globe. Axon fibers pass through a sievelike connective tissue, *lamina cribrosa* of the sclera, where the *optic nerve* begins acquiring myelin. Up to this point myelin is absent. The diameter of the optic nerve increases about twofold beyond this point (Fig. 34–56). With the acquisition of myelin, the optic nerve becomes a tract comparable to white matter of the brain. It is surrounded by meningeal

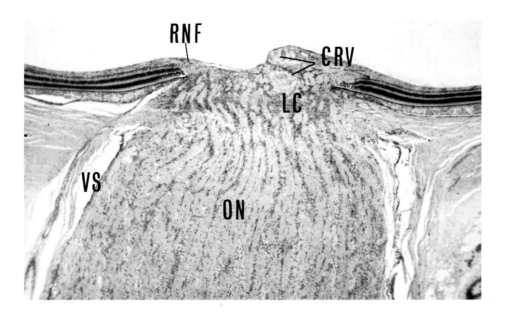

34–56 Cross section through the nerve head. **ON,** myelinated optic nerve; **VS,** vaginal space; **LC,** lamina cribrosa; **CRV,** central retinal vessels; **RNF,** retinal nerve fibers that are nonmyelinated. × 60.

sheaths: a robust dura (continuous with the sclera), a delicate arachnoid, and a thin pia. The subdural and subarachnoid spaces, called collectively the vaginal spaces of the optic nerve, are continuous with those of the intracranial spaces.

The optic nerve contains approximately a million axon fibers, which are strikingly irregular in size and are grouped into small bundles by *astrocytes*. These bundles are then grouped by the connective tissue, *septa*, which contains blood vessels.

34–57 Glial cells of the optic nerve. **As,** astrocyte; **Ol,** oligodendroglial cell. × 19,300.

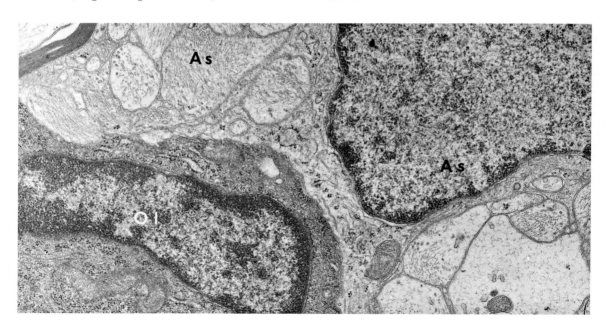

Axons consist of electron-lucent cytoplasm (axoplasm) with regularly spaced microtubules and occasional mitochondria. Smooth endoplasmic reticulum is sparsely distributed in the axon.

The cytoplasm of the astrocyte is electron-lucent and is rich in neurofilaments. Other microorganelles are sparse. Fine processes of this cell extend among axon bundles and become the background tissue of the optic nerve (Fig. 34–57). Cell processes are joined to each other by gap junctions and desmosomes in several locations. The astrocytes form thick basement membranes where the cells attach to the connective tissue of the lamina cribrosa and septa.

Each axon fiber is surrounded by five to 10 layers of the myelin membrane, which is believed to be produced by the *oligodendroglial cell*. The *oligodendroglial* cells have electron-dense cytoplasm that contains rich rough endoplasmic reticulum and Golgi apparatus (Fig. 34–57). Nodes of Ranvier are present regularly.

Glial cells that have very little cytoplasm are infrequently present in the optic nerve. These glial cells are *microglia* and they may have a phagocytic function in a certain pathological condition.

Ocular Adnexa and Orbit

Surrounding the eye is a sheath of connective tissue called *Tenon's capsule*. Although it is often considered a socket within which the eye rotates, it has no synovial membrane and no other resemblance to joint structures.

The orbital cavity contains extraocular muscles, optic nerves, blood vessels, and ciliary nerve elements. The rest is filled with adipose and loose connective tissue. The *ciliary ganglion* and plexuses of the ciliary nerves are present medial and inferior to the optic nerve.

Lacrimal Gland

The *lacrimal gland* is an acinous structure similar to salivary glands, situated in the upper outer portion of the orbit and opening onto the conjunctiva by 10 to 20 separate ducts. The gland consists of serous glandular cells, surrounded by myoepithelial elements, and ducts containing mucus-forming cells.

The cytoplasm of the gland cell contains mucoid granules and electron-dense secretory substances. Rough endoplasmic reticulum and Golgi apparatus are abundant. Well-developed myoepithelial cells are present at the basal portion of the gland (Fig. 34–58).

Nasolacrimal Canal

The *nasolacrimal canal* is situated in the bony fossa at the side of the nose. It consists of stratified epithelium, about 10 cells thick, connected with canaliculi from the upper and lower lids and with a nasolacrimal duct that opens into the middle meatus of the nose. The epithelium of the canaliculi consists of columunar ciliated cells. The canaliculi, sac, and duct constitute the effluent channels for tears.

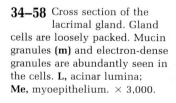

34–58 Cross section of the lacrimal gland. Gland cells are loosely packed. Mucin granules **(m)** and electron-dense granules are abundantly seen in the cells. **L,** acinar lumina; **Me,** myoepithelium. × 3,000.

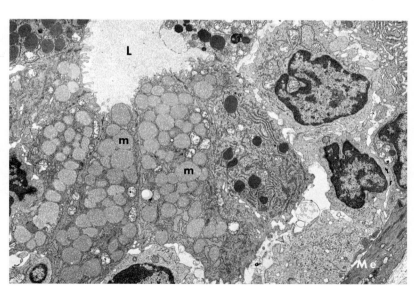

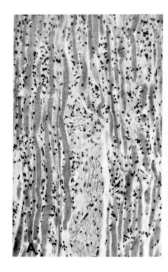
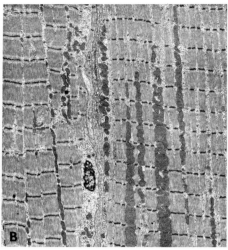

34–59 Rectus muscle. **A.** The muscle consists of fine muscle fibers, abundant nerves, and considerable connective tissue. × 160. **B.** Portions of two muscle fibers. Muscle fiber on the left has large myofibrils and sparse mitochondria, whereas the one on the right has fine myofibrils and abundant mitochondria. × 2,400.

Extraocular Muscles

There are seven *extraocular muscles:* the *levator*, the four *recti* (medial, superior, lateral, and inferior), and the two *obliques* (superior and inferior) (Fig. 34–4).

Fibers of the extraocular muscle are considerably small and irregular in size (10–30 μm in diameter). Richly vascularized connective tissue and abundant nerve fibers are present among loosely packed muscle fibers (Fig. 34–59A). Two distinct kinds of muscle fiber are intermingled within a muscle bundle; small fibers consisting of well-defined myofibrils and rich mitochondria, and large fibers with fused myofibrils and sparse mitochondria (Fig. 34–59B). The fine structure of the individual muscle fiber is not different from that of other striated muscles.

Regular Changes with Age

Certain changes occur with age so regularly that they may be considered normal. They will be mentioned briefly.

1. Sudanophilia of the circumferential portions of Descemet's membrane and, to a lesser extent, of the circumferential stroma of the cornea and of Bowman's membrane. This causes an opacity of the cornea that is known clinically as arcus lipoides.
2. Hyalinization of the stroma in the ciliary processes and between the ciliary muscle and epithelium. Also, the number of the pigmented epithelial cells decreases and the basement membrane of the nonpigmented ciliary epithelium increases in thickness.
3. Condensation of the lens fibers with loss of malleability of the lens substance. This results in a progressive decrease of accommodative power (presbyopia), becoming so marked in middle age that supplementary glasses are needed for near focusing.
4. Occlusion of the capillaries with cyst formation in the most anterior portions of the retina. The number of endothelial cells of the retinal capillary decreases considerably.
5. Sudanophilia and basophilia of Bruch's membrane in the posterior portions of the eye.

References and Selected Bibliography

Duke-Elder, S., and Wybar, K. C. 1961. *In* S. Duke-Elder, (ed.), The Anatomy of the Visual System, System of Ophthalmology, vol. 2. St. Louis: The C. V. Mosby Company.

Eisler, P. 1930. Die Anatomie des menschen Auges. *In* F. Schieck and A. Brückner (eds.), Kurzes Handbuch der Ophthalmologie, vol. 1. Berlin: Springer-Verlag OHG.

Fine, B. S., and Yanoff, M. 1972. Ocular Histology. New York: Harper & Row, Publishers, Inc.

Hogan, M. J., Alvarado, J. A., and Weddell, J. E. 1971. Histology of the Human Eye. Philadelphia: W. B. Saunders Company.

Mann, I. 1950. The Development of the Human Eye, 2nd ed. New York: Grune & Stratton, Inc.

Polyak, S. 1941. The Retina. Chicago: University of Chicago Press.

Smelser, G. K. (ed.). 1961. The Structure of the Eye. New York: Academic Press, Inc.

Wolff, E. 1961. The Anatomy of the Eye and Orbit, 5th ed. New York: McGraw-Hill Book Company.

Young, R. W. 1967. The renewal of photoreceptor cell outer segments. J. Cell Biol. 33:61.

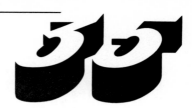

The Ear

Åke Flock

General Structure

The ear is composed of three parts, which are illustrated schematically in Fig. 35–1:

1. The external ear, which includes the auricle, or pinna, projecting from the head and the external auditory meatus leading from the surface to the ear drum;
2. The middle ear, including the tympanic cavity, the drum, and the chain of three bones extending from the drum to the medial wall of the tympanic cavity, which communicates with the nasopharynx by means of the auditory (eustachian) tube;
3. The internal ear, which consists of the membranous labyrinth containing the organs of hearing and equilibrium, the bone surrounding these sense organs, and the acoustic nerve.

External Ear

Auricle

The *auricle* consists of an irregular flap of elastic cartilage. On the lateral surface, the skin adheres tightly to the perichondrium, which contains abundant elastic fibers, whereas on the posterior surface a subcutaneous layer is present. Sebaceous glands are often quite large and are associated with small hairs.

External Auditory Meatus

The *external meatus* is lined with skin continuous with the cutaneous layer of the tympanic membrane. In the deep or osseous portion, the

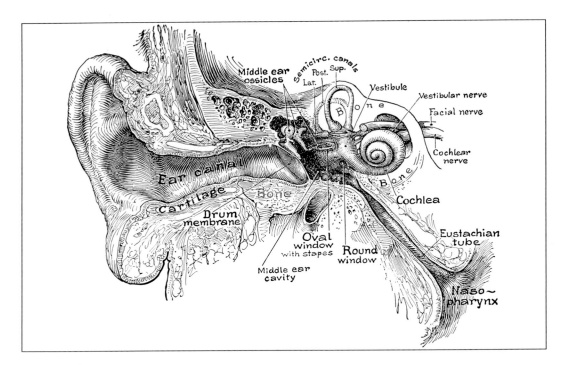

35–1 Schematic drawing of the human ear, illustrating the anatomic relationships of the various parts of the ear and the surrounding and connecting structures. M. Brödel, three unpublished drawings of the anatomy of the human ear. (Courtesy of W. B. Saunders Company, Philadelphia.)

skin is very thin and without hairs or glands except along its upper wall. There, and in the outer or cartilaginous part, ceruminous glands that secrete a wax (cerumen) are abundant. They are branched, tubuloalveolar glands that in many respects resemble large sweat glands. Their ducts are lined with stratified epithelium, and their coils consist of a single layer of secreting cells, generally cuboid, surrounded by smooth muscle fibers and a well-defined basement membrane. They differ from sweat glands in that their coils have a very large lumen, especially in the adult, and their gland cells, often with a distinct cuticular border, contain many pigment granules and lipid droplets. Their narrow ducts end on the surface of the skin or they open together with sebaceous glands into the neck of hair follicles.

Middle Ear

Tympanic Cavity

The air-filled *tympanic cavity,* or *tympanum,* is lined with a mucous membrane closely connected with the surrounding periosteum. It consists of a thin layer of connective tissue covered generally with simple cuboidal epithelium. In places the epithelial cells may be flat or tall, with nuclei in two rows. Cilia are sometimes widely distributed and are usually found on the floor of the cavity. In the anterior part of the tympanic cavity, small alveolar mucous glands occur very sparingly. Capillaries form wide-meshed networks in the connective tissue, and lymphatic vessels are found in the periosteum.

Tympanic Membrane

The tympanic cavity is separated from the external auditory canal by the *tympanic membrane* or *eardrum,* which consists of the following strata: the outermost cutaneum, the radiatum, the circulare, and the innermost mucosum. The stratum cutaneum is a thin skin without papillae in its corium, except along the handle or manubrium of the malleus. There it is a thicker layer, containing the vessels and nerves that descend along the manubrium and spread from it radially. In addition to the venous plexus that accompanies the artery there, a plexus of veins at the periphery of the membrane receives tributaries from both the stratum cutaneum and the less vascular stratum mucosum. The radiate and circular strata consist of compact bundles of fibrous and elastic tissue that are so arranged as to suggest tendon. The fibers of the radial layer blend with the perichondrium of the hyaline cartilage covering the manubrium. Peripherally the fiber layers form a fibrocartilaginous ring that connects with the surrounding bone. The stratum mucosum is a thin layer of connective tissue covered with a simple, nonciliated, flat epithelium continuous with the lining of the tympanic cavity. Peripherally, in children, its cells may be taller and ciliated. As a whole, the tympanic membrane is divided into tense and flaccid portions. The latter is a relatively small upper part in which the fibrous layers are deficient. The tensor tympani muscle is attached by a tendon to the center of the tympanic membrane.

Auditory Ossicles

The tympanic membrane is connected to the inner ear through a chain of three small bones, the *malleus, incus,* and *stapes* (Fig. 35–1). They articulate against each other by regular joints and are supported in the middle ear cavity by connective tissue strands. The *manubrium* of the malleus attaches to the tympanic membrane; the footplate of the stapes is held by an annular fibrous ligament in the *fenestra vestibuli,* or oval window, which opens into the inner ear. The *stapedius muscle* attaches to the head of the stapes (Fig. 35–2).

Auditory Tube

The *auditory,* or *eustachian tube* (Fig. 35–1), includes an osseous part toward the tympanum and a cartilaginous part toward the pharynx. Its mucosa consists of fibrillar connective tissue, with a ciliated columnar epithelium that becomes stratified as it approaches the pharynx. The stroke of the cilia is toward the pharyngeal orifice. In the osseous portion, the mucosa is without glands and very thin; it adheres closely to the surrounding bone. Along its floor there are pockets containing air, the cellulae pneumaticae. In the cartilaginous part the mucosa is thicker; near the pharynx it contains many mixed glands. Lymphocytes are abundant in the surrounding connective tissue, forming nodules near the end of the tube that blend with the pharyngeal tonsil. The cartilage, which only partly surrounds the auditory tube, is hyaline near its junction with the bone of the osseous portion. Here and there are coarse nonelastic fibers. Toward the pharynx the matrix contains thick nets of elastic tissue, so the cartilage there is elastic.

35–2 Cat stapes with stapedius muscle. The stapes is in the oval window. The stapedius muscle is attached to the head of the stapes. Note the sesamoid bone between the head of the stapes and the incus. The facial nerve is cut in cross section. **TC,** tympanic cavity; **FN,** facial nerve; **SB,** sesamoid bone; **I,** incus; **HS,** head of stapes; **FS,** footplate of stapes; **CS,** crura of stapes; **V,** vestibule; **SM,** stapedius muscle. × 15. (Courtesy of M. Lurie.)

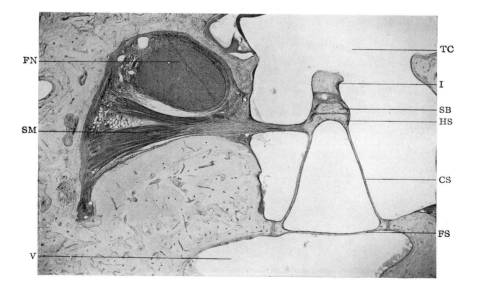

Inner Ear

Bony and Membranous Labyrinth

The inner ear is located in the pars petrosus of the temporal bone. The bone is pierced by a system of tortuous canals and cavities, the *bony labyrinth*, which is shaped to lodge the *membranous labyrinth*. The bony labyrinth is filled with a fluid, *perilymph*, and communicates with the cerebrospinal space by a narrow canal, the *vestibular aqueduct*.

The membranous labyrinth (Fig. 35–3) has two subdivisions. The *vestibular labyrinth* contains the organs of equilibrium: the *semicircular canals*, the *utricle*, and the *saccule*. The *cochlea* contains the organ of hearing: the *organ of Corti*. The membranous labyrinth is filled with a fluid called *endolymph*.

Vestibular Labyrinth

The *utricle* is an elliptical sac that lies in the upper posterior part of the bony vestibule, a cavity on the bony labyrinth. The spherical saccule lies anterior and medial to the utricle and is connected to it by the utriculosaccular duct. From the utriculosaccular duct arises the endolymphatic duct. The three membranous semicircular canals communicate with the utricle. These three canals lie at right angles in the three dimensions of space. Each one has an ampullated end. The ampullae of the anterior (vertical) and lateral (horizontal) canals lie close to each other and open into the superior end of the utricle, whereas the ampulla of the posterior (vertical) canal opens into its inferior end. The common end of the two vertical canals, the *crus commune*, enters the midportion of the utricle, as does also the nonampullated end of the horizontal canal.

The connective tissue layer of the utricle, saccule, and membranous canals consists of a finely fibrillated intercelluar substance and spindle-shaped or stellate fibroblastic cells (Fig. 35–4). From its outer surface, trabeculae run through the perilymphatic spaces to the inner periosteum of the osseous vestibule and the bony semicircular canals. These trabeculae support the semicircular canals, utricle, and saccule. The spaces and periosteum are lined with a layer of flattened connective tissue cells, which is a mesothelium.

35–3 Schematic drawing of the membranous labyrinth. (Reproduced with permission of C. V. Mosby.)

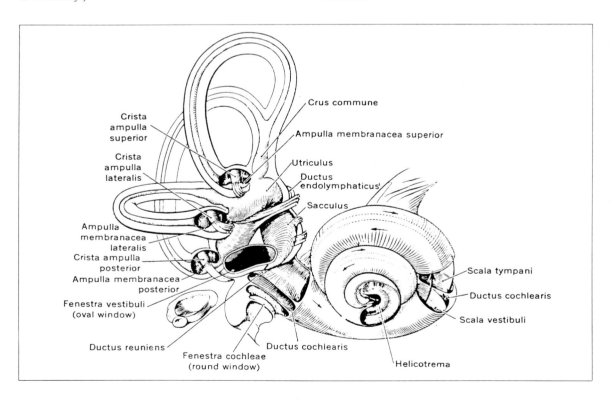

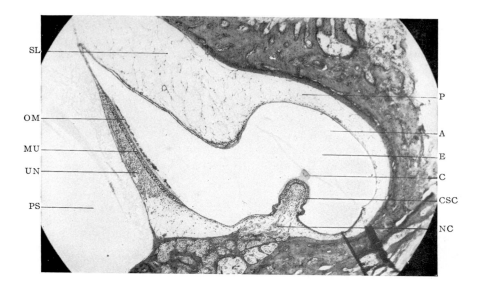

The neuroepithelial areas of the utricle and saccule are called *maculae*. The macula of the utricle, which is about 2 × 2 mm, lies in the superior anterior part of the utricle, approximately in the plane of the base of the skull and also in the plane of the horizontal semicircular canal. The macula of the saccule, which is about 2 × 3 mm, lies in a sagittal plane of the head, so the two maculae are perpendicular to each other.

Semicircular Canals. Each semicircular canal is provided with a sense organ responding to angular acceleration in the plane of the canal. This organ is the *crista ampullaris* (Figs. 35–4 to 35–6), a ridge of connective tissue that projects into the ampulla of the canal and is covered by a neuroepithelium consisting of sensory *hair cells* and supporting cells (Fig. 35–7). At both ends, where the crista joins the wall of the ampulla, is a region of tall cylindrical cells called *planum semilunatum*. Each hair cell has a bundle of sensory hairs that project from the luminal surface (Figs. 35–7 and 35–8) and are attached to a gelatinous structure, the *cupula*, which rides on top of the crista and reaches to the roof of the ampulla. The cupula acts as a swinging door to the motion of endolymph and excites the sensory cells by displacing the sensory hairs.

Two types of hair cells are distinguished in vestibular sensory epithelia (Fig. 35–7). *Type I cells* have a constricted neck and a round cell body, most of which is enclosed in a chalice-like afferent nerve terminal. The nerve chalice, in turn, is contacted by endings of efferent nerve fibers that contain abundant vesicles and probably

35–4 Macula utriculi and the ampulla of a semicircular canal. Supporting ligaments run from the membranous semicircular canal and utricle to the bony walls of the cavity. The utricle is suspended in the vestibule. **PS,** perilymphatic space; **SL,** supporting ligaments; **MU,** macula utriculi; **UN,** utricular nerve; **OM,** otolithic membrane; **A,** ampulla; **CSC,** crista, semicircular canal; **C,** cupula; **NC,** nerve to crista; **E,** endolymph; **P,** perilymph. Guinea pig. × 40. (Courtesy of M. Lurie.)

35–5 Ampulla of the semicircular canal cut open to expose the sensory epithelium of the crista. The cupula has been removed during dissection. **A,** ampulla; **C,** crista; **P,** planum semilunatum. Scanning microscopy. (Courtesy of Wersäll, Björkroth, Flock, and Lundquist. With permission of Springer-Verlag.)

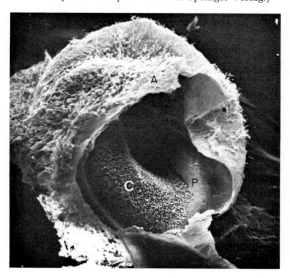

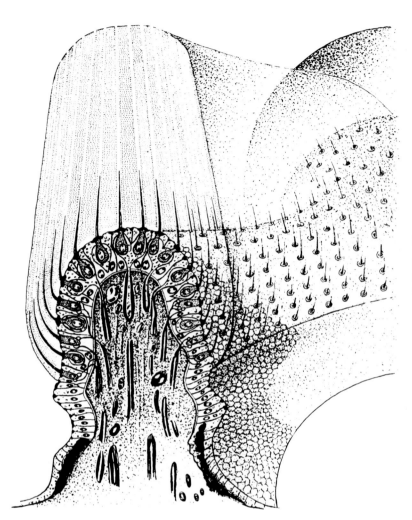

35–6 Sensory epithelium of the crista ampullaris contains hair cells with apical sensory hairs coupled to the cupula. (Courtesy of J. Wersäll.)

have an inhibitory function. *Type II cells* are cylindrical cells innervated at their base by terminals of afferent and efferent fibers. At the afferent synapse of both types of cells are regions of ultrastructural specialization with a presynaptic dense bar surrounded by vesicles similar to those seen where neurochemical synaptic transmission occurs.

Each sensory hair bundle is composed of 40 to 80 *stereocilia*, which progressively increase in length toward one pole of the cell (Fig. 35–7). These sensory hairs are modified microvilli with a core of fibrils, 60 Å in diameter (Fig. 35–9), which continue as a rootlet into a *cuticular plate* in the apical cytoplasm (Fig. 35–10). The cuticular plate is absent near the longest stereocilia, where a single *kinocilium* that has the "9 + 2" pattern of microtubules seen elsewhere is situated, although motility is not expected in this cilium. Each hair cell can thus be given a direction in which the kinocilium is facing. This arrangement is functionally important because the sensory nerve fiber connected to that cell increases its firing rate when the sensory hairs are bent in the direction of the kinocilium, whereas opposite displacement causes a decrease in firing frequency. The transducing elements of the hair cell are the stereocilia. Their inside core filaments are composed of actin and so is the cuticular plate. The organization and functional polarity of the actin filaments is seen in Fig. 35–11.

The supporting cells have basal nuclei, an apical cytoplasm containing secretory granules, and a luminal surface provided with microvilli. Their secretory product forms the matrix of the cupula.

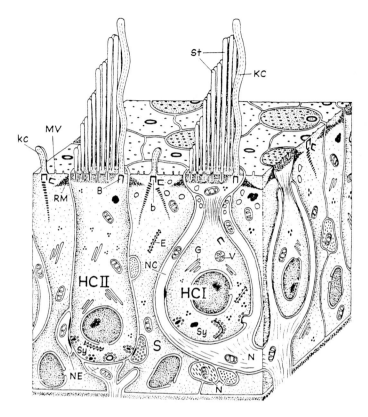

35–7 Schematic drawing of vestibular
sensory cells. **HC I,** hair cell type I;
HC II, hair cell type II; **NC,** nerve chalice;
N, nerve fiber; **NE,** nerve endings; **St,**
stereocilia; **KC,** kinocilium; **RM,** reticular
membrane; **G,** golgi complex; **V,** vesicles;
Sy, synaptic ribbons; **E,** endoplasmic
reticulum; **S,** supporting cell. (Courtesy of
Spoendlin.)

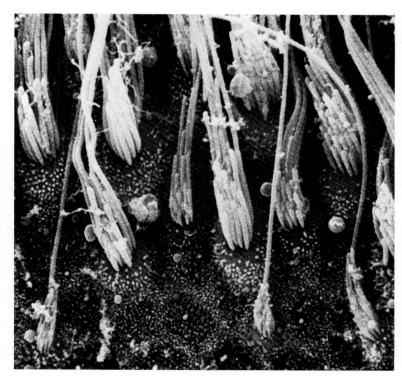

35–8 Scanning picture showing
sensory hair bundles
projecting from the
neuroepithelium. The cupula has
been removed. There are bundles
with different architecture, some
have large massive stereocilia,
others have small stereocilia and a
tall kinocilium rising in solitude.

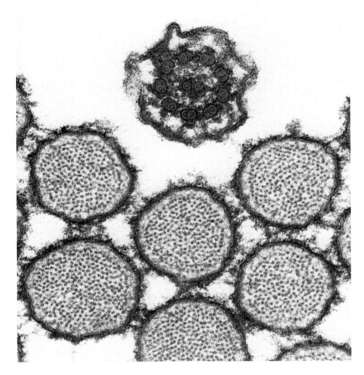

35–9 Transverse section through stereocilia and kinocilium.

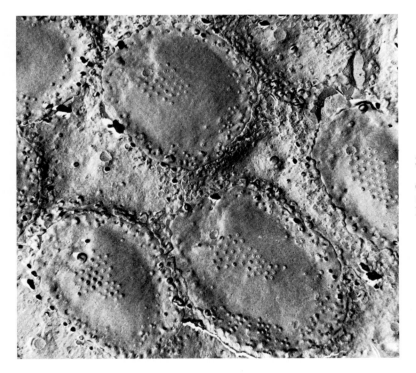

35–10 Freeze-fracture replica showing the surface of the crista ampullaris. Cuticular plates display insertion points of sensory hairs.

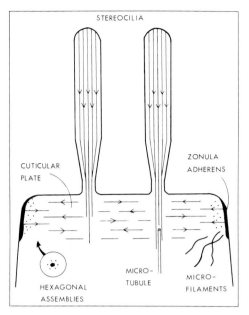

STEREOCILIA

CUTICULAR
PLATE

ZONULA
ADHERENS

HEXAGONAL
ASSEMBLIES

MICRO-
TUBULE

MICRO-
FILAMENTS

35–11 Schematic drawing showing the arrangement of actin filaments in the mechanoreceptor region. (Courtesy of Flock, Cheung, Flock, and Utter. Reproduced with permission of Chapman and Hall.)

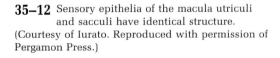

35–12 Sensory epithelia of the macula utriculi and sacculi have identical structure. (Courtesy of Iurato. Reproduced with permission of Pergamon Press.)

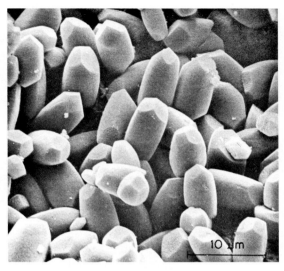

35–13 Otoconia from the human utricle.

Utricle and Saccule. The sensory epithelium of the macula utriculi and macula sacculi has the same structure as that of the crista (Figs. 35–7 and 35–12). The surfaces of the maculae are covered with a layer of gelatinous substance, the *otolithic membrane*, into which the sensory hair bundles penetrate. In the free surface of the otolithic membrane lie many crystals of calcium carbonate, called *otoconia* (Fig. 35–13). Because the otoconia are denser than endolymph, gravitational forces can cause a shear motion of the otolith membrane relative to the sensory epithelium and thus excite or inhibit the sensory cells.

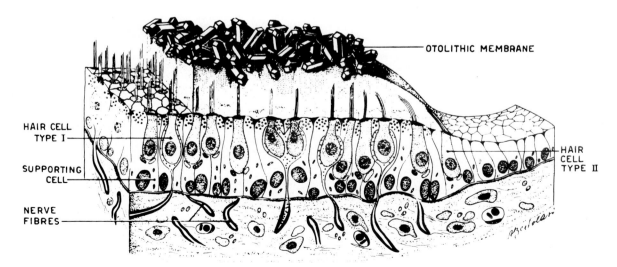

OTOLITHIC MEMBRANE

HAIR CELL
TYPE I

SUPPORTING
CELL

NERVE
FIBRES

HAIR
CELL
TYPE II

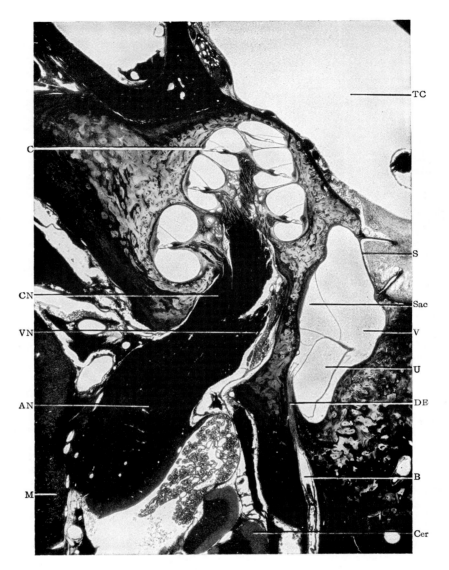

35–14 Cochlea and vestibule of a cat. Horizontal section shows the footplate of the stapes in the oval window, the vestibule showing the relationship of saccule and utricle to the oval window, and the large perilymphatic space around the footplate of the stapes. The ductus endolymphaticus can be followed in the aquaeductus vestibuli. The bulb of the ductus lymphaticus can be seen. The cochlea is cut to show three turns. The cochlear nerve and vestibular nerve can be seen in their course from the spiral and Scarpa's ganglia into the medulla. **TC**, tympanic cavity; **S**, stapes; **V**, vestibule; **Sac**, saccule; **U**, utricle; **DE**, ductus endolymphaticus; **B**, bulb (sarcus) of ductus endolymphaticus; **C**, cochlea; **CN**, cochlear nerve and spiral ganglion; **VN**, vestibular nerve, Scarpa's ganglion; **AN**, auditory nerve; **Cer**, cerebellum. × 12. (Courtesy of M. Lurie.)

Linear acceleration and changes of the position of the head are adequate stimuli.

Cochlea

The bony cochlea provides a rigid protective covering for the membranous cochlea (ductus cochlearis) with its delicate sense organ for hearing. The canal of the bony cochlea makes 2.5 turns around its axis, which is a pillar of spongy bone called the *modiolus* (Figs. 35–3 and 35–14). The base of the modiolus (the largest turn) forms the anterior wall of the internal acoustic meatus. The cochlear nerve and blood vessels enter the cochlea through the base of the

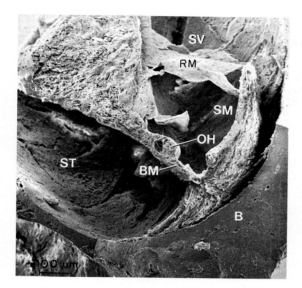

35–15 Freeze-fracture through the cochlear portion shows the scala vestibuli **(SV)**, scala media **(SM)**, scala tympani **(ST)** separated by Reissner's membrane **(RM)**, and the basilar membrane **(BM). O,** organ of Corti; **S,** spiral ganglion; **B,** bone; **V,** stria vascularis.

Attached to the osseous lamina and the outer wall of the canal lies the membranous cochlea, which separates the bony cochlear canal into two partitions: the *scala vestibuli,* which opens into the vestibule, and the *scala tympani,* which ends basally at the *round window.* The round window faces the middle ear cavity. The lumen of the membranous cochlea is referred to as the *scala media.* It is delimited toward the scala vestibuli by the *Reissner's membrane* and toward the scala tympani by the *basilar membrane.* The membranous cochlea filled with endolymph ends as a blind sac (lagena or cecum cupulare) at the apex of the cochlea. Just beyond this point the scala vestibuli and scala tympani, which had been separated by the membranous cochlea, join; this structure is called the *helicotrema.* The aquaeductus cochleae stems from the scala tympani at the base of the cochlea near the round window and passes to the subarachnoid space near the jugular fossa.

The membranous cochlea, which is triangular when seen in cross section, is attached inwardly

modiolus. The bony canal is partially divided by a projection of bone from the modiolus, called the *lamina spiralis ossea.* In radial section of the cochlea through the modiolus, this projection looks like the thread of a screw. The lamina spiralis ossea has two lips separated by a sulcus, an upper vestibular lip, or *limbus spiralis,* and a lower tympanic lip (Figs. 35–15 and 35–16).

35–16 Organ of Corti of a mouse. First turn of the cochlea, showing the relationship of scala vestibuli, scala media, and scala tympani. **SV,** scala vestibuli; **RM,** Reissner's membrane; **STV,** stria vascularis; **SPL,** spiral ligament; **LSO,** lamina spiralis ossea; **VL,** vestibular lip; **TL,** tympanic lip; **TM,** tectorial membrane, **ISC,** inner sulcus cells; **IHC,** inner hair cell; **EHC,** external hair cells; **BM,** basilar membrane; **ST,** scala tympani; **SpG,** spiral ganglia. × 120. (Courtesy of M. Lurie.)

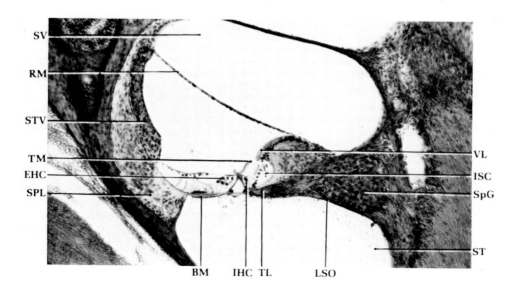

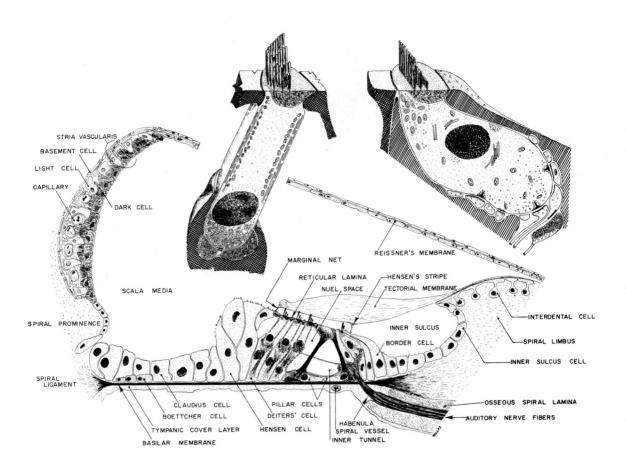

STRIA VASCULARIS
BASEMENT CELL
LIGHT CELL
CAPILLARY
DARK CELL
SCALA MEDIA
SPIRAL PROMINENCE
SPIRAL LIGAMENT
REISSNER'S MEMBRANE
MARGINAL NET
RETICULAR LAMINA
NUEL SPACE
HENSEN'S STRIPE
TECTORIAL MEMBRANE
INNER SULCUS
BORDER CELL
INTERDENTAL CELL
SPIRAL LIMBUS
INNER SULCUS CELL
CLAUDIUS CELL
BOETTCHER CELL
TYMPANIC COVER LAYER
BASILAR MEMBRANE
PILLAR CELLS
DEITERS' CELL
HENSEN CELL
HABENULA
SPIRAL VESSEL
INNER TUNNEL
OSSEOUS SPIRAL LAMINA
AUDITORY NERVE FIBERS

35–17 The organ of Corti. (Courtesy of Dallos. Reproduced with permission of McGraw-Hill.)

to the lamina spiralis ossea and outwardly by the *spiral ligament* to the outer wall of the bony canal. The base of the membranous cochlea is made of the tympanic lip of the lamina spiralis ossea and the basilar membrane, which connects the tympanic lip with the spiral ligament. At the attachment of the basilar membrane to the spiral ligament there is a small sulcus called the *external sulcus*. Attached to the vestibular lip of the lamina spiralis ossea are Reissner's membrane and the *tectorial membrane*. The space between the limbus and the tympanic lip is called the *internal sulcus*.

The basilar membrane is sometimes considered to have two parts, the zona arcuata (inner zone) and the zona pectoralis (outer zone). Its middle layer is formed by fibers that run through both zones. The basilar membrane varies in width from the basal coil at the round window to the apex. It is smallest at the round window, 0.16 mm, and widest at the helicotrema, 0.52 mm. The length of the basilar membrane in humans is about 31 mm. On its scala tympani aspect, mesothelial cells and connective tissue line the basilar membrane. There is a small artery running under it, the *vas spirale*. On the upper surface of the basilar membrane in the scala media rests the organ of Corti. Reissner's membrane is attached to the inner superior surface of the vestibular lip of the lamina spiralis ossea and goes to the outer wall of the bony cochlea at the upper end of the spiral ligament. It is two cell layers in thickness and is lined with epithelium on its surface facing the scala media and with mesothelium on its surface facing the scala vestibuli.

The third wall of the scala media is called the *stria vascularis*. It runs from the attachment of Reissner's membrane to the external sulcus. It has a low pseudostratified epithelium in intimate

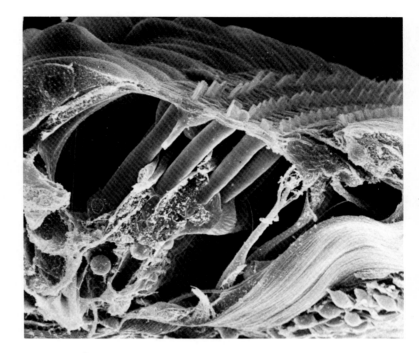

35–18 Scanning micrograph of the organ of Corti. (Courtesy of Bredberg.)

contact with the capillaries. The stria vascularis is believed to secrete the endolymph that fills the membranous cochlea. It runs the whole length of the scala media.

Organ of Corti. On the basilar membrane lies the organ of Corti, which is built up by hair cells and supporting cells arranged in a complicated manner (Figs. 35–17 and 35–18). It runs from the round window to the helicotrema of the cochlea. There are no blood vessels in the organ of Corti. A portion of it rests on the tympanic lip of the lamina spiralis ossea, but most of it lies on the basilar membrane. Between these parts is a free triangular space called the *tunnel,* which is delimited by two rows of supporting cells, the *inner pillar cells* resting on or near the tip of the tympanic lip and the *outer pillar cells* on the basilar membrane. The pillar cells have a broad base in which the nucleus lies. The body of the pillar cell contains rigid tonofibrils. The top of the pillar cell is enlarged and covered on its free surface with a cuticular plate. The head of the inner pillar cell is concave so that the rounded head of the outer pillar cell can fit into it, like a ball-and-socket joint. There are about 6,000 inner pillar cells and about 4,000 outer pillar cells, so that three inner cells articulate with two outer cells.

The sensory cells are in two groups: the *inner hair cells,* a single row of about 3,500 cells close to the inner pillar cells, and the *outer hair cells,* about 20,000 cells in three to four rows external to the outer pillar cells. The outer hair cells are cylindrical with a rounded lower end (Fig. 35–19). They are slanted relative to the surface of the organ of Corti. From the apical end of each outer hair cell a bundle of about 100 stereocilia (Figs. 35–19 to 35–21) projects from a cuticular plate in a **W** pattern (Fig. 35–22), with the row of tallest hairs facing away from the modiolus toward the stria vascularis. The cuticular plate is absent in that part of the cell that is near the stria vascularis. Here is a centriole that sits with its axis perpendicular to the cell membrane and with its upper end close to the membrane (Figs. 35–19 and 35–22). Consequently, the hair cells in the organ of Corti are morphologically polarized like the vestibular hair cells, with similar functional implications. The stereocilia contain actin filaments cross-linked by a protein named fimbrin (Fig. 35–23). The cuticular plate is a dense meshwork of actin and fimbrin and also contains myosin. At their base the outer hair cells are innervated by a few afferent nerve endings and several large efferent nerve endings containing abundant vesicles.

The inner hair cells have a roundish cell body

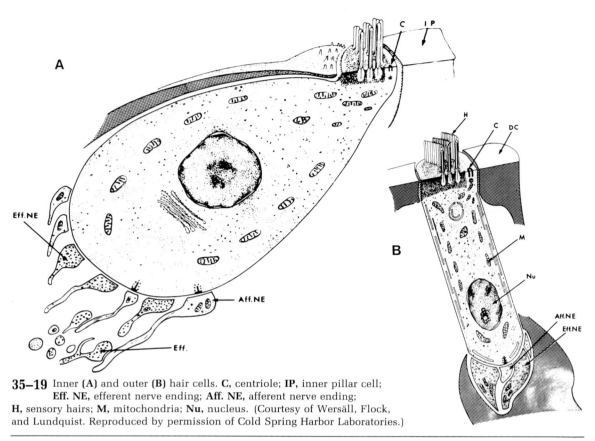

35–19 Inner **(A)** and outer **(B)** hair cells. **C,** centriole; **IP,** inner pillar cell; **Eff. NE,** efferent nerve ending; **Aff. NE,** afferent nerve ending; **H,** sensory hairs; **M,** mitochondria; **Nu,** nucleus. (Courtesy of Wersäll, Flock, and Lundquist. Reproduced by permission of Cold Spring Harbor Laboratories.)

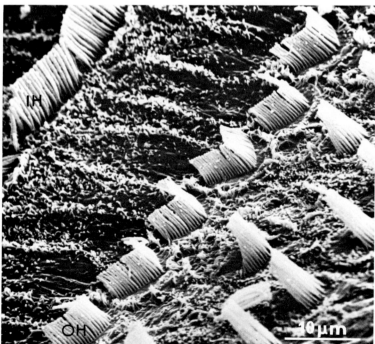

35–20 Sensory hair bundles of inner **(IH)** and outer **(OH)** hair cells project from the surface of the organ of Corti. Supporting cells of the reticular lamina have microvilli.

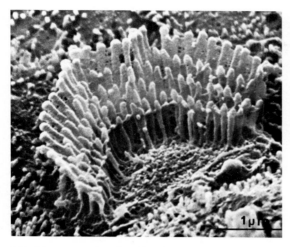

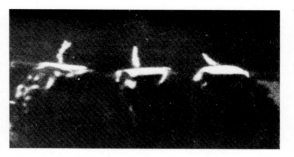

35–23 The stereocilia and cuticular plate contain actin and also a cross-linking protein fimbrin, demonstrated here by immunofluorescence. (Courtesy Flock, Bretscher, and Weber. Reproduced with permission of Elsevier North-Holland.)

35–21 Sensory hair bundle of an outer hair cell seen from the modiolus side. Human. (Courtesy of P.-G. Lundquist, Å. Flock, and J. Wersäll. 1971. Österreich Monatsschr. HNO 105:285. Reprinted with permission from Urban & Schwarzenberg, Vienna.)

35–22 Section through the sensory hairs of one outer hair cell and through part of the cuticular plate **(Cu)** and the centriole **(C)** of its neighbor. (Courtesy of Å. Flock, R. Kimura, P.-G. Lundquist, and J. Wersäll. 1962. J. Acoust. Soc. Am. 34:1351.)

(Fig. 35–19), their sensory hairs are lined up in straight rows, and their centriole also faces the stria vascularis. They are innervated by several afferent and a few efferent terminals. The inner hair cells are totally enclosed by supporting cells called *inner phalangeal cells,* and the outer hair cells are held by supporting *outer phalangeal cells.* These cells extend as a slender curved process toward the surface of the organ of Corti (Fig. 35–24). At the surface they form a rhomboid plate that interlocks with its neighbors to form the *reticular membrane* that holds the apical ends of the hair cells. Outwardly the phalangeal

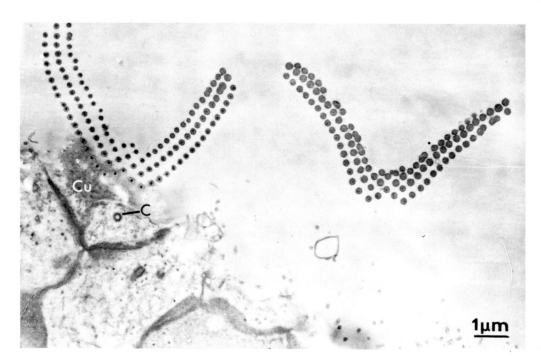

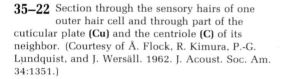

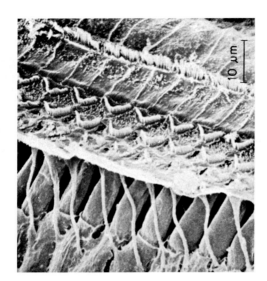

10 μm

35–24 Phalangeal cells have slender twisted processes that reach the surface of the organ of Corti where their heads form the reticular lamina. (Courtesy of J. Wersäll, Å. Flock, and P.-G. Lundquist. 1970. Z. Hörgeräte Akustik 9:56. Reproduced with permission from Killisch-Horn Verlag.)

cells are succeeded by tall *Hensen's cells*. Hensen's cells then pass into a layer of cuboidal *cells of Claudius,* which terminate in the external sulcus just under the spiral prominence.

Lying above the organ of Corti is a gelatinous *tectorial membrane* whose lower surface rests on the tips of the tallest row of stereocilia in each hair bundle (Fig. 35–17). It is attached to the limbus spiralis, which contains the *interdental cells* that secrete the substance of the membrane.

Nerve Supply

The VIIIth cranial (auditory) nerve supplies the sensory areas of the membranous labyrinth. It divides into a superior posterior part, the *vestibular nerve,* and an inferior anterior part, the *cochlear nerve.*

The vestibular nerve has a superior portion that supplies the macula of the utricle and the cristae of the anterior vertical and the horizontal canals, and an inferior portion that supplies the macula of the saccule and the cristae of the posterior semicircular canals. The ganglion of the vestibular nerve, called the *vestibular ganglion* or *Scarpa's ganglion,* lies in the internal auditory canal. There is also a small branch from the inferior portion of the vestibular nerve that joins

the cochlear nerve and is called the *nerve of Oort.* Scarpa's ganglion cells are bipolar. The axons of the ganglion cells enter the medulla and end in the vestibular nuclei of the medulla in the region of the fourth ventricle. The vestibular nuclei have connections with the cerebellum and the third, fourth, and sixth eye nuclei, through the posterior longitudinal bundle. They then send axons down the spinal cord through the vestibular spinal tracts.

The cochlear nerve enters the cochlea through the modiolus, and its ganglion *(the spiral ganglion)* lies in the lamina spiralis ossea. The sensory neurons are bipolar. The nerve fibers go to the hair cell through canals in the lamina spiralis ossea and enter the organ of Corti through small openings called the *foramina nervosa.* When the nerve fibers leave the foramina nervosa, they lose their myelin sheaths.

The pattern of innervation is very complex and is not yet fully understood. It seems that several afferent neurons innervate each inner hair cell, to which they take a direct course (Fig. 35–25). Other fibers cross the tunnel of Corti, turn toward the base of the cochlea, and run as outer spiral fibers to innervate several outer hair cells.

The cochlear nerve enters the medulla and terminates in the cochlear nuclei. From the cochlear nuclei there are connections with other nuclei; most of the cochlear nuclei fibers go to the medial geniculate of the thalamus and then radiate to the auditory centers of the brain, which lie in the temporal lobe.

The organ of Corti also receives an efferent innervation, as does the vestibular apparatus (Fig. 35–26). These fibers, the olivocochlear bundle, have their cell bodies in the superior olivary nucleus. Fibers from the contralateral side cross the midline of the medulla at the bottom of the fourth ventricle. The efferent fibers leave the medulla with the vestibular nerve and then pass over to the cochlear nerve in Oort's anastomosis. Within the cochlea they travel along a spiral course in the spiral ganglion. Efferent fibers pass the tunnel of Corti to innervate several outer hair cells. Inner hair cells are not as well supplied with efferents.

Sympathetic fibers innervate the blood vessels of the inner ear and also form a plexus of fibers independent of blood vessels. These free fibers have terminals in the vestibular ganglion and in the peripheral vestibular nerve branches. Terminals are seen also in the spiral ganglion and are

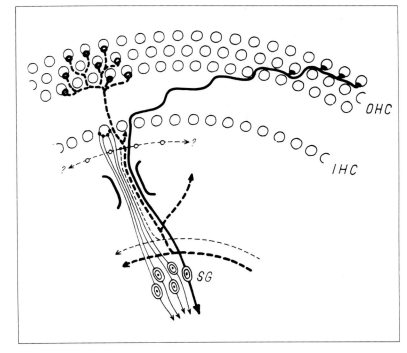

35–25 Innervation pattern of the organ of Corti in the cat. **Dashed lines** are afferent fibers; **solid lines** are efferent fibers. **OHC,** outer hair cells; **IHC,** inner hair cells; **SG,** spiral ganglion. (Courtesy of H. Spoendlin. 1966. *In* Advances in Oto-Rhino-Laryngology, vol. 13. Basel: S. Karger. Reprinted with permission from Karger.)

35–26 Efferent nerve supply to the inner ear. (Modified by Iurato from Rossi and Cortesina. Reproduced with permission from Pergamon Press.)

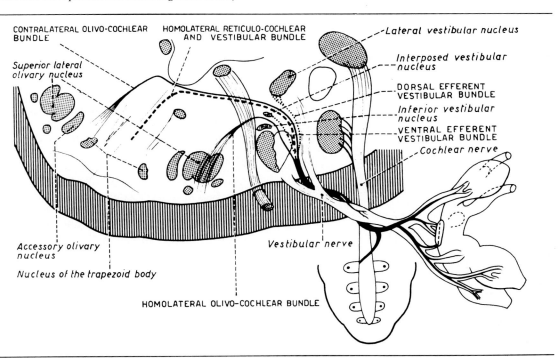

conspicuous at the point of demyelinization of cochlear nerve fibers in the foramina nervosa of the lamina spiralis ossea. The sympathetic fibers originate in the superior cervical ganglion and reach the inner ear via arteries and via the plexus tympanicus. Their function is as yet unknown.

Endolymphatic Sac

Utriculus and sacculus are joined by a short duct, the *ductus utriculo saccularis*, from which springs the *ductus endolymphaticus*, which terminates as the endolymphatic sac under the dura. The epithelium outlining the endolymphatic sac is specialized for absorption. The sac often contains cellular debris, and active phagocytosis has been demonstrated.

Vessels of the Labyrinth

The internal auditory artery is a branch of the basilar artery. It arises along with branches that are distributed to the underside of the cerebellum and the neighboring cerebral nerves, and it passes through the internal acoustic meatus to the ear. It divides into vestibular and cochlear branches. The *vestibular artery* supplies the vestibular nerve and the upper lateral portion of the sacculus, utriculus, and semicircular ducts. The *cochlear artery* sends a vestibulocochlear branch to the lower and medial portion of the sacculus, utriculus, and ducts. This branch also supplies the first third of the first turn of the cochlea. The capillaries formed by the vestibular branches are generally wide-meshed, but near the maculae and cristae the meshes are narrower. The terminal portion of the cochlear artery enters the modiolus and forms three or four spirally ascending branches that divide into about 30 radial branches distributed to three sets of capillaries—to the spiral ganglion, to the lamina spiralis, and to the outer walls of the scalae and the stria vascularis of the cochlear duct.

The veins of the labyrinth form the following three groups.

1. The *vena aquaeductus vestibuli*, which receives blood from the semicircular ducts and a part of the utriculus. It passes toward the brain in a bony canal along with the ductus endolymphaticus and empties into the superior petrosal sinus.
2. The *vena aquaeductus cochleae*, which receives blood from parts of the utriculus, sac-

culus, and cochlea. It passes through a bony canal to the internal jugular vein. It arises from small vessels, including the vas prominens and the vas spirale. Branches derived from these veins pass toward the modiolus. There are no vessels in Reissner's membrane of the adult, and the vessels in the wall of the scala tympani are arranged so that only veins occur in the part toward the membranous spiral lamina. Thus the latter is not affected by arterial pulsation. Within the modiolus the veins unite in an inferior spiral vein, which receives blood from the basal and a part of a second turn of the cochlea, and a superior spiral vein, which proceeds from the apical portion. These two spiral veins unite with vestibular branches to form the vena aquaeductus cochleae.
3. The *internal auditory vein*, which arises within the modiolus from the veins of the spiral lamina. These veins anastomose with the spiral veins. It receives branches also from the acoustic nerve and from the bones and empties into the *vena spiralis anterior*.

Lymphatic spaces within the internal ear are represented by the perilymph spaces, which communicate through the aquaeductus cochleae with the arachnoid space. The connecting structure, or *ductus perilymphaticus*, is described as a lymphatic vessel.

Embryological Development

The sense organs are derivatives of the ectoderm. The internal ear first appears as a bilateral local thickening of ectoderm opposite that part of the medullary tube destined to become the pons. The thickened areas invaginate, as shown in Fig. 35–27, and the pockets thus formed separate from the ectoderm and develop into auditory vesicles (*otocysts*). The point where they become detached from the epidermis is marked by an elevation on the medial side of the vesicle, which elongates and produces the endolymphatic duct.

In two places the medial and lateral walls of the auditory vesicle approach one another and fuse, and the epithelial plates thus formed become thin and are absorbed, leaving two loops, each attached at both ends to the parent vesicle. These loops are the vertical semicircular canals. Similarly, a third canal forms soon afterward. The lower portion of the otocyst elongates and coils to make 2.5 revolutions, forming the ductus

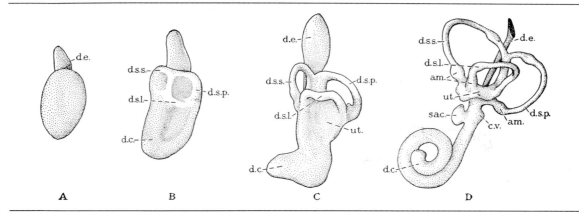

cochlearis. A constriction separates the sacculus from the utricle and the cochlea. The surrounding mesenchyme becomes cartilage and then bone.

The middle ear develops from the first pharyngeal pouch and the external ear from the first branchial cleft. At an early stage the ectoderm of the branchial cleft and the endoderm of the pharyngeal pouch meet and fuse to form the tympanic membrane.

35–27 Lateral or external surfaces of models of the membranous portion of the left internal ear from human embryos. Different enlargements. **A,** From an embryo of 6.9 mm; **B,** 10.2 mm; **C,** 13.5 mm; **D,** 22 mm. **am,** ampulla; **cv,** cecum vestibulare of **dc,** cochlear duct; **de,** endolymphatic duct; **dsl, dsp,** and **dss,** horizontal, posterior vertical, and anterior vertical semicircular ducts; **sac,** sacculus; **ut,** utriculus. (Courtesy of His, Jr.)

Physiology of the Ear

Middle Ear

The ossicles of the middle ear transfer motion of the ear drum to motion of the fluids in the cochlear partition. This change of sound conduction in fluid rather than in air calls for matching of mechanical impedance and is met by the change in size from the large ear drum to the small footplate of the stapes. The stapedius muscle improves detectibility of speech in a noisy surrounding.

Vestibular System

The semicircular canals control the position of the eye-bulbs in relation to the visual field through what is called the nystagmus reflex. This has a slow phase that turns the eyes left if the head is rotated to the right and vice versa. The image of the visual field is thus held stationary on the retina in a highly precise manner so that the image is not blurred. It is controlled by the motion of the cupula due to inertial movement of endolymph. Nerve fibers from the crista ampullaris inform about the position of the cupula by the frequency with which they fire nerve impulses. Other fibers detect changes in the speed of rotation. The two types of fiber may be related to different types of hair cell in terms of structure of sensory hair bundles or innervation pattern. The efferent nerve fibers can influence the level of activity in the afferent nerve fibers by changing the rate of release of a neurotransmitter at the afferent synapse.

The Cochlea

Motion of the stapes in response to sound produces pressure fluctuations across the scala media, the pressure being released through the round window. As a result, a wave develops in the basilar membrane starting at the apex and traveling toward the base. For low-frequency tones the wave does not travel far but has its maximum at the apex. For high-frequency tones it travels further down toward the base. For different frequencies the traveling wave reaches a maximum amplitude at different points along the basilar membrane. This phenomenon is the basis for frequency selectivity in the cochlea. According to the "place principle," different nerve fibers along the coils become engaged at different frequencies. At low frequencies information about the frequency of a tone can also be carried in individual nerve fibers that fire nerve impulses in synchrony with the period of the tone.

References and Selected Bibliography

Bast, T. H., and Anson, B. J. 1949. The Temporal Bone and the Ear. Springfield, Ill.: Charles C. Thomas, Publisher.

Békésy, G. von. 1960. Experiments in Hearing. New York: McGraw-Hill Book Company.

Dallos, P. 1973. The Auditory Periphery. New York: Academic Press, Inc.

Davis, H. 1965. A model for transducer action in the cochlea. Cold Spring Harbor Symp. Quant. Biol. 30:181.

Engström, H., Ades, H., and Anderson, A. 1966. Structural Pattern of the Organ of Corti. Stockholm: Almqvist and Wiksell.

Flock, Å. 1971. Transduction in hair cells. In W. R. Loewenstein (ed.), Handbook of Sensory Physiology, Vol. 1, Principles of Receptor Physiology. Berlin: Spring-Verlag OHG, p. 396.

Iurato, S. (ed.). 1967. Submicroscopic Structure of the Inner Ear. New York: Pergamon Press.

Kimura, R. S., Schuknecht, H. F., and Sundo, I. 1965. Fine morphology of the sensory cells in the organ of Corti in Man. Acta Otolaryngol. (Stockh.) 58:390.

Kolmer, W. 1927. Gehörorgan. In W. von Möllendorff and W. Bargmann (eds.), Handbüch der mikroskopischen Anatomie des Menschen, Vol. 3. Berlin: Springer-Verlag OHG, p. 250.

Lindeman, H. 1969. Studies on the morphology of the sensory regions of the vestibular apparatus. Adv. Anat. Embryol. Cell Biol. 42:1.

Lundquist, P.-G. 1965. The endolymphatic duct and sac in the guinea pig. Acta Otolaryngol. (Suppl.) (Stockh.) 201:1.

Spoendlin, H. 1966. The organization of the cochlear receptor. In Advances in Oto-Rhino-Laryngology, Vol. 13. Basel: S. Karger.

Takasaka, T., and Smith C. 1971. The structure and innervation of the pigeon's basilar papilla. J. Ultrastruct. Res. 35:20.

Wersäll, J. 1956. Studies on the structure and innervation of the sensory epithelium of the cristae ampullares in the guinea pig. Acta Otolaryngol. (Suppl.) (Stockh.) 126.

Index